VASCULAR SURGERY

A Comprehensive Review

VASCULAR SURGERY

A Comprehensive Review

Edited by

WESLEY S. MOORE, M.D.

Professor of Surgery and Chief
Section of Vascular Surgery
University of California at Los Angeles
Los Angeles, California

W. B. SAUNDERS COMPANY
A Division of Harcourt Brace & Company

Philadelphia / London / Toronto / Montreal / Sydney / Tokyo

W. B. SAUNDERS COMPANY
A Division of Harcourt Brace & Company

The Curtis Center
Independence Square West
Philadelphia, PA 19106

Library of Congress Cataloging-in-Publication Data

Vascular surgery : a comprehensive review / [edited by] Wesley S.
   Moore. — 4th ed.
        p.   cm.
     Includes bibliographical references and index.
     ISBN 0-7216-4841-X
     1. Blood-vessels—Surgery. I. Moore, Wesley S.
     [DNLM: 1. Vascular Surgery.   WG 170 V3313]
   RD598.5.V374   1993
   617.4′13059—dc20
   DNLM/DLC   92-49116

CONTRIBUTORS

SAMY ABDOU, M.D.

Plastic and Reconstructive Surgery Research Fellow, UCLA School of Medicine, Los Angeles, California
Lympedema and Tumors of the Lymphatics

SAMUEL S. AHN, M.D.

Assistant Professor of Surgery, Department of Surgery, UCLA School of Medicine, Center for the Health Sciences, Los Angeles, California
Endovascular Surgery

BENJAMIN O. ANDERSON, M.D.

Fellow in Surgical Oncology, Department of Surgery, Memorial Sloan-Kettering Cancer Center, New York, New York
Congenital Vascular Malformations of the Extremities

ERIC R. ASHBY, M.D.

Plastic and Reconstructive Surgery Research Fellow, UCLA School of Medicine, Los Angeles, California
Lymphedema and Tumors of the Lymphatics

J. DENNIS BAKER, M.D.

Professor of Surgery, UCLA School of Medicine, Los Angeles, California; Chief, Vascular Surgery Section, Sepulveda V.A. Medical Center, Sepulveda, California
The Vascular Laboratory

WILEY F. BARKER, M.D.

Professor Emeritus, Department of Surgery, UCLA School of Medicine, Los Angeles, California
A History of Vascular Surgery

ROBERT S. BENNION, M.D.

Associate Professor of Surgery, UCLA School of Medicine, Los Angeles, California
Hemodialysis and Vascular Access

JOHN J. BERGAN, M.D.

Scripps Memorial Hospital, La Jolla, California; Clinical Professor of Surgery, UCSD, San Diego; Clinical Professor of Surgery, USUHS, Bethesda, Maryland
Visceral Ischemic Syndromes; Varicose Veins: Chronic Venous Insufficiency

RAMON BERGUER, M.D., Ph.D.

Professor, Division of Vascular Surgery, Wayne State University, School of Medicine, Detroit, Michigan; Chief, Division of Vascular Surgery, Harper Hospital

Reconstruction of the Supra-aortic Trunks and Vertebrobasilar System

VICTOR M. BERNHARD, M.D.

Professor of Surgery, University of Arizona College of Medicine; Chief, Section of Vascular Surgery, University of Arizona Health Sciences Center, Staff Surgeon-Veterans Administration Hospital, Tucson, Arizona

Noninfectious Complications in Vascular Surgery

DAVID A. BULL, M.D.

Fellow-Cardiothoracic Surgery, University of Utah Medical Center, Salt Lake City, Utah

Noninfectious Complications in Vascular Surgery

RONALD W. BUSUTTIL, M.D., Ph.D.

Professor of Surgery, Department of Surgery, Liver Transplantation Program, Center for the Health Sciences, Los Angeles, California

Portal Hypertension

JOE A. CATES, M.D.

Resident, UCLA Medical Center, Los Angeles, California

Primary Arterial Infections

ALEXANDER W. CLOWES, M.D.

Professor of Surgery, University of Washington School of Medicine, Department of Surgery, Seattle, Washington

Anatomy, Physiology, and Pharmacology of the Vascular Wall

MICHAEL D. COLBURN, M.D.

Resident in General Surgery, Department of Surgery, UCLA School of Medicine, Los Angeles, California

Myointimal Hyperplasia

JACK L. CRONENWETT, M.D.

Professor of Surgery, Dartmouth Medical School; Chairman, Section of Vascular Surgery, Dartmouth-Hitchcock Medical Center, Hanover, New Hampshire

Biologic and Synthetic Vascular Grafts

RICHARD H. DEAN, M.D.

Professor and Director, Division of Surgical Sciences, Bowman Gray School of Medicine, Wake Forest University, Winston-Salem, North Carolina

Renovascular Hypertension

DAVID H. DEATON, M.D.

Fellow in Vascular Surgery, Adjunct Assistant Professor of Surgery, UCLA Center for the Health Sciences, Los Angeles, California

Infection in Prosthetic Vascular Grafts

RALPH G. DePALMA, M.D.

Lewis B. Saltz Professor of Surgery, George Washington University School of Medicine, Washington, D.C.

Vasculogenic Impotence

MAGRUDER C. DONALDSON, M.D.

Assistant Professor, Harvard Medical School; Surgeon, Brigham and Women's Hospital, Boston, Massachusetts

Evaluation of Cardiac Risk in the Patient with Vascular Disease; Aortoiliac Occlusive Disease

JANETTE D. DURHAM, M.D.

Assistant Professor of Radiology, University of Colorado Health Sciences Center, Denver, Colorado

Congenital Vascular Malformations of the Extremities

PETER A. EDWARDS, Ph.D.

Professor of Biological Chemistry and Medicine, UCLA School of Medicine, Los Angeles, California

Atherosclerosis; Pathology, Pathogenesis, and Medical Management

D. PRESTON FLANIGAN, M.D.

Visiting Professor of Surgery, University of Illinois College of Medicine, Chicago, Illinois

Aneurysms of the Peripheral Arteries

ALAN M. FOGELMAN, M.D.

Professor of Medicine, UCLA School of Medicine, Division of Cardiology, Los Angeles, California

Atherosclerosis; Pathology, Pathogenesis, and Medical Management

HUGH A. GELABERT, M.D.

Assistant Professor of Surgery, UCLA School of Medicine, Los Angeles, California

Primary Arterial Infections; Antibiotic Prophylaxis of Vascular Graft Infection; Portal Hypertension

JERRY GOLDSTONE, M.D.

Professor and Vice Chairman, Department of Surgery, Chief, Division of Vascular Surgery, University of California, San Francisco, San Francisco, California

Aneurysms of the Aorta and Iliac Arteries

ANTOINETTE S. GOMES, M.D.

Associate Professor of Radiology and Medicine, UCLA, Medical Center, Los Angeles, California

Principles of Angiography and Interventional Radiology

LINDA M. GRAHAM, M.D.

Professor of Surgery, Case Western Reserve University; Chief, Vascular Surgery Service, Veterans Administration Hospital, Cleveland, Ohio

Biologic and Synthetic Vascular Grafts

LAZAR J. GREENFIELD, M.D.

Frederick A. Collar Professor and Chairman, Department of Surgery, University of Michigan, Ann Arbor, Michigan

Venous Thromboembolic Disease

MARGARET E. HABERLAND, Ph.D.

Associate Professor of Medicine, UCLA School of Medicine, Los Angeles, California

Atherosclerosis; Pathology, Pathogenesis, and Medical Management

E. JOHN HARRIS, JR., M.D.

Assistant Professor of Surgery, Division of Vascular Surgery, Stanford University School of Medicine, Stanford, California

Nonatherosclerotic Vascular Disease

JOHN R. HOCH, M.D.
Assistant Professor, Section of Vascular Surgery, University of Wisconsin–Madison, Madison, Wisconsin
Hemostasis and Thrombosis

LARRY H. HOLLIER, M.D.
Chairman, Department of Surgery, Ochsner Clinic and Alton Ochsner Medical Foundation; Clinical Professor of Surgery, Tulane Medical Center and LSU School of Medicine, New Orleans, Louisiana
Thoracoabdominal Aortic Aneurysms

PAUL W. HUMPHREY, M.D.
Fellow in Vascular Surgery, University of Missouri Hospital and Clinics, Columbia, Missouri
Hemostasis and Thrombosis

GLENN C. HUNTER, M.D.
Associate Professor of Surgery, University of Arizona Health Sciences Center, Tucson, Arizona
Noninfectious Complications in Vascular Surgery

FRANCIS J. KAZMIER, M.D.
Chairman, Vascular Medicine, Ochsner Clinic and Alton Ochsner Medical Foundation, New Orleans, Louisiana
Thoracoabdominal Aortic Aneurysms

J. DAVID KILLEEN, JR., M.D.
Associate Professor of Surgery, Loma Linda University School of Medicine; Chief, Division of Vascular Surgery, Loma Linda University Medical Center, Loma Linda, California
Surgical Anatomy and Exposure of the Vascular Wall

TED R. KOHLER, M.D.
Associate Professor of Surgery, University of Washington School of Medicine, Seattle, Washington
Anatomy, Physiology, and Pharmacology of the Vascular Wall

MICHAEL M. LAW, M.D.
Research Fellow, Department of Surgery, UCLA School of Medicine, Los Angeles, California
Antibiotic Prophylaxis of Vascular Graft Infection

S. MARTIN LINDENAUER, M.D.
Professor of Surgery, University of Michigan Medical School, Attending Surgeon, Section of Vascular Surgery, University Hospital, Ann Arbor, Michigan
Biologic and Synthetic Vascular Grafts

HERBERT I. MACHLEDER, M.D.
Professor of Surgery, Department of Surgery, UCLA Medical Center, UCLA, Los Angeles, California
Vascular Disease of the Upper Extremity and the Thoracic Outlet Syndrome

JAMES M. MALONE, M.D.
Chairman, Department of Surgery, Maricopa Medical Center, Phoenix, Arizona
Lower Extremity Amputation

JOHN A. MANNICK, M.D.
Moseley Professor of Surgery, Harvard Medical School, Brigham and Women's Hospital, Boston, Massachusetts
Evaluation of Cardiac Risk in the Patient with Vascular Risk; Aortoiliac Occlusive Disease

ROBERT J. MARINO, M.D.

Associate Chairman, Department of Anesthesiology, Oschner Foundation Hospital, New Orleans, Louisiana

Thoracoabdominal Aortic Aneurysms

DAVID S. MAXWELL, Ph.D.*

Professor of Anatomy and Cell Biology, UCLA School of Medicine; and Professor of Surgery and Anatomy, Charles Drew Medical School, Los Angeles, California

Embryology of the Vascular System

LOUIS M. MESSINA, M.D.

Associate Professor of Surgery, University of Michigan Medical School, Ann Arbor, Michigan

Splanchnic and Renal Artery Aneurysms

TIMOTHY A. MILLER, M.D.

Professor of Surgery, UCLA School of Medicine; Chief, Plastic Surgery Section, VA Medical Center, West Los Angeles, California

Lymphedema and Tumors of the Lymphatics

WESLEY S. MOORE, M.D.

Professor of Surgery, UCLA School of Medicine; Chief, Section of Vascular Surgery, UCLA Center for the Health Sciences, Los Angeles, California

Extracranial Cerebrovascular Disease—The Cartoid Artery; Myointimal Hyperplasia; Infection in Prosthetic Vascular Grafts

MALCOLM O. PERRY, M.D.

Professor and Chief of Vascular Surgery, Texas Tech University Health Sciences Center, Lubbock, Texas

Vascular Trauma

JOHN M. PORTER, M.D.

Professor of Surgery, Head, Division of Vascular Surgery, Oregon Health Sciences University, Portland, Oregon

Nonatherosclerotic Vascular Disease; Natural History and Nonoperative Treatment of Chronic Lower Extremity Ischemia

WILLIAM J. QUIÑONES-BALDRICH, M.D.

Associate Professor of Surgery, UCLA School of Medicine, Los Angeles, California

Thrombolytic Therapy for Vascular Disease; Acute Arterial and Graft Occlusion

ROBERT B. RUTHERFORD, M.D.

Professor of Surgery, University of Colorado School of Medicine; Chief, Vascular Surgery Section, University Hospital, Denver, Colorado

Congenital Vascular Malformations of the Extremities; Role of Sympathectomy in the Management of Vascular Disease

DONALD SILVER, M.D.

W. Alton Jones Distinguished Professor and Chairman, Department of Surgery, Chief of Vascular Surgery, University of Missouri Medical Center, Columbia, Missouri

Hemostasis and Thrombosis

---

*Deceased.

LOUIS L. SMITH, M.D.

Professor of Surgery, Loma Linda University Medical Center, Loma Linda, California

Surgical Anatomy and Exposure of the Vascular System

JAMES C. STANLEY, M.D.

Professor of Surgery, University of Michigan Medical School; Head, Section of Vascular Surgery, University Hospital

Biologic and Synthetic Vascular Grafts; Splanchnic and Renal Artery Aneurysms

EDWARD A. STEMMER, M.D.

Professor of Surgery, University of California, Irvine, California; Chief, Surgical Service, Veterans Affairs Medical Center, Long Beach, California

Influence of Diabetes Mellitus on the Patterns and Complications of Vascular Occlusive Disease

D. EUGENE STRANDNESS, JR., M.D.

Professor of Surgery; Head, Division of Vascular Surgery, Department of Surgery, University of Washington School of Medicine, Seattle, Washington

Hemodynamics for the Vascular Surgeon

LLOYD M. TAYLOR, JR., M.D.

Professor of Surgery, Division of Vascular Surgery, Oregon Health Sciences University, Portland, Oregon

Nonatherosclerotic Vascular Disease; Natural History and Nonoperative Treatment of Chronic Lower Extremity Ischemia

FRANK J. VEITH, M.D.

Professor of Surgery, Albert Einstein College of Medicine; Professor and Chief, Vascular Surgical Services, Montefiore Medical Center, Bronx, New York

Femoral-Popliteal-Tibial Occlusive Disease

THOMAS W. WAKEFIELD, M.D.

Associate Professor of Surgery, University of Michigan Medical Center, Co-Chief, Vascular Surgery Service, Veterans Administration Hospital; Attending Surgeon, Section of Vascular Surgery, University Hospital, Ann Arbor, Michigan

Biologic and Synthetic Vascular Grafts

ANTHONY D. WHITTEMORE, M.D.

Associate Professor of Surgery, Harvard Medical School; Surgeon, Brigham and Women's Hospital, Boston, Massachusetts

Evaluation of Cardiac Risk in the Patient with Vascular Disease; Aortoiliac Occlusive Disease

SAMUEL E. WILSON, M.D.

Professor of Surgery, University of California, Irvine; Chairman, Department of Surgery, UCI Medical Center, Torrance, California

Hemodialysis and Vascular Access

CHRISTOPHER K. ZARINS, M.D.

Chidester Professor of Surgery, Stanford University; Chairman, Division of Vascular Surgery, Stanford University Medical Center, Stanford, California

Hemodynamic Factors in Atherosclerosis

GERALD B. ZELENOCK, M.D.

Professor of Surgery, University of Michigan Medical School; Attending Surgeon, Section of Vascular Surgery, University Hospital; Attending Surgeon, Veterans Administration Hospital, Ann Arbor, Michigan

Biologic and Synthetic Vascular Grafts; Splanchnic and Renal Artery Aneurysms

R. EUGENE ZIERLER, M.D.

Associate Professor of Surgery, University of Washington School of Medicine, Seattle, Washington

Hemodynamics for the Vascular Surgeon

PREFACE

As this text enters the fourth edition, our original objective of presenting the topics in a complete manner and at the same time keeping the book manageable in size remains an important part of editorial planning. Since vascular surgery is a rapidly evolving and changing field, both with respect to new technology as well as outcome data, the frequency of new editions is crucial to keeping the textbook up to date. For that reason, we have settled on a three-year revision cycle in order to provide the reader with current information. All of the original chapters have either been thoroughly revised or replaced in order to provide current information.

In the three years that have elapsed since the last edition, we have added five new chapters. The topics of "Primary Vascular Infection" and "Antibiotics in Vascular Surgery" are each presented in a separate and dedicated chapter.

The diagnosis and management of patients with *vasculogenic impotence* is a difficult and demanding endeavor. A new chapter on this topic covers, in detail, the important elements of history and physical examination, laboratory and noninvasive testing, as well as therapeutic options.

A chapter on "Evaluation of Cardiac Risk of the Patient with Vascular Disease" has been added. Coexistent coronary artery disease in patients with peripheral vascular disease is relatively frequent. However, the extent of preoperative screening and the nature of screening tests continue to be controversial. This chapter establishes the rationale for patient evaluation and presents a logical approach to preoperative assessment and management of the vascular patient with concomitant cardiac disease.

Myointimal hyperplasia has emerged as one of the most important pathologic responses to vessel wall injury and reconstruction that ultimately leads to failure of surgical intervention. The prominence of this diagnosis is now highlighted in a chapter that is dedicated to the discussion of pathophysiology, pathology, incidence, and pharmacologic approach to modulating this response.

Finally, we continue to believe in the importance of offering challenging questions at the end of crucial chapters in order to provide the opportunity to the reader for self-assessment.

WESLEY S. MOORE, M.D.

PREFACE
to the Third Edition

Vascular Surgery: A Comprehensive Review has evolved into a standard textbook of vascular surgery. Our objectives of both completeness and manageable size continue to be paramount in editorial planning. All of the original chapters have either been revised to reflect new and updated information or replaced by new manuscripts. Instructions for revision have included the efficient and limited length of each chapter.

In the four years that have elapsed since the last edition, a number of new and important developments have taken place in the management of patients with vascular disease. These are reflected in new chapters and include the following:

• "Anatomy, Physiology, and Pharmacology of the Vessel Wall." It is clear that the blood vessel is no longer considered a passive conduit for arterial and venous circulation. Rather, there is a complex interaction, both on a physiologic and pharmacologic basis, that takes place between flowing blood and its individual elements. This chapter details the current level of knowledge concerning these relationships.

• "Natural History and Nonoperative Treatment of Chronic Lower Extremity Ischemia." Recognition of the fact that many patients will do quite well with nonoperative management has led to the development of the material in this chapter. Information concerning the natural history of chronic arterial occlusive disease of the lower extremities as well as conservative methods of management are outlined in detail.

• "Reconstruction of the Supra-aortic Trunks and Vertebrobasilar System." The section on cerebrovascular disease has been expanded to include, as a separate chapter, these important areas. Details concerning patterns of disease, diagnosis, and surgical intervention have been expanded in this important area.

• "Endovascular Surgery." An entirely new subject in the field of peripheral vascular disease management has been the evolution of endovascular surgery to include the imaging techniques of vascular endoscopy and intra-arterial ultrasound as well as the therapeutic measures of balloon angioplasty, atherectomy, and laser assisted angioplasty. All of these techniques are reviewed in detail, and the reader is updated concerning the current status of these important new developments.

• "Acute Arterial Occlusion." The topic of acute arterial occlusion has been expanded to cover those areas of the failing vascular graft, management of acute graft failure, and an extended discussion of the reperfusion injury phenomenon.

Finally, we continue to provide questions at the end of each chapter for self-assessment of the material presented.

PREFACE
to the Second Edition

Vascular Surgery: A Comprehensive Review was originally conceived as a text, of manageable size, that would provide current and complete information to those individuals preparing for examinations in vascular surgery.

Our original objective was achieved and, in addition, the book has taken on the stature of becoming a standard text in vascular surgery. For this reason, the Second Edition has been expanded to achieve the completeness required of a standard textbook while keeping in mind the importance of maintaining a manageable size for our readers.

New chapters include the following:

• "Embryology of the Vascular System." This chapter is designed to provide the basic science background for understanding the origins of the vascular system as well as presenting a basis for the understanding of developmental anomalies that the vascular surgeon may be required to treat.

• "Hemodynamics in Atherogenesis." This represents an expansion of the text on atherogenesis that explores not only the biochemical aspects but also other theories and contributors to the basic disease process that we are required to manage.

• "Preoperative Evaluation of the Vascular Surgery Patient." This chapter explores the medical evaluation of patients with vascular disease with respect to coexisting risk factors and their management.

• "Cardiovascular Monitoring and Perioperative Management of the Vascular Surgery Patient." This chapter reviews the types of invasive monitoring used pre- and intra-operatively for the management of complex surgical procedures required on this high risk group of patients.

• "Antibiotics in Vascular Surgery." This represents an emerging area of importance in the surgical management of patients with vascular disease and presents an expanded discussion on the appropriate use of antibiotics in treatment of primary vascular infection, infection prophylaxis, and management of acquired sepsis.

• "The Role of Sympathectomy in the Management of Vascular Disease." While sympathectomy has generally been eclipsed by direct arterial repair, there are many areas in which sympathectomy represents an important form of primary or adjunctive treatment. This chapter surveys the current role of sympathectomy in managing vascular disease.

• "Thrombolytic Therapy for Vascular Disease." Over the past few years, thrombolytic therapy has emerged as an important adjunct in the management of arterial and venous thrombotic problems.

• "Etiology, Diagnosis, and Management of Vascular Graft Infection." This area was previously covered in a chapter on complications in vascular surgery. Because of the importance of graft infection and its management, however, we have expanded this into a separate chapter in order to permit the original complications chapter to focus on non-infectious problems. The expanded chapter on vascular graft infection deals, in depth, with the complex problems presented by patients with vascular graft sepsis.

Finally, each of the original chapters has been thoroughly revised by its authors and brought up to date with respect to new information, statistics, and methods of management. Questions are presented at the end of each chapter to enable readers to test their knowledge of the material presented.

PREFACE
to the First Edition

During the past 20 years of rapid growth and development in vascular surgery, many graduates of general surgery programs found that their training in vascular surgery represented a valuable new resource for their hospital and practice communities. That training in vascular surgery often provided an important edge in establishing a new practice led to the widespread use of the term *general and vascular surgery* on the community announcements and business cards of new surgeons.

Yet in 1969 a survey conducted by a committee composed of James A. DeWeese, F. William Blaisdell, and John H. Foster discovered that among the 83 residents graduating from the 22 general surgery training programs surveyed, only 19 had performed more than 40 arterial reconstructive procedures during the course of their training, and more than half of the graduating residents had performed fewer than 20 arterial reconstructive procedures. The DeWeese committee, which had been established in 1969 to develop a document on optimal resources in vascular surgery, thus concluded that there was considerable suboptimal vascular surgery being performed in the United States, owing to a combination of both inadequate training and continued deficiencies in vascular surgery experience following training. A survey of the frequency of vascular operations in 1143 hospitals across the United States had revealed that in over 75 percent of these hospitals fewer than 10 aneurysm resections and 10 femoropopliteal arterial reconstructions were conducted annually. This discovery led to the unfortunate conclusion that many surgeons were performing only occasional vascular operations, often leading to poor results.

The substance of the DeWeese report was reviewed by the two national vascular societies and their responsible leadership. This paved the way for, among other things, the definition of adequate training in vascular surgery and the recommendation that physicians who wish to practice vascular surgery spend an additional year of training to guarantee adequate experience in the specialty. In order to ensure prospective candidates that a given fellowship program in vascular surgery would provide a broad and responsible experience, the vascular societies established a committee for program evaluation and endorsement from which program directors could request review. Programs reviewed and found to meet the criteria of appropriate education as established by the committee would be announced annually.

Program evaluation by the joint council of the two national vascular societies was taken on as a temporary responsibility because the role would ultimately become the purview of the Residency Review Committee and the Liaison Committee for Graduate Medical Education. It was recognized that once adequate training programs were developed, the certification of candidates successfully completing training rested with the American Board of Surgery.

After approximately 10 years of experience, debate, and review, the American Board of Medical Specialties approved an application by the American Board of Surgery to grant

"Certification of Special Competence in General Vascular Surgery." The first examination for certification was given to qualified members of the American Board of Surgery and Thoracic Surgery in June 1982. The second written examination is being held in November 1983 in several centers across the United States.

The intent of this textbook is to provide a comprehensive review of vascular surgery together with the related medical and basic science disciplines. This edition of the text has been developed to accompany a postgraduate course designed to help candidates prepare for the examination leading to certification in general vascular surgery. Accordingly, a list of questions designed to aid the reader in self-examination completes each chapter. All question sets simply represent the authors' opinion, a fair and adequate survey of the material covered since none of the chapter authors is a member of the American Board of Surgery (this would be a conflict of interest).

Although chapter outlines were suggested by an editorial committee, the final chapter text represents, in the opinion of its authors, core material in each subject. Particular effort to identify and separate generally accepted concepts from new or controversial material was made. Though this book was designed as a comprehensive review to prepare for an examination, it is also in view of its organization and content, a comprehensive text of vascular surgery.

CONTENTS

1
A HISTORY OF VASCULAR SURGERY

WILEY F. BARKER

History is not unchanging, for it is only that which has been written down or remembered. Much personal interpretation of such material is necessarily involved, and this is especially true the closer the observer is to the scene and time of the action. A historical view needs some distance for proper perspective and little will therefore be said in this chapter concerning the last few years: Hence there will be only minor additions and changes based on new information and new interpretations of old information as well as updating of the bibliography since the first edition of this volume.

This history will be presented as a series of scenes and acts; and, as with many modern stage plays, different actors will appear in different scenes in different roles. It must also be recognized that many scenes are occurring at the same time and yet must be observed from different points of view, depending upon the immediate subject at hand. Finally, the whole will ultimately fit together, as one scene prepares the reader to understand either the scene just past or that to come.

PROLOGUE

Although some might argue that Guy de Chauliac or Ambroise Paré should properly be called the sire of surgery, John Hunter appears above all others as the prototype of the vascular surgeon. He was an unbelievably productive and tireless worker, cut from the same Scottish mold as his brother William, who was 10 years older. John, however, was largely unlettered, whereas William had become sophisticated through the elegance of an education at Glasgow. Yet they shared a frenetic capacity for work and an incurable curiosity.

To place the Hunters in a clear perspective with regard to nonmedical history, one should remember that they were contemporaries of George Washington and Benjamin Franklin. William was born in Scotland in 1718, his brother John 10 years later; William died in 1783, John in 1793.[1,2]

William had preceded John to London, and there became interested in many medical subjects, including aneurysms. In fact, he proposed the concept that a carelessly used lancet during bloodletting might enter both artery and vein, and that healing might occur such that the two channels might be connected, and thus imagined an arteriovenous fistula; imagination not being enough, he soon found just such a patient,[3] and described the clinical manifestations with great accuracy. William's primary activity, however, was focused on obstetrics, and on the teaching of anatomy; in this latter project John became at first his assistant.

Mr. John Hunter is remembered for many things, but most especially for his studies of the dynamics and efficiency of collateral arterial circulation in the vessels feeding the antlers of a stag after he had interrupted the major arteries in the neck, and for the ligation of the femoral artery at a distance from a popliteal aneurysm—in "Hunter's canal."[1,2]

To be sure, others had preceded him. In the third century, a Roman surgeon, Antyllus, had described proximal and distal ligation of the artery followed by incision of the aneurysm and removal of its contents, a formidable operation without either anesthesia or asepsis.[4] In 1680, Mathaeus Purmann,[5] faced with a large aneurysm in the antecubital space, carried out ligation of the vessels and excision of the aneurysmal mass. Shortly thereafter, Anel,[6] in 1714, had described an operation in which he placed *one* ligature on the artery just at the proximal extent of the aneurysm. The disagreement between these several surgical approaches is not so great as it seems. Hunter had seen that the ligature at times would cut through the artery when placed too close to the popliteal aneurysm and so he chose a site more remote, one easily reached by the surgeon, one that would preserve collaterals; but most of Anel's patients suffered from a false aneurysm caused by bloodletting in an otherwise healthy artery as opposed to the femoropopliteal aneurysms treated by Hunter, which were due to degenerative processes, probably a mixture of lues and trauma.[1,6,7]

Many other surgeons were ligating aneurysms in various anatomical sites at this time. Sir Astley Cooper soon ligated the carotid for aneurysm in 1805,[8] as well as the aorta for iliac artery aneurysm,[9] but it is only these few important names that have remained with us from before the latter part of the 19th century.

Ligation was substantially the only procedure that could be used at this time in the management of arterial problems. To be sure, Hallowell in Newcastle-on-Tyne had carried out one arterial repair of an artery torn during bloodletting.[10] The laceration was a short one, and at the suggestion of Richard Lambert, he placed a short (1/4–inch) steel pin through the edges of the wound and looped a ligature around it, approximating the edges of the wound with apparent success. Hallowell wrote to Dr. William Hunter concerning this in 1761, foreseeing that if this were a successful technique, "we might be able to cure wounds of some arteries that would otherwise require amputation, or be altogether incurable." Twelve years later (1773) Conradus Asman[11] reviewed the work, attempted some experiments himself that were disastrous, and soon concluded that such a procedure could not work and that Lambert and Hallowell's efforts had probably also failed. Asman's work was contemporaneous with that of Hunter, and after Asman's criticism the matter of arterial repair rested quietly for nearly another hundred years.

John Hunter's less well known contributions are scattered through the immense museum he left to the Royal College of Surgeons of England, and they hint at a greater understanding of arterial pathology than would be generally known for half a century. They include dissections of several atherosclerotic aortic bifurcations (specimens P.1177 and P.1178) showing the lesion Leriche was to describe 150 years later; a carotid bifurcation with an ulcerated atheroma from a patient who died of a ruptured luetic thoracic aneurysm (specimen P.1171) and an extracranial internal carotid aneurysm (specimen P.282) in a patient whose neatly described symptoms appear as almost typical classical transient ischemic episodes.[12] To cap it all, in a postmortem specimen, Hunter had dissected the atheromatous layers (although the term "atheroma" had not yet come into use) from the remaining healthy wall of an atherosclerotic terminal aorta (specimen P.1176), foreshadowing dos Santos by more than 150 years. Regrettably, most of Hunter's notes have not survived to give us more than this fragmentary view of his understanding of vascular disease.

Hunter and his student, later to become *Sir* Astley Cooper, both seemed to hold with the teleological belief of the times that in "senile" or "spontaneous gangrene" in older persons, thrombosis of the major vessels supervened so that the patient would not bleed to death when the gangrenous part separated.[13] It was Cruveilhier[14] who first clearly stated that the term "gangrene due to obstruction of the arteries" by thickening and by thrombosis should replace the terms "spontaneous" and "senile" gangrene, but he attributes the concept to Dupuytren.

Thus gangrene due to occlusion of the arteries was recognized by the early 19th century, but the understanding that there were symptoms of a functional nature less dramatic than the terminal morphological changes of gangrene was not expressed clearly until Barth[15] described in 1835 a patient who manifested classical claudication—complicated by heart failure due to mitral valvular disease, which caused her demise. Barth's report included a description of thrombosis of the terminal aorta with a sketch that suggests the lesion was either a thrombosed hypoplastic terminal aorta or a contracted atherosclerotic lesion, or a combination of both. Barth repeated Hunter's observation that the obstructing material could easily be separated from the residual arterial wall.

Although Charcot has most commonly been credited with the description of "intermittent claudication in the horse and in man,"[16] his 1858 report cited Barth as having observed and described claudication very precisely in man 20 years earlier. Charcot, however, details the vanishing pulses, the cold extremity, and the loss of sympathetic tone in a horse in the throes of a spasm of severe claudication. In his human patient, Charcot related the functional symptoms to an occlusion of the common iliac artery distal to a traumatic aneurysm, itself secondary to a bullet wound suffered 20 years before. In this patient he described symptoms similar to those seen in the horse, but in addition he delineated the "herald" hemorrhage of an aortoenteric fistula.

Such information was of little utility to the surgeon, however, until arterial repair became a reality. In consistency with the observations of Asman, several German masters had *ex cathedra* defined attempts at arterial repair (as opposed to ligation) as impossible. Langenbeck[17] had stated in 1825 that since the primary requirement for healing is perfect rest, so long as the movements of the arterial wall continued, the wound could never heal. Heinecke[18] had been certain that the subject would bleed to death through the suture holes and the apposed edges of the arterial wall.

Repair of venous injuries, however, was becoming an established procedure: the lateral ligature, in which a clamp is placed on the defect in the venous wall and ligature tied around the puckered wall, had been performed in 1816 (Travers, cited by Jassinowsky[19]). The first lateral suture of a venous defect (an erosion of the common jugular vein from an infected neck wound) was undertaken by Czerny[20] in 1881, but the patient died of sepsis and hemorrhage. Schede[21] is credited by Jassinowsky[19] with the first successful repair of a large venous injury (one to the common femoral vein). Furthermore, Eck[22] had reported the experimental creation of a portocaval fistula. The original description hints he had little to confirm his success. Among a series of eight dogs, one did not survive 24 hours, six lived 2 to 6 days, and the one survivor "tired of life in the laboratory and ran away after two months." The doctoral dissertation of Jassinowsky,[19] written in 1889 as purely library research work, reviews the published information on arterial suture and concludes that it could not be successful at that moment but that there might be hope in the future.

Only 2 years later, however, Jassinowsky himself did succeed and in 1891 he reported his successful animal experiments on arterial suture.[23] The suture he described was passed carefully two thirds of the way through the media: he tried to avoid penetrating the intima except in very thin-walled vessels. Dörfler[24] modified Jassinowsky's method, and passed the suture through all thicknesses of the arterial wall, and recognized that the arterial suture in the lumen of the vessel did no harm if uninfected: he said that it soon became covered with a glistening membrane. Shortly thereafter, in 1896, Jaboulay and Briau[25] described successful end-to-end carotid arterial anastomoses using an everting "U"-shaped suture. Successful arterial suture is thus barely a century old!

Jaboulay was one of the surgeons at Lyon under whose influence Alexis Carrel studied. When Sadi Carnot, the President of the Republic of France, was assassinated and died because no one dared to try to repair his wounded portal vein, Carrel was highly critical, for he believed the blood vessels could be sutured as well as any other tissue.[26] He soon began to undertake experimental arterial anastomoses. Some of the earliest of these were arteriovenous communications in which the high-flow system assured patency. Carrel's contributions to technical arterial surgery included methods that vascular surgeons use routinely today.[27,28] He devised the triangulation suture to facilitate end-to-end anastomosis; he described the patch technique to anastomose a small vessel to the side of a larger one; and he pioneered the use of vessel grafts and organ transplantation. His work, however, was not fully accepted in the United States for many years. Part of this stemmed from disputations that arose between him and his coworker for a year, E. A. Guthrie.[29]

Nonetheless, European surgeons not only accepted but began to follow Carrel's lead. In 1906, Goyanes[30] of Madrid resected a popliteal aneurysm, then restored arterial continuity with an in situ venous graft using the popliteal vein, probably the first successful clinical vascular replacement.

Surgeons in America were at this time beginning vascular surgery in their own way. In New Orleans in 1888 Rudolph Matas[31] had described a landmark operation. He had stumbled into the surgical procedure for which he is commonly remembered, endoaneurysmorrhaphy, when the aneurysm for which he had ligated the brachial artery with apparent success began to pulsate again 10 days later. He chose to reoperate, and to ligate the brachial artery distally. Even after this distal ligation, the pulsation remained and he was forced to open the aneurysm, clean out the sac (the Antyllian operation), and oversew the other arteries feeding the aneurysm from inside the sac. Matas differed from Antyllus in that he used a suture to obliterate the feeding vessels from within the sac instead of ligating them after extensive dis-

section outside the sac and risking interference with collateral circulation and other adherent anatomical structures. It was many years before he again performed an endoaneurysmorrhaphy, for most patients were treated successfully by simple proximal ligation.[32] Matas ultimately expanded his technique to include "restorative" and "reconstructive" modifications, and to report an approach to the arteriovenous fistula through the venous component,[33] as had been proposed by Bickham.[34]

J. B. Murphy[35] of Chicago had performed a series of experiments on animals in which he successfully restored flow by invagination of the proximal into the distal vessel; then in 1897 he presented a successful human case. Sterling Edwards revived this anastomic technique of invagination briefly in his recommendations for the use of the first braided nylon grafts.[36]

Murphy's invagination techniques were reflected in other nonsuture methods of anastomosis: Nitze[37] and Payr[38] used small metal or ivory rings through which the vessel was drawn, everted, and tied in place; this unit was then inserted into the mouth of the distal vessel and another ligature secured it there. This is quickly recognized as the Blakemore tube,[39] used, but without signal success, in World War II.[40]

During the same period William Stewart Halsted was beginning his tenure at Johns Hopkins Hospital, with an abundance of vascular trauma and of leutic aneurysms commanding his attention. In the early 1900s Carrel visited Halsted and described his work, including his early arteriovenous anastomoses. As a result, Halsted *almost* made history in 1907[41] when, faced with the dilemma of a patient whose popliteal artery and vein had been sacrificed during an *en bloc* dissection of a sarcoma of the popliteal space, Halsted went to the other leg, took the saphenous vein, reversed it, and anastomosed the distal saphenous vein to the proximal femoral artery. For his distal anastomosis, however, he chose the popliteal *vein*, and although the graft pulsated for 40 minutes, it soon thrombosed. One can only imagine what a dramatic leap forward vascular surgery would have made then if Halsted, with his superb surrounding cast, had chosen the popliteal artery for the distal anastomosis and had achieved in 1907 a truly successful arterial reconstruction!

During this same period of time, German surgeons such as Höpfner,[42] Lexer,[43,44] and Jeger[45] had become familiar with the use of vein grafts. Höpfner had described the bypass procedure, which was illustrated in an encyclopedic book by Jeger. Jeger's book, as republished posthumously in 1937, included a foreword that described Jeger's replantation of the completely severed arm of a German soldier, which he had performed in 1914. A year later, Jeger came to an untimely death from typhus, while on the Russian front.

Lexer[44] collected and reported on 65 vein transplants, of which some 13 were his personal cases. In eight of these 13 cases, Lexer had obtained a distal pulse. This report prompted a Polish surgeon, Weg-lowski,[46] to present his own personal series of 51 cases, mostly traumatic in origin, operated upon between 1914 and 1921; in 40 patients he could document good distal pulses and normal arterial tracings. Yet all this seemed forgotten in the next 25 years, as Germany suffered in the agonies of the interbellum years, and as the forceful and charismatic personality of René Leriche appeared on the scene. We will pick up his role in a later section.

ABDOMINAL AORTIC ANEURYSM

Beyond the management of trauma to the arteries, the aneurysm is one of the great themes that has bound vascular surgeons together for many years, and the management of the abdominal aneurysm is certainly one of vascular surgery's major accomplishments. Vesalius is said to have been the first to describe an abdominal aneurysm.[47]

The technical maneuvers that have been described concerning the ligation of aneurysms in various anatomical sites usually involved aneurysms of the peripheral vessels; aneurysms of the trunk were sacrosanct, for proximal control was not feasible. Sir Astley Cooper (1768–1849), a student of John Hunter, had continued many of Hunter's studies, including evaluation of collateral arterial supplies. In 1805 he ligated the common carotid for aneurysm,[8] but he opened the door for even wider surgical applications when in 1818 he ligated the abdominal aorta to control external hemorrhage from an aneurysm of the external iliac artery that had eroded to the surface of the skin of the flank, bleeding openly at that site.[9]

Various other methods to accomplish obstruction of an aneurysm have been attempted: Colt, at the end of the 19th century, used wire to pack the aneurysm, and then heated the wire.[48] Blakemore and King[49] revived interest in this in 1938, and many surgeons undertook modifications of the wiring technique—largely without success.

The major actors in the next scene are again Rudolph Matas of New Orleans and William Stewart Halsted of Baltimore. Their interest in the management of trauma to the vessels, and in the management of the late sequelae of trauma, provided material for the fertile imaginations of the many surgeons who were emboldened to follow their footsteps. Reid[50] reported the experience of the Johns Hopkins Hospital, which is properly that of its chief, Halsted, with aneurysms in 1926; but although these aneurysms included many varieties, both anatomical and etiological, the treatment of the abdominal aneurysms was substantially a failure.

These operations were only preparation for the last gasp of treatment by ligation for aneurysms of the abdominal aorta. Matas finally accomplished a successful aortic ligation (just below the renal arteries). He reported it first in 1923,[51] but later in the *Annals of Surgery* in 1940.[52] In the same issue of the *Annals*

of Surgery was a similar paper by Elkin,[53] as well as the hint of a coming era of vascular reconstruction in the report by I. A. Bigger[54] of Virginia. He had ligated the neck of an abdominal aneurysm using fascia that he expected to loosen gradually and allow restoration of flow; with the protection of this temporary control, he performed a plication of the aneurysm, restoring the aorta to its proper caliber. The patient had a protracted survival not only without recurrence of the aneurysm but also with restoration of femoral pulses.

Other experiences with the aorta were preparing the way for present-day management of the abdominal aneurysm. Alexander and Byron[55] had resected a thoracic aneurysm associated with coarctation of the aorta, and successfully oversewn the ends of the vessel, although that patient ultimately died of renovascular hypertension.[56] Various attempts were made to utilize either reactive cellophane[57] or the irritating plasticizer in it, diacetyl phosphate,[58] as a means of inducing sclerosis that might restrain the dilatation of the aneurysm. Again, results were poor.

About this time, however, cardiac surgery began to emerge. During the first decade of the century Jeger[45] had proposed valved venous bypasses from the left pulmonary veins to the left ventricle to bypass mitral stenosis, and a valved venous graft from the left ventricle to the innominate artery to bypass aortic stenosis. In the mid-1920s, Cutler, Levine, and Beck[59] had attempted to treat mitral stenosis surgically, but with minimal success. A valvulotome was used through a ventricular approach. Nonetheless, the influence of these attempts led Gross to the successful ligation[60] and then division[61] of the patent ductus arteriosus. In Baltimore, Blalock and Taussig[62] began their series of pioneering surgical procedures upon various cardiac anomalies, of which the first and most dramatic was the "blue baby" operation, the creation of a systemic shunt from the subclavian artery to the pulmonary artery in congenital pulmonic stenosis. Crafoord and Nylin[63] reported the successful end-to-end anastomosis of the aorta after resection of an aortic coarctation at the same time that Gross and Hufnagel[64] carried out their first case. This last operation demonstrated that lesions of the thoracic and abdominal segments of the aorta were amenable to surgical approach.

In 1947 Hufnagel had reported on the use of rapid freezing for the preservation of arterial homografts[65] for use in the repair of long aortic coarctations. Gross,[66] who at first seemed to fear that frozen vessels could not survive, published a laboratory and clinical report on his experiences with homografts preserved in electrolyte solutions for use in various cardiac operations, but particularly for the management of coarctation of the aorta. Swan[67] soon used a homograft for a thoracic aneurysm associated with a coarctation. The report of Estes[68] that defined the grave risk to life for the patient who had an abdominal aneurysm provided the surgeon with justification to consider *elective* resection of the aneurysm instead of attempting treatment only after it was too late in the game, when the odds were hopeless. In 1951 Oudot[69] reported the use of an aortic homograft to treat an aortic obstruction (Leriche syndrome) after resecting the bifurcation, and set the stage for the successful resection of an abdominal aortic aneurysm and replacement with a homograft by Charles Dubost[70] on the 19th of March, 1951. Schaffer and Hardin[71] had actually preceded Dubost by 4 weeks, but their publication appeared considerably later. Dubost's operation was then followed by those of Julian,[72] Brock,[73] DeBakey,[74] and Bahnson.[75] It is a curious twist of fate to find that Dubost had left the practice of colorectal surgery to become a cardiac surgeon after he had seen Blalock and Bahnson perform cardiac operations while they were visiting France in the late 1940s. Szilagyi's[76] classical study of the benefits of the operation provided a confirmation and justification of the procedure that thoroughly confirmed the surgical treatment of the material that Estes had presented.

The arterial homograft seemed at first to be a quite successful substitute for the thoracic or the abdominal aorta. Initially fresh grafts were used, then they were preserved in Tyrode's solution.[65,66] The techniques of freezing[77] and then lyophilization[78] allowed the development of artery banks. Early successes were soon erased by late failures of the homografts, and a truly satisfactory aortic substitute was clearly needed.

The complicated abdominal aneurysm still posed a major problem. Ellis[79] was one of the first to implant the renal arteries into the graft when the aneurysm was found to include their orifices. Etheredge[80] extended this operation to resect a major thoracoabdominal aortic aneurysm. He used a heparinized plastic shunt of the type described in Schaffer's resection and replacement of an abdominal aneurysm with a homograft in March of 1951. Etheredge established the shunt, divided the aorta, and performed the proximal anastomosis; he then moved the clamp down the graft after each successive visceral anastomosis was completed, then finished with the lower aortic anastomosis to the graft. Schumacker[81] modified Etheredge's operation slightly, placing the graft as a permanent bypass, dividing the aorta just below the anastomosis and continuing with attachment of the individual visceral branches, and finally performing an obliterative endoaneurysmorrhaphy.

DeBakey[82] reported in 1956 a series of complicated abdominal aneurysms that were resected by a technique similar to that of Shumacker. Stoney and Wylie[83] popularized the long thoracoabdominal incision for the approach to this lesion in 1973. The great advance in the management of these complicated lesions was made by Stanley Crawford,[84] who introduced a direct approach to the aneurysm in which the aorta is clamped above and below and then opened throughout the length of the aneurysm. A fabric graft is sewn into the proximal aorta, then the major groups of arteries, including the lower intercostals, are sewn into the wall of the fabric tube using the expeditious

Carrel patch method of anastomosis; then the distal anastomosis is completed. This direct method has greatly simplified the approach to lesions that might otherwise have been considered irresectable.

PERIPHERAL ARTERIAL ANEURYSMS

The peripheral arterial aneurysm was one of the first arterial lesions treated by the surgeon, but its importance paled beside the advances made in the management of the aortic aneurysm described above. The history of treatment by ligation has been detailed above.

In 1949, Linton[85] had utilized Leriche's principle of arteriectomy and sympathectomy for the management of a series of 14 patients who had popliteal aneurysm—an ingenious approach that in his series resulted in no amputations. The patient received a preliminary sympathectomy, then shortly—although sometimes at the same séance—underwent resection of the aneurysm with ligation of the vessels.

The ability to replace vessels of the size of the popliteal artery promptly brought to the fore the concept that the popliteal aneurysm had a risk-benefit pattern similar to the abdominal aneurysm; if operations were done electively the results were excellent, but once thrombosis occurred the risk to the limb was grave, as Whychulis and his associates[86] and Gifford and his associates[87] demonstrated. Wylie (in discussion of Whychullis[86]) and Edwards[88] introduced the procedure of exclusion of the aneurysm and restoration of flow through a bypass technique.

ARTERIAL SUBSTITUTES

It was mentioned in a previous paragraph that the arterial homograft had functioned fairly well in the aorta, but it was material that was difficult to obtain, harvest, sterilize, and store, and grafts other than those of the aorta fared poorly. The use of an artificial arterial substitute was to allow the great expansion of arterial reconstruction. Homografts of smaller vessels containing a higher proportion of smooth muscle were even less satisfactory.

Following the experience in the laboratory reported by Abbe,[89] Tuffier[90] had used rigid tubes of metal and of paraffined glass in World War I, but without much success. Similar tubes were used in World War II, but the results were no better than in immediate ligation of the artery.[40] Hufnagel chose a more inert surface, methylmethacrylate,[91,92] and designed a better hemodynamic tube. These functioned very well except for the difficulties in securing them within a major artery such as the aorta without the risk of ultimate erosion, but the use of the pliable plastic fabrics substantially eliminated the use of the rigid tube.

In 1952, Voorhees, Jaretzki, and Blakemore[93] observed that fabric threads in the heart soon became covered with endothelium. Dörfler[24] had made a similar gross observation 60 years earlier but had not carried the observation to its conclusion. Voorhees and his associates at Columbia experimented not only with Vinyon-N, but with parachute silk and other materials. Many fabrics were tried, and most were quickly discarded; braided and crimped nylon tubes were introduced by Edwards and Tapp,[36] but nylon rapidly lost strength and was shown to be unsatisfactory. Orlon[92] and Teflon[94] were both used, and Teflon remains in use by many surgeons today. Szilagyi[95] and Julian[96] introduced variations of Dacron. The transcripts of the vascular surgery meetings of the late 1950s might be mistaken for a textile journal, as various weaves, deniers, calendarizing, and the advantages of braid versus knit versus taffeta weaves were discussed. The summation of the principles of vascular grafting by Wesolowski and Dennis[97] and by Deterling[98] and the definition of the importance of porosity by Wesolowski[99] were all important landmarks.

It was the knitted Dacron introduced by DeBakey,[100] however, that placed a successful graft in the hands of every surgeon. Subsequent modifications by the addition of velour to the surface by Sauvage[101] and by Cooley[102] have been refinements in this outstanding contribution. The concept that the fabric tube would become "encapsulated" and might develop a firm new endothelial surface has been pursued as a goal, but has not been achieved.

The immediate porosity of the grafts has been troublesome, especially in patients whose situation requires heparinization, or in whom even minor blood loss from a weeping graft is intolerable. Impregnation of grafts with either collagen[103] or albumin[104] have been dramatic steps forward, as has been the use of expanded polytetrafluoroethylene, a flexible nonfabric material that is substantially nonporous. It was introduced by Soyer[105] for use as a venous substitute, but it has come to be used extensively in distal arterial reconstructions as a second choice after the autologous saphenous vein.[106]

Other biological substitutes than the arterial homograft have been used, however. Rosenberg and his associates[107] used bovine carotid arteries that were subjected to enzymatic treatment to remove all of the tissue-specific protein except the basic structural collagen of the bovine artery. Sawyer and his associates[108] modified the bovine heterograft by inducing a negatively charged lining in an effort to inhibit thrombosis; and Dardik[109] used treated umbilical vein grafts supported with a mesh of Dacron as a peripheral arterial substitute.

OCCLUSIVE ARTERIAL DISEASE

As mentioned earlier, it was not until the middle of the last century that the relationship between arterial occlusions and either clinical symptoms or gangrene had clearly become established. Repair of acute injuries had been accomplished, but the management of more chronic arterial obstructions had not become a surgical problem.

René Leriche, born in 1879, had been educated and trained at Lyon, where he had known Jaboulay and Carrel. After completing his training, Leriche stayed on the service of Professor Poncet, until the latter died, and shortly thereafter Jaboulay was killed; "Surgery in Lyon was decimated," said Leriche.[110] Then came World War I, with its forced dislocations and peregrinations. After he was demobilized Leriche worked in a trauma hospital in Lyon for several years; he saw many patients with posttraumatic neuralgias and confirmed the concepts of the role of the sympathetic nervous system in this problem, and the possible treatment by periarterial sympathectomy, about which he had first published in 1916.[111] Then, seeing patients with arterial thrombosis due to "artérite," a loose and nonspecific term used to describe arterial occlusion in general, Leriche came to the conclusion that if the patient was seen before the occluding thrombosis was too widespread, a local resection of the thrombosed artery provided relief. Since many patients did well after this simple procedure and soon developed relatively warm feet, he concluded that the collateral circulation in these patients must usually have been satisfactory and that the coldness of the extremity must be due to vasospasm instead of insufficient arterial flow. He therefore applied the principle of sympathectomy, first as a periarterial operation, then as an arteriectomy (excising the obstructed segment), and then as a division of the sympathetic rami.

Dietz,[112] dissatisfied with the results of periarterial sympathectomy, modified that operation into the lumbar ganglionectomy. At nearly the same time Royle[113] and Hunger[114] introduced the same operation for the fruitless management of spasm in striated muscle. The use of this operation for the management of pain syndromes, and for the management of ischemic extremities, remains controversial.

It seems likely that the force of Leriche's personality led European surgical thought along lines that diverged from the known techniques of vascular grafting; this is not to say that he actively spoke against the use of grafts. In fact, it is commonly stated that he often said it would have been ideal to connect the two ends of a severed artery by a graft but the distance always seemed too great; instead, he chose to offer arterial excision and sympathectomy, an approach that had benefit but less risk.

One of Leriche's most important early observations included the definition of the syndrome to which we have attached his name, the atherosclerotic obliteration of the terminal aorta and the iliac arteries. He described this in 1923,[115] during the period in which he was beginning to evaluate arteriectomy. It was 17 years, however, before he found a suitable case in which he could perform the resection of the aortic bifurcation and lumbar sympathectomy.[116] His surgical clinic became famous, and he collected around him a great series of surgeons who came to learn: DeBakey, Learmonth, dos Santos, and Kunlin to name only a few.

The possibility of effective arterial suture *anastomosis* had been developed through the ideas of Jaboulay, and of Carrel, at Lyon. After World War I another surgeon from Lyon assumed a major role in vascular surgery. Here it will be necessary to flash back briefly to 1909, for in that year Murphy[117] removed an embolus from the common iliac artery and restored flow into the femoral system. Although locally successful, distal thrombosis required a distal amputation. Two years later, Labey, as cited by Mosney and Dumont,[118] removed an embolus from the artery of a patient with full success. Embolectomy was thereafter performed with occasional success world wide, but it had not become a fully satisfactory procedure because of the need for great haste in operating before extensive distal thrombosis supervened. After the clinical introduction of heparin by Murray,[119] it became possible to extend the indications and limiting time restrictions for embolectomy and to improve the results.

Surgeons such as João Cid dos Santos[120] and his father Reynaldo undertook the use of heparin in order to prevent thrombosis after the old Matas endoaneurysmorrhaphy. The younger dos Santos believed that with the protection of heparin he might be able to remove chronically adherent arterial emboli and their associated thrombus and have healing without rethrombosis. Finding such a patient with advanced renal disease and a seriously ischemic extremity, dos Santos removed the clot and reestablished flow, but was chided by the pathologist for having removed the intima as well. After another successful case, in which he removed a chronic thrombosis of the subclavian, axillary, and brachial arteries secondary to the scalenus anticus syndrome, he sent his report to René Leriche. Leriche presented the work in the name of dos Santos to the French Academy of Surgery,[121] and endarterectomy was underway. It is interesting to note that neither of these patients suffered from primarily atherosclerotic thrombosis.

Subsequently, Freeman,[122] Wylie,[123] and others in this country adopted the operation, using the open technique that was primarily claimed by Reboul.[124] Wylie's work was reported in September of 1951, and described endoaneurysmectomy and endarterectomy of the aorta. We had undertaken six procedures without success, but in the summer of 1951 Wylie had visited us and in October, 1951, we performed the first successful endarterectomy in our series.[125] The operation consisted of a combination of the Matas endoaneurysmorrhaphy and the dos Santos endarterectomy (or, rather, the technique as revised by Reboul): an abdominal aneurysm was endarterectomized, tailored to a proper size, and wrapped with fascia lata, and endarterectomy in continuity was performed throughout the length of the left iliofemoral-popliteal system. In fact, these operations were only

extensions of the repair of an aneurysm performed by Bigger[54] in 1940.

Cannon and Barker later introduced the long closed endarterectomy using intraluminal strippers,[126] which was a modification of the original method of dos Santos. Several varieties of endarterectomy loops were devised, by Butcher,[127] and by Vollmar,[128] among others. A period of early successes was followed by disenchantment with the difficulty of the operation in comparison to the increasingly popular grafting procedures.

Leriche and his close associate, Jean Kunlin, had not had great technical success with the operation of endarterectomy, especially in the femoral artery system. Kunlin[129,130] revived the vein graft in the form of a *long* venous bypass graft. Veins had been used for very short (4- to 8-cm) replacements on rare occasions during the prior 40 years. This is the technique that has persisted as the basic method of arterial reconstruction ever since.

Saphenous vein grafting was useful only in the femoral and iliofemoral system, however, and it remained for Jacques Oudot to perform a comparable operation upon the aorta[69] using an aortic homograft, which thoracic and cardiac surgeons were already using as a graft in segments of the thoracic aorta for coarctation and for other thoracic aortic lesions. Oudot was presented with a 51-year-old patient, claudicating as a result of a proximal iliac and distal aortic occlusion. The anatomical lesion is commonly represented in descriptions of Oudot's operation as a simple bifurcation graft, common iliac to common iliac, but in fact it was a much more complicated procedure. He approached the bifurcation through a left flank incision and resected the bifurcation. The patient's internal iliacs were found to be thrombosed and were ligated. The external iliac arteries of the graft were very small, but the graft's internal iliacs were large; Oudot therefore anastomosed the graft's internal iliacs to the patient's external iliacs. However, he did the left-sided anastomosis first and then found it obstructed his view and manipulations of the right-sided anastomosis. This difficult anastomosis thrombosed promptly. Oudot made the best of a bad situation and pointed out that he had done a perfect experiment; there was still some argument from the camp of Leriche as to whether grafting at this level would be worthwhile. On the right side Oudot had performed substantially nothing more than an arteriectomy; on the left he had a reconstitution of the lumen. The right side was warm but pulseless and fatigued easily, whereas the left side had a pulse and did not tire.

Six months later Oudot[131] reoperated upon the patient, who was still complaining of right-sided claudication; he performed an iliac-to-iliac "extraanatomical" bypass, even as had been suggested by Kunlin in 1951.[130] A few months later Oudot climbed Anapurna with the French team, and shortly after his return to France he was killed in an automobile accident at the age of 40.

The saga of the treatment of arterial disease continues with the development and then the failure of artery banks, and then with the introduction of the plastic prosthesis, but by 1952 the stage was set for nearly everything that is done today. Robert Linton's espousal[132] of the reversed saphenous vein confirmed the approach of Kunlin, and established the procedure of choice for peripheral reconstruction for many years.

Endarterectomy did not die: it persists in carotid operations, but only occasionally is it used in the aorta. Edwards[133] made one important attempt to utilize it in the femoral artery by means of the use of a long patch; the procedure worked well unless the patch was so wide it created a stagnant column of blood in the femoral artery. Its use was limited to the distal portion of the popliteal artery and it was exceedingly tedious, and the procedure fell out of favor. In recent years, however, closed endarterial procedures have become commonplace. Dotter and Judkins[134] have used a stiff dilator, a procedure that was not widely accepted. Gruntzig[135] modified this method by using a balloon that could distend and fracture the stenotic plaque. Others, injecting drugs or small emboli of biological and nonbiological materials, have been able to control arterial or venous hemorrhage, thrombose small aneurysms, and control the multiple arteriovenous connections of vascular malformations.

Endarterial manipulations have been extended to include not only dilatations and placement of emboli of several kinds in bleeding arteries, but also, by development of newer methods, to attempts at removal of the atherosclerotic lesion by endarterial manipulations through a percutaneous route. A major requirement for endarterial procedures was believed to be endarterial visualization, beyond that given by contrast radiography. Visualization began effectively with the work of Greenstone.[136] Actual removal of the plaque by several mechanical means has followed: Simpson[137] used a side-biting forceps in a catheter, Kensey[138] a catheter through which is passed a rapidly rotating auger-like tip, and Ahn[139] advocated a high-speed rotary burr. Others have used various forms of laser energy to destroy the plaque,[140] one that recognizes the difference between plaque and normal arterial wall,[141] or a laser-heated probe that "melts" the atheroma.[142] Further mechanical dilatation often accompanies these initial coring methods. Appraisal of these methods, however, belongs in the clinical rather than the historical section of this volume, for they appear to offer only limited removal of the atheromatous material and much less satisfactory results than the classical techniques of endarterectomy.

Two further important extensions of the distal femoral reconstruction have come onto the scene; the first is the introduction of the graft to the infrapopliteal artery. Palma[143] published in 1960 descriptions of vein graft insertions into the tibial arteries. More recent communication from Palma (personal communication, September 16, 1988) indicates that these were performed as early as 1956. McCaughan[144] described the exposure of the distal popliteal artery in 1958, but his terminology included a description of the artery usually known as the tibioperoneal trunk as the "distal popliteal artery." In that paper McCaughan had described a successful graft into the tibial vessels in July of 1957, using an exposure in the upper third of the calf. He presented six further patients with grafts into the tibial segment in 1960.[145] In 1966, McCaughan[146] went one step further when he reported four grafts in which the distal site of the graft was the posterior tibial artery at the ankle. George Morris[147] in 1959, and Tyson[148] were other pioneers in the infrapopliteal procedures.

The other extension of distal femoral reconstruction was the application of the in situ vein graft with destruction of valvular competence within the vein by Karl Victor Hall.[149] The procedure did not receive much attention until revitalized by Leather and his associates[150] in 1981. Many variations on the theme of the distal bypass have been introduced combining free grafts and in situ methods: Dardik[109,151] introduced not only the use of the tanned human umbilical vein, but also a distal arteriovenous fistula; this was not so much a revival of Carrel's earlier attempts to revascularize an extremity through the veins, but rather an attempt to provide a sufficient outflow for a long graft to assure its patency while some of the graft flow would still be directed through the distal arterial tree. DeLaurentis[152] introduced a method of sequential multiple bypasses in the extremity, and Veith and his associates[153] have carried this to extremes with bypasses from one tibial artery to another, even with bypasses beginning and ending below the malleolus. Dalman and his associates[154] have applied this small vessel bypass technique to management of small vessel disease in the hand.

A different approach to the ischemic limb was advocated by Peter Martin,[155] who introduced an extended form of profundaplasty. His work was preceded by earlier contributions by French surgeons Oudot and Cormier,[156] but since that time Miller,[157] Cohn,[158] and Towne and Bernhard[159] have added useful concepts to the management of ischemia with the help of the profunda femoris artery.

None of this great advance of reconstructive surgery, however, has been helpful in the management of the frustrating syndrome of thromboangiitis obliterans. It is likely that von Winiwarter did describe the pathological process, but his description is ambiguous.[160] Certainly, Leo Buerger[161] described the clinical picture, although neither von Winiwarter nor Buerger noted the association with tobacco, nor the involvement of the upper extremities.

One major contribution rounds out this section. In 1963 Thomas Fogarty[162] devised one of the most useful technical methods for the management of occlusive arterial disease when he introduced the balloon embolectomy catheter for the extraction of clot in the treatment of embolization. This technique has been modified for use in many other arterial and venous operations, and has even been adapted to many general surgical uses.

ARTERIAL TRAUMA

Arterial injuries have always been a challenge to the surgeon. Trauma was the source of Hallowell's first arterial repair. During the years that followed the Civil War, Weir Mitchell[163] described the syndrome of burning pain ("causalgia") that followed many arterial injuries, and it was this lesion that intrigued Leriche and led him to his interest in the sympathetic nervous system.[111] Halsted had remarked upon the fascination that arterial injuries held for the surgeon. During World War I, Makins[164] surveyed the injuries to blood vessels incurred by the British forces. DeBakey and Simeone[165] provided a similar service for the United States forces after World War II and noted almost no benefit from the vascular surgical techniques then available, because of the incidental and associated surgical problems and the matters of delay.

So it was that few arterial injuries were treated definitively—except for ligation—until the Korean War. Before that time the main interest in arterial injuries seemed to lie in the estimation of the prognosis for survival of the limb, and for the selection of the appropriate level for ligation of the artery.

During the Korean War, however, Jahnke,[166] Hughes,[167] and Spencer[168] participated in a program in which acute vascular injuries were treated by the use of fresh vein grafts. Whelan[169] and Rich[170] continued this use of the techniques of arterial repair in Vietnam. The Registry of Vascular Injuries from Vietnam as maintained at the Walter Reed Army Medical Center under the direction of Rich has continued to yield a monumental body of information concerning acute vascular repair. Civilian medical centers have continued the applications of these techniques to the everyday pattern of injuries to the vessels.

The arteriovenous fistula is one of the sequelae of trauma to the major vessels that poses a special challenge to surgeons. Its acute effects on the distal circulation, its systemic effects as a major left-to-right shunt, and its local changes, which result in increased blood flow through the feeding arterial supply, have all been intriguing examples of the body's adaptability—or lack of it.

The arteriovenous fistula was first described by William Hunter.[3] The lesion did not become common until the end of the 19th century, as the patterns of weapons changed. Volumes have been written in interpretation of the diverse physiological parameters involved in this lesion, but, as early as 1913, Soubbotitich[171] noted that simple ligation of the proximal artery should never be done. Not long after, Lexer[43] introduced the "ideal" operation, consisting of resection of the aneurysmal sac and restoration of flow through the artery with a short venous graft if the ends of the artery could not be brought back

together. Reconstruction of the vein was desirable but not mandatory. Bickham[34] had suggested approaching the repair of the artery through the venous component of the sac, with repair of the vein if possible, a modification of the Matas endoaneurysmorraphy. For the most part, however, until the era of the Korean War in the 1950s and even later, the commonest form of surgical management was quadruple ligation and excision of the sac and fistula. Such an operation depends upon the development of sufficient collateral circulation to the distal limb to allow the limb to survive after arterial interruption, but must occur before the extra load placed upon the heart by left-to-right shunt caused serious cardiac disability; the timing became a matter of most delicate clinical judgment. Emile Holman, who had developed a lifelong interest in the arteriovenous fistula during his training at Johns Hopkins, was the most eminent contributor to the understanding of the physiology of the arteriovenous fistula.[172] With the advent of prompt exploration and repair of acute arterial injuries, it was anticipated that the number of late arteriovenous fistulas would be greatly reduced, but this has not been the case.

EXTRACRANIAL CEREBROVASCULAR ARTERIAL OCCLUSIONS

The critical nature of the blood flow to the brain through the great arteries of the neck was recognized by the ancient Greeks, who named the carotid artery after the symptoms that followed its occlusion—asphyxia, or stupor. The clinical importance of carotid artery obstruction has been only slowly accepted by the neurological community in general, however, despite the fact that eminent neurologists such as Savory,[173] Hunt,[174] and Fisher[175,176] had made the critical clinical observations relating arterial lesions and atheroembolic phenomena many years before surgical treatment became accepted.

The first elective attempt to restore flow to the ischemic brain was made by Carrea and his associates[177] in 1951 (reported in 1955), and was identical to the reconstruction accomplished by Lefèvre[178] in a case of trauma in 1918; the carotid bulb was resected, the common carotid ligated, and the internal and external carotid arteries anastomosed to provide to the brain the arterial supply from the rich anastomoses of the external carotid. The most widely acclaimed carotid early reconstruction and the one that truly began the phase of modern carotid surgery was the resection of the carotid bifurcation and restoration of carotid flow by anastomosis of the common carotid to the internal carotid artery by Eastcott, Pickering, and Rob[179] in 1954. It now appears that others, including Denton Cooley[180] and Michael DeBakey,[181] separately had preceded this operation with isolated carotid endarterectomy. As was the case with Estes and his paper justifying the approach to the abdominal aneurysm, so the report to the National Research Council of Great Britain by Yates and Hutchinson[182] indicated the importance of occlusive disease of the carotid and vertebral arteries. Whisnant and his associates[183] in Rochester (Minnesota) identified the risk of stroke in the presence of transient ischemic attacks and provided the solid basis for operation upon the carotid artery. Hollenhorst[184] called attention to the bright cholesterol emboli that are pathognomonic of atherosclerotic embolization, but Julian and his associates[185] and Moore and Hall[186] clearly identified the role of embolization as the major cause of transient cerebral ischemic symptoms. Further landmark studies of the morphology of the carotid plaque and its evolution were presented by Imparato[187] and by Lusby.[188] Moore and Hall[189] and other of Wylie's associates called attention to the role of carotid back-pressure in identifying those patients whose brains need protection during the period of operative occlusion.

Operation for the symptomatic patient was soon relatively well accepted, but operation to prevent stroke by the identification of patients who have a carotid stenosis manifesting itself either by a bruit or by a measurable change in retinal artery pressure or some other laboratory noninvasive test remains controversial. Thompson's work[190] is the predominant authoritative source in spite of criticism concerning lack of perfect controls; recently Dixon and his associates[191] have brought forth further evidence concerning the role of large and asymptomatic ulcerations of the carotid bifurcation. Berguer[192] has shown that many "asymptomatic" patients with carotid lesions actually demonstrate multiple small cerebral infarcts that have not been clearly reflected in the patient's symptoms.

An immense body of controversial literature has been published concerning the use of anticoagulant or antiplatelet agents to prevent thrombosis or thromboembolization, but these modalities remain an adjunct to the highly effective operation of carotid endarterectomy when performed by trained surgeons.

Moore[193] has recently summarized elsewhere in this volume the several multicenter randomized trials of carotid endarterectomy that have been performed for comparison of carotid endarterectomy with nonsurgical methods. These have shown such an excellence of effectiveness that many criticisms of the operation have been quieted.

The inability of the surgeon to clear the totally occluded bifurcation safely and effectively has been addressed by the use of microsurgical techniques. Yasargil and Jacobson[194] first popularized this technique, and since then many neurosurgeons have become skillful in the performance of extracranial-to-intracranial bypass. Most recently, however, a randomized study has indicated serious doubts about the value of this technique in preventing strokes.[195]

VISCERAL VASCULAR OCCLUSIONS

One of the most important lesions in relatively small arteries has been the occlusive lesion in the coronary arteries. Longmire, Cannon, and Kattus[196] carried out a few successful coronary endarterectomies in 1958. The difficulties associated with endarterectomy in small vessels led others to the use of the vein graft, first as a replacement by Favoloro[197] and then as a bypass by Johnson and his associates[198] in 1969.

Renal arterial insufficiency has been treated successfully for many years. Goldblatt[199] recognized the importance of renal ischemia, and others came to explain the details of the deranged physiology. Freeman and his associates[200] were among the first to treat this lesion successfully, and they opened a vast area of renovascular hypertension to successful surgical management. Decamp,[201] Poutasse,[202] and Foster and his associates[203] have been leaders in the perfection of these techniques.

The recognition of the several forms of fibromuscular hyperplasia in the renal artery was followed by its discovery in the internal carotid artery by Connett and Lansche.[204] Ehrenfeld and his associates[205] put the surgical management of this lesion on a firm footing.

Occlusive disease occurs much less commonly in the mesenteric vessels than in most other visceral beds, but is nonetheless a frequently lethal lesion. It is commonly recognized only when it has reached an advanced stage and has occasioned extensive intestinal necrosis. Dunphy,[206] however, in 1936 related the progression of symptoms of mesenteric ischemia to the status of frank intestinal infarction. Fifteen years later Klass[207] removed an embolus from the superior mesenteric artery successfully, although the patient died of his primary cardiovascular disease, and in 1957 Shaw[208] carried out an embolectomy of the superior mesenteric artery without concomitant bowel resection. The following year saw Shaw and his associates[209] identify two patients who had both malabsorption and mesenteric ischemia and treat them successfully with endarterectomy. In the meantime Mikkelsen[210] reported similar experiences from California, and he clarifed the term "intestinal angina."

The meandering mesenteric collaterals so well described by Kountz and Connolly[211] provided a radiographic sign suggesting the presence of serious stenosis of the celiac axis and superior mesenteric vessels, which should be cause for careful evaluation of these vessels, whether found at operation or in the radiological suite.

One of the important nonsurgical lesions that mimics obstructive mesenteric vascular disease is the nonocclusive form of mesenteric vascular insufficiency identified by Heer and his associates,[212] which occurs in forms of cardiogenic shock in which cardiac output is low and mesenteric vascular resistance is high.

The extrinsic compression syndrome of the celiac axis is a subject capable of generating considerable discussion. Marable and his associates[213] first described this as compression by the arcuate ligament of the diaphragm. Other authors have believed that other anatomical structures such as the neural components of the celiac ganglion may also be involved. Many support the existence of this lesion as a cause of serious symptoms, and others forcefully deny its existence.[214]

EXTRAANATOMICAL BYPASS AND VASCULAR INFECTIONS

There are many technical and mechanical advances that cannot properly be placed in any one of the above compartments of the history of vascular surgery; one of these is the concept of the *extraanatomical bypass*. The term itself is controversial: it has been suggested that this implies a bypass outside of the body instead of outside classical anatomical routes, but its usage is so well established that it will be retained here. It was proposed by Kunlin,[130] and actually carried out as a femorofemoral bypass by Oudot in 1951.[131] Although rerouting of flow through short shunts for one reason or another had been done by many surgeons, the first dramatic step was taken by Blaisdell, DeMattei, and Gauder,[215] who led a graft from the thoracic aorta extraperitoneally to the femoral artery. Shortly thereafter this anatomical arrangement was modified as the axillofemoral and then the axillobifemoral graft in 1963.[216]

The axillofemoral bypass was first advised as a means of establishing flow to the extremity in the presence of an infected aortic reconstruction that had to be removed; similarly, in 1969 Guida and Moore[217] introduced the obturator bypass to avoid infection in the groin: Shaw and Baue[218] expanded this concept 2 years later. Vetto[219] reported the femorofemoral bypass in 1962, 11 years after Oudot's ilioiliac operation. Today the pattern of unusual anatomical configurations seems limited only by the patient's needs and the surgeon's ingenuity.[169]

One of the important indications for replacement of the classical aortic prosthesis is the development of an aortoenteric fistula. These lesions have plagued surgeons since the first aortic grafts were performed. Elliott, Smith, and Szilagyi[220] contributed one of the first important papers to the understanding of this problem. More recently Busutill and his associates[221] have defined the common primary role of a false aneurysm at the aortic suture line and clarified the management.

VENOUS DISEASE

The history of venous surgery is in one sense older and in another sense newer than arterial surgery. Venous repairs were undertaken before arterial repairs were generally successful. Most of the first generation of arterial surgeons learned about the vagaries of the venous system as their first experiences in vascular surgery. Varicose veins, venous thrombosis, pulmonary embolism, and the postphlebitic extremity have been the four major topics.

Varicose veins were treated surgically by surgeons of Da Costa's era by extensive local resection. Homans[222] is given credit for the introduction of the concept of interruption of the saphenous vein in the groin to control regurgitant flow, but Trendelenberg[223] had performed a similar operation in 1890. Babcock[224] had devised techniques to strip or avulse veins by means of extraluminal strippers; the Mayo external stripper has been for many years a useful instrument to facilitate dissection of the vein.[225]

Pulmonary embolism has long been a major problem for physicians in all areas of medical practice. In 1908 Trendelenberg[226] introduced the operation of pulmonary embolectomy. This operation was infrequently undertaken, and usually unsuccessful, but its rare successes have continued to challenge surgeons to improve it. It is an operation that can be applied more frequently today because of the ability to support the patient's cardiovascular system until the operation can be performed, but its role may be threatened by the ability of the radiologist to place catheters in the pulmonary artery and dissolve the clot with thrombolytic agents.

In 1934 the true relationship between deep, bland venous thrombosis of the leg veins and pulmonary embolism was clarified by John Homans[227,228] of Boston, who matched the ends of a thrombus taken from the pulmonary artery at autopsy with residual clot in the popliteal vein, and then indicated that this must have been the source of the embolus. Homans recognized that the great venous sinuses in the soleal veins were capable of returning large quantities of blood during exercise, but that at other times blood might indeed be stagnant there. Thus, given the other factors of Virchow's triad (stagnant flow, endothelial injury, increased coagulability) one might anticipate spontaneous thrombosis at this site. In fact, subsequent studies with radioiodinated fibrinogen have shown an alarming rate of thrombosis here; fortunately only a very small proportion of these thromboses yield thrombi that propagate into the mainline channels and produce serious clinical problems.

The next step in the management of the patient with venous thrombosis was also made by Homans,[227,229] who introduced the ligation of the femoral (superficial) vein where it joins the deep femoral system in the groin. This procedure must be viewed in the context of the times; there was no practical anticoagulant commonly in use. Allen,[230] Veal,[231] and others quickly took up this operation. Disappointment came to Homans; a patient, whose femoral vein he and I had ligated, propagated a clot through the deep femoral system and into the common femoral vein and suffered a fatal embolism in spite of superficial femoral interruption.

The level of venous ligation was moved upward because of similar failures of superficial femoral vein interruption. First the common femoral, then the iliacs were ligated bilaterally; these operations could be performed under local anesthesia through groin incisions, but since it was soon recognized that bilateral ligation of the iliac veins was indicated, the level was soon raised to the vena cava. It is hard to identify who first did ligate the vena cava for pulmonary embolism, but Buxton,[232] O'Neill,[233] and Collins[234] are all credited with early reports.

It seems unfortunate that as anticoagulants became commonly available—first Coumadin (Endo Labs) and then heparin—their combination with ligation was not common; ligation and anticoagulation were on an "either one or the other" basis. Simple ligation without anticoagulant therapy was associated with a serious frequency of increased thrombosis in the stagnant systems below the ligature, which often led to severe postphlebitic symptoms. Anlyan,[235] Bowers,[236] and others seriously criticized interruption, and in fact gave rise to a school that treated venous thrombosis with increasingly large doses of heparin.[237] The extent of the postphlebitic syndrome, however, seems to be more clearly related to the extent of the inflammatory thrombophlebitic process and its destruction of the valves than it does to ligation, or to the level of ligation.[238] The successful use of large doses of heparin has greatly diminished the need for venous interruption.

Another approach to venous interruption, however, was the suggestion that some flow could be maintained through the cava and still prevent the passage of emboli to the lungs by plication of the cava with sutures.[239] Other occlusive devices were suggested by Moretz,[240] by Miles[241] and by Adams and DeWeese.[242] Mobin-Uddin's invention of a transvenous umbrella,[243] and Greenfield's transvenous wire clip[244] have reduced the need for major venous interruption by open surgical methods even further.

The problems of the postphlebitic extremity remain. This syndrome was well described by Homans,[245] but his contributions to its therapy were not particularly fruitful except that they represent the culmination of the best forms of nonoperative therapy. Trout,[246] Linton,[247] and Dodd and Cockett[248] separately advocated methods which accomplish subfascial interruption of the communicating veins in the lower leg; this procedure remains a surgical standard.

The recreation of a venous drainage channel which is protected from regurgitant flow has offered a new approach to this old problem. Kistner[249] demonstrated the technique of making an incompetent valve into a competent one. Venous transposition is another approach,[250,251] and Taheri[252] has published the results of a free graft of a valved segment of the axillary vein into the diseased femoral system. Taheri's interests have gone in further with the attempts to develop prosthetic venous valves.[253]

HIGHLIGHTS IN DIAGNOSIS

The diagnosis of both arterial and venous diseases has long depended on the use of contrast radiography. One of the first to use this successfully in the living patient was Brooks,[254] who injected sodium iodide to demonstrate the lesions of Buerger's disease in digital vessels. Moniz[255] described "arterial encephalography" for neurological lesions in 1927. His presentation was not only a seminal paper; it defined the needs of the radiographer in terms that are pertinent 60 years later.

In the audience at Moniz' presentation were Reynaldo dos Santos and his son João Cid dos Santos. The father soon published the basic technical approach to the arteriography of the vessels of the abdomen and their branches.[256] Each of these foresaw the great advances in the development of rapid cassette changers and contrast media with less toxicity, but the techniques of image enhancement and subtraction by electronic means have been more recent contributions.[257]

One of the major technical advances was Seldinger's technique,[258] which, instead of using a single needle for the injection of the contrast material, used a catheter that was passed over a wire that in turn had been introduced through the primary arterial puncture. The wire was first advanced to the desired site, then the appropriate catheter was advanced over the wire. Wire and catheter could be alternated so that injections could be made at different sites and at different rates; this method has allowed the radiologist to place a catheter at almost any site in the body. The culmination of these technical advances has been intravenous injection, digitalization of the signal from the fluoroscopic screen, and enhancement of the output and its clarification by subtraction. The ultimate utilization of the ramifications of this technique promises great advantages.

A totally different aspect of radiology was signaled by such work as that of Dotter,[134] who used a rigid dilator passed through a large needle under fluoroscopic guidance to dilate narrowed arteries; this has led to the burgeoning field of *interventional* rather than purely diagnostic radiology.

The growth of vascular surgery has in recent years been almost synonymous with the development of methods of noninvasive diagnosis of peripheral vascular disease. This is an outgrowth of those methods commonly taken for granted, which had their humble beginnings in the stethoscope, the sphygmomanometer,[259] and the ophthalmoscope.

The measurement of many physiological parameters in the laboratory was brought to bear on the patient by such physicians as Winsor,[260] whose evaluation of pressure gradients remains a critical basis for the clinical estimation of the severity of arterial obstruction. Other parameters commonly measured in the early vascular diagnostic laboratories included digital and segmental plethysmography, and skin temperature and resistance studies both before and after sympathetic blockade.

Pachon[261] introduced a modification of the sphygmomanometer and the segmental plethysmograph as the oscillometer, which provided a very rough measure of the volume of the distensile arterial pulse wave;

the figures obtained bear no physiological definition, but comparisons at different levels in one extremity, of comparable levels in different extremities, and of one site on successive occasions did provide the surgeon with some objective evidence of change.

Although used by all physicians, the role of the stethoscope in the evaluation of murmurs over the peripheral arteries was clarified and codified by Edwards and Levine[262] and then by Wylie and his associates.[263]

One of the interesting early techniques was that of Baillart,[264] who used the ophthalmoscope and ophthalmodynamometry to evaluate lesions of the eye. Operator sensitivity and reproducibility, a critical aspect of many such techniques, was such that its utility was not great. Kartchner,[265] however, introduced a recording device to reproduce relative pressure curves within the ocular globe, and to compare the peak time of the retinal artery pulse wave, which is reflected in the globe's pressure, on each side as well as with the arrival of the pulse wave in the ear lobe, which enabled estimation of the severity of obstruction in the carotid system. Gee[266] developed a method to evaluate the back-pressure in the totally occluded carotid in order to predict the necessity for the use of shunt during operative carotid occlusion. His method has, however, come to be of greater value in the evaluation of the forward pressure beyond the stenotic carotid, for it provides more precise measurement of the pressures, but it does not provide such accurate time relationships as does Kartchner's system.

The use of ultrasound has been one of the most popular modalities in its many ramifications. Leopold and his associates[267] used classical ultrasonic imaging (B mode) techniques to outline the aorta as well as other abdominal viscera. Ultrasound in another form (i.e., in either the continuous or the gated Doppler mode that measures the shift in frequency of the ultrasonic signal reflected from moving red blood cells) was introduced by Strandness.[268,269] Combined with a sphygmomanometer, this method has become one of the most useful and standard methods of evaluating peripheral arterial disease, and of identifying segmental pressure differences just as Winsor had done with less satisfactory methods. The use of

the ultrasonic flow detector was soon modified by Brockenbrough[270] to determine the direction of flow through the supraorbital artery, which is reversed in the presence of high-grade obstruction of the ipsilateral carotid artery; Machleder[271] dramatized the technique, but the extreme operator sensitivity limits its use considerably. Technical improvements have made it possible to use this method to evaluate intracranial flow at the base of the brain.[272–274]

Imaging of the crude Doppler signal was introduced by Thomas,[275] who simply mounted a Doppler probe on a scanning device. Sophistication of these scanning methods with a combination of the regular ultrasonic B mode scanning to define the anatomy and to obtain a reference point from which pulsed Doppler reflections can be read allows exact identification of blood flow patterns at the site within the lumen near apparent anatomical irregularities in arteries that can be "reached" by the Doppler signal.[276] This method was at first used in the carotid bifurcation but it has now been extended to common use in peripheral arterial sites, in the mesenteric vessels,[273] and as a monitoring device[277] at the operating table.

Evaluation of the venous side of the circulation has not provided such exact information. Cranley[278] introduced "phleborheography," which evaluates the changes in venous pulse, outflow, and respiratory excursions in the diagnosis of deep venous disease of the legs. Less sophisticated, easier to handle, but perhaps less informative is Wheeler's impedance plethysmography.[279]

The Doppler velocity probe, in spite of some drawbacks of operator sensitivity, remains a useful method for identifying obstruction in the available superficial major veins, such as in the groin, the popliteal space, and the axilla. It can also be used in the postphlebitic extremity to identify both regurgitant flow in superficial channels and flow from communicating veins, and can be used even in the presence of brawny edema that otherwise obscures much of the venous system from sight and palpation.

As might be predicted from the historical evolution of these noninvasive tests, Comerota[280] has now suggested that duplex venous scanning is the preferred method for the diagnosis of deep venous thrombosis.

REFERENCES

1. Dobson J: John Hunter. Edinburgh, E & S Livingstone Ltd, 1969.
2. Gray EA: Portrait of a Surgeon. A Biography of John Hunter. London, Robert Hale Ltd, 1952.
3. Hunter W: A history of aneurism of the aorta with some remarks on aneurisms in general. Med Obs Inquiries 1:323, 1757.
4. Cames C: Wörtliche Uebersetzung des Werkes des römischen Artzes Antyllus. Düsseldorf, Michael Trilitsch Verlag, 1941, p 107.
5. Purmann MG: Chirurgia Curiosa, Edition of 1716, p 612.
6. Erichsen Sir JE: Observation on Aneurism (Anel). London, Sydenham Society, 1844, p 216.
7. Erichsen Sir JE: Observation on Aneurism (Hunter). London, Sydenham Society, 1844, p 404.
8. Brock RC: Astley Cooper and carotid artery ligation. Guy's Hospital Reports (Special Number) 117:219–224, 1968.
9. Tyrell FG: The lectures of Sir Astley Cooper, Bart, FRCS, on the principles and practice of surgery (4th American edition from the last London edition). Philadelphia, Carey EL, Hart A, 1835, pp 212–214.
10. Lambert R: Letter from Mr Lambert to Dr Hunter: Giving an account of a new method of treating an aneurism. Med Obs Inquiries, June 15, 1761.
11. Asman C: Inaugural dissertation. Groningen, 1773.

12. Blane G: (Communication without title). *In*: Transactions of a Society for the Improvement of Medical and Chirurgical Knowledge 2:1, 1800.

13. Cooper Sir A: The lectures of Sir Astley Cooper, Bart, FRCS, On the principles and practice of surgery (2nd ed). London, FC Westley, 1830, p 98.

14. Cruveilhier J: Senile Gangrene. Anatomie Pathologique du Corps Humain, Section 27 (Malades des Artères, 1–8, Plate v. 27) Paris, 1835–42.

15. Barth (No initial): Observation d'une oblitération complète de l'aorte abdominale, recuillie dans le service de M. Louis, suivie de réflections. Arch Gen Med, Second Series, 8:26–53, 1835.

16. Charcot J-M: Obstruction artérielle et claudication intermittente dans le cheval et dans l'homme. Mem Soc Biol 1:225–238, 1858.

17. Langenbeck CJM: Pathology and Therapy of Surgical Illnesses. Göttingen, Heimatsverlag, 1825, vol III, p 414.

18. Heinecke W: Blutung, Blutstillung, Transfusion nebst Luftentritt und Infusion. *In* Billroth T, Luecke H (eds): Deutsche Chirurgie. Stuttgart, Verlag von Ferdinand Enke, 1885.

19. Jassinowsky A: Die Arteriennaht: Eine experimentelle Studie. Inaugural dissertation for the Degree of Doctor of Medicine, Dorpat, 1889.

20. Czerny V: On lateral closure of vein wounds. Langenbeck's Arch Chir 28:671, 1881.

21. Schede M: Einege Bemerkungen über de Naht von Venenwunden. Arch Klin Chir 43:548, 1883.

22. Eck NV: K. voprosu o perevyazkie vorotnoi veni. Prevaritelnoye soobshtshjenye. Voen Med J (St Petersburg) 130:1–2, 1877 (as cited by Child CG III: Eck's fistula. Surg Gynecol Obstet 96:375–376, 1953).

23. Jassinowsky A: Ein Beitrag zur Lehre von der Gefässnaht. Arch Klin Chir 42:816–841, 1891.

24. Dörfler J: Ueber Arteriennaht. Beitr Klin Chir 22:781–825, 1899.

25. Jaboulay M, Briau E: Recherches expérimentales sur la suture et la greffe arterielles. Bull Lyon Med 81:97–99, 1896.

26. Edwards P, Edwards WS: Alexis Carrel, Visionary Surgeon, Springfield, IL, Charles C Thomas, 1974.

27. Carrel A: Les anastomoses vasculaires et leur technique opératoire. Union Med Can 33:521–527, 1904.

28. Carrel A: The surgery of blood vessels, etc. Johns Hopkins Hosp Bull 18:18–28, 1907.

29. Harbison SP: The origins of vascular surgery: The Carrel-Guthrie letters. Surgery 52:406–418, 1962.

30. Goyanes J: Nuevos trabajos de chirurgia vascular, substitucion plastica de los arterios por las venas o arterioplatica venosa, applicada comon nuevo metodo al tratamiento de los aneurismas. El Siglo Med 53:546–549, 561–568, 1906.

31. Matas R: Traumatic aneurism of the left brachial artery. Med News 53:462–466, 1888.

32. Cohn I Sr: Rudolph Matas. New York, Doubleday and Company Inc, 1960.

33. Matas R: Some experiences and observations in the treatment of arteriovenous aneurisms by the intrasaccular method of suture (endoaneurismorrhaphy) with special reference to the transvenous route. Ann Surg 71:403–427, 1920.

34. Bickham WS: Arteriovenous aneurisms. A case of traumatic arteriovenous aneurism of the common femoral artery and vein—unsuccessfully treated by a new method of compression—and finally cured by the proximal ligation of the external iliac artery extraperitoneally—with the suggestion that the application to these aneurisms of the Matas method of operation used for ordinary aneurisms—and the mention of some other recent methods of operating. Ann Surg 39:767–775, 1904.

35. Murphy JB: Resection of arteries and veins injured in continuity—end-to-end suture—experimental and clinical research. Med Rec 51:73–88, 1897.

36. Edwards WS, Tapp JS: Chemically treated nylon tubes as arterial grafts. Surgery 38:61–76, 1955.

37. Nitze F: Kleinere Mittheilungen Kongres im Moskau. Zentralbl Chir 24:1042, 1897.

38. Payr E: Beiträge zur Technik der Blutgefässe und der Nervennaht nebst Mittheilungen die Verwundung eines resorbibaren Metalles in der Chirurgie. Arch Klin Chir 62:67–93, 1900.

39. Blakemore AH, Lord JW Jr, Stefko PL: The severed primary artery in war wounded: A nonsuture method of bridging arterial defects. Surgery 12:488–508, 1942.

40. Elkin ED, DeBakey ME: Vascular Surgery (Surgery in World War II, vol IV). Washington, DC, Office of the Surgeon General, 1955.

41. Halsted WS: (in discussion of a paper by Matas R) Some of the problems related to the surgery of the vascular system: Testing the efficiency of the collateral circulation as a preliminary to the occlusion of the great surgical arteries. Trans Am Surg Assoc 28:49–51, 1910.

42. Höpfner E: Ueber Gefässnaht, Gefässtransplantionen und Replantationen von amputieren Extremitäten. Arch Klin Chir 70:417–471, 1903.

43. Lexer E: Die ideale Operation des arteriellen und des arteriell-venösen Aneurysma. Arch Klin Chir 83:459–477, 1907.

44. Lexer E: 20 Jahre Transplantionsforschung in der Chirurgie. Arch Klin Chir 138:251–302, 1925.

45. Jeger E: Die Chirurgie der Blutgefässe und des Herzens (Republication of 1913 edition). Berlin, Springer-Verlag, 1973.

46. Weglowski R: Ueber de Gefässtransplantation. Zentralbl Chir 52:2241–2243, 1925.

47. Leonardo RA: History of Surgery. New York, Froben Press, 1943, p 139.

48. Power DA: The palliative treatment of aneurysms by "wiring" with Colt's apparatus. Br J Surg 9:27–36, 1921.

49. Blakemore AH, King BG: Electrothermic coagulation of aortic aneurysms. JAMA 111:1821–1827, 1938.

50. Reid M: Aneurysms in the Johns Hopkins Hospital. All cases treated in the surgical service from the opening of the hospital to January 1922. Arch Surg 12:1–73, 1926.

51. Matas R: Ligation of the abdominal aorta: Report of the ultimate result, one year, five months and nine days after the ligation of the abdominal aorta for aneurysm of the bifurcation. Ann Surg 81:457–464, 1925.

52. Matas R: Aneurysm of the abdominal aorta at its bifurcation into the common iliac arteries. Ann Surg 112:909–922, 1940.

53. Elkin DC: Aneurysm of the abdominal aorta: Treatment by ligation. Ann Surg 112:895–905, 1940.

54. Bigger IA: Surgical treatment of aneurysm of the aorta: Review of literature and report of two cases, one apparently successful. Ann Surg 112:879–894, 1940.

55. Alexander J, Byron FX: Aortectomy for thoracic aneurysm. JAMA 126:1139–1145, 1944.

56. Alexander JT, Byron FX: Aortectomy for thoracic aneurysm: A supplemental report. JAMA 132:22, 1946.

57. Pearse HE: Experimental studies on the gradual occlusion of large arteries. Ann Surg 122:923–937, 1940.

58. Yeager G, Cowley RA: Studies on the use of polythene as a fibrous tissue stimulant. Ann Surg 128:509–920, 1948.

59. Cutler EC, Levine SA, Beck CC: The surgical treatment of mitral stenosis. Arch Surg 9:689–821, 1924.

60. Gross RE: A surgical approach for ligation of a patent ductus arteriosus. N Engl J Med 220:510–514, 1939.

61. Gross RE: Complete surgical division of the patent ductus arteriosus. Surg Gynecol Obstet 78:36–43, 1944.

62. Blalock A, Taussig HB: The surgical treatment of malformations of the heart in which there is pulmonary stenosis or pulmonary atresia. JAMA 128:189–202, 1945.

63. Crafoord C, Nylin G: Congenital coarctation of the aorta and its surgical treatment. J Thorac Surg 14:347–361, 1945.

64. Gross, RE, Hufnagel CA: Coarctation of the aorta. Experimental studies regarding its correction. N Engl J Med 233:287–293, 1945.

65. Hufnagel CA: Preserved homologous arterial transplants. Bull Am Coll Surg 32:231, 1947.

66. Gross RE, Hurwitt ES, Bill AH Jr, Peirce EC II: Preliminary observations on the use of human arterial grafts in the treatment of certain cardiovascular defects. N Engl J Med 239:578–579, 1948.

67. Swan H, Maaske C, Johnson M, et al: Arterial homografts: II. Resection of thoracic aneurysm using a stored human arterial transplant. Arch Surg 61:732–737, 1950.

68. Estes JE Jr: Abdominal aortic aneurysm: A study of 102 cases. Circulation 2:258–264, 1950.

69. Oudot J: La greffe vasculaire dans les thromboses due carrefour aortique. Presse Med 59:234–236, 1951.

70. Dubost C, Allary M, Oeconomos N: Resection of an aneurysm of the abdominal aorta: Reestablishment of the continuity by a preserved human arterial graft, with result after five months. Arch Surg 64:405–408, 1952.

71. Schaffer PW, Hardin CW: The use of temporary and polythene shunts to permit occlusion, resection and frozen homologous artery graft replacement of vital vessel segments. Surgery 31:186–199, 1952.

72. Julian OC, Grove WJ, Dye WS, et al: Direct surgery of arteriosclerosis. Resection of abdominal aorta with homologous aortic graft replacement. Ann Surg 138:387–403, 1953.

73. Brock RC: Reconstructive arterial surgery. Proc Soc Med 46:115–130, 1953.

74. DeBakey ME, Cooley DA: Surgical treatment of aneurysm of abdominal aorta by resection and restoration of continuity with homograft. Surg Gynecol Obstet 97:257–266, 1953.

75. Bahnson HT: Considerations in the excision of aortic aneurysms. Ann Surg 138:377–386, 1953.

76. Szilagyi DE, Smith RE, DeRusso FJ, et al: Contribution of abdominal aortic aneurysmectomy to prolongation of life. Ann Surg 164:678–699, 1966.

77. Deterling RA Jr, Coleman CC, Parshley MS: Experimental studies on the frozen homologous aortic graft. Surgery 29:419–439, 1951.

78. Marangoni AG, Cecchini LP: Homotransplantation of arterial segments by the freeze-drying method. Ann Surg 134:977–983, 1951.

79. Ellis FH Jr, Helden RA, Hines EA Jr: Aneurysm of the abdominal aorta involving the right renal artery: Report of a case with preservation of renal function after resection and grafting. Ann Surg 142:992–995, 1955.

80. Etheredge SN, Yee JY, Smith JV, Schonberger S, Goldman MJ: Successful resection of a large aneurysm of the upper abdominal aorta and replacement with homograft. Surgery 38:1071–1081, 1955.

81. Shumacker HB Jr: Innovation in the operative management of the thoracoabdominal aneurysm. Surg Gynecol Obstet 136:763–794, 1973.

82. DeBakey ME, Creech O, Morris GC: Aneurysm of the thoracoabdominal aorta involving the celiac, mesenteric and renal arteries. Report of four cases treated by resection and homograft replacement. Ann Surg 144:549–573, 1956.

83. Stoney RJ, Wylie EJ: Surgical management of arterial lesions of the thoracoabdominal aorta. Am J Surg 126:157–164, 1973.

84. Crawford ES: Thoraco-abdominal aortic aneurysms involving renal, superior mesenteric and celiac arteries. Ann Surg 179:763–772, 1974.

85. Linton RR: The arteriosclerotic popliteal aneurysm. A report of 14 patients treated by preliminary lumbar sympathectomy and aneurysmectomy. Surgery 26:41–58, 1949.

86. Whychullis AR, Spittel JS Jr, Wallace RB: Popliteal aneurysms. Surgery 68:942–952, 1970.

87. Gifford RW Jr, Hines EA Jr, Janes JM: An analysis and follow-up study of one hundred popliteal aneurysms. Surgery 33:284–293, 1953.

88. Edwards WS: Exclusion and saphenous bypass of popliteal aneurysm. Surg Gynecol Obstet 128:829–830, 1969.

89. Abbe R: The surgery of the hand. NY Med J 59:33–40, 1894.

90. Tuffer M: De l'intubation dans les plaies des grosses artères. Bull Acad Med 74:455–460, 1915.

91. Hufnagel CA: Permanent intubation of the thoracic aorta. Arch Surg 54:382–389, 1947.

92. Hufnagel CA: The use of rigid and flexible plastic prosthesis for arterial replacement. Surgery 37:165–174, 1955.

93. Voorhees AB Jr, Jaretzki A III, Blakemore AH: Use of tubes constructed of Vinyon-"N" cloth in bridging arterial defects. Ann Surg 135:332–336, 1952.

94. Girvin GW, Wilhelm MC, Merendino KA: The use of Teflon fabric as arterial grafts. An experimental study in dogs. Am J Surg 92:240–247, 1966.

95. Szilagyi DE, France LC, Smith RF, et al: Clinical use of an elastic Dacron prosthesis, Arch Surg 77:538–551, 1958.

96. Julian OC, Deterling RA, Dye WS, et al: Dacron tube and bifurcation prosthesis produced to specification: II. Continued clinical use and the addition of microcrimping. Arch Surg 78:260–270, 1957.

97. Weslowski SA, Dennis CA (eds): Fundamentals of Vascular Grafting. New York, The Blakiston Division, McGraw-Hill Book Company, 1963.

98. Deterling RA, Bhonslay SB: An evaluation of synthetic materials and fabrics suitable for blood vessel replacement. Surgery 38:71–89, 1955.

99. Wesolowski SA, Fries CC, Karlson KE, et al: Porosity: Primary determinant of ultimate fate of synthetic vascular grafts. Surgery 50:91–96, 1961.

100. DeBakey ME, Cooley DA, Crawford ES, Morris GC Jr: Clinical application of a new flexible knitted Dacron arterial substitute. Arch Surg 74:713–724, 1957.

101. Sauvage G, Berger KE, Wood SJ, et al: An external velour surface for porous arterial prosthesis. Surgery 70:940–953, 1971.

102. Cooley DA, Wukasch DC, Bennet JC, et al: Double velour knitted grafts for aorto-iliac replacement. *In* Sawyer PN, Kaplitt MJ (eds): Vascular Grafts. New York, Appleton-Century-Crofts, 1978.

103. Quiñones-Baldrich WJ, Moore WS, Ziomek S, Chvapil M: Development of a "leak-proof" knitted Dacron vascular prosthesis. J Vasc Surg 3:895–903, 1986.

104. Guidion R, Snyder R, Martin L, et al: Albumin coating of a knitted polyester arterial prosthesis: An alternative to preclotting. Ann Thorac Surg 37:457–465, 1984.

105. Soyer T, Lempinen M, Cooper P, Norton L, Eiseman B: A new venous prosthesis. Surgery 72:864–872, 1972.

106. Veith FJ, Gupta SK, Ascer E, et al: Six-year prospective multicenter randomized comparison of autologous saphenous vein and expanded polytetrafluoroethylene grafts in infrainguinal arterial reconstructions. J Vasc Surg 3:104–114, 1986.

107. Rosenberg NL, Henderson J, Lord GW, et al: Use of enzyme treated heterografts as arterial substitutes. Arch Surg 85:192–197, 1969.

108. Sawyer PN, Stancezewski B, Lucas TR, et al: Experimental and clinical evaluation of a new negatively charged bovine heterograft for use in peripheral and coronary revascularization. *In* Sawyer PN, Kaplitt MJ (eds): Vascular Grafts. New York, Appleton-Century-Crofts, 1978.

109. Dardik H, Ibrahim IM, Sprayregan S, et al: Clinical experiences with modified human umbilical cord vein for arterial bypass. Surgery 79:618–624, 1976.

110. Leriche R: Souvenirs de ma Vie Mort. Paris, Editions du Seuil, 1956.

111. Leriche R: De la causalgie envisagée comme une névrite du sympathetique et de son traitement par la dénudation et l'excision des plexus nerveux périartèriels. Presse Med 25:178–180, 1916.

112. Diez J: Le traitement des affections trophiques et gangréneuses des membres inférieurs par la résection du sympathique lombo-sacré. Rev Neurol 33:184–192, 1926.

113. Royle N: A new operative procedure in the treatment of spastic paralysis and its experimental basis. Med J Aust 1:77–86, 1924.

114. Hunter JI: The influence of the sympathetic nervous system

in the genesis of rigidity in striated muscle in spastic paralysis. Surg Gynecol Obstet *39*:721–743, 1924.

115. Leriche R: Des obliterations artèrielles hautes (obliteration de la terminacion de l'aorte) comme causes des insuffisances circulatoires des membres inférieurs. Bull Mem Soc Chir (Paris) *49*:1404–1406, 1923.

116. Leriche R: De la résection du carrefour aortico-iliaque avec double sympathectomie lombaire pour thrombose artéritique de l'aorte. Le syndrome de l'oblitération terminoaortique par artérite. Presse Med *48*:601–604, 1940.

117. Murphy JB: Removal of an embolus from the common iliac artery, with re-establishment of circulation in the femoral. JAMA *52*:1661–1663, 1909.

118. Mosney N, Dumont MJ: Embolie fémorale au cours d'un rétrécissement mitral pur. Artèriotomie. Guérison. Bull Acad Natl Med (Paris) *66*:358–361, 1908.

119. Murray GDW: Heparin in thrombosis and embolism. Br J Surg *27*:567–598, 1939.

120. dos Santos JC: From embolectomy to endarterectomy or the fall of a myth. J Cardiovasc Surg *17*:113–128, 1976.

121. dos Santos JC: Sur la désobstruction des thromboses artérielles anciennes. Mem Acad Chir *73*:409–411, 1947.

122. Freeman NE, Leeds FH: Vein inlay graft in treatment of aneurysm and thrombosis of abdominal aorta: Preliminary communication with report of 3 cases. Angiology *2*:579–587, 1951.

123. Wylie EJ Jr, Kerr E, Davies O: Experimental and clinical experiences with use of fascia lata applied as a graft about major arteries after thromboendarterectomy and aneurysmorrhaphy. Surg Gynecol Obstet *93*:2–272, 1951.

124. Bazy L, Hugier J, Reboul H, et al: Technique des "endartérectomies" or artérities oblitérantes chroniques des membres inférieures, des iliaques, et de l'aorte abdominale inférieur. J Chir *65*:196–210, 1949.

125. Barker WF, Cannon JA: An evaluation of endarterectomy. Arch Surg *38*:488–495, 1953.

126. Cannon JA, Barker WF: Successful management of obstructive femoral arteriosclerosis by endarterectomy. Surgery *38*:48–60, 1955.

127. Butcher HR Jr: A simple technique for endarterectomy. Surgery *44*:984–989, 1958.

128. Vollmar J, Trede BA, Laubach K, Forrest H: Principles of reconstructive procedures for chronic femoropopliteal occlusions: Report on 546 operations. Ann Surg *168*:215–223, 1968.

129. Kunlin J: Le traitement de l'artérite oblitérante par la greffe veineuse longue. Arch Mal Coeur *42*:371–372, 1949.

130. Kunlin J: Le traitement de l'artérite oblitérante par la greffe veineuse longue. Rev Chir *70*:207–238, 1951.

131. Oudot J: Un deuxième cas de greffe de la bifurcation aortique pour thrombose de la fourche aortique. Mem Acad Chir *77*:644–645, 1951.

132. Linton RR: Some practical considerations in surgery of blood vessel grafts. Surgery *38*:817–834, 1955.

133. Edwards WS: Composite reconstruction of the femoral artery with saphenous vein after endarterectomy. Surg Gynecol Obstet *111*:651–653, 1960.

134. Dotter CT, Judkins MP: Percutaneous transluminal treatment of arteriosclerotic obstruction. Radiology *84*:631–643, 1956.

135. Gruntzig A, Hopff H: Perkutane Recanalisation chronischer arterieller Arterienverschlusse mit einem neuen Dilatations-katheter: Modification der Dotter-Technik. Dtsch Med Wochenschr *99*:2502–2505, 1974.

136. Greenstone SM, Shore JM, Heringman EC, Massell TB: Arterial endoscopy (arterioscopy). Arch Surg *93*:811–812, 1966.

137. Simpson JB, Selmon MR, Robertson GC, et al: Transluminal atherectomy for occlusive peripheral vascular disease. Am J Cardiol *61*:91G–101G, 1988.

138. Kensey KR, Nash JE, Abrahams C, Zarins CK: Recanalization of obstructed arteries with a flexible, rotating tip catheter. Radiology *165*:387–389, 1987.

139. Ahn SS, Auth DC, Marcus DR, Moore WS: Removal of focal

atheromatous lesions by angioscopically guided high-speed rotary atherectomy: Preliminary experimental observations. J Vasc Surg *7*:292–300, 1988.

140. Grundfest WS, Litvack F, Forrester JS, et al: Laser ablation of human atherosclerotic plaque without adjacent tissue injury. J Am Coll Cardiol *5*:929–933, 1985.

141. Murphy-Chetorian D, Kosek J, Mok W, et al: Selective absorption of ultraviolet laser energy by human atherosclerotic plaque treated with tetracycline. Am J Cardiol *55*:1293–1297, 1985.

142. Abela GS, Fenech A, Crea F, Conti CR: "Hot-tip": Another method of laser vascular recanalization. Lasers Surg Med *5*:327–225, 1985.

143. Palma EC: Treatment of arteritis of the lower limbs by autogenous vein grafts. Minerva Cardioangiol Eur *8*:36–49, 1960.

144. McCaughan JJ Jr: Surgical exposure of the distal popliteal artery. Surgery *44*:536–539, 1958.

145. McCaughan JJ Jr: Study of 100 consecutive bypass grafts of the femoral artery. Memphis Med J *35*:227–237, 1960.

146. McCaughan JJ Jr: Bypass graft to the posterior tibial artery at the ankle: Case reports. Am Surg *32*:126–130, 1966.

147. Morris GC Jr, DeBakey ME, Cooley DA, Crawford ES: Arterial bypass below the knee. Surg Gynecol Obstet *108*:321–332, 1959.

148. Tyson RR, DeLaurentis DA: Femorotibial bypass. Circulation *33–34*(suppl I):I-183–I-188, 1966.

149. Hall KV: The great saphenous vein used in situ as in arterial shunt after extirpation of the vein valves. Surgery *51*:492–495, 1962.

150. Leather RP, Shah DM, Karmody AM: Infrapopliteal bypass for limb salvage: Increased patency and utilization of the saphenous vein "in situ." Surgery *90*:1000–1008, 1981.

151. Dardik H, Sussman B, Ibrahim IM, et al: Distal arteriovenous fistula as an adjunct to maintaining arterial graft patency for limb salvage. Surgery *94*:478–486, 1983.

152. DeLaurentis DA, Friedman P: Segmental femorotibial bypass: Another approach to the inadequate saphenous vein problem. Surgery *71*:400–404, 1972.

153. Veith FJ, Ascer E, Gupta SJ, et al: Tibiotibial vein bypass grafts: A new operation for limb salvage. J Vasc Surg *2*:552–557, 1985.

154. Nehler MR, Dalman RL, Harris EJ: Upper extremity arterial bypass distal to the wrist. J Vasc Surg *16*:633–642, 1992.

155. Martin P, Renwick S, Stephenson C: On the surgery of the profunda femoris artery. Br J Surg *55*:539–542, 1971.

156. Oudot J, Cormier JM: La localization la plus fréquente de l'artérite segmentaire celle de l'artére fémorale superficielle. Presse Med *61*:1361–1364, 1953.

157. Miller T, Niazmand R, Barker WF: Femoral artery reconstruction under local anesthesia: Maximal results from minimal risks. Am J Surg *122*:513–516, 1971.

158. Cohn LH, Trueblood W, Crowley LG: Profunda femoris reconstruction in the treatment of femoropopliteal occlusive disease. Arch Surg *103*:475–479, 1971.

159. Towne JB, Bernhard VM, Rollins DL, et al: Profundaplasty in perspective: Limitations in the long-term management of limb ischemia. Surgery *90*:1037–1046, 1981.

160. Von Winiwarter F: Ueber eine eigenthümliche Form von Endarteritis und Endophlebitis mit Gangrän des Fusses. Arch Klin Chir *23*:202–225, 1879.

161. Buerger L: Thrombo-angiitis obliterans: A study of the vascular lesions leading to presenile spontaneous gangrene. Am J Med Sci *136*:567–580, 1908.

162. Fogarty TJ, Cranley JJ, Krause RJ, Strasser ES, Hafner CD: A method of extraction of arterial emboli and thrombi. Surg Gynecol Obstet *116*:241–244, 1963.

163. Mitchell SW: Injuries of the Nerves and Their Consequences. Philadelphia, JP Lippincott, 1872.

164. Makins GH: On Gunshot Wounds to the Blood-Vessels. Bristol, John Wright and Sons Ltd, 1919.

165. DeBakey ME, Simeone FA: Battle injuries of the arteries in World War II. Ann Surg *123*:534–579, 1958.

166. Jahnke EJ Jr, Howard JM: Primary repair of major arterial injuries. Arch Surg 66:646–649, 1953.
167. Hughes CW: Acute vascular trauma in Korean War casualties. An analysis of 180 cases. Surg Gynecol Obstet 99:91–100, 1954.
168. Spencer FC, Grewe RV: The management of arterial injuries in battle casualties. Ann Surg 141:304–313, 1955.
169. Whelan TJ, Burkholder WE, Gomez CA: Management of war wounds. Adv Surg 3:227–350, 1968.
170. Rich NL, Hughes CW: Vietnam Vascular Registry: A preliminary report. Surgery 65:218–226, 1969.
171. Soubbotitich V: Military experience of traumatic aneurysms. Lancet 2:720–721, 1913.
172. Holman E: Arteriovenous Aneurysms: Abnormal Communication between the Arterial and Venous Circulation. New York, Macmillan Publishing Company, Inc, 1937.
173. Savory WS: Case of a young woman in whom the main arteries of both upper extremities and of the left side of the neck were throughout completely obliterated. Med Chir Trans London 39:205–235, 1856.
174. Hunt JR: The role of the carotid arteries in the causation of vascular lesions of the brain with remarks on certain special features of the symptomatology. Am J Med Sci 147:704–713, 1914.
175. Fisher M: Occlusion of the internal carotid artery. Arch Neurol Psychiatry 65:346–377, 1951.
176. Fisher M: Occlusion of the carotid arteries: Further experiences. Arch Neurol Psychiatry 72:187–204, 1954.
177. Carrea R, Mollins M, Murphy G: Surgical treatment of spontaneous thrombosis of the internal carotid artery in the neck. Carotid-carotideal anastomosis. Report of a case. Acta Neurol Latinoam 1:71–78, 1955.
178. Lefèvre MH: Sur un cas de plaie du bulbe carotidien per balle, traitée par ligature de la carotid primitive et l'anastomose bout à bout de la carotid externe avec la carotid interne. Bull Mem Soc Chir 44:923–928, 1918.
179. Eastcott HHG, Pickering GW, Rob C: Reconstruction of internal carotid artery in a patient with intermittent attacks of hemiplegia. Lancet 2:994–996, 1954.
180. Cooley DA, Al-Naaman YD, Carton CA: Surgical treatment of arteriosclerotic occlusion of common carotid artery. J Neurosurg 13:500–506, 1956.
181. DeBakey ME: Successful carotid endarterectomy for cerebrovascular insufficiency: Nineteen year followup, JAMA 233:1083–1085, 1975.
182. Yates PO, Hutchinson EC: Cerebral infarction: The role of stenosis of the extracranial arteries. Med Res Council Spec Report (London) 300:1–95, 1961.
183. Whisnant JP, Matsumoto N, Eleback LR: Transient cerebral ischemic attacks in a community: Rochester, Minnesota, 1955 through 1969. Mayo Clin Proc 48:195–198, 1973.
184. Hollenhorst RW: Significance of bright plaques in the retinal arterioles. JAMA 183:23–29, 1961.
185. Julian OC, Dye WS, Javid H, Hunter JA: Ulcerative lesions of the carotid artery bifurcation. Arch Surg 86:803–809, 1963.
186. Moore WS, Hall AD: Ulcerated atheroma of the carotid artery: A cause of transient cerebral ischemia. Am J Surg 116:237–242, 1969.
187. Imparato AM, Riles TJ, Gorstein F: The carotid bifurcation plaque: Pathologic findings associated with cerebral ischemia. Stroke 10:238–245, 1979.
188. Lusby RJ, Ferrell LD, Ehrenfeld WA, et al: Carotid plaque hemorrhage: Its role in production of cerebral ischemia. Arch Surg 117:147–148, 1982.
189. Moore WS, Hall AD: Carotid artery back pressure: A test of cerebral tolerance to temporary carotid artery occlusion. Arch Surg 99:702–710, 1969.
190. Thompson JE, Patman RD, Talkington CM: Asymptomatic carotid bruit. Ann Surg 188:308–316, 1978.
191. Dixon S, Pais SO, Raviola C, et al: Natural history of nonstenotic, asymptomatic ulcerations of the carotid artery: A further analysis. Arch Surg 117:1493–1498, 1982.
192. Berguer R, Sieggreen MY, Lazo VA, Hodakowski GT: The silent brain infarct in carotid surgery. J Vasc Surg 3:442–447, 1986.
193. Moore WS: Indications for carotid endarterectomy. Results of randomized trials. Presented at the 29th Annual "Controversial Areas in General Surgery", UCLA Extension Program, Palm Springs, CA, April 2, 1992 (summarized in Chapter 31 of this volume).
194. Yasargil MG, Krayenbuhl KA, Jacobson JH II: Microneurosurgical arterial reconstruction. Surgery 67:221–223, 1970.
195. EC/IC Bypass Group: Failure of extracranial-intracranial bypass to reduce the risk of ischemic stroke; Results of an international randomized trial. N Engl J Med 313:1191–1200, 1985.
196. Longmire WP Jr, Cannon JA, Kattus HA: Direct-vision coronary endarterectomy for angina pectoris. N Engl J Med 259:993–999, 1958.
197. Favoloro RG: Saphenous vein autograft replacement of severe segmental coronary artery occlusion. Ann Thorac Surg 5:334–339, 1968.
198. Johnson WD, Flemma RJ, Lepley D Jr, et al: Extended treatment of severe coronary artery disease: A total surgical approach. Ann Surg 170:460–470, 1969.
199. Goldblatt H, Lynch J, Hanzal RF, et al: Studies on experimental hypertension. J Exp Med 59:347–379, 1934.
200. Freeman NE, Leeds FH, Elliott WG, Roland SI: Thromboendarterectomy for hypertension due to renal artery occlusion. JAMA 156:1077–1079, 1954.
201 DeCamp P, Birchall R: Recognition and treatment of renal arterial stenosis associated with hypertension. Surgery 43:134–152, 1958.
202. Poutasse EF: Surgical treatment of renal hypertension: Results in patients with occlusive lesions of renal arteries. J Urol 82:403–411, 1959.
203. Foster JH, Dean RH, Pinkerton JA, et al: Ten years' experience with renovascular hypertension. Ann Surg 177:755–766, 1973.
204. Connett MC, Lansche JM: Fibromuscular hyperplasia of the internal carotid artery. Report of a case. Ann Surg 162:59–62, 1965.
205. Ehrenfeld WK, Stoney RJ, Wylie EJ: Fibromuscular hyperplasia of the internal carotid artery. Arch Surg 95:284–287, 1967.
206. Dunphy JE: Abdominal pain of vascular origin. Am J Med Sci 192:109–113, 1936.
207. Klass J: Embolectomy in acute mesenteric occlusion. Ann Surg 134:913–917, 1951.
208. Shaw RS, Rutledge RH: Superior-mesenteric-artery embolectomy in treatment of massive mesenteric infarction. N Engl J Med 257:595–598, 1957.
209. Shaw RS, Maynard EP: Acute and chronic thrombosis of the mesenteric arteries associated with malabsorption. Report of two cases successfully treated by thromboendarterectomy. N Engl J Med 258:874–878, 1958.
210. Mikkelsen WP, Zaro JA: Intestinal angina: Report of a case with preoperative diagnosis and surgical relief. N Engl J Med 260:912–914, 1959.
211. Kountz SL, Laub DR, Connolly JE: "Aortoiliac steal" syndrome. Arch Surg 92:490–497, 1966.
212. Heer FW, Silen W, French WS: Intestinal gangrene without apparent vascular occlusion. Am J Surg 110:231–238, 1965.
213. Marable SA, Molnar E, Beman FJ: Abdominal pains secondary to celiac axis compression. Am J Surg 111:493–495, 1966.
214. Szilagyi DE, Rion RL, Elliott JP, et al: The celiac artery compression syndrome: Does it exist? Surgery 178:232–246, 1973.
215. Blaisdell FW, DeMattei GA, Gauder PJ: Extraperitoneal thoracic aorta to femoral bypass graft as replacement for an infected aortic bifurcation prosthesis. Am J Surg 102:583–585, 1961.
216. Blaisdell FW, Hall AD: Axillary-femoral artery bypass for lower extremity ischemia. Surgery 54:563–568, 1963.
217. Guida PM, Moore SW: Obturator bypass technique. Surg Gynecol Obstet 128:1307–1316, 1969.

218. Shaw RS, Baue AE: Management of sepsis complicating arterial reconstructive surgery. Surgery 53:75–86, 1963.
219. Vetto RM: The treatment of unilateral iliac artery obstruction with a transabdominal subcutaneous femorofemoral graft. Surgery 52:342–345, 1962.
220. Elliott JP, Smith RF, Szilagyi DE: Aorto-enteric and para-prosthetic-enteric fistulas: Problems of diagnosis and management. Arch Surg 108:479–490, 1974.
221. Busuttil RW, Rees W, Baker JD, et al: Pathogenesis of aortoduodenal fistula. Surgery 85:1–13, 1979.
222. Homans J: The etiology and treatment of varicose ulcer of the leg. Surg Gynecol Obstet 24:300–311, 1917.
223. Trendelenberg F: Ueber die Unterbindung der Vena saphena magna bei Unterschenkelvaricen. Beitr Klin Chir 7:195–210, 1890.
224. Babcock WW: A new operation for the extirpation of varicose veins. NY Med J 86:153–156, 1907.
225. Mayo CH: The surgical treatment of varicose veins. St Paul Med J 6:695–699, 1904.
226. Trendelenberg F: Ueber die operative Behandlung der Embolie der Lungenarterie. Arch Klin Chir 86:686–700, 1908.
227. Homans J: Thrombosis of the deep veins of the lower leg causing pulmonary embolism. N Engl J Med 211:933–997, 1934.
228. Homans J: Venous thrombosis in the lower extremity: Its relation to pulmonary embolism. Am J Surg 38:316–326, 1937.
229. Homans J: Deep quiet thrombosis in the lower limbs: Preferred levels for interruption of the veins: Iliac section or ligation. Surg Gynecol Obstet 79:70–82, 1944.
230. Allen AW: Management of thromboembolic disease in surgical patients. Surg Gynecol Obstet 96:107–114, 1953.
231. Veal JR: Prevention of pulmonary complications by high ligation of the femoral vein. JAMA 121:240–244, 1943.
232. Northway O, Buxton RW: Ligation of the inferior vena cava. Surgery 18:85–94, 1945.
233. O'Neill EE: Ligation of the inferior vena cava in the prevention and treatment of pulmonary embolism. N Engl J Med 232:641–646, 1945.
234. Collins CG, Jones JR, Nelson WE: Surgical treatment of pelvic thrombophlebitis. New Orleans Med Surg J 95:324–329, 1943.
235. Anlyan WG, Campbell FH, Shingleton WW, et al: Pulmonary embolism following venous ligation. Arch Surg 64:200–207, 1952.
236. Bowers RF, Leb SM: Late results of inferior vena cava ligation. Surgery 37:622–628, 1955.
237. Conti S, Daschbach M, Blaisdell FW: A comparison of high-dose versus conventional-dose heparin therapy for deep vein thrombosis. Surgery 92:972–980, 1982.
238. Barker WF, Mandiola S: Postphlebitic syndrome after vena caval interruption. In Foley WT (ed): Advances in the Management of Cardiovascular Disease. Chicago, Year Book Publishers, Inc, 1980, pp 31–42.
239. Spencer FC: Plication of the inferior vena cava for pulmonary embolism. Surgery 62:388–392, 1955.
240. Moretz WH, Rhode CM, Shepherd MH, et al: Prevention of pulmonary emboli by partial occlusion of the inferior vena cava. Am Surg 25:617–626, 1959.
241. Miles RM, Richardson RR, Wayne L, et al: Long-term results with the serrated Teflon vena cava clip in the prevention of pulmonary embolism. Ann Surg 169:881–991, 1969.
242. Adams JT, DeWeese JA: Partial interruption of the inferior vena cava with a new plastic clip. Surg Gynecol Obstet 123:1087–1088, 1966.
243. Mobin-Uddin K, Smith PE, Martinez LD, et al: A vena cava filter for the prevention of pulmonary embolus. Surg Forum 18:209–211, 1967.
244. Greenfield LJ, Peyton MD, Brown PP, et al: Transvenous management of pulmonary embolic disease. Ann Surg 180:461–468, 1974.
245. Homans J: The late results of femoral thrombophlebitis and their treatment. N Engl J Med 235:249–253, 1934.
246. Trout H: Ulcers due to varicose veins and lymphatic blockage. W Va Med J 34:54–60, 1938.
247. Linton RR: The communicating veins of the lower leg and the technique for their ligation. Ann Surg 107:582–593, 1938.
248. Dodd K, Cockett FB: The Pathology and Surgery of the Veins of the Lower Limb. Edinburgh, E & S Livingstone Ltd, 1956.
249. Kistner RL: Surgical repair of the incompetent vein valve. Arch Surg 110:1336–1342, 1975.
250. Dale WA: Venous crossover grafts for the relief of iliofemoral venous block. Surgery 57:608–612, 1976.
251. Palma EC, Esperoń R: Vein transplants and grafts in the surgical treatment of the postphlebitic syndrome. J Cardiovasc Surg 1:94–107, 1960.
252. Taheri SA, Lazar L, Elias S, et al: Surgical treatment of postphlebitic syndrome with vein valve transplant. Am J Surg 144:221–224, 1982.
253. Taheri SA, Rigan D, Wels P, Mentzsner R, Shores RM: Experimental prosthetic vein valve. Am J Surg 156:111–114.
254. Brooks B: Intra-arterial injection of sodium iodide. JAMA 82:1016–1019, 1924.
255. Moniz E: L'encéphalographie artérielle, son importance dans la localization des tumeurs cérébrales. Rev Neurol (Paris) 2:72–90, 1927.
256. dos Santos R, Lamas A, Caldas P: L'artériographie des membres, de l'aorte et des ses branches abdominales. Bull Mem Soc Natl Chir 55:587–601, 1929.
257. Kruger RA, Mistretta CA, Crummy AB, et al: Digital K-edge subtraction radiography. Radiology 125:243–245, 1951.
258. Seldinger SI: Catheter replacement of the needle in percutaneous angiography. Acta Radiol 39:368–376, 1953.
259. Erlanger J: Blood pressure estimations by indirect methods: I. The mechanisms of the oscillatory criteria. Am J Physiol 39:401–446, 1915–16.
260. Winsor T: Pressure gradients. Influence of arterial disease on the systolic blood pressure gradients of the extremity. Am J Med Sci 220:117–126, 1950.
261. Pachon V: Sur la méthode des oscillations et les conditions correctes de son emploi en sphygomanométrie clinique. C R Soc Biol (Paris) 66:733–735, 1909.
262. Edwards EA, Levine HD: Peripheral vascular murmurs. Mechanisms of production and diagnostic significance. Arch Intern Med 90:284–300, 1952.
263. Wylie EJ, McGuiness JS: The recognition and treatment of arteriosclerotic stenosis of major arteries. Surg Gynecol Obstet 97:425–433, 1953.
264. Baillart P: La pression artérielle dans les branches de l'artère centrale de la retine: Nouvelle technique pour la determiner. Ann d'Occul 154:648–666, 1917.
265. Kartchner MM, McRaw LP, Crain V, et al: Oculoplethysmography: An adjunct to arteriography in the diagnosis of extracranial occlusive disease. Am J Surg 106:528–535, 1973.
266. Gee WG, Mehigan JI, Wylie EJ: Measurement of collateral hemispheric blood pressure by ocular pneumoplethysmography. Am J Surg 130:121–127, 1975.
267. Leopold GR, Goldberger LE, Bernstein EF: Ultrasonic detection and evaluation of abdominal aortic aneurysm. Surgery 72:939–945, 1972.
268. Strandness DE, Schultz RD, Sumner DS, et al: Ultrasonic flow detection: A useful technique in the evaluation of peripheral vascular disease. Am J Surg 113:311–320, 1967.
269. Sumner DS, Strandness DE Jr: The relationship between calf blood flow and ankle blood pressure in patients with intermittent claudication. Surgery 65:763–771, 1969.
270. Brockenbrough EC: Screening for Prevention of Stroke: Use of a Doppler Flowmeter. Washington/Alaska Regional Medical Program, Information and Education Resource Unit, 1969.
271. Machleder HI, Barker WF: The stroke on the wrong side:

Use of the Doppler ophthalmic test in cerebrovascular screening. Arch Surg *105*:943–947, 1972.

272. Bendick PJ, Jackson VP: Evaluation of vertebral arteries by duplex sonography. J Vasc Surg *3*:523–530, 1986.

273. Jäger K, Bollinger A, Valli C, Amman R: Measurement of mesenteric blood flow by duplex scanning. J Vasc Surg *3*:462–469, 1986.

274. Lindegaard KF, Bakke SJ, Grolimund P, et al: Assessment of intracranial hemodynamics in carotid artery by transcranial Doppler ultrasound. J Neurosurg *63*:890–898, 1985.

275. Thomas GI, Spencer MD, Jones TW, et al: Non-invasive carotid bifurcation mapping: Its relation to carotid surgery. Am J Surg *128*:168–174, 1974.

276. Barber FE, Baker DW, Arthur CW, et al: Ultrasonic duplex echo-Doppler scanner. IEEE Trans Biomed Eng *21*:109–113, 1974.

277. Flanigan DP, Douglas DJ, Mach I, et al: Intraoperative ultrasonic imaging of the carotid artery during carotid endarterectomy. Surgery *100*:893–899, 1986.

278. Cranley JJ, Canos JJ, Sull WF, et al: Phleborheographic technique for diagnosing deep venous thrombosis of the lower extremities. Surg Gynecol Obstet *141*:331–339, 1975.

279. Wheeler HB, Pearson D, O'Connell D: Impedance plethysmography: Technique, interpretation and results. Arch Surg *104*:164–169, 1972.

280. Comerota AJ, Katz ML, Greenwald L, et al: Should venous duplex imaging replace hemodynamic tests? J Vasc Surg *11*:53–61, 1990.

2

EMBRYOLOGY OF THE VASCULAR SYSTEM

DAVID S. MAXWELL

It is quite evident that the vascular apparatus does not independently and by itself "unfold" into the adult pattern. On the contrary, it reacts continuously in a most sensitive way to the factors of its environment, the pattern in the adult being the result of the sum of the environmental influences that have played upon it throughout the embryonic period. We thus find that this apparatus is continuously adequate and complete for the structures as they exist at any particular stage as the environmental structures progressively change; the vascular apparatus also changes and thereby is always adapted to the newer conditions. Furthermore, there are no apparent ulterior preparations at any time for the supply and drainage of other structures which have not yet made their appearance. For each stage it is an efficient and complete going-mechanism, apparently uninfluenced by the nature of its subsequent morphology.

George L. Streeter (1918)

In the above quotation from George Streeter over 70 years ago, we see exemplified the finest tradition of the working scientist: years of attention to the most minute details of his subject, which eventuate in the broadest and most comprehensive view of the fundamental issues. In this statement, Streeter says in summary all that needs to be said and virtually all that can be said about the development of the vascular system, save for some specific details that only serve to embellish the theme he has laid out.

The story of the development of the vascular system encompasses the life span of the organism. This system retains the ability to grow, change, regenerate, and add on in response to changing needs on the part of tissues, from the earliest stages of embryonic life to the final breath. Thus it supports normal growth, wound healing, and revascularization of tissues endangered by restricted flow in existing vessels, just as it supports the new growth of tumors, and transiently develops a highly efficient transport and exchange system through the uteroplacental circulation of pregnancy. All this is accomplished by the opening of, and enlargement of preexisting, vessels and the budding of new vascular growth from preexisting stem vessels. That it may fail eventually

to respond in some instances to adequately supply myocardium or the central nervous system is not as remarkable as that it does respond so well for so long. It must seem that in the embryonic and fetal history of the vascular system there would be clues to the mysteries that surround this responsiveness throughout life. Furthermore, in the prenatal unfolding of the vascular system lie the origins of the various cardiovascular malformations to which the human organism is subject. We do not yet know if the mechanisms of growth and the stimuli to vascularization of the embryo and fetus are the same as those that encourage and sustain the responsiveness of the vasculature in the postnatal organism.

In this summary chapter I shall not attempt to review the enormous literature on the subject, and I shall sacrifice many exciting details in the interest of a simple narrative exposition of the high points. The organizational scheme will take us first to a short history of the heart, which is simply a greatly modified blood vessel, followed by descriptions of the development of the large arteries and veins. I shall conclude with some comments on the growth of small vessels, which like acorns must appear and flourish first, to produce the mighty trunk and branches of the vascular tree.

EARLY HISTORY

An organism of a cubic millimeter or so in volume (depending on the surface area and other factors related to the effectiveness of diffusion) may thrive without a vascular system. The human embryo enjoys the elaboration of a vascular system from its earliest stages, almost as if it anticipated that its bulk would soon require a highly sophisticated transport system. As the embryonic disk becomes recognizable, a rapid accumulation of blood islands occurs around the periphery of the disk. These isolated "puddles" begin to coalesce and communicate with one another until the embryo resembles a bloody sponge. Most prominent is the precephalic region in which the seemingly random coalescence of blood islands forms a network in the region soon to be identified as the *cardiogenic plate* (Fig. 2–1A).

In these earliest stages of development the vascular system manifests one of its greatest mysteries: to what extent is the developmental pattern dictated by tissue needs and demands (possibly through the re-

lease of angiogenic factors, or through stimulus provided by metabolic products), and to what extent by factors such as extravascular pressures restricting flow in one set of possible blood channels and forcing enlargement of adjacent alternate routes of blood flow? And to what extent is the overall pattern dictated genetically? The *similarity* of the vascular tree from one individual to another urges the speculative fa-

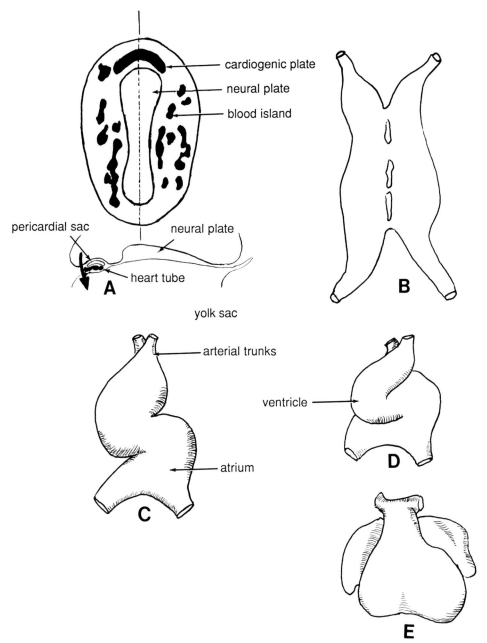

FIGURE 2–1. *A,* Embryonic disk from above, head of embryo up. Dotted line indicates plane of longitudinal section below, cranial end to the left. In the section the pericardial sac is above the heart tube, but as the head folds under the forebrain (direction of the large arrow), the positions of the heart and sac will be reversed, with the heart invaginating from above the pericardial sac. *B,* The two parallel primitive heart tubes (from dorsal view) fusing in the midline to form a single heart tube and a single-chambered heart. *C–E,* Successive stages of the folding of the heart tube, viewed from the front. The venous end of the tube swings posteriorly to form the atria while the arterial end (ventricles) remains anterior. *C, D,* and *E* represent the "loop stage" (see Delacruz et al.[1]). (Adapted from Moore KL: The Developing Human, 3rd ed. Philadelphia, WB Saunders Company, 1982; and Rushmer RF: Cardiovascular Dynamics, 2nd ed. Philadelphia, WB Saunders Company, 1961.)

voring of a detailed genetic code. The *variability* from one to the other, each pattern seemingly equally efficient in supporting tissues and organs, argues for development according to need and use, and to mechanical and other adventitious factors.

In the case of the heart a detailed genetic code is surely the guiding factor. Here, curiously, we begin with a parallel pair of cardiac tubes that fuse into one large tube, and then the latter divides internally into the right and left hearts. At first glance, this seems inefficient; why not simply have each original tube of the pair form a right or left heart? The reason is clear when we examine the details of internal division of the heart, in which the single outflow tract is divided in such a way as to connect the right heart to the primitive vessels supplying the pulmonary circuit, and connecting the remaining members of the branchial arch arteries to the left heart.

HEART

Our interest in the heart in this chapter shall be restricted to its development as that bears on the origins of the great vessels. The heart is simply a highly modified artery from both the histological and the embryological viewpoint. Histologically it resembles a muscular artery, because it has three layers to its walls: *adventitia* (epicardium), *tunica media* (myocardium), and *tunica intima* (endocardium). At the beginning the heart tubes are simply a parallel pair of vessels, seemingly little different from the other components of the random network of primitive blood vessels. Nonetheless, the fusion of these two tubes, and the development of a feeble myocardial investment around the endothelium, leads quickly to irregular contractions of the musculature with feeble and inefficient ejection of blood. Subsequent events display the development of septa, dividing the single-chambered heart into right and left halves, and the appearance of valves that dictate unidirectional flow. The heart is beating with increasing regularity and with an efficiency-improving peristalsis and force as the myocardial element thickens and cytodifferentiates; and presumably from these first feeble sporadic beats, there is a stirring of the blood contents of the primitive vessels, perhaps with some benefit to the growing tissues around them, and perhaps beginning to stimulate the enlargement of those channels that will survive into later embryonic stages. Beginning to channel blood through preferred pathways leads to closure and disappearance of less satisfactory routes, and enlargement of the more successful channels into definitive blood vessels soon worthy of names recognizable in terms of the adult circulatory pattern. Channel formation from blood islands might be influenced simply by the choice of the lowest resistance of the available pathways.

The now-fused heart tube (Fig. 2–1B) begins to invaginate the presumptive pericardial cavity, acquiring its visceral and parietal layers of pericardium while still a single-chambered heart configured as a simple, relatively straight tube. As the somites begin to appear in the neck and trunk region, the heart tube begins to fold on itself, first bulging ventrally, further invaginating the pericardial sac. The heart that is now swinging ventrocaudally comes to lie in front of the head and will continue its descent down the front of the neck and into the anterior chest. The ventrally directed bulge created by the "U"-shaped fold of the heart characterizes the "loop stage."[1] The ventral limb of the "U" is the arterial outflow path, and the dorsal limb of the "U" will become the venous inflow tract (Fig. 2–1C through E). By the 10-somite stage, approximately 3 weeks' ovulation age, the heart has begun to fold in a coronal plane as well, directing the ventricular region to the left, and forming a recognizable outflow tract, now termed the *bulbus cordis*, whose distal part is called the *truncus arteriosus* (Fig. 2–1C). At this stage, the heart is still a single-chambered structure innocent of valves, but rather completely enclosed in a pericardial sac, and demonstrably beating, albeit irregularly. There is no single primordium, no segment of the primitive heart tube, that can be identified as leading to a specific cardiac cavity in the early postloop stage. Instead, there are microscopically and experimentally identifiable zones, each of which gives origin to a specific anatomical region of a definitive "cardiac cavity." These primordia are most accurately termed "primitive cardiac regions"; thus referring to segments of the heart tube as forerunners of the chambers of the fully formed heart is misleading.[1] The folds in the heart tube, and the peristaltic nature of myocardial contraction lead to a predetermined direction of flow out through the *bulbus cordis*, the folds acting as inefficient "valves" to so direct the flow. Such early vitality is not surprising, because the cardiovascular system is the earliest formed and functional of the organ systems of the body. The heart is disproportionately large for the size of the embryo at this stage and this disproportion remains until birth, with only a modest decline in heart-body ratio toward birth. This obviously is due to the fact that the heart must support not only the growing tissue of the organism, but the embryo's share of the enormous placental circulation as well.

It is worth digressing for a moment at this time to emphasize the functional problems faced by the developing heart. It is required to form and to function in such a way as to support the growth of and to maintain the developing organism in an intrauterine (aquatic) environment; that is, to support an organism incapable of independent gas exchange itself and dependent upon the placenta for oxygen and nutriment, and for other metabolic exchange. Its lungs are developed rather late, and require only to be supplied with enough blood to support their growth. To perfuse the embryonic lungs with a rate of blood flow commensurate with an air-breathing existence would be energetically inefficient, and perhaps an impediment to their growth and development, but during the early stages of development of the cardiovascular system, the lungs are simply not sufficiently developed to be called anything other than buds, volumetrically incapable of containing any significant quantity of blood. So the heart must develop a mechanism whereby it can support the organism in an aquatic environment with extensive exchange across a placenta and provide adequate distribution of blood throughout the growing body of the embryo, yet it must simultaneously develop a configuration that will enable it to shift its mode of function instantly at birth to the support of the organism by way of pulmonary gas exchange. Simply put, in fetal and embryonic life the two sides of the heart may function as two pumps operating "in parallel," with the output of both ventricles distributed to the placenta and to the growing tissues of the body, and with no interdependence of the output. Yet the two hearts must have the means to shift from functioning "in parallel" to "in tandem" at birth, wherein the outflow of one heart becomes the inflow of the other, and blood is obligated to first perfuse the pulmonary circuit, to return to the heart, and then to perfuse the systemic circuit, and so on. One emphasis of this survey is to focus upon the development of this organ's features that render it capable of these sequential and different modes of function.

ARTERIES

During the early folding of the heart and with identification of a bulbus cordis and truncus arteriosus as an outflow tract, the aortic arches are beginning to form. The truncus arteriosus is continuous with a ventral aorta. This large, single-channeled artery is connected to a pair of dorsal aortae through a series of branchial (pharyngeal) arch arteries. The developing pharynx passes through a period in its development in which it is said to mimic the development of the gill apparatus of fish. Outpouchings of the pharyngeal wall grow as pockets toward the surface, where they are met or at least approached by corresponding infoldings of the ectodermal surface. Normally, these outpouchings and infoldings neither meet nor coalesce to form gill slits or fistulae. The supporting tissue on either side of the pouches is endowed with a cartilaginous supporting bar, a nerve, and a blood vessel, respectively known as the branchial arch (pharyngeal) cartilage, branchial arch nerve, and branchial arch artery. The first such cartilaginous bar is Meckel's cartilage, in front of the first pharyngeal pouch; the second, Reichert's cartilage, lies between the first and second pouches, and so on. The pharynx is supported by six arch complexes, surrounding and intervening between the pharyngeal pouches. The arteries of these arches are the connectives from the ventral aorta to the dorsal aortae, and they appear in sequence from cranial to caudal. Rarely are more than three such arch arteries identifiable at one time; in this case as elsewhere in

the embryo the cranial development leads or precedes that occurring more caudally. As the fourth arch artery appears, the first is being transformed into its successor structures, and ceases to be identifiable as an arch artery. In man, it seems there are five such arch arteries, numbered 1, 2, 3, 4, and 6, in recognition of the dropping out in phylogeny of the fifth arch artery, which plays no significant role in human development (the fifth pharyngeal pouch becomes fused with the fourth at its opening into the pharynx; its rudimentary arch between the fourth and fifth pouches contributes to the formation of the larynx). In contrast to the constancy of innervation of the derivatives of the pharyngeal arches, the vascular supply to the arches is subject to later, often extensive modification. The motor nerve to an arch persists throughout phylogeny and throughout ontogenetic development in supplying the derivatives of that arch (first arch, mandibular nerve; second arch, facial nerve; third arch, glossopharyngeal nerve; fourth through sixth arches, recurrent and superior laryngeal nerves and vagal pharyngeal nerve). The geometric representation of the arch artery pattern and the fate of those arteries is summarized in Figure 2–2. The paired dorsal aortae sweep posteriorly, and fuse in the midline to form a single dorsal aorta (Fig. 2–2 inset) posterior to entry points of the arch arteries.

The lungs begin their development as a ventrally directed outgrowth from the pharynx, and the single tube that will become the trachea descends into the presumptive chest cavity, where it branches into a pair of lung buds. These buds from the beginning receive a small blood supply from branches of the sixth aortic arch arteries (see Fig. 2–2A). Clearly the sixth arch arteries will play a role in the development of the pulmonary arterial tree. The developmental problem posed here is that the sixth arch arteries are initially part of the systemic circulation, simply representing the caudalmost of the branchial arch arteries springing from the truncus arteriosus, and uniting with the dorsal aortae. In the division of the heart tube into right and left hearts, some provision must be made for joining the right ventricular outflow tract to the sixth arch arteries, and the remainder of the great branchial arch system and aortae with the left ventricle. The rationale for fusion of primitive heart tubes into a single channel and subsequent division is now clear in this need to divide the bulbus cordis and truncus arteriosus into a pulmonary and an aortic artery. In the manner of that division we shall see the solution to the problem of connecting the right ventricle and the developing pulmonary artery to the lungs, and the remainder of the arch arteries to the systemic circulation and to the left ventricle. The interested reader is encouraged to examine the beautifully illustrated paper of Congdon[2] for further clarification of this point.

We shall turn now to the division of the heart into four chambers comprising two separate hearts, with provision for a parallel mode of function before birth and a tandem mode after birth. The umbilical veins

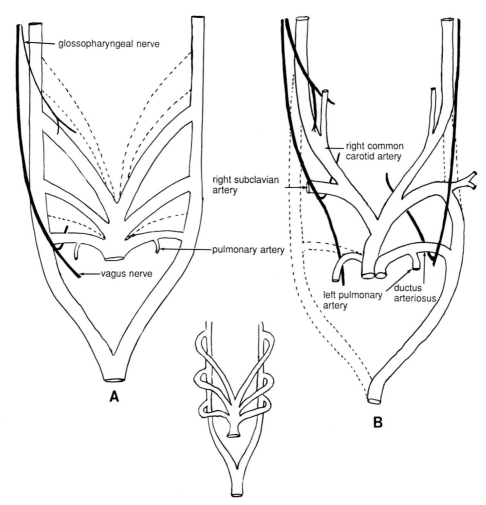

FIGURE 2–2.   The fate of the branchial arch arteries. *A,* The primitive arrangement of six arch arteries. Arches 1 and 2 have formed and been accommodated into the vessels of the head (dotted lines indicate arteries that are no longer "arches," i.e., 1, 2, and 5; see text). Arches 3, 4, and 6 connect the ventral aorta (aortic sac and truncus arteriosus) with the paired dorsal aortae. These latter fuse posteriorly to form a single dorsal aorta. *B,* The subsequent disposition of these vessels. The dotted lines indicate vessels that normally disappear, and include the right sixth arch beyond the right pulmonary artery. The glossopharyngeal nerve (motor to the third arch) and the recurrent laryngeal nerve (motor to the sixth arch derivatives) are shown. The recurrent is a branch of the vagus "recurring" around the sixth arch in *A,* and in *B,* these nerves recur around the ductus arteriosus and around the right subclavian. *Inset,* The first three aortic arch arteries from the front (ventral) view, during the branchial period (schematic: at no time are all arch arteries evident at the same time). The paired dorsal aortae unite into a single dorsal aorta posterior to the entry of the arch arteries. The postbranchial period, during which time the heart descends from the branchial region into the chest, is characterized by the modification of the arch system into the adult disposition of the derived arteries.

(after the sixth week, a single left umbilical vein) return blood to the fetal heart by their union with the inferior vena cava. This return route sees the umbilical vein enter the liver, where a shunt, the *ductus venosus,* bypasses the complex hepatic circulation and shunts the blood directly into the inferior vena cava. Thus the right atrium receives a supply of freshly oxygenated blood, in contrast to the adult condition. Before separation of the right and left atrium that placental return is into the single atrial chamber, which is diagrammatically depicted in Figure 2–3A. The single chamber undergoes a constriction in the plane of the atrioventricular orifices (and the *atrioventricular sulcus* on the exterior of the heart). From

the margins of this constriction, endocardial cushions grow inward to begin the formation of the tricuspid and mitral valves. The single atrium begins its separation into two halves by the downgrowth from the dorsocranial wall of a filmy crescentic curtain, the *septum primum* (Fig. 2–3B). The leading invaginated edge of the crescent grows down toward the floor of the single atrium, that floor now forming by virtue of the growth of the atrioventricular valve primordia. Figure 2–3B shows the septum primum from the right side as it progresses toward complete closure of the single atrial chamber in its midline, and we see that just before the *foramen primum* closes, a group of perforations in the dorsocranial part of the parti-

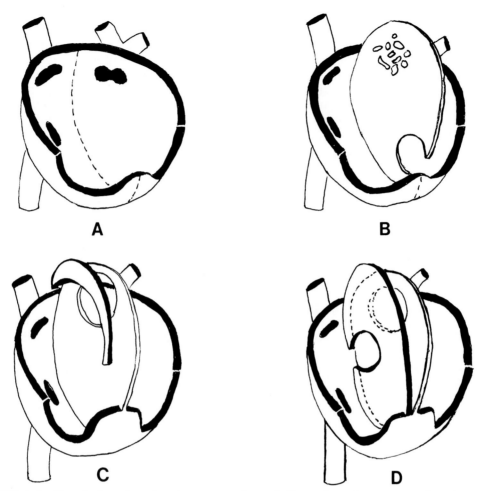

FIGURE 2–3. The single early atrium is represented as a hollow sphere, from an anterolateral view. The atrioventricular canals are the lower part of the cutaway sphere. *A,* The dotted line indicates the plane of division into right and left atria. The entry of the superior and inferior venae cavae (right atrial segment of the sphere) and the pulmonary arteries (left segment of the sphere) are indicated by entering tubes. *B–D,* Successive stages in development of interatrial septum. *B,* the septum primum grows down, leaving a free margin as the ostium primum. As this ostium prepares to close, holes appear in the upper posterior part of the septum, which in C have coalesced into an ostium secundum. *C,* The septum secundum begins to grow down to the right of the septum primum, covering over the ostium secundum on that side. The free margin of the septum secundum does not close over D, leaving the foramen ovale open. The right atrial contents flow into the left atrium, via the foramen ovale and ostium secundum. (Adapted from Tuchmann-Duplessis H, David HG, Haegel P: Illustrated Human Embryology. New York, Springer-Verlag, 1972.)

tion form (Fig. 2–3B) and then coalesce into a *foramen secundum* (Fig. 2–3C). This is necessary, inasmuch as throughout this developmental sequence, the heart is pumping blood to and returning it from the placenta, and the returning blood must be shunted from the right side of the heart into the left atrium in large volume to sustain the systemic circulation. *Thus at no point in fetal life may the right and left atria be functionally separate.* During the time when the placental circulation is intact, the pressure in the right atrium will exceed that in the left atrium, and a right-to-left shunt will be operative. Thus the foramen secundum opens just in time to continue that shunt as the foramen primum closes. Now, on the right side of the septum primum, a much more robust and rigid septum secundum begins its downgrowth following the same

pattern as that of the septum primum (Fig. 2–3C), a crescent-shaped leading edge growing down from above toward the endocardial cushions that will finally separate the atria from the ventricles. This downgrowth of the septum secundum comes to overlie the orifice of the foramen secundum. Fortunately, the septum secundum is sturdy and relatively unyielding, while the septum primum is thin and curtain-like. As long as the free lower edge of the septum secundum fails to reach the floor of the atrium, thus forming the *foramen ovale*, the elevated pressure in the right atrium will push blood through the ovale, deflecting the septum primum and allowing blood to pass through the foramen secundum into the left atrium and permitting continuation of the obligatory right-to-left shunt. Inasmuch as the downgrowth of the septum secundum is arrested, leaving a fixed foramen ovale, such a shunt operates throughout the intrauterine life of the organism. The orifice of the foramen ovale is just above and medial to the orifice of the inferior vena cava (Fig. 2–3D), so inferior caval (i.e., placental) blood is preferentially directed into that foramen, and thence into the left atrium, with remarkably little mixing of this oxygenated blood with the oxygen-poor blood returning via the superior vena cava.

The division of the ventricles and the single aortic outflow path is, at the same time, simpler to understand but more critically complex. The ventricle begins to divide by the upward growth of a muscular partition of myocardium from the cardiac apex toward the truncus arteriosus (Fig. 2–4A). This will form the muscular part of the interventricular septum. At the same time, a pair of ridges, the spiral ridges, grow toward each other as outgrowths of the walls of the truncus arteriosus. These will fuse together to form a *spiral septum*, dividing the septum from above down. The lower ends of the spiral ridges contribute to the formation of the final septal closure (Fig. 2–4B). This is an extraordinarily complex phenomenon involving early histological changes and probably initiated by hemodynamic influences and subsequently controlled by genetic factors (see the careful analysis by Fanapazir and Kaufman[3]). Where the three cushions meet the membranous interventricular septum is formed. Figures 2–4C and 2–4D schematically depict the spiral arrangement of the division of the truncus arteriosus whereby the single outflow tract is divided into pulmonary and aortic tubes, each connected to its corresponding ventricular cavity. The complexity of the closure lies in the precise pitch of the spiral septum, which must occur to align its lower end with the upthrusting muscular cushion to meet accurately in a single plane, or other interference in the fusion of those cushions into a complete membranous septum will lead to a membranous interventricular septal defect. Misalignment of the spiral ridges may result in failure of the great arteries to form and to function independently through the accident of a pulmonary-aortic fistula. Misalignment of the lower end of the dividing arteries, and asymmetry in the positioning of the spiral ridges could lead to such errors as overriding aorta with right ventricular contents partially ejected into the aorta. The features of the tetralogy of Fallot can be readily interpreted as a result of such misalignment in the truncus division: the tetralogy consists of *overriding aorta*, *pulmonary stenosis*, and *membranous septal defect* (due presumably to asymmetrical division of the proximal truncus arteriosus), and *right ventricular hypertrophy* (secondary to the right-to-left shunt through the overriding aorta and to the stenotic pulmonary artery).

A superbly illustrated and truly classical account of early experimental findings and an excellent historical review of the anatomy and physiology of fetal circulation is to be found in Barclay et al.[4] and more recent summaries may be obtained in standard works (Arey,[5] Clemente,[6] Hamilton and Mossman,[7] Moore,[8] Sabin,[9] and Tuchmann-Duplessis et al.[10]).

The original plan of five pairs of aortic arch arteries (Fig. 2–2) becomes modified by incorporation of the first two arch arteries into the internal carotid system, dropping out of the paired dorsal aortae between the third and fourth arches, and participation in the formation of the common carotid arteries by the third arches. Caudal to the lost segments of dorsal aortae, the fourth arches become the roots of the subclavian arteries, the right sixth is lost distal to its pulmonary branch, and the left sixth becomes the left pulmonary, with the segment distal to the pulmonary "branch" serving as the *ductus arteriosus* (see Fig. 2–2B). This arterial shunt vessel develops specialized muscle in its tunica media, which is stimulated to contract and shut down the shunt vessel after birth. It is believed that abnormal migration of some of this specialized smooth muscle into the aortic wall accounts for aortic stenosis, the stricture having developed in the aorta at the site of this ectopic "ductus" muscle after birth.

The closure of this right-to-left shunt on the arterial side at birth results in a great increase in pulmonary blood flow (the resistance of pulmonary vessels drops dramatically with inflation of the lungs and elongation of *helicine* arteries). On the venous side, the rise in left atrial pressure and loss of umbilical venous return arrests the interatrial right-to-left shunt. Elevated left atrial pressure results in the two interatrial septa operating as a flap valve, closing the foramen ovale by applying the curtain-like septum primum against the left (Fig. 2–3D).

Certainty in the derivation of the arteries of the head is not easy to achieve. The vessels form from a loose network of interconnected vessels, in which it is often not possible even to distinguish between arteries and veins.[11] The artery of the first arch becomes a part of the internal carotid artery, which also forms in part from persistence of the rostral parts of the dorsal aortae. The second arch artery appears in the form of the *stapedial artery*. This artery of the tympanic cavity passes through the annulus (obturator foramen) in the stapes and in some mammals it persists in this form. In man, this form of stapedial artery may remain into adulthood as a surgically troublesome vascular anomaly. This artery of the second arch for a time supplies three branches (supraorbital, infraorbital, and mandibular), distributed with the divisions of the trigeminal nerve. An anastomosis between the infraorbital and mandibular branches of the stapedial artery and the external carotid is said to give rise to the maxillary artery and its middle meningeal branch. It is further argued that the orbital anastomotic branch of the middle meningeal artery is the remnant of the original supraorbital branch of the stapedial artery. Some information is indicated in the phylogenetic history of the artery. In most mammals the originally small external carotid artery, as it grows forward, taps the origin of the stapedial artery and appropriates its branches, which at one

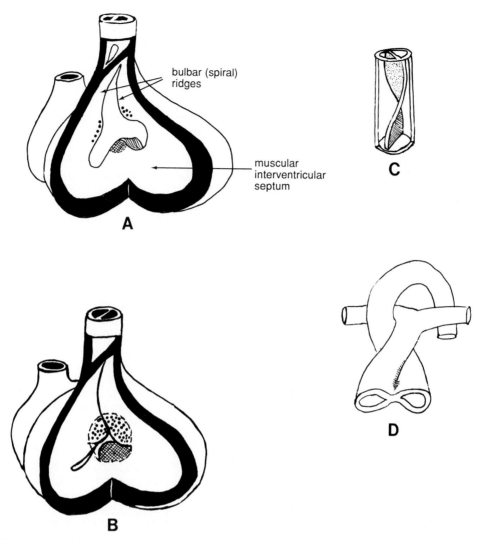

FIGURE 2–4. Stages in the division of the ventricle and the formation of the great arteries from the truncus arteriosus and bulbus cordis. *A*, The ventricle has begun to divide by formation of the muscular part of the interventricular septum by growth of the musculature of the ventricular wall. The bulbus cordis is dividing into two vessels, beginning with the growing together of two spiral ridges. *B*, The two spiral ridges meet and fuse to divide the bulbus cordis into two outflow tracts: the pulmonary artery and the ascending aorta. The ridges at their lower extremities (stippled cushions) meet a muscular cushion derived from the muscular interventricular septum (hatched), to form the membranous part of the interventricular septum (outlined in dotted lines). The spiral character of the arterial division connects the sixth arch arteries to the right ventricle, and the left ventricle to the other arch arteries and their derivatives. *C*, Spiral septum shown diagrammatically, in a cutaway cylinder representing the single bulbus cordis. The hatched surface of the septum may be taken as the aortic side of the division, and the stippled side as the pulmonary surface of the septum. The two resulting arteries must spiral around one another as in D; derived from a single tube, they are constrained to remain wrapped in a single pericardial sleeve. (Adapted from Tuchmann-Duplessis H, David HG, Haegel P: Illustrated Human Embryology. New York, Springer-Verlag, 1972; and Moore KL: The Developing Human. Philadelphia, WB Saunders Company, 1982.)

stroke reduces the size and causes the disappearance of the original stapedial artery, and extends the distribution of the external carotid. As Romer[12] colorfully put it, "the process is analogous to 'stream piracy,' whereby one river taps the headwaters of another." Padget[13] offers a detailed discussion and critical appraisal of the literature of the general mammalian stapedial artery and of the human artery, and her discussion is recommended to the interested reader.

The third arch artery forms the common carotid arteries, and the first segments of the internal carotid arteries. Thus it is probable that portions of the first three arches all contribute to the external carotid arteries. The left fourth arch forms the arch of the aorta, and the left dorsal aorta distal to the point of union of this arch forms the descending aorta along with the single dorsal aorta more caudally (Fig. 2–2B). The entirety of the right dorsal aorta is lost. The right horn of the aortic sac forms the brachiocephalic artery, from which the right common carotid and subclavian arteries spring.

The sixth arches are associated with the pulmonary blood supply, first as the source of the small twigs to the lung buds. Those twigs and their parent stems from the truncus arteriosus become the definitive pulmonary arteries. Now it should be clear why the complex twist of the spiral septum dividing the truncus arteriosus is necessary. In dividing the truncus, it is essential to connect the right ventricle to the origins of the sixth arches from the truncus, while leaving the more rostral arch arteries connected to the part of the truncus connected to the left ventricle. The arch arteries spring from a single vessel, the truncus, and must end as arteries arising from separate arteries: the sixth arising from the pulmonary artery and the first through fourth from the aortic component of the truncus. The twisting division of the truncus accounts also for the intertwined course of the pulmonary artery and the ascending aorta, and their derivation from a single vessel, the truncus, accounts for these great arteries being wrapped in a single pericardial sleeve (Fig. 2–4D).

The branchial arches develop nerve supplies along with their vascular supplies, and it is an axiom of anatomy that once nerve supply is established it is never lost. The motor nerves of the branchial arches supply the structures derived from those arches henceforth, no matter what developmental events ensue. In Figure 2–2 we see the position of the glossopharyngeal nerve as the motor nerve of the third arch, and the recurrent laryngeal branch of the vagus as the motor nerve of the sixth arch, as these nerves are drawn caudally by the descent of the heart and growth of the branchial arch system. The "recurrent" branch of the vagus is in fact the motor nerve derived from the *nucleus ambiguus* of the brainstem, which happens to distribute by way of the vagus, having emerged from the brainstem as the cranial root of the spinal accessory nerve (XI). The recurring course of the nerve is accounted for by its inherited requirement of lying caudal to the sixth arch artery. The distal part of the left sixth arch artery becomes the ductus arteriosus (the *ligamentum arteriosum* after birth). Thus arises the asymmetry in the courses of the two recurrent laryngeal nerves. The left nerve is constrained to occupy its original relationship to its arch artery, as that artery is drawn down into the chest by the descent of the heart. The right nerve loses that constraint, as the sixth arch drops out distal to the origin of the pulmonary artery. The only persisting arch to prevent the nerve's remaining in the neck as the heart descends is the fourth arch on the right side (the right subclavian artery), around which we find the nerve "recurring" in the adult human (Fig. 2–2B). The surgeon who finds in thyroid surgery that the right recurrent nerve does not recur around the subclavian artery should take that as a warning that a developmental abnormality in the formation of the right subclavian artery might be expected (e.g., a retroesophageal right subclavian). In

that event the right subclavian forms from the right seventh intersegmental artery and part of the right dorsal aorta, the right fourth arch artery and right dorsal aorta having involuted cranial to the origin of the seventh intersegmental artery (see Moore's[8] figures 14 through 37, and other embryology texts).

The developing embryo in its earliest stages is supported by a yolk sac of nutriment, sustaining growth until the placenta is sufficiently developed to assume those duties. The embryo lies on the surface of the yolk sac, the interior of the latter in continuity with the developing gastrointestinal tract. The digestive tract cranial to the yolk sac is termed the "foregut," that caudal to the yolk sac is termed the "hindgut," and that directly connected to the yolk sac is termed the "midgut." Three aortic branches, midline and unpaired, arise to supply each of these segments of the digestive tract, and these arteries remain the source of arterial blood for those portions of the tract and their derivatives. Thus, the celiac artery is the artery of the foregut and the derivatives of the foregut, including the liver and spleen. The artery of the midgut is the superior mesenteric artery; the artery of the hindgut is the inferior mesenteric artery. During development the digestive tract outgrows the room available for it in the abdominal cavity, and temporarily "herniates" out into the umbilical cord. Its return from this extraabdominal sojourn is accompanied by a rotation that accounts for the disposition of the stomach, duodenum, and the bowel in the adult. The axis of rotation around which this reentry into the abdomen occurs is the superior mesenteric artery (see the exquisitely illustrated account of Dott[14]).

The kidneys begin their development in the pelvis and migrate cranially to their final position on the posterior abdominal wall. The pelvic kidneys derive their arterial blood supply from the iliac system, and as they ascend, the previous arterial supply drops out and new vessels from the aorta are established. The ascent and the history of the previous blood supply is to be read in the sources of small vessels supplying the ureter, the origins of these indicating the stems of vessels formerly supplying the kidney. Should the "ascent" of the kidney be arrested, the blood supply at the time, of course, remains the supply into adulthood. So the ascent of the horseshoe kidney is arrested by the overhanging inferior mesenteric artery, and the horseshoe kidney has arterial blood supplied from common iliac vessels or the aorta at a level lower than the origin of the normal renal arteries. So, too, accessory renal arteries usually arise below the renal arteries, and enter the inferior pole of the kidney, attesting to a previous source of blood that did not entirely disappear with ascent to the final renal destination.

The limbs seem to be organized around a central arterial stem, so from the beginning an axial artery is identifiable. Figure 2–5 depicts the changes in circulatory pattern for the two limbs. Generally, the axial artery in large part disappears, and certainly ceases to be the principal source of limb blood.

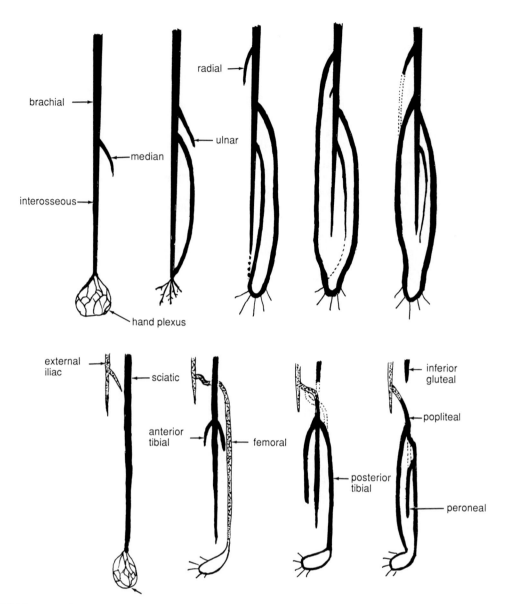

FIGURE 2–5. The development of the arterial pattern of the limbs; top row (left to right), upper limb; lower row, lower limb. *Upper limb,* Initially the limb is organized around a single axial artery, the brachial and its interosseous continuation, terminating in a hand plexus. The hand plexus will develop into the palmar arches. The stem artery gives rise in succession to the median, ulnar, and radial arteries. The median normally has an evanescent existence as a major vessel, losing its connection with the hand plexus, which it usurped from the axial vessel. See text for details. *Lower limb,* The axial vessel for the lower limb is the sciatic, which remains in the adult as the inferior gluteal, and portions of the popliteal and peroneal arteries. The femoral arises from the external iliac, and appropriates the distal part of the sciatic to dominate the vascular distribution of the limb. The anterior tibial arises as a branch of the popliteal; the posterior tibial is developed from the union of the femoral with the popliteal. Notice, in the third figure from the left, an upper segment of the femoral is lost, allowing the popliteal to become interposed. See text for details. (Adapted from Arey LB: Developmental Anatomy, 7th ed. Philadelphia, WB Saunders Company, 1965.)

In the upper limb, the axial artery passes down the core of the limb to the hand plexus. It is a continuation of the subclavian and axillary system, already established in the 5-mm embryo, and is the forerunner of the brachial and, more distally, the interosseous arteries. The upper limb axial artery sprouts a median and an ulnar arterial branch on the medial side of the stem artery. The median temporarily joins with the ulnar in the volar arch. A radial sprout follows on the preaxial side of the limb, and this new branch usurps the median's connection with the volar arch. The distal axial artery persists as the anterior interosseous. This pattern is completed before the end of the second month, and the early dominance of the axial and the median arteries is permanently lost. The median artery persists as a branch of the anterior interosseous artery, serving as the nutrient artery of the median nerve. It may persist in a much enlarged form as an anomaly, accompanying the median nerve into the palm, and retaining its connection with and contribution to the palmar arterial arches.

Figure 2–5 shows the steps by which the adult pattern of arterial supply to the lower limb is derived from the axial artery of the limb bud. The axial vessel is the sciatic artery, a direct branch of the umbilical. It is the primary source of the blood for the limb bud in the 9-mm embryo. The major stem artery for the limb becomes the femoral as the latter continues the course of the external iliac. The femoral annexes the foot plexus of the sciatic, and the origin of this axial vessel. The remaining proximal "stump" of the once dominant sciatic artery persists as the inferior gluteal artery. A branch of the latter, the artery of the sciatic nerve, is all that remains of the former glory of the sciatic artery. The distal parts of the sciatic stem, appropriated by the femoral near its origin from the external iliac, give rise to the anterior tibial artery, which connects with the plantar arch distally. The newer, more distal femoral establishes a new connection to the distal sciatic so it and the plantar arch come to branch from the sciatic. The most distal segment of the sciatic shifts its origin to the posterior tibial as the peroneal, and the adult pattern is established. The remnants of the sciatic persist (from above down) as the inferior gluteal with its small artery of the sciatic nerve, the popliteal artery, and the peroneal artery. In the adult arterial plan these persisting segments of the original sciatic artery no longer have any continuity with each other in any significant way.

The umbilical arteries, carrying blood to the placenta for gas and metabolite exchange, appear as large branches of the internal iliac arteries and persist unmodified throughout gestation. These arteries develop robust branches to the upper surface of the urinary bladder. At birth the segments of the umbilical arteries distal to the origin of the arteries to the bladder are obliterated, and remain as fibrous cords, the medial umbilical ligaments. The stem of these arteries and the branches to the bladder are henceforth known as the *superior vesicle arteries*.

VEINS

As the arterial distribution system develops, appropriate return pathways arise simultaneously. The venous system is extensively interconnected, with great capacity for collateral routes of venous return, and arteries generally are accompanied by corresponding veins. The short review of the venous system here will focus only on the great systems of veins that arise early in embryonic life and that give rise to the major collecting pathways recognizable in the normal adult. Thus even such important, but developmentally simple systems as the pulmonary venous system will not be subjects of discussion here.

A passing comment on venous valves is appropriate here, however, to draw attention to a provocative analysis and comparative study of superficial veins in the limbs of primates.[15] The number and spacing of venous valves is dictated genetically, and is relevant to the need to maintain optimum pressures within capillary beds to ensure a balance in fluid exchange in tissues. The distance between venous valves in the limbs is just that needed to provide the transcapillary pressure gradients required for an equilibrium in fluid efflux and return to the vascular bed, and is not, as previously supposed, an adaptation to counter the effects of gravity in the bipedal posture.

The veins of the embryo fall into three major groups: vitelline (omphalomesenteric) veins, umbilical veins, and the cardinal system of veins. The coalesced blood islands that give rise to undifferentiated blood networks develop a venous side, as they do an arterial side, as directions of blood flow become established through them. Preferential pathways emerge on the venous side, giving rise to larger and more dominant veins that undergo modification as regional or organ-specific changes occur. Many of the venous channels developed in support of fetal life disappear as the need for them vanishes through subsequent development.

The vitelline veins are the veins of the yolk sac. They pass through the intestinal portal of the umbilical cord, alongside the (at first) wide channel of communication between the sac and the midgut region of the alimentary canal. A vitelline plexus is formed of communicating venous channels between the vitelline veins in the *septum transversum*, and as the liver develops in this septum it infringes upon the vitelline plexus, breaking it up into hepatic sinusoids. The vitelline pathway from the septum transversum into the heart persists in spite of this encroachment, as hepaticocardiac channels. The right channel of this return persists as the terminal segment of the inferior vena cava (Fig. 2–6). The vitelline plexus also surrounds the duodenum during the stage of hepatic growth, and the plexus is further distorted when the herniated midgut returns in a spiraling motion into the abdominal cavity. It is this rotation during the return that brings the duodenum into its transverse position, and fixes this position of the duodenum by peritonealization. This position forces the blood in the surrounding plexus to shunt from the right to the left vitelline vein, which is the segment of the vitelline system lying just caudal to the transversely oriented duodenum. The left vitelline vein then sends its blood directly across to the liver by way of its dorsal anastomosis with the persistent cranial end of the right vitelline vein.

The portal vein thus formed does not spiral around the duodenum as so commonly described and illustrated, but instead is short and straight, with the duodenum spiralling around it. The ease with which these changes take place may be readily understood if the two following basic facts are appreciated: (1) the essentially plexiform nature of the embryonic vascular system, and (2) the natural tendency for blood to seek the most direct route of flow because of hy-

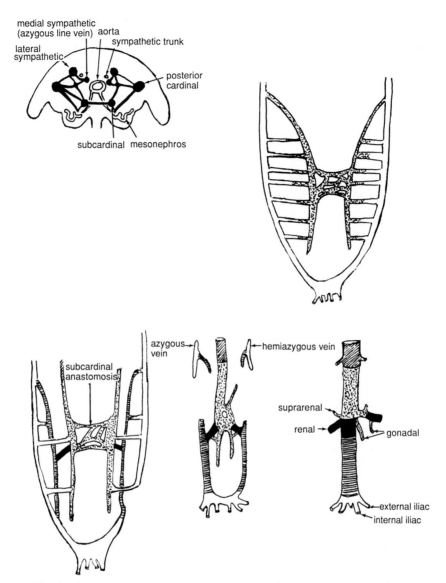

FIGURE 2–6. The development of the large veins. *Upper left,* A schematic cross-section of the embryo to show the relative positions and extensive interconnections of the major body wall veins. *Upper right* and *lower row* (left to right), succession of stages in the development of the inferior vena cava and the related body wall veins. See key below for identification of the component veins, making up the inferior vena cava (lower right). For simplicity, the azygos and hemiazygos veins are depicted as if they arose from the lateral sympathetic veins, while in fact they arise as derivatives from the parallel medial sympathetic (azygous line) veins. See text for details. (Adapted from Williams PL, Wendell-Smith CP, Treadgold S: Basic Human Embryology, 2nd ed. Philadelphia, JB Lippincott Co, 1969; and Hollinshead WH, Rosse L: Textbook of Anatomy, 4th ed. Philadelphia, Harper & Row, 1985.)

drodynamic factors. (Refer to the clear sequence of illustrations of this development in Figs. 225 through 230 of the fourth edition of "Hamilton, Boyd and Mossman's Human Embryology,"[7] p. 274.)

The umbilical veins, entering the abdominal cavity by way of the umbilicus, must also traverse the septum transversum to arrive at the heart, and their septal segments within the septum also become enmeshed with the vitelline veins in the hepatic plexus of sinusoids. In the 5-mm embryo, the umbilical veins communicate extensively with the vitelline plexus in the liver. Two days later, the right umbilical vein undergoes atrophy, and all placental blood returns to the fetal heart via the left vein. The left vein's channel through the liver enlarges to accommodate this enhanced flow and forms the *ductus venosus*, a direct channel through the liver between the left umbilical vein and the inferior vena cava. This channel, of course, obliterates at birth with cessation of flow through the umbilical system, and the intrahepatic shunt is replaced by the *ligamentum venosum*. There thus is said to be a sphincter in this shunt that regulates umbilical flow, a particularly important feature during uterine contractions to prevent overloading the fetal heart. This sphincter's closure at birth contributes to the prompt obliteration of the shunt. The course of the left umbilical vein caudal to the liver is in the free margin of the ventral mesentery. The obliterated umbilical vein between umbilicus and liver is the *ligamentum teres hepatis* of the adult, lying in the free margin of the falciform ligament; the latter is the adult counterpart of the ventral mesentery between the liver and the anterior abdominal wall.

The cardinal veins are the body wall veins of the embryo and fetus. There are several sets designated by distinguishing names: a source of considerable confusion for the student of human anatomy. The *anterior cardinal veins* (also termed "precardinal" veins) drain the cranial region of the early embryo. The *posterior cardinal veins* drain the caudal portion, and arise slightly later than the anterior cardinals. The *subcardinal veins* appear shortly after the posterior cardinal veins, and are derived in conjunction with the rapidly growing progenitor of the kidney, the *mesonephros*. The term "*supracardinal*" *veins* is sometimes employed to designate lateral sympathetic, or thoracolumbar line veins, or paraureteric veins. To limit the number of "cardinal veins" one must attend to, I shall avoid use of "supracardinal veins" here in discussing the veins of the posterior body wall anterior to the segmental vessels, using instead "*lateral sympathetic*."

The primary head vein of the embryo evolves into the complex system of dural sinuses and venous pathways of the head and the reader is referred to the classical accounts of Streeter[16] and Padget,[11,13] whose illustrations make amply clear the changes leading to the adult pattern. The anterior and posterior cardinal veins unite behind the heart to form the common cardinal veins, or ducts of Cuvier (right and left). The union of the ducts of Cuvier is the ductus venosus at the venous end of the heart. Part of the ductus venosus becomes incorporated into the walls of the atria, most notably the right atrium.

The posterior cardinal veins are the first of a series of caudal longitudinal body wall veins, which form an interconnected system (Fig. 2–6) giving rise to the caudal body wall venous drainage, and to the inferior vena cava and azygous system of veins.

The subcardinal veins appear soon after the posterior cardinal veins, as a pair of veins along the medial side of the urogenital folds. They are associated with the mesonephros, and probably arise as a series of longitudinal anastomoses for the plexuses of the mesonephroi. They drain the mesonephroi and the germinal epithelium and terminate cranially and caudally by connecting with the posterior cardinal veins (Fig. 2–6). The subcardinal veins unite with each other, and along their lengths with the posterior cardinal veins through anastomoses; the multiple transverse anastomoses of these veins is probably their most distinctive feature. One of these anastomoses is the intersubcardinal anastomosis between the two veins ventral to the aorta. The right subcardinal vein establishes a communication with the liver sinusoids and that segment becomes the hepatic segment of the inferior vena cava (Fig. 2–6). The preaortic anastomosis comes into play in the establishment of the vena cava inferior to that segment.

The lateral sympathetic ("supracardinal") veins appear soon after the hepatic segment of the inferior vena cava, anterior to the segmental vessels. They appear first as a plexus, but quickly become a longitudinal trunk, ending cranially in the posterior cardinal vein, and posteriorly anastomosing with the subcardinal vein, especially strongly on the right side. The part caudal to that latter anastomosis persists, and most of the remainder of the lateral sympathetic veins regress, the persisting right caudal segment surviving as the infrarenal part of the inferior vena cava (Fig. 2–6). As the lateral sympathetic veins appear, a medial pair (medial sympathetic or azygous line veins) also arise, but medial to the sympathetic trunk in the abdominal wall. These link across the midline, and by the dropping out of an intermediate segment on the left side, form the azygous system of veins.

The adult pattern is completed by the emerging dominance of the right common cardinal vein. The left upper intercostal spaces drain into the remainder of the left common cardinal vein, which connects with the left brachiocephalic vein after the lateral part of the left common cardinal is lost. The left superior intercostal vein is formed in part by the left posterior and anterior cardinal veins. The potential communication between the two may persist as a left superior vena cava; and the latter's position may be identified in the normal adult as the oblique cardiac vein (of Marshall), which in the adult may be traced at times to the left superior intercostal vein as a reminder of that origin.

The inferior vena cava has a complex origin. The hepatic segment, it was noted above, is derived from the cranial segment of the right vitelline vein and the hepatic sinusoids. A prerenal segment forms distal to this as an anastomosis between the hepatic segment and the right subcardinal vein. This latter vein forms the prerenal segment (down to the junction of the renal veins). A renal segment is formed from a renal collar (note the preaortic anastomosis between the subcardinals described above). The renal collar is an anastomosis involving this preaortic anastomosis, and anastomoses between the right subcardinal and lateral sympathetic veins. A postrenal segment forms from the lumbar part of the right lateral sympathetic vein down to the level of the common iliac veins. The common iliacs join with the lower part of the inferior vena cava as the postcardinal veins degenerate, forcing the iliacs to find this secondary route of venous return to the heart. The definitive renal veins, as the kidneys come to rest in the adult position, are formed as connections to the inferior vena cava through the anastomoses between subcardinals and lateral lumbar veins. On the left side, the longer path to the inferior vena cava is accomplished through recruitment of this anastomosis between the subcardinal veins. On the right this anastomosis is incorporated into the formation of the renal segment of the inferior vena cava, and the situation is less complex.

The multiple sources incorporated into the inferior vena cava, including anastomoses across the midline, may lead to some bizarre malformations. Most dramatic of these may be the retrocaval ureter, which is clearly not a malformation of the ureter or a misguided path of ascent of the kidney, but must be interpreted as incorporation of unusual components of the renal collar into the inferior vena cava. Fortunately, this is a very rare occurrence, but accounts in the literature agree on this interpretation as a caval rather than a ureteric malformation.[17-19]

GROWTH OF NEW VESSELS

It would be helpful to know if the development of new blood vessels in the fetus and during postnatal growth of the organism were a model for vascular proliferation under other circumstances. It is very likely that this is so, although the factors that might serve to stimulate and direct such growth might be quite different. The central nervous system (CNS) provides a model that has been much studied by a variety of means. The relative maturity of the brain at birth provides an existing and fully functional vascular tree that might be taken as a model of a relatively mature vascular system. The further growth and development of the CNS dictates the need for postnatal neovascularization to support the further maturation of the tissue.

Examination of the vascularization of the CNS, in addition to the interest derived in relation to vascular proliferation, addresses a fundamental issue in vascular growth during development: To what extent is development of a vascular bed a permissive condition for the subsequent onset of function; that is, to what extent is it anticipatory of and necessary for function? Or, conversely, to what extent is the development of a vasculature the response to the greater metabolic demands of a tissue that is increasing in or beginning to achieve the functional levels expected of it at full maturation?

Study of CNS regions at the time of onset of measurable function (e.g., auditory system) reveals that vascular sprouting parallels such events in their time courses (Skolnik and Maxwell, unpublished). Such observations cannot distinguish cause and effect, and perhaps they must go hand in hand, functional and vascular maturation identically timed or responsive to some common signal from yet another source. Greater temporal resolution would have to be applied than we have been able to bring to bear on this question to date.

It is possible to describe the manner of new vessel growth in the CNS, and to derive some quantitative information therefrom. Rowan and Maxwell[20] studied the postnatal rat cerebral cortex, which is structurally and cytologically quite immature at birth and undergoes a remarkable degree of postnatal matur-

ation in the first 3 weeks after birth. CNS blood vessels display alkaline phosphatase activity alone among CNS tissue elements. Using a simple histochemical procedure it is possible to visualize small vessels in the light and electron microscopes, relying on the enzyme reaction to label vessels, and those cells that are in the process of becoming vessels through cytodifferentiation, with no ambiguity whatsoever.[21] It has been a matter of widely accepted dogma that new vessels in the CNS and perhaps elsewhere begin as a proliferation of solid cords of cells that later "canalize" (develop lumens). Such a mechanism seems improbable on purely mechanistic grounds, and this does not seem to be the case in the CNS. In this tissue, postnatal growth of new vessels seems to occur by budding from preexisting vessels, the buds recognizable by their enzyme content, and by the presence of lumens, although collapsed and empty. The lumens are not identifiable by light microscopy, so the interpretation of solid cords of cells is quite understandable. The buds or sprouts have characteristic cytoplasmic protuberances or fingers that "explore" in advance of the growth of the sprout, seeming to seek the most appropriate path, or perhaps sensing the direction where vessel growth will best satisfy the perceived need. Figures 2–7, 2–8, 2–9, and 2–10 show a series of such sprouts from the rat cerebral cortex. These sprouts presumably link up with a venous channel, and hemodynamics should serve to open the lumen as a capillary link is thus established. Figure 2–11 is an electron micrograph of such a sprout, in which the unopened state of the lumen is evident. Inasmuch as it is CNS arteries that prominently display alkaline phosphatase activity, and the sprouts at the earliest detectable stages also dis-

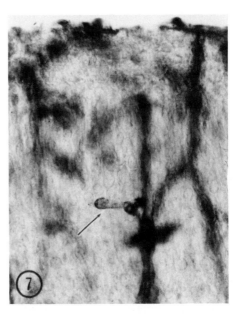

FIGURE 2–7. Light micrographs of rat cerebral cortex, reacted for alkaline phosphatase. A vascular sprout (arrow) is seen in the superficial cortex 2 days postnatal, cortical surface at the top. ×1548. (Reproduced with permission of Dr. R. Rowan.)

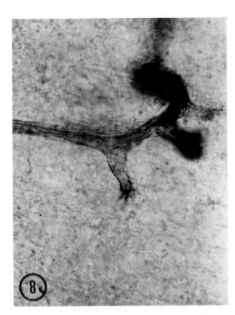

FIGURE 2–8. Light micrographs of rat cerebral cortex, reacted for alkaline phosphatase. A vascular sprout in middle third of the rat cortex, 7 days postnatal. Delicate exploratory fingers, or pseudopodia, are seen at the tip of the sprout. ×3148. (Reproduced with permission of Dr. R. Rowan.)

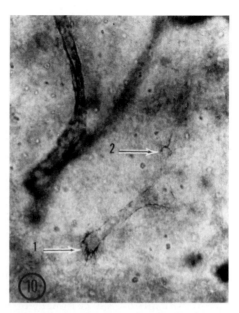

FIGURE 2–10. Light micrographs of rat cerebral cortex, reacted for alkaline phosphatase. A branched sprout with two tips (arrows). A larger tip (*1*) extends down and to the left of the stem vessel; a smaller tip extends upward (*2*). The parent sprout and the two sprout tips are much less intensely stained than the mature vessels dominating the upper and left parts of the photograph. ×3148. (Reproduced with permission of Dr. R. Rowan.)

play this enzyme, we presume that postnatal vascularization proceeds by arteriolar sprouting, with subsequent linkage with the venous bed. An excellent historical review of the study of growth and differentiation of blood vessels, and statement of the current status of the field, is to be found in Eriksson and Zarem.[22]

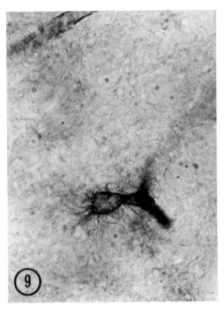

FIGURE 2–9. Light micrographs of rat cerebral cortex, reacted for alkaline phosphatase. Vascular sprout, middle third of the cortex, 8 days postnatal. Pseudopodia are evident at the tip. ×3148. (Reproduced with permission of Dr. R. Rowan.)

The factors that may induce an arteriole to sprout may be multiple, possibly legion. An enormous literature on angiogenic factors is available for the CNS and for other tissues, including tumors. Attention must be drawn here, however, to a recent series of papers announcing a major achievement by Vallee's group at Harvard.[23–25] These investigators isolated and analyzed an angiogenic factor from human carcinoma cells, and for the first time an angiogenic factor has been isolated, its amino acid sequence determined, and its genetic code identified. Curiously, this factor, "angiogenin," is remarkably similar in its amino acid sequence to a ribonuclease, and the unraveling of the biological meaning of this similarity and possible relationship will be fascinating to watch in the literature. This is not to say that only one angiogenic protein is the cause of neovascularization. There may be many, perhaps different ones operating in the embryo and fetus compared to the adult in wound healing, and perhaps again even another set operating in neoplasms. There is abundant evidence that tissue metabolites are capable of stimulating vascular development (e.g., high carbon dioxide and low oxygen content in tissue fluids). A complex list of possibilities will have to be sorted out to determine which of such factors act to stimulate production and/or release of specific angiogenic factors from cells (and which cells), and which are sufficient factors in their own right, acting directly on preexisting vessels.

It may not be satisfying to conclude a survey such as this with a dismaying array of presently unan-

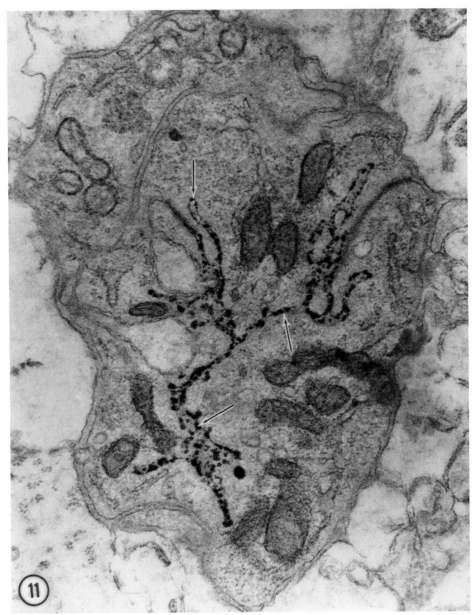

FIGURE 2–11. Electron micrograph of a sprout in the middle third of the cortex 8 days postnatal. The unopened lumen is delicately outlined by deposition of enzyme (alkaline phosphatase) reaction product and is indicated by arrows. ×42,200. (Reproduced with permission of Dr. R. Rowan.)

swered questions. It is compelling evidence, however, that the questions are there, and that the vigorous activity in laboratories around the world will yield some answers. The control of neovascularization, of which the embryo is such a master, may allow us to apply the lessons the embryo has to teach us to a wide spectrum of problems afflicting the adults in our clinics and hospitals.

REFERENCES

1. Delacruz M, Sanchez-Gomez C, Palomino MA: The primitive cardiac regions in the straight tube heart (stage 9) and their anatomical expression in the mature heart: An experimental study in the chick embryo. J Anat *165*:121–131, 1989.
2. Congdon ED: Transformation of the aortic-arch system during the development of the human embryo. Carnegie Contr Embryol *14(68)*:47–110, 1922.
3. Fanapazir K, Kaufman MH: Observations on the development of the aorticopulmonary spiral septum in the mouse. J Anat *158*:157–172, 1988.

4. Barclay AE, Franklin KJ, Prichard MML: The Foetal Circulation. Oxford, Blackwell Scientific Publ, 1946.
5. Arey LB: Developmental Anatomy, 7th ed. Philadelphia, WB Saunders Company, 1965.
6. Clemente CD: Gray's Anatomy, 30th American ed. Philadelphia, Lea & Febiger, 1985.
7. Hamilton WJ, Mossman HW: Hamilton, Boyd and Mossman's Human Embryology, 4th ed. Baltimore, Williams & Wilkins, 1972.
8. Moore KL: The Developing Human, 3rd ed. Philadelphia, WB Saunders Company, 1982.
9. Sabin FR: Origin and development of the primitive vessels of the chick and pig. Carnegie Contr Embryol 6(18):63–124, 1917.
10. Tuchmann-Duplessis H, David HG, Haegel P: Illustrated Human Embryology. New York, Springer-Verlag, 1972.
11. Padget DH: Development of the cranial venous system in man, from the viewpoint of comparative anatomy. Carnegie Contr Embryol 36(247):79–140, 1957.
12. Romer AS: The Vertebrate Body, 4th ed. Philadelphia, WB Saunders Company, 1970.
13. Padget DH: The development of the cranial arteries in the human embryo. Carnegie Contr Embryol 32(212):205–261, 1948.
14. Dott NM: Anomalies of intestinal rotation: Their embryology and surgical aspects: With report of five cases. Br J Surg 11:252–286, 1923.
15. Thiranagama R, Chamberlain AT, Wood BA: Valves in superficial limb veins of humans and nonhuman primates. Clin Anat 2:135–145, 1989.
16. Streeter GL: The developmental alterations in the vascular system of the brain of the human embryo. Carnegie Contr Embryol 9(24):5–38, 1918.
17. Derbes VJ, Dial WA: Postcaval ureter. J Urol 36:226–233, 1936.
18. Gruenwald P, Surks SN: Pre-ureteric vena cava and its embryological explanation. J Urol 49:195–261, 1943.
19. Randall A, Campbell EW: Anomalous relationship of the right ureter to the vena cava. J Urol 34:565–583, 1935.
20. Rowan RA, Maxwell DS: Patterns of vascular sprouting in the postnatal development of the cerebral cortex of the rat. Am J Anat 160:246–255, 1981.
21. Rowan RA, Maxwell DS: An ultrastructural study of vascular proliferation and vascular alkaline phosphatase activity in the developing cerebral cortex of the rat. Am J Anat 160:257–265, 1981.
22. Eriksson E, Zarem HA: Growth and differentiation of blood vessels. In Kaley G, Altura BM (eds): Microcirculation, vol I. Baltimore, University Park Press, 1977, pp 393–419.
23. Fett JW, Strydom DJ, Lobb RR, et al: Isolation and characterization of angiogenin, an angiogenic protein from human carcinoma cells. Biochemistry 24:5480–5486, 1985.
24. Kurachi K, Davie CW, Strydom DJ, et al: Sequence of the cDNA and gene for angiogenin, a human angiogenesis factor. Biochemistry 24:5494–5499, 1985.
25. Strydom DJ, Fett JW, Lobb RR, et al: Amino acid sequence of human derived angiogenin. Biochemistry 24:5486–5494, 1985.

3

ANATOMY, PHYSIOLOGY, AND PHARMACOLOGY OF THE VASCULAR WALL

ALEXANDER W. CLOWES and TED R. KOHLER

NORMAL ANATOMY

Although the vasculature is a series of tubes whose primary function is to act as nonthrombogenic conduits for blood, in fact it is quite diverse in structure and function. Not only do the vessels act as conduits, but they act as capacitors, and they regulate the molecular and cellular traffic between the vascular and extravascular spaces. This latter function is largely a property of small vessels (particularly postcapillary venules), since the cellular elements (endothelium and smooth muscle cells) in the microvasculature are the same as in the large vessels. We might expect the cells to have some of the same regulatory properties when located in arteries and veins as when they are located in the arterioles and venules. As we shall see later on, the similar properties of the endothelium and smooth muscle cells in large and small vessels may account for some of the abnormal properties of vessels undergoing atherosclerotic change or thickening after transplantation (transplant atherosclerosis).

The vasculature has distinct anatomical and physiological features. Arteries are divided into three categories: large elastic arteries, medium-sized muscular arteries, and small arteries. All arteries possess three layers or tunics called the intima, media, and adventitia. The intima, the innermost layer of the wall lying inside the internal elastic lamina and directly adjacent to the flowing blood, is composed of endothelium at the luminal surface and subendothelial extracellular matrix. In some vessels, one or more layers of smooth muscle cells are present; this so-called intimal cushion of smooth muscle cells might in some circumstances be the progenitor of the fibrous intimal plaque.

The media, bounded by the internal and external elastic laminae, contains smooth muscle cells embedded in a matrix of collagen, elastin, and proteoglycans. The adventitia lies outside the external elastic lamina and is composed of loose connective tissue, fibroblasts, capillaries, occasional leukocytes (particularly mast cells), and small nerve fibers.

The large elastic arteries of the body include the aorta and its major branches, while the medium-sized muscular arteries include most of the distributing vessels to the organs. These two classes of arteries, like all vessels, have all three layers represented in the wall. They differ principally in the amount of elastic tissue present in the media. The aortic wall is composed of well-defined lamellar units consisting of commonly oriented and elongated smooth muscle cells with their surrounding matrix, including a meshwork of collagen, and a layer of elastin.[1,2] The number of lamellar units in the aortae of various mammalian species, encompassing a wide range of body sizes, is proportional to the radius, regardless of variations in wall thickness.[1] As a result, the average tension per lammellar unit is remarkably constant. This lamellar unit represents the structural and functional unit of the aortic wall. Wall stress, which is pressure times radius divided by thickness, is fairly constant as a result of the linear relationship between wall thickness and radius and the fact that blood pressure is independent of species and size. This results in a good match between the strength of the wall and the tangential distending force within it. Increases in pressure, as occurs in hypertension or in the wall of thin vein grafts placed in the arterial circulation, or vessel diameter, as occurs when vessels dilate in response to increased flow, result in increased stress and compensatory increases in wall thickness.

In the elastic arteries, the media is composed of layers of smooth muscle cells interspersed with clearly

From Clowes AW: Series of atherosclerosis. *In* White RA (ed): Atherosclerosis: Human Pathology and Experimental Animal Methods and Models. Boca Raton, FL, CRC Press, 1989, pp 3–15.

defined lamellae of elastin. The media of muscular arteries is also composed of smooth muscle cells but lacks discrete elastic lamellae, except for the internal and external elastic layers (Fig. 3–1). The elastin is present only as thin fibers. In the largest elastic arteries with greater than 28 elastic layers, a microvasculature (vasa vasorum) penetrates the media from the adventitial side and provides a nutrient supply to the deep layers of the wall.[3] The inner layers depend on direct imbibition of nutrients from the lumen.

As arteries become smaller there is a progressive loss of elastic tissue to the point that the internal and external elastic lamellae become discontinuous and fragmented, and the clear distinction between the various layers is lost. At the arteriolar level the wall is composed of an endothelium, a layer of smooth muscle, and a filamentous collagenous adventitia.

Compared to other arteries in the body the small arteries have a relatively thick media and a large ratio of media to lumen, in keeping with their function as resistance vessels.

As has been pointed out by others,[4] the differentiation of these three types of arteries is of great pathological significance, since each class of vessels is subject to particular types of disease. Atherosclerosis is confined to elastic and muscular arteries and medial calcific sclerosis to muscular arteries. Small arteries develop diffuse fibromuscular thickening and hyalinization.

Veins tend to be much larger and more thin walled than arteries. The intima contains only an endothelial layer. The internal elastic layer is clearly evident only in the larger veins, and the media contains relatively few smooth muscle cells, collagen, and little elastin.

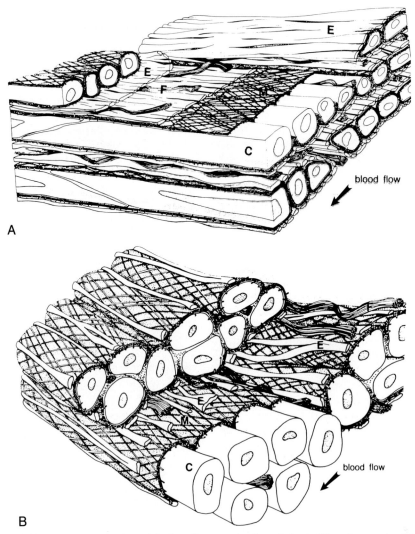

FIGURE 3–1. Schematic representation of the lamellar organization of elastic (*A*) and muscular (*B*) arteries. The transverse (circumferential) plane of section is indicated by *C* and the longitudinal axis by *L*. Each unit is composed of a group of commonly oriented smooth muscle cells (*Ce*) surrounded by matrix (*M*) consisting of basal lamina and a fine meshwork of collagen and surrounded by elastic fibers (*E*) oriented in the same direction as the long axes of the cells. Wavy collagen bundles (*F*) lie between the elastic fibers. The elastic lamellae are much better defined in the elastic arteries (*A*) than in the muscular arteries (*B*). (From Clark JM, Glagov S: Transmural organization of the arterial media: The lamellar unit revisited. Arteriosclerosis 5:19–34, 1985. By permission of the American Heart Association, Inc.)

In the veins of the extremities, there are thin bicuspid valves containing mainly endothelium and connective tissue.

REGULATION OF LUMINAL AREA

Although a description of the structures of the normal vasculature underscores the point that endothelial and smooth muscle cells are the principal cellular elements, such a description does not provide any insight into the mechanisms that regulate wall structure and function under normal circumstances or during the development of pathological lesions. Furthermore, such a description does not give a clue to how a vessel adjusts its mass and dimensions in response to external stimuli (hypertension, increased blood flow, vascular injury) nor to how it maintains a nonthrombogenic state. To understand these physiological responses, we must consider the functions of the individual cellular elements and the activities of these cells when they exist together as an organ in the fully formed vessel.

Both developing and mature vessels respond to changes in blood flow by adjusting their diameter in a manner that maintains constant shear. A striking example of this change is found in an artery proximal to an arteriovenous fistula.[5] The vessel enlarges and can, over the course of a lifetime, become aneurysmal. Conversely, diameter is reduced when outflow is diminished. This has been observed in mature and developing arteries and in vessels where flow is reduced by a proximal obstruction.[6-8] Diseased arterial segments themselves also can respond to changes in flow. A coronary artery with an enlarging atherosclerotic intima will presumably develop luminal stenosis and therefore the blood velocity in that stenosis should increase. This increase in blood velocity should, in turn, cause vasodilatation. In fact, a diseased coronary artery can dilate and can maintain normal luminal dimensions despite changes in wall structure as long as the intimal lesion does not exceed 40 per cent of the area inside the internal elastic lamina.[9] At this point pathological narrowing begins. Why vessels should dilate in each of these instances when the velocity of flow increases has not been determined. One possibility is that the cells in the wall, particularly the endothelium, are somehow capable of sensing changes in blood velocity and shear and can translate this biomechanical information into biochemical signals that then regulate the contractile state of the underlying smooth muscle cells.[10] One of the principal functions of the smooth muscle cells is to maintain vascular tone as well as to synthesize structural matrix components. These activities can be modulated by factors internal as well as external to the vascular wall.

Because of recent findings in vascular physiology, it is convenient to classify pharmacological agents regulating vascular wall contraction as endothelial and nonendothelial dependent.[11] Furchgott and Zawadzki reported in 1980 that the relaxation of isolated rabbit aorta and other arteries induced by acetylcholine and other agonists for muscarinic receptors depended on the presence of endothelial cells. After removal of the endothelial cells, acetylcholine no longer induced relaxation; instead, it caused contraction. A large number of agents, including acetylcholine, arachidonic acid, adenosine triphosphate (ATP) and adenosine diphosphate (ADP), bradykinin, histamine, norepinephrine, serotonin, thrombin, and vasopressin, have been shown to produce an endothelium-dependent relaxation of arteries. Other substances, such as adenosine and adenosine monophosphate (AMP), papaverine, isoproterenol, nitrovasodilators (such as sodium nitroprusside), and prostacyclin, do not require the presence of endothelial cells to elicit relaxation. The endothelial-dependent relaxation results from release of a very labile, nonprostanoid endothelial factor that stimulates guanylate cyclase of the underlying smooth muscle cells and causes an increase in cyclic guanosine monophosphate (cGMP). There is good evidence that the endothelial-relaxant factor is nitric oxide and that it is derived from L-arginine.[12] The factor is present in higher concentrations in small resistance vessels than in larger conduit arteries.

In addition to expressing a relaxing factor, endothelium can express contracting factors.[11,13] The contracting factors appear to be responsible for contractions in some systemic vessels induced by arachidonic acid and hypoxia and in isolated cerebral vessels by stretch. One of these factors is peptide, endothelin, that has been isolated from cultured endothelial cells and is a potent vasoconstrictor. It is of physiological interest that increase in shear stress suppresses the expression of the gene for endothelin while causing the increased production of the relaxant factor from endothelial cells. Whether these endothelial-derived relaxing and constricting factors are expressed and are directly responsible for the long-term vascular adaptation in response to increased blood flow is not known. Certain pathological conditions in which endothelium is either missing or abnormal are associated with acute and chronic vasospasm; it is quite possible that the acute problems of atypical angina (coronary vasospasm) and cerebrovasospasm after cerebral hemorrhage are in part manifestations of abnormal endothelial function and abnormal secretion of these factors.[14]

REGULATION OF MEDIAL AND INTIMAL THICKENING

Arterial wall thickening is a prominent feature of most pathologic processes. In hypertensive animals and man arteries exhibit medial thickening, whereas after endothelial denudation or in the presence of hypercholesterolemia they develop a thick intima.[15-17] Exactly how these responses are regulated is not clear, although it is certain that in each instance proliferation of smooth muscle cells and accumulation of extracellular matrix are important components. In addition, in hypercholesterolemic subjects, the accumulation of lipid and lipid-filled macrophages contributes to the intimal lesion.

Since smooth muscle accumulation is a central feature of most forms of vascular thickening, it is worth discussing the mechanisms of growth control as we presently understand them.[18] During growth and development smooth muscle cells proliferate; they revert spontaneously to a quiescent state in adult vessels. In the adult rat smooth muscle cells turn over at the rate of 0.06 per cent per day, a number barely detectable with available methodology.[19] How the early rapid growth and late quiescence are regulated is not known, but this must be of importance to the problem of primary hypertension and local susceptibility to atherosclerotic change.

Of the models of smooth muscle growth in vivo perhaps the best characterized is the balloon injury model.[20] In this model, smooth muscle proliferation is stimulated by the passage of an inflated balloon catheter along an artery. The artery is at once stretched and denuded of its endothelium. Immediately thereafter platelets begin to adhere to the wall wherever endothelium is missing; they then spread and degranulate.

In most situations endothelial denudation and platelet adherence are followed 1 to 2 days later by the onset of medial smooth muscle proliferation and migration of these cells across the internal elastic lamina to form a neointima.[19] In the ballooned rat carotid this can be a most dramatic response, with a marked increase in the thymidine labeling index (a measure of proliferation) (Fig. 3–2). A link between smooth muscle proliferation and earlier platelet granule release has been proposed based on studies characterizing the proteins within the granules.[16] Among them are several growth factors, including platelet-derived growth factor (PDGF), transforming growth factor β, and an epidermal growth factor-like protein.[21] Where these granule proteins go after being released from the platelets is not known. One hypothesis suggests that these factors accumulate in the artery wall and stimulate subsequent smooth muscle growth. This hypothesis (the reaction-to-injury hypothesis) was first proposed many decades ago as a general mechanism for atherogenesis and has been refined in view of recent information.[16] Although attractive in theory, it is based on rather slim evidence mainly derived from experiments in thrombocytopenic animals. Injured arteries in these animals showed very little intimal thickening.[22] More recent work using thrombocytopenic rats suggests that platelets may be more important in stimulating migration than cell proliferation.[23] These animals had reduced intimal thickening even though smooth muscle cell proliferation was not measurably altered. Additional work using anti-PDGF antibodies or infusion of PDGF following balloon injury supports this concept.[24,25]

This early proliferation in the media of the injured

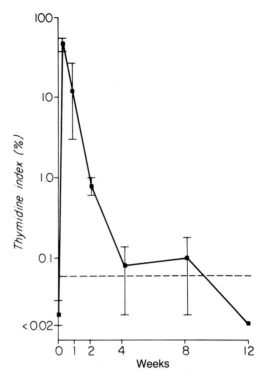

FIGURE 3–2. Smooth muscle cell proliferation rates following balloon catheter injury of the rat carotid artery as measured by the percentage of cells that incorporate thymidine. Proliferation is greatest at 48 hours and falls rapidly thereafter. (Adapted from Clowes AW, Reidy MA, Clowes MM: Kinetics of cellular proliferation after arterial injury: I. Smooth muscle growth in the absence of endothelium. Lab Invest 49:327–333, 1983.)

artery does not lead to an increase in wall thickness; the wall thickens only after smooth muscle cells migrate from the media and proliferate in the intima. This process persists for a period of time and subsides spontaneously whether or not endothelium reappears at the luminal surface. The intimal mass is further increased by the accumulation of extracellular matrix synthesized by the smooth muscle cells (Fig. 3–3).[26]

Although little is known of what starts or stops the intimal thickening process, there are several observations that are interesting and perhaps important. The first is that the surface of the injured artery accumulates a single layer of platelets. Fibrin and microthrombi are only seen at the luminal surface when the artery is reinjured after an intimal thickening has formed, or in small craters in association with adherent macrophages in hypercholesterolemic animals. Thus active, fulminant thrombosis is not a usual feature of injured vessels; when it occurs it must represent a major aberration of vessel function.[27] Second, in models demonstrating early reendothelialization or partial deendothelialization without medial injury, intimal thickening does not develop, although one or two rounds of medial smooth muscle proliferation can occur. This result suggests that endothelium might play a role in suppressing smooth muscle growth and migration from the media to the

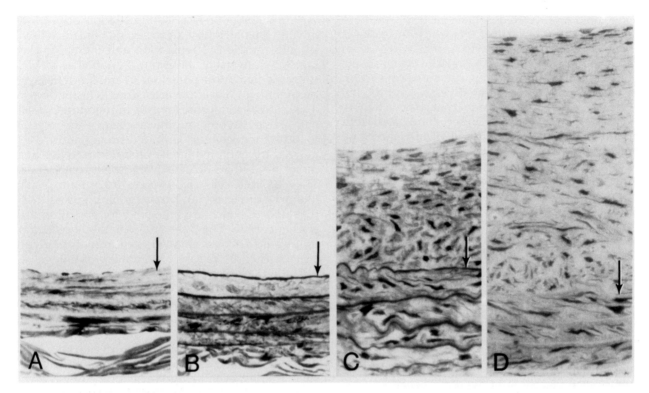

FIGURE 3–3. Histologic cross-sections of the region lacking endothelium of injured left carotid arteries. *A*, Normal vessel. Note single layer of endothelium in intima. *B*, Denuded vessel at 2 days. Note loss of endothelium. *C*, Denuded vessel at 2 weeks. Intima is now markedly thickened because of smooth muscle proliferation. *D*, Denuded vessel at 12 weeks. Further intimal thickening has occurred. Internal elastic lamina indicated by arrow. Lumen is at the top. (From Clowes AW, Reidy MA, Clowes MM: Kinetics of cellular proliferation after arterial injury: I. Smooth muscle growth in the absence of endothelium. Lab Invest 49:327–333, 1983.)

intima. We know that smooth muscle growth inhibitors can be extracted from the vessel wall, that endothelium can synthesize a heparin-like molecule that inhibits smooth muscle cell growth in vitro, and that heparin itself can suppress both proliferation and migration of smooth muscle cells in vitro and in vivo.[28] Taken together, these findings suggest that endothelium can inhibit smooth muscle proliferation and that the quiescent state of smooth muscle cells in the normal arteries of adult animals might be an actively maintained one rather than one attributable to the lack of growth factors. Finally, there is the more general concept emerging that the cells of the vascular wall "speak" to each other and regulate the function of one another.

The possibility of cell-cell communication has now been considered briefly twice: in regard to chronic vasodilatation in response to increased blood velocity and in regard to control of smooth muscle cell proliferation and migration. Let us examine the kinds of messages and the participants in more detail, particularly with regard to growth control and the maintenance of the antithrombotic state. At the outset, we can state that at least in vitro there is evidence for direct cell-cell communication by means of intercellular junctions; there is also evidence for communication by means of molecules secreted into the extracellular space and acting at a distance.

Direct cell-cell junctional communication has been demonstrated in monolayers of endothelium[29] and in mixed cell populations between endothelium and smooth muscle cells.[30] Gap junctions have been demonstrated morphologically between endothelial cells and between endothelium and smooth muscle cells in vivo and in vitro. The significance of these direct links has in general not been defined, although in culture pericytes and smooth muscle cells can inhibit endothelial growth when the cells are in contact with one another.[30] Plasma membrane preparations from confluent large vessel endothelium also actively inhibit growing endothelial cells.[31] In vivo capillary endothelial growth is associated with absence of pericytes, and cessation of growth with their reappearance. In addition, the intercellular links might help to regulate endothelial proliferation and endothelial-mediated vascular relaxation in collateral vessels by propagating signals from one cell to the next upstream from a large vessel occlusion. They would also provide a mechanism for a local response in a vessel without the need for the release and wide dissemination of potent vasoactive or growth-regulatory substances.

Cell-cell communication at a distance is likely to

be mediated by secreted soluble factors. As mentioned above, the blood platelet, which in reality is a fragment of a megakaryocyte, carries within it an array of potent mitogens. The notion that platelets are involved in wound healing processes came from morphological studies of injured vessels and the observation that whole blood serum contains much more growth-promoting activity than serum prepared from blood depleted of all cellular elements, including platelets (plasma-derived serum). These findings led to the discovery of PDGF, a basic dimeric protein[32] with a molecular weight of approximately 30,000. It is transported in the blood in the alpha granule of the platelet and is released along with other alpha granule proteins. PDGF is by itself extremely potent and is active as a smooth muscle mitogen in trace amounts (nanograms per milliliter). It also exhibits a range of other activities (stimulates smooth muscle migration, contraction, and matrix synthesis) on smooth muscle and other types of cells, although it is not a mitogen for endothelium. When placed in a wound chamber in vivo, it induces a granulation tissue response.[33]

Perhaps the most exciting development in regard to the growth factor field in the last decade was the demonstration that the structure of the gene for PDGF was nearly identical to that of the oncogene v-*sis*, a gene associated with cellular transformation by the simian sarcoma virus.[34,35] This discovery, coupled with the finding that a variety of cells (including normal cells) synthesize and secrete active PDGF, raises the possibility that normal wound healing and malignant, unscheduled growth of tumor cells might have striking similarities with subtle differences in gene regulation. It also led to a search for growth factors in vascular wall cells. We now have solid evidence that endothelium, smooth muscle cells, and leukocytes, including macrophages, can express the PDGF gene (c-*sis*) in vitro and in vivo.[32] What role the gene product, the PDGF protein, plays in wall function remains to be resolved. The work mentioned above using anti-PDGF antibodies or infusion of PDGF in animals undergoing carotid injury by balloon catheter suggests that the primary role of PDGF is to stimulate smooth muscle cell migration rather than proliferation.[24,25]

Recent work suggests that intracellular mitogens released from injured medial smooth muscle cells are primarily responsible for stimulating cell proliferation. First, smooth muscle cell proliferation occurs when arteries are injured by hydrostatic distention that does not cause significant endothelial injury.[36] In this case, there is very little smooth muscle cell migration, probably because of the lack of platelet factor release.[36] Second, very little smooth muscle cell proliferation is observed when the endothelium is injured using a fine nylon loop that does not damage the media.[37,38] Basic fibroblast growth factor (bFGF) may be the principle mitogen responsible for smooth muscle cell proliferation following injury. Both bFGF mRNA and protein are found in the uninjured vessel wall.[39] Infusion or local administration of bFGF following arterial injury causes a marked increase in smooth muscle cell replication and intimal thickening.[39,40] Conversely, infusion of antibodies to bFGF causes a significant reduction in smooth muscle cell proliferation.[41] Basic fibroblast growth factor does not appear to be mitogenic for cells in uninjured vessels, suggesting that other products of injury are necessary to induce mitogenesis. Cultured smooth muscle cells derived from injured media produce up to five times more PDGF than do cells from uninjured arteries.[42] These injured cells also express mRNA for insulin-like growth factor[43] and transforming growth factor β,[44] both of which are mitogenic for smooth muscle cells in culture. Thus, the smooth muscle cells in the injured media may stimulate cell growth in a paracrine fashion by release of a number of mitogens.

The rate of blood flow, which affects diameter in developing and mature arteries, also influences intimal hyperplasia in injured vessels and vascular grafts. Wall thickening of vein and synthetic grafts is increased in areas of reduced flow[45,46] and is reduced by high flow (Fig. 3–4).[47,48] Flow also appears to affect intimal hyperplasia in balloon-injured rat carotid arteries, even though the endothelium is absent in this model.[49] This implies that surface smooth muscle cells can respond to flow in a manner similar to that of endothelium.

There are several interesting preliminary observations that permit us now to outline a rather rough theory of growth control in the wall. Endothelial cells in vitro can condition the tissue culture medium with growth-promoting factors for smooth muscle cells; a portion of this activity is due to PDGF-like proteins and perhaps to other characterized factors like bFGF. Production of the PDGF is increased when the cells are exposed to endotoxin or phorbol esters and is decreased when the cells are exposed to oxidized low-density lipoprotein.[50] Smooth muscle cells make PDGF in vitro as well; in particular, cells derived from neonatal as opposed to adult aortas and proliferating cells derived from injury-induced intimal thickenings as opposed to quiescent media are prone to do this.[18] Macrophages, when stimulated, increase their production of PDGF. Finally, injured vascular wall cells release intracellular mitogens (e.g., bFGF). These fragmentary results support the concept that "activated" vascular wall cells can amplify the initial stimulus (perhaps an influx of platelet-derived factors) by producing PDGF and other growth-promoting factors that would then act on the cells. Furthermore, these factors might also act to regulate the traffic of leukocytes in and out of the wall; the activated leukocytes could in turn reciprocate by the production of factors affecting the function of the vascular wall cells. What emerges here is the notion that there might be a great deal of cross-talk between the cells of the wall and the blood, with many complex feedback loops (Fig. 3–5).[51]

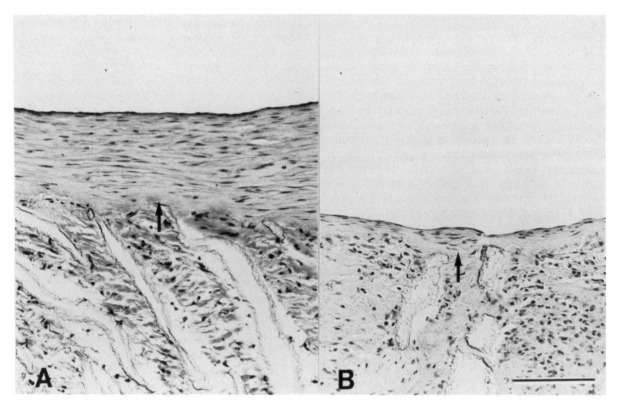

FIGURE 3–4. Cross-sections of polytetrafluoroethylene grafts 3 months after placement in the aortoiliac circulation in baboons. *A,* Control side with normal flow. *B,* Experimental side with a distal arteriovenous fistula causing increased flow. The arrows indicate the junction of the graft and neointima. Bar, 100 μm. (From Kohler TR, Kirkman TR, Kraiss LW, Zierler BK, Clowes AW: Increased blood flow inhibits neointimal hyperplasia in endothelialized vascular grafts. Circ Res *69:*1557–1565, 1991. By permission of the American Heart Association, Inc.)

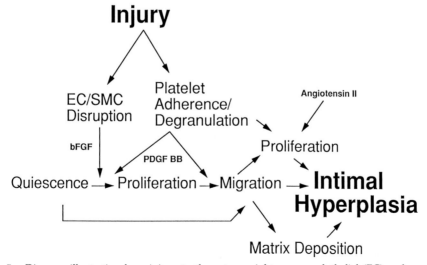

FIGURE 3–5. Diagram illustrating how injury to the artery might cause endothelial (EC) and smooth muscle cell (SMC) disruption and release of intracellular mitogens such as basic fibroblast growth factor (bFGF). FGF then stimulates medial smooth muscle proliferation. Factors from platelets (PDGF) regulate movement of the smooth muscle cells from the media to the intima. Angiotensin II also affects the intimal thickening process. (From Clowes AW, Reidy MA: Prevention of stenosis after vascular reconstruction: Pharmacologic control of intimal hyperplasia—a review. J Vasc Surg *13:*885–891, 1991.)

REGULATION OF THROMBOSIS BY THE ENDOTHELIUM

Empirical observation demonstrates quite clearly that a normal endothelial-lined artery is resistant to thrombosis. Even with complete cessation of blood flow for a prolonged period of time clotting does not occur, although blood in a damaged vessel clots rather readily. It would seem that endothelium must make one or more antithrombotic or anticoagulant molecules, and this has proven to be true. What is the more striking is that the endothelium expresses an extensive array of procoagulant functions as well. Like the growth factors, these procoagulant-anticoagulant functions are regulated by messages coming from the blood or from neighboring cells.[52]

On the anticoagulant side of the balance, the endothelium synthesizes a membrane-associated heparan sulfate that, like heparin, increases the affinity of antithrombin III for thrombin.[53] Since this interaction requires the binding of heparan sulfate to the antithrombin III, the complex must be active at the level of the endothelial surface. Heparan–antithrombin III then rapidly inactivates circulating thrombin and other activated serine proteases in the clotting cascade, including factors VII, IX, and X. Thus endothelial-derived heparan sulfate can act to impede two aspects of the injury response: the activation of the clotting cascade and the stimulation of smooth muscle proliferation that we referred to earlier.[28] In addition, endothelial cells can inhibit clotting by means of the protein C pathway.[54] Endothelium synthesizes and secretes a protein called thrombomodulin, which in turn is bound to a surface receptor. The receptor-thrombomodulin complex binds thrombin and in so doing inactivates the proteolytic activity for fibrinogen. The thrombomodulin-thrombin complex activates protein C, and the activated protein C binds to protein S on the endothelial surface. The protein C–protein S complex then can inactivate factor Va, thereby inhibiting the clotting cascade. That this pathway is important is amply demonstrated in homozygous-deficient patients, who develop spontaneous thrombosis. Finally, endothelial cells can inhibit platelet adhesion and aggregation through the synthesis of prostaglandin I_2 and can degrade formed fibrin by activating plasminogen to plasmin.

On the procoagulant side, endothelial cells synthesize and secrete tissue factor, a plasminogen activator inhibitor, and von Willebrand factor, and they express a number of receptors for factors of the clotting cascade. When the cells are exposed to a variety of inflammatory mediators derived from the blood or from resident macrophages [e.g., endotoxin, interleukin 1 (IL 1), tumor necrosis factor] endothelial cells respond by changing the balance of anticoagulant-procoagulant activities to favor coagulation. Also, the cells synthesize and express IL 1, which potentially could affect the underlying smooth muscle cells.[55] At present these conclusions are largely based on in vitro experiments; although they have relevance mainly for the microvasculature, they also may prove to be important for large vessels in view of the recent evidence that not only macrophages but also different populations of lymphocytes are present in the atherosclerotic plaque. Furthermore, the ability of the vascular wall cells to maintain the anticoagulant state at the luminal surface must have a direct bearing on the thrombotic complications associated with end-stage atherosclerosis.

SUMMARY

The normal blood vessel must be viewed not only as a conduit but also as an organ containing endothelial and smooth muscle cells that can respond to physical and chemical stimuli in the blood by adjusting vascular diameter and thickness. Furthermore, vascular wall cells can communicate among themselves and express factors that can regulate cell proliferation and coagulation as well as allow the cells to participate in local inflammatory reactions.

REFERENCES

1. Wolinsky H, Glagov S: A lamellar unit of aortic medial structure and function in mammals. Circ Res 20:99, 1967.
2. Clark JM, Glagov S: Transmural organization of the arterial media: The lamellar unit revisited. Arteriosclerosis 5:19, 1985.
3. Wolinsky H, Glagov S: Nature of species differences in the medial distribution of aortic vasa vasorum in mammals. Circ Res 20:409, 1967.
4. Cotran RS, Kumar V, Robbins SL: Pathologic Basis of Disease. Philadelphia, WB Saunders Company, 1989, p 553.
5. Zarins CK, Zatina MA, Giddens DP, Ku DN, Glagov S: Shear stress regulation of artery lumen diameter in experimental atherogenesis. J Vasc Surg 5:413, 1987.
6. Langille BL, O'Donnell F: Reductions in arterial diameter produced by chronic decreases in blood flow are endothelium-dependent. Science 231:405, 1986.
7. Guyton JR, Hartley CJ: Flow restriction of one carotid artery in juvenile rats inhibits growth of arterial diameter. Am J Physiol 248:H540, 1985.
8. Brownlee RD, Langille BL: Arterial adaptations to altered blood flow. Can J Physiol Pharmacol 69:978, 1991.
9. Glagov S, Weisenberg E, Zarins CK, Stankunavicius R, Kollettis GJ: Compensatory enlargement of human atherosclerotic coronary arteries. N Engl J Med 316:1371, 1987.
10. Frangos JA, Eskin SG, McIntire LV, Ives CL: Flow effect on prostacyclin production by cultured human endothelial cells. Science 227:1477, 1985.
11. Furchgott RF, Vanhoutte PM: Endothelium-derived relaxing and contracting factors. FASEB J 3:2007, 1989.
12. Moncada S, Higgs EA, Hodson HF, et al: EDRF and EDRF-related substances. The L-arginine:nitric oxide pathway. J Cardiovasc Pharmacol 17(Suppl 3):S1–S9, 1991.
13. Furchgott RF, Zawadzki JV: The obligatory role of endothelial cells in the relaxation of arterial smooth muscle by acetylcholine. Nature 288:373–376, 1980.

14. Freiman PC, Mitchell GG, Heistad DD, Armstrong ML, Harrison DG: Atherosclerosis impairs endothelium-dependent vascular relaxation to acetylcholine and thrombin in primates. Circ Res 58:783, 1986.

15. Wolinsky H: Long-term effects of hypertension on the rat aortic wall and their relation to concurrent aging changes: Morphological and chemical studies. Circ Res 30:301, 1972.

16. Ross R: Pathogenesis of atherosclerosis—an update. N Engl J Med 314:488, 1986.

17. Steinberg D: Lipoproteins and the pathogenesis of atherosclerosis. Circulation 76:508, 1987.

18. Schwartz SM, Campbell GR, Campbell JH: Replication of smooth muscle cells in vascular disease. Circ Res 58:427, 1986.

19. Clowes AW, Reidy MA, Clowes MM: Kinetics of cellular proliferation after arterial injury: 1. Smooth muscle growth in the absence of endothelium. Lab Invest 49:327, 1983.

20. Baumgartner HR, Studer A: Consequences of vessel catheterization in normal and hypercholesterolemic rabbits [German]. Pathol Microbiol 29:393, 1966.

21. Bowen-Pope DF, Ross R, Seifert RA: Locally acting growth factors for vascular smooth muscle cells: Endogenous synthesis and release from platelets. Circulation 72:735, 1985.

22. Friedman RJ, Stemerman MB, Wenz B, Moore S, Gauldie J: The effect of thrombocytopenia on experimental arteriosclerotic lesion formation in rabbits, smooth muscle cell proliferation and re-endothelialization. J Clin Invest 60:1191, 1977.

23. Fingerle J, Johnson R, Clowes AW, Majesky MW, Reidy MA: Role of platelets in smooth muscle cell proliferation and migration after vascular injury in rat carotid artery. Proc Natl Acad Sci USA 86:8412, 1989.

24. Ferns GAA, Raines EW, Sprugel KH, Motani AS, Reidy MA, Ross R: Inhibition of neointimal smooth muscle accumulation after angioplasty by an antibody to PDGF. Science 253:1129, 1991.

25. Jawien A, Bowen-Pope DF, Lindner V, Schwartz SM, Clowes AW: Platelet-derived growth factor promotes smooth muscle migration and intimal thickening in a rat model of balloon angioplasty. J Clin Invest 89:507, 1992.

26. Clowes AW, Reidy MA, Clowes MM: Mechanisms of stenosis after arterial injury. Lab Invest 49:208, 1983.

27. Reidy MA: A reassessment of endothelial injury and arterial lesion formation. Lab Invest 53:513, 1985.

28. Clowes AW, Clowes MM: Regulation of smooth muscle proliferation by heparin in vitro and in vivo. Int Angiol 6:45, 1987.

29. Larson DM, Carson MP, Haudenschild CC: Junctional transfer of small molecules in cultured bovine brain microvascular endothelial cells and pericytes. Microvasc Res 34:184–199, 1987.

30. Orlidge A, D'Amore PA: Inhibition of capillary endothelial cell growth by pericytes and smooth muscle cells. J Cell Biol 105:1455, 1987.

31. Heimark RL, Schwartz SM: The role of membrane-membrane interactions in the regulation of endothelial cell growth. J Cell Biol 100:1934, 1985.

32. Ross R, Raines EW, Bowen-Pope DF: The biology of PDGF. Cell 46:155, 1986.

33. Sprugel KH, McPherson JM, Clowes AW, Ross R: Effects of growth factors in vivo. I. Cell ingrowth into porous subcutaneous chambers. Am J Pathol 129:601, 1987.

34. Doolittle RF, Hunkapillar MW, Hood LE, Aaronson SA, Antoniades HN: Simian sarcoma virus oncogene, v-sis, is derived from the gene (or genes) encoding a platelet-derived growth factor. Science 221:275, 1983.

35. Waterfield MD, Scrace GT, Whittle N, Stroobant P, Johnsson H, Wasteson A, Westermark B, Heldin CH, Huang JS, Deuel TF: Platelet-derived growth factor is structurally related to the putative transforming protein p28-sis of simian sarcoma virus. Nature 304:35, 1983.

36. Clowes AW, Clowes MM, Fingerle J, Reidy MA: Kinetics of cellular proliferation after arterial injury. V. Role of acute distention in the induction of smooth muscle proliferation. Lab Invest 60:360–364, 1989.

37. Tada T, Reidy MA: Endothelial regeneration. IX. Arterial injury followed by rapid endothelial repair induces smooth-muscle-cell proliferation but not intimal thickening. Am J Pathol 129:429, 1987.

38. Fingerle J, Au YPT, Clowes AW, Reidy MA: Intimal lesion formation in rat carotid arteries after endothelial denudation in absence of medial injury. Arteriosclerosis 10:1082, 1990.

39. Lindner V, Lappi DA, Baird A, Majack RA, Reidy MA: Role of basic fibroblast growth factor in vascular lesion formation. Circ Res 68:106, 1991.

40. Edelman ER, Nugent MA, Smith LT, Karnovsky MJ: Basic fibroblast growth factor enhances the coupling of intimal hyperplasia and proliferation of vasa vasorum in injured rat arteries. J Clin Invest 89:465, 1992.

41. Lindner V, Reidy MA: Proliferation of smooth muscle cells after vascular injury is inhibited by an antibody against basic fibroblast growth factor. Proc Natl Acad Sci USA 88:3739, 1991.

42. Walker LN, Bowen-Pope DF, Reidy MA: Production of platelet-derived growth factor-like molecules by cultured arterial smooth muscle cells accompanies proliferation after arterial injury. Proc Natl Acad Sci USA 83:7311, 1986.

43. Cercek B, Fishbein MC, Forrester JS, Helfant RH, Fagin JA: Induction of insulin-like growth factor I messenger RNA in rat aorta after balloon denudation. Circ Res 66:1755, 1990.

44. Majesky MW, Lindner V, Twardzik DR, Schwartz SM, Reidy MA: Production of transforming growth factor b₁ during repair of arterial injury. J Clin Invest 88:904–910, 1991.

45. Berguer R, Higgins RF, Reddy DJ: Intimal hyperplasia. Arch Surg 115:332, 1980.

46. Rittgers SE, Karayannacos PE, Guy JF: Velocity distribution and intimal proliferation in autologous vein grafts in dogs. Circ Res 42:792, 1978.

47. Kohler TR, Kirkman TR, Kraiss LW, Zierler BK, Clowes AW: Increased blood flow inhibits neointimal hyperplasia in endothelialized vascular grafts. Circ Res 69:1557, 1991.

48. Kraiss LW, Kirkman TR, Kohler TR, Zierler B, Clowes AW: Shear stress regulates smooth muscle proliferation and neointimal thickening in porous polytetrafluoroethylene grafts. Arterioscler Thromb 11:1844, 1991.

49. Kohler TR, Jawien A: Flow affects development of intimal hyperplasia following arterial injury in rats. Arterioscler Thromb 12:963, 1992.

50. DiCorleto PE, Bowen-Pope DF: Cultured endothelial cells produce a platelet-derived growth factor-like protein. Proc Natl Acad Sci USA 80:1919, 1983.

51. Libby P, Salomon RN, Payne DO, Schoen FJ, Pober JS: Functions of vascular wall cells related to development of transplantation-associated coronary arteriosclerosis. Transplant Proc 21:1, 1989.

52. Hawiger JJ: Hemostasis, bleeding, and thromboembolic complications of trauma and infection. In Clowes GHA Jr (ed): Trauma, Sepsis and Shock. The Physiological Basis of Therapy. New York, Marcel Dekker, 1988, p 123.

53. Marcum J, McKenney J, Rosenberg R: The acceleration of thrombin-antithrombin III complex formation in rat hind quarters via heparin-like molecules bound to endothelium. J Clin Invest 74:341, 1984.

54. Esmon CT: Protein C. In Spaet TH (ed): Progress in Hemostasis and Thrombosis, vol 7. New York, Grune & Stratton, 1984.

55. Libby P, Ordovas JM, Auger KH, Robbins AH, Birinyi LK, Dinarello CA: Endotoxin and tumor necrosis factor induce interleukin-1 beta gene expression in adult human vascular endothelial cells. Am J Pathol 124:179, 1986.

REVIEW QUESTIONS

1. In normal arteries, most of the smooth muscle cells are found in:
   (a) the intima
   (b) the media
   (c) the adventitia
   (d) none of the above

2. Arteries respond to an increase in blood flow by:
   (a) contracting
   (b) dilating
   (c) intermittently contracting
   (d) intermittently dilating

3. Endothelial cells synthesize and secrete substances that cause:
   (a) vasodilatation
   (b) vasoconstriction
   (c) both vasodilatation and vasoconstriction
   (d) none of the above

4. Injured arteries thicken on account of:
   (a) medial smooth muscle hyperplasia
   (b) intimal smooth muscle hyperplasia
   (c) intimal endothelial hyperplasia
   (d) none of the above

5. The "reaction to injury hypothesis" was proposed to explain the initial stages of atherosclerosis. Which element of this hypothesis has not been proven?
   (a) smooth muscle cells are important components of the plaque
   (b) thrombus can accumulate on atherosclerotic lesions
   (c) platelets contain potent growth factors
   (d) growth factors released from platelets stimulate smooth muscle growth in vivo

6. Platelet-derived growth factor (PDGF) is found in:
   (a) platelets
   (b) smooth muscle cells
   (c) endothelium
   (d) all of the above

7. Smooth muscle cells respond to PDGF by:
   (a) proliferating
   (b) synthesizing matrix
   (c) migrating
   (d) all of the above

8. Based on in vitro studies, endothelial cells appear to express molecules that regulate the behavior of the blood at the luminal surface. Which of the following endothelial-derived molecules act to sustain the anticoagulant state?
   (a) heparan sulfate
   (b) von Willebrand factor
   (c) plasminogen activator inhibitor
   (d) thrombomodulin
   (e) prostacyclin

9. Which of the molecules listed in question #8 are procoagulants?

10. In general, inflammatory mediators (e.g., interleukin 1) cause endothelial cells to express:
    (a) increased procoagulant activities
    (b) increased anticoagulant activities
    (c) increased endothelial-derived relaxing factor
    (d) none of the above

ANSWERS

1. b	2. b	3. c	4. b	5. d	6. d	7. d
8. a,d,e	9. b,c	10. a				

4
SURGICAL ANATOMY AND EXPOSURE OF THE VASCULAR SYSTEM

LOUIS L. SMITH and J. DAVID KILLEEN, Jr.

A well-planned surgical exposure facilitates even the most difficult surgical procedure. Awareness of the relationship of surface anatomy to underlying vascular structure makes possible the precise placement of the incision, thus minimizing tissue trauma and reducing the likelihood of infection. Detailed knowledge of the anatomy involved helps to prevent injury to vital structures in the operative field.

The authors will emphasize surface anatomy in relation to underlying vascular structure. We will stress anatomic relationships and emphasize vascular variations that may be encountered during common vascular exposures. Several uncommonly used surgical approaches will be described for the sake of completeness. Sources given in the reference list will supply the reader with any desired additional detailed information.

Since carotid endarterectomy is one of the most commonly performed surgical procedures in the United States, we will begin with the exposure of the carotid bifurcation and systematically discuss exposure of the circulatory system, ending with commonly used approaches to the arterial circulation in the leg.

EXPOSURE OF THE CAROTID BIFURCATION

The common carotid artery bifurcates approximately 2.5 cm below the angle of the mandible. The carotid bifurcation moves upward with age; consequently the precise location of the bifurcation must be determined from the lateral selective carotid angiogram. Digital subtraction angiography does not provide this information, since bony structure has been subtracted.

We employ a flexion crease incision, since this gives good exposure with the best cosmetic appearance of the postoperative scar. Should atherosclerotic disease extensively involve the common carotid artery, an incision along the anterior border of the sternocleidomastoid muscle is preferred in this situation.

The surgeon must be constantly aware of the location of important cranial and somatic nerves during carotid endarterectomy. The mandibular ramus of the facial nerve is vulnerable to injury during this operation; damage by a metal retractor or surgical dissection can cause temporary or permanent nerve dysfunction. Turning the head toward the opposite side draws the mandibular ramus well below the mandible, so that the possibility of facial nerve injury is increased.

The great auricular nerve (C2,C3) should be protected in its location on the sternocleidomastoid muscle just anterior to and below the ear. Damage to this nerve can cause a distressing postoperative occipital headache on the operated side.

The common facial vein will come into view as the incision is deepened. This vessel courses superficial to the carotid bifurcation to join the internal jugular vein. It serves as an important landmark during the dissection. Several small vessels coursing toward the sternocleidomastoid muscle are nutrient branches from the superior thyroid artery and vein and must be divided and ligated.

The descending branch of the hypoglossal nerve is located anterior to the sternocleidomastoid muscle and parallel to it. If this branch is followed upward, the main hypoglossal nerve trunk can usually be located with ease. A nutrient vein and artery to the sternocleidomastoid muscle course in immediate relation to this nerve and care should be taken to avoid injury to the underlying hypoglossal nerve.

Division of the descending branch of the hypoglossal nerve near its origin allows the main nerve trunk to be displaced upward and forward, thus providing higher exposure of the internal carotid artery. Dissection in the crotch of the carotid bifurcation should be avoided, since this area is extremely vascular. It is much easier to encircle the internal carotid artery 1 to 2 cm above the bifurcation and thereby avoid troublesome bleeding from the very vascular carotid sinus tissue.

The surgeon must be constantly aware of the location of the vagus nerve and its branches. It lies within the carotid sheath between the common carotid artery and the internal jugular vein and is directly behind the internal carotid artery at its origin. Care must be taken to prevent injury to the nerve at this vulnerable location. The superior laryngeal nerve arises from the vagus nerve above the carotid bifurcation, passes behind the internal carotid artery, and descends medial to the superior thyroid artery. Care must be taken during mobilization of this vessel not to injure the superior laryngeal nerve or its external branch (Fig. 4–1). The external laryngeal nerve may sometimes pass between branches of the superior thyroid artery or be adherent to it.

Table 4–1 lists the important nerves encountered during carotid endarterectomy, their location, tests for function, and remarks. The importance of cranial nerve protection during carotid surgery is emphasized by the reports of Evans et al.[1] and Hertzer et al.[2] Both of these reports record both preoperative and postoperative evaluation of cranial nerve function.

The vagus nerve is the cranial nerve most commonly damaged during carotid endarterectomy. Evans and associates[1] have made an important prospective study of cranial nerve injury during carotid surgery. Their study group included surgeons as well as a speech pathologist. Observations were made prior to and following operations. They found a 4 per cent incidence of vagus nerve dysfunction preoperatively when the evaluation was made by a clinician, but a 30 per cent incidence of tenth cranial nerve dysfunction preoperatively when the evaluation was made by a speech pathologist. Two days

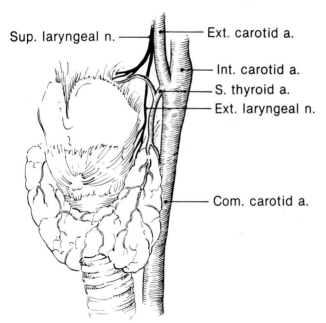

Sup. laryngeal n. ——
—— Ext. carotid a.
—— Int. carotid a.
—— S. thyroid a.
—— Ext. laryngeal n.

—— Com. carotid a.

FIGURE 4–1. Note the vulnerable location of the external laryngeal branch of the superior laryngeal nerve to the superior thyroid artery.

postendarterectomy, clinical evaluation revealed a 14.6 per cent vagal nerve deficit, whereas the speech pathologist's evaluation reported a 35 per cent incidence of superior or recurrent nerve dysfunction!

The data cited indicate the wisdom of doing a vocal cord check prior to performing carotid endarterectomy because of the high incidence of unrecognized vagal nerve dysfunction. Examination of vocal cord function is of particular importance when carotid reoperation is planned or when operating on the second side soon after the first, at which time paresis of cord function may still persist.

The reader is referred to the *Manual of Vascular Surgery—Volume I*[3] for very nice color illustrations of the steps in performing a carotid endarterectomy.

EXPOSURE OF THE HIGH INTERNAL CAROTID ARTERY

One of the most difficult surgical exposures is the high internal carotid artery. The surgeon must contend with vital nerve structures within a confined space, frequently made more difficult by a space-occupying vascular lesion or the presence of vascular injury with hemorrhagic staining and displacement of the tissues. Structures that overlie the high internal carotid artery in the neck include the facial nerve, the parotid gland, the ramus of the mandible, and the mastoid and styloid processes. It is crossed by the hypoglossal nerve, the digastric and stylohyoid muscles, and the occipital and posterior auricular arteries. The internal carotid artery courses progressively deeper to enter the petrous canal of the temporal bone.

Exposure routinely begins at the carotid bifurcation and the dissection continues distally, protecting the vagus nerve, which lies immediately behind the internal carotid artery. Division of the descending branch of the hypoglossal nerve allows displacement of this structure forward out of the way. It becomes evident that one is now working in a progressively narrowing triangle with inadequate space to perform any surgical reconstructive procedure.

Fisher and associates[4] described a useful maneuver to increase exposure by subluxation of the mandible. They have described a unique technique of wire fixation of the mandible to hold this position during the operative procedure. The 12 to 15 mm of space obtained converts the triangle described above into a narrow rectangle (Fig. 4–2). They stress the importance of not dislocating the mandible, since serious injury can occur to the temporomandibular joint and even to the contralateral internal carotid artery.

The digastric and stylohyoid muscles are divided. The styloid process and the stylohyoid ligament are excised. The glossopharyngeal and the superior laryngeal nerves must be identified and preserved. Stanley, in discussing Fisher's paper, has suggested an operative modification, that of using a special towel clip placed on the angle of the mandible through two small

TABLE 4-1. CAROTID ENDARTERECTOMY AND THE REGIONAL NERVES ENCOUNTERED

Nerve Branch	Location Encountered	Test for Function	Remarks
Mandibular ramus of facial nerve (cranial nerve VII)	Deep to platysma muscle; can be 5–10 mm below inferior margin mandible	Ask patient to show teeth—check for paralysis of lower lip	Gentle use of metal retractors on mandible; nerve is pulled down when head is rotated to opposite side for operative exposure
Great auricular nerve (C2 and C3)	Anteromedial surface of sternocleidomastoid muscle anterior and below ear	Anesthesia of ear and adjacent scalp	Causes disturbing occipital headache when damaged
Cutaneous cervical nerve (C2 and C3)	Subcutaneous on deep fascia	Anesthesia of skin below mandible	Should warn patient preop regarding possible sensory loss
Glossopharyngeal nerve branch (cranial nerve IX)	Between external and internal carotid arteries ("carotid sinus nerve")		Manipulation of nerve may cause bradycardia and/or hypotension; atropine IV or local infiltration of nerve with Xylocaine will relieve circulatory changes
Vagus nerve (cranial nerve X)	Within carotid sheath; between internal jugular vein and common carotid artery; directly behind internal carotid artery	Indirect laryngoscopy for vocal cord function	Dissect "right on" distal common and internal carotid arteries; while mobilizing these vessels, avoid "past pointing" with vascular occluding clamps
Superior laryngeal nerve (branch of cranial nerve X)	Adjacent and medial to superior thyroid artery	Loss of function of cricothyroid muscle	Inability to reproduce high tones
Hypoglossal nerve (cranial nerve XII)	Descending branch visualized; first crosses about I cm above carotid bifurcation; sternocleidomastoid artery and ventricular branches overlie nerve	Extended tongue deviates to side of injured nerve	Visualize descending branch first and follow up to main nerve trunk; careful individual ligation of sternocleidomastoid muscular arterial and venous branches to preserve dry operative field

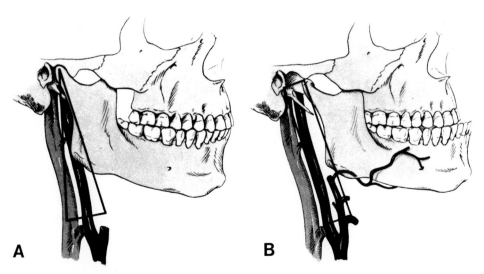

A   **B**

FIGURE 4–2. These diagrams show how the narrow triangle of exposure (*A*) for the high internal carotid artery is expanded to a narrow rectangle (*B*) by anterior subluxation of the condyle of the mandible. (From Fisher DF Jr, Clagett GP, Parker JI, et al: Mandibular subluxation for high carotid exposure. J Vasc Surg *1*:727, 1984.)

stab incisions, allowing the subluxation to be fixed by minimal retraction. Thus arch bars or wiring are not required. Figure 4–3 shows a diagram of the location of the condyle of the mandible during subluxation.

In those situations in which there is a high internal carotid artery aneurysm requiring more room for reconstruction, we favor transection of the mandibular ramus with either translocation or temporary removal of the condyle and ramus fragment for wider exposure. Wylie and associates[5] have described this approach with detailed color illustrations of the anatomy involved.

Following the induction of anesthesia, the mandible is immobilized by arch bars and wires. The incision involved is a long flexion crease incision in the upper neck extending posteriorly to a point behind the ear. The carotid bifurcation is exposed as described previously for carotid endarterectomy. The mandibular ramus of the facial nerve is protected. The hypoglossal nerve is exposed and the descending branch is divided in order to displace the hypoglossal nerve forward. The angle of the mandible is exposed and the periosteum elevated toward the mandibular notch anteriorly and posteriorly. The mandibular ramus is divided vertically using a power saw posterior to the foramen of the inferior alveolar artery and nerve. The posterior bone fragment is gently rotated out and upward as the pterygoid muscles are divided, thus allowing removal of this fragment, which is preserved in chilled lactated Ringer's solution until replaced following the arterial reconstruction.

Once the mandibular ramus is removed, the digastric and stylohyoid muscles are divided and the dissection is continued to the base of the skull if need be. Care should be taken to protect the hypoglossal, glossopharyngeal, and vagal nerves, which are in immediate relation to the high internal carotid artery.

Following completion of the internal carotid reconstruction, the mandibular fragment is returned to its anatomic location and the temporomandibular joint capsule is closed by interrupted nonabsorbable sutures. The mandibular fragment is fixed in place by a thin titanium plate. The cervical fascia and platysma muscle are closed in layers, followed by routine skin closure.

EXPOSURE OF THE AORTIC ARCH BRANCHES AND ASSOCIATED VEINS

Brachiocephalic and Proximal Common Carotid Arteries and Superior Vena Cava

The incision most commonly employed for the exposure of the brachiocephalic and proximal common carotid arteries, as well as the superior vena cava and its confluent brachiocephalic veins, is the median sternotomy (Fig. 4–4). This surgical approach provides excellent exposure of the great vessels with the exception of the left subclavian artery. The aortic arch passes obliquely posterior and to the left after its origin from the base of the heart, thus making the first portion of the left subclavian artery inaccessible from this anterior approach.

The two lobes of the thymus gland are separated in the midline, and if the surgeon carefully observes the pleural bulge during positive pressure inspiration, entry into either pleural cavity can be avoided. Nutrient vessels to the thymus gland are carefully ligated and divided, keeping a dry field for visibility. These vessels arise from the internal thoracic artery and drain into the internal thoracic or brachiocephalic veins. The left brachiocephalic vein will be visualized in the upper portion of the wound. A thymic vein may join this vessel inferiorly and an inferior thyroid vein may require ligation and division as it joins the brachiocephalic vein superiorly. Following complete mobilization of the left brachiocephalic vein, the anterior surface of the aortic arch will be visualized, as well as the origin of the brachiocephalic artery.

The recurrent laryngeal nerve must be protected

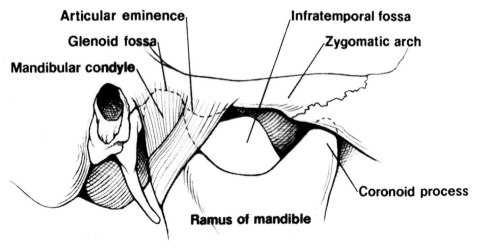

FIGURE 4–3.   Anterior subluxation moves the condyle of the mandible to the articular eminence, but not to the infratemporal fossa as would occur with dislocation of the mandible. (From Fisher DF Jr, Clagett GP, Parker JI, et al: Mandibular subluxation for high carotid exposure. J Vasc Surg 1:727, 1984.)

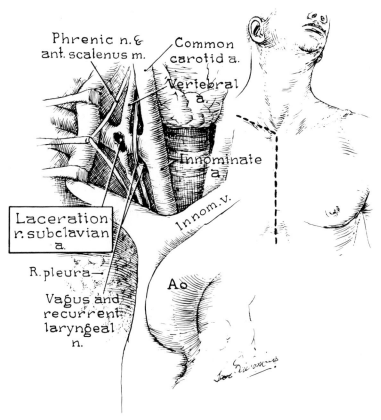

FIGURE 4–4. Exposure of the anterior aortic arch branches through a median sternotomy incision. Note the location of the phrenic, vagus, and recurrent laryngeal nerves, which must be identified and protected. (From Ernst C: Exposure of the subclavian arteries. Semin Vasc Surg 2:202, 1989.)

during exposure of the bifurcation of the brachiocephalic artery. It courses from the vagus nerve anteriorly around the origin of the subclavian artery to return in the tracheoesophageal groove to its termination in the larynx. Should additional exposure of the proximal common carotid artery be necessary, the skin incision should be extended upward along the anterior border of the sternocleidomastoid muscle, with division of the strap muscles on the right. The carotid bifurcation can thus be easily exposed by this extension if need be.

Origin of the Right Subclavian Artery and Vein

The origin of the right subclavian vessels are easily exposed through a median sternotomy incision with an extension above and parallel to the clavicle. The right sternohyoid and sternothyroid muscles are divided, followed by exposure of the scalene fat pad. Branches of the thyrocervical trunk are divided, followed by exposure of the anterior scalene muscle. The phrenic nerve should be identified as it courses from lateral to medial across the anterior surface of the anterior scalene muscle to pass into the superior

mediastinum. Care should be taken to protect this important structure.

A traumatic vascular injury at the confluence of the internal jugular and subclavian veins is most difficult to manage through a supraclavicular approach. Extension of this incision should be made via a median sternotomy incision while an assistant maintains compression of the veins against the sternum to temporarily control exigent hemorrhage (Fig. 4–4).

Origin of the Left Subclavian Artery

The origin of the left subclavian artery arises from the aortic arch posteriorly and to the left side of the mediastinum and cannot be adequately exposed through a median sternotomy incision. Traumatic injuries and aneurysms of the proximal left subclavian artery and proximal to the sternoclavicular joint should be approached through the left chest. The preferred exposure is a posterolateral fifth intercostal incision. If the injury or aneurysm is extensive, it is wise to prep the arm free so that it can be positioned for a second supraclavicular incision, should this be necessary, in order to expose the second portion of the subclavian artery and thus gain distal control. The posterolateral exposure allows partial occlusion of the aortic arch in lesions involving the origin of the subclavian artery. The phrenic and vagus nerves must be identified and preserved following opening the pleura prior to dissecting free the first portion of the subclavian artery.

In situations where there is exigent bleeding from a traumatic injury of the proximal left subclavian artery into the pleural space, prompt control can be obtained by an anterior thoracotomy in the third or fourth intercostal space and the placement of an occluding vascular clamp across the origin of the bleeding subclavian artery (Fig. 4–5). An inframammary incision is used in the female and the breast is mobilized superiorly for the above exposure.

Subclavian and Vertebral Arteries

Exposure of the second portion of the subclavian artery is most easily accomplished through a supraclavicular incision beginning over the tendon of the sternocleidomastoid muscle and extending laterally for 8 to 10 cm. The platysma muscle is divided, as is the scalene fat pad. It is well to save as much of the fat pad as possible to preserve neck contour and to act as "filling" for hemostasis following wound closure. Thyrocervical vessels are ligated and divided as encountered, with exposure of the anterior surface of the anterior scalene muscle. The phrenic nerve can be seen coursing from lateral to medial over this muscle and should be gently mobilized and preserved. The anterior scalene muscle is divided, following which the subclavian artery can be palpated

just above the clavicle. The origin of the left vertebral artery arises from the medial surface of the subclavian artery and behind the sternoclavicular joint. The internal thoracic artery may be ligated and divided at its origin to provide more mobility of the proximal subclavian artery. Figure 4–6 is a diagram of the essential anatomy in this exposure.

Resection of subclavian aneurysms and emergency exposure for vascular injury involving the second and third portions of this vessel require wide exposure. This can be most easily accomplished by resecting the clavicle, including the periosteum. The latter structure, when preserved, results in the reossification of a deformed clavicle.

The surgical exposure of the vertebral artery is described in detail in Chapter 27 of this book and in the surgical literature.[6] Injuries to the intraosseous portion of the vertebral artery with associated hemorrhage are best managed by embolic occlusion in the angiography suite.

AXILLARY VESSEL EXPOSURE

The proximal axillary artery is exposed by a short incision made between the clavicular and sternal portions of the pectoralis major muscle. Branches of the thoracoacromial vessels are divided to expose the axillary vein first and then the axillary artery above and posterior to the vein. If additional exposure is required laterally, a portion of the pectoralis minor muscle can be divided near its insertion into the coracoid process of the scapula.

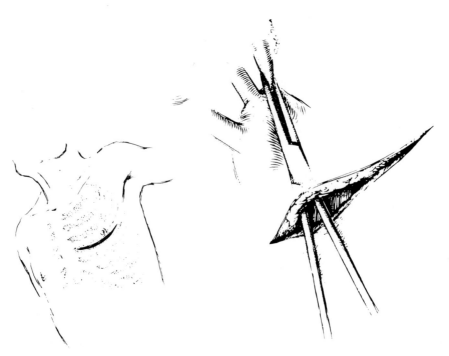

FIGURE 4–5.   Anterior thoracotomy with placement of an occluding vascular clamp for control of exigent bleeding from the proximal left subclavian artery. (From Trunkey D: Great vessel injury. *In* Blaisdell F, Trunkey D (eds): Trauma Management, Vol III: Cervicothoracic Trauma. New York, Thieme, Inc, 1986, p 255.)

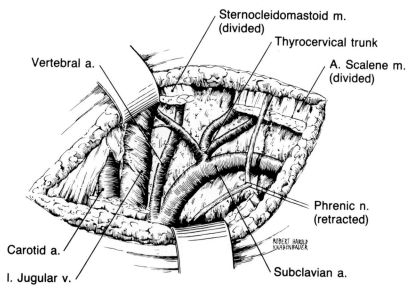

FIGURE 4–6. Exposure of the second portion of the left subclavian artery via a supraclavicular incision. Note that both the sternocleidomastoid and the anterior scalene muscles are divided for this exposure.

The second portion of the axillary artery is more difficult to expose, since it lies directly behind the pectoralis major muscle. The incision is begun in the groove between the clavicular and sternal portions of the pectoralis major muscle and continues across the distal portion of this muscle at the anterior axillary fold and out onto the midline of the proximal medial surface of the arm (Fig. 4–7). The tendinous portion of the muscle is divided near its insertion to expose the axillary contents. The pectoralis minor muscle can also be divided if more medial exposure is desired.

FIRST RIB EXPOSURE

Roos[7] in 1966 described the transaxillary approach for resection of the first rib in management of the

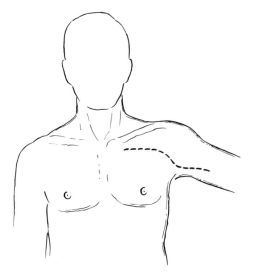

FIGURE 4–7. Incision employed for the exposure of the axillary artery.

thoracic outlet compression syndrome. This is currently the most common approach to decompress the thoracic outlet. The patient is placed in the lateral position and the involved arm is prepped and draped free for mobility. The shoulder is elevated by the assistant using a double wristlock maneuver and a transverse incision is made below the hairline (Fig. 4–8). The lateral thoracic artery and the thoracoepigastric vein are divided in their location deep to the subcutaneous fascia. Dissection is continued up to the level of the first rib, taking care to preserve the intercostal brachial nerve emerging from the second intercostal space. The pulse of the subclavian artery can be felt and the tendon of the subclavius muscle palpated anteriorly at the costoclavicular junction. The anterior scalene tendon is isolated and this structure dissected off the first rib extraperiosteally to reduce the likelihood of recurrent bone formation and nerve or vascular entrapment with recurrence of symptoms.

The tendon of the subclavius muscle is incised and the costochondral junction identified. The first rib is divided anteriorly at this junction. The dissection is carried posteriorly extraperiosteally, taking care not to enter the pleural space. The scalenus medius muscle is pushed posteriorly using a dull periosteal elevator, and by now the nerve trunk C8/T1 can be identified. Extreme care should be taken to retract this nerve trunk away from the first rib using the Roos nerve retractor. The first rib is transected posteriorly at its articulation with the transverse process of the vertebra using an angled Roos first rib cutter. During this maneuver, the C8/T1 nerve trunk must be protected by the assistant using the nerve retractor. Additional rib segments can be rongeured to leave smooth ends that do not impinge upon the adjacent nerve trunk.

The pleura is tested for air leaks and, if any are

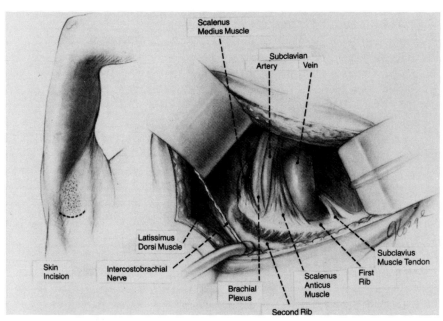

FIGURE 4–8. *Left*, The incision for first rib exposure. *Right*, The anatomy for first rib exposure. See text for details. (From Kunkel JM, Machleder HI: Treatment of Paget-Schroetter syndrome. Arch Surg *124*:1153, 1989.)

present, a small Robinson catheter is placed into the pleural cavity for the aspiration of air following wound closure. Roos[8] has recently described his procedure for first rib resection, including excellent illustrations of anatomic relationships.

EXPOSURE OF THE DESCENDING THORACIC AND PROXIMAL ABDOMINAL AORTA

No single approach lends itself so well to extensive exposure of the thoracic and abdominal aorta as a properly positioned thoracoabdominal incision. The interspace chosen depends on the extent of thoracic aorta to be exposed. A sixth intercostal space incision is used when the proximal descending thoracic aorta is to be exposed, whereas a ninth intercostal space incision allows terminal thoracic aortic exposure plus wide abdominal aortic visualization.

Exposure is gained by unwinding the torso as described by Stoney and Wylie.[9] The patient is placed in the right lateral position on the operating table with the hips rotated 45 degrees from horizontal. The left arm is passed across the upper chest and suspended by a specially made forearm support (Fig. 4–9).

An intercostal incision is made in the sixth to the ninth intercostal space depending on the level of the aortic involvement and is continued across the costal margin and obliquely across the abdomen to the anterior superior iliac spine on the right. If the terminal aorta and iliac vessels are to be exposed, the incision is extended down the linea alba to the symphysis pubis. A segment of the cartilaginous costal arch is

excised to provide a stable approximation of the costal arch following wound closure.

The diaphragm is incised circumferentially at a distance of approximately 2.5 cm from the chest wall to avoid injury to the phrenic nerve branches. The left crus of the diaphragm is incised to expose the terminal descending thoracic aorta. The shelf of diaphragm still attached to the chest wall simplifies reapproximation of this structure.

If a transaortic endarterectomy is contemplated, the left kidney will be left undisturbed and aortic exposure developed laterally by incising the celiac and superior mesenteric autonomic nerve plexi. The left inferior phrenic artery will be ligated and divided and the left adrenal gland exposed during this dissection. The origins of the celiac and superior mesenteric vessels can be palpated and dissected free as indicated by the disease process present. Figure 4–9 shows the excellent exposure of the proximal aorta and its branches.

Surgical exposure for a thoracoabdominal aneurysm is best performed by mobilizing the left kidney forward and clearing the posterior lateral surface of the aneurysm for aortotomy and graft inclusion by suturing the graft within the aortic lumen.

If more extensive exposure is required about the renal arteries, the left renal vein can be divided in its midportion anterior to the aorta; however, the large lumbar communicating vein must be saved for collateral circulation via the hemiazygos vein. Continued dissection is carried out behind the pancreas and through the transverse mesocolon to expose the proximal portion of the infrarenal abdominal aorta. In the event more distal exposure is required, the posterior parietal peritoneum should be opened im-

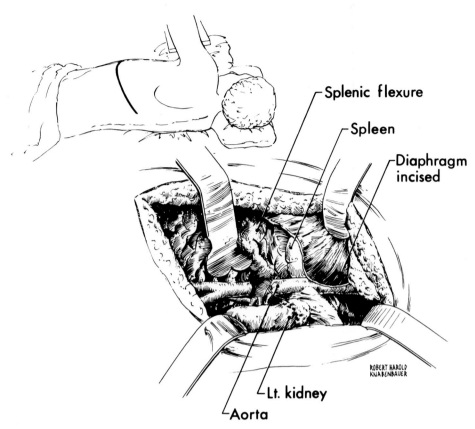

FIGURE 4–9.   The position for exposure of the thoracoabdominal aorta is shown above. The excellent exposure gained by this incision is shown below.

mediately adjacent to the fourth portion of the duodenum and the aorta exposed in a routine fashion with the transverse colon and mesocolon retracted upward.

Preservation of the blood supply to the spinal cord is critical in this extensive operation. Szilagy and associates[10] have stressed the importance of the arteria radicularis magna (artery of Adamkiewicz) in providing circulation to the anterior spinal artery. This vessel is a branch of either a distal intercostal or a proximal lumbar artery at the T8 to L1 level (Fig. 4–10). This vessel may supply up to two thirds of the spinal cord blood supply, according to *Gray's Anatomy*.[11]

ALTERNATE EXPOSURE OF THE HIGH ABDOMINAL AORTA

A helpful modification of the midline abdominal incision can be used to expose the proximal abdominal aorta without entering the chest. An inverted hockey-stick incision is employed beginning at the ninth intercostal space at the costal margin. The left rectus muscle is transected and the oblique and transversus muscles are divided in the direction of the skin exposure. The incision is continued down the linea alba to the symphysis pubis. The spleen is gently mobilized and brought forward toward the midline by incising the posterior parietal peritoneum of the

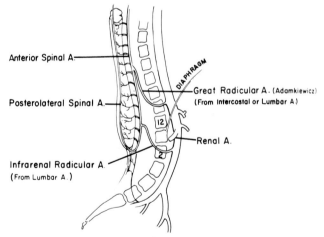

FIGURE 4–10.   Diagram of the great and infrarenal radicular arteries supplying the anterior spinal artery. (From Szilagy DG, Hageman JH, Smith RF, et al: Spinal damage in surgery of the abdominal aorta. Surgery *83*:38, 1979.)

phrenicocolic ligament. The dissection is continued by forward mobilization of the spleen, pancreatic tail, and splenic flexure of the colon between the transverse mesocolon and Gerota's fascia, taking care not to damage the adrenal gland medially or the adrenal vein at its junction with the left renal vein. This approach gives good exposure of the suprarenal aorta and its branches, including the left renal artery. It can be used in slender or elderly individuals, and in patients with chronic obstructive pulmonary disease.

EXPOSURE OF THE ABDOMINAL AORTA AND ITS BRANCHES

A midline abdominal incision from the xiphoid to the symphysis pubis is the most commonly used incision for the exposure of the infrarenal aorta and its branches. A common problem of exposure is the visualization of the proximal abdominal aorta and/or the renal artery origins through this incision. This lack of exposure is usually due to a failure to make the incision up to the xiphoid process and to make a lateral extension across the upper rectus muscle to the costal margin if additional exposure is needed.

A second error in exposure is the improper mobilization of the third and fourth portions of the duodenum when exposing the infrarenal aorta. It is easy to damage the circulation to the left colon or sigmoid unless the surgeon hugs the lateral surface of the duodenum. This is particularly important in dealing with ruptured abdominal aortic aneurysms, where landmarks are frequently obscured by an extensive retroperitoneal hematoma. The duodenum can nearly always be visualized and used as a "fix" during exposure of a ruptured infrarenal aortic aneurysm.

When dissecting aortic aneurysms, the proximal portion of the inferior mesenteric artery is frequently covered by dense preaortic fascia that obscures the origin of this vessel. It is easy to injure the ascending branch of the left colic artery, and in patients with an incomplete or occluded marginal vessel this can result in left colic or sigmoid colon ischemia.

It is wise to palpate the aortic bifurcation and expose the iliac vessels from the midline, thereby avoiding injury to the ureters. Fibers of the sympathetic nerves arch over the left iliac artery in the male, and damage to these sympathetic fibers can result in loss of potency. Figure 4–11 shows the relationship of the infrarenal sympathetics to the aorta and the iliac arteries.

EXPOSURE OF THE ABDOMINAL AORTA AT THE DIAPHRAGMATIC HIATUS

One of the truly useful maneuvers for the vascular surgeon is the prompt control of the abdominal aorta at the diaphragmatic hiatus. Exposure of the supraceliac aorta is life saving for early control of exigent hemorrhage in ruptured abdominal aortic aneurysms. It is also useful for the temporary control of the aorta in aortocaval fistulae and in infected infrarenal aortic grafts. Less frequently this exposure is useful in revascularizing the celiac axis or superior mesenteric artery.

The stomach is retracted down and the lesser sac opened in the midline. The aortic pulse is palpated

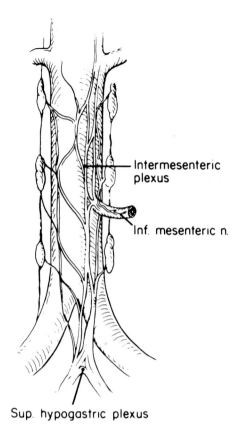

FIGURE 4–11. Relationship of the infrarenal sympathetic nerves to the aorta and iliac arteries. Note the condensation of nerve elements coursing over the left common iliac artery origin. (From Weinstein MH, Machleder HI: Sexual function after aortoiliac surgery. *Ann Surg 181*:787, 1975.)

and the arching fibers of the diaphragm at the aortic hiatus are divided directly over the aorta. The periaortic fascia is opened and the index finger passed medially and then laterally to the aorta. No effort is made to completely encircle the aorta, since a lumbar artery or vein can be avulsed with troublesome bleeding. At this point the opened aortic clamp is slid over the aorta, with interruption of blood flow. Figure 4–12 illustrates this exposure.

In cases in which a celiac artery reconstruction is planned, a more generous incision is made in the posterior parietal peritoneum and the arcuate fibers of the right crus of the diaphragm. The inferior phrenic arteries should be isolated, divided, and ligated. The aortic branch to the left adrenal gland is also usually visualized and sacrificed. Dissection is continued distally to expose the celiac artery, which can be easily palpated at its origin from the aorta. The dense fibers of the arcuate ligament are divided along with the neural elements forming the celiac plexus. This neural tissue is vascular and stick ties and cautery are employed for hemostasis. Once the main celiac trunk has been exposed, the hepatic artery is usually easily palpated as it courses toward the hilum of the liver. Sympathetic nerve fibers can be seen to entwine on the surface of this vessel. There is usually a 3- to

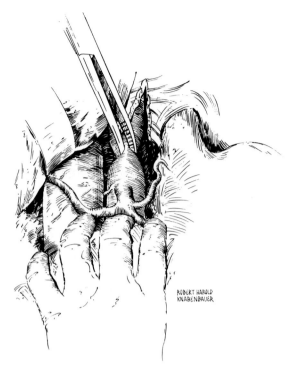

FIGURE 4–12. Exposure of the abdominal aorta at the diaphragm. See text for details.

4-cm segment that is free of branches and therefore useful as a site for vascular anastomosis.

The left gastric artery is the smallest of the three main branches of the celiac artery and courses anteriorly to follow the lesser curvature of the stomach. The splenic artery is palpable at the superior border of the pancreas gland and courses to the left toward the splenic hilum. Here again there is a 4- to 5-cm segment free of branches and again useful for the placement of a distal bypass anastomosis.

The supraceliac aorta can be useful as a bypass source for superior mesenteric artery reconstructions. The proximal anastomosis is made on the anterior surface of the aorta after opening the aortic hiatus as described above. A tunnel is made behind the pancreas using careful finger dissection. The bypass is passed through the tunnel and anastomosed to the distal patent superior mesenteric artery. Kinking of the bypass is unlikely with replacement of the bowel into the abdomen, as can occur with an infrarenal aortic-to-superior mesenteric bypass graft.

EXPOSURE OF THE SUPERIOR MESENTERIC ARTERY

Exposure of the superior mesenteric artery requires opening the posterior parietal peritoneum lateral to the third and fourth portions of the duodenum. The anterior and lateral aspect of the aorta is exposed and the left renal vein identified and mobilized as described above for exposure of the renal arteries. The left renal vein is retracted downward and the dis-

section carried upward on the aorta until the superior mesenteric artery origin can be palpated. It usually arises from the left side of the anterior surface of the aorta and is immediately encased by the superior mesenteric sympathetic nerve plexus, which must be incised for exposure. Bleeding from the vascular plexus tissue is controlled by cautery and suture ligatures.

There are no branches from the superior mesenteric artery for a distance of up to 5 cm. The first branch is usually the middle colic artery, which arises from the anterior and right lateral surface of the superior mesenteric artery. This first branch of the superior mesenteric artery is the usual site for an embolus to lodge. It is important to remember that the common hepatic artery arises from the superior mesenteric artery in 4 per cent of cases according to Luzsa.[12] Figure 4–13 shows the exposure of the vessel by this approach after the posterior parietal peritoneum has been incised and the proximal infrarenal aorta exposed.

EXPOSURE OF THE RENAL ARTERIES

The left main renal artery usually arises from the posterior lateral surface of the aorta at the level of the upper border of the left renal vein as it crosses the abdominal aorta. The right renal artery usually arises at a slightly lower level. Exposure of the origin of either renal artery involves incision of the posterior parietal peritoneum just lateral to the fourth portion of the duodenum. Additional exposure is obtained by continuing this incision along the distal third portion of the duodenum.

The renal vein is next identified and carefully mo-

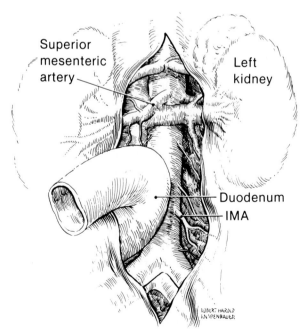

FIGURE 4–13. Exposure of the superior mesenteric artery via the infracolic approach. The pancreas and transverse colon are not shown but are retracted upward and forward. See text for details.

bilized. Frequently there is a small parietal vein that terminates in the inferior margin of the left renal vein over the aorta. Otherwise there are only two major venous tributaries to be identified, ligated, and divided. The first is located by following the inferior margin of the left renal vein laterally; the termination of the left gonadal vein will be easily identified, ligated, and divided. Next the dissection is carried laterally along the superior surface of the left renal vein until the confluence of the left adrenal vein is identified. It should be ligated flush with the renal vein and divided. The entire left renal vein can then be mobilized on a Silastic vascular loop.

A word of caution here. There is an important large communicating vein arising from the posterior surface of the proximal left renal vein that communicates with the adjacent lumbar vein and thence to the hemiazygous system and the superior vena cava. The presence of this venous collateral makes possible the acute ligation of the left renal vein without impairment of renal function. This lumbar venous communication should be preserved if at all possible.

Once the left renal vein is mobilized, attention should be directed to exposing the left lateral surface of the inferior vena cava above and below the level of the left renal vein. Once this has been done, the surgeon can feel the right renal artery arising from the posterior lateral surface of the aorta. Autonomic nerve elements will be encountered on the renal artery but can be divided without concern. The gentle placement of a vein retractor under the left renal vein with upward retraction by an assistant greatly facilitates mobilization of the left renal artery. Here again, a Silastic loop placed about the renal artery aids in the exposure of this vessel.

The right renal artery is more difficult to expose, since it passes directly behind the vena cava on its course to the right renal hilum. The origin of this artery is palpated as it emerges from the right posterior aspect of the aorta. Care should be taken not to injure the right adrenal branch. This vessel arises 5 to 10 mm from the origin of the right renal artery, and in cases in which there is a distal stenosis, the size of this vessel may be 2 to 3 mm, since it becomes a very important collateral to the distal right renal artery via capsular branches. In the event that the entire right renal artery and its branches must be exposed, the surgeon must carefully expose, ligate, and divide all adjacent lumbar veins as they enter the vena cava to completely mobilize this structure.

The subhepatic space is next entered and the duodenum kocherized to allow exposure of the right renal vein as it joins the inferior vena cava. The renal vein is mobilized on a Silastic tape to aid in identification of the main renal artery lying beneath. This latter structure can usually be palpated and then isolated, and mobilized on a Silastic tape. Exposure of this vessel is completed when this distal dissection joins the medial exposure already described.

Bilateral transaortic endarterectomy includes not only exposure of the origins of both renal arteries, but mobilization of the aorta with control of any lumbar arteries in the segment of the aorta to be isolated. The proximal exposure of the aorta should include the origin of the superior mesenteric artery as well so that the proximal aortic clamp can be placed at that level.

ALTERNATE RENAL ARTERY EXPOSURES

The following exposures are helpful when prior aortic or proximal renal artery procedures are likely to have caused extensive adhesion, making the previously described renal artery exposures difficult and bloody. The distal right renal artery can be exposed through a right-sided retroperitoneal incision, which is a "mirror image" of the incision described in the section on retroperitoneal exposure of the aorta. The patient is positioned for an incision in the right flank. The muscles of the abdominal wall are divided and the retroperitoneal space entered. The peritoneum and contents are gently mobilized anteriorly and medially, including the right kidney enclosed in Gerota's fascia. The renal artery is palpated distally and carefully dissected free. The vena cava is identified and dissected free, including the ligation of two or three paired lumbar veins. The cava is gently elevated to expose the side of the aorta for the application of a side-biting vascular clamp for anastomosis of the proximal bypass graft. Thereafter, the distal anastomosis is complete for revascularization of the kidney.

An alternate revascularization procedure for the right kidney is described by Moncure and associates[13] and employs a right subcostal incision extending into the flank. The hepatic flexure of the colon is mobilized and rotated to the left. The duodenum is kocherized toward the midline to expose the right kidney. The renal artery is located behind and just above the right renal vein. Next, the hepatic artery is palpated in the hepatoduodenal ligament and the gastroduodenal artery identified. The hepatic artery proximal to the gastroduodenal artery is dissected free. The distal anastomosis of the bypass graft to the side of the renal artery is made first. The bypass is brought over the hepatoduodenal ligament and anastomosed to the side of the hepatic artery for vascularization of the kidney (Fig. 4–14).

The left renal artery can be exposed peripherally by the same incision described later in this chapter for the retroperitoneal exposure of the aorta. Once the left renal artery is exposed distally, the peritoneal cavity is opened and the splenic flexure of the colon is mobilized to the right by dividing the phrenicocolic ligament. The tail of the pancreas is separated from the left adrenal to expose the splenic artery for bypass to the left renal artery as described by Moncure and associates (see Fig. 4–15). An alternate source for blood supply can be obtained from the aorta distal to the renal artery. Once the aorta is exposed, a bypass can be placed from the aorta to the transected distal renal artery.

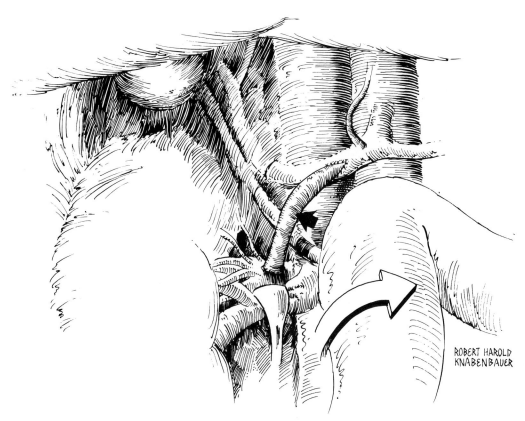

FIGURE 4–14. Illustration of hepatic-to-right renal artery bypass. The duodenum is kocherized (open arrow) for exposure. The reverse saphenous vein bypass is identified by the solid arrow. Note the retraction of the right renal vein for exposure.

EXPOSURE OF THE INFERIOR MESENTERIC ARTERY

The inferior mesenteric artery is easily located by incising the posterior parietal peritoneum immediately to the left of the infrarenal aorta. Care must be taken not to divide this mesenteric vessel distal to the left colic branch during the resection of an abdominal aortic aneurysm. The ascending branch of the left colic artery becomes the central anastomotic artery or the arc of Riolan and provides collateral circulation between the superior and the inferior mesenteric arteries and vice versa.

In some large aneurysms the thickened wall of the

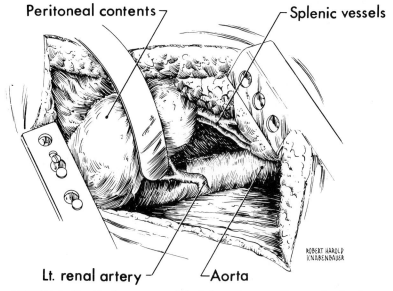

FIGURE 4–15. Flank exposure of the left renal artery. See text for details.

aorta obscures the actual origin of the inferior mesenteric artery, and division distal to the left colic branch of this vessel may result in sigmoid colon infarction. This complication is much more likely to occur when there is an arteriosclerotic occlusion of the marginal artery of Drummond. Figure 4–16 is a reproduction of an aortogram showing a patent central anastomotic artery (arc of Riolan) and also a patent marginal artery of Drummond.

RETROPERITONEAL EXPOSURE OF THE AORTA

This exposure is not new; Rob[14] in 1963 reported on a very large series of aortic resections performed through this exposure. However, there is a renewed interest in this approach, particularly if there is involvement of the renal or proximal aortic vessels, or if multiple previous intraperitoneal surgeries would hinder exposure by the conventional transperitoneal approach.

Shepard and associates[15] have described and illustrated the retroperitoneal approach to the abdominal aorta. The patient is positioned in the lateral position with right side down, but with the pelvis allowed to rotate posteriorly to allow exposure of both groins (Fig. 4–17). The incision begins at the lateral border of the rectus muscle 4 to 5 cm below the umbilicus and ends at the most posterior portion of the 11th or 12th rib. The retroperitoneal space is entered laterally and, using gentle finger dissection, the peritoneum and its contents are displaced forward as

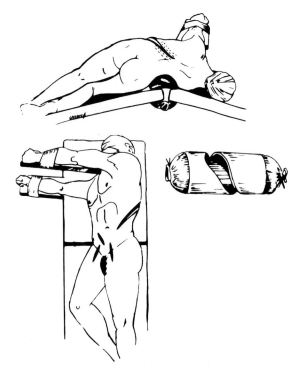

FIGURE 4–17. Positioning for exposure of the retroperitoneal aorta. *Top,* Flexion of table increases exposure. *Bottom left,* The hips are positioned at a 45-degree angle with the table and the left arm is passed across the chest. *Bottom right,* The position unwinds the torso for greater exposure. Incisions for exposure of the right iliac and common femoral arteries are shown in the bottom left. (From Shepard A, Scott G, Mackey W, et al: Retroperitoneal approach to high-risk abdominal aortic aneurysms. Arch Surg 126:157, 1973.)

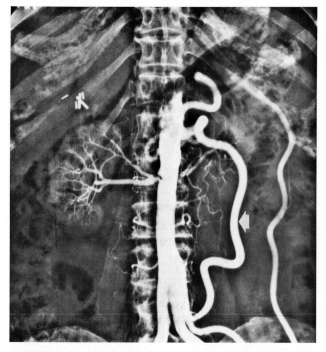

FIGURE 4–16. Angiogram from a patient with occlusion of the celiac and superior mesenteric arteries. Note the large inferior mesenteric artery with a central anastomotic artery (arrow) and a large marginal artery (lateral position) providing collateral circulation.

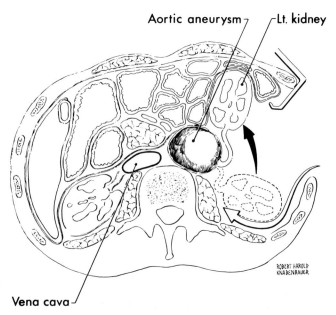

FIGURE 4–18. Retroperitoneal approach to an aortic aneurysm. The open arrow shows mobilization of the left kidney, which is displaced anteriorly (solid arrow).

illustrated in Figure 4–18. Gerota's fascia with the contained left kidney is elevated anteriorly and medially. The renal artery is identified by noting the large communicating vein connecting the renal to the hemiazygos vein. The renal artery is adjacent to this vessel. The superior, anterior, and left lateral surface of the aorta 1.5 to 2 cm above the left renal artery is exposed. The left iliac artery is easily isolated for control; however, the right iliac artery is best controlled by a balloon catheter placed into this vessel after the aorta is controlled proximally and opened posteriorly and laterally. The proximal aorta is easily isolated by gentle finger dissection, since the inferior vena cava lies at a distance from this vessel in the upper abdomen and is therefore not easily injured.

The inferior mesenteric artery must be ligated and divided to gain adequate exposure of the anterior surface of the aorta. Should additional exposure be necessary proximally, the aortic hiatus can be opened by dividing the left lateral crus of the diaphragm. The pleura is gently pushed away by blunt dissection. This approach is not advised in obese patients, when a large aneurysm is present, or when there is extensive iliac artery occlusive disease or aneurysmal change.

EMERGENCY EXPOSURE OF VISCERAL VASCULAR TRAUMA

Vascular exposure of the injured vessels within the abdomen is best carried out through a generous midline abdominal incision. The location of the hematoma encountered determines the exposure to be employed. Since the abdominal circulation arises in a retroperitoneal location, the overlying viscera will have to be rotated to the left or to the right or elevated superiorly in order to expose the aorta and its major branches or the caval or portal venous circulation.

Kudsk and Sheldon[16] have classified the retroperitoneal space into three zones (Fig. 4–19). The presence of a central hematoma (zone 1) indicates injury to the aorta, vena cava, proximal renal, mesenteric, celiac, or portal vein. Lateral hematomas (zone 2) indicate injury to distal visceral vessels. Retroperitoneal pelvic hematomas (zone 3) usually indicate torn branches of the iliac vessels associated with pelvic fractures and may not require exploration unless the hematoma is expanding or there is evidence of large-vessel injury demonstrated by angiography.

Exposure of the Proximal Aorta

The exposure of choice in emergency abdominal exploration is a generous midline incision, usually from xyphoid to symphysis pubis. An expanding central upper abdominal hematoma with extension to the left indicates a proximal aortic or adjacent major branch injury. Exposure can be facilitated by division of the left rectus muscle transversely in the left upper quadrant. The splenic flexure is mobilized

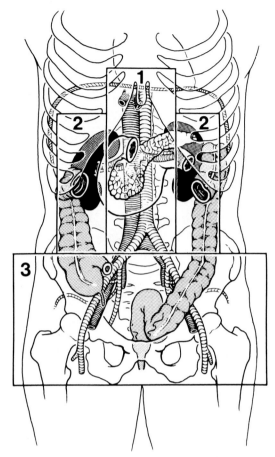

FIGURE 4–19.   Anatomic zones for exploration of retroperitoneal hematomas. See text for details. (From Kudsk KA, Sheldon GF: Retroperitoneal hematoma. *In* Blaisdell FW, Trunkey DD (eds): Trauma Management, Vol 1: Abdominal Trauma, 2nd ed. New York, Thieme Medical Publishers, Inc., 1993, p 400.)

including the spleen and the left kidney with rotation of these viscera to the right (rotation right). This gives excellent exposure of the proximal aorta from the aortic hiatus to the bifurcation. The origins of the celiac, superior mesenteric, and left renal arteries are likewise exposed (Fig. 4–20).

Exposure of the Infrahepatic Vena Cava and Portal Vein

The presence of a large upper abdominal hematoma with extension into the right flank is indicative of major caval, portal venous, or proximal injury to a major arterial branch in the right upper quadrant. Exposure is gained by incising the peritoneum lateral to the ascending colon followed by reflecting this structure medially followed by kocherizing the duodenum by sharp and blunt dissection and then rotating the right colon and duodenum to the left (rotation left) (Fig. 4–21). The entire vena cava from the iliac confluence to the liver can thus be exposed.

The portal vein can be inspected by incising the hepatoduodenal ligament above the duodenum. The

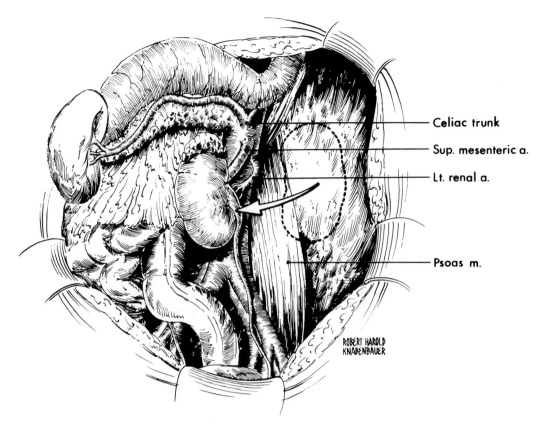

Celiac trunk

Sup. mesenteric a.

Lt. renal a.

Psoas m.

ROBERT HAROLD
KNABENBAUER

FIGURE 4–20.   Rotation right of intraabdominal contents including the left kidney for complete visualization of the abdominal aorta. The arrow indicates rotation of the kidney forward and to the right from the renal fossa indicated by the dotted outline. (From Smith LL, Catalano RD: Exposure of vascular injuries. *In* Bongard FS, Wilson SE, Perry MO (eds): Vascular Injuries in Surgical Practice. Norwalk, CT, Appleton & Lange, 1991, p 18.)

common bile duct is retracted laterally and the hepatic artery can be palpated and isolated for inspection. Thereafter the portal vein can be exposed by retracting the hepatic artery toward the midline. The right side of the aorta can be inspected as well as the proximal right renal artery if the rotation and mobilization of the overlying bowel is continued to the midline.

EXTRAPERITONEAL EXPOSURE OF THE EXTERNAL ILIAC ARTERIES

The external iliac arteries are easily exposed extraperitoneally. An oblique incision is made in either lower quadrant of the abdomen depending on the side of involvement. This incision begins near the pubic tubercle and extends up and back, staying medial to the anterior superior spine of the pubis. The external oblique aponeurosis is opened in the direction of its fibers and the incision continued into the fleshy portion of this muscle. The internal oblique and transversus muscles are divided in the direction of the incision and the preperitoneal space entered. The peritoneum is gently pushed medially and a small Deaver retractor is placed to expose the external iliac artery. Care should be taken not to injure the ilioinguinal or genitofemoral nerves during exposure or retraction. Their

location on the anterior surface of the psoas muscle is vulnerable. Combination of this incision with a vertical incision over the common femoral artery allows exposure of the terminal common iliac artery to the proximal superficial or deep femoral arteries.

EXPOSURE OF THE COMMON FEMORAL ARTERY

A vertically placed incision centered over the palpable pulse provides the best exposure of the common femoral artery. In the absence of a pulse, the diseased artery can frequently be rolled beneath the index finger. Lacking either of these aids, the femoral artery is located one third of the distance from the pubic tubercle to the anterior superior iliac spine. This point lies just lateral to the pubic hair escutcheon.

It is important to check for posterior branches, since an aberrant medial femoral circumflex artery can arise anywhere along the posterior surface of the common femoral artery. Failure to do this can result in troublesome bleeding upon opening the common femoral artery. The combination of careful posterior dissection and palpation while elevating the common femoral artery with a Silastic loop results in the early discovery of this important branch.

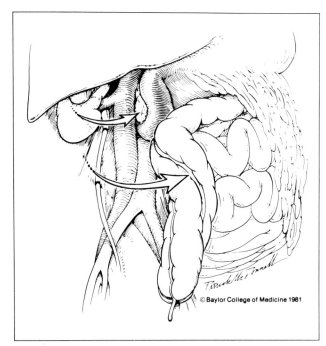

FIGURE 4–21. Rotation left of intraabdominal viscera by mobilization of the right colon and by kocherization of the duodenum. The right kidney can also be mobilized to inspect the posterior surface of the vena cava if necessary. (Reproduced with the permission of Dohrmann M, original illustrator.)

The lateral femoral circumflex artery arises from the lateral side of the profunda femoral artery. It is well to isolate this vessel for subsequent control should this be necessary. Care should be taken to identify the lateral femoral circumflex vein, which courses from medial to lateral in the crotch between the superficial and deep femoral arteries. Failure to identify this vein can result in troublesome bleeding. Once the lateral femoral circumflex vein is ligated and divided, the dissection can be continued down the deep femoral artery with relative ease.

EXPOSURE OF THE PROFUNDA FEMORAL ARTERY

Occasionally the deep femoral artery must be located in a patient with a badly scarred groin following prior operations. Nunez and associates[17] have described an approach lateral to the sartorius muscle. Figure 4–22 shows the location of the incision over the branches of the lateral femoral circumflex artery. These branches are followed medially to the profunda femoral artery.

In cases in which the deep femoral artery is being exposed as an initial procedure, Hershey and Auer[18] have stressed the importance of flexing and externally rotating the thigh to relax the involved muscles and thereby aid the dissection. The profunda femoral artery is located 1.5 cm medial to the femur and lies on the pectineus and adductor brevis muscles. King and associates[19] have described the anatomy, including measurements of the profunda femoral artery

branches. The reader is well advised to consult this excellent and well-illustrated article.

EXPOSURE OF THE POPLITEAL ARTERY

The popliteal artery is exposed from a medial approach with few exceptions. The proximal and distal portions of this vessel are easily exposed; however, the midportion of the artery at the level of the joint space of the knee is obscured by the medial head of the gastrocnemius muscle and the tendinous insertions of the long adductor muscles.

The proximal popliteal artery is exposed through an incision placed in the groove between the vastus medialis and sartorius muscles. The greater saphenous vein lies just posterior to this incision and care must be taken to preserve this structure during the dissection. The sartorius muscle is retracted posteriorly and the investing fascia incised longitudinally, preserving the saphenous nerve, which is usually seen lying on the deep fascial surface. Once the fascia is opened, the popliteal artery can be palpated in its location under the adductor magnus tendon.

Additional exposure can be obtained distally by dividing the tendon of the medial head of the gastrocnemius muscle. The gentle insertion of the left index finger behind this tendinous origin aids in isolating this structure and protecting the underlying neurovascular bundle. Should additional distal exposure be necessary, the tendinous insertions of the sartorius, semimembranosis, semitendinosis, and gracilis muscles may be divided. It is well to mark these tendons with identifying sutures to aid in their subsequent repair.

The terminal popliteal artery and the tibial peroneal arterial trunk are exposed through an incision placed 1 cm posterior to the medial margin of the tibia. Once again the surgeon must be aware of the greater saphenous vein and protect it in its subcutaneous location. The thick muscular fascia overlying the gastrocnemius muscle is incised and the popliteal space entered. The large popliteal vein is usually encountered first and gently retracted superiorly using a vein retractor. The artery is easily felt by its pulse, or if absent as a cord structure beneath the vein. The dissection can be carried distally until the anterior tibial artery origin is located arising anteriorly and laterally from the terminal popliteal artery. This distal dissection requires the division of the soleus muscle fibers arising from the medial margin of the tibia.

LATERAL EXPOSURE OF THE POPLITEAL ARTERY

The lateral approach to the popliteal artery can be employed when prior medical exposure has resulted in dense scarring of the tissues. Repeat procedures using the medial exposure may be extremely difficult. Consequently, the lateral exposure of the popliteal

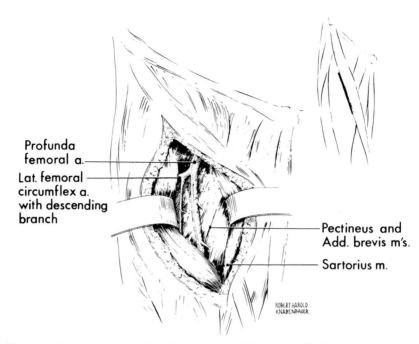

FIGURE 4–22. Lateral approach to the deep femoral artery. *Upper right*, The incision is lateral to the sartorius muscle. *Lower left*, The exposure of the profunda femoral vessel. See text for details.

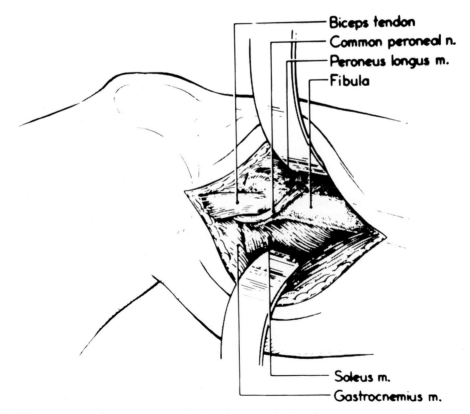

FIGURE 4–23. Lateral approach to the distal popliteal artery. Note the common peroneal nerve coursing around the neck of the fibula. (From Veith F, Ascer E, Gupta S: Lateral approach to the popliteal artery. J Vasc Surg 6:119, 1987.)

artery as described in detail by Veith and associates[20] may be employed.

Above-Knee Popliteal Artery

The lateral incision for this portion of the popliteal artery is placed between the iliotibial tract and the biceps femoris muscle. The dissection is deepened through the lateral intramuscular septum to enter the popliteal space. The neurovascular bundle is then easily identified within the popliteal fat.

Below-Knee Popliteal Artery

The below-knee popliteal artery is approached by an incision over the head and proximal one fourth of the fibula. As the incision is deepened, care must be taken to preserve the common peroneal nerve as it courses around the neck of the fibula (Fig. 4–23). The biceps femoris tendon is divided. The ligamentous attachments to the head of the fibula are divided and the proximal fibula is removed. Following removal of this bone, the entire below-knee popliteal artery, tibioperoneal trunk, anterior tibial artery, and the origins of the posterior tibial and peroneal arteries are accessible (Fig. 4–24).

EXPOSURE OF THE TIBIAL AND PERONEAL ARTERIES

The increased use of long leg bypass grafts in managing ischemic vascular disease of the leg makes an accurate knowledge of the circulation of the leg of utmost importance. We have already discussed the approach to the tibial peroneal trunk vessel and will now describe the usual approaches used in exposing the tibial and peroneal arteries in the leg.

Anterior Tibial Artery

The skin incision is made approximately 2.5 cm lateral to the anterior border of the tibia. The anterior tibial artery courses between the tibialis anterior and the extensor digitorum longus muscles in the upper portion of the anterior compartment of the leg. Dorsiflexion and internal rotation of the foot aid in the identification of the groove between these two muscles. The extensor digitorum hallucis muscle crosses over the artery from lateral to medial in the distal leg. The muscles are gently separated down to the anterior tibial artery, which lies between its two accompanying veins on the interosseous membrane.

It is important to keep in mind the relationship of the three major leg arteries to the tibia and fibula, as well as the compartments of the leg. Figure 4–25 shows these important relationships. Note the ante-

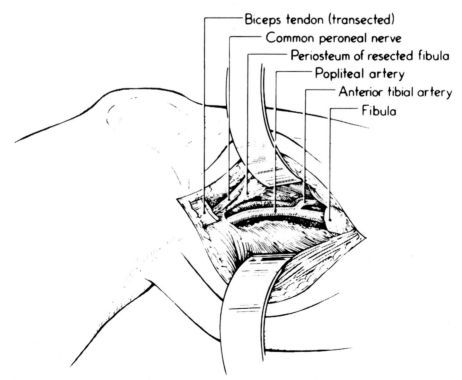

FIGURE 4–24. Lateral approach to the distal popliteal artery following the removal of the proximal fibula. Note the transected tendon of the biceps muscle and the intact common peroneal nerve. (From Veith F, Ascer E, Gupta S: Lateral approach to the popliteal artery. J Vasc Surg 6:119, 1987.)

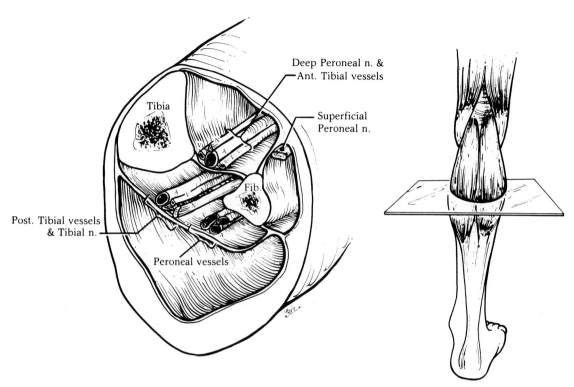

FIGURE 4–25. Cross-section of the leg showing the location of the anterior tibial artery in the anterior compartment of the leg and the posterior tibial and peroneal arteries in the deep portion of the posterior compartment. (From Briggs S, Seligson D: Management of extremity trauma. *In* Richardson D, Polk H, Flint M (eds): Trauma: Clinical Care and Pathophysiology. Chicago, Year Book Medical Publishers, Inc, 1987, p 544.)

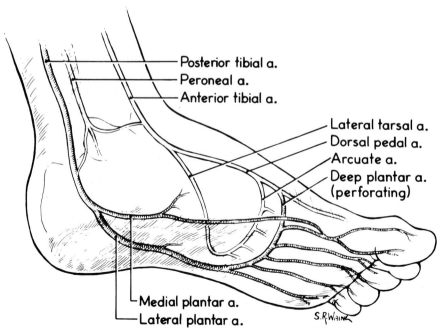

FIGURE 4–26. Anatomy of the arterial circulation of the foot. (From Ascer E, Veith F, Gupta S: Bypasses to plantar arteries and other tibial branches: An extended approach to limb salvage. J Vasc Surg 8:434, 1985.)

rior tibial vessels lying on the interosseous membrane in the anterior compartment. Also observe the peroneal artery coursing just medial to the medial margin of the fibula in the posterior compartment, just deep to the intermuscular septum. Also observe that the posterior tibial vessels lie medial to the peroneal artery and veins, but also deep to the intermuscular septum and in the posterior compartment of the leg as well.

Posterior Tibial Artery

We have already described the proximal exposure of the tibial artery by extending the incision used for the exposure of the distal popliteal artery. It is necessary to incise the origin of the soleus muscle from the medial border of the tibia in order to gain exposure of the intermuscular septum. Once this structure is opened, the posterior tibial vessels will be observed coursing between the tibialis posterior and the flexor digitorum longus muscles. The posterior tibial nerve crosses the artery posteriorly from medial to a lateral position and must be protected.

Peroneal Artery

The peroneal artery can be exposed by resecting a short segment of the fibula through a lateral incision over this bone. This incision should be placed below the entrance of the peroneal nerve into the anterior compartment of the leg. The peroneal vessels lie just deep to the medial border of the fibula, and once the short segment of bone is removed, the vessels are easily exposed.

An easier exposure of the peroneal artery uses a medial incision as described for exposure of the posterior tibial artery above. Once this latter artery is exposed, the dissection is continued to a deeper level, staying on the intermuscular septum. The peroneal artery is located adjacent to the medial border of the fibula. This exposure is deep and therefore more difficult in a large leg.

Mobilization of the crural vessels requires patience and great care. There are numerous small muscular branches and each artery has two accompanying veins with their respective tributaries to protect. Carelessness during this dissection leads to bleeding that obscures the field and increases the likelihood of injury to these delicate vascular structures.

EXPOSURE OF THE PLANTAR ARTERIES

A detailed understanding of the arterial circulation of the foot has become important, since distal bypass sites in the foot are used for limb salvage. Ascer, Veith, and Gupta[20] have described the surgical approaches employed as well as the results of these distal lower extremity bypass procedures. Figure 4–26 shows the branches and distribution of the anterior and posterior tibial arteries in the foot.

Posterior Tibial Artery and the Plantar Branches

Exposure of the terminal posterior tibial artery is accomplished by a retromalleolar incision to expose the artery and its concomitant veins. The dissection is continued distally by division of the lacunate ligament should the proximal artery be unsatisfactory as an anastomotic site. Further distal dissection may require sequential incisions in order to accurately follow the course of the terminal posterior tibial artery into the plantar surface of the foot. Direct exposure of the terminal posterior tibial artery and the plantar branches may invite a difficult retraction problem in locating these vessels due to the thickness and rigidity of the overlying plantar tissues. Should more distal exposure be necessary, the plantar aponeurosis and the flexor digitorum brevis muscle can be incised to more adequately expose the medial plantar artery as well as the larger lateral plantar vessel (Fig. 4–27). This latter vessel continues distally into the foot to form the deep plantar arch.

Distal Dorsal Pedal Artery and the Lateral Tarsal Branch

These vessels are approached through a longitudinal incision just lateral to the extensor hallucis ten-

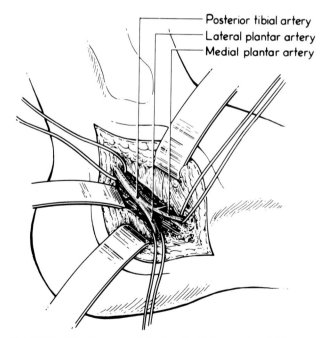

FIGURE 4–27. Exposure of the terminal left posterior tibial artery using a retromalleolar incision. The terminal branches of this vessel are shown, the larger being the lateral plantar branch. See text for details. (From Ascer E, Veith F, Gupta S: Bypass to plantar arteries and other tibial branches: An extended approach to limb salvage. J Vasc Surg 8:436, 1988.)

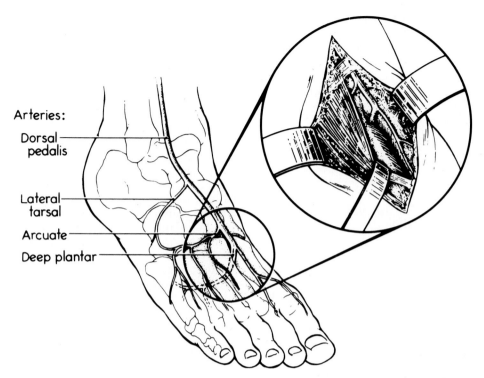

Arteries:

Dorsal pedalis

Lateral tarsal

Arcuate

Deep plantar

FIGURE 4–28. Diagram of the arterial circulation on the dorsum of the foot. The insert shows the origin of the deep plantar branch as it courses between the two heads of the first dorsal interosseous vessel. See text for details. (From Ascer E, Veith F, Gupta S: Bypass to plantar arteries and other tibial branches: An extended approach to limb salvage. J Vasc Surg *8*:437, 1988.)

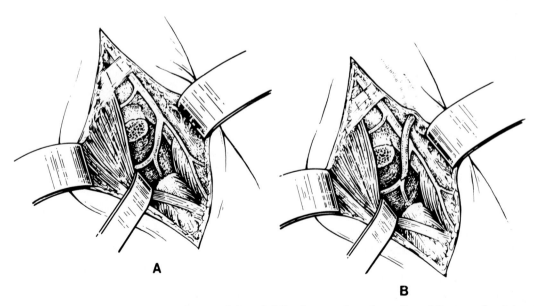

A

B

FIGURE 4–29. *A*, Shows the deep plantar arch branch following resection of a portion of the second metatarsal bone. *B*, Shows the distal anastomosis of a bypass to this vessel. (From Ascer E, Veith F, Gupta S: Bypass to plantar arteries and other tibial branches: An extended approach to limb salvage. J Vasc Surg *8*:437, 1988.)

don. The inferior extensor retinaculum is divided at the level of the ankle joint to expose this vessel. The lateral tarsal branch of the dorsal pedal artery usually arises at the level of the navicular bone and beneath the extensor digitorum brevis muscle. This artery is of importance, since it communicates with the arcuate artery and is thereby an important collateral blood supply to the dorsum of the foot.

Deep Plantar Artery

This vessel is the main continuation of the dorsalis pedis artery at the level of the metatarsal bones and is approached through a curvilinear incision over the dorsum of the foot lateral to the extensor hallucis tendon. The artery is followed distally until it divides into the first dorsal metatarsal and deep plantar branches. The latter vessel descends between the two heads of the first dorsal interosseous muscle to anastomose with the lateral plantar branch to form the deep plantar arch of the foot (Fig. 4–28). Adequate exposure of the deep plantar branch requires retraction or transection of the extensor hallucis brevis muscle. The periosteum of the second metatarsal bone is then carefully elevated and a portion of the bone is removed by a rongeur to provide adequate exposure for distal arterial anastomosis (Fig. 4–29). This exposure requires delicate dissection in order not to injure adjacent arterial branches or venous tributaries.

REFERENCES

1. Evans W, Mendelowitz D, Liapis C, et al: Motor speech deficit following carotid endarterectomy. Ann Surg *196*:461, 1982.
2. Hertzer N, Feldman B, Beven E, et al: A prospective study of the incidence of injury to the cranial nerves during carotid endarterectomy. Surg Gynecol Obstet *151*:781, 1980.
3. Wylie E, Stoney R, Ehrenfeld W: Carotid atherosclerosis. *In* Egdahl R (ed): Manual of Vascular Surgery, Vol I. New York, Springer-Verlag, 1980.
4. Fisher D, Clagett G, Parker J, et al: Mandibular subluxation for high carotid exposure. J Vasc Surg *1*:727, 1984.
5. Wylie E, Stoney R, Ehrenfeld W, Effeney D: Nonatherosclerotic disease of the extracranial carotid arteries. *In* Egdahl R (ed): Manual of Vascular Surgery, Vol II. New York, Springer-Verlag, 1986.
6. Berguer R: Distal vertebral artery bypass: Technique, the "occipital connection," and potential uses. J Vasc Surg *2*:621, 1985.
7. Roos D: Transaxillary approach for first rib resection to relieve thoracic outlet syndrome. Ann Surg *163*:354, 1966.
8. Roos D: Surgical treatment of the thoracic outlet syndromes. *In* Jamison CW (ed): Current Operative Surgery: Vascular Surgery. London, Bailliere & Tindall, 1985.
9. Stoney R, Wylie E: Surgical management of arterial lesions of the thoracolumbar aorta. Am J Surg *126*:157, 1973.
10. Szilagy D, Hageman J, Smith R, et al: Spinal cord damage in surgery of the abdominal aorta. Surgery *83*:38, 1979.
11. Williams PL, Warwick R: Gray's Anatomy, 36th British ed. Philadelphia, WB Saunders Company, 1980, p 896.
12. Luzsa G: X-Ray Anatomy of the Vascular System. Philadelphia, JB Lippincott Company, 1974, p 232.
13. Moncure A, Brewster D, Darling R, et al: Use of the splenic and hepatic arteries for renal revascularization. J Vasc Surg *3*:196, 1986.
14. Rob C: Extraperitoneal approach to the abdominal aorta. Surgery *53*:87, 1963.
15. Shepard A, Scott G, Mackey W, et al: Retroperitoneal approach to high-risk abdominal aortic aneurysms. Arch Surg *121*:444, 1986.
16. Kudsk KA, Sheldon GF: Retroperitoneal Hematoma. *In* Blaisdell FW, Trunkey DD (eds): Trauma Management, Vol I: Abdominal Trauma. New York, Thieme-Stratton, Inc, 1982, p 281.
17. Nunez A, Veith F, Gupta S, et al: Direct approaches to the distal portions of the deep femoral artery for limb salvage bypasses. J Vasc Surg *8*:576, 1988.
18. Hershey F, Auer A: Extended surgical approach to the profunda femoris artery. Surg Gynecol Obstet *138*:88, 1974.
19. King T, Rhodes R, DePalma R: Use of the profunda femoris artery for secondary revascularization. *In* Bergan JJ, Yao JST (eds): Operative Techniques in Vascular Surgery. New York, Grune & Stratton, 1980, p 233.
20. Veith F, Ascer E, Gupta S: Lateral approach to the popliteal artery. J Vasc Surg *6*:119, 1987.
21. Ascer E, Veith F, Gupta S: Bypasses to plantar arteries and other tibial branches: An extended approach to limb salvage. J Vasc Surg *8*:434, 1985.

REVIEW QUESTIONS

1. Of the following nerves, the one most likely to be injured during carotid endarterectomy is:
   (a) recurrent laryngeal nerve
   (b) vagus nerve (X)
   (c) hypoglossal nerve (XII)
   (d) superior laryngeal nerve
   (e) glossopharyngeal nerve (IX)

2. Structures contributing to thoracic outlet compression syndrome may include: (true or false)
   (a) subclavius muscle
   (b) first rib
   (c) scalenus anticus
   (d) congenital cervical rib
   (e) sternocleidomastoid muscle

3. Concerning the lower extremity circulation: (true or false)
   (a) the deep femoral artery is accessible only to the lateral aspect of the sartorious muscle
   (b) lateral or medial approaches are possible to expose the popliteal artery above or below the knee
   (c) the lateral tarsal artery is the largest distal branch of the posterior tibial artery
   (d) the deep plantar arch is formed by the deep plantar artery and the lateral plantar artery

4. During repair of an infrarenal abdominal aortic aneurysm: (true or false)

    (a) autonomic nerve fibers crossing the left common iliac artery should be protected to preserve sexual potency

    (b) a large anastomotic artery appearing on arteriography between the superior and inferior mesenteric arteries indicates satisfactory perfusion of the left colon with little risk of ischemia if inferior mesenteric artery ligation is performed

    (c) a large lumbar artery near the renal arteries should be preserved because this may represent significant contribution to the anterior spinal artery

    (d) the left renal vein may be safely ligated and divided to facilitate aortic exposure if the lumbar and adrenal tributaries are maintained for collateral circulation

    (e) initial aortic control at the diaphragm will safely facilitate infrarenal control in the patient with a ruptured or juxtarenal abdominal aortic aneurysm

5. Patients with a superior mesenteric artery occlusion or stenosis would be expected to have: (true or false)

    (a) a large central anastomotic artery

    (b) retrograde filling of the superior mesenteric artery

    (c) a large marginal artery of Drummond

    (d) low incidence of left colon ischemia following inferior mesenteric artery ligation

    (e) multiple visceral artery occlusions are rarely required to produce intestinal "angina"

6. Renal artery reconstruction:

    (a) may be performed via a left or right retroperitoneal approach

    (b) may be difficult in the obese or previously operated patient if the anterior transabdominal approach is used

    (c) is facilitated in the high-risk patient using splenic artery-to-left renal artery bypass; or hepatic artery-to-right renal artery bypass

    (d) exposure and revascularization of right renal arteries is more difficult because of its retro-vena cava position

    (e) all of the above

7. The distal internal carotid artery: (true or false)

    (a) is crossed posteriorly by the hypoglossal nerve (XII)

    (b) vagus nerve (X) passes posterior lateral to the carotid bifurcation

    (c) exposure is safely facilitated by anterior dislocation of the mandible

    (d) distal exposure may be facilitated by division of the digastric muscle and the stylohyoid muscle

    (e) anteriorly, is covered by the parotid gland, angle of the mandible, and the styloid process

8. Regarding trauma to the great vessels: (true or false)

    (a) exposure of the left subclavian artery is best accomplished via median sternotomy

    (b) temporary right third interspace thoracotomy may be used to control exigent hemorrhage from the brachiocephalic artery

    (c) right subclavian exposure via a simple supraclavicular incision is adequate

    (d) exposure of either common carotid artery origin is best accomplished via a sternal splitting incision extended along the anterior border of the appropriate sternocleidomastoid muscle

    (e) all of the above

9. Exposure of the infrapopliteal arteries involves the following anatomic relationships: (true or false)

    (a) the anterior tibial artery passes posterior to the interosseous membrane

    (b) exposure of the peroneal artery laterally requires segmental fibular resection

    (c) the posterior tibial nerve crosses the artery anteriorly

    (d) the posterior tibial artery lies deep to the intermuscular septum

    (e) all of the above

10. The arteria radicularis magna (artery of Adamkiewicz):

    (a) is important in providing circulation to the anterior spinal artery

    (b) may supply up to two thirds of the spinal cord

    (c) presents as a branch of either a distal intercostal or proximal lumbar artery (T8/L1)

    (d) is rarely identified via arteriography preoperatively

    (e) all of the above

ANSWERS

1. b

2. (a) T
   (b) T
   (c) T
   (d) T
   (e) F

3. (a) F
   (b) T
   (c) F
   (d) T

4. (a) T
   (b) F
   (c) T
   (d) T
   (e) T

5. (a) T
   (b) T
   (c) T
   (d) F
   (e) F

6. e

7. (a) F
   (b) T
   (c) F
   (d) T
   (e) T

8. (a) F
   (b) F
   (c) F
   (d) T
   (e) F

9. (a) F
   (b) T
   (c) F
   (d) T
   (e) F

10. e

5

HEMOSTASIS AND THROMBOSIS

PAUL W. HUMPHREY, JOHN R. HOCH, and DONALD SILVER

Most of the bleeding that occurs during surgery or in association with trauma is mechanical and can usually be controlled. Occasionally a patient's bleeding will be caused or accelerated by congenital or acquired defects of the hemostatic mechanisms. The vascular surgeon's knowledge of the hemostatic mechanisms must be sufficient to allow him to stop and/or restore hemostasis according to the needs of his patients. In addition, the vascular surgeon must be able to restore arterial and venous blood flow not only by mechanical means but also by pharmacologic means.

This chapter will review the pathophysiology, diagnosis, and management of disorders of hemostasis and thrombosis. The endothelium's expanding role in these disorders is emphasized.

HEMOSTASIS

Hemostasis, the process by which bleeding from injured tissue is controlled, requires the interaction of the blood vessel wall, platelets, coagulation, and fibrinolytic proteins. Although hemostasis is a dynamic process, it can be divided into four components: vessel reaction to injury, platelet response, activation of coagulation with clot stabilization, and mobilization of the fibrinolytic pathway.

Components of Hemostasis

Vessel Response

When a vessel is injured, the interaction of humoral, neurogenic, and myogenic events leads to smooth muscle cell (SMC) contraction and vasoconstriction in the muscular arteries and arterioles.[1] Vasoconstriction has less of a role in obtaining hemostasis in veins and venules. Platelet adherence to the injured vessel wall is followed by release of adenosine diphosphate (ADP) and serotonin from the platelet's dense granules. These dense granule products, together with the thromboxane A_2 released by platelets, potentiate SMC contraction. Local production of thrombin also contributes to SMC contraction. Loss of endothelium potentiates vasoconstriction by eliminating the vasodilating stimuli provided by prostacyclin (PGI_2) and the endothelial-derived relaxing factor (EDRF).[2]

In normal vessels, endothelial cells cover the luminal surface by forming a monolayer with a cobblestone morphology. This monolayer exhibits tight cell-cell interaction and is quiescent, with a low rate of replication. The endothelium weighs approximately 1.5 to 2.0 kg and has a volume equal to that of the liver.[3] Once regarded as a passive barrier between the blood and the underlying thrombogenic subendothelium, the endothelium is now recognized as a biologically active organ that participates in and modulates various physiologic processes, including hemostasis and thrombosis.

In their normal quiescent state, endothelial cells are actively antithrombogenic (Table 5–1). Endothelial cells synthesize and secrete PGI_2, a potent vasodilator and inhibitor of platelet aggregation. PGI_2 stimulates adenylate cyclase, increasing cyclic adenosine monophosphate (cAMP) levels within platelets, thus blocking platelet activation.[4] Stimulants to endothelial cell production of PGI_2 include thrombin, ADP, adenosine triphosphate (ATP), kallikrein, and histamine.[5,6]

Endothelial cells synthesize heparin-like substances, heparan sulfates, which possess anticoagulant properties and act as cofactors for antithrombin III (AT III).[7,8] AT III, also synthesized by endothelial cells, inactivates thrombin. The inactivation of thrombin is greatly accelerated by the heparan sulfates.[9]

Protein C is activated when thrombin becomes bound to the endothelial cell membrane protein thrombomodulin. Thrombomodulin is synthesized by endothelial cells.[10] A second cofactor, protein S, is synthesized by both endothelial cells and the liver.[11,12] Protein S is also expressed on the endothelial cell surface.

Endothelium synthesizes tissue-type plasminogen activator (t-PA) and urokinase. Both are serine proteases that bind to fibrinogen and remain bound to fibrin. These proteases convert plasminogen to plas-

71

TABLE 5–1. THE ENDOTHELIAL CELL AS MODULATOR OF HEMOSTASIS

	Hemostatic Effect
Thrombogenic Function	
Loss of EDRF[a] and PGI$_2$ following injury	Loss of vasodilating stimulus
VIII:vWF synthesis	↑ Platelet adhesion
Factor V synthesis	↑ Thrombin
Expression of tissue factor	↑ Thrombin
Binds factors VIIa and IXa	↑ Thrombin
Surface membrane site for prothrombinase complex	↑ Thrombin
Plasminogen activator inhibitor synthesis	↓ t-PA
Antithrombogenic Function	
EDRF and PGI$_2$ synthesis	Vasodilating stimulus
PGI$_2$ synthesis and granule release	↓ Platelet aggregation
Thrombomodulin synthesis	↓ Factors Va and VIIIa
Protein S synthesis	↓ Factors Va and VIIIa
Heparin sulfates synthesis	↓ Thrombin
Tissue-type plasminogen activator (t-PA) and urokinase synthesis	↑ Plasmin

[a]EDRF, endothelial-derived relaxing factor; PGI$_2$, prostacyclin; VII: vWF, von Willebrand's factor.

min, the enzyme responsible for fibrinolysis. Endothelial cells also synthesize a plasminogen activator inhibitor (PAI-1), which rapidly inactivates circulating t-PA. When the plasminogen activator becomes incorporated within a thrombus or hemostatic plug, it is more slowly inactivated by PAI-1.[3,13]

The endothelium possesses substantial procoagulant activity and acts as a template for hemostasis when stimulated following vessel injury (Table 5–1). Endothelial cells express tissue factor (thromboplastin) on their surfaces when stimulated by agonists such as interleukin 1 (IL 1), thrombin, or endotoxin.[3] Thromboplastin may serve as a cofactor to allow activated coagulation factor VII to bind to the cell surface and catalyze conversion of factor IX to activated factor IX, leading to thrombin formation via the intrinsic pathway.[14]

Endothelial cells, in addition to the liver, synthesize factor V, which promotes the binding of activated factor X to the endothelial cell's surface, leading to the formation of the prothrombinase complex, once thought only to form on platelets.[15] The prothrombinase complex accelerates the conversion of prothrombin to thrombin.

Endothelial cells and the liver synthesize and secrete von Willebrand's factor (VIII:vWF) into the circulation and subendothelial matrix. Von Willebrand's factor is necessary for platelet adherence following endothelial disruption.[2]

The endothelium's complex role in hemostasis is determined by the balance between the endothelium's procoagulant and anticoagulant attributes. The balance is modulated by other cells and circulating proteins.

Platelet Activities

Platelets are small, discoid-shaped, anuclear cells with an average circulatory life span of 8 to 12 days. There are usually 200,000 to 400,000 platelets/cu mm in human blood. Platelets are released as cytoplasmic fragments of megakaryocytes within bone marrow.

The platelet's surface membrane is a bilayer of glycoproteins, phospholipids, and proteins. Carbohydrate moieties of the glycoproteins make up the outer layer, known as the glycocalyx, with which circulating proteins interact. Surface receptors are known to exist for thrombin, serotonin, fibrinogen, fibronectin, ADP, epinephrine, collagen, vasopressin, thromboxane A$_2$, platelet activating factor, and coagulation proteins, especially activated factor X and factor V.[16]

Platelets contain three types of storage granules: (1) amine storage or *dense* granules, which contain serotonin, ADP, ATP, and calcium; (2) protein storage or *alpha* granules, which contain coagulation factors, including high-molecular-weight kininogen (HMWK), fibrinogen, fibronectin, factor V, and factor VIII:vWF, as well as other proteins, including platelet-derived growth factor, platelet factor 4, β-thromboglobulin, and thrombospondin; and (3) *lysosomes*, which contain numerous proteases, glycosidases, and acid hydrolases.[17,18]

Platelets usually do not adhere to each other or to the endothelium. Following vascular injury, platelets are activated and adhere within seconds to the injured vessel wall, lose their discoid shape, and spread onto the subendothelial matrix. The initial stimulus to adherence is probably the exposed collagen fibrils. Platelets will not adhere to injury sites unless sufficient and functionally normal VIII:vWF is present within the subendothelium.[13] Platelets possess two different membrane glycoprotein binding sites for VIII:vWF. The clinically relevant receptor is glycoprotein Ib.[19] Following adhesion, collagen, ADP, thrombin, and epinephrine, which interact with specific platelet membrane receptors, stimulate platelets to release their granule contents. Alpha granule release provides additional VIII:vWF, as well as fibronectin, which promotes additional platelet adherence.

ADP released from dense granules initiates platelet-platelet interaction, leading to a loose aggregation. A second wave of aggregation is induced by the stimulation of membrane phospholipase A$_2$, resulting in the release of arachidonic acid. Arachidonic acid is converted by cyclooxygenase to the prostaglandin endoperoxides PGG$_2$ and PGH$_2$. PGG$_2$ is then converted to thromboxane A$_2$ by thromboxane synthetase. Thromboxane A$_2$, PGG$_2$, and PGH$_2$ stimulate further aggregation and platelet granule release.[20]

Thrombin is known to stimulate release of ADP from dense granules and to activate the arachidonic pathway, but it can also induce aggregation without these mediators. Thrombin activates a phospholipase C, causing the cleavage of inositol lipids to form inositol triphosphate and 1,2-diacylglycerol.

Diacylgylcerol activates protein kinase C, which then phosphorylates proteins necessary for the release reaction. Inositol triphosphate causes increased mobilization of intracellular calcium, leading to platelet aggregation.[21]

Regardless of the stimulant, aggregation involves the reversible expression of fibrinogen receptors on the platelet surface. Circulating fibrinogen and fibrinogen released from alpha granules form bridges between adjacent platelets. The binding sites are composed of glycoproteins IIb and IIIa on the platelet surface.[22] The initial stage of hemostasis, consisting of vasoconstriction and platelet plug formation, is called "primary hemostasis."

Platelets are dynamically involved in the coagulation cascade. Procoagulant phospholipids (platelet factor 3) are exposed on the platelet membrane following stimulation by thrombin and collagen. These phospholipids provide a binding site for the prothrombinase complex.[23] Platelets also release factor V from alpha granules. Factor V becomes activated and membrane bound, acting as a receptor for the binding of activated factor X. Additionally, platelets have surface receptors for factors XI and activated XI and HMWK. There is evidence that platelets may activate factor XI in the presence of kallikrein and HMWK, initiating the intrinsic pathway without the activation of factor XII.[24]

Coagulation Process

Coagulation Activation. The platelet plug, required for normal hemostasis, will deaggregate as its fibrinogen bridges dissociate unless thrombin is generated and fibrin stabilization of the plug occurs. The formation of fibrin requires the interaction of platelet aggregates, endothelial cells, and plasma coagulation proteins.

Thirteen plasma coagulation proteins have been designated by the Roman numerals I through XIII (an "a" follows the Roman numeral when the factor has been activated). Hepatocytes synthesize all factors except VIII:C and III. Factor VIII:C, the antihemophilic factor, is synthesized by endothelial cells. Vascular endothelium is the primary source of VIII:vWF, but platelets and megakaryocytes may also release it. Although synthesized at separate sites, factors VIII:C and VIII:vWF interact in plasma and circulate as a complex. Tissue factor (factor III) is a lipoprotein found in many tissues. Endothelial cells also may express tissue factor when activated by IL 1, thrombin, or endotoxin.[25]

The hepatic synthesis of factors II, VII, IX, and X is vitamin K dependent. When vitamin K is not available, these factors are synthesized and released, but are not biologically active.

The sequence of enzymatic events leading to thrombin formation has been termed the "coagulation cascade" (Fig. 5–1). Classically, it has been taught that two pathways of coagulation capable of initiating thrombin formation exist. This division of the pathways is helpful for understanding coagulation; however, it must be emphasized that the coagulation pathways frequently function in tandem.

The intrinsic pathway is activated when plasma is exposed to a negatively charged surface such as subendothelium, collagen, or endotoxin. Factor XII is activated to XIIa by the interaction of HMWK, prekallikrein, and the negatively charged surface. Factor XIIa activates factor XI (XIa), which then proteolytically activates factor IX (IXa). Deficiencies of factor XII, HMWK, and prekallikrein do not cause hemorrhagic disorders. A deficiency of factor XI, however, can lead to a significant bleeding diathesis. This implies the existence of alternative pathways capable of activating the intrinsic pathway without factor XII.[14]

The next step takes place on the activated platelet membrane, where a specific phospholipid moiety (platelet factor 3) becomes exposed upon stimulation by thrombin or collagen. Factor IXa, thrombin-activated VIII:C, and calcium interact with factor X on the platelet surface, converting it to factor Xa. With the production of factor Xa, the two coagulation pathways merge into a final "common pathway."

The extrinsic pathway to thrombin production is initiated by the release of tissue factor (TF) from injured tissues. TF binds to factor VII in the presence of calcium (TF.VII). This complex will activate factor X to Xa. Factor VII also stimulates the activation of factor IX in the presence of phospholipid and calcium. Therefore, tissue factor initiates factor Xa formation and links the extrinsic to the intrinsic pathway. Additionally, factors IXa, Xa, and XIIa can feed back and activate factor VII (TF.VIIa). The TF.VIIa complex possesses a 100-fold greater proteolytic potential than does TF.VII.[26]

Factor Xa, factor Va, prothrombin, and calcium are brought into the correct spatial configuration on the platelet membrane. This prothrombinase complex greatly accelerates the production of thrombin.

Thrombin's primary action is to proteolytically cleave fibrinopeptides A and B from the fibrinogen molecule. The resulting fibrin monomers polymerize and propagate to form a gel. Factor XIII is activated by thrombin to covalently cross-link adjacent fibrin monomers within the fibrin polymer. Crosslinking forms a stable clot that is more resistant to lysis by plasmin. Thrombin also stimulates further platelet aggregation and activates factors VIII and V and protein C. Thrombin stimulates IL 1 secretion by the endothelium, leading to the expression of TF on endothelial surfaces. The events of thrombin generation and the subsequent fibrin stabilization of the platelet plug are termed "secondary hemostasis."

Coagulation Inhibition. Two major systems have evolved to control thrombin formation. The major physiologic inhibitor of thrombin is the glycoprotein AT III, which is synthesized in the liver and endothelial cells. AT III also inhibits factors IXa, Xa, XIa, and XIIa. The inactivation of the activated coagulation factors is enhanced at least 1000-fold whenever AT III binds to circulating heparin or endothelial-bound heparin-like molecules. After the AT III–heparin

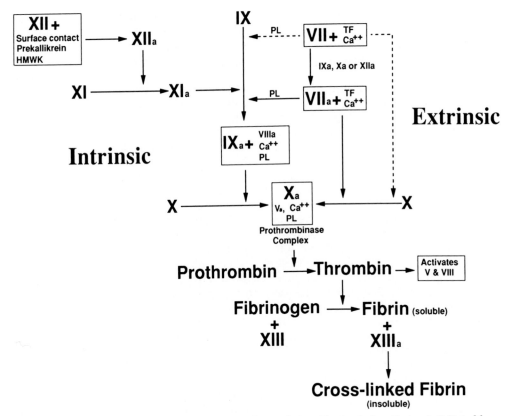

FIGURE 5–1. The intrinsic and extrinsic pathways of coagulation. The intrinsic pathway is initiated by surface contact while the extrinsic pathway is initiated by the release of tissue factor (TF) from tissues injured during surgery or trauma. Factor VIIa possesses a 100-fold greater activity than factor VII. The pathways are interrelated and operate in tandem to achieve hemostasis. PL, phospholipid from activated platelet or endothelial membranes.

complex binds to an activated coagulation factor, the heparin dissociates and continues to act as a catalyst for the formation of other AT III–serine enzyme complexes.

Heparin cofactor II is another specific inhibitor of thrombin. It is a glycoprotein that acts as a heparin cofactor to form a stable 1:1 complex with thrombin, inhibiting its activity. Unlike AT III, heparin cofactor II cannot inhibit other clotting factors. The plasma concentration of heparin cofactor II is approximately one half that of AT III and it is unlikely that heparin cofactor II plays a major role in the regulation of hemostasis.[27]

The second major system to control thrombus formation involves protein C and protein S. Thrombin binds to thrombomodulin on endothelial surfaces, catalyzing the activation of protein C in the presence of protein S. Activated protein C cleaves coagulation factors Va and VIIIa, thus inhibiting thrombin formation. It also stimulates the release of tissue plasminogen activator.[10]

Fibrinolysis

Plasminogen is bound to fibrinogen and remains bound to fibrin. t-PA, a protease released from endothelial cells during thrombin generation, also binds to fibrin, thus enhancing the proteolytic activation of plasminogen to plasmin.[28] Plasmin, a serine protease, digests fibrin as well as the coagulation and other plasma proteins. The fibrin degradation products released have an inhibitory effect on fibrin polymerization and platelet aggregation. Plasmin released into plasma is rapidly inhibited by α_2-plasmin inhibitor.[28] This specific inhibitor of plasmin also binds to cross-linked fibrin and to fibrin-bound plasminogen. Thus within the fibrin clot, mechanisms exist to both degrade fibrin and limit its degradation. The outcome depends on the relative concentrations of activators and inhibitors. Several less specific proteases that inhibit fibrinolysis are α_1-protease inhibitor and α_2-macroglobulin.

Recently, several t-PA inhibitors (PAI) have been identified. PAI-1, the most common inactivator of plasminogen, is released by endothelial cells and platelets. This inhibitor efficiently inactivates t-PA in plasma. PAI-2 is a specific inhibitor of urokinase and t-PA. It is released into the circulation during pregnancy by the placenta. PAI-3, found in urine and plasma, is an inhibitor of the activation of plasminogen by urokinase. Additional roles for the plasminogen activator inhibitors remain to be defined.[13,29]

Preoperative Evaluation

A good history and a thorough physical exam will detect the majority of bleeding disorders preoperatively. Laboratory testing is warranted if a bleeding disorder is present or suspected. Careful questioning should distinguish a congenital bleeding disorder from an acquired one. Determining the pattern of inheritance may further aid in identifying a congenital deficiency. A history of bleeding problems beginning in childhood or at the beginning of menses implies an inherited bleeding disorder. A history of postoperative or spontaneous bleeding in a family member is important because many patients with inherited disorders will not experience serious bleeding until challenged by an operative procedure or trauma. All patients should be asked about bleeding following tooth extraction, minor trauma, circumcision, and other surgical procedures.

An acquired hemostatic disorder should be suspected in adults who bleed during or following surgery or trauma but have no previous history of bleeding disorders. However, some patients with congenital disorders, such as von Willebrand's disease, may not demonstrate their bleeding diatheses until challenged. Patients with liver disease are at increased risk for developing a coagulopathy during surgery, after trauma, and after massive transfusion. Patients resuscitated with greater than 20 ml/kg of hetastarch in 24 hours are at risk for bleeding from decreased platelet adhesiveness and deficiencies in coagulation proteins. Patients receiving greater than 1.5 mg/kg of dextran in 24 hours are also at increased risk for bleeding as a result of impaired platelet function and reduced plasma concentration of vWF. A detailed history of drug use is also important because many drugs alter platelet function and predispose patients to bleeding complications.

Physical examination should include a thorough inspection for ecchymoses, petechiae, purpura, hemangiomas, jaundice, hematomas, and hemarthroses. Petechiae are frequently associated with platelet dysfunction, while ecchymoses may be due to a variety of vascular, platelet, or coagulation abnormalities. Hemarthroses and frequently hematomas are associated with congenital bleeding disorders. Splenomegaly may be associated with thrombocytopenia. Signs of hepatic insufficiency should be noted because these patients may have decreased production of coagulation proteins. Patients suffering from myeloproliferative disorders, some malignant neoplasms, collagen disorders, or renal insufficiency are at increased risk for bleeding complications.

The "screening" laboratory tests include: platelet count and examination of peripheral blood smear; bleeding time; and prothrombin time (PT), activated partial thromboplastin time (aPTT), and thrombin time. The bleeding time, a very sensitive test for hemosta-sis, is prolonged with qualitative platelet deficiencies as well as with decreased levels of fibrinogen and factors V and VIII:vWF. The PT assesses the extrinsic pathway and is prolonged by deficiencies of prothrombin, fibrinogen, and factors V, VII, and X. The aPTT is prolonged by deficiencies of factors in the intrinsic pathway, including VIII, IX, XI, and XII, and to a lesser extent detects factor deficiencies in the common pathway: V, X, prothrombin, and fibrinogen. The aPTT is also prolonged by heparin and by the lupus anticoagulant. The lupus anticoagulant binds to phospholipids and inhibits the formation of the prothrombinase complex in vitro; it does not cause clinical bleeding. The thrombin time is prolonged by hypofibrinogenemia, fibrin abnormalities, and heparin.

Hemorrhagic Disorders of the Vascular Wall

Congenital and acquired disorders of vessels are infrequently responsible for severe hemorrhage in surgical or trauma patients (Table 5–2). The congenital disorders include the Ehlers-Danlos syndrome, pseudoxanthoma elasticum, and Marfan's syndrome. Bleeding in these patients with inherent vessel wall structural defects may be very difficult or impossible to control.

Patients with *Ehlers-Danlos syndrome* present with fragile tissues, hypermobile and hyperextendable joints, and bleeding diatheses. This syndrome may be transmitted as an autosomal dominant, recessive, or X-linked trait. Type IV Ehlers-Danlos patients have decreased amounts of type III collagen in their vessels. We have experienced a 40 per cent mortality and a 60 per cent recurrent bleed rate in five of these patients.[30] Seventy per cent of patients with type IV Ehlers-Danlos syndrome have been reported to die of spontaneous arterial rupture. Aneurysms and aortic dissections are also common. Patients with type IV Ehlers-Danlos syndrome should avoid elective surgery because of the risk of hemorrhage and the known delay in wound healing. Arteriography is contraindicated in most patients with type IV Ehlers-Danlos syndrome.

Patients with *pseudoxanthoma elasticum*, inherited as an autosomal recessive trait, suffer from a defect in elastic fibers causing them to have a characteristic

TABLE 5–2. VASCULAR DISORDERS ASSOCIATED WITH BLEEDING

Congenital Disorders	Acquired Disorders
Ehlers-Danlos syndrome	Purpura
Marfan's syndrome	Inflammatory
Hereditary hemorrhagic telangiectasia	Drug induced
Pseudoxanthoma elasticum	Amyloidosis
Osteogenesis imperfecta	Diabetes
	Macroglobulinemia

facies, redundant folds of skin, and weakened vessel walls. These patients are predisposed to develop early atheromatous changes and have an increased tendency for thrombosis of their major arteries. Spontaneous hemorrhage may occur, most commonly in the gastrointestinal tract or subarachnoid space. No prolongation of bleeding times or delays in wound healing have been reported.[31]

Marfan's syndrome is transmitted as an autosomal dominant trait characterized by arachnodactyly, long limbs, ocular defects, and cardiovascular abnormalities. The principle causes of death for these patients are aortic insufficiency and dissection. However, these patients may also bleed excessively while undergoing elective surgery.[32]

Acquired disorders of vessel walls are more common than congenital defects. Scurvy causes decreased vascular collagen and decreased platelet adherence. Amyloidosis may result in purpura, ecchymoses, and spontaneous bleeding. Cushing's syndrome has a characteristic purpura that is secondary to the loss of dermal connective tissues. Inflammatory disorders, diabetes mellitus, infectious diseases, and drug reactions may be responsible for acquired vascular disorders. In both congenital and acquired coagulation disorders, awareness and correction of any coagulation deficit and meticulous attention to hemostasis intraoperatively may minimize hemorrhagic complications.

Platelet Disorders

Hemorrhagic complications may occur because of quantitative or qualitative platelet disorders that are acquired or congenital in origin. Thrombocytopenia and qualitative platelet defects are among the commonest causes of bleeding in surgical patients. Spontaneous bleeding may occur when platelet counts fall below 20,000/cu mm. Platelet counts between 30,000 and 50,000/cu mm are adequate to assure hemostasis provided that there are no associated functional platelet or coagulation disorders. Platelet counts of 50,000 to 100,000/cu mm are required to restore hemostasis during bleeding. Thrombocytopenia may occur from increased platelet destruction, abnormal production, or temporary sequestration.

Thrombocytopenia

Platelets may be "consumed" at regions of endothelial damage. This mechanism has been proposed to explain the thrombocytopenia seen in patients with thrombotic thrombocytopenic purpura, some vasculitides, and the hemolytic-uremic syndrome. In these syndromes, platelets are stimulated to aggregate and become trapped in the microcirculation. These processes are difficult to detect; their management is empirical. Early plasma exchange or transfusion has been of benefit. The use of platelet inhibiting medications to decrease platelet aggregation has been proposed.[33,34]

Immune platelet destruction may occur with primary disease processes or may be drug induced. Platelets are destroyed in the spleen following antibody binding to platelets in both acute and chronic idiopathic thrombocytopenic purpura. In emergency settings, patients are managed by platelet transfusion, plasma exchange, or intravenous gamma globulin.[35] Long-term therapy consists of treatment with corticosteroids, followed by splenectomy in nonresponders. Certain drugs (e.g., quinidine and sulfonamides) act as haptens to form antibody-antigen complexes that bind to platelet membranes. Therapy includes halting the use of the offending drug.

Deficient production of platelets occurs in patients with Fanconi's anemia, a congenital disorder characterized by bone marrow aplasia. The toxic effects of radiation or drugs such as busulfan, thiazides, and chloramphenicol lead to decreases in platelet production. Infections may cause thrombocytopenia as a result of decreased platelet production as well as by causing endothelial damage, which leads to increased platelet consumption. Finally, thrombocytopenia may be due to the redistribution of platelets by sequestration or by dilution.

Thrombocytopenia commonly follows massive transfusions of banked blood. Only 10 per cent of platelets remain viable in blood held in cold storage for longer than 24 hours. The percentage of functionally normal platelets is even less. Dilutional thrombocytopenia following massive transfusion in surgical patients is further amplified by consumption of platelets by the coagulation process initiated by operative trauma.

Hypothermia (less than 32° C) may also cause thrombocytopenia. The mechanisms of the hypothermia-induced bleeding diathesis is unclear.[36] However, sequestration of platelets during hypothermia is well documented. Platelets appear to become activated, release alpha granule products, aggregate, and become sequestered in the portal circulation. Rewarming causes a return of up to 80 per cent of the circulating platelets in animal studies.[37] Recently, investigators have also described cases of apparent hypothermia-induced disseminated intravascular coagulation (DIC), perhaps caused by the release of tissue thromboplastin from cold-injured tissue.[38] The cold-induced coagulopathy is best prevented by transfusing warmed blood products and maintaining the core body temperature above 32° C.

When quantitative deficiencies of platelets are present intraoperatively, platelet transfusions are necessary to increase the platelet count to greater than 50,000 platelets/cu mm to ensure hemostasis. Postoperatively, platelets should be transfused in any bleeding patient with less than 50,000 platelets/cu mm. Nonbleeding patients with less than 20,000 platelets/cu mm should be followed closely for signs of spontaneous bleeding and transfused if bleeding occurs. One unit of single donor platelets will usually increase a patient's platelet count by 10,000 platelets/cu mm.

Qualitative Platelet Disorders

Qualitative platelet disorders should be suspected when bleeding occurs in patients with normal coagulation studies and platelet counts. Qualitative disorders may be congenital or acquired; acquired disorders are much more common. Disturbances of platelet adherence and aggregation rarely cause bleeding spontaneously but certainly exacerbate bleeding secondary to surgery and trauma. Congenital qualitative platelet disorders include von Willebrand's disease, Bernard-Soulier syndrome, thrombasthenia (Glanzmann's disease), and "storage pool" diseases.

Von Willebrand's disease is characterized by decreased platelet adherence resulting from a deficiency in factor VIII:vWF or the presence of abnormal variants of VIII:vWF. Von Willebrand's disease is usually transmitted as an autosomal dominant trait. Heterozygotes may have minimal symptoms, such as excessive ecchymosis and menorrhagia, and may also bleed following minor surgery. Homozygotes, however, exhibit severe bleeding during surgery and may have histories of hemarthroses and spontaneous bleeding. Decreased platelet adherence causes prolongation of the bleeding time. The PT and aPTT are normal. Ristocetine aggregation of platelets is impaired but can be corrected with the addition of factor VIII:vWF–rich cryoprecipitate. Patients scheduled for surgery should have their factor VIII levels adjusted to above 40 to 50 per cent of normal to assure adequate hemostasis.[39] Purified factor VIII contains little factor VIII:vWF; therefore cryoprecipitate, which contains high concentrations of factors VIII:vWF and VIII:C, should be used. Factor VIII levels should be followed closely postoperatively and transfusions of cryoprecipitate used as necessary until the wound is healed.

Patients with type I von Willebrand's disease, the most common type of vWD (80 per cent), may benefit from infusion of deamino(-D-arginine) vasopressin (DDAVP), which will decrease the bleeding time and frequently obviate the need for transfusion of blood products.[40] DDAVP causes an increase in plasma factor VIII:C and VIII:vWF activity that shortens the bleeding time in 60 per cent of patients with type I von Willebrand's disease. Some patients with type IIa vWD may also have DDAVP-induced correction of the bleeding time. DDAVP is contraindicated in patients with type IIb von Willebrand's disease because it will not correct the bleeding time and may cause platelet aggregation and thrombocytopenia in these patients. If DDAVP is ineffective in types I and IIa vWD, cryoprecipitate should be administered to replace the vWF.

Bernard-Soulier syndrome is transmitted as an autosomal recessive trait and is characterized by the lack of glycoprotein Ib in platelet membranes. These patients have prolonged bleeding times, mild to moderate thrombocytopenia, and giant platelets. Without glycoprotein Ib, platelets cannot adhere to subendothelial connective tissue.[19] Normal platelets should be transfused to assure proper primary hemostasis.

Thrombasthenia, or Glanzmann's disease, is a rare autosomal recessive trait in which platelet membranes lack glycoproteins IIb and IIIa, leading to failure of platelet aggregation after initial adherence. These patients experience serious bleeding during surgery or after trauma and should be managed by platelet transfusions.

"Storage pool" diseases are a group of rare hereditary disorders characterized by defects in platelet granule content such that aggregation following granule release is minimized. Platelet transfusion is recommended prior to surgery.

Acquired qualitative abnormalities are commonly caused by the effects of drugs. Aspirin is probably the commonest cause of abnormal platelet aggregation. Aspirin acetylates cyclooxygenase, inhibiting the synthesis of the prostaglandin endoperoxides and thromboxane. This irreversible event inhibits platelet aggregation and granule release by the thromboxane A_2/endoperoxide pathway for the life of the platelet. Aspirin also blocks the synthesis of PGI_2 by endothelial cells, but this effect is short lived and reversible. Other nonsteroidal antiinflammatory drugs, such as indomethacin, phenylbutazone, and ibuprofen, reversibly inhibit cyclooxygenase. Dipyridamole has been shown to inhibit platelet aggregation by increasing platelet phosphodiesterase. Certain antibiotics, including carbenicillin, ticarcillin, mezlocillin, piperacillin, and moxalactam, have been shown to prolong bleeding times and impair platelet aggregation because they coat platelet membrane receptors.

Uremia, cirrhosis, myeloproliferative disorders, leukemia, and dysproteinemias may result in qualitative platelet disorders. Uremia appears to cause decreased platelet adherence and aggregation in response to thrombin and arachidonic acid. Uremic patients have prolonged bleeding times. DDAVP has been shown to reverse prolonged bleeding times preoperatively in uremic patients.[40] DDAVP, 0.3 to 0.4 μg/kg, is given intravenously; bleeding times have been normalized in up to 75 per cent of patients within 1 hour.

Coagulation Disorders

Defects in secondary hemostasis may be due to congenital or acquired disorders of coagulation factors.

Congenital Disorders

Congenital disorders of coagulation usually involve a single factor. Preoperative transfusion of the appropriate factor is necessary and may be required during surgery and postoperatively. Deficiencies of factor XII, HMWK, and prekallikrein cause prolongation of the aPTT, but do not cause significant bleeding diatheses. Deficiencies of the remaining factors (except III and IV) may result in serious bleeding following surgery or trauma.

Hemophilia A is the commonest of the inherited coagulation defects. It is due to a deficiency of factor VIII. *Hemophilia B* (Christmas disease) is clinically indistinguishable from hemophilia A and is due to a deficiency of factor IX. Both hemophilia A and B are sex-linked recessive disorders, but hemophilia A is seven times more frequent (1:10,000). Deficient amounts of factors VIII and IX result in failures of secondary hemostasis and are frequently associated with episodic bleeding into deep tissues, with resultant hematomas or hemarthroses. Excessive bleeding frequently follows trauma or surgery. The severity of these disorders depends upon the amount of plasma factor VIII or IX activity that is present; the presence of greater than 5 per cent of normal plasma factor activity will prevent spontaneous bleeding. Factor VIII:C plasma activity should be 50 per cent of normal for most elective surgical procedures; patients undergoing cardiac, vascular, and neurosurgical procedures require 80 to 100 per cent of normal VIII:C activity.[41]

Appropriate levels of factor VIII may be restored by transfusing fresh-frozen plasma, cryoprecipitate, or purified factor VIII. Fresh-frozen plasma or purified factor IX may be used in patients with Christmas disease. Plasma factor activity should be followed postoperatively and maintained above 25 per cent until adequate wound healing occurs. Patients may require transfusions for 7 to 21 days. Up to 10 per cent of patients with factor VIII deficiencies will develop antibodies to factor VIII. These patients will require larger amounts of factor VIII to maintain adequate plasma activity.[41] Factor VIII levels may be sufficiently increased by DDAVP in patients with mild hemophilia A to allow safe elective surgery.[40] Bleeding from superficial wounds or intraoperative surfaces may be controlled with the combination of pressure or topical thrombin.

Abnormalities of fibrinogen may also be inherited. Afibrinogenemia is inherited as an autosomal recessive trait and is very rare. Dysfibrinogenemia refers to autosomal dominant traits characterized by synthesis of structurally abnormal fibrinogens. Patients with these disorders may develop hemorrhagic complications. The level of normal fibrinogen necessary for hemostasis is 100 mg/dl. This level may be obtained by transfusion of cryoprecipitate or fresh-frozen plasma.

Congenital hyperfibrinolytic states have recently been described that may result in bleeding. The congenital hyperfibrinolytic states include heterozygous and homozygous α_2-antiplasmin deficiencies, elevated levels of t-PA, and functionally abnormal PAI-1.[42] Epsilon aminocaproic acid (EACA) is recommended for managing patients who bleed from their congenital hyperfibrinolytic state.[29]

Acquired Disorders

Patients develop acquired coagulation disorders because of deficiencies of coagulation proteins, synthesis of nonfunctioning coagulation factors, and consumption or inadequate replacement of coagulation proteins. Hepatic insufficiency may contribute to significant bleeding in surgical patients as a result of reductions in factors II, V, VII, IX, X, XIII, and fibrinogen. However, levels of factors VIII:C and VIII:vWF may be elevated in these patients. The presence of subclinical DIC in patients with longstanding or severe hepatic insufficiency has been postulated.[43] Correction of a coagulopathy in patients with advanced liver failure may not be possible except by replacement therapy. Replacement of coagulation proteins with fresh-frozen plasma is recommended because vitamin K_1 administration alone may not, especially with advanced liver failure, reverse the coagulopathy. The thrombocytopenia associated with hepatic insufficiency should be treated by platelet transfusions.

Vitamin K deficiency may cause a bleeding diathesis as a result of the synthesis of nonfunctional forms of the vitamin K–dependent coagulation factors II, VII, IX, and X. Vitamin K deficiency may be caused by poor dietary intake, antibiotic therapy, abnormal liver function, and biliary obstruction. Administration of vitamin K_1, 10 to 20 mg subcutaneously or intramuscularly, will correct the hemostatic defect, if liver function is adequate, in 24 to 48 hours. Intravenous vitamin K_1 (2.5 mg) will help restore the clotting defect more quickly. Fresh-frozen plasma may be used to promptly correct the coagulation defect and is preferable if the patient is to be anticoagulated with warfarin again. Vitamin K_1 should be administered preoperatively to patients with hepatic insufficiency, obstructive jaundice, and malabsorption states or malnutrition in order to increase their level of vitamin K–dependent coagulation proteins.

The banked blood used for massive transfusion not only contains few, if any, functional platelets, but may be deficient in factors V and VIII. The dilution of circulating factors V and VIII by massive transfusion may cause bleeding; however, more significantly, it potentiates the posttransfusion bleeding diatheses often associated with long operations complicated by hypotension and massive blood loss.

Vascular patients may have bleeding complications secondary to excessive anticoagulation. Heparin has a short half-life of 90 minutes; therefore, heparin infusion should be stopped 1 to 2 hours preoperatively to assure hemostasis. Bleeding from excessive heparin may be neutralized by administering dilute protamine sulfate, 1 mg/100 units of heparin, slowly to avoid hypotension. Patients should wait 2 to 4 days after stopping warfarin anticoagulation prior to elective surgery. Deficiencies of vitamin K–dependent coagulation factors can be corrected slowly with the administration of vitamin K and more rapidly with fresh-frozen plasma.

Disseminated intravascular coagulation is characterized by intravascular coagulation with consumption of coagulation factors and platelets and secondary activation of the fibrinolytic system. Its etiology may be attributed to massive tissue destruction, sepsis, hypotension, trauma, transfusion reaction, arteriovenous fistula, cavernous hemangioma, vasculitis, hepatic insufficiency, and aneurysm.[43-45] Fibrin and platelet deposition occurs in the microcirculation while plasminogen is converted to plasmin, which initiates fibrinolysis and maintains patency of the microcirculation. Hemorrhage is associated with severe DIC because deficiencies of coagulation factors and platelets develop as a result of their continued intravascular consumption. The fibrin degradation products produced by secondary fibrinolysis possess a strong anticoagulant effect and potentiate the bleeding diathesis.

A DIC may exist in which coagulation factors and platelets are replaced as they are consumed—a compensated DIC. This type of DIC is diagnosed only by laboratory testing. The presence of ecchymoses and petechiae in patients should alert the surgeon to the possibility of a low-grade DIC. During surgery, DIC may be accelerated by tissue trauma, hypotension, and/or transfusion reactions, with the consumption of coagulation factors and platelets now occurring faster than they can be replaced, leading to excessive bleeding. Regardless of the etiology, the surgeon should be alerted to the development of DIC either by persistent bleeding from newly incised surfaces, indicating a failure of hemostasis, or by fresh bleeding from previously dry areas, indicating lysis of previously formed clots.

A combination of abnormal laboratory test results, including thrombocytopenia, prolongation of the PT and aPTT, hypofibrinogenemia, and increased fibrin degradation products, confirms the clinical diagnosis of DIC. At the time of surgery a whole-blood clotting test may be performed by placing 1 ml of blood in a glass tube and assessing clot formation. Failure of the blood to clot or the formation of a friable clot that undergoes lysis within 1 hour suggests the presence of DIC.[46]

The first goal of management is the elimination of the cause of the DIC. When this is possible, the intravascular coagulation ceases with the return of normal hemostasis. In severe DIC, with ongoing blood loss, patients are best managed by replacement of deficient blood elements using whole blood, fresh-frozen plasma, and platelets while the precipitating cause of the DIC is eliminated. If the cause of the DIC cannot be eliminated, transfusion of blood elements may increase the consumption of coagulation factors.

Some investigators have proposed that heparin may be beneficial in halting the consumptive process of DIC.[44] Heparin administration is occasionally beneficial in those patients with active bleeding in whom blood product replacement is unable to restore hemostatic levels of coagulation factors. Heparin should be used cautiously, in a loading dose of 3000 units intravenously followed by 300 to 500 units/hour, with careful clinical observation and laboratory monitoring. EACA, which inhibits clot lysis by preventing the binding of plasminogen to fibrin, should not be used early in DIC because the fibrinolysis is necessary to prevent excessive fibrin deposition in the microcirculation. However, after the stimulus to intravascular coagulation is removed and the DIC is controlled, EACA may be used to treat any persistent secondary hyperfibrinolysis. The usual adult dose of EACA is 5 g intravenously as a loading dose and 1 g/hour until excessive lysis is controlled, usually in 3 to 6 hours.[46]

Primary hyperfibrinolysis is a rare cause of clinical bleeding and is often difficult to distinguish from the secondary hyperfibrinolysis of DIC. Both conditions are characterized by reduced coagulation proteins. Platelet counts are normal in patients with primary hyperfibrinolysis and are decreased in patients with DIC. Primary hyperfibrinolysis is associated with conditions that cause excessive fibrinolytic activation, such as electric shock, extracorporeal circulation, acute hypoxemia, severe acidosis, and leukemia. Management consists of removing (i.e., extracorporeal circulation) or improving the conditions (i.e., hypoxemia, acidosis, leukemia) that led to the primary hyperfibrinolysis. EACA is offered if the hyperfibrinolytic states persist.

THROMBOSIS

Virchow suggested, in 1856, that thrombus formation was the result of an interaction between an injured surface, stasis, and the hypercoagulability of blood. One or more components of Virchow's triad can be invoked when determining the etiology of an in vivo thrombosis. The only major process that contributes to intravascular thrombosis not recognized by Virchow is that of hypofibrinolysis.

Venous Thrombosis

Venous thromboses form under conditions of low or disturbed flow and are composed of red cells and fibrin with relatively few platelets.[47] The thromboses usually begin as small platelet aggregates in vein valve pockets where areas of maximum stasis occur or on injured vein walls. Venostasis allows high concentrations of activated clotting factors to remain in proximity to vessel walls and reduces the rate at which activated clotting factors are exposed to circulating anticoagulants. Many of these thromboses are asymptomatic and undergo spontaneous lysis. However, activation of coagulation, by release of tissue factor by surgery, trauma, or other stimuli, accelerates the coagulation process and increases the rate of thrombus formation beyond that which can be controlled by the anticoagulants and/or the fibrinolytic system.

Inherited Prethrombotic Conditions

Deficiencies of anticoagulant proteins are inherited as autosomal dominant traits. Patients with such deficiencies have an increased tendency to develop thrombosis; a homozygote condition may be incompatible with life.

Antithrombin III Deficiency. The most prevalent inherited hypercoagulable state, with an incidence of 1:5000 of the population, is caused by a deficiency of AT III. AT III is the major plasma inhibitor of thrombin and also inhibits factors IXa, Xa, XIa, and XIIa. Patients with congenitally low levels of AT III are predisposed primarily to venous thrombosis. The risk of thromboembolism increases as functional AT III activity decreases below 80 per cent of normal, with the highest risk occurring when the AT III levels drop below 60 per cent of normal.[48] The level of AT III in heterozygotes is usually 40 to 70 per cent of normal. The development of thromboembolism usually begins during the second decade. While thromboembolism may occur spontaneously, it is usually associated with a precipitating event, such as surgery, trauma, or pregnancy. Arterial thrombosis, although less common than venous thrombosis, also occurs. AT III levels may be reduced to less than 80 per cent of normal in other disease states, including hepatic insufficiency, DIC, venous thrombosis, sepsis, and in women on oral contraceptives. The minimum level of AT III necessary to prevent thrombosis is unknown; however, it is suggested that levels be adjusted to greater than 80 per cent of normal activity prior to surgery in patients with acquired or congenital AT III deficiency. AT III may be replaced by transfusion of fresh-frozen plasma or cryoprecipitate. AT III concentrate is available in limited quantities. Long-term warfarin therapy is recommended for patients with AT III deficiencies who have experienced thrombotic events.

Protein C and Protein S Deficiencies. More than half of heterozygotes with protein C deficiency develop a pulmonary embolism or deep vein thrombosis before their fifth decade.[49] Homozygotes often die early in life from thrombotic complications; however, if protein C levels are greater than 5 per cent, they may survive to adulthood. Functional and immunologic assays are available to establish the diagnosis of protein C deficiencies. Histories of patients with congenital protein S deficiencies are very similar to those of patients with low levels of protein C.[50] The plasma concentration of protein S that is necessary to avoid life-threatening thrombotic events appears to be lower than 5 per cent. Arterial thrombosis is uncommon. However, protein C and S deficiencies have been found in 15 to 20 per cent of patients less than 50 years old with peripheral vascular occlusive disease.[51]

Both protein C and protein S are vitamin K–dependent proteins synthesized in the liver. Consequently, their plasma levels are decreased in patients with hepatic insufficiency. Patients with chronic renal failure, vitamin K deficiency (malabsorption, biliary obstruction), DIC, and patients undergoing major operative procedures may also have decreased protein C and S levels.

Fresh-frozen plasma may restore functional levels of protein C and protein S. Life-long warfarin anticoagulation has been recommended for patients with deficiencies of these proteins; however, warfarin should be used selectively because many patients never develop thrombosis. Cutaneous necrosis is more likely to occur when warfarin anticoagulation is used in protein C–deficient patients. Consequently, all patients, and especially those with protein C deficiency, should receive heparin for the first 3 or 4 days of warfarin therapy because protein C levels are depressed more rapidly than are coagulation factors II, IX, and X.

Heparin Cofactor II Deficiency. Heparin cofactor II is produced by the liver and is a specific inhibitor of thrombin. Heparin cofactor II deficiency is a rare condition that is transmitted in an autosomal dominant fashion. Heparin cofactor II inactivates thrombin by binding to it in a 1:1 stoichiometric relationship. Heparin dramatically enhances the rate of thrombin inactivation by heparin cofactor II. Patients with heparin cofactor II deficiency are at risk for thrombosis when their cofactor II level becomes 50 per cent or less of normal.[52] Of 41 patients identified to have congenital heparin cofactor II deficiency, 15 had thrombotic events.[53] Heparin cofactor II deficiency should be considered a risk factor for thrombosis. However, conclusive evidence of a causal relationship between heparin cofactor II deficiency and thrombosis has not been proven.

Deficient Plasminogen and Plasminogen Activator Activity. Increased thrombotic tendencies have also been reported in patients with defects in plasminogen or the plasminogen activator system. Patients have been reported possessing functional deficiencies of plasminogen as a result of the production of 12 variant forms of the plasminogen molecule.[54] Functional abnormalities of plasminogen have included altered active sites and inability of the molecule to form activator complexes. Patients with recurrent thromboembolism have been identified who have decreased production of plasminogen activator by venous endothelial cells obtained by biopsy. Patients affected by these deficiencies may suffer arterial and venous thromboses, and are treated with long-term warfarin therapy.[55]

Homocysteinemia. Homocysteinemia is due to an inborn error of metabolism related to the deficiency of several enzymes. Homocysteine accumulates in plasma and tissues resulting in many clinical abnormalities. Homocysteinemia is associated with early onset atherosclerosis and thrombosis. Thrombosis is thought to be related to the circulating homocysteine, which damages endothelial cells and causes platelet aggregation. The elevated homocysteine levels and associated atherosclerotic and thrombotic tendencies may be prevented by pyridoxine (300 mg/day) and antiplatelet drugs (dipyridamole 100 mg/day and acetylsalicylic acid 1 gm/day).[56] Folic acid (10 mg/day), cobalamin (0.3 mg/day), and riboflavin (9 mg/day) also lower plasma homocysteine levels.[57]

Acquired Prethrombotic Conditions

Thromboses are frequently caused by acquired disorders that affect coagulation. *Endarterectomy and balloon angioplasty* expose deep layers of the arterial wall, which initiates platelet interaction and activation of coagulation. All synthetic grafts develop a limited mural thrombus after implantation. Endothelial cells usually cover the synthetic graft for only 1 to 2 cm from either anastomosis. The pseudointima that forms on the remainder of the graft surface is composed of fibrin, collagen, fibroblasts, and smooth muscle–like cells. Large-diameter grafts interposed in high-flow conditions will remain patent despite the absence of an endothelial lining. However, small-diameter prosthetic grafts (less than 6 mm) or grafts placed in low-flow conditions have less satisfactory patency rates.

Many *clinical disorders* predispose to thrombosis by activating the coagulation system or causing platelet aggregation. Soft tissue trauma, thermal injuries, and operative dissection all predispose to thrombosis through activation of the extrinsic coagulation pathway by releasing tissue thromboplastin.

Sepsis predisposes to thrombosis via multiple mechanisms. Gram-positive bacteria may directly cause platelet aggregation and subsequent thrombosis. Gram-negative bacterial endotoxin may stimulate platelet aggregation but may also, through interaction with leukocytes and endothelial cells, cause tissue factor–like activation of the coagulation system. Endotoxin is known to be a major stimuli for the development of DIC.

Malignancies are associated with an increased incidence of venous thrombosis.[58,59] Some, such as multiple myeloma, promyelocytic leukemia, and mucin-secreting adenocarcinomas, are known to secrete tissue thromboplastin. Colonic, vaginal, and breast cancers are known to release proteases capable of activating factor X. Many patients with malignancies have increased concentrations of factors V, VIII, IX, and X and fibrinogen and decreased AT III, which increases their risk for thrombosis.

Pregnant women and those on exogenous estrogens have an increased tendency to develop venous thrombosis. Although the exact mechanism is unclear, these women demonstrate increased levels of factors II, VII, VIII, IX, and X with low levels of AT III and decreased activity of the plasminogen activator system.[60]

Intravascular hemolysis may promote thrombosis by making available phospholipid that activates the intrinsic coagulation pathway. Transfusion of incompatible blood, hemolytic anemias, paroxysmal nocturnal hemoglobinuria, and cardiopulmonary bypass all may cause hemolysis.

Circulating *lupus anticoagulants* are IgG or IgM immunoglobulins to platelet and endothelial cell membrane phospholipids that cause prolongation of affected patients' aPTTs. These patients also have a striking predisposition for thrombosis. The mechanism is unclear. However, patients with systemic lupus erythematosus, malignancies, and peripheral vascular occlusive disease who have circulating lupus anticoagulants and anticardiolipin antibodies have a high incidence of pulmonary embolism, venous thrombosis, myocardial infarction, acute peripheral arterial occlusion, and abortions.[51] Patients suspected of having the lupus anticoagulant are not only tested for this, but also for anticardiolipin antibodies, because 15 per cent of patients may not have a functional lupus anticoagulant. Long-term warfarin therapy is recommended for these patients. Warfarin may be discontinued when the IgM and/or IgG immunoglobulins are no longer detectable.

Hyperlipidemia, myeloproliferative diseases (e.g., polycythemia vera, chronic myelogenous leukemia, myeloid metaplasia), diabetes mellitus, sepsis, hemolytic-uremic syndrome, and thrombotic thrombocytopenic purpura predispose to thrombosis because of their effect on platelets. Hyperlipidemia may activate platelets, by modulating adenylate cyclase activity or increasing thromboxane A_2.[61,62] Diabetes mellitus affects platelets and the vessel wall by increasing thromboxane A_2, factor VIII:vWF, and fibrinogen while decreasing platelet sensitivity to PGI_2.[63,64] Both thrombotic thrombocytopenic purpura and the hemolytic-uremic syndrome are characterized by the deposition of platelet-fibrin aggregates in the microcirculation. Smoking is associated with an increased risk of arterial thrombosis. Platelets of smokers exhibit hypersensitivity to aggregatory agents. Smoking may also damage endothelium and subendothelial structures and decrease PGI_2 production.

Venous Thromboembolism Prophylaxis

The incidence of venous thrombosis and pulmonary embolism may be reduced by limiting venous stasis and/or administering drugs to inhibit coagulation. Stasis is reduced by ambulation or other forms of muscle activity, compressive hose, and pneumatic compression of the lower extremities. A review of four randomized trials evaluating the effects of elastic stockings revealed a 9.3 per cent incidence of deep vein thrombosis in patients wearing stockings and a 24.5 per cent incidence in the controls.[65]

Pneumatic compression has proven benefit in lowering rates of lower extremity venous thrombosis. The rhythmic alteration of pressure within the leg compartments increases venous return and augments fibrinolysis. External pneumatic compression has proven as effective as low-dose subcutaneous heparin in preventing venous thrombosis in surgical patients.[66] Pneumatic compression may be more effective in patients undergoing open prostatectomy and neurosurgical patients than is low-dose subcutaneous heparin.[67,68] A combination of low-dose heparin and pneumatic compression stockings may be more effective in preventing venous thrombosis than either alone.[69] The efficacy of external pneumatic compression in preventing pulmonary embolism has been demonstrated.[66,70]

Anticoagulant drugs effectively prevent venous

thrombosis when properly administered. Antiplatelet drugs are less effective in preventing venous thrombosis.

Warfarin.   Warfarin has a proven role in the prevention of venous thromboembolism. Warfarin inhibits the synthesis of the vitamin K–dependent coagulation factors II, VII, IX, and X. Warfarin also decreases the production of vitamin K–dependent anticoagulant protein C and protein S, a cofactor for C. Decreases in factor activity are dependent on the circulating half-lives of the factors; factor VII reaches a steady state after 1 to 2 days, whereas prothrombin (factor II) takes up to 10 days. Patients with liver disease or vitamin K deficiency (malnourished condition or receiving long-term intravenous alimentation without vitamin K supplementation) or the elderly should receive reduced initial dosages. Daily loading doses greater than 10 mg are not indicated. Numerous drugs may affect the actions of warfarin (Table 5–3). The maintenance dose is the daily dose that keeps the prothrombin time 1.5 to 1.7 times the control.[71] The primary complication of warfarin's use is hemorrhage. Less common complications include alopecia, urticaria, dermatitis, fever, nausea, diarrhea, abdominal cramping, and hypersensitivity reactions. Dermal gangrene of the thigh, breast, and/ or buttocks is a rare complication. It is felt to result from a rapid decrease in protein C levels, producing a transient hypercoagulable state and dermal venous thrombosis. This complication is prevented by the simultaneous administration of heparin during the first 3 to 4 days of warfarin therapy.

Numerous studies have established the efficacy of warfarin in preventing venous thrombosis and embolism, but most emphasize limiting its use to high-risk patients because of the risk of hemorrhage. Sevitt and Gallagher found that the incidence of clinical venous thrombosis in patients with hip fractures decreased from 28.7 per cent in the control group to 2.7 per cent in the group treated with oral anticoagulation. At autopsy, the incidence of thrombosis in the two groups was 83 and 14 per cent, respectively.[72] In other studies, the incidence of pulmonary embolism in patients while on warfarin therapy averaged 1.2 per cent compared to 8.4 per cent in untreated patients; the risk of serious hemorrhage ranged between 3 and 7 per cent and fatal hemorrhages occurred in an average of 0.3 per cent of patients receiving warfarin.[72–74] The frequency of hemorrhagic complications increases as the prothrombin time increases.

The prophylactic use of warfarin seems justified in certain groups; for example, patients with recent femur or hip fractures, hip surgery, or malignancies capable of inducing a prethrombotic state, in which low-dose subcutaneous heparin has proven less efficacious.

Subcutaneous Heparin.   Heparin is a glycosaminoglycan with a molecular weight between 5000 and 48,000. Commercial heparin is derived from beef and pork lung or intestine. The AT III binding site of heparin has been identified as a pentasaccharide that is present in only one third of heparin's saccharide chains. Heparin combines with AT III in a 1:1 stoichiometric ratio. This creates a conformational change in AT III, which makes its active centers more available for binding to thrombin and other serine proteases of the coagulation cascade. The heparin–AT III complex irreversibly inhibits factors IIa, IXa, Xa, XIa, and XIIa. Heparin dissociates after the serine protease is bound and can then combine with another AT III binding site.

Small doses of heparin administered subcutaneously prevent thrombosis in low- to moderate-risk patients with normal levels of AT III. Low-dose heparin is less effective in high-risk patients and in patients with activated coagulation systems. In pooled data from randomized clinical trials evaluating venous thrombosis prophylaxis in general surgery patients, the incidence of thrombosis diagnosed by fibrinogen scan and phlebogram was reduced from 19.1 per cent (288/1507) in controls to 6 per cent (50/831) in patients receiving low-dose subcutaneous heparin.[65] The incidence of serious complications with low-dose heparin prophylaxis is low, with fatal hemorrhage occurring in 0.2 per cent of patients in an international, multicenter clinical trial.[75] The low-dose subcutaneous heparin regimen consists of administering 5000 units subcutaneously 2 hours preoperatively, followed by 5000 units every 8 to 12 hours postoperatively. Laboratory monitoring of the aPTT is usually not needed. Patients may develop the heparin-induced thrombocytopenia syndrome from low doses of heparin. Therefore, patients receiving subcutaneous heparin should have daily platelet counts.

Several investigators have advocated the use of low-molecular-weight (LMW) heparin for prophylaxis of venous thrombosis. The LMW heparins have smaller pentasaccharide units (less than 18 to 20 saccharides) and therefore can't simultaneously bind AT III and thrombin. Compared to standard heparin, LMW heparins have decreased anticoagulant activity

TABLE 5–3.   DRUG INTERACTIONS WITH ORAL ANTICOAGULANTS

Potentiate	Antagonize
Allopurinol	Antihistamines
Aminoglycosides	Carbamazepine
Anabolic steroids	Cholestyramine
Chloramphenicol	Glutethimide
Chlorpromazine	Griseofulvin
Cimetidine	Haloperidol
Chlofibrate	Oral contraceptives
Co-trimoxazole	Phenobarbital
Dipyridamole	Phenytoin
Disulfiram	Spironolactone
Metronidazole	Vitamin K
Phenylbutazone	
Quinidine	
Oral hypoglycemic drugs	
Salicylates	
Tricyclic antidepressants	

as measured by the aPTT and maintain anti-Xa activity. Theoretically, LMW heparins might prevent thrombosis, may have a lower incidence of hemorrhagic side effects, and possibly are less antigenic. Kakkar and Murray compared LMW heparin with standard heparin in a controlled trial of patients undergoing abdominal surgery.[76] Patients received either 1850 units of LMW heparin once daily and a placebo or 5000 units of standard heparin twice a day. No difference was reported in the incidence of wound hematomas or serious bleeding episodes in the groups. The LMW heparin group had a 2.5 per cent incidence of venous thrombosis, which was significantly lower than the 7.5 per cent of patients in the standard heparin group. The incidence of bleeding complications with LMW heparin have been reported to be higher[77] and lower[78] than unfractionated heparin.

Low-dose heparin administration effectively prevents fatal pulmonary embolism in general surgical patients. A large multicenter trial compared the low-dose heparin regimen with controls in 4121 randomized patients (2076 controls; 2045 heparin). One hundred-eighty patients, 100 controls and 80 patients receiving heparin, died. Only two deaths in the heparin group were directly attributed to pulmonary embolism, compared to 16 deaths among the controls.[75] This significantly lower incidence of fatal pulmonary embolism in patients receiving heparin has been demonstrated by others.[69]

A combination of 5000 units of heparin and 0.5 mg of dihydroergotamine has been used for venous thromboembolism prophylaxis. Dihydroergotamine increases venous flow by constricting capacitance vessels and, to a lesser degree, the resistance vessels. The effects of dihydroergotamine appear not to be limited to increasing venous flow; the vasoconstriction may stimulate plasminogen activator activity, thereby promoting fibrinolysis. The effectiveness of heparin with dihydroergotamine was compared to low-dose heparin in nine randomized trials, including over 1600 general surgical patients.[65] Fibrinogen scanning found the incidence of deep venous thrombosis was 9.0 per cent among dihydroergotamine-treated patients and 14.5 per cent in patients treated with low-dose standard heparin. There was no difference in the incidence of pulmonary embolism in the groups. However, there were significantly fewer major bleeding complications in the dihydroergotamine-treated patients (0.26 versus 1.6 per cent). Dihydroergotamine may cause severe arterial vasoconstriction and clinical ergotism. Although the incidence of this complication is around 0.2 per cent, it has slowed the acceptance of dihydroergotamine for venous thromboembolism prophylaxis.[79]

Dextran. Dextran has been used prophylactically to prevent both venous and arterial thromboses. Dextran appears to decrease platelet adhesiveness and alter the release reaction, which results in decreased aggregation. Dextran also decreases plasma VIII:vWF. High concentrations (10 mg/ml plasma) interfere with the polymerization of fibrinogen, so that clots that form are more susceptible to lysis by plasmin. The plasma volume-expander action of dextran also increases blood flow and thus reduces venostasis.

Results from several studies reveal that venous thrombosis developed in 15.6 per cent (115/738) of patients receiving dextran and 24.2 per cent (193/799) of controls.[65] Dextran has been reported to reduce by half the incidence of venous thrombosis following femur fractures or hip surgery.[80,81] However, Brisman et al. prospectively examined the use of dextran 70 in high-risk surgical patients and found no improvement in mortality or incidence of pulmonary embolism compared to controls.[82] Gruber et al. compared dextran 70 infusion with low-dose heparin in a multicenter, prospective study; the incidence of fatal pulmonary embolism was the same for each group.[83]

The amount of dextran proven effective in clinical trials has varied between 500 ml of a 6 per cent solution to 1000 ml of a 10 per cent solution of either dextran 40 or dextran 70 over 24 hours. Hemorrhagic complications are increased if greater than 10 per cent of a patient's blood volume is replaced by dextran. Dextran infusion may be associated with other serious complications, including pulmonary edema secondary to plasma volume expansion, renal failure, allergic reactions, and rare anaphylactoid reactions. Many clinicians prefer alternative measures for preventing deep venous thrombosis because of these potential complications.

Ancrod. Ancrod, the venom of the Malayan pit viper (*Agkistrodon rhodostoma*), cleaves fibrinopeptides-A from circulating fibrinogen, rendering the resultant molecule incapable of forming clot. Ancrod is administered by the subcutaneous or intravenous route. The level of hypofibrinogenemia can be more effectively titrated with intravenous administration. Anticoagulation can be achieved in 6 to 12 hours after the administration of 1 unit/kg over 2 to 4 hours. Serum fibrinogen levels are measured every 12 hours for 48 hours, then daily. Fibrinogen levels can usually be maintained in the 20 to 40 mg/ml range by the administration of 1 to 2 units/kg of ancrod every 24 hours. Ancrod may be beneficial in patients with heparin-induced thrombocytopenia and/or other complications of heparin. AT III–deficient patients who are resistant to heparin anticoagulation may be effectively treated with ancrod.[84] Uncommon complications related to ancrod use include fever, minor allergic reactions, and hemorrhage. Resistance to ancrod developed in 4 (three intramuscular and one intravenous administration) of 16 patients in one series.[85] Antibody production to ancrod is the likely cause for the resistance. The intravenous route is the preferred route for the administration of ancrod.

Arterial Thrombosis

Arterial thrombosis occurs in regions of disturbed flow (e.g., with stasis or turbulence) and in vessels with altered endothelial coverage (e.g., following endothelial ulceration and/or endarterectomy). Arterial thromboses contain relatively higher concentrations of platelets than do venous thromboses.[47] Vessel wall injury is more important in the pathogenesis of arterial thrombosis than venous thrombosis. In regions of high shear stress, endothelial cells may be denuded, allowing platelet adherence and aggregation to occur on the exposed subendothelium. Rupture of atherosclerotic plaques also exposes surfaces capable of initiating thrombosis. Following platelet adhesion and aggregation, coagulation is activated, leading to the formation of a mature thrombus. Vessel spasm may contribute to thrombosis in small muscular arteries. Thromboses are especially prone to develop in atherosclerotic vessels with altered endothelium and reduced flow. The thrombus size is limited by arterial shear force; an occlusive thrombosis will develop if the flow is sufficiently compromised.

Platelet Function—Inhibiting Drugs

Aspirin decreases platelet aggregation by acetylating cyclooxygenase and blocking the conversion of arachidonic acid to the prostaglandin endoperoxides PGH_2 and PGG_2. This effectively inhibits the synthesis of thromboxane A_2 for the lifespan of the acetylated platelet. Aspirin also inhibits PGI_2 synthesis by endothelial cells; however, the endothelial cells have nuclei and can synthesize new prostacyclin synthetase and reverse the effects of aspirin. As little as 160 mg of aspirin is capable of inhibiting 80 per cent of platelet cyclooxygenase activity.[86] The aspirin doses recommended have ranged between 80 and 1300 mg/day in clinical trials. We recommend that one aspirin (325 mg) be taken once daily with a meal. Aspirin is contraindicated in patients with aspirin hypersensitivity, active peptic ulceration, or bleeding diatheses.

Nonsteroidal antiinflammatory drugs, such as sulfinpyrazone, indomethacin, ibuprofen, and phenylbutazone, reversibly inhibit cyclooxygenase and cause decreased platelet aggregation.[87,88] Dipyridamole suppresses platelet aggregation by inhibiting platelet phosphodiesterase, causing a rise in intracellular cAMP. The elevation of cAMP levels causes a fall in cytoplasmic calcium, resulting in the inhibition of platelet aggregation. It also potentiates adenosine's inhibition of platelet function and may act synergistically with PGI_2. Dipyridamole has not proven effective alone and is used relatively infrequently at present.[89]

Ticlopidine is an antiplatelet drug currently undergoing clinical trials. Its platelet function—inhibiting effect appears to be secondary to an irreversible platelet membrane alteration and its effect lasts 5 to 7 days after discontinuing the drug. Adverse side effects have been described in approximately 2 per cent of patients and include pancytopenia, neutropenia, and agranulocytosis. Ticlopidine prophylactic effectiveness remains to be determined; however, early studies are encouraging. In one study, ticlopidine reduced the risk of stroke, myocardial infarction, and

vascular death by 23 per cent in patients who had had a previous stroke.[90]

Cerebrovascular Disease

Platelet function—inhibiting drugs have been extensively evaluated as prophylactic agents in patients who have suffered transient ischemic attacks (TIAs) and cerebral infarctions. Bousser et al. studied 604 patients with histories of TIAs and assigned them to receive either aspirin (990 mg/day), aspirin plus dipyridamole (325 mg aspirin/day), or placebo.[91] Seventeen patients in the aspirin group, 18 in the aspirin/dipyridamole group, and 31 in the placebo group developed cerebral infarctions during the 3 years of the study. The differences between the aspirin and placebo groups were significant; the addition of dipyridamole did not enhance the effects of aspirin alone. No sex differences were noted.

The Canadian Co-Operative Study Group examined the effects of aspirin, sulfinpyrazone, aspirin plus sulfinpyrazone, and placebo.[92] The aspirin-treated men had a significant reduction in the incidence of TIAs, stroke, or death. Sulfinpyrazone alone achieved no significant beneficial effect. Why women failed to benefit from aspirin therapy in this study but not in others is unclear.

These studies and others have effectively established that aspirin therapy results in a 20 to 30 per cent reduction in the incidence of stroke among patients with TIAs and minor strokes.[93,94] The generally accepted dose of aspirin varies from 325 to 1300 mg/day (the authors use 325 mg once daily with meals). Preliminary results from a study in Britain suggest that 325 mg/day offers equal protection with few side effects.[94]

Anticoagulants are of unproved value in patients who have suffered a major stroke. They are clearly contraindicated following hemorrhagic stroke. Many authors continue to recommend heparin therapy for patients with progressing strokes. Although this is a common practice, there have been no well-controlled randomized clinical trials proving the efficacy of anticoagulation in this setting. An exception may be the use of heparin in patients with cerebral emboli of cardiogenic origin, who have a 14 to 16 per cent incidence of repeat embolism within 2 weeks of their ischemic events. Early heparin therapy followed by 3 to 6 months of warfarin therapy have reduced the incidence of recurring embolism by 66 per cent.[94–96] If a brain scan reveals cerebral hemorrhage, anticoagulant therapy should be delayed.

Many clinicians have advocated the use of anticoagulation after TIAs because the risk of stroke is highest in the month following a TIA. No randomized controlled trial has proven the efficacy of heparin in preventing subsequent stroke following TIA. A recent population-based retrospective study of the initial management of patients with TIAs of recent onset found no differences in the incidence of stroke, death, or recurrent TIAs between patients treated with heparin and a control group that did not receive heparin during a 30-day period.[97] Despite the absence of evidence proving anticoagulant therapy efficacy, many clinicians continue to administer heparin to patients with focal cerebral ischemia, exposing them to the risk of hemorrhagic complications. Only appropriately designed randomized clinical trials can settle the debate over the role of anticoagulant therapy in the management of cerebrovascular disease.

Vascular Grafts

Recent clinical trials have examined the efficacy of antiplatelet drugs in maintaining the patency of saphenous vein aortocoronary artery bypass grafts. Chesebro et al. randomized patients to receive dipyridamole for 48 hours preoperatively and aspirin daily beginning 7 hours after aortocoronary artery bypass.[98] Thrombosis occurred in grafts of 10 per cent of patients receiving the placebo but only 3 per cent of the treated patients. One-year follow-up revealed a 25 per cent occlusion rate among the placebo group but only an 11 per cent rate in the treated group. Other investigators have demonstrated a similar effect with aspirin.[99]

Several studies have demonstrated the efficacy of aspirin in reducing lower extremity graft thrombosis when aspirin administration was begun within 24 hours of operation. Others have reported significant improvement in early patency of both saphenous vein and prosthetic grafts when the aspirin and dipyridamole were begun preoperatively.[100,101] However, Kohler et al. reported a large prospective trial in which no improvement in femoropopliteal bypass graft patency occurred when aspirin and dipyridamole were administered 24 hours postoperatively.[102] Platelet function–inhibiting therapy following peripheral vascular surgery is being used with increased frequency. We recommend that aspirin administration begin several days preoperatively (325 mg once daily) and that it be continued indefinitely. Aspirin can be given by suppository, if necessary, postoperatively.

The role of dextran in preventing arterial thrombosis has been studied. A recent clinical trial of dextran 40 in patients undergoing difficult lower extremity bypass procedures resulted in improved early graft patency.[103] Further clinical trials of dextran are necessary before its role as an arterial, antithrombotic, prophylactic agent can be defined.

Warfarin anticoagulation remains the prophylactic agent of choice for patients with prosthetic heart valves. Investigators have reported a lower incidence of embolic events when antiplatelet drugs, such as aspirin or dipyridamole, are added to the warfarin therapy.[104,105] However, there is an increase in hemorrhagic complications when the antiplatelet drugs are added.

Treatment of Established Thrombosis

Thrombolytic agents have an increasingly important role in the management of arterial and venous thromboses. Thrombolytic therapy is discussed in Chapter 18. Although the management of venous thromboembolic disorders is presented in Chapter 41, we emphasize here one of the potential complications of heparin therapy, that of heparin-induced thrombosis.

Heparin-Induced Thrombosis

Heparin-induced thrombocytopenia has two distinct patterns of presentation. The first is more common, occurring in 5 to 30 per cent of patients within 2 to 3 days of the onset of heparin therapy; the thrombocytopenia is transient and its sequelae are not clinically significant. The second type of thrombocytopenia has a delayed onset, occurring usually after 5 to 7 days of therapy, and is not dependent on dose or route of administration. All types of heparin can induce this second type of thrombocytopenia; the patients develop a heparin-dependent antibody that initiates platelet aggregation in the presence of heparin. This syndrome is associated with heparin-initiated thrombosis, thromboembolism, and rarely hemorrhage. A 61 per cent morbidity and a 23 per cent mortality rate have been reported in this syndrome.[106] The mortality and morbidity can be reduced to 22.5 and 12 per cent, respectively, with early recognition and treatment of the disorder.[107] Heparin-induced thrombocytopenia should be suspected in all patients receiving heparin who have falling platelet counts, increased resistance to heparin therapy, or new thrombohemorrhagic events. The diagnosis is established by platelet aggregometry studies. Management includes the prompt cessation of the administration of any form of heparin and the use of platelet function–inhibiting drugs. If anticoagulation is needed, alternate forms of anticoagulation should be used, such as warfarin, dextran, and hetastarch. It is recommended that all patients receiving heparin be monitored with daily platelet counts in order that the syndrome be recognized early.

Acute Peripheral Arterial Occlusion

The initial therapy for patients presenting with the signs and symptoms of acute peripheral arterial occlusion is prompt initiation of heparin therapy. Heparin arrests the thrombotic process and protects collateral flow by preventing clot propagation. The majority of patients should undergo thromboembolectomy using the techniques first described by Fogarty. Limb salvage rates of 95 per cent with 12 per cent mortality rates have been reported if balloon embolectomy is performed promptly and followed by anticoagulation.[108] Postoperative heparinization benefits the patient by lowering the incidence of recurrent thromboembolism and improving vessel patency. There is a 20 per cent incidence of wound hematomas among patients receiving heparin postoperatively. If arterial occlusion is due to emboli of cardiac origin, the patient should receive warfarin while the intracardiac thrombus is present.

Thrombolytic therapy has been successfully used

in the management of acute arterial occlusion (Chapter 36). The advantage of lytic therapy is the complete lysis of thrombus without the risks of surgery. Lytic therapy, however, may take from 12 to 72 hours to achieve this goal; therefore, the patient must be hemodynamically stable and the extremity viable. Lytic therapy frequently restores flow in the primary vessels and grafts and allows subsequent operative, balloon, or laser reconstruction of the graft and/or vessel segment responsible for the thrombosis. Thrombolytic therapy may be associated with hemorrhage, distal embolization, allergic reactions, and pericatheter thrombosis. Thrombolytic therapy should be used selectively after carefully weighing the morbidity, mortality, and anticipated difficulty of the surgical alternatives.

REFERENCES

1. Vanhoutte PM: Platelets, endothelium and vasospasm (abstr). Thromb Haemost 58:252, 1987.
2. Chesterman CN: Vascular endothelium, haemostasis and thrombosis. Blood Rev 2:88–94, 1988.
3. Engleberg H: Endothelium in health and disease. Semin Thromb Hemost 14:1–11, 1988.
4. Gorman RR, Bunting S, Miller OV: Modulation of human platelet adenylate cyclase by prostacyclin. Prostaglandins 13:377–378, 1977.
5. Pearson JD, Carlton JS, Hutchings A: Prostacyclin release stimulated by thrombin or bradykinin in porcine endothelial cells cultured from aorta and umbilical vein. Thromb Res 29:115–124, 1983.
6. Levin RI, Weksler BB, Marcus AJ, et al: Prostacyclin production by endothelial cells. In Jaffe EA (ed): Biology of Endothelial Cells. Boston, Martinus Nijhoff, 1984, pp 228–247.
7. Rosenberg RD, Rosenberg JS: Natural anticoagulant mechanisms. J Clin Invest 74:1–6, 1984.
8. Marcum JA, Atha DH, Fritze LMS, et al: Cloned bovine endothelial cells synthesize anticoagulantly active heparin sulfate proteoglycans. J Biol Chem 261:7505–7517, 1986.
9. Chan TK, Chan V: Antithrombin III, the major modulator of intravascular coagulation, is synthesized by human endothelial cells. Thromb Haemost 46:504–506, 1981.
10. Esmon CT, Owen WG: Identification of an endothelial cell cofactor for thrombin-catalyzed activation of protein C. Proc Natl Acad Sci USA 78:2249–2252, 1981.
11. Naworth PP, Brett J, Steinberg S, et al: Endothelium and protein S: Synthesis, release and regulation of anticoagulant activity (abstr). Thromb Haemost 58:49, 1987.
12. Stern D, Brett J, Hams K, et al: Participation of endothelial cells in the protein C–protein S anticoagulant pathway: The synthesis and release of protein S. J Cell Biol 102:1971–1978, 1986.
13. Kun-yu Wu K, Frasier-Scott K, Hatzakis H: Endothelial cell function in hemostasis and thrombosis. Adv Exp Med Biol 242:127–133, 1987.
14. Marlar RA, Kleiss AJ, Griffin JH: An alternative extrinsic pathway of human blood coagulation. Blood 60:1353–1358, 1982.
15. Rodgers GM, Shuman MA: Enhancement of prothrombin activation on platelets by endothelial cells and mechanism of activation of factor V. Thromb Res 45:145–152, 1987.
16. Miletich J, Kane W, Hofmann S, et al: Deficiency of factor Xa–factor Va binding sites on the platelets of a patient with a bleeding disorder. Blood 54:1015–1022, 1979.
17. Kaplan KL: Platelet granule proteins: Localization and secretion. In Gordon JL (ed): Platelets in Biology and Pathology. Amsterdam, Elsevier/North Holland, 1981, pp 77–90.
18. George JN, Nurden AT, Phillips DR: Molecular defects in interactions of platelets with the vessel wall. N Engl J Med 311:1084–1098, 1984.
19. Hagen I, Nurden A, Bjerrum OJ, et al: Immunochemical evidence for protein abnormalities in platelets from patients with Glanzmann's thrombasthenia and Bernard-Soulier syndrome. J Clin Invest 65:845–855, 1980.
20. Silver MJ, Smith JB, Ingerman CM, et al: Arachidonic acid–induced human platelet aggregation and prostaglandin formation. Prostaglandins 4:863–875, 1973.
21. Berridge MJ: Inositol triphosphate and diacyglycerol as second messengers. Biochem J 220:345–360, 1984.
22. Nachman RL, Leung LLK: Complex formation of platelet membrane glycoproteins IIb and IIIa with fibrinogen. J Clin Invest 69:263–269, 1982.
23. Walsh PN: The role of platelets in the contact phase of blood coagulation. Br J Haematol 22:237–254, 1972.
24. Walsh PN, Griffin JH: Contributions of human platelets to the proteolytic activation of blood coagulation factors XII and XI. Blood 57:106–118, 1981.
25. Stern DM, Bank I, Nawroth PP, et al: Self-regulation of procoagulant events on the endothelial cell surface. J Exp Med 162:1223–1235, 1985.
26. Zur M, Radcliffe RD, Oberdick J, et al: The dual role of factor VII in blood coagulation. Initiation and inhibition of a proteolytic system by a zymogen. J Biol Chem 257:5623–5631, 1982.
27. Tollefsen DM, Blank MK: Detection of a new heparin-dependent inhibitor of thrombin in plasma. J Clin Invest 68:589–596, 1982.
28. Collen D: On the regulation and control of fibrinolysis. Thromb Haemost 43:77–89, 1980.
29. Stump DS, Fletcher BT, Nesheim ME, et al: Pathologic fibrinolysis as a cause of clinical bleeding. Semin Thromb Hemost 16(3):260–273, 1990.
30. Cikrit DF, Miles JH, Silver D: Spontaneous arterial perforation: The Ehlers-Danlos specter. J Vasc Surg 5:248–255, 1987.
31. Scully RE, Mark EJ, McNeely BU: Case records of Massachusetts General Hospital. Weekly clinicopathologic exercises. N Engl J Med 308:579–578, 1983.
32. Bick RL: Vascular disorders associated with thrombohemorrhagic phenomena. Semin Thromb Hemost 5:167–183, 1979.
33. Thorsen CA, Rossi EC, Green D, et al: The treatment of the hemolytic-uremic syndrome with inhibitors of platelet function. Am J Med 66:711–716, 1979.
34. Brain MC, Neame PB: Thrombotic thrombocytopenic purpura and the hemolytic-uremic syndrome. Semin Thromb Hemost 8:186–197, 1982.
35. Imbach P, Barandun S, d'Apuzzo V: High-dose intravenous gammaglobulin for idiopathic thrombocytopenic purpura in childhood. Lancet 1:1228–1231, 1981.
36. Yoshihara H, Yamamoto T, Mihara H: Changes in coagulation and fibrinolysis occurring in dogs during hypothermia. Thromb Res 37:503–512, 1985.
37. Villalobos TJ, Adelson E, Riley PA, et al: A cause of the thrombocytopenia and leukopenia that occur in dogs during deep hypothermia. J Clin Invest 37:1–7, 1958.
38. Mahajan SL, Myer TJ, Baldini MG: Disseminated intravascular coagulation during rewarming following hypothermia. JAMA 245:2517–2518, 1981.
39. Biggs R, Matthews JM: The treatment of haemorrhage in von Willebrand's disease and the blood level of factor VIII. Br J Haematol 9:203–214, 1963.

40. Mannucci PM: Desmopressin (DDAVP) for treatment of disorders of hemostasis. Prog Hemost Thromb 8:19–45, 1986.
41. Bick RL: Congenital coagulation factor defects and von Willebrand's disease. In Disorders of Hemostasis and Thrombosis. New York, Thieme, Inc, 1985, pp 127–156.
42. Schleef RR, Higgins DL, Kellemer E, et al: Bleeding diathesis due to decreased functional activity of type I plasminogen activator inhibitor. J Clin Invest 83:1747, 1989.
43. Baker WF: Clinical aspects of disseminated intravascular coagulation: A clinician's point of view. Semin Thromb Hemost 15:1–57, 1989.
44. Feinstein DI: Treatment of disseminated intravascular coagulation. Semin Thromb Hemost 14:351–362, 1988.
45. Thompson RW, Adams DH, Cohen JR, et al: Disseminated intravascular coagulation caused by abdominal aortic aneurysm. J Vasc Surg 4:184–186, 1986.
46. Silver D: Sudden unexpected bleeding in critically ill surgical patients. Probl Gen Surg 4:512–520, 1987.
47. Hirsh J, Buchanan MR, Ofosu FA, et al: Evolution of thrombosis. Ann NY Acad Sci 516:586–604, 1987.
48. Sager S, Nairn D, Stamatakis JD, et al: Efficacy of low-dose heparin in prevention of extensive deep-vein thrombosis in patients undergoing hip replacement. Lancet 1:1151–1154, 1976.
49. Broekmans AW, Veltcamp JJ, Bertina RM: Congenital protein C deficiency and venous thromboembolism: A study of three Dutch families. N Engl J Med 309:340–344, 1983.
50. Broekmans AW, Bertina RM, Reinalda-Poot J, et al: Hereditary protein S deficiency and venous thromboembolism. Thromb Haemost 52:273–277, 1985.
51. Eldrup-Jorgensen J, Flanigan DP, Brace L, et al: Hypercoagulable states and lower limb ischemia in young adults. Vasc Surg 9:334–341, 1989.
52. Tollefsen DM: Laboratory diagnosis of antithrombin and heparin cofactor II deficiency. Semin Thromb Hemost 16(2):162–168, 1990.
53. Vinazzer H, Stocker K: Heparin cofactor II: Experimental approach to a new assay and clinical results. Thromb Res 61:235–241, 1991.
54. Robbins KC: Classification of abnormal plasminogens: Dysplasminogenemias. Semin Thromb Hemost 3:217–220, 1990.
55. Korninger C, Lechner K, Niessner H, et al: Impaired fibrinolytic capacity predisposes for recurrence of venous thrombosis. Thromb Haemost 52:127–130, 1984.
56. Harkar LA, Schicter SJ, Scott CR, et al: Homocystinemia: Vascular injury and arterial thrombosis. N Engl J Med 291:537–543, 1974.
57. Olszewski AJ, Szostak WB, Bialkowska M, et al: Reduction of plasma lipid and homocysteine levels by pyridoxine, folate, cobalamin choline, riboflavin and troxerutin in atherosclerosis. Atherosclerosis 75:1–6, 1989.
58. Kies MS, Posch JJ, Giolma JP, et al: Hemostatic function in cancer patients. Cancer 46:831–837, 1980.
59. Pineo GF, Brain MC, Gallus AS, et al: Tumors, mucus production and hypercoagulability. Ann NY Acad Sci 230:262–270, 1974.
60. Tooke JE, McNichol GP: Thrombotic disorders associated with pregnancy and the pill. Clin Haematol 10:613–630, 1981.
61. Sinha AK, Shattil SJ, Colman RW: Cyclic AMP metabolism in cholesterol-rich platelets. J Biol Chem 252:3310–3314, 1977.
62. Stuart MJ, Gerrard JM, White JG: Effect of cholesterol on production of TXB_2 by platelets in vitro. N Engl J Med 302:6–10, 1980.
63. Betteridge DJ, El Tahir KEH, Reckless JPD, et al: Platelets from diabetic subjects show diminished sensitivity to prostacyclin. Eur J Clin Invest 12:395–398, 1982.
64. Cowell JA, Winocour PD, Lopes-Virella M, et al: New concepts about the pathogenesis of atherosclerosis in diabetes mellitus. Am J Med 75:67–80, 1983.
65. Clagett GP, Reisch JS: Prevention of venous thromboembolism in general surgical patients. Ann Surg 208:227–240, 1988.
66. Salzman EW, Davies GC: Prophylaxis of venous thromboembolism: Analysis of cost effectiveness. Ann Surg 191:207–218, 1980.
67. Coe N, Collins RE, Klein L, et al: Prevention of deep vein thrombosis in urological patients: A controlled randomized trial of low dose heparin and external pneumatic compression boots. Surgery 83:230–234, 1978.
68. Black PMcL, Baker MF, Snook CP: Experience with external pneumatic calf compression in neurology and neurosurgery. Neurosurgery 18:440–444, 1986.
69. Torngren S: Optimal regimen of low dose heparin prophylaxis in gastrointestinal surgery. Acta Chir Scand 145:87–93, 1979.
70. Flanc C, Kakkar VV, Tuttle RJ, et al: Post-operative deep vein thrombosis: Effect of intensive prophylaxis. Lancet 1:477–478, 1969.
71. Hull R, Raskob G, Hirsch J, et al: A cost-effectiveness analysis of alternative approaches for long-term treatment of proximal venous thrombosis. JAMA 252:235–239, 1984.
72. Sevitt S, Gallagher NG: Prevention of venous thrombosis and pulmonary embolism in injured patients. Lancet 2:974–980, 1959.
73. Skinner DB, Salzman EW: Anticoagulant prophylaxis in surgical patients. Surg Gynecol Obstet 125:741–746, 1967.
74. Sevitt S: Venous thrombosis and pulmonary embolism: Their prevention by oral anticoagulants. Am J Med 33:703–716, 1967.
75. International Multicentre Trial: Prevention of fatal postoperative pulmonary embolism by low doses of heparin. Lancet 1:45–51, 1975.
76. Kakkar VV, Murray WJG: Efficacy and safety of low-molecular-weight heparin (CY216) in preventing postoperative venous thromboembolism: A co-operative study. Br J Surg 72:786–791, 1985.
77. Bergqvist D, Burmark US, Frisell J, et al: Low molecular weight heparin once daily compared with conventional low dose heparin twice daily. Br J Surg 73:204–208, 1986.
78. Hirsch J: Rationale for development of low molecular weight heparins and their clinical potential in the prevention of postoperative venous thrombosis. Am J Surg 161:512, 1991.
79. Gatterer R: Ergotism as complication of thromboembolic prophylaxis with heparin and dihydroergotamine. Lancet 2:638–639, 1986.
80. Harris WH, Salzman EW, DeSantis RW, et al: Prevention of venous thromboembolism following total hip replacement: Warfarin vs dextran 40. JAMA 220:1319–1322, 1972.
81. Ahlberg A, Nylander G, Robertson B, et al: Dextran in prophylaxis of thrombosis in fractures of the hip. Acta Chir Scand (Suppl) 387:83–85, 1968.
82. Brisman R, Parks LC, Haller JA: Dextran prophylaxis in surgery. Ann Surg 174:137–141, 1971.
83. Gruber UF, Saldeen T, Brokop T, et al: Incidences of fatal post-operative pulmonary embolism after prophylaxis with dextran 70 and low-dose heparin: An international multicentre study. Br Med J 280:69–72, 1980.
84. Cole CW, Brumanis J: Ancrod: A practical alternative to heparin. J Vasc Surg 8:59–63, 1988.
85. Pitney WR, Bray C, Holt PJL, Bolton G: Acquired resistance to treatment with arvin. Lancet 00:79–81, 1969.
86. Burch JW, Stanford N, Majerus PW: Inhibition of platelet prostaglandin synthetase by oral aspirin. J Clin Invest 61:314–319, 1978.
87. Steele P, Carroll J, Overfield D, et al: Effect of sulphinpyrazone on platelet survival time in patients with transient cerebral ischemic attacks. Stroke 8:396–398, 1977.
88. Weily HS, Genton E: Altered platelet function in patients with prosthetic mitral valves. Effects of sulphinpyrazone therapy. Circulation 42:967–972, 1970.
89. Chesebro JH, Fuster V, Elveback LR, et al: Trial of combined warfarin plus dipyridamole or aspirin therapy in prosthetic heart valves: Danger of aspirin compared with dipyridamole. Am J Cardiol 51:209–214, 1983.
90. Gent M, Blakely JA, Easton JO, et al: The Canadian Amer-

88   *Chapter 5*—HEMOSTASIS AND THROMBOSIS

ican Ticlopidine Study (CATS) in thromboembolic stroke. Lancet 1:1215–1220, 1989.
91. Bousser MG, Eschwege E, Haguenau M, et al: "AICLA" controlled trial of aspirin and dipyridamole in the secondary prevention of athero-thrombotic cerebral ischemia. Stroke 14:5–14, 1983.
92. Canadian Co-Operative Study Group: A randomized trial of aspirin and sulphinpyrazone in threatened stroke. N Engl J Med 299:53–59, 1978.
93. Riekkinen RJ, Lowenthal A, Googers FA: Main results of the European stroke prevention study. Neurology 37 (suppl 1):103, 1987.
94. Grotta JC: Current medical and surgical therapy for cerebrovascular disease. N Engl J Med 317:1505–1516, 1987.
95. Cerebral Embolism Task Force: Cardiogenic brain embolism. Arch Neurol 43:71–84, 1986.
96. Cerebral Embolism Study Group: Immediate anticoagulation of embolic stroke: A randomized trial. Stroke 14:668–676, 1983.
97. Keith DS, Phillips SJ, Whisnant JP, et al: Heparin therapy for recent transient focal cerebral ischemia. Mayo Clin Proc 62:1101–1106, 1987.
98. Chesebro JH, Fuster V, Elvback LR, et al: Effect of dipyridamole and aspirin on late vein-graft patency after coronary bypass operation. N Engl J Med 310:209–214, 1984.
99. Lorenz RL, Weber M, Kotzur J, et al: Improved aortocoronary bypass patency by low-dose aspirin (100 mg daily). Lancet 1:1261–1264, 1984.
100. Green RM, Roedersheimer R, DeWeese JA: Effects of aspirin and dipyridamole on expanded PTFE graft patency. Surgery 92:1016–1026, 1982.
101. Goldman M, Hall C, Dykes J, et al: Does 111-indium-platelet deposition predict patency in prosthetic arterial grafts? Br J Surg 70:635–638, 1983.
102. Kohler TR, Kaufman JL, Kacoyanis G, et al: Effect of aspirin and dipyridamole on the patency of lower extremity bypass grafts. Surgery 96:462–466, 1984.
103. Rutherford RB, Jones DN, Bergentz SE, et al: The efficacy of dextran 40 in preventing early postoperative thrombus following difficult lower extremity bypass. J Vasc Surg 1:765–773, 1984.
104. Arrants JE, Hairston P: Use of persantine in preventing thromboembolism following valve replacement. Am Surg 38:432–435, 1972.
105. Silver D, Kapsch D, Tsoi E: Heparin-induced thrombocytopenia thrombosis and hemorrhage. Ann Surg 198:301–306, 1983.
106. Dale J, Myhre E, Storstein O, et al: Prevention of arterial thromboembolism with acetylsalicylic acid. A controlled clinical study in patients with aortic ball valves. Am Heart J 94:101–111, 1977.
107. Laster J, Cikrit D, Walter N, et al: The heparin-induced thrombocytopenia syndrome: An update. Surgery 102:763–767, 1987.
108. Tawes RL, Harris EJ, Brown WH, et al: Acute limb ischemia: Thromboembolism. J Vasc Surg 5:901–903, 1987.

REVIEW QUESTIONS

1. The following are examples of endothelium's procoagulant nature except:
   (a) expression of tissue factor (thromboplastin)
   (b) expression of thrombomodulin
   (c) synthesis of factor V
   (d) synthesis of von Willebrand's factor
   (e) synthesis of plasminogen activator inhibitor

2. Which of the following is not true regarding platelet aggregation?
   (a) ADP released from dense granules initiates platelet-platelet interaction leading to loose aggregation
   (b) thromboxane A_2 stimulates platelet aggregation and granule release
   (c) von Willebrand's factor is essential for normal platelet aggregation
   (d) thrombin can induce platelet aggregation by activating phospholipase, leading to activation of protein kinase C
   (e) regardless of the stimulant, aggregation involves the reversible expression of fibrinogen receptors on the platelet surface

3. Which of the following is not a vitamin K–dependent coagulation factor?
   (a) factor II   (c) factor VII   (e) factor X
   (b) factor V   (d) factor IX

4. The extrinsic pathway to thrombin formation is initiated by:
   (a) platelet aggregation and release of dense granule contents
   (b) exposed subendothelial collagen
   (c) tissue factor, a phospholipid released by injured tissues
   (d) the activation of factor XII
   (e) the combined interaction of HMWK, prekallikrein, and a negatively charged surface

5. The major physiologic inhibitor of thrombin is:
   (a) heparin   (d) protein S
   (b) urokinase   (e) antithrombin III
   (c) tissue plasminogen activator

6. What is the maximum volume of hetastarch that can be used in a 24-hour period without dangerously decreasing platelet adhesiveness?
   (a) 5 ml/kg   (c) 15 ml/kg   (e) 30 ml/kg
   (b) 10 ml/kg   (d) 20 ml/kg

7. Type IV Ehlers-Danlos syndrome patients are characterized by all of the following except:
   (a) extremely low amounts of elastin
   (b) spontaneous arterial rupture
   (c) increased incidence of aortic aneurysms and dissections
   (d) hypermobile and hyperextensible joints
   (e) patients should avoid elective surgery because of the risk of hemorrhage

8. One unit of single donor platelets will usually raise a patients' platelet count by:
   (a) 1000 platelets/cu mm   (c) 10,000 platelets/cu mm
   (b) 5000 platelets/cu mm   (d) 15,000 platelets/cu mm

(e) 25,000 platelets/cu
  mm

(d) increased PTT
(e) prolonged bleeding times

9. Patients with von Willebrand's disease are characterized by:
   (a) increased fibrin degradation products
   (b) thrombocytopenia
   (c) increased PT

10. For most elective surgical procedures, factor VIII:C
    plasma activity should be at least:
    (a) 5 per cent of normal   (d) 75 per cent of normal
    (b) 25 per cent of normal   (e) 100 per cent of nor-
                                    mal
    (c) 50 per cent of normal

ANSWERS

1. b	2. c	3. b	4. c	5. e	6. d	7. a
8. c	9. e	10. c				

6

ATHEROSCLEROSIS: Pathology, Pathogenesis, and Medical Management

ALAN M. FOGELMAN, PETER A. EDWARDS, and
MARGARET E. HABERLAND

The major problems facing the vascular surgeon are the consequences of atherosclerosis. The lesions of atherosclerosis are characterized by intimal proliferation of smooth muscle cells, invasion of the damaged intimal layer by macrophages derived from blood-borne monocytes, and accumulation of large amounts of connective tissue matrix, together with large amounts of lipid. Early lesions are known as fatty streaks and are composed of cells filled with cholesteryl esters that give the cells a vacuolated appearance. Because of this appearance, these have been named foam cells. Some of these fatty streak lesions will disappear, and others will progress to fibromuscular lesions and, eventually, to complex lesions that consist of necrotic cells and intra- and extracellular lipids, including cholesterol crystals.

Risk factors for atherosclerosis include (1) low levels of high-density lipoprotein (HDL), (2) hyperlipidemia, (3) hypertension, (4) diabetes mellitus, (5) other genetic factors, and (6) gender.

THE RESPONSE TO INJURY HYPOTHESIS

The naturally occurring atherosclerotic lesions look very much like those that occur in experimental animals after endothelial injury. Ross[1] proposed that atherosclerosis results from a continuing repair process of the arterial wall, which is a response to continuing injury of the arterial intima. According to this hypothesis, the endothelial lining of arteries can be damaged by a number of factors, including hyperlipidemia, increased shear stress in hypertension, and hormone dysfunction.

Gerrity[2,3] and Faggiato, Ross, and Harker[4,5] have established that the earliest events in the development of atherosclerotic lesions involve recruitment of blood-borne monocytes into the subendothelial space.

Here the monocytes convert into cholesteryl ester–laden foam cells.[6] Additionally, some lymphocytes also migrate into the subendothelial space. The accumulation of foam cells in this space distorts the overlying single layer of endothelial cells. Eventually this distortion produces microseparations between the endothelial cells, and platelets adhere and release a number of factors, including a mitogen and thromboxane A_2 (TxA_2). The mitogen (platelet-derived growth factor) is essential for the division and growth of smooth muscle cells in tissue culture. The smooth muscle cells migrate into the subendothelial space and some convert into foam cells. As the accumulation of cells and lipid proceeds some cells die and release their contents into the artery wall. The process continues to expand from the subintimal space toward the adventitia. When expansion in an adventitial direction is no longer possible the process encroaches on the lumen, leading to obstruction to flow. Neovascularization of the plaque develops from adventitial vessels and in later lesions extracellular calcium deposition occurs. After many months the pathologic picture will vary considerably within the same vessel. Some plaque will demonstrate a predominance of foam cells; others will have only an occasional nest of foam cells and the predominant picture will be that of a smooth muscle cell lesion. More complicated lesions will contain a necrotic core covered by a fibrous plaque with or without ulceration, hemorrhage, calcification, and nests of foam cells.

PROSTAGLANDINS

The ability of platelets to aggregate at the endothelial cell surface is partially controlled by two prostaglandins with opposing effects. TxA_2 is synthesized by platelets from endogenous arachidonic acid and is released upon platelet aggregation. Released TxA_2 stimulates further platelet aggregation and also results in vasoconstriction. The endothelial cells and the underlying cells of the intima and media synthesize a prostaglandin different from arachidonic acid, prostacyclin [prostaglandin I_2 (PGI_2)]. However, PGI_2 prevents platelet aggregation and also acts as a vasodilator. Presumably, under normal conditions, the degree of vasoconstriction and aggregation of platelets is at least partly controlled by the relative amounts of TxA_2 and PGI_2. Aspirin in the usual therapeutic dosage (650 mg every 4 hours) is absorbed into the systemic circulation and therefore can inhibit the synthesis of both TxA_2 and PGI_2. However, low-dose aspirin (80 mg/day) acetylates the cyclooxygenase of platelets as they pass through the portal circulation and prevents TxA_2 formation. However, at this low dose little or no aspirin escapes from the liver and hence arterial PGI_2 synthesis is not inhibited.

Arachidonic acid is an essential fatty acid. It must be obtained from the diet directly or from linoleic acid, which can be converted to arachidonic acid. Eicosapentaenoic acid, another fatty acid, is also obtained from the diet primarily in fish, marine mammals, and other seafood. Eskimos who eat a diet rich in eicosapentaenoic acid have a low incidence of coronary atherosclerosis. This may in part be due to decreased platelet deposition on their artery walls.

Platelets from hypercholesterolemic patients have an increased tendency to aggregate and release more TxA_2 than platelets of normolipidemic patients.

LOW-DENSITY LIPOPROTEIN RECEPTORS

Our understanding of the mechanism by which hyperlipidemia contributes to the atherosclerotic disease process has come from the pioneering work of Brown and Goldstein.[7] These workers demonstrated that normal human cells in tissue culture have a cell surface receptor that recognizes plasma low-density lipoprotein (LDL). Once bound to the receptor, the LDL is internalized and transported to a compartment where proteolysis occurs, releasing amino acids into the medium. The cholesterol ester core of LDL is also hydrolyzed to unesterified cholesterol and a fatty acid. The cholesterol is released into the cell, where it brings about a number of metabolic changes:

1. It decreases the rate of endogenous cholesterol synthesis by inhibition of the rate-limiting enzyme in cholesterol biosynthesis, HMG-CoA reductase.

2. It stimulates the activity of the enzyme (ACAT) responsible for reesterifying the cholesterol.

3. It results in a reduction in the number of cell surface LDL receptors, which in turn leads to a decrease in the subsequent rate of uptake of LDL.

Brown and Goldstein and their colleagues have cloned the gene for the LDL receptor and have sequenced it. The structure of the receptor protein has thus been deduced. Normally, the receptor is synthesized in the endoplasmic reticulum, processed through the Golgi apparatus, and inserted into the plasma membrane. The inserted receptors are then concentrated in active regions of endocytosis called coated pits. Genetic abnormalities have been identified that result in no recognizable protein or an abnormal receptor protein that does not bind LDL normally. Rarely an abnormality occurs in which the receptor is inserted properly into the cell membrane and binds LDL normally. However, because of a defect in the cytoplasmic tail of the receptor the receptor-LDL complex is not clustered into the coated pits and internalized. Cells from heterozygous familial hypercholesterolemia patients have half the normal amount of receptors and demonstrate regulation of cellular metabolic functions intermediate between normal subjects and homozygotes.

Approximately 75 per cent of the degradation of LDL in humans and animals occurs by the LDL pathway. Hence, in these patients (hypercholesterolemia type IIa) with a defect in the LDL receptor, there is a decrease in the amount of LDL taken up and degraded by the receptor-mediated mechanism. Consequently, an increase is observed in the plasma LDL concentrations of such patients to levels as high as 1000 mg/dl LDL in homozygotes compared to the normal value of 120 mg/dl. Clinically, the patient with familial hypercholesterolemia is at a high risk for the development of atherosclerosis; the incidence of clinical atherosclerosis in males affected with the heterozygous form is 40 times normal.

HYPERLIPIDEMIA

Diagnosis

Diagnosis of hyperlipidemia requires a fasting blood sample (12- to 14-hour fast and not during the course of an acute myocardial infarction). If the cholesterol concentration in such a sample exceeds 260 mg/dl or the triglyceride concentration exceeds 150 mg/dl, hyperlipidemia is likely. A recent consensus panel of the National Institutes of Health has recommended that cholesterol levels should be below 200 mg/dl. Cholesterol and triglycerides are virtually insoluble in aqueous solutions. Their transport is dependent on their inclusion in water-soluble molecules called lipoproteins. Plasma lipoproteins may be grouped into five major classes according to their density in the ultracentrifuge: chylomicrons, very low-density lipoproteins (VLDLs), LDLs, intermediate-density lipoproteins (IDLs), and HDLs.

In some individuals (usually women), an elevated cholesterol level may be due to an elevation of HDL. While it is not necessary to measure the LDL concentration directly because of the high correlation with the total plasma cholesterol concentration, it is necessary to measure HDL separately. This is particularly important because of the inverse relationship between HDL levels and the risk for coronary heart disease. The triglyceride concentration reflects the VLDL and chylomicron content of the plasma. The presence of chylomicrons can be detected by allowing the plasma to stand overnight in the refrigerator. Chylomicrons will float to the top and form a cream layer. VLDLs will not float to the top but will remain in the infranatant, causing turbidity. There is no need to perform lipoprotein electrophoresis in the usual clinical setting. Determination of the fasting cholesterol, triglyceride, and HDL levels, together with the appearance of the plasma after an overnight stay in the refrigerator, is all that is required. If type III hyperlipoproteinemia (broad beta disease) is suspected, one must resort to ultracentrifugal analysis or determination of apoprotein E phenotypes.

Classification

Hyperlipidemias can be divided into those that are primary and those that are secondary.[8] In cases of the latter, discontinuing an offending drug may be all that is required.

Secondary Hyperlipidemias

In diabetic patients, there are two recognized causes of hyperlipidemia: overproduction of lipids and removal defects. A significant fraction of obese persons with adult-onset diabetes have hyperlipidemia caused by overproduction related to their hyperinsulinemia. When these individuals lose weight, their insulin levels and their lipid levels decline. Other diabetic persons have a removal defect due to an insulin deficiency, which causes their lipoprotein lipase activity to be subnormal; they may benefit from insulin therapy.

Primary Hyperlipidemias

Primary hyperlipidemias can be divided into those that have a genetic component and those that do not (often called sporadic hyperlipidemias). Genetic hyperlipidemias can be further divided into those that are monogenic (due to the action of a single gene) and those that are polygenic (due to multiple genes interacting with environmental factors).

Polygenic Hyperlipidemia. Polygenic hyperlipidemia occurs in 3 to 4 per cent of the population. It is characterized by an elevation in cholesterol and/or triglyceride levels in families such that the distribution of these levels is unimodal but shifted to a higher mean value. The risk for atherosclerosis is increased but not to the degree seen in the monogenic disorders, and the onset of clinical disease is often after age 60. Tendon xanthomas are rarely found in this disorder.

The relative risk ratio for coronary artery disease of sporadic hyperlipidemia is probably greater than normal but much less than that of monogenic hyperlipidemia.

Monogenic Hyperlipidemia. Monogenic disorders include familial hypercholesterolemia, familial hy-pertriglyceridemia, familial combined hyperlipidemia, broad beta disease, and lipoprotein lipase deficiency.

Familial hypercholesterolemia is an autosomal dominant disorder that has complete penetrance in childhood. By 1 year of age, 50 per cent of the children will have hypercholesterolemia with normal triglyceride levels. Both the cholesterol and triglyceride levels are normal in the other 50 per cent of the family members. This disorder has been classified based on the function of the receptor for LDL at the surface of cultured cells. The homozygous form of this disease is very rare and is characterized by plasma cholesterol levels of 800 to 1000 mg/dl. Children with this illness have xanthomas and coronary artery disease, which frequently leads to death before the age of 20. The heterozygous form occurs in 1 to 5 of every 1000 persons. The cholesterol levels typically range between 300 and 600 mg/dl. The triglyceride levels are typically normal or low; in some instances they are elevated, but the ratio of cholesterol to triglycerides is greater than or equal to 2:1. Half of the families carrying the gene for this disorder have at least one member with tendon xanthomas. The average age of myocardial infarction is in the early 40s. By age 40, approximately 40 per cent of those who require cardiac catheterization will have left main coronary artery disease.

Familial hypertriglyceridemia is an autosomal dominant disorder with incomplete penetrance in childhood. Only 10 per cent of the children will have hypertriglyceridemia. However, by age 30 half of the family members will have hypertriglyceridemia with normal cholesterol levels, whereas the other half will have normal lipid levels. As many as 1 per cent of the population may carry the gene for this disorder. Ordinarily, triglyceride levels are in the range of 250 to 300 mg/dl and the physical examination is not remarkable. However, oral contraceptives, estrogen treatment, alcohol, or untreated diabetes can lead to high triglyceride concentrations and even chylomicronemia. When the triglyceride level reaches 1500 mg/dl, eruptive xanthomas may appear, and there is risk of pancreatitis. The relative risk ratio for coronary heart disease is somewhere between two and five times normal in some families and is not increased above normal in other families.

Familial combined hyperlipidemia is also an autosomal dominant disorder with incomplete penetrance in childhood. Approximately 1 per cent of the population carries the gene for this disease. By age 30, half the family members will have abnormal lipid levels, whereas the other half will be normal. Of those that are affected, approximately one third will have hypertriglyceridemia (on the order of 250 mg/dl) but with normal cholesterol levels. Another third of the affected members will have normal triglyceride levels but elevated cholesterol levels (on the order of 300 mg/dl). The remaining third of the affected members will have an elevation in both cholesterol and triglyceride levels. These patients often have an excess of apolipoprotein B in their LDL relative to their LDL cholesterol content. The physical examination is not remarkable. Tendon xanthomas are rarely if ever found in this disorder. The relative risk ratio for coronary artery disease is 10 times normal, and the average age at which myocardial infarction occurs is 55 or less.

The incidence of *broad beta disease* (type III hyperlipoproteinemia) is no more than 1 in 5000 of the general population. It is characterized by the presence of increased circulating levels of IDL (the cholesterol-rich remnant created by the action of lipoprotein lipase on VLDL); IDLs are rarely, if ever, found in children, although 4 per cent of children from affected families may have hypertriglyceridemia. The usual lipid levels are about 450 mg/dl for cholesterol and 600 mg/dl for triglycerides. Frequently, there are swings in the lipid levels in these patients, but the ratio of the cholesterol concentration to the triglyceride concentration usually remains 1:1 regardless of the absolute lipid levels. The diagnosis of this disorder requires ultracentrifugal analysis or measurement of apoprotein E (apo E) phenotype. The most common form of this disorder requires the presence of an apo E phenotype designated E2:E2. The abnormality involves the substitution of a cysteine residue for an arginine residue in a critical area of apolipoprotein E. The incidence of premature atherosclerosis is clearly elevated in affected family members. Although peripheral vascular disease is relatively uncommon in familial hypercholesterolemia, it is present in more than a quarter of persons with broad beta disease. Xanthomas (palmar, tendinous, tuberous, or eruptive) are found in approximately three quarters of affected persons. More than half have xanthoma striata palmaris.

Lipoprotein lipase deficiency is a rare group of diseases that includes a form that has its onset in childhood and is characterized by eruptive xanthomas, lipemia retinalis, hepatosplenomegaly, episodic abdominal pain, and bouts of pancreatitis. This disease is often called type I hyperlipoproteinemia. The plasma looks like cream of tomato soup, the plasma triglyceride concentrations are often in the range of 3000 to 7000 mg/dl, and the cholesterol concentrations are in the range of 300 to 450 mg/dl. After the plasma has been left in the refrigerator overnight, a cream layer is seen on top of a clear infranatant layer. The disease appears to be due to a deficiency in lipoprotein lipase activity, which results in a failure to remove chylomicrons from the circulation. The most common clinical measurements of lipoprotein lipase activity are made after the administration of heparin—the postheparin lipolytic activity (PHLA). In normal persons, lipoprotein lipase activity increases; in this disorder, it remains low even after heparin administration. A less well-defined variant of lipoprotein lipase deficiency begins in the third decade of life and may be characterized by bouts of abdominal pain, pancreatitis, hepatosplenomegaly, lipemia retinalis, eruptive xanthomas (when the triglyceride concentrations exceed

1500 mg/dl), a higher than normal prevalence of diabetes, and hyperuricemia. The PHLA is usually not as low as that seen in type I hyperlipoproteinemia. When the plasma is left in the refrigerator overnight, a cream layer appears above a turbid infranatant layer. This disorder is frequently called type V hyperlipoproteinemia. The mode of inheritance is not clear and is often difficult to ascertain because of the frequent appearance of this phenotype in persons with diabetes, alcoholism, renal disease, hypothyroidism, and dysglobulinemia, and in persons on estrogen treatment or high-dose corticosteroid therapy. One cause for this disorder is a lack of apolipoprotein C-II, which is required for normal lipoprotein lipase activity. The gene for lipoprotein lipase has recently been cloned and sequenced and an explanation for many of the clinical syndromes associated with disorders of this enzyme should be forthcoming.

General Treatment Measures

Cigarette Smoking

Even in the genetically accelerated forms of atherosclerosis (e.g., familial hypercholesterolemia), cigarette smoking has been shown to dramatically increase the rate of progression of atherosclerosis. This increased rate of progression has been measured in terms of the onset of clinically evident disease and has been found to be on the order of one decade. Women with familial hypercholesterolemia who did not smoke on the average suffered a myocardial infarction in their 50s, whereas others with the same disease, even from the same family, who did smoke were found to have myocardial infarctions 10 years earlier. Persons with these disorders absolutely must not smoke.

Exercise

Exercise has been shown to decrease VLDL and LDL levels in persons with hyperlipidemia and to raise the HDL levels in some. These changes have been modest, but they may be quite important and are worthy of pursuing, because exercise also reduces the mortality from myocardial infarction (probably through an effect on peripheral resistance).

Blood Pressure

Hypertension adds to the accelerated atherosclerosis associated with hyperlipidemias and therefore should be controlled.

Dietary Management

Calories. Weight reduction is important in all forms of hyperlipidemia, even homozygous familial hypercholesterolemia. The goal is to reduce weight to the point of eliminating all excess fat. A simple device for determining the true lean body mass is to ask the patient what his or her weight was upon graduation from high school or college. If there was no gain in height after that time, in almost all cases the weight gained is fat. It is unusual in our society to gain muscle mass over that which was present at graduation. Having decided on the ideal body weight, the physician must prescribe caloric restrictions that will produce the desired weight loss. One of the major problems will be convincing the patient to ignore the remarks of others that he/she will "not look well" at the weight decided on. The importance of the weight loss may be realized only if the ideal body weight is actually achieved. Often, the decline in the lipid levels is minimal until all excess fat is lost. Exercise, together with the diet, will improve the patient's sense of well-being.

Saturated Fat. One of the main determinants of cholesterol synthesis and LDL receptor activity is the intake of saturated fatty acids. These should be reduced to the lowest possible level. A reduction from the usual 40 per cent of total calories to 25 to 30 per cent is not sufficient. Foods rich in saturated fatty acids include all dairy products except for skim milk and cheese made from skim milk, fatty plants such as avocados and nuts, and all red meats. Coconut and palm oil are also rich in saturated fatty acids.

Polyunsaturated Fat. The diet should not be greatly enriched with omega-6 polyunsaturates, such as corn oil, even though this produces a lowering of the plasma cholesterol concentration on the order of 10 per cent. There is evidence in animals and some epidemiologic data to suggest that a diet high in polyunsaturates may accelerate the development of cancer, and we advise our patients to reduce their total fat intake and to use polyunsaturates only as needed. Recent evidence suggests that a diet rich in omega-3 fatty acids (e.g., eicosapentaenoic acid), as are contained in fish oils (e.g., salmon), will lower triglyceride levels and decrease platelet aggregation. The decrease in VLDL and LDL by omega-3 fatty acids appears to be mediated by a decrease in the synthesis of apolipoprotein B. This beneficial effect may be offset in some patients by the absorption of cholesterol. Fish such as salmon are very rich in cholesterol and some patients will increase their cholesterol levels on such a diet. Frequent measurements of serum lipids are therefore indicated. Vitamin E supplementation (400 I.U./day) is also recommended when diets rich in omega-3 fatty acids are prescribed.

Monounsaturated Fat. Recent studies suggest that monounsaturated fat such as that contained in olive oil may lower LDL levels while modestly raising HDL levels.

Cholesterol. The vast majority of the cholesterol carried in the plasma is synthesized in the body. However, dietary cholesterol increases cholesterol levels in many patients with hyperlipidemia. Moreover, there is evidence suggesting that dietary cholesterol alters the composition of HDL, causing it to behave more like LDL. Therefore, we restrict the cholesterol intake in our patients with hyperlipidemia to less than 200 mg/day. Foods rich in cholesterol include egg yolks, crab, lobster, and shrimp. Other shellfish may contain as little as 40 per cent of their total sterols as cholesterol. The atherogenicity of the other marine sterols remains to be determined.

Alcohol. Alcohol has been shown to increase HDL levels, and its use has been shown to be inversely related to the risk for coronary artery disease. However, in patients with hypertriglyceridemia, particularly type V, alcohol may increase VLDL levels and lower HDL levels. For such patients, it should be restricted. It is our experience that unrestricted alcohol intake makes it impossible for patients to determine their caloric intake accurately; hence, we frequently limit alcohol intake to 8 oz of white wine (200 calories) each day.

Drug Therapy

There is now evidence that lowering plasma lipid levels by drug therapy will reduce the risk for atherosclerosis. We reserve these agents for persons who have failed to normalize their lipid levels on diet alone and who are at high risk for premature atherosclerosis (e.g., familial hypercholesterolemia, familial combined hyperlipidemia, broad beta disease), for those who already have evidence of premature atherosclerosis and hyperlipidemia, and for those who are symptomatic (e.g., eruptive xanthoma) or who are at risk for pancreatitis.

Since it has recently been found that Atromid-S (Ayerst) may be associated with reduced life expectancy, we now reserve this drug only for persons who are at risk for pancreatitis or for cases in which some other extenuating circumstance warrants its use.

Lovastatin (which inhibits HMG-CoA reductase) is usually well tolerated and is often effective in lowering LDL levels. The major side effects seem to be elevations in liver enzymes and in muscle enzymes in a minority of patients. Therefore blood tests need to be performed every 4 to 6 weeks during the first year of therapy and every 8 weeks afterward. Together with a bile acid sequestrant, lovastatin will lower LDL levels dramatically in many heterozygous familial hypercholesterolemics. The combination of nicotinic acid and a bile acid sequestrant is also often effective.[9] However, lovastatin, when used with niacin or gemfibrozil, is associated with an increased incidence of myositis. Bile acid sequestrants will lower LDL levels but may raise VLDL levels. Gemfibrozil will produce a modest lowering of LDL and a lowering of VLDL, and will raise HDL levels. Nicotinic acid may lower VLDL and LDL levels and may increase HDL levels. All of these agents have potential side effects and therefore they should only be used in appropriate cases and by experienced physicians.

Aspirin has been shown to reduce the risk for stroke and heart attack in males. We currently recommend 160 mg daily taken on a full stomach.

REFERENCES

1. Ross R: The pathogenesis of atherosclerosis—an update. N Engl J Med *314*:488–500, 1986.
2. Gerrity RG: The role of the monocyte in atherogenesis. I. Transition of bloodborne monocytes into foam cells in fatty lesions. Am J Pathol *103*:181–190, 1981.
3. Gerrity RG: The role of the monocyte in atherogenesis. II. Migration of foam cells from atherosclerotic lesions. Am J Pathol *130*:191–200, 1981.
4. Faggiotto A, Ross R: Studies of hypercholesterolemia in the nonhuman primate. II. Fatty streak conversion to fibrous plaque. Arteriosclerosis *4*:341–366, 1984.
5. Faggiotto A, Ross R, Harker L: Studies of hypercholesterole- mia in the nonhuman primate. I. Changes that lead to fatty streak formation. Arteriosclerosis *4*:323–340, 1984.
6. Brown MS, Goldstein JL: Lipoprotein metabolism in the macrophage: Implications for cholesterol deposition in atherosclerosis. Annu Rev Biochem *52*:223–261, 1983.
7. Brown MS, Goldstein JL: A receptor mediated pathway for cholesterol hemostasis. Science *232*:34–47, 1986.
8. Fogelman AM: Hyperlipidemia. *In* Hershman JM (ed): Management of Endocrine Disorders. Philadelphia, Lea & Febiger, 1980, pp 214–225.
9. Havel RJ, Kane JP: Therapy of hyperlipidemic states. Annu Rev Med *33*:417–433, 1982.

REVIEW QUESTIONS

1. The initial lesion in atherosclerosis is currently thought to involve:
   (a) monocytes
   (b) granulocytes
   (c) adipocytes
   (d) all of the above

2. A factor released from platelets that may be important in atherogenesis is:
   (a) glucose
   (b) cholesterol
   (c) platelet-derived growth factor
   (d) serotonin

3. The balance between thromboxane A_2 and which of the following may be important in determining platelet aggregation in vivo?
   (a) cholesterol
   (b) triglycerides
   (c) prostacyclin
   (d) prostaglandin E_2

4. Which fatty acid prolongs the bleeding time?
   (a) arachidonic acid
   (b) oleic acid
   (c) eicosapentaenoic acid
   (d) palmitic acid

5. Cholesterol primarily enters cells by:
   (a) diffusion through membranes
   (b) phagocytosis
   (c) cytosis
   (d) LDL receptor

6. High-density lipoprotein cholesterol is:
   (a) inversely correlated with risk for atherosclerosis
   (b) directly correlated with risk for atherosclerosis

7. Tendon xanthomas are found in patients with:
   (a) familial hypercholesterolemia
   (b) familial combined hyperlipidemia
   (c) familial triglyceridemia

8. Familial hypercholesterolemia is due to:
   (a) increased cholesterol absorption
   (b) lack of LDL receptors
   (c) overproduction of bile acids

9. The current treatment of choice for heterozygous familial hypercholesterolemia is:
   (a) cholestyramine or coestipol
   (b) lovastatin
   (c) both of the above

10. The dietary treatment of hyperlipidemia should emphasize:
    (a) avoidance of saturated fat
    (b) high consumption of unsaturated fat
    (c) both of the above

ANSWERS

1. a   2. c   3. c   4. c   5. d   6. a   7. a
8. b   9. c   10. a

7

HEMODYNAMIC FACTORS IN ATHEROSCLEROSIS

CHRISTOPHER K. ZARINS

Atherosclerosis is a degenerative process of the artery wall with well-recognized systemic risk factors such as hyperlipidemia, hypertension, and cigarette smoking. However, many individuals at high risk for atherosclerosis are free of significant plaque formation, while others with no recognized risk factors develop extensive lesions. Furthermore, morbidity and mortality usually result from localized plaque deposition rather than diffuse disease. Certain vessels, such as the abdominal aorta, carotid arteries, coronary arteries, and peripheral arteries, are particularly susceptible to plaque formation, while others, such as upper extremity vessels, are rarely involved. Even in susceptible arteries, plaque deposition is focal. The distal internal carotid is almost always free of disease despite marked atherosclerosis in the adjacent carotid bifurcation.

Several hypotheses have been proposed to account for the unique and focal pattern of atherosclerotic plaque formation. The knowledge that blood flow exerts stresses on vessel walls and affects mass transport to arterial tissue has led to the hypothesis that fluid dynamic forces are localizing factors in atherogenesis. Differences in local susceptibility and reactivity of the artery wall may also play a significant role. The purpose of this chapter is to examine both hemodynamic and artery wall factors that may determine the focal nature of plaque deposition and to consider the specific conditions that promote atherosclerosis in several highly vulnerable sites in the arterial tree.

HEMODYNAMIC FACTORS IN PLAQUE LOCALIZATION

Blood does not flow uniformly in the arterial tree because of variations in geometric configuration and resistance to flow. Differing lumen diameters, curvatures, branchings, and angles produce local disturbances in the primary flow field, resulting in regions of altered shear stress and boundary conditions with areas of separation, secondary flow patterns, and turbulence. Characterization of these conditions at specific sites becomes much more complex when the pulsatile nature of blood flow is taken into consideration. Branch points are known to be particularly vulnerable to plaque formation and are subject to wide variation in hemodynamic conditions. Thus, it is not surprising that a wide variety of hemodynamic factors have been implicated in plaque pathogenesis, including high and low wall shear stress, flow separation and stasis, oscillation of flow, turbulence, and hypertension.[1]

Wall Shear Stress

Wall shear stress (π_w) in arteries is the tangential drag force produced by blood moving across the endothelial surface. It is described by the Hagen-Poiseuille formula:

$$\pi_w = \frac{4\,\mu Q}{\pi r^3}$$

where μ = viscosity of blood, Q = blood flow, and r = radius. Wall shear stress is a function of the velocity gradient of blood near the endothelial surface and is directly proportional to blood flow and blood viscosity and inversely proportional to the cube of the vessel radius. Thus, a small change in vessel radius will have a large effect on wall shear stress.

High Shear Stress

High shear stress has been thought to potentiate plaque formation by producing endothelial injury and disruption, thereby exposing the underlying artery wall to circulating platelets and lipids.[2,3] Areas of high shear stress can be produced in the aorta of experimental animals by constricting the lumen. This reduces radius and increases flow velocity and results in marked elevations in wall shear. In 1968 Fry constricted the canine aorta with a mechanical intraluminal device and increased wall shear stress to approximately 400 dynes/sq cm.[4] This represented a 20-fold increase above the normal level of 15 to 20 dynes/sq cm,[5] and resulted in endothelial damage and an increase in endothelial permeability. Other studies reported the in vivo finding of damaged and disrupted endothelial cells in high shear stress areas such as aortic ostial flow dividers.[6] Together, these findings were taken as evidence that high shear stress was an initiating factor in atherogenesis.

It is now recognized that the reported in vivo endothelial abnormalities were due to experimental artifacts and that under normal circumstances there is no morphologic evidence of endothelial denudation or disruption either in high- or low-shear areas in the arterial tree.[7] Furthermore, when shear stress was elevated by aortic coarctation and studied after 10 days to 9 months rather than acutely, there was no evidence of endothelial damage or denudation in the high-shear coarctation channel[8] (Fig. 7–1). Thus, if endothelial damage occurred acutely as a result of very high shear, it healed rapidly with no scarring or residual intimal thickening. Specific injury to the endothelium and aortic wall by clamping and suturing to produce a constriction also healed without evidence of endothelial abnormality or intimal thickening in the high shear stress area (Fig. 7–2).

The relationship between high shear stress and plaque formation has been studied in monkeys with aortic coarctation that were fed an atherogenic diet. Extensive intimal plaques formed in the aorta prox-

imal to the coarctation, but within the high shear stress coarctation channel, plaque formation was inhibited[8] (Fig. 7–3). Thus, there is no evidence that high shear stress results in endothelial damage, and rather than promoting plaque formation, high shear appears to inhibit plaque deposition.[9] Such a feedback inhibition may serve to limit the rate of plaque deposition in developing stenoses, which produce local elevations in wall shear stress.

Low Shear Stress

The earliest atherosclerotic lesions in experimental atherosclerosis develop at the upstream rims of aortic ostia, which are regions of low shear stress. Similar plaque localization has been noted in humans (Fig. 7–4), and Caro et al. have suggested that low wall shear rates may retard the mass transport of atherogenic substances away from the wall, resulting in increased intimal accumulation of lipids.[10] In addition, low shear stress may interfere with turnover at the endothelial surface of substances essential both to artery wall nutrition and to the maintenance of optimal endothelial metabolic function.[11]

Correlative studies of plaque localization in the human carotid bifurcation with quantitative model flow studies have shown that intimal plaques form in the low shear stress region of the carotid sinus opposite the flow divider and not in the high shear stress region along the inner wall of the internal carotid artery.[12,13] Shear stress values of zero and below were recorded in the region most likely to develop plaque,[13] and it has been suggested that a threshold value below which plaque deposition occurs may exist.[12] Similar quantitative correlative studies of the human aortic bifurcation have also shown that plaques localize in regions of low shear stress rather than high shear stress.[14]

Flow Field Changes

A number of flow field alterations other than shear stress changes occur at branch points and have been implicated in plaque localization.[5] These changes are particularly prominent in the carotid bifurcation because of the presence of the carotid sinus, and may account for the marked vulnerability of this site to atherosclerosis. The carotid sinus has twice the cross-sectional area of the distal internal carotid artery and this, together with the effects of branching and angulation, results in a large area of *flow separation and stasis* along the outer wall of the carotid sinus (Fig. 7–5). Flow visualization studies demonstrate that as flow from the common carotid artery enters the bifurcation, flow streamlines are compressed toward the flow divider and inner wall of the internal carotid artery, where flow is rapid and laminar and shear stress is high. Plaques do not form in this area. Along the outer wall of the sinus, a large area of flow separation develops in which flow velocity and shear stress are low. The earliest intimal plaques develop

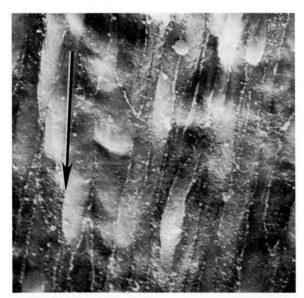

FIGURE 7–1. Scanning electron micrograph of endothelial surface of a coarcted monkey aorta. Six months after coarctation, there was a 70 per cent lumen stenosis, a 15 mm Hg pressure gradient, and high flow velocity and shear stress within the coarctation channel. The endothelial surface in the center of the coarctation channel, as well as elsewhere in the aorta, was intact with no evidence of endothelial disruption or damage. Arrow denotes direction of blood flow. (From Zarins CK, Bomberger RA, Glagov S: Local effects of stenosis: Increased flow velocity inhibits atherogenesis. *Circulation 64* (suppl II):II-221, 1981.)

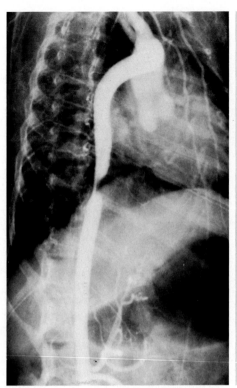
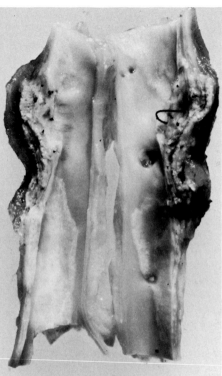

FIGURE 7–2.   Coarctation of aorta in monkey fed atherogenic diet for 6 months. The coarctation was produced by suture. The prior arterial wall injury has healed fully and there is no evidence of endothelial disruption or plaque formation within the stenosis. Intimal plaque formed proximal and distal to the stenosis, suggesting that plaque formation was inhibited in the high shear stress area. (From Zarins CK, Bomberger RA, Glagov S: Local effects of stenosis: Increased flow velocity inhibits atherogenesis. Circulation *64* (suppl II):II-221, 1981.)

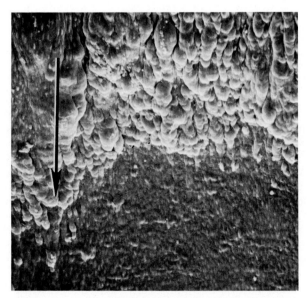

FIGURE 7–3.   Scanning electron micrograph of intimal surface of coarctation channel of a monkey fed an atherogenic diet. Note the abrupt cessation of intimal plaque at the entry into the stenotic area. The inhibition of plaque formation coincides with the area of increased shear stress. (From Zarins CK, Bomberger RA, Glagov S: Local effects of stenosis: Increased flow velocity inhibits atherogenesis. Circulation *64* (suppl II):II-221, 1981.)

in this region, as do late, complicated, and clinically significant lesions.[13] In the region of flow separation there is a reversal of axial flow and slow fluid movement upstream. However, the region of separation is not simply a zone of stasis and recirculation but is a zone of complex secondary flow patterns, including counterrotating helical trajectories (Fig. 7–6). Flow reattaches distally in the sinus, and the distal internal carotid, which is almost always free of plaque, has relatively rapid axial flow throughout its cross-section.

Particles of dye are carried rapidly along the inner wall but are cleared very slowly from the outer region of flow separation and low flow velocity. Particles in the region of flow separation have an *increased residence time* and would have greater opportunity to interact with the vessel wall. Time-dependent lipid particle–vessel wall interactions would thus be facilitated in the slow flow region, making it more likely for plaque formation to occur. In addition, blood-borne cellular elements that may play a role in atherogenesis are likely to have an increased probability of deposition or adhesion to the vessel wall in regions of increased residence time.[15] Flow separation has been shown to favor deposition of platelets in vitro,[16] which may stimulate cell proliferation and induce intimal thickening and plaque formation. Radiographic and ultrasound studies have confirmed the

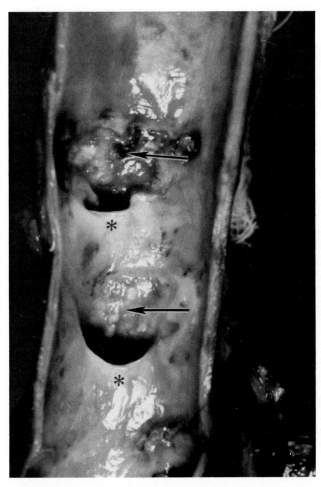

FIGURE 7–4. Human aorta demonstrating plaque deposition at upstream rim of celiac and superior mesenteric ostia (arrow). These are areas of low shear stress. The flow divider (asterisk) is exposed to high shear stress and is free of plaque.

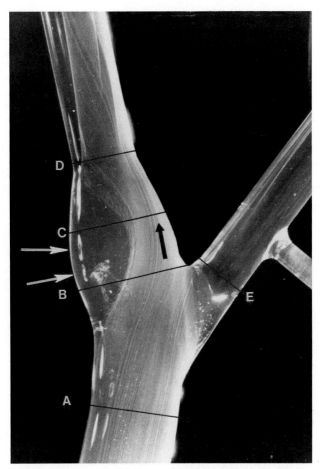

FIGURE 7–5. Hydrogen bubble flow visualization studies in a glass model human carotid bifurcation under steady flow conditions. Flow is rapid, laminar, and longitudinal along the inner wall of the carotid sinus (black arrow). Along the outer wall there is a large area of flow separation (white arrows). The letters A–E refer to tissue sections taken in a corresponding human carotid bifurcation that demonstrated that early intimal plaques form in the area of flow separation. (From Zarins CK, Giddens DP, Bharadvaj BK, et al: Carotid bifurcation atherosclerosis: Quantitative correlation of plaque localization with flow velocity profiles and wall shear stress. Circ Res 53:502, 1983.)

presence of flow separation and stasis in patients in this outer wall region of the carotid bifurcation.[17] Not only do early plaques localize in this region, but extensive, complicated, stenotic, and ulcerated lesions have the same pattern of distribution along the outer wall of the carotid sinus.

Oscillation of Flow

Under conditions of *pulsatile* flow, the flow field considerations are more complex. Conditions along the inner wall of the carotid sinus are similar to those seen under steady flow conditions.[18] Flow velocity and shear stress are high and flow remains laminar. There are fluctuations in magnitude of velocity and shear, but no change in velocity or shear stress direction.

Along the outer wall, where plaque forms, pulsatile flow produces an *oscillating shear* stress pattern (Fig. 7–7). During early systole, the region of flow separation disappears with forward flow throughout the cross-sectional area of the sinus. During late sys-

tole, however, the region of separation and flow reversal becomes prominent along the outer wall and there is a reversal in the shear stress directional vector.[18] During diastole, conditions are similar to those seen under steady flow conditions. The magnitudes of velocity and shear are low in this region and correlate strongly to plaque localization. Alternating positive and negative shear stress vectors (oscillations) along the outer wall of the carotid sinus have also been shown to correlate strongly with early plaque deposition.[12]

Particle tracking studies reveal *increased residence time* along the outer wall, which is caused by oscillation of fluid velocity about a mean value close to zero. This delays the convection of fluid and traps fluid elements near the outer wall for several cycles despite the absence of a clear region of stasis or of an area of permanent boundary layer separation (Fig.

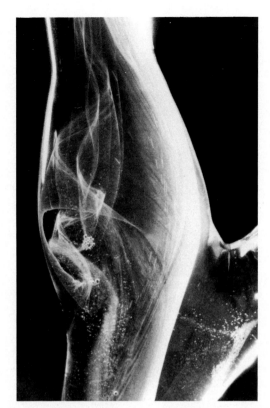

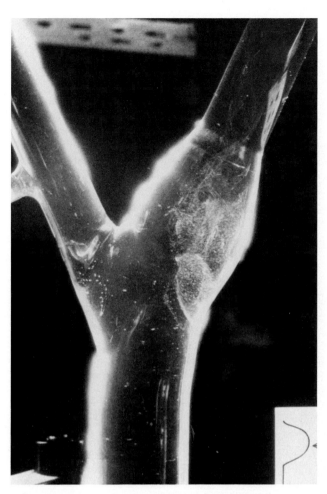

FIGURE 7–6. Hydrogen bubble flow visualization study in a glass model human carotid bifurcation demonstrating complex helical flow patterns within the area of flow separation. There is a reversal of axial flow, slow fluid movement upstream, and increased fluid residence time. (From Zarins CK, Giddens DP, Bharadvaj BK, et al: Carotid bifurcation atherosclerosis: Quantitative correlation of plaque localization with flow velocity profiles and wall shear stress. Circ Res 53:502, 1983.)

FIGURE 7–8. Hydrogen bubble flow visualization study under conditions of pulsatile flow demonstrating persistence of bubbles in the region of flow separation. The bubbles have remained for two pulse cycles after clearance of the mainstream bubbles, indicating increased residence time of fluid elements in the region of the outer sinus wall where plaques form. (From Ku DN, Giddens DP: Pulsatile flow in a model carotid bifurcation. Arteriosclerosis 3:31, 1983.)

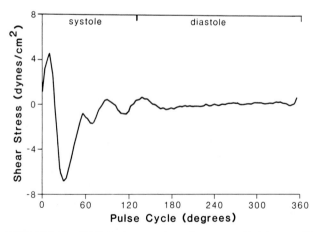

FIGURE 7–7. Wall shear stress along the outer wall of the carotid sinus measured in a glass model human carotid bifurcation under conditions of pulsatile flow. Wall shear stress oscillates from positive to negative values during systole but has very little oscillation during diastole. Shear stress oscillation occurs in areas of the carotid sinus in which there is intimal plaque deposition. (From Ku DN, Giddens DP, Zarins CK, et al: Pulsatile flow and atherosclerosis in the human bifurcation: Positive correlation between plaque location and low and oscillating shear stress. Arteriosclerosis 5:293, 1985.)

7–8). Increased residence time increases the duration of exposure of the lumen surface to circulating atherogenic agents and favors time-dependent transendothelial diffusion as well as intimal entrapment of atherogenic particles.[1]

Thus, variations in shear stress direction associated with pulsatile flow may lead to increased endothelial permeability, whereas even relatively high shear stresses that remain unidirectional may not be injurious.[19] The oscillating shear stress pattern may cause an increased ingress of plasma constituents through the endothelial monolayer by effects on the stability of intercellular junctions. Endothelial cells normally align in the direction of flow[20] in an overlapping arrangement. Changing shear stress may cause cyclic shifts in the relationship between shear stress direction and the orientation of intercellular overlapping borders. This hypothesis agrees well with reports of increased permeability of cultured, confluent endothelial cells subjected to changes in shear stress[22] and increased Evans blue dye staining in relation to differences in endothelial organization[23] that may be attributable to changing flow patterns.

Since oscillation of shear stress direction is a systolic event, the number of such oscillations is directly related to the number of systoles, or heart rate. *Heart rate* has been implicated as an independent risk factor in coronary atherosclerosis and will be discussed further in the section dealing with the coronary arteries.

Turbulence

Turbulence implies random movement of elements in a flow field. Whether or not blood flow will be turbulent depends on blood flow velocity, artery diameter, and blood viscosity. Extreme or abrupt changes in geometry due to intraluminal projections, severe stenoses, or other obstacles in the flow stream can cause focal turbulence.[24] Although turbulent flow has often been implicated as a factor in plaque pathogenesis, [25,26] both experimental atherosclerosis studies and in vitro observations in the model carotid bifurcation fail to support this suggestion.

Flow field disturbances such as flow separation, recirculation, and vortex formation may occur in various regions of the arterial tree under normal and abnormal conditions. However, turbulence does not develop in the absence of abnormal geometry such as stenoses or shunts. Experimentally induced arteriovenous anastomoses,[27] stenoses,[28,29] or aneurysms[30] can produce intimal thickenings with some features of atherosclerosis. However, regions immediately distal to severe stenoses, where significant turbulence has been demonstrated,[31,32] are free of atherosclerotic lesions.[33-35]

In the human carotid bifurcation, in the region where plaques form, although there is a zone of complex secondary and tertiary flow patterns, including counterrotating helical trajectories (Fig. 7–6), there is no turbulence.[36] This is true under a wide range of Reynolds numbers and flow conditions, including both steady and pulsatile flow. Furthermore, in vivo noninvasive pulsed Doppler ultrasound studies of carotid arteries in normal human subjects do not exhibit turbulence.[37] Thus, while it is clear that strong secondary flow patterns exist in the normal carotid bifurcation in areas of early plaque formation, turbulence does not. Turbulence may develop late, however, as a result of severe carotid stenosis and thus would be a result of, rather than a cause of, atherosclerotic plaques.

Hypertension

Postmortem studies have revealed that hypertension is associated with an increase in both the extent and severity of atherosclerosis.[38] Numerous epidemiologic studies have identified hypertension as an important risk factor for the development of clinical complications of atherosclerosis, such as myocardial infarction and stroke.[39-41] Yet, recent clinical data comparing the development of myocardial infarction or stroke in persons with and without control of mild to moderate hypertension revealed no significant difference, suggesting that other factors, possibly interacting with hypertension, may be important.[42]

Thus, the effects of hypertension may be different in different portions of the arterial tree as a result of other local hemodynamic variables. It is well known, for example, that hypertension is a more important factor in cerebrovascular disease and stroke than in coronary artery or peripheral occlusive disease.[40] The occurrence of severe atherosclerosis in clinically normotensive individuals and the sparing of vessels distal to stenoses, even in the presence of elevated blood pressure, indicate that although hypertension may potentiate or enhance atherogenesis, it may not be in itself a necessary atherogenic factor.

Experimentally, hypertension has been implicated as an important etiologic factor in plaque pathogenesis.[43] When hypertension was induced by midthoracic aortic coarctation in atherosclerotic primates, there was increased plaque deposition in the aorta proximal to the coarctation.[44,45] However, other hemodynamic conditions also existed in the region proximal to the coarctation, including decreased flow velocity, decreased shear stress, increased pulse pressure and wall motion, and increased wall tension. In the aorta distal to the coarctation mean blood pressure was also elevated because of the presence of renovascular hypertension, but plaque deposition in the distal aorta was almost entirely absent[35] (Table 7–1). Inhibition of plaque deposition despite the presence of hypertension and marked hyperlipidemia was associated with a decreased pulse pressure,[8,35] decreased wall motion,[46] and decreased arterial wall metabolism.[47] Hypertension enhanced experimental plaque formation but inhibited plaque regression[48] and enhanced plaque progression,[49] despite reduction of hypercholesterolemia. These observations suggest that factors other than blood pressure per se may be of primary importance in atherogenesis. Thus although hypertension is important in the clinical complication of atherosclerosis, the nature of its role in plaque pathogenesis remains unclear.

ARTERY WALL SUSCEPTIBILITY

In addition to the interaction of intraluminal hemodynamic conditions with the systemic and lipid environment, local susceptibility and responses of the artery wall are important in the development of atherosclerotic lesions. The artery wall is composed of the intima, which is covered on the luminal surface by a monolayer of endothelial cells; the media, which contains smooth muscle cells, collagen, and elastin;

TABLE 7–1.   EFFECT OF COARCTATION ON ATHEROSCLEROSIS IN CYNOMOLGUS MONKEYS

Stenosis	Proximal Aorta		Distal Aorta	
	No Stenosis	70% Stenosis	No Stenosis	70% Stenosis
Surface atherosclerosis (%)	56 ± 7	74 ± 8	54 ± 9	12 ± 4[a]
Mural cholesterol (mg/sq mm)	9.1 ± 4.1	9.7 ± 1.7	4.6 ± 0.8	2.1 ± 0.6[a]
DNA content (mg/sq mm)	0.77 ± 0.07	0.75 ± 0.10	0.50 ± 0.07	0.23 ± 0.03[a]
Collagen content (mg/sq mm)	23 ± 3	27 ± 1	22 ± 2	15 ± 2[a]
Elastin content (mg/sq mm)	42 ± 2	56 ± 5[a]	29 ± 1	29 ± 6

Adapted from Bomberger RA, Zarins CK, Taylor KE, et al: Effect of hypotension on atherosclerosis and aortic wall composition. J Surg Res 28:402–409, 1980.
[a]Statistically significantly different.

and the adventitia, which contains a network of vasa vasorum.

Endothelial Injury

Endothelial injury and the response to endothelial injury have been implicated in plaque pathogenesis. According to this hypothesis,[50] the endothelial lining of arteries is damaged by one of several factors, including mechanical forces such as shear stress and hypertension, chemical agents such as hyperlipidemia or homocysteine, immunologic reactions, or hormonal dysfunction. The injury hypothesis also encompasses the response to such injury, including platelet deposition, release of platelet-derived growth factor, leukocyte adhesion and diapedesis, cellular proliferation, and lipid deposition.[51–53] Focal, repeated endothelial injury would account for the localized nature of plaque deposition.

Although widely quoted, direct evidence for this hypothesis is lacking. There is no in vivo evidence of spontaneous endothelial injury or disruption, with or without platelet adherence, in areas at risk for future lesion development.[54,55] In addition, there is no direct evidence that experimentally induced endothelial damage or removal results in eventual sustained lesion formation[7] On the contrary, evidence has been advanced that the formation of experimental intimal plaques may require the presence of a continuous endothelial covering.[7,54] Moreover, the role of platelets in atherogenesis remains unclear, and platelet-derived growth factor has now been isolated from tissue other than platelets.[56] Recent studies have been aimed at the study of functional alterations in intact endothelium.[57–59] Activated endothelial cells become permeable to low-density lipoprotein (LDL), have higher replication rates, and develop prothrombotic properties. They express surface glycoproteins that promote the adhesion of neutrophils, monocytes, and platelets. Activated endothelium also promotes the transition of smooth muscle cells from the contractile to the synthetic phenotype, which promotes smooth muscle cell proliferation and cholesterol accumulation.[59] Thus, although mechanical endothelial injury is unlikely to be a significant contributing factor to plaque initiation, endothelial cell

function plays an important role in the responses and functions of the artery wall.

Medial Functional State and Metabolism

The functional state of the media appears to be important in plaque pathogenesis. Under conditions in which there is increased pulse pressure, increased wall motion, and increased wall tension, such as exist proximal to aortic coarctation, there is smooth muscle cell proliferation, increased biosynthetic activity, and plaque formation.[35] Similar increases in metabolic activity of medial smooth muscle cells can be demonstrated in vitro.[60] Cyclic stretching of elastin membranes on which were grown smooth muscle cells resulted in increased biosynthesis of collagen, hyaluronate, and chondroitin-6-sulfate.[61] Thus, plaques form readily in areas where medial smooth muscle cells are metabolically active.

Conversely, distal to severe aortic coarctations, despite an increase in mean pressure, pulse pressure is decreased and aortic wall motion is diminished.[46] This is accompanied by atrophy of the media with loss of smooth muscle cells and a significant reduction in DNA content[35] (Table 7–1). Metabolic function is diminished with decreased glycolysis[47] and decreased collagen synthesis. Under these conditions, intimal plaque did not form despite a high mean blood pressure and marked hypercholesterolemia, with total serum cholesterol levels of 700 to 900 mg/dl.

Further evidence for the importance of the media in plaque formation can be found in the healing of arterial injuries in the presence of marked hypercholesterolemia. Standard, focal, transmural necrotizing injuries were produced in hypercholesterolemic rabbits. Despite endothelial sloughing at the time of injury, the endothelium was completely regenerated after 4 days. After 30 days, however, in many instances the media had not healed. Those injury sites with a healed, intact media developed intimal thickening at the site of injury. However, those in which the media failed to heal and became atrophic had no intimal thickening but rather became aneurysmal.[62] These observations suggest that an intact, metabolically active media is necessary for intimal plaque formation.

ARTERY WALL ADAPTATION

Artery walls can adapt to enlarging intimal plaques by dilating in order to maintain a normal lumen diameter. Hemodynamic forces appear to be important in this adaptation.[63] Vessels in high-flow positions, such as arteries feeding an arteriovenous fistula,[64] autogenous aortorenal bypass grafts,[65] and collateral arteries carrying increased flow about an obstruction, tend to enlarge. Conversely, lumen diameter is reduced in arteries with low flow, distal to arteriovenous fistulae, in arteries supplying atrophic or amputated extremities, or in vascular bypass grafts that are too large in relationship to the runoff bed.

Arteries proximal to a chronic arteriovenous fistula have markedly increased blood flow and flow velocity. However, there is no increase in wall shear stress due to artery dilatation and increase in lumen radius.[66,67] Kamiya and Togawa have suggested that shear stress acts to regulate lumen diameter through an alteration in protein flux in the artery wall. Guyton and Hartley[68] have suggested that arteries dilate as a result of an increase in flow pulsatility and peak velocity, which are sensed by endothelial cells and signaled to medial smooth muscle cells. The response appears to be dependent on the presence of an intact endothelial surface[69] and may be mediated through endothelial-derived vasoactive agents.

Atherosclerotic Artery Enlargement

In experimental diet-induced atherosclerosis in monkeys, coronary arteries[70] and carotid arteries[71] have been noted to enlarge as intimal plaques increase in size. Atherosclerotic artery enlargement has also been demonstrated in human coronary,[72,73] carotid, and superficial femoral arteries[74] as well as in the abdominal aorta. Artery enlargement can compensate for the enlarging intimal plaque and prevent lumen encroachment or stenosis[72] (Fig. 7–9). However, this compensatory mechanism appears to be effective in preventing stenosis for relatively small plaques that occupy less than 40 per cent of internal elastic lamina cross-sectional area.[72] Larger plaques result in lumen encroachment and stenosis. Compensatory enlargement to intimal plaques can be excessive in certain arterial segments, resulting in a larger than normal caliber.[73] This may predispose to aneurysmal enlargement. Thus, the development of stenosis may be a balance between plaque deposition on the one hand (which tends to narrow the lumen) and artery enlargement on the other (which can maintain a normal lumen caliber or predispose to aneurysm formation). Hemodynamic forces may play a role in the size regulation of atherosclerotic arteries through normal endothelial-dependent artery wall

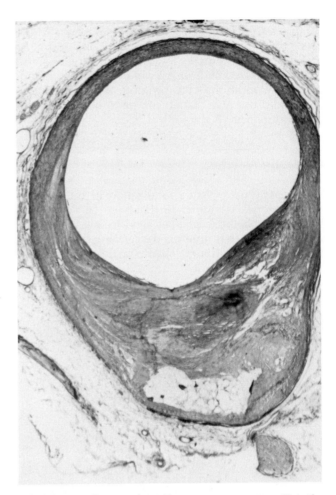

FIGURE 7–9. Cross-section of human coronary artery. Note the eccentric plaque deposition, oval contour of the external surface of the artery, and relatively rounded contour of the lumen. Arteries with enlarging intimal plaques tend to enlarge in order to maintain lumen diameter. This adaptive response of the artery wall is important in maintaining lumen patency.

responses or through direct effects of the plaque on the underlying artery wall.

PLAQUE LOCALIZATION

Carotid Bifurcation

Carotid bifurcation atherosclerosis occurs primarily along the outer wall of the internal carotid artery in the area of the carotid sinus. This has been noted on postmortem specimens,[75,76] on angiograms of patients with severe carotid stenosis,[77] in carotid bifurcation plaques removed during carotid endarterectomy,[75] and in experimental carotid plaques.[71] Angiographic studies in patients have demonstrated static zones and boundary layer separation at the outer wall of the carotid sinus in the region where plaques form,[17] and Doppler spectrum analyses have confirmed flow separation and stasis in this area of the carotid bifurcation in patients.[40] Quantitative correlative studies demonstrate that the earliest carotid plaques form in the area subjected to low shear stress, oscillating shear stress, flow separation, and flow stasis.[12,13] Late, complex lesions and ulcerations also occur in this region, and it is possible that the hemodynamic conditions may promote not only plaque formation, but also plaque complication, ulceration, and thrombosis (Fig. 7–10).

Coronary Arteries

The pattern of plaque localization in human coronary arteries is similar to that seen at the carotid bifurcation, because plaques tend to localize preferentially in the left anterior descending coronary artery just distal to the major proximal branch point.[79]

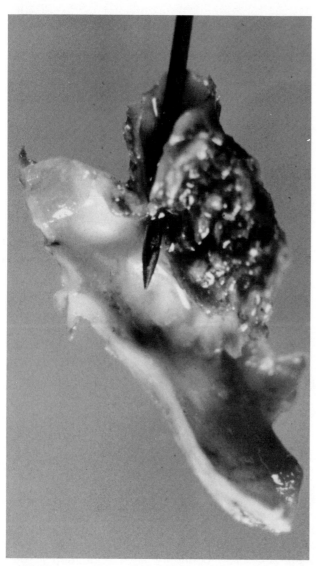

FIGURE 7–10. Sagittal section of plaque removed during carotid endarterectomy. Probe is in the lumen of the internal carotid artery. Note prominent complex plaque along the outer wall of the carotid sinus. This is the same region in which flow separation, low shear stress, and oscillation of shear stress occurred in model flow studies (see Figs. 7–5 through 7–8.)

This is a region of low flow velocity and low and oscillating wall shear stress opposite the flow divider.[80] If oscillation of shear stress direction, which occurs mainly during systole, is a major factor in plaque localization, coronary arteries may be at greater risk than other systemic arteries, because the coronary arteries are subjected to two systolic episodes and one diastolic episode of flow acceleration and deceleration during each cardiac cycle. Coronary arterial flow decreases initially in systole during the isovolumetric contraction and rapid ejection phases, increases briefly when peak systolic aortic pressure exceeds intracoronary pressure, and decreases again during the remainder of systole as intramyocardial pressure increases the resistance to flow.[81] Flow reversal during systole has been demonstrated with tachycardia and in concentric left ventricular hypertrophy. During isovolumetric relaxation, as intramyocardial and intraventricular pressure decline, coronary flow accelerates rapidly, then decreases slowly as aortic pressure falls and intraventricular pressure builds again late in diastole.

If other determinants of coronary flow are held constant, net coronary flow is directly proportional to heart rate.[82] Conversely, the diastolic time interval is inversely related to heart rate.[83] As heart rate increases, the time spent in diastole when flow is greatest decreases markedly. Since phasic fluctuation in coronary flow is predominantly a systolic occurrence, both the frequency and magnitude of oscillations in shear stress direction should be directly dependent on heart rate. Thus, the frequent preferential localization of plaques in the coronary arteries compared to the renal or other peripheral arteries may be related to the fact that the coronary arteries experience at least twice as many oscillations of flow velocity over time as other major arteries. Thus, during a 1-year period a resting heart rate of 80 results in 10.5 million more systoles than a resting heart rate of 60, emphasizing the remarkable cumulative effect of a modest change in heart rate on flow conditions in the coronary arteries.

In order to test the hypothesis that heart rate is an important risk factor in coronary atherosclerosis, we produced sinoatrial node ablation in cynomolgus monkeys. This resulted in a 20 per cent reduction in mean heart rate and a reduction in the magnitude of heart rate fluctuation. After 6 months on an atherogenic diet, animals with a low heart rate had a 50 per cent reduction in intimal plaque area, a 50 per cent reduction in maximum lesion size, and a 50 per cent reduction in percentage stenosis.[84] Similarly, there was a significant reduction in carotid bifurcation atherosclerosis.[71] Thus heart rate reduction had a protective effect on both coronary and carotid atherosclerosis in monkeys.

Heart rate has also been directly implicated as an independent risk factor in human coronary atherosclerosis. A number of major prospective clinical studies have found high heart rates in men at rest to be predictive of future manifestations of coronary heart disease.[85,86] Conversely, low heart rates are thought to protect against the development of coronary atherosclerosis.[87] Although increased resting heart rate seems to correlate significantly with an atherogenic lipid profile in sedentary men, suggesting a possible metabolic pathway for the effect of heart rate on coronary artery disease,[88] both theoretical and experimental evidence suggests that hemodynamic factors associated with cyclic myocardial contraction predisposes the coronary arteries selectively to atherosclerosis. Hemodynamic factors such as hypertension, altered shear stress, and flow disturbances have also been implicated in plaque localization and progression in several locations in the coronary arteries,[19] but a selective effect in the coronary tree has not been emphasized.

Abdominal Aorta

Human and experimental atherosclerotic lesions are prone to localize in regions of the arterial tree exposed to relatively low flow rates. The human abdominal aorta may be particularly vulnerable to early and rapid development of atherosclerosis because of relatively low flow velocities compared to the remainder of the aorta. One quarter of the cardiac output is delivered to the renal arteries at rest.[89] Renal artery flow, together with celiac and superior mesenteric artery flow, thus ensure a relatively constant high-volume flow through the proximal aorta. In contrast, the volume of flow in the aorta below the renal arteries is greatly dependent on the muscular activity of lower extremities. The infrarenal abdominal aorta may be the appropriate size for a physically active bipedal existence, but with an increasingly sedentary life-style, the infrarenal human abdominal aorta may be subjected to relatively slower flow velocities than the suprarenal aorta during a major portion of the day. This effect may be further accentuated by the tendency of the aorta to dilate with age. Thus, a slower flow pattern in the abdominal aorta may tend to favor intimal proliferation and the ingress of lipids, with the formation of atherosclerotic plaques.

Model flow studies of the aorta confirm that under resting and postprandial conditions, the infrarenal aorta experiences velocity direction oscillation, vortex formation, and increased fluid residence time, whereas the suprarenal aorta has laminar flow. Under conditions of increased flow, such as occurs during exercise, flow in the infrarenal aorta becomes laminar and the adverse hemodynamic conditions disappear.[90] These data support the clinical observations that an active life-style limits the manifestations of atherosclerosis and prolongs life expectancy.

Aneurysm Formation

Hemodynamic factors are important in both plaque localization and adaptive enlargement of athero-

sclerotic arteries. These processes may also play a role in aneurysm formation. The association between atherosclerosis and abdominal aortic aneurysms has long been recognized and it is well known that patients undergoing operation for aortic aneurysmal disease are generally 8 to 10 years older than patients undergoing operation for aortoiliac occlusive disease. This suggests that aortic aneurysm formation may be a later stage of atherosclerotic aortic degeneration.[91] Intimal plaque formation in the aorta stimulates adaptive enlargement of the aorta and is usually associated with atrophy and degeneration of the aortic wall underlying the plaque. If plaque degeneration, ulceration, or atrophy were to subsequently develop, this would leave an enlarged thin-walled aorta prone to progressive aneurysmal enlargement. Experimental studies from our laboratory have demonstrated that aneurysms form in diet-induced atherosclerosis with prolonged atherogenic regimens associated with plaque and artery wall atrophy.[92] A controlled trial of lesion regression by lowering of serum cholesterol in experimental animals resulted in aneurysmal enlargement of the abdominal aorta.[93] These findings suggest that the interaction between the plaque and artery wall and evolution of the plaque over time may be important in the pathogenesis of aneurysms.

Alterations in blood flow in the aorta may also influence aneurysm pathogenesis by local alterations in wall shear. An increased incidence of abdominal aortic aneurysms as a very late finding in World War II amputees supports this hypothesis.[94]

CLINICAL IMPLICATIONS

Clinical efforts to control systemic risk factors such as hyperlipidemia, smoking, and hypertension have been shown to be effective in limiting morbidity and mortality due to atherosclerotic plaques. Control of localizing hemodynamic factors is also possible and may be important in inhibiting plaque formation, enhancing artery wall adaptation, and, perhaps, promoting regression of established plaques. Increased cardiac output and blood flow brought on by increased flow velocity and increased wall shear stress would tend to limit plaque formation and promote artery lumen dilation. Experimental[95] as well as clinical[87] evidence supports the beneficial effects of exercise on coronary atherosclerosis. Increased flow with excercise would also serve to limit flow stasis and particle residence time, thus limiting time-dependent lipid–vessel wall interaction. Significant benefit in coronary atherosclerosis can also be anticipated by reduction in heart rate by exercise,[95] modification of psychosocial stress,[96] and drug therapy. Thus, a comprehensive approach to controlling clinical complications of atherosclerosis should address not only systemic but also local factors in plaque pathogenesis.

REFERENCES

1. Glagov S, Zarins CK, Giddens DP, Ku DN: Hemodynamics and atherosclerosis. Arch Pathol Lab Med *112*:1018–1031, 1988.

2. Ross R, Harker L: Hyperlipidemia and atherosclerosis. Science *193*:1094, 1976.

3. Ross R: The pathogenesis of atherosclerosis: An update. N Engl J Med *314*:488–500, 1986.

4. Fry DL: Acute vascular endothelial changes associated with increased blood velocity gradients. Circ Res *22*:165, 1968.

5. Giddens DP, Zarins CK, Glagov S: Response of arteries to near-wall fluid dynamic behavior. Appl Mech Rev *43*:(5):S96–S102, 1990.

6. Reidy MA, Bowyer DE: Scanning electron microscopy of arteries. The morphology of aortic endothelium in haemodynamically stressed areas associated with branches. Atherosclerosis *26*:181–194, 1977.

7. Reidy MA: Biology of disease: A reassessment of endothelial injury and arterial lesion formation. Lab Invest *53*:513–520, 1985.

8. Zarins CK, Bomberger RA, Glagov S: Local effects of stenosis: Increased flow velocity inhibits atherogenesis. Circulation *64*(suppl II):II-221–II-227, 1981.

9. Bassiouny HS, Lieber BB, Giddens DP, Xu CP, Glagov S, Zarins CK: Quantitative inverse correlation of wall shear stress with experimental intimal thickening. Surg Forum *39*:328–330, 1988.

10. Caro CG, Fitz-Gerald JM, Schroter RC: Atheroma and arterial wall shear: Observation, correlation and proposal of a shear dependent mass transfer mechanism for atherogenesis. Proc R Soc Lond (Biol) *117*:109–159, 1971.

11. Robertson AJ Jr: Oxygen requirements of the human arterial intima in atherogenesis. Prog Biochem Pharmacol *4*:305–316, 1968.

12. Ku DN, Giddens DP, Zarins CK, et al: Pulsatile flow and atherosclerosis in the human carotid bifurcation: Positive correlation between plaque location and low and oscillating shear stress. Arteriosclerosis *5*:293–302, 1985.

13. Zarins CK, Giddens DP, Bharadvaj BK, et al: Carotid bifurcation atherosclerosis: Quantitative correlation of plaque localization with flow velocity profiles and wall shear stress. Circ Res *53*:502–514, 1983.

14. Friedman MH, Hutchins GM, Bargeron CB, et al: Correlation between intimal thickness and fluid shear in human arteries. Atherosclerosis *39*:425–436, 1981.

15. Gerrity RG, Goss JA, Soby L: Control of monocyte recruitment by chemotactic factor(s) in lesion-prone areas of swine aorta. Arteriosclerosis *5*:55–66, 1985.

16. Parmentier EM, Morton WA, Petschek HE: Platelet aggregate formation in a region of separated blood flow. Phys Fluids *20*:2012–2021, 1981.

17. Fox JA, Hugh AE: Static zones in the internal carotid artery: Correlation with boundary layer separation and stasis in model flows. Br J Radiol *43*:370–376, 1976.

18. Ku DN, Giddens DP: Pulsatile flow in a model carotid bifurcation. Arteriosclerosis *3*:31–39, 1983.

19. Fry DL: Hemodynamic forces in atherogenesis. *In* Scheinberg P (ed): Cerebrovascular Disease. New York, Raven Press, 1976, pp 77–95.

20. Nerem RM, Levesque MJ, Cornhill JF: Vascular endothelial morphology as an indicator of the pattern of blood flow. J Biomech Eng *103*:171–176, 1981.

21. Clark JM, Glagov S: Luminal surface of distended arteries by scanning electron microscopy. Eliminating configurational artifacts. Br J Exp Pathol *57*:129–135, 1976.

22. Dewey CF, Bussolari SR, Gimbrone MA, et al: The dynamic response of vascular endothelial cells to fluid shear stress. J Biomech Eng *103*:177–185, 1981.

23. Fry DL: Responses of the arterial wall to certain physical factors. Ciba Found Symp *12*:93–125, 1973.

24. Giddens DP, Khalifa AMA: Turbulence measurements with pulsed Doppler ultrasound employing a frequency tracking method. Ultrasound Med Biol *8*:427–437, 1982.

25. Davies PF, Remuzzi A, Gordon EJ, et al: Turbulent fluid shear stress induces vascular endothelial cell turnover in vitro. Proc Natl Acad Sci USA *83*:2114–2117, 1986.

26. Gutstein WH, Farrell GA, Armellini C: Blood flow disturbance and endothelial cell injury in pre-atherosclerotic swine. Lab Invest *29*:134–149, 1973.

27. Davis PF, Stehbens WE: The biochemical composition of haemodynamically stressed vascular tissue: I. The lipid, calcium, and DNA concentration in experimental arteriovenous fistulae. Atherosclerosis *56*:27–37, 1985.

28. Schneiderman G, Ellis CG, Goldstick TK: Mass transport to walls stenosed arteries: Variation with Reynolds number and blood flow separation. J Biomech *12*:869–877, 1979.

29. Subbiah MTR, Kottke IA, Kottke BA, et al: Regional differences in cholesterol content of aorta in response to experimental coarctation in spontaneously atherosclerosis-susceptible pigeons. Basic Res Cardiol *75*:589–583, 1980.

30. Stehbens WE: Predilection of experimental arterial aneurysms for dietary-induced lipid deposition. Pathology *13*:735–747, 1981.

31. Lieber BB: Ordered and random structures in pulsatile flow through constricted tubes. Thesis. Georgia Institute of Technology, Atlanta, 1985.

32. Khalifa AMA, Giddens DP: Characterization and evolution of post-stenotic flow disturbances. J Biomech *14*:279–296, 1981.

33. Ku DN, Zarins CK, Giddens DP, et al: Reduced atherogenesis distal to stenosis despite turbulence and hypertension (abstr). Circulation *74*(suppl 2):II-334, 1986.

34. Coutard M, Osborne-Pellegrin MJ: Decreased dietary lipid deposition in spontaneous lesions distal to a stenosis in the rat caudal artery. Artery *12*:82–98, 1983.

35. Bomberger RA, Zarins CK, Taylor KE, et al: Effect of hypotension on atherogenesis and aortic wall composition. J Surg Res *28*:402–409, 1980.

36. Bharadvaj BK, Mabon RF, Giddens DP: Steady flow in a model of the human carotid bifurcation: Part II. Laser Doppler anemometer measurements. J Biomech Eng *15*:363–378, 1982.

37. Ku DN, Giddens DP, Phillips DJ, et al: Hemodynamics of the normal human carotid bifurcation: In vitro and in vivo studies. Ultrasound Med Biol *11*:13–26, 1985.

38. Glagov S, Rowley DA, Kohut R: Atherosclerosis of human aorta and its coronary and renal arteries. Arch Pathol Lab Med *72*:558–571, 1961.

39. Chabanian AV: The influence of hypertension and other hemodynamic factors in atherogenesis. Cardiovasc Dis *26*:177–196, 1983.

40. Kannel WB, Schwartz MJ, McNamara PM: Blood pressure and risk of coronary heart disease: The Framingham Study. Dis Chest *56*:43–52, 1969.

41. Robertson WB, Strong JP: Atherosclerosis in persons with hypertension and diabetes mellitus. Lab Invest *18*:538, 1969.

42. Medical Research Council Working party: MCR trial of treatment of mild hypertension: Principal results. Br Med J *291*:97–104, 1985.

43. Breterton KN, Day AJ, Skinner SL: Hypertension-accelerated atherogenesis in cholesterol-fed rabbits. Atherosclerosis *27*:79–87, 1977.

44. Bomberger RA, Zarins CK, Glagov S: Subcritical arterial stenosis enhances distal atherosclerosis. Resident Research Award. J Surg Res *30*:205–212, 1981.

45. Hollander W, Madoff I, Paddock J, Kirkpatrick B: Aggravation of atherosclerosis by hypertension in a subhuman primate model with coarctation of the aorta. Circ Res *38* (suppl 2): 63, 1976.

46. Lyon RT, Runyon-Hass A, Davis HR, Glagov X, Zarins CK: Protection from atherosclerotic lesion formation by reduction of artery wall motion. J Vasc Surg *5*(3):413–420, 1987.

47. Cozzi PJ, Lyon RT, Davis HR, Glagov S, Zarins CK: Aortic wall metabolism in relation to susceptibility and resistance to experimental atherosclerosis. J Vasc Surg *7*(5):706–714, 1988.

48. Zarins CK, Bomberger RA, Taylor KE, et al: Artery stenosis

inhibits regression of diet-induced atherosclerosis. Surgery *88*:86–92, 1980.

49. Xu C-P, Glagov S, Zatina MA, Zarins CK: Hypertension sustains plaque progression despite reduction of hypercholesterolemia. Hypertension *18*(2):123–129, 1991.
50. Ross R, Glomset J: The pathogenesis of atherosclerosis. N Engl J Med *295*:369, 1976.
51. Ross R: Atherosclerosis: A problem of the biology of arterial wall cells and their interactions with blood components. Arteriosclerosis *1*:293, 1981.
52. Ip JH, Fuster V, Badimon L, Badimon J, Taubman MB, Chesebro JH: Syndromes of accelerated atherosclerosis: Role of vascular injury and smooth muscle proliferation. J Am Coll Cardiol *15*:1667–1687, 1990.
53. Schwartz S, Heimark R, Majesky M: Developmental mechanisms underlying pathology of arteries. Physiol Rev *70*:1177–1209, 1990.
54. Zarins CK, Taylor KE, Bomberger RA, et al: Endothelial integrity at aortic ostial flow dividers. SEM *3*:249–254, 1980.
55. Taylor KE, Glagov S, Zarins CK: Preservation and structural adaptation of endothelium over experimental foam cell lesions. Arteriosclerosis *9*:881–894, 1989.
56. Di Corleto PE, Bowen-Pope DF: Cultured endothelial cells produce a platelet-derived growth-like factor protein. Proc Natl Acad Sci USA *80*:1919, 1983.
57. Bevilacqua MP, Pober JS, Majeau GR, et al: Interleukin 1 (IL-1) induces biosynthesis and cell surface expression of procoagulant activity in human vascular endothelial cells. J Exp Med *160*:618, 1984.
58. Einhorn S, Eldor A, Vladavsky I, et al: Production and characterization of interferon from endothelial cells. J Cell Physiol *122*:200, 1985.
59. Whatley R, Zimmerman G, McIntyre T, Prescott S: Lipid metabolism and signal transduction in endothelial cells. Prog Lipid Res *29*:45–63, 1990.
60. Glagov S, Grande JP, Xu C-P, Giddens DP, Zarins CK: Limited effects of hyperlipidemia on the arterial smooth muscle response to mechanical stress. J Cardiovasc Pharmacol *14* (suppl 6):S90–S97, 1989.
61. Leung DYM, Glagov S, Mathews MU: Cyclic stretching stimulates synthesis of matrix components by arterial smooth muscle cells in vitro. Science *191*:475–477, 1976.
62. Bomberger RA, Zarins CK, Glagov S: Medial injury and hyperlipidemia in development of aneurysms or atherosclerotic plaques. Surg Forum *31*:338–340, 1980.
63. Zarins CK: Adaptive responses of arteries. J Vasc Surg *9*:382, 1989.
64. Schumacker HB Jr: Aneurysm development and degenerative changes in dilated artery proximal to arteriovenous fistula. Surg Gynecol Obstet *130*:636, 1970.
65. Szilagyi DE, Elliott JP, Hagerman JH, et al: Biologic fate of autogenous vein implants as arterial substitutes. Surgery *178*:232, 1973.
66. Zarins CK, Zatina MA, Giddens DP, et al: Shear stress regulation of artery lumen diameter in experimental atherogenesis. J Vasc Surg *5*(3):413–420, 1987.
67. Masuda H, Bassiouny HS, Glagov S, Zarins CK: Artery wall restructuring in response to increased flow. Surg Forum *40*:285–286, 1989.
68. Guyton JH, Hartley CJ: Flow restriction of one carotid artery in juvenile rats inhibits growth of arterial diameter. Am J Physiol *248*(Heart Circ Physiol 17):H540–H546, 1985.
69. Langille BL, O'Donnell F: Reductions in arterial diameter produced by chronic diseases in blood flow are endothelial-dependent. Science *231*:405–407, 1986.
70. Bond MD, Adams MR, Bullock BC: Complicating factor in evaluating coronary artery atherosclerosis. Artery *9*:21, 1981.
71. Beere PA, Glagov S, Zarins CK: Experimental atherosclerosis at the carotid bifurcation of the cynomolgus monkey: Localization compensatory enlargement and the sparing effect of lowered heart rate. Atheroscler Thromb *12*:1245–1253, 1992.
72. Glagov S, Weisenberg E, Kolletis G, et al: Compensatory enlargement of human atherosclerotic coronary arteries. N Engl J Med *316*:1371–1375, 1987.

73. Zarins CK, Weisenberg E, Kolettis G, et al: Differential enlargement of artery segments in response to enlarging atherosclerotic plaques. J Vasc Surg *7*(3):386–394, 1988.
74. Blair JM, Glagov S, Zarins CK: Mechanism of superficial femoral artery adductor canal stenosis. Surg Forum *41*:359–360, 1990.
75. Imparato AM, Riles TS, Gorstein F: The carotid bifurcation plaques: Pathologic findings associated with cerebral ischemia. Stroke *10*:238–245, 1979.
76. Solbert LA, Eggen DA: Localization and sequence of development of atherosclerotic lesions in the carotid and vertebral arteries. Circulation *43*:711–724, 1971.
77. Bauer RB, Sheehan S, Weehsler N, et al: Arteriographic study of sites, incidence and treatment of arteriosclerotic cerebrovascular lesions. Neurology *12*:698–711, 1962.
78. Bassiouny HS, Davis H, Masawa N, Gewertz BL, Glagov S, Zarins CK: Critical carotid stenoses: Morphologic and biochemical similarity of symptomatic and asymptomatic plaques. J Vasc Surg *9*(2):202–212, 1989.
79. Montenegro MR, Eggen DA: Topography of atherosclerosis in the coronary arteries. Lab Invest *18*:586–593, 1968.
80. Tang TD, Giddens DP, Zarins CK, Glagov S: Velocity profile and wall shear measurements in a model human coronary artery. Adv Bio Eng ASME *17*:261–263, 1990.
81. Granata L, Olsson RA, Huvos A, et al: Coronary inflow and oxygen usage following cardiac sympathetic nerve stimulator in unanesthetized dogs. Circ Res *16*:114, 1965.
82. Laurent D, Bolenc-Williams C, Williams FL, et al: Effects of heart rate on coronary flow and cardiac oxygen consumption. Am J Physiol *185*:355–364, 1956.
83. Boudoulas H, Rittgers SE, Lewis RP, et al: Changes in diastolic time with various pharmacologic agents. Circulation *60*:164–169, 1979.
84. Beere PA, Glagov S, Zarins CK: Retarding effect of lowered heart rate on coronary atherosclerosis. Science *226*:180–182, 1984.
85. Schroll M, Hagerup LM: Risk factors of myocardial infarction and death in men aged 50 at entry. Dan Med Bull *24*:252, 1977.
86. Dyer AR, Persky V, Stamler J, et al: Heart rate as a prognostic factor for coronary heart disease and mortality: Findings in three Chicago epidemiologic studies. Am J Epidemiol *112*:736, 1980.
87. Williams PT, Wood PD, Haskell WL, et al: The effects of running mileage and duration on plasma lipoprotein levels. JAMA *247*:2674, 1982.
88. Williams PT, Haskell WL, Vranizan KM, et al: Associations of resting heart rate with concentrations of lipoprotein subfractions in sedentary men. Circulation *71*:441, 1985.
89. Guyton AC: Textbook of Medical Physiology, 2nd ed. Philadelphia, WB Saunders Company, 1961, p 356.
90. Ku DN, Glagov S, Moore JE Jr, Zarins CK: Flow patterns in the abdominal aorta under simulated post prandial and exercise conditions: An experimental study. J Vasc Surg *9*:309–316, 1989.
91. Zarins CK, Glagov S: Aneurysms and obstructive plaques: Differing local responses to atherosclerosis. Aneurysms: Diagnosis and Treatment. Bergan JJ, Yao JST (eds): New York, Grune & Stratton, Inc., 1982, pp 61–82.
92. Zarins CK, Glagov S, Wissler RW, Vesselinovitch D: Aneurysm formation in experimental atherosclersis: Relationship to plaque evolution. J Vasc Surg *12*(3):246–256, 1990.
93. Zarins CK, Xu C-P, Glagov S: Aneurysmal enlargement of the aorta during regression of experimental atherosclerosis. J Vasc Surg *15*:90–101, 1992.
94. Vollmar JF, Pauschinger P, Paes E, Henze E, Friesch A: Aortic aneurysms as late sequelae of above-knee amputation. Lancet *iii*, 834–835, 1989.
95. Kramsch D, Aspen AJ, Abramowitz BM, et al: Reduction of coronary atherosclerosis by moderate conditioning exercise in monkeys on an atherogenic diet. N Engl J Med *305*:1483, 1981.
96. Kaplan JR, Manuck SB, Clarkson TB, et al: Social stress and atherosclerosis in normocholesterolemic monkeys. Science *220*:733, 1983.

8

NONATHEROSCLEROTIC VASCULAR DISEASE

JOHN M. PORTER, LLOYD M. TAYLOR, JR., and E. JOHN HARRIS, JR.

While a large majority of the arterial abnormalities occupying the interest of vascular surgeons are caused by atherosclerosis, a significant minority results from a variety of congenital and developmental abnormalities. The medical specialties that may be expected to be familiar with the diagnosis and treatment of these conditions are generally found to rely on vascular surgeons for this function. As the specialty of vascular surgery matures, the vascular surgeon obviously must become familiar with the spectrum of vascular disease, not just that resulting from atherosclerosis.

This chapter will describe briefly the pathogenesis, symptoms, diagnosis, and treatment of a variety of nonatherosclerotic arterial diseases. The topics covered will include immune as well as infectious and radiation arteritis, fibromuscular dysplasia, compartment and entrapment syndromes, a variety of congenital and developmental arterial abnormalities, a number of which are caused by known or suspected hereditary biochemical disorders, and the hyperviscosity syndromes.

SYSTEMIC VASCULITIS

Vasculitis has a deceptively simple definition—inflammation, often with necrosis and occlusive changes of the blood vessels—but its clinical manifestations are diverse and complex.[1] All students of vasculitis agree that our knowledge of this condition is incomplete and that the currently used classification systems are chaotic and filled with exceptions and overlap syndromes. The term "arteritis" has been used to describe many of these syndromes, yet vasculitis is a more precise term, as many of the entities involve veins as well as arteries. Vasculitis may be generalized or localized. The term vasculitis properly only applies to a pathologic process that occurs in a variety of syndromes or diseases, some of unknown origin (idiopathic vasculitis) and others associated with established underlying diseases (secondary vasculitis).

The etiology and pathogenesis of most vasculitides are quite complex and either unknown or incompletely understood. Earlier attempts to associate vasculitis only with the single mechanism of immune complex–induced injury has not been substantiated in the majority of vasculitides.[2] The prevailing theory is that most vasculitides are caused by immune-mediated injury, either humoral or cellular. The inciting antigen has been detected in very few instances. Rheumatoid vasculitis appears to develop from immune complex deposition along the vascular wall, but most other idiopathic vasculitides are lacking evidence supporting immune complex deposition (Fig. 8–1).

In the majority of idiopathic vasculitides, a cellular immune reaction is suggested, with associated production of soluble mediators such as cytokines, arachidonic acid metabolites, and fibrinolytic and coagulation by-products. With the production of cytokines, there also is the recruitment of an inflammatory response with neutrophilic, eosinophilic, monocytic, and lymphocytic interactions at the inflammatory site. Endothelial cells are also involved in the inflammatory response. Endothelial cells produce cytokines that attract the inflammatory cells and express cell membrane receptors specific for many of these inflammatory cells. Binding of the inflammatory cells to the endothelial cell triggers intracellular production of additional endothelial cytokines that affect the local inflammatory environment. Platelet interactions with the intact and injured endothelium may contribute to the inflammatory process through stimulation of the coagulation pathways and release of cytokines capable of stimulating and modifying immune responses.

A complete description of the recognized and potential interactions of these cellular immune and inflammatory activities is beyond the scope of this chapter and the interest of most vascular surgeons. The interested reader is directed to the excellent summary of current information by Savage.[2]

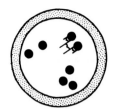

1) Circulating soluble immune complexes in antigen excess

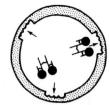

2) Increased vascular permeability via platelet derived vasoactive amines and IgE mediated reactions

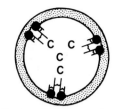

3) Trapping of immune complexes along basement membrane of vessel wall and activation of complement components (C)

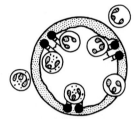

4) Complement derived chemotactic factors (C3 a, C5a, C567) cause accumulation of PMNs

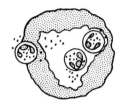

5) PMNs release lysosomal enzymes (collagenase, elastase)

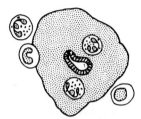

6) Damage and necrosis of vessel wall, thrombosis, occlusion, hemorrhage

FIGURE 8–1. Diagram showing the mechanism of arterial injury in immune arteritis. The key steps are immune complex deposition, complement activation, and lysosomal enzyme release from leukocytes. *PMN,* polymorphonuclear leukocyte. (From Fauci AS, Haynes BF, Katz P: The spectrum of vasculitis. Ann Intern Med *89:*660–676, 1978.)

The histology of the inflammatory cell infiltrate has been used to categorize the vasculitides, although overlaps are frequent. The type of inflammatory cell infiltrate is independent of the size of the blood vessels involved with vasculitis. A mixed inflammatory cell infiltrate is more frequently identified than a single type of infiltrate. Often, the type of infiltrate will change during the evolution from an acute to chronic phase of the disease. The histologic types of vasculitis currently are categorized into six types: (1) necrotizing angiitis; (2) granulomatous (giant-cell) angiitis; (3) thromboangiitis obliterans; (4) eosinophilic (allergic) angiitis; (5) leukocytoclastic vasculitis; and (6) lymphocytic vasculitis. Although there is some overlap, the different histologic types of vasculitis tend to affect blood vessels of different diameters, as presented in Table 8–1.

Thrombosis, aneurysm formation, hemorrhage, or arterial occlusion may all follow or accompany the transmural damage created by the mixture of immune and inflammatory reactions on the vascular wall. The sequelae of vasculitic injury occupies the attention of the vascular surgeon in these diseases. An abbreviated list of recognized types of vasculitis based on pathologic findings, each of which has potential vascular surgical significance, is presented in Table 8–2. Only aspects of the diseases of vascular surgical significance will be considered in this section.

Polyarteritis Nodosa

Polyarteritis nodosa (PAN) is a disseminated disease characterized by focal necrotizing lesions involving primarily small- and medium-sized muscular arteries. A characteristic crescent-forming glomerulonephritis is also observed frequently. This disease has a male-to-female preponderance of 2:1, with a peak incidence in the fifth decade. Due to the variety of organs involved with PAN, the clinical manifestations are varied. PAN may involve only one organ, or may involve multiple organs simultaneously or sequentially over time. The most frequently observed features of PAN have been renal disease, polyarteritis, polymyositis, and abdominal pain, classically described by Arkin in 1930.[3] The presence of pulmonary involvement in PAN remains uncertain. Most cases of systemic vasculitis accompanied by pulmonary infiltrates and nodules are better classified as Churg-Strauss granulomatosis or Wegener's granulomatosis.[4,5]

The essential pathologic feature of PAN is focal transmural arterial inflammatory necrosis. Light microscopy suggests the process begins with medial destruction, followed by a sequential acute inflammatory response and fibroblastic proliferation. This injury is resolved as intimal proliferation, thrombosis, or aneurysm formation, all of which may culminate in luminal occlusion with consequent organ ischemia and infarction.[6] With further investigation using electron microscopy, it appears the initial injury is within the intima and includes endothelial damage. Interestingly, immune complexes do not appear to be involved in the endothelial degeneration.[7]

Nonspecific serologic markers of inflammation are elevated in PAN: specifically, the erythrocyte sedimentation rate, C-reactive protein, and factor XIII–

TABLE 8–1.   HISTOPATHOLOGY OF VASCULITIDES: MORPHOLOGY TYPE VERSUS VESSEL SIZE[a]

Histopathology	Prototype Example	Large Arteries	Medium-Sized Arteries	Small Arteries and Arterioles	Veins and Venules
Necrotizing angiitis	Polyarteritis nodosa	0	+ + +	+ + +	+
Granulomatous (giant cell) angiitis	Temporal and Takayasu arteritides	+ + +	+ + +	+	+
Thromboangiitis obliterans	Buerger's disease	+	+ + +	+ + +	+ + +
Eosinophilic angiitis	Churg-Strauss syndrome	+	+ +	+ + +	+ +
Leukocytoclastic vasculitis	Urticarial vasculitis	0	0	+ + +	+ + +
Lymphocytic vasculitis	Erythema nodosum	+ +	+ +	+ + +	+ +

[a]Modified from Lie JT: Vasculitis, 1815 to 1991: Classification and diagnostic specificity. J Rheumatol *19*:83–89, 1992.

related protein.[6] Mild anemia and a leukocytosis are frequent. Antineutrophil cytoplasmic antibodies (ANCA) have been detected in patients with systemic vasculitis, including PAN, but are largely absent in patients with immune-mediated vascular injury.[8] Although cytoplasmic and perinuclear staining patterns have been recognized, these patterns do not presently permit stratification of the systemic vasculitides by ANCA patterns.

The hallmark of PAN is the formation of aneurysms associated with inflammatory destruction of the media. Among the most frequently involved organs are the kidney, heart, liver, and gastrointestinal tract. A detailed arteriographic study of 17 patients with PAN reported that 10 of the patients had multiple arterial aneurysms involving the hepatic, renal, and mesenteric circulations.[9] Ruptured PAN aneurysms have been reported often and may contribute to death. Visceral PAN lesions may also lead to visceral artery narrowing incident to the inflammatory process which may process to occlusion. The visceral ischemia may be manifested as cholecystitis, appendicitis, or more commonly with enteric perforation, gastrointestinal hemorrhage, or ischemic stricture formation with bowel obstruction.[10,11] Rupture of intraabdominal PAN aneurysms has been well described and may represent a surgical emergency.[12]

TABLE 8–2.   IMMUNE ARTERITIS OF POTENTIAL VASCULAR SURGICAL SIGNIFICANCE

Polyarteritis nodosa group
  Classic polyarteritis nodosa
  Kawasaki disease
  Drug abuse arteritis
  Cogan's syndrome
  Behçet's syndrome
Hypersensitivity arteritis group
  Hypersensitivity arteritis
  Arteritis of collagen vascular disease
  Mixed cryoglobulinemia with vasculitis
  Arteritis associated with malignancy
Giant cell arteritis
  Temporal arteritis
  Takayasu's arteritis
Buerger's disease

Curiously, these aneurysms have been clearly documented to regress on occasion after vigorous steroid and cyclophosphamide therapy, which should be recommended for all asymptomatic visceral aneurysms.[13,14] An arteriogram of a patient with PAN showing the typical visceral and renal artery aneurysms is shown in Figure 8–2.

To date, little vascular surgical experience has been reported. The multiplicity of diseased areas renders elective vascular repair of all lesions impossible, and there is no accurate way to recognize the dangerous ones. Likewise, the role of vascular surgery in intestinal revascularization in PAN is presently undefined.

Steroid therapy has become therapeutically important in PAN, improving 5-year survival from 15 per cent before routine use of steroids to the current 50 per cent 5-year survival in steroid-treated patients.[15] Cyclophosphamide may be added to the steroid regimen in acute, severe cases.[14] During the acute phase of PAN, renal and gastrointestinal lesions account for the majority of the mortality, whereas cardiovascular and cerebral events account for the mortality in chronic cases of PAN.[15]

Kawasaki Disease

In the 1960s an unusual febrile exanthematous illness swept Japan. Tomisaku Kawasaki observed 50 cases in the Department of Pediatrics at the Japan Red Cross Medical Center and termed the disease the mucocutaneous lymph node syndrome (MCLS).[16,17] Over the next decade, the spread of the disease was noted worldwide and it came to be known as Kawasaki disease.[18,19] The disease had been described sporadically before, usually as juvenile polyarteritis nodosa because of associated arterial aneurysms. The first reports of this disease in the United States appeared in 1976, and within the next 5 years over 500 cases had been reported to the Centers for Disease Control.[20]

The disease is not limited to those of Asian descent and occurs in all ethnic groups, although children of Japanese or mixed Japanese ancestry appear to be most susceptible. Although many suspect an infec-

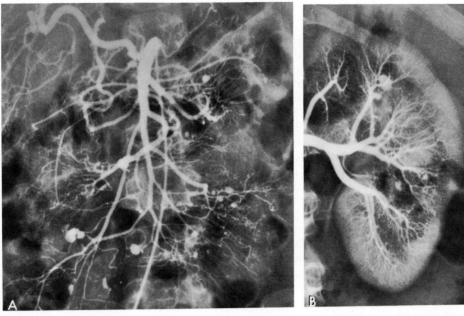

FIGURE 8–2. *A*, Arteriogram showing multiple visceral aneurysms in a patient with polyarteritis nodosa. *B*, Same patient showing multiple renal artery aneurysms.

tious etiology, numerous microbiological and epidemiological studies have not defined the etiology of this disease. As the disease has become better known, strict clinical criteria have evolved for the diagnosis of Kawasaki disease: (1) high fever present for 5 or more days; (2) bilateral congestion of ocular conjunctiva; (3) changes of the mucous membranes of the oral cavity including erythema, dryness, and fissuring of the lips and/or diffuse reddening of the oropharyngeal mucosa; (4) changes of the peripheral portions of the extremities including reddening and induration of the hands and feet and periungual desquamation; (5) polymorphous exanthem; and (6) acute nonsuppurative swelling of the cervical lymph nodes. The presence of a prolonged high fever and any four of the five remaining criteria, in the absence of concurrent evidence of bacterial or viral infection, establishes the diagnosis.[17,21]

Kawasaki disease affects young children, with a peak incidence from 1 to 2 years of age; it has not been described in neonates and is rarely seen for the first time in those over the age of 5.[22] The acute symptoms may persist for 7 to 14 days before improvement as the fever subsides. Notable laboratory features include a high erythrocyte sedimentation rate and thrombocythemia. A small proportion of patients with acute Kawasaki disease will show exacerbation or recrudescence of symptoms and signs during the convalescent phase of the disease within 1 to 3 weeks after initial clinical onset.[23] Some feel this biphasic pattern represents a more severe form of Kawasaki disease with a higher incidence of arterial lesions and a worse prognosis.[24]

Coronary arteritis is most likely present in all children with Kawasaki disease. The spectrum of documented coronary artery pathology consists of active arteritis, thrombosis, calcification, and stenosis, although the distinguishing feature of Kawasaki disease is the formation of diffuse fusiform and saccular coronary artery aneurysms.

Previous reports employing routine echocardiography in patients with Kawasaki disease have demonstrated coronary artery aneurysms in 20 per cent, with the aneurysms typically appearing in the second week of illness and reaching maximum size from the third to eighth week after the onset of fever.[25,26] Cross-sectional echocardiography may show the fusiform or saccular dilation of the right, left, or anterior descending coronary arteries. The circumflex coronary artery is rarely affected by aneurysmal degeneration.[27]

Stenotic lesions may also occur as a result of the arteritic process and tend to be multiple, of varying degree up to complete occlusion, and are only demonstrated by coronary arteriography. Stenotic lesions are most frequently seen in the left anterior descending artery.[28] Patients with fever lasting longer than 14 days, older than 2 years of age, with pericardial effusion, and those not treated with anticoagulant agents appear to have a higher incidence of aneurysm formation.[25] Recently, patients treated with gamma globulin have shown a decreased incidence of aneurysm formation.[28]

Serial arteriographic studies have shown a considerable capacity for all types of coronary arterial lesions to evolve. The aneurysms may regress, leaving a patent arterial lumen, or less favorably the arterial segment may become stenotic. In patients treated with low-dose aspirin (5 to 10 mg/kg) daily during a mean follow-up of 26 months, several factors favoring aneurysmal regression have been noted: an age of less than 1 year at time of onset of Kawasaki disease, female sex, and fusiform aneurysm morphology.[29] Most stenotic lesions also regress with maintenance of a patent lumen, but a few do progress to occlusion. New coronary arterial lesions are infrequent after 2 weeks. Regression of the coronary arterial lesions is usually completed over a 2-month period, although some lesions have remained unchanged for more than a year before regression was observed.[30] The healing phase of the arteritis involves medial fibrosis and intimal thickening, with the later stages involving medial replacement by fibrous scar.[28]

Systemic arteritis also occurs in Kawasaki disease, with iliac arteritis as prevalent as coronary arteritis. Aneurysm formation is far less common in the systemic arteries than in the coronary arteries, with one report identifying systemic arterial aneurysms in 3.3 per cent of 662 Kawasaki disease patients, all of whom had coronary artery aneurysms.[31] The axillary and iliac arteries are the most frequent sites for extracoronary aneurysm formation in these patients. The healing process in the systemic arterial lesions may lead to focal arterial stenoses from fibrotic changes in the area of the initial arteritis or aneurysm, just as in the coronary arteries. A typical coronary arteriogram of such a patient is seen in Figure 8–3A. Peripheral arterial involvement is seen in angiograms in Figure 8–3A and B, showing both subclavian and axillary artery aneurysms.

Thrombosis of coronary artery aneurysms is the overwhelming cause of death in the earlier stages of Kawasaki disease, causing acute myocardial infarction or arrhythmia. Coronary aneurysm rupture has also been described. With the initiation of antithrombotic agents—namely, aspirin—and more recently, immunoglobulin therapy, the mortality from Kawasaki disease has decreased from 2 to 3 per cent, to 0.3 to 0.5 per cent over the past two decades.[28] Currently there is a consensus that aspirin and immunoglobulin therapy should be initiated in the acute phase of the disease, at least for all children less than 12 months of age. Gamma globulin is given intravenously for 4 days, a dose of 400 mg/kg/day. Aspirin is given orally for 14 days at a dose of 100 mg/kg/day, then continued in low-dose form, 3 to 5 mg/kg/day for an additional 8 weeks.[32–34]

Coronary insufficiency has been reported in patients with Kawasaki disease, ranging from angina pectoris to sudden cardiac death. Coronary artery bypass grafting was first used in Kawasaki disease in 1976.[35] The first procedure used saphenous vein as conduit, and several more reports followed.[36,37] Concerns over the use of saphenous vein and its potential for growth with the child have been raised. Few long-term follow-up studies exist, yet the preliminary evidence suggests inferior 5-year patency for saphenous vein grafts with Kawasaki disease. These results have led to the use of the internal mammary artery,[38] bilateral internal mammary arteries,[39] and more recently the right gastroepiploic artery[40] for cor-

onary revascularization in patients with Kawasaki disease. Although these grafts are living and should theoretically grow with the child and his/her heart, long-term results are not currently available.

Aneurysms of the abdominal aorta and iliac, axillary, brachial, mesenteric, and renal arteries have been observed as late sequelae of the systemic vasculitis. When these lesions become symptomatic from occlusion, expansion, or embolization, most surgeons would proceed with standard repair techniques with interposition grafting. Although experience to date is limited, surgical repair of the aneurysms has been accomplished safely, with long-term outcomes uncertain.[41,42]

Citron and associates in 1970 published an important report describing the occurrence of necrotizing arteritis indistinguishable from PAN in a group of addicts with intravenous drug abuse habits.[43] Although many drugs were abused by the patients, methamphetamine was the one most commonly used. These patients developed multiple arterial aneurysms and areas of arterial stenosis that appeared to result from fibrosis occurring in areas of previous arterial necrosis. Four of these 14 patients died of acute disease, with combinations of renal failure, central nervous system dysfunction, and localized intestinal necrosis and perforation. Isolated cerebral angiitis has also been reported in the setting of methamphetamine abuse.[44] No medical therapy is of proven effectiveness for this condition.

A second type of arterial obstruction has been reported in drug abuse patients that has nothing to do with immune complex arteritis. Rather, this represents arterial damage following the accidental intraarterial injection of drugs during attempted intravenous injections. The most frequently reported drugs have been parenteral barbiturates intended for intravenous injection, in which case arterial injury and thrombosis appear to result from chemical damage, perhaps related to the low pH of the injectate.[45,46] Another pattern of arterial damage results from the accidental injection of drug preparations intended for oral use. Certain drug abusers dissolve tablets in water and then inject the solution intravenously. This practice is enormously harmful because of the large number of substances (such as silica and tragacanth) in tablets that facilitate their dissolution. When this material is accidentally injected intraarterially, significant distal arterial obstruction occurs. In this situation the distal ischemia results from obstruction of the small arteries by the inert materials.[47] Illustrative material from such a patient is seen in Figure 8–4.

No convincing evidence has been presented demonstrating the value of any specific treatment in these patients. A variety of therapeutic efforts have been tried, including anticoagulation, regional sympathetic block, and the administration of vasodilators, without any convincing proof of efficacy. In large measure the outcome appears determined at the time of injection by the quantity and concentration of injectate reaching the distal arterial bed, and this out-

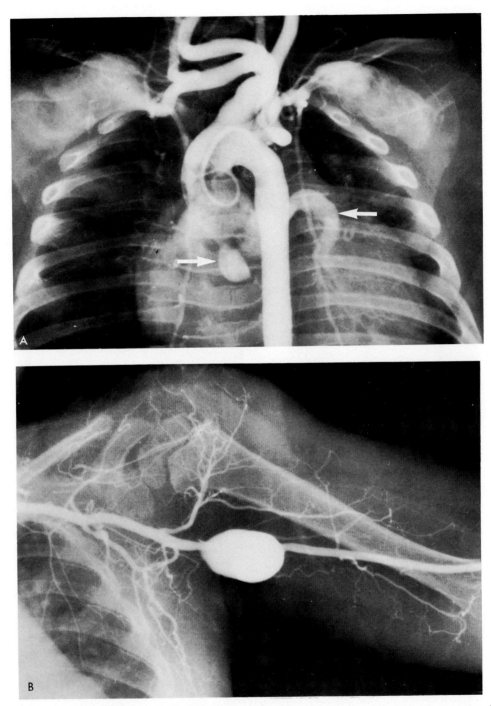

FIGURE 8–3. *A,* Arteriogram of an infant with Kawasaki disease showing coronary artery aneurysms (white arrows) and massive subclavian artery aneurysms. *B,* Arteriogram of a 2-year-old child showing a large axillary artery aneurysm resulting from Kawasaki disease.

come has never been convincingly shown to be modified by subsequent treatment. Nonetheless, we favor heparin anticoagulation if the patient is seen acutely and has no contraindications to this treatment.

Two additional syndromes have been described that appear to be uncommon variants of PAN and may require vascular surgery: Cogan's syndrome and Behçet's syndrome. Cogan's syndrome is a rare condition consisting of nonsyphilitic interstitial keratitis associated with bilateral deafness.[48] Recent evidence has shown that Cogan's syndrome may appear as a component of systemic vasculitis that is similar to PAN.[49] Aortic valve insufficiency and mesenteric ischemia may occur in patients with Cogan's syndrome, apparently resulting from arteritic involvement. Both successful valve replacement and mesenteric revascularization have been performed in these patients.[50]

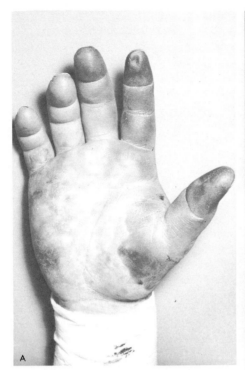
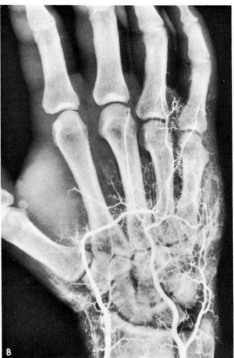

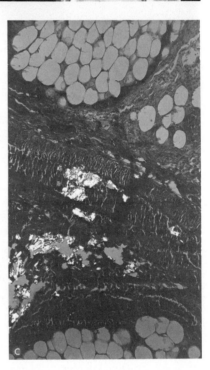

FIGURE 8–4. *A*, Hand photograph of a 22-year-old man who injected a pentazocine tablet dissolved in tap water into his radial artery. The hand was severely ischemic, with gangrenous changes of the radial side. *B*, Arteriogram showing massive arterial obstruction of the common and proper digital arteries to the thumb, index, and long fingers. *C*, Slide from amputation specimen under polarized light showing bright refractile silica particles in the hand arteries.

Behçet's Syndrome

In 1937, Behçet described three patients with iritis and associated oral and genital mucocutaneous ulcerations, an association subsequently termed "Behçet's disease."[51] The underlying pathologic lesion is a vasculitis, which results in both venous thromboses and specific arterial lesions.[52] The latter include occlusive and aneurysmal disease, which when present has a very high mortality rate (up to 20 per cent).[53] This systemic disease largely affects individuals from the Mediterranean area as well as the Far East. Infectious etiologies have been proposed, both bacterial and viral, although definitive evidence is lacking for the implication of infections in the etiology of Behçet's syndrome.[54–58]

Autoimmune dysfunction is the likely cause of this condition. Several investigators have identified circulating immune complexes in affected patients and have suggested autoimmunity because of the observed abnormalities, including the diffuse vasculitis.[59,61] Immune complexes and complement have been demonstrated in the arterial wall and surrounding tissues. The activation of complement within the vascular wall may lead to destruction of the media and subsequent aneurysm formation, possibly through complement fixation to immune complexes within the vasa vasorum of the arterial wall with subsequent occlusion of these nutrient arteries.[60] Vasa vasorum occlusion may in turn lead to transmural necrosis of the large muscular arterial walls, with perforation and ultimately pseudoaneurysm formation following vessel perforation.[61,62]

Behçet's syndrome may also have a genetic component, because there is an increased incidence of certain histocompatibility antigens in patients with this condition.[63] Interestingly, human leukocyte antigen (HLA) genetic markers have been identified with the clinical subtypes of Behçet's syndrome: HLA-B5 with ocular symptoms, HLA-B27 with arthritic symptoms, and HLA-B12 with mucocutaneous lesions.[63]

The pathologic lesion in Behçet's syndrome is a nonspecific panarteritis. Thickening of the endothelium is accompanied by disorganization of the elastic fibers of the media and perivascular round cell infiltration.[64] The perivascular infiltration is often accompanied by luminal thrombosis. Symptomatic arterial involvement, while uncommon, may result in aneurysmal or occlusive disease, although the latter is rare.[64]

Venous involvement is prominent, and lower extremity superficial or deep vein thrombosis occurs in 12 to 27 per cent of patients.[65] Large artery involvement is an uncommon but serious complication of Behçet's syndrome. Arterial aneurysms, while distinctly less common than the mucocutaneous, ophthalmic, or arthritic lesions, are the most frequent cause of death in patients with Behçet's syndrome.[53] Although aneurysms have been described in numerous arteries, including the carotid, popliteal, femoral, iliac, and subclavian, the aorta is the most frequent site of aneurysm formation in this disease.[60,64,66,67] Curiously, the aneurysms frequently appear phlegmonous, suggesting acute bacterial infection, although the cultures are invariably negative. Because of the vascular wall disruption and associated arterial wall fragility, aneurysms frequently recur at anastomotic sites following arterial grafting.[61,68,69] Arterial puncture may lead to the development of pseudoaneurysms in Behçet's syndrome, rendering diagnostic arteriography hazardous. The arterial aneurysms are frequently multiple and may occur dyssynchronously. Unfortunately, interposition bypass grafts have a high incidence of thrombosis in addition to the propensity to develop anastomotic pseudoaneurysms, with long-term graft patencies the exception rather than the norm.[52,65,70]

Immunosuppressive agents, including azathioprine, have been used with some success for nonarterial symptoms, as have corticosteroids.[71,72] Although corticosteroids may suppress symptoms, especially arthritic and ophthalmic ones, they unfortunately do not appear to alter the progression or course of the underlying disease.[72,73] Reports of corticosteroid prevention of pseudoaneurysm recurrence must be viewed as unproven.[60]

Although currently no uniformly satisfactory therapy exists for Behçet's syndrome, early diagnosis and meticulous reconstructive management of identified arterial aneurysms has provided long-term limb salvage in some patients despite the well-recognized propensity for arterial graft complications.[61] Vigilant follow-up is required once large-artery disease is recognized in a patient with Behçet's syndrome. Because this population is at high risk for arteriographic complications, periodic noninvasive imaging and hemodynamic assessment of the arterial system appears prudent.

Hypersensitivity Angiitis Group

This classification incorporates a large and heterogeneous group of clinical syndromes that have in common the predominant involvement of small arteries, contrasted to the medium-sized muscular artery involvement in PAN or the large artery involvement in giant cell arteritis. The entities in this section include classic hypersensitivity angiitis, arteritis of collagen vascular disease,[74] mixed cryoglobulinemia arteritis,[75,76] and arteritis associated with malignancy.[77,78] A semantic discussion continues as to the proper categorization of sclerodermatous arteriopathy. In this condition the arteries show basement membrane thickening, swelling of the collagenous connective tissues, and swelling and fragmentation of the elastic fibers. The end result is vascular occlusion and regional ischemia, just as occurs in the other conditions, although the usual pathologic changes of inflammatory arteritis are not seen.

With the exception of scleroderma, all of these conditions appear to result from antigen exposure followed by the formation of antigen-antibody immune complexes with small artery localization and production of arterial damage. In certain of these conditions a drug or environmental chemical may be implicated as the inciting antigen. In others it may be the hepatitis B virus or possibly a specific tumor antigen protein. In certain of the autoimmune diseases the inciting antigen appears to be fragments of cellular DNA or RNA with an accompanying nucleoprotein, although in most of the autoimmune diseases the identity of the inciting antigen is not known with certainty.

The clinical syndromes typically associated with this group of diseases include skin rash, fever, and evidence of organ dysfunction, none of which specifically concern vascular surgery or the vascular surgeon. It is clear, however, that certain of these syndromes may present with arteritic involvement substantially limited to the hands and fingers. In these patients the clinical picture is typically that of severe and widespread palmar and digital arterial occlusions and digital ischemia. In our ongoing study of Raynaud's disease and digital ischemia, we have encountered 45 patients with ischemic digital ulceration resulting from one of the conditions in this group.[79] A photograph of a painful finger ulcer in one of these patients, accompanied by the hand angiogram, is seen in Figure 8–5.

After detailed clinical and serologic studies, certain of these patients were found to have systemic autoimmune diseases, including scleroderma, rheumatoid arteritis, Sjögren's syndrome, and lupus. Of great interest was the finding that fully two thirds of these patients had no evidence of any systemic disease process and presented with only the acute onset of hand arterial occlusion and finger ischemia.[80,81] None of these patients had any serologic evidence of autoimmune disease. While a few of the patients had a history of a new drug or environmental chemical exposure, the majority did not. Each of these patients showed extensive occlusion of the palmar and digital arteries on arteriography.

Each patient experienced healing of the digital ulceration on a conservative program of scrubs of the open ulcers, conservative surgical débridement, and drug treatment with guanethidine, 10 mg daily, for any vasodilatory effect obtainable. Of interest is the observation that each patient has remained healed and none has experienced any recurrent acute episodes. This condition appears to represent a new type of hypersensitivity angiitis. Judging from personal communications with vascular surgeons, the condition is not rare.

Despite a lack of evidence that vasospasm accompanies ischemic digital ulcerations, vasodilators frequently result in anecdotal improvement. This may be related in part to the remarkable ability of the forearm and hand to increase arteriovenous shunt flow, apparently as a phylogenetic heat-conservation technique. The drugs that appear most useful in this area are nifedipine, 10 mg three times daily, accompanied by guanethidine, 10 mg daily.[82] Acute digital ischemia may be improved in many patients in our experience with tourniquet-controlled intravenous reserpine injection—the Bier block technique, which appears to achieve a complete regional medical sympathectomy.[83] We find no persuasive evidence that either surgical sympathectomy or such unconventional treatment as prostaglandin E infusion or plasmapheresis results in any benefit in these patients over that achieved through the conservative treatment methods described above.[84]

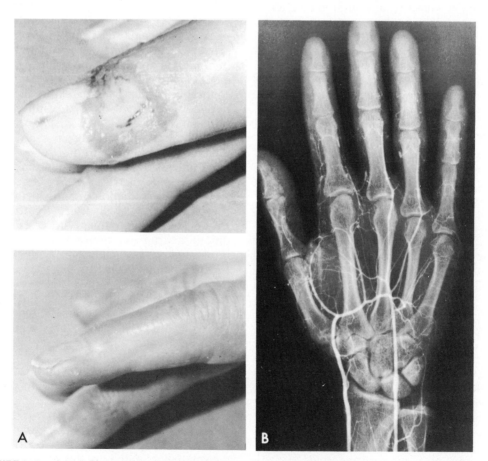

FIGURE 8–5. *A (top),* Photograph of a very painful ischemic finger ulcer resulting from widespread digital artery occlusion caused by arteritis. *(bottom),* Same area showing healing after conservative treatment described in the text. *B,* Arteriogram of same patient showing massive digital artery obstruction.

Giant Cell Arteritis Group

The two conditions included in this group are systemic giant cell, or temporal, arteritis and Takayasu's arteritis. While these do segregate themselves into fairly distinctive clinical patterns, as noted in Table 8–3, there is evidence that the two entities may represent different manifestations of the same disease process.[74] The microscopic pathology of the conditions differs overall, but individual slides are frequently impossible to categorize as clearly one or the other. Both conditions consist of localized periarteritis with inflammatory mononuclear infiltrates and giant cells, along with disruption and fragmentation of the elastic fibers of the arterial wall.

Systemic Giant Cell Arteritis (Temporal Arteritis)

This disease is essentially limited to patients more than 55 years of age, occurs three times as frequently in women as men, and is much more prominent in whites. A recent epidemiologic survey found the annual incidence in white females greater than 50 years of age to be more than 16 cases/100,000.[85] The condition is a systemic disease process characterized by chronic inflammation of the aorta and its major branches. The usual symptoms are headache accompanied by severe pain in the pelvic and shoulder girdle regions, a condition termed "polymyalgia rheumatica." Detailed reviews of the subject have been published.[86]

Systemic giant cell arteritis may involve any large artery of the body, although it does have a propensity to involve branches of the carotid artery. The clinical history usually begins with a febrile myalgic process involving primarily the back, shoulder, and pelvic regions. The most characteristic complaint is severe pain along the course of the temporal artery accompanied by tenderness and nodularity of the artery together with overlying skin erythema. The involvement is frequently bilateral.

TABLE 8–3. CLINICAL PATTERNS IN GIANT CELL ARTERITIS

	Temporal Arteritis	Takayasu's Arteritis
Age/sex	Elderly Caucasian females	Young females
Pathology	Inflammatory cellular infiltrates; giant cells	Same
Area of involvement	Branches of carotid usually; may involve any artery	Aortic arch and branches; pulmonary artery
Complications	Blindness	Hypertension, stroke
Response to steroids	Excellent	Unpredictable—unproven

One of the frequent and severe complications of this disease is visual disturbance, which occurs in over 50 per cent of patients. The mechanism of the visual alterations may be either ischemic optic or retrobulbar neuritis, or occlusions of the central retinal artery. In one large clinical series, 42 per cent of all patients with symptomatic giant cell arteritis experienced a permanent loss of part or all of their vision.[87]

The diagnosis of this condition is suspected clinically and confirmed by the finding of an elevated erythrocyte sedimentation rate and a temporal artery biopsy showing the typical pathologic changes.[88] The importance of a precise and early diagnosis lies in the early initiation of steroid therapy, which has been of great value in preventing the devastating visual complications of the disease.

Systemic giant cell arteritis is of concern to cardiac and vascular surgeons because it may cause aneurysms or stenoses of the aorta or its main branches. As noted, both true thoracic aortic aneurysms and dissecting aneurysms may occur. Some have speculated that early and adequate steroid therapy will minimize the likelihood of these serious complications, although convincing evidence of this presumption seems wanting.[74] Successful cardiovascular surgery has occasionally been performed for the thoracic aortic complications.[89,90]

Peripheral arterial involvement in giant cell arteritis was once thought to be a pathologic curiosity. More recent reviews, however, have noted a significant incidence of symptomatic peripheral arterial occlusions or stenoses in these patients. Klein and associates[91] found that 34 of 248 patients had evidence of symptomatic large-artery involvement, while Swinson and associates[92] recently reported two patients with subclavian artery obstruction. Rivers et al. recently described our experiences with six patients with symptomatic giant cell arteritis who presented with subclavian-axillary occlusion.[93] The angiographic features most suggestive of arteritis include long segments of smooth stenosis interspersed with normal segments, smoothly tapered occlusions, absence of irregular plaques and ulcerations, and distribution of these abnormalities among the subclavian, axillary, and brachial arteries.[91] A representative angiogram is seen in Figure 8–6.

The importance of an early diagnosis is twofold: prompt steroid therapy will frequently result in a restoration of pulses, a finding noted by us and others, which is probably dependent upon a reversal of the inflammatory process; and, most important, vascular reconstructive surgery is relatively contraindicated in these patients. Surgical procedures fail in a high percentage of patients unless accompanied by high-dose steroid administration.[93] One must have a high level of suspicion that the underlying condition may be giant cell arteritis in an elderly white female who presents with the recent onset of upper extremity ischemia. Four of our six patients had no myalgias, fever, or headaches to suggest a systemic disease

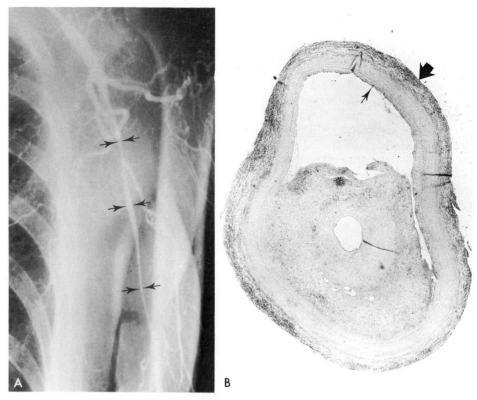

FIGURE 8–6. *A,* Typical giant cell arteritis showing smooth tapering of axillary artery (arrows). *B,* Photomicrograph of axillary artery involved with giant cell arteritis showing transmural inflammation. (From Rivers SP, Baur GM, Inahara T, Porter JM: Arm ischemia secondary to giant cell arteritis. Am J Surg *143:*554–558, 1982.)

process. An underlying arteritis would have been missed in the absence of a high index of suspicion.

Takayasu's Disease

As seen in Table 8–3, Takayasu's disease differs clinically from systemic giant cell arteritis, although the microscopic picture may be similar. A large majority of the patients reported to date have been Asian. About 85 per cent of all patients are female, with the age at onset between 3 and 35 years. The early symptoms in about two thirds of patients are quite nonspecific, consisting of fever, myalgia, and anorexia. These symptoms may be followed shortly thereafter by cardiovascular symptoms depending on disease location. The cardiovascular areas of involvement have been characterized as types I, II, III, and IV and are shown diagrammatically in Figure 8–7.

Type I is limited to involvement of the arch and arch vessels and occurs in 8.4 per cent of patients. Type II involves the descending thoracic and abdominal aorta and accounts for 11.2 per cent of cases. Type III has involvement of the arch vessels and the abdominal aorta and its branches and accounts for 65.4 per cent of cases. Type IV has primarily pulmonary artery involvement with or without the other types and accounts for 15 per cent of patients.[94] Most of the lesions are stenotic, although localized aneurysms have been reported.

Patients may develop cardiovascular or neurologic symptoms. The predominant cardiovascular findings are diminished peripheral arterial pulsations and hypertension. The hypertension may be due to aortic coarctation or renal artery stenosis. The possible relationship of this disease to the middle aortic, or abdominal coarctation, syndrome will be described in a subsequent section. Neurologic symptoms may result from hypertension or central nervous system ischemia associated with large artery occlusion or stenosis. Heart failure occurs in these patients as a consequence of systemic hypertension and in some patients from pulmonary hypertension. Coronary artery involvement in Takayasu's disease is rare. The cardiac pathology most frequently found is nonspecific and appears to result from heart failure associated with systemic and pulmonary hypertension.

The role of vascular surgery in the treatment of Takayasu's arteritis is not well defined. Certainly, isolated cases have been described in which such procedures as repair of a descending thoracic aortic coarctation have given satisfactory short-term results.[95]

The role of surgery in lesions of the arch vessels, visceral arteries, and renal arteries is uncertain. Endarterectomy has resulted in early failure and generally is not recommended.[96] Visceral artery surgical results were so poor in the past that some internists condemned the role of reconstructive vascular surgery.[94]

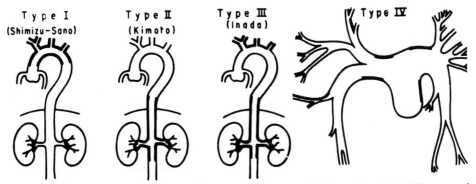

FIGURE 8–7.   Diagrammatic representation of the recognized types of Takayasu's arteritis. The areas of arterial involvement are shown in heavy lines. (From Lupi-Herrera E, Sanchez-Torres G, Marcustiamer J, et al: Takayasu's arteritis: Clinical study of 107 cases. Am Heart J 93:94–103, 1977.)

Available information suggests a conservative surgical approach to these patients. Aneurysms of the aorta or branch arteries should be treated on their own merits just as are atherosclerotic aneurysms in the same location. Patients probably should have a course of steroids prior to surgery. Visceral and arch vessel lesions appear to be best managed with bypass grafts. It is important to note that these statements regarding the role of surgery are based on only a few published reports, many of which are more than 10 years old. It is clear, however, that optimal treatment of these difficult patients requires judicious adherence to vascular surgical principles, as well as close cooperation between the vascular surgeon and the internist.

Buerger's Disease

Few conditions in vascular surgery have created more controversy than has Buerger's disease. Scholarly denials of the existence of the condition have been met by equally scholarly advocates.[97,98] There currently appears to be a consensus that the condition does exist as a distinct clinical entity with objective diagnostic criteria. The condition appears clinically and pathologically distinct from both atherosclerosis and various forms of immune arteritis.

Buerger's disease, also known as thromboangiitis obliterans, is a clinical syndrome characterized by the occurrence of segmental thrombotic occlusions of small- and medium-sized arteries in the lower, and frequently the upper, extremities, accompanied by a prominent arterial wall inflammatory cell infiltration.[99] Affected patients are predominantly young male smokers, who usually present with distal limb ischemia, frequently accompanied by localized digital gangrene. Interestingly, the life expectancy for patients with Buerger's disease appears near normal when compared with age-matched controls, in distinct contrast to the shortened life spans seen in individuals with atherosclerosis.[100–102]

While Buerger's disease appears definitely on the decline in North America, a large volume of patients continue to be reported from the Far East, Middle East, and Asia.[102–106] This peculiar geographic distribution remains unexplained.

Approximately 40 to 50 per cent of patients with Buerger's disease have a history of superficial migratory thrombophlebitis, Raynaud's syndrome, or both. The arterial lesions of Buerger's disease usually occur in the distal portions of both upper and lower extremities and may be accompanied by digital gangrene, especially of the toes. Descriptions of cerebral, coronary, and visceral artery involvement with Buerger's disease are controversial. The available reports are not well supported by pathologic data and must be regarded as unproven.[107,108] However, there have been several well-documented reports, both arteriographically and pathologically, of iliac artery involvement.[105,109] Without question, however, the large majority of patients with thromboangiitis obliterans have disease limited to the extremity arteries distal to the elbow and knee. In North America, about 50 per cent of patients with Buerger's disease have isolated lower extremity involvement, 30 to 40 per cent have upper and lower extremity involvement, and about 10 per cent have isolated upper extremity involvement.[104,110] Although males are more commonly affected, women constitute up to 20 per cent of the patients reported in the largest North American series.[101,103]

The acute lesion of Buerger's disease is a nonnecrotizing panarteritis with a prominent component of intraluminal thrombosis. This lesion may be differentiated from both immune arteritis and atherosclerosis by the presence of an intact or minimally disrupted internal elastic lamina, with a conspicuous absence of arterial wall necrosis, and preservation of normal vascular wall architecture.

The intraluminal thrombosis in Buerger's disease leads to an intense hypercellular inflammatory cell infiltration of both the arterial wall and the thrombus itself, with prominent fibroblast proliferation, frequently accompanied by giant cell development. Progression of the lesion to a subacute phase is signified by a shift in the infiltrating cells to a predominantly mononuclear form with more giant cells. As the lesion progresses to a chronic phase, the hypercellularity of the thrombus resolves with the production of perivascular fibrosis, with recanalization of the luminal thrombus. As with the acute lesion, the layers of the arterial wall remain recognizable. Adjacent veins and nerves are often involved in a prominent contiguous perivascular inflammatory process.

From a careful examination of our recently reported patients, as well as a review of published experience, we propose the following diagnostic criteria for Buerger's disease.[104,111,112] These include onset of distal extremity ischemic symptoms before 45 years of age; a uniform history of tobacco abuse; the absence of an underlying proximal embolic source; the absence of trauma, autoimmune disease, diabetes, or hyperlipidemia; the presence of undiseased arteries proximal to the popliteal or distal brachial level; and the presence of distal occlusive disease with distinctive plethysmographic, arteriographic, and pathologic findings consistent with Buerger's disease. We recognized that these criteria are so restrictive that some patients with Buerger's disease will be excluded, but we believe these strict criteria are necessary to eliminate the diagnostic uncertainty obvious in many publications of purported Buerger's disease.

Buerger's disease is accompanied by distinctive arteriographic findings.[97,113,114] The extremity arteries proximal to the popliteal and distal brachial levels are arteriographically normal, at least in North American reports. Proximal atherosclerosis is absent. The typical finding is an abrupt transition from a normal, smooth proximal vessel to an area of occlusion. Involvement tends to be segmental rather than diffuse and is commonly symmetric. Extensive digital, palmar, and plantar arterial occlusions are common. Tortuous "corkscrew" collaterals frequently reconstitute patent distal arterial segments. The typical corkscrew appearance of distal collateral sites, while not pathognomonic, is suggestive of Buerger's disease. A typical arteriogram is seen in Figure 8–8.

Arteriography, while desirable, is not essential for the diagnosis of every case of Buerger's disease.[112] Arteriography may be omitted when a patient's history is typical for Buerger's disease, there are no associated atherogenic risk factors such as hyperlipidemia or diabetes mellitus, the serologic tests for autoimmune disease (as previously described) are negative, and vascular lab exam reveals diffusively abnormal digital plethysmographic tracings in all four extremities accompanied by a conspicuous absence of proximal large artery occlusive disease.[112]

Digital plethysmography frequently provides especially important diagnostic information in this condition. In the typical Buerger's patient, obstructive arterial waveforms are present in all digits, providing objective evidence of widespread digital arterial occlusion or stenosis. Patients with unilateral digital plethysmographic abnormalities should undergo arteriography to rule out a proximal potentially surgically correctable arterial lesion causing the digital ischemia. Additionally, patients with symptoms and objective findings localizing their disease to the distal

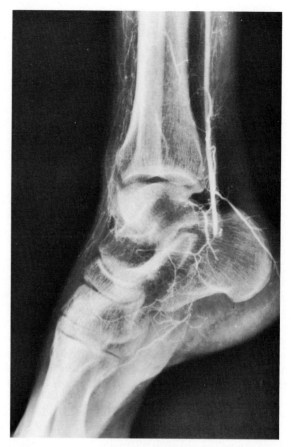

FIGURE 8–8. Arteriogram of patient with Buerger's disease showing occlusion of the posterior tibial artery at the ankle, total occlusion of the anterior tibial artery, and numerous small collateral vessels.

feet and toes, and who have normal hand and finger plethysmography, should undergo arteriography to rule out a proximal embolic source for their ischemia.

The etiology of Buerger's disease remains unknown. Although a strong association with cigarette smoking has been clinically recognized, a causal relationship has not been conclusively demonstrated.[115–117] Nonetheless, we and others have never recognized Buerger's disease in a nonsmoker. Abnormal coagulation profiles have been described in Buerger's disease, but closer scrutiny suggests these mild abnormalities are more likely secondary to the underlying thrombotic process rather than causative.[118] Considerable evidence indicates that an autoimmune process is central to Buerger's disease. Several independent investigators have identified elevated levels of anticollagen antibodies in certain patients with Buerger's disease.[100,119,120] It remains unclear at this point whether the finding of elevated anticollagen antibodies is specific for Buerger's disease, or merely a nonspecific finding associated with a variety of inflammatory conditions of the vascular wall. An association of Buerger's disease with HLA-A9 and HLA-B5 has been reported, but we have been unable to confirm this finding in our patients.[112,121,122]

The cornerstone of treatment for patients with Buerger's disease is tobacco abstinence. The disease typically undergoes remissions and relapses that correlate closely with the cessation and resumption of cigarette smoking.[103,112,116,123,124] In our clinical series, no patient has sustained further tissue loss following cessation of smoking.[112] Unfortunately, tobacco addiction is a notoriously difficult condition to treat, with prolonged abstinence the exception rather than the norm in patients with Buerger's disease.

We use a prolonged conservative local treatment program for areas of finger ulceration and gangrene, with the primary goal being a clean, dry digit.[125] Ischemic ulcer débridement, often including nail removal, is used frequently, accompanied by minimal ronguer removal of exposed phalangeal bone as needed. Proximal finger amputations are rarely required and wrist or forearm amputations have never been necessary in our patients with Buerger's disease. Prolonged conservative management is usually rewarded by healing with preservation of maximal digital length, providing smoking has been discontinued. We have found thoracic sympathectomy ineffectual in this setting, and we find no convincing evidence that this procedure is of any benefit in these patients. Sympathectomy is not recommended.[126]

The course of lower extremity Buerger's disease stands in marked contrast to that observed with upper extremity involvement. Several large series have reported a 12 to 31 per cent incidence of major leg amputation over a 5- to 10-year period.[102,127] Our own recent experience revealed a 31 per cent incidence of major leg amputation.[112] In the past we occasionally performed lumbar sympathectomy in patients in whom foot rest pain persisted despite optimal medical management. It now appears clear from our experience and that of others that lumbar sympathectomy for Buerger's disease is not beneficial, and we no longer perform or recommend the procedure.

If arteriography reveals a patent distal vessel, and if autogenous vein is available, a distal arterial bypass may be considered.[117,128,129] The use of autogenous vein is mandatory. Distal bypass is rarely feasible because of the diffuse nature of the arterial occlusive disease process. In our experience and that of others, the long-term results of reconstruction are poor; only a small number of patients with Buerger's disease can undergo lower extremity bypass, and even with optimal patient selection the intermediate patency is disappointing.[112] We no longer recommend bypass to segmentally patent distal arteries because none of these have remained patent.

Many medications have been recommended in the treatment of Buerger's disease, including corticosteroids, prostaglandin E_1 infusion, vasodilators, hemorrheologic agents, antiplatelet agents, and anticoagulants.[97,112,116,130–135] None of these has ever been subjected to a randomized, controlled clinical trial in patients with Buerger's disease, and there is no evidence that any are effective. We have noted anecdotal improvement in pain control with the use of either nifedipine or diltiazem in patients with Buerger's disease accompanied by severe Raynaud's syndrome.[112] We have noted similar anecdotal benefits from pentoxifylline in patients with rest pain or digital ulceration, especially of the fingers. We often empirically place Buerger's disease patients on antiplatelet therapy because this appears reasonable for the treatment of a disease characterized by widespread, segmental arterial and superficial venous thromboses. Thus we treat many of our Buerger's disease patients with a combination of nifedipine, pentoxifylline, and aspirin, although we clearly recognize an absence of objective evidence supporting the use of these agents.

RADIATION-INDUCED ARTERIAL DAMAGE

Irradiation given in treatment of regional malignancy causes well-recognized changes in arteries in the radiation field. The primary changes consist of intimal thickening and proliferation, medial hyalinization, and cellular infiltration of the adventitia. The endothelial cells are sloughed if the radiation intensity is sufficient. Small arteries are more likely to occlude, but even large arteries may show narrowing or occlusion.[136] Numerous reports describe arterial stenosis as a consequence of radiation.[137–140] A typical arteriogram is seen in Figure 8–9.

Of considerable importance is the reported tendency of arteries in an irradiated area to show stenosis years later. Several recent papers have described an unusually large incidence of carotid artery stenosis in patients years after neck irradiation, as well as an increased likelihood of stroke.[140,141] The lesions found vary between diffuse scarring and areas of typical atheromatous narrowing, with a preponderance of the latter. Radiation may stimulate the development of atherosclerosis, although the experimental evidence is inconclusive.[142] Whatever the mechanism of arterial injury, patients who have had neck area irradiation should have careful vascular follow-up, probably with repeated vascular laboratory examinations.

Vascular surgery on irradiated arteries may be performed with standard techniques. Prosthetic and autogenous bypass grafts as well as endarterectomy have all been performed satisfactorily. Prudence would suggest avoidance of a prosthetic graft in a field in which infection may be expected, such as a radical neck dissection following irradiation.

ARTERIAL INFECTIONS

Infection occurring in an arterial aneurysm was first described by Koch in 1851, and the first use of the term "mycotic aneurysm" was by Osler in 1885.[143] Osler's use of the term "mycotic" was understood to mean any infection caused by microorganisms. Since that time the word "mycotic" has been applied specifically to fungal infections, although the term

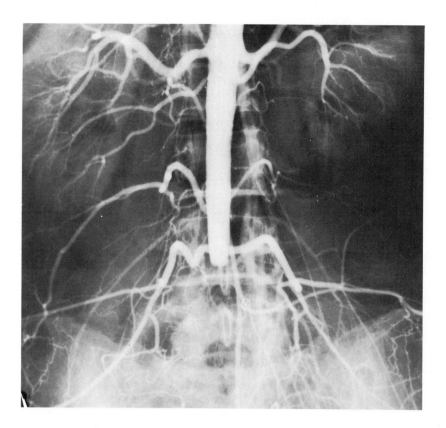

FIGURE 8–9. Radiation arteritis. Arteriograms in a 40-year-old woman who had received extensive internal and external irradiation for treatment of carcinoma of the cervix. There is a typical absence of atherosclerotic disease of the infrarenal aorta.

"mycotic aneurysm" has persisted. There now is general agreement that this semantic confusion is best avoided by abandoning the term and substituting the term "arterial infection" or "infected arterial aneurysm." A large majority of arterial infections as well as infected arterial aneurysms occur in relationship to prosthetic arterial grafts, and are described in Chapter 34. Only primary arterial infections will be considered in this section. In the modern world, discussion of arterial infection must be categorized into illicit drug–related infection and non–drug-related, or primary, arterial infections.

Primary (Non–Drug-Related) Arterial Infections

The infrequency of infected arterial aneurysms can be readily appreciated because a widely quoted review[144] in the preantibiotic era found only 66 cases reported prior to 1923. Over the 14-year period 1961 to 1974, only 17 infected abdominal aortic aneurysms were seen at the Massachusetts General Hospital.[143]

The pathogenesis of non–drug-related arterial infections has changed remarkably since the advent of antibiotics. In the preantibiotic era, the usual etiology was septic embolization from bacterial endocarditis.[145] The propensity of small fragments of embolic material to pass distally accounted for the large incidence of peripheral infected arterial aneurysms. At the present time, the most common etiology is hematogenous seeding of the arterial wall during episodes

of bacteremia. Bacterial localization in the arterial wall vasa vasorum has been postulated, although the importance of this proposed cryptogenic mechanism is unknown.[146] Arterial infection may also occur through direct extension or through lymphatics from a contiguous area of infection, or following trauma, but these mechanisms appear distinctly less frequently than bacteremic seeding. At the present time, no precise source or mechanism of infection can be identified in 50 per cent of patients with primary arterial infection.[147] Arterial infection in these patients presumably results from transient bacteremia.

Considerable evidence indicates that bacteremia rarely causes infection in a normal artery, with the exception of particulate embolization from an identified proximal septic focus. Rather, bacteria appear to localize preferentially on diseased and roughened atherosclerotic surfaces. Once a local bacterial inflammatory process is established, the development of the infectious process may follow several courses. One uncommon but well-recognized course is the development of a virulent suppurative arteritis with necrosis of the arterial wall and rupture.[147] Another possibility is a less virulent septic arteritis with progression to a localized or controlled rupture and formation of a pseudoaneurysm. This may be differentiated from an atherosclerotic aneurysm in that it lacks arterial wall layers and usually presents as an eccentric, or saccular, process rather than as a fusiform dilation typical of an atherosclerotic aneurysm.[148]

Recent investigations have shown that positive arterial wall bacterial cultures can be obtained in 40 to

50 per cent of all atherosclerotic vessels, none of which have gross evidence of infection.[149] The organism most commonly cultured has been *Staphylococcus epidermidis*, which comprises 70 per cent of the positive arterial wall cultures. *S. epidermidis* tends to be a less virulent organism than *Staphylococcus aureus*, producing a chronic, indolent infection. *S. epidermidis* has displaced *S. aureus* as the most prevalent organism identified in infected arterial biomaterials.[150–152] Newer culture techniques employing tissue sonication have yielded even higher percentages of positive arterial wall cultures with *S. epidermidis*.[153]

The bacteriology of arterial infections has changed with antibiotics. In the preantibiotic era when the most frequent cause of arterial infections was embolization, the most commonly isolated organisms were *Streptococcus*, *Pneumococcus*, *Haemophilus*, and occasionally *Staphylococcus*.[144,145,154] At the present time, the organisms most frequently found in infected arterial aneurysms are *Salmonella*, *Staphylococcus aureus* and *albus*, *Escherichia coli*, and a mixture of gram-negative organisms. Interestingly, bacterial colonization of noninfected abdominal aortic aneurysms as determined by routine culture at surgery has been found in 15 per cent of patients, with over 80 per cent of the organisms being gram-positive cocci.[155]

Salmonella appears to be an especially virulent organism causing arterial infection and is occurring with increasing frequency, accounting for 30 to 50 per cent of recently reported cases of infected arterial aneurysms.[147,156,157] Although distinctly uncommon, arterial infections may be caused by fungi, as summarized in an excellent review by Miller and associates.[158] Most patients with fungal arterial infections either are immunosuppressed or have established fungal infections elsewhere.

The recent improvement in transplant graft survival associated with cyclosporine immunosuppression has led to an increasing population of immunosuppressed patients. Immunosuppressed patients clearly have an increased risk for developing infections. Infected arterial aneurysms of the donor organ arterial anastomosis have been reported for renal, hepatic, pancreatic, and heart-lung transplants.[159–165] Infected arterial aneurysms in this setting frequently prove to be infected pseudoaneurysms. This lesion typically develops at potentially weakened sites, including arterial suture lines and cannulation and clamp sites. Transient bacteremia from even minor events may be sufficient to seed an injured endothelial surface in the setting of profound immunosuppression. The culture-isolated organisms from a number of these case reports support this hypothesis because normal human flora have been isolated frequently, including gram-negative bacilli, gram-positive cocci, and yeast.[160,163–166] Allograft anastomotic infection is a devastating complication frequently requiring allograft removal, even when the organ is functioning well. Delayed native arterial stump rupture has been described following allograft removal and ligation.[163]

The triad of back pain, pulsatile abdominal mass,

and fever suggests the presence of an infected arterial aneurysm. Several investigators have observed that over 50 per cent of patients with infected arterial aneurysms will have positive blood cultures.[148,167] Other features suggesting infection include the finding of saccular aneurysms or noncalcified aortic aneurysms.[168]

The arteriogram may be quite suggestive if it reveals a saccular or lobulated aneurysm with otherwise normal vasculature.[169] However, the angiogram may reveal only a typical atherosclerotic aneurysm if the infectious process involves a preexisting atherosclerotic aneurysm.

There is general agreement that the optimal treatment of infected arterial aneurysms is excision and remote grafting through a clean field, accompanied by a prolonged course of antibiotics. This principle of remote grafting is difficult or impossible to apply to suprarenal infected aortic aneurysms. In these patients, in situ aortic and visceral prosthetic reconstruction has been successfully performed when accompanied by long-term antibiotic therapy.[166] A few patients have survived excision of infected infrarenal aneurysms with interposition grafting directly in the same field. This favorable outcome, however, appears to reflect the presence of infecting organisms of low virulence or a limited infection treated by thorough débridement prior to graft placement.[170,171] Interposition grafting in the same field seems especially prone to failure in the presence of *Salmonella*,[156] although exceptions have been described.[170,172]

Illicit Drug-Related Arterial Infections

The recent increase in the use of illicit street drugs has predictably been accompanied by a commensurate increase in the incidence of cardiovascular morbidity resulting from drug injections with a contaminated needle and syringe. Contaminated injections into veins and/or arteries have resulted in a variety of cardiovascular injuries, including infective endocarditis, chronic venous thrombosis, local sepsis, and pseudoaneurysms of the femoral artery.[173] Huebl and Read were the first to describe the development of arterial aneurysmal abscesses as a complication of intraarterial or periarterial injections of illicit street drugs.[174] Over the past 20 years, the incidence of this lesion has increased to a point where it is now one of the most common sequelae of drug abuse requiring surgical intervention.[175]

Three approaches to treatment have been proposed: ligation and excision of the infected pseudoaneurysm with immediate arterial reconstruction; ligation and excision alone with subsequent amputation as needed for the development of gangrene; and ligation, excision, and delayed reconstruction for persistent ischemia. Feldman et al.[176] found that immediate reconstruction had a high rate of graft infection and that those patients treated with ligation and excision alone did not have a higher rate of limb loss.

Their best results were reported in a group of six patients treated by excision and ligation, followed by delayed extraanatomic bypass 5 days to 20 months postoperatively for persistent ischemia.[176]

Fromm and Lucas pointed out that critical ischemia often developed after excision and ligation of a femoral pseudoaneurysm when the pseudoaneurysm involved the femoral bifurcation.[177] These authors recommended iliofemoral bypass through the obturator foramen prior to excision of the infected arterial aneurysm. Initially this group believed they could predict limbs at risk for ischemia by careful review of the arteriograms prior to excision and ligation of the infected arterial aneurysm. However, a more recent review of their experience has led the authors to conclude that no preoperative tests can accurately predict those limbs at risk for ischemia following excision and ligation of an infected arterial aneurysm.[178]

The controversy over routine versus selective revascularization persists. Reddy et al. have followed a selective approach to revascularization in their series of 54 infected femoral pseudoaneurysms.[179] Pseudoaneurysms involving the common femoral bifurcation were the most problematic, because those treated with ligation and excision alone suffered an amputation rate of 21 per cent, and all synthetic grafts placed for revascularization became infected, eventually requiring graft removal. Abscess formation limited to the common femoral artery did well with excision and ligation alone, and those common femoral bifurcation revascularizations utilizing autogenous conduit suffered no infectious complications. On the basis of this experience, the authors recommend ligation and excision without concomitant revascularization for arterial infection proximal to the femoral bifurcation, and immediate autogenous conduit reconstruction for selected common femoral bifurcation lesions.[179,180]

Patel et al. recently reviewed their experience with routine revascularization along with resection of the infected femoral pseudoaneurysm in 15 patients with a history of drug abuse.[181] All pseudoaneurysms resulted from drug injections in the groin. All patients had extraanatomic bypass grafts placed prior to excision and ligation of the pseudoaneurysm, with polytetrafluoroethylene the graft conduit in all cases. *S. aureus* was by far the most predominant organism. There were no graft infections through a follow-up period ranging from 1 to 44 months, with a 13 per cent amputation rate.

A synthesis of this information indicates that acute arterial reconstruction may not be required following excision of infected femoral artery pseudoaneurysms when the femoral artery bifurcation is not involved. If the femoral bifurcation is involved, arterial reconstruction is frequently necessary to prevent limb loss, and appears best accomplished with autogenous reconstruction through a clean field.

FIBROMUSCULAR DYSPLASIA

Fibromuscular dysplasia (FMD) is the term applied to an arterial developmental abnormality character-

ized generally by a series of eccentric stenoses with intervening areas of dilation, although rare variants may have only a single area of stenosis. Detailed histologic studies have resulted in the recognition of at least four distinct pathologic types: intimal fibroplasia, medial fibroplasia, medial hyperplasia, and perimedial dysplasia.[182]

The first case report of FMD was by Leadbetter and Burkland in 1938, describing a patient with renal artery involvement.[183] By far the majority of cases involve the renal artery, with the carotid and iliac arteries representing distant second and third most likely areas of involvement.[184] Other arteries that may be involved with FMD include the mesenteric, subclavian, axillary, vertebral, and coronary. Ninety per cent of adult patients with FMD are female, and, curiously, 80 per cent of renal artery involvement affects the right side. A typical renal arteriogram of FMD appears in Figure 8–10.

Medial fibroplasia accounts for 85 per cent of renal artery involvement and perimedial dysplasia accounts for 10 per cent. The groups are distinguished from each other by the vessel wall layer primarily affected and by the tissue components that predominate. An increase of fibrous connective tissue, collagen, and ground substance within the media is characteristic of medial fibroplasia, whereas an excess of medial smooth muscle is present in medial hyperplasia. The smooth muscle cell is clearly multipotential and appears to be the stem from which the proliferative changes in FMD are derived. The etiology of FMD is unknown. Several theories have been advanced, including (1) arterial stretching, (2) mural ischemia secondary to an abnormal distribution of vasa vasorum, (3) estrogenic (or other hormonal) effect on the arterial wall, (4) immunologic insult, or (5) embryologic maldevelopment.[185]

Symptoms produced by FMD are generally secondary to the associated arterial stenosis and are generally indistinguishable from those caused by atherosclerosis. The two most frequently seen clinical syndromes are renovascular hypertension and transient cerebral ischemic attacks. The disease may occur without symptoms, as shown by Youngberg and associates, who found only four of nine patients with renal artery FMD to have diastolic blood pressure greater than 100 mm Hg.[186]

Fibromuscular dysplasia of the renal artery may be associated with the formation of renal artery aneurysms. The indications for resection of visceral aneurysms are described in Chapter 20. Treatment is generally recommended for arterial stenotic lesions only when they produce significant symptoms. Renovascular hypertension caused by FMD has historically been treated by bypass grafting, or occasionally by open graduated internal dilatation. Renovascular hypertension caused by FMD has generally responded more favorably to surgery than has that caused by atherosclerosis.[187] Recently percutaneous transluminal angioplasty has been shown to be effective in selected patients.[188]

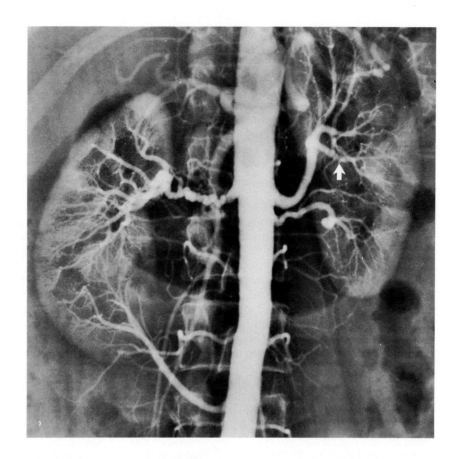

FIGURE 8–10. Fibromuscular dysplasia. The superior right renal artery shows typical involvement extending beyond the primary branching. Moderate left kidney segmental artery FMD is present (white arrow).

Carotid artery FMD causes symptoms identical to atherosclerosis and, like atherosclerosis, the disease usually stops before the internal carotid artery enters the base of the skull. Fewer than 1 per cent of patients undergoing carotid arteriography have FMD.[185] Treatment of symptomatic patients by graduated internal dilation at the time of surgery is preferred, but patch angioplasty or interposition grafting may be required, depending on the location and extent of involvement.[189] Iliac and femoral artery FMD have been successfully treated by graduated internal dilation with long-term success.[190]

ADVENTITIAL CYSTIC DISEASE

Adventitial cystic disease is a rare condition in which arterial stenosis is caused by single or multiple synovial-like cysts in the subadventitial layer of the arterial wall. The cysts are similar to ganglion cysts and are filled with mucin. Eighty per cent of patients with this condition are male, and the median age at presentation is 40 years. Both legs are equally affected.

The first case report describing operative management was in 1954.[191] Since then fewer than 150 cases have been reported. The popliteal artery has been by far the most frequently involved artery, with the femoral and iliac arteries being the next most frequent areas of involvement.[192] An excellent summary of this condition was published by Flanigan and associates in 1979.[193]

The etiology of adventitial cystic disease is unknown. Three theories have been presented, including (1) repeated arterial microtrauma, (2) the presence within the arterial wall of mucin-secreting cell rests derived embryologically from the synovial anlage of the knee joint, and (3) the development of true ganglia in the adventia.

The condition, along with the popliteal entrapment syndrome and thromboangiitis obliterans, should be considered in young people who present with claudication. On examination, the finding of a popliteal bruit and the absence of palpable pulses with knee flexion have been noted in a number of patients with popliteal artery involvement with adventitial cystic disease.[194,195] Arteriography may be helpful in demonstrating a "scimitar" sign of luminal encroachment by the cyst in a normally placed vessel that has no other signs of occlusive disease.

Several methods of treatment have been described. Arteries with a small cyst have been successfully treated with simple needle aspiration or cyst enucleation, although approximately 10 per cent recur following this treatment. In more severely involved patients, segmental arterial replacement may be required. Patients presenting with popliteal occlusion require bypass grafting. Treatment has been successful in over 90 per cent of reported cases.[193]

POPLITEAL ENTRAPMENT SYNDROMES

Stuart[196] in 1879 was the first to describe the anatomic abnormality associated with popliteal entrapment, and Hamming[197] in 1959 reported the first successful treatment of the condition. Love and Whelan[198] coined the term "popliteal artery entrapment syndrome" in 1965.

The anatomic basis of the syndrome has its origins in the anomalous embryonic development of two independent structures, the popliteal artery and the gastrocnemius muscle.[199] Development of a mature popliteal artery requires the successful union of two embryonic vessels; the poplitea profunda artery forming the proximal segment and the superficialis poplitea artery forming the lower segment. The deeper vessel is a continuation of the primitive axial/ischiadic artery running posteriorly along the developing leg, deep to the popliteus muscle. The poplitea profunda artery gives rise to the anterior tibial, posterior tibial, and peroneal arteries. The more superficial vessel enlarges with the development of the superficial femoral artery, eventually becoming the dominant vessel now coursing superficial to the popliteus muscle. The poplitea profunda artery usually disappears with successful development of the superficial system.[200] The anlage of the gastrocnemius muscle develops as a single muscle migrating cephalad from its development on the calcaneus. As it matures, it divides into larger medial and smaller lateral heads that gain their final attachments on the femoral epicondyles.[201] The medial head of the gastrocnemius migrates from its lateral origin toward the medial epicondyle at the same developmental stage at which the popliteal artery is undergoing its transition from a deep to superficial structure.

The exact etiology of popliteal artery entrapment remains unknown. The various anomalies primarily arise from variations in the relationship of the popliteal artery and the medial head of the gastrocnemius muscle itself, or a muscular slip. Less frequently, the popliteus, the plantaris, or the semimembranosus muscles provide the constriction.[202] Insua and associates[203] classified the variants into four groups, and Rich and associates[204] added an additional category. A diagram of these types is seen in Figure 8–11. About half of the cases involve the popliteal artery deviating medial to the normally placed medial head of the gastrocnemius muscle (type 1). Type 2 (25 per cent) lesions involve an abnormal attachment of the medial head of the gastrocnemius with the popliteal artery passing medially, but with less deviation than in type 1. In type 3 (6 per cent) the normally situated popliteal artery is compressed by muscle slips of the medial head of the gastrocnemius. Type 4 lesions have associated fibrous bands on the popliteus muscle compressing the popliteal artery. Compressions of the artery by other structures have been described, but these are rare.[202,205] Rich et al. added type 5 lesions, in which the popliteal vein accompanies the artery in its abnormal course.[204] Additionally, iatrogenic or acquired popliteal artery entrapment syndromes have been described where an autogenous vein graft has been improperly tunneled either medial to the medial head of the gastrocnemius or through the medial head of the muscle rather than between the medial and lateral heads.[206,207]

The true incidence of popliteal artery entrapment syndrome is unknown. The reported incidence is increasing coincidentally with the development of more sophisticated diagnostic tests. A recent review of 20,000 patients screened with routine vascular lab testing identified verifiable popliteal artery entrapment syndrome in less than 1 per cent.[202] However, in a recent autopsy series, Gibson et al. found an incidence of anatomic abnormality consistent with popliteal artery entrapment in 3.5 per cent of the 86 postmortem examinations.[199] Interestingly, the patients all died past their seventh decade of life, and the popliteal arteries showed no histological abnormalities. Clearly, not all entrapped popliteal arteries will become symptomatic.

Most of the information published on the popliteal artery entrapment syndrome have been retrospective reviews of the diagnosis and treatment of symptomatic popliteal artery entrapment. About 90 per cent of reported cases have occurred in men; more than half have become symptomatic below the age of 30. Twenty per cent of patients have the defect bilaterally.[205]

Symptoms are due to obstruction of the popliteal artery with gastrocnemius contraction. Premature atherosclerotic changes occur, presumably in relation to repeated microtrauma.[208] Thrombosis, embolus, or aneurysm formation may ensue. Symptomatic patients may present with acute popliteal artery occlusion (10 per cent) with resultant severe ischemia or with progressive intermittent claudication. Calf claudication in patients less than 40 years of age is sufficiently uncommon that its presence should suggest the possibility of popliteal artery entrapment syndrome.

Diagnosis of popliteal artery entrapment syndrome has been difficult, as most patients are asymptomatic at rest. Symptomatic patients may have normal, reduced, or absent pulses of the lower leg. Ankle dorsiflexion or plantar flexion or knee extension may diminish or occlude the pulses. Recently, continuous-wave Doppler, photoplethysmography, and arterial duplex scanning have been used with these same maneuvers of the leg to provide objective confirmation of popliteal artery entrapment.[209–211] Others have used progressively more challenging treadmill exercise regimens to elicit symptoms and objective decline in the ankle brachial index for patients suspected of having popliteal artery entrapment syndrome.[212] Computed tomography (CT) scanning has received some attention as an adjunct for diagnosis of entrapment of the popliteal artery.[213,214] CT scans with intravenous contrast can define the course of the popliteal artery through the popliteal fossa, its relationship to adjacent musculoskeletal structures,

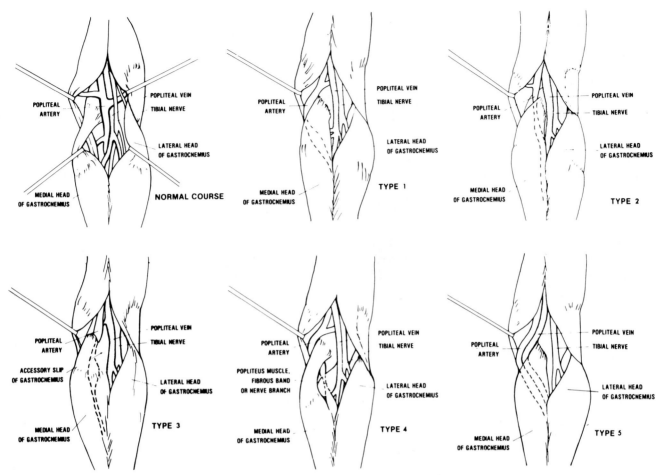

FIGURE 8–11.   Diagram of the types of popliteal artery entrapment. (From Rich NM, Collins G Jr, McDonald PT, et al: Popliteal vascular entrapment: Its increasing interest. Arch Surg *114*:1377–1384, 1979.)

and the patency of the artery. Furthermore, one exam gives bilateral detail. As magnetic resonance imaging (MRI) continues to mature, its role in the diagnosis of popliteal artery entrapment will surely grow. Although both CT and MRI may define the entrapment, MRI provides better soft-tissue contrast and does not require the use of intravenous contrast to localize the vascular structures or define their patency status.[215] Unlike conventional CT scans, MRI can also provide longitudinal views of the popliteal fossa. Figure 8–12 shows an MRI of a patient with bilateral popliteal artery entrapment.

Arteriography has been the "gold standard" for the diagnosis of the popliteal artery entrapment syndrome but may be replaced by MRI. The diagnosis is confirmed by angiography with the leg in a position of stress, which should demonstrate midpopliteal artery compression or medial deviation.

The treatment of this condition is surgical. Identifying the specific type of entrapment preoperatively is both difficult and unnecessary, as the surgical management will only be influenced by the patency of the popliteal artery. If diagnosed early and if minimal arterial changes are present, section of the medial gastrocnemius head may be sufficient. Bypass graft-

ing is required in patients with significant arterial stenosis, occlusion, or aneurysm formation. Without question autogenous vein is the only acceptable graft across the knee. Prosthetic grafting should never be used at this site. The original descriptions of the surgical technique for this condition favored a posterior approach to the popliteal fossa.[197] Later, a medial approach was emphasized as a means to assure total division of the medial head of the gastrocnemius and as a safeguard against iatrogenic popliteal artery entrapment, as the entire length of the popliteal artery is easily exposed.[216] To date, similar results have been obtained with both techniques, but we currently favor the medial approach.

Another arterial compression syndrome in the leg was described by Lee and associates[217] in 1972 and termed the "adductor canal syndrome." This anomaly involves the compression of the junction of the superficial femoral artery and popliteal artery as it passes through the tendinous insertion of the adductor magnus to the femur (Hunter's canal). Treatment consists of lysis of the tendinous insertion of the adductor magnus muscle or segmental arterial bypass.

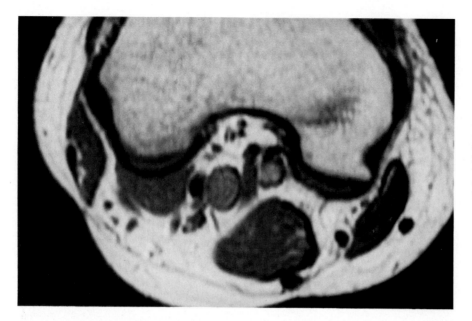

FIGURE 8–12. MRI scan showing the abnormal insertion of the medial head of the gastrocnemius muscle (large arrow) between the popliteal artery and vein. The popliteal artery (small arrow) ends up medial to the medial head of the gastrocnemius muscle.

COMPARTMENT SYNDROMES

Compartment syndromes occur whenever tissue pressure within a confined space becomes sufficiently elevated to impair blood flow. If untreated, diminished nutritive blood flow results in limb dysfunction secondary to ischemic muscle contracture.[218] The first clinical description of this syndrome was by von Volkman over a century ago in a report on contracture involving the arm following trauma. He attributed the deformity to a prolonged interruption of the vascular supply to the muscle.[219] Jepson[220] in 1926 reported successful experimental reproduction of the syndrome and demonstrated that early compartment decompression may prevent ischemic muscle paralysis and contracture.

The multiple clinical etiologies for compartment syndromes have been well described by Matsen[221] and are listed in Table 8–4. Although Matsen used the term "compartmental syndrome," current convention favors the term "compartment syndrome." Pivotal to the development of the syndrome, whether from external compression or internal tissue swelling, is the production of sufficient intracompartmental pressure to impair blood flow to the tissues of the compartment. There is no absolute pressure above which the syndrome will invariably occur, although tissue blood flow diminishes rapidly as intracompartmental pressure approaches the level of the diastolic blood pressure. Additionally, conditions such as hypotension or vasoconstriction may lead to the production of the syndrome at lower intracompartmental pressures.[222] In addition to the absolute and relative intracompartmental pressures, the length of ischemia is an important causative factor. Nerve tissue appears to be most susceptible to ischemia, with symptoms occurring within minutes and permanent damage at about 2 hours or less. Muscle death begins

TABLE 8–4.   ETIOLOGIES OF COMPARTMENTAL SYNDROMES

Decreased compartmental volume	Closure of fascial defects Application of excessive traction to fractured limbs

Increased compartmental content	Bleeding
	Major vascular injury
	Coagulation defect
	  Bleeding disorder
	  Anticoagulant therapy

Increased compartmental content	Increased capillary filtration
	Increased capillary permeability
	  Reperfusion after arterial revascularization
	  Trauma
	    Fracture
	    Contusion (crush)
	  Intensive use of muscles
	    Exercise
	    Seizures
	  Burns
	  Intraarterial drug injection
	  Cold
	  Orthopedic surgery
	  Snakebite
	Increased capillary pressure
	  Intensive use of muscles
	  Venous obstruction
	Diminished serum osmolarity–nephrotic syndrome

Externally applied pressure	Tight casts, dressings, or air splints Lying on limb

at approximately 4 hours. Maximal muscle contracture appears to require about 12 hours of ischemia.[221] Skin and subcutaneous tissues are capable of tolerating periods of ischemia that will not be tolerated by skeletal muscle or peripheral nerves.[223–225]

Recent interest in experimental models of compartment syndromes and reperfusion injury has provided some insights. Short periods of ischemia can cause cell damage that may not be apparent when overall function of the organ is assessed. Eklof identified metabolic changes in the skeletal muscle of the legs, persisting for 16 hours, following short periods of aortic cross-clamping during routine vascular surgical procedures.[226] It appears that partial ischemia, as is more common in clinical vascular surgery, is capable of causing cell damage. In a recent experimental model, Perry identified more severe cell membrane dysfunction, persisting for more prolonged periods when dogs subjected to 3 hours of partial limb ischemia were compared with dogs subjected to 3 hours of tourniquet ischemia.[227]

Ischemic injury and reperfusion injury in clinical practice are best thought of as a continuum. The role of oxygen-derived free radicals in the pathogenesis of ischemic injury in multiple organ systems is well established. The common link appears to be increased capillary permeability caused, at least to some degree, by oxygen-derived free radical–mediated endothelial injury.[228] Oxygen can be metabolized to any of several toxic metabolites, including hydrogen peroxide (H_2O_2) and the superoxide (O_2^-) and hydroxyl (OH) free radicals, all of which are highly reactive molecules. These toxic metabolites, normally produced in small amounts during oxidative metabolism, are detoxified by endogenous free radical scavengers such as superoxide dismutase and catalase.[229] Accumulation of these toxic metabolites may occur following ischemic/reperfusion injury overwhelming the normal scavenging systems. Recent experimentation in animal models of ischemic/reperfusion injury suggests a favorable role for pretreatment of patients with free-radical scavengers prior to reperfusion.[230] Perhaps this is an added beneficial effect of mannitol, a known free-radical scavenger, when it is used in the treatment of the compartment syndrome.[231]

Because diminished function of the extremity precedes nerve and muscle necrosis by several hours, the accurate diagnosis of compartment syndrome leading to successful treatment is based on the recognition of the early signs and symptoms of increased compartmental pressure. Clinical signs include fullness and tenderness of the compartment, pain disproportionate to the physical findings, paresthesias of the compartmental nerves, and weakness and pain of the involved muscles.

In questionable clinical situations or when the patient is unable to adequately communicate, objective data reflecting either intracompartmental pressure or nerve function may be monitored. Continuous or intermittent compartmental pressure determinations may be made by the Wick catheter technique described by Mubarek and associates[232] or Matsen and associates,[223] in which a plastic catheter is placed percutaneously and is connected to a pressure transducer as well as a low-volume continuous heparinized saline infusion. More recently, a solid-state transducer has been developed to fit within a catheter tip in a hand-held unit, the "solid-state transducer in catheter" (STIC) monitor. The artifacts introduced by pressure lines and dome transducers are effectively eliminated by the STIC monitors with improved reproducibility. Continuous and intermittent measurements are possible, although STIC-measured values tend to be lower than those obtained with older catheter techniques.[233]

Surgical decompression is generally recommended in patients who have a compartment pressure of 40 mm Hg or greater, or for patients who have had a compartment pressure above 30 mm Hg for 4 hours. Nerve conduction velocity is a second method of monitoring the adequacy of compartmental blood flow and appears to be a very accurate method, if somewhat cumbersome.[223,234] As mentioned before, the absolute compartmental pressure is not the only factor affecting neuromuscular function. A noninvasive method of anterior tibial compartment pressure determination using positional Doppler pressure measurements has been described.[235] Ultrasonography may play an expanded diagnostic role in the future.[236]

The palpable pulse status and Doppler pressures are unreliable reflections of intracompartmental pressures. They diminish only in the late stages of compartmental ischemia or not at all. Palpable pulses may be present at the ankle when anterior tibial compartment pressure is sufficiently high to have caused muscle necrosis.[237] As tissue pressures exceed capillary perfusion pressure, cell damage may occur despite continued arterial inflow.[238] With compression of postcapillary venules and a continued fall in the arteriovenous perfusion gradient, tissue damage occurs before the compartmental pressure exceeds the arterial pressure.

Once a compartment syndrome occurs, the time delay before treatment becomes the critical factor in determining outcome. Twelve hours appears to be the point beyond which significant residual dysfunction will likely occur despite adequate surgical decompression.[239] All circumferential bandages or casts should be removed on suspicion of increased compartmental pressure to allow a complete examination of the extremity. The extremity should be placed at the level of the heart and not elevated because elevation may further jeopardize marginally ischemic compartment components.[240] If physical examination, pressure measurements, or nerve conduction studies suggest a compartment syndrome, immediate surgical decompression is indicated. Our choice of a decompressive technique is shown in Figure 8–13. Routine fibulectomy has not been used as a standard treatment.[241]

Of particular interest to the vascular surgeon are those clinical situations in which an acute compartment syndrome is likely to develop following extremity vascular injury or disease. In patients with acute interruption of arterial blood flow, the likelihood of the need for fasciotomy following restoration of flow is increased if more than 6 hours of ischemia have

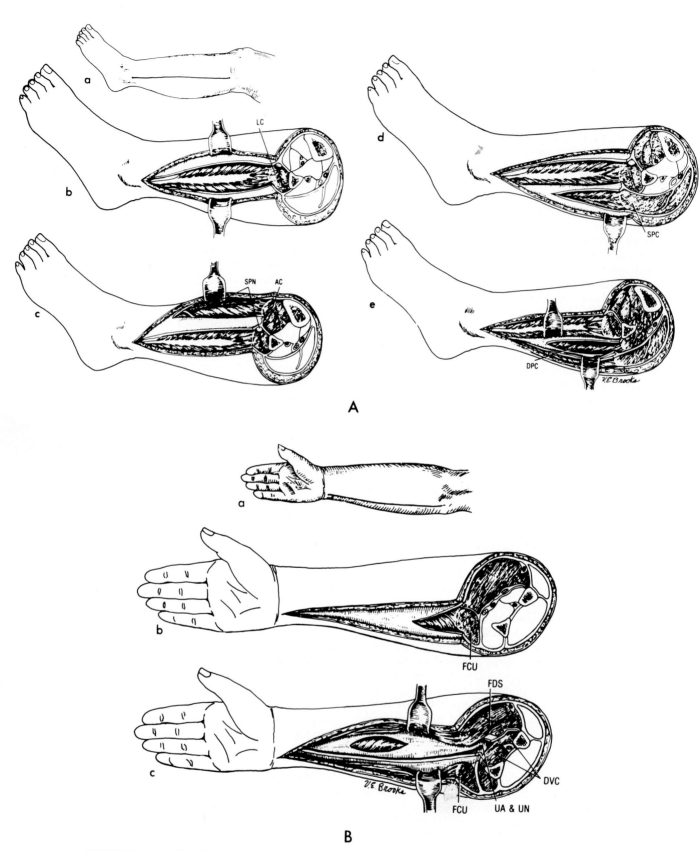

FIGURE 8–13. *A,* Parafibular decompression of all four compartments of the leg. (a) The skin incision runs the length of the fibula. (b) The lateral compartment (*LC*) is opened directly beneath the skin incision. (c) The anterior compartment (*AC*) is exposed by retracting the anterior skin flap and is opened over the entire length. Care is taken to preserve the superficial peroneal nerve (*SPN*). (d) The superficial posterior compartment (*SPC*) is exposed

occurred or if there has been a substantial period of shock in association with the arterial injury. Other circumstances increasing the need for fasciotomy include the occurrence of a tight swelling of the extremity preoperatively or intraoperatively, the combination of arterial and venous injury, and the presence of concomitant soft-tissue crush injury. Acute treatment with intravenous mannitol may be of value.[242] Osmotic diuretics have been advocated by many surgeons as adjunctive therapy for the compartment syndrome. Prevention of the reperfusion syndrome has been shown in selective patients following the administration of hypertonic mannitol.[243]

Compartment syndromes may occur in any closed space, but most commonly occur in a few well-recognized areas. In the upper extremity, the volar forearm compartment is the most frequently involved, but the dorsal forearm as well as the biceps, deltoid, and hand interossei have also been reported. In the lower leg, the anterior compartment is most commonly involved, followed by the lateral, deep posterior, and superficial posterior compartments. In the thigh, the quadriceps compartment, and in the buttock the gluteal compartment may be involved.

Anterior tibial compartment syndrome may occur without antecedent trauma or arterial obstruction and may occur with acute or chronic systems. Simple overexercise resulting in muscle swelling within the confines of the compartment may cause the condition. Local erythema, muscle tenderness, and muscle pain with ankle motion are typically present. Patients with the severe form of spontaneous compartment syndrome require urgent decompression of the anterior tibial compartment to reverse the cycle of ischemia. Those with the chronic variety of this syndrome may be relieved by anterior tibial compartment fasciotomy on an elective basis.[235] Chronic compartment syndrome (CCS) has also been described as a cause of claudication. CCS is usually observed in well-conditioned athletes, particularly runners, who overuse the affected muscle group. CCS may cause claudication, tightness of the compartment, or even paresthesias. The diagnosis of CCS is confirmed by the finding of mildly elevated compartment pressures (normal, less than 15 mm Hg; CCS, greater than 20 mm Hg). The only effective treatment has been surgical decompression of the involved compartment.[244]

Untreated compartment syndrome results in direct neurologic dysfunction or the development of contractures following fibrous replacement of myonecrosis. Symptomatic severity ranges from mild to critical, and amputation may be required. Frequent examination of the blood from patients with critical compartment syndrome may reveal elevated levels of creatinine phosphokinase as well as hyperkalemia. Subsequently, there may be myoglobinuria.[243] Renal failure secondary to myoglobinuria has been reported.[234,241] In such patients, restoration of normal hemodynamics, the administration of mannitol to enhance urine flow and improve intrarenal blood distribution, and alkalinization of the urine to prevent precipitation of myoglobin within the renal tubules, are specific therapeutic measures.[245] Deep muscle infections are uncommon but potentially life threatening.[234]

CONGENITAL CONDITIONS AFFECTING THE ARTERIES

Abdominal Coarctation

Coarctation of the aorta below the diaphragm is a rare but well-recognized condition. Quain described a stricture of the abdominal aorta in 1846 that he believed as congenital in origin.[246] Glenn et al. in 1952 reported the first successful surgical repair, which consisted of bypassing the coarctation with a splenic artery graft.[247] Since that time many cases have been treated, and several authors have reported the surgical treatments and clinical courses of a large number of patients.[248–252] The clinical manifestations are predictable, and surgical treatment has become standardized, although considerable uncertainty remains regarding the etiology of the condition.

Clinical Manifestations

Abdominal coarctation is usually discovered during an evaluation for hypertension. Most patients with abdominal coarctation become symptomatic during the second decade, with the complaints usually being those associated with hypertension, including headache, fatigue, shortness of breath, and palpitations. Severe leg ischemia is distinctly unusual, although moderate claudication is common. Involvement of the superior mesenteric arteries occurs frequently, although symptoms of visceral ischemia have not been reported. Patients may on occasion present with severe congestive heart failure or intracranial hemorrhage, both of which are secondary to hypertension.

---

by retracting the posterior skin flap and is opened over its entire length. (e) The lateral compartment is retracted anteriorly, and the superficial posterior compartment is retracted posteriorly after the fibular origin of the soleus muscle is released (not shown). This exposes the deep posterior compartment (*DPC*), which is opened over its entire length. (From Matsen FA, Winquist RA, Krugmire RB: Diagnosis and management of compartmental syndromes. J Bone Joint Surg 62:286–291, 1980.) *B*, Decompression of the volar compartment of the forearm. (a) The skin incision is over the volar-ulnar aspect of the forearm. (b) The superficial volar compartment is opened over the length of the forearm, exposing the flexor carpi ulnaris muscle (*FCU*). (c) The interval between the flexor carpi ulnaris muscle (*FCU*) and the flexor digitorum sublimis muscle (*FDS*) is opened to reveal the muscles of the deep volar compartment (*DVC*). This compartment is opened over its entire length, care being taken to avoid the ulnar artery (*UA*) and nerve (*UN*). (From Matsen FA, Winquist FA, Krugmire RB: Diagnosis and management of compartmental syndromes. J Bone Joint Surg 62:286–291, 1980.)

Physical findings in these patients are similar to those associated with the more common thoracic coarctation. Lower extremity pulses are reduced or absent, with a noticeable radial/femoral pulse delay in many patients. All patients have prominent abdominal systolic bruits, and many have systolic bruits in the lumbar region or lower posterior thoracic area, rather than the interscapular bruit commonly associated with thoracic coarctation.

The natural history of untreated abdominal coarctation is that of severe hypertension, with death from either renal or cardiac failure within a few years of the onset of symptoms.[253] Limb-threatening lower extremity ischemia has not been reported.

Pathology

Multiple variants of abdominal coarctation have been described, with the variable factors being the precise location and length of the aortic involvement and the number of visceral branches affected. The origins of the visceral arteries may be involved even when originating from an area of relatively uninvolved aorta. Stenosis or occlusion of the visceral arteries usually does not extend beyond a few millimeters from the origin, emphasizing that the process is primarily aortic.[249]

Two primary pathogenetic theories have been presented, and available evidence suggests that both may be correct, with different patients having abdominal coarctation caused by different mechanisms. The first proposes a congenital anomaly representing a failure of normal fusion of the two dorsal aortae of the embryo, with resultant aortic narrowing. The existence of multiple renal arteries in a large number of these patients supports this theory because the formation of a single renal artery is a developmental step that coincides in both location and timing with fusion of the dorsal aortae.[249] The congenital origin of abdominal coarctation in some of these patients may be related to intrauterine injury, because the anomaly has been reported in association with the maternal rubella syndrome.[254] In all these patients in whom the lesion is congenital, the involved vessels are hypoplastic, without gross or microscopic inflammatory reaction.[255]

In the second group of patients with lesions quite similar in hemodynamic effect, anatomic location, and clinical manifestations, examination reveals pronounced inflammatory changes in the involved arteries. Some have named the lesion the "middle aortic syndrome" to indicate its acquired etiology and distinguish it from congenital abdominal coarctation.[256] This inflammatory middle aortic narrowing is likely a variant of Takayasu's arteritis and appears to occur with a frequency reflecting the primarily Asian distribution of that disease.[257] Although this arteritis can be successfully treated with corticosteroids during the acute stage, diagnosis is most often made after this stage has passed and the chronic fibrotic and stenotic lesions, which are amenable only to surgical treatment, are present.

The etiology of the hypertension associated with abdominal coarctation has been intensively studied. A renovascular mechanism acting through the renin-angiotensin system is clearly responsible both in experimental models[252,258] and in patients who have undergone appropriate testing.[249,259]

Diagnostic Studies

Arteriography is necessary to define the extent of the lesion and plan treatment. Lateral and oblique views are helpful in detecting the extent of visceral vessel involvement. In some patients with very high-grade stenosis or with aortic occlusion, combined retrograde (transfemoral) and antegrade (transaxillary, brachial, or carotid) catheter insertion may be needed to provide complete angiographic visualization. Renovascular hypertension may be accurately assumed, and renin studies or split renal function studies are not necessary unless the potential viability of a poorly visualized kidney (i.e., nephrectomy versus renal revascularization) is questionable. An arteriogram in a child with abdominal coarctation is shown in Figure 8–14.

Treatment

Many authors have reported successful surgical treatment of abdominal coarctation by a variety of methods including aortoaortic bypass, iliac or femoral bypass, prosthetic patch aortoplasty, and splenoaortic anastomosis.[247–253,255] In contrast to thoracic coarctation, prosthetic bypass grafting from the descending thoracic aorta to an uninvolved area of the infrarenal aorta, or iliac or femoral arteries has emerged as the procedure of choice.[253] This operation may be performed through a thoracoabdominal incision[249] or through separate laparotomy and thoracotomy incisions.[248] Complete revascularization has been reported as a staged procedure.[260] However, because most of these patients are young and do not have the major cardiopulmonary risk factors associated with an older atherosclerotic population, extensive vascular reconstruction is usually well tolerated, as has been emphasized recently.[249] Most authorities now recommend single-stage repair. In very small children operation may be delayed to an age (5 to 6 years) at which increased vessel size allows greater chance of successful repair, as long as cardiac and renal function can be preserved by medical management of hypertension.

Renal vascularization is most often performed by bypass grafts originating from the thoracoabdominal graft. Autogenous vein and artery and prosthetic tube have all been used successfully.[248,249,252] Unsuspected proximal stenosis of a visceral artery (splenic) used for renal revascularization has been reported as a cause of failure.[253]

Indications for visceral revascularization are unclear because no patients with visceral ischemia have been reported. Several prophylactic visceral revascularizations have been performed.[249,261–263] The interesting speculation that unrecognized preexisting visceral orificial stenosis related to abdominal coarctation may explain the marked female predominance

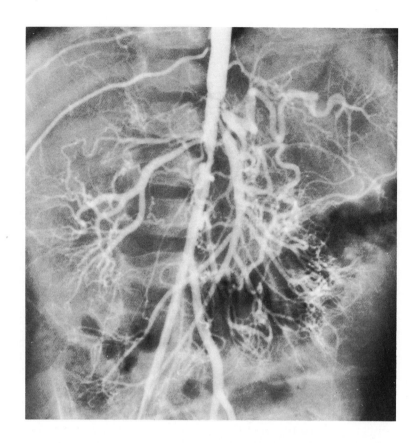

FIGURE 8–14. Abdominal aortic coarctation in a 2-year-old child showing infrarenal aortic narrowing and high-grade stenoses at the origins of the celiac, superior mesenteric, and right renal arteries. Near-total occlusion of the left renal artery.

in most atherosclerotic visceral ischemic series remains unproven.[253]

Results of surgical treatment of abdominal coarctation have been good. Stanley and associates,[253] reviewed the results of 73 reported cases and found an 8 per cent operative mortality and 80 per cent excellent or good results.

Persistent Sciatic Artery

In the embryo, the axial or sciatic artery arises from the umbilical artery and supplies blood to the lower limb, following a dorsal course to the popliteal area and then proceeding through the midcalf to the ankle. As development proceeds this artery is replaced in its upper part by the femoral artery developing from the external iliac. By the third month of gestation, the femoral artery predominates and the vestiges of the sciatic artery remain only as the inferior gluteal artery, the distal popliteal artery, and the peroneal artery.[264]

Rarely, part of all of the sciatic artery may persist into postnatal life as a large artery originating from the hypogastric, following a course through the buttock and posterior thigh and ending at the popliteal artery. The artery may coexist with a normal superficial femoral artery,[265] or the superficial femoral artery may be hypoplastic.[266] In some patients the entire superficial femoral may be absent, with the sciatic artery being the only vessel in the limb in continuity with the popliteal artery.[267] A sciatic artery is complete if there is direct continuity with the popliteal

and incomplete if the connection to the popliteal is by way of collaterals.[268] This anomaly is reported to occur with an incidence of 0.03 to 0.06 per cent in large series of femoral arteriograms.[264,269]

The surgical importance of persistent sciatic artery lies in the propensity of this vessel to develop aneurysms,[270] which classically present as pulsatile buttock masses. The necessity for complete angiographic evaluation of these lesions is obvious. Treatment has usually consisted of aneurysm ligation or excision with femoral-to-popliteal or iliac-to-popliteal bypass grafting.[266,269,270]

DISEASES AFFECTING THE ARTERIAL MEDIA

A variety of conditions known to affect the strength or stability of collagen or elastin result in arterial abnormalities of surgical importance. These conditions all have in common the presence of medial defects, because the collagen and elastin fibers essential for normal arterial strength and resilience lie in the arterial media.

Cystic Medial Necrosis

Cystic medial necrosis is the name given by Erdheim to a condition associated with aortic dissection and manifested pathologically by uniform hyaline degeneration of the media and replacement by a mucoid-appearing basophilic substance.[271] Erdheim believed that the disease was the result of medial replacement by overproduction of mucoid ground substance. Subsequently, numerous studies have shown that the pathologic changes of cystic medial necrosis, with the resultant clinical problems of aortic dissection, spontaneous arterial rupture, and disseminated aneurysm formation, result from a variety of metabolic conditions and syndromes affecting the composition and structure of collagen, elastin, and mucopolysaccharide ground substance. Thus, Marfan's syndrome, Ehlers-Danlos syndrome, any of the mucopolysaccharidoses (Hunter's, Hurler's, Morquio's, Sanfilippo's, etc.), and occasionally neurofibromatosis may all present with the typical arterial lesions and pathologic changes identified as cystic medial necrosis. Although the specific biochemical alterations for certain of these syndromes have been discovered, for others they remain obscure. The most common arterial condition resulting from cystic medial necrosis is aortic dissection, the treatment of which is discussed in Chapter 11.

Aortic dissection from cystic medial necrosis has been reported as a cause of superior vena cava syndrome.[272] Although unusual, the condition has also been reported to involve the pulmonary arteries[273] and the superficial temporal artery.[274] Rarely, patients have been reported with a rapidly progressive syndrome of disseminated arterial dissection, spontaneous arterial rupture, and aneurysm formation in which the only discernible lesion has been cystic medial necrosis.[275] The angiograms of such a patient are seen in Figure 8–15.

Most patients with cystic medial necrosis have an identifiable clinical syndrome, the most common of which are Marfan's syndrome and Ehlers-Danlos syndrome.

Marfan's Syndrome

Marfan's syndrome is an inherited disorder of connective tissue characterized by a panoply of anatomic disorders with variable phenotypic expression, serious largely because of its cardiovascular complications. Until recently, the precise nature of the biochemical defect was unknown. The clinical features of the disease suggested an abnormality in collagen, or perhaps elastin, yet detailed analysis of the structural collagen genes and less intensive evaluation of the elastin genes in patients suffering from the disorder failed to yield any clues.[276–279]

Attention then turned to the microfibrillar system, which often is associated with elastin, is widely distributed in the extracellular space, but is very prominent in the ciliary zonule containing the suspensory ligament of the lens.[280,281] The microfibrils have also been detected in the aortic media, and in the periosteum of bone.[282,283] Fibrillin, a large glycoprotein (350 kd), is one of the structural components of the elastin-associated microfibrils.

Hollister and colleagues began to investigate fibrillin levels in patients with Marfan's syndrome,

initially detecting diminished levels of fibrillin in skin biopsies and cultured fibroblasts in the Marfan group with an immunoassay technique.[284,285] Subsequently, genetic linkage studies identified the abnormal fibrillin gene on chromosome 15 in a group of patients with Marfan's syndrome.[286,287] Dietz further identified the same missense mutation on chromosome 15 in two sporadic cases of Marfan's syndrome.[288] It is probable that a variety of mutations of the fibrillin gene on chromosome 15 will be detected among patients with Marfan's syndrome. A second fibrillin gene has been located on chromosome 5, although abnormalities of this gene appear in patients with congenital contractural arachnodactyly and not Marfan's syndrome.[289,290] Congenital contractural arachnodactyly is a mild disorder whose clinical phenotype overlaps with that of Marfan's syndrome, without cardiovascular or ocular abnormalities.[291] Perhaps a class of fibrillins exists with several subtypes, similar to collagen, and the abnormal type will determine the phenotypic expression much the same way as the different collagen abnormalities determine the types of Ehlers-Danlos syndromes.

The incidence of Marfan's syndrome is estimated at 1 in 10,000, and there has been no tendency to inordinately affect members of any race or sex.[292] Inheritance is by an autosomal dominant pattern. In its classic form the syndrome is easily recognizable and consists of abnormalities of the eye (subluxation of the lens), skeleton (arachnodactyly, extreme limb length, pectus excavatum or carinatum, and joint laxity), and cardiovascular system (aortic dilation and aortic valvular incompetence).[293]

The cardiovascular abnormalities of surgical importance in Marfan's syndrome have been well studied. Almost all patients with the condition develop progressive dilation of the aortic root with a resultant ascending aortic aneurysm and aortic valve incompetence. A smaller number have mitral valve prolapse and mitral insufficiency. If untreated, the life expectancy of a patient with Marfan's syndrome is about 40 years, with 95 per cent of deaths related to cardiovascular causes.

Histopathologic evaluation of aortic segments of Marfan's syndrome patients has revealed cystic medial necrosis, disruption of collagen fibers, with fibrosis of the media.[294] Decreased tensile strength has also been demonstrated in the aortic segments obtained after death from Marfan's syndrome patients dying from cardiovascular complications.[295] A recent study measured aortic distensibility and aortic stiffness indices of the ascending aorta and the midabdominal aorta in Marfan's syndrome patients and age-matched controls. The values were determined indirectly measuring changes in echocardiographic diameter and pulse pressure. Compared to the normal subjects, the Marfan's syndrome patients had decreased aortic distensibility and increased aortic stiffness indices in both aortic segments, irrespective of the aortic diameter.[296]

Because of the predictably progressive nature of the aortic dilation, all patients with Marfan's syndrome

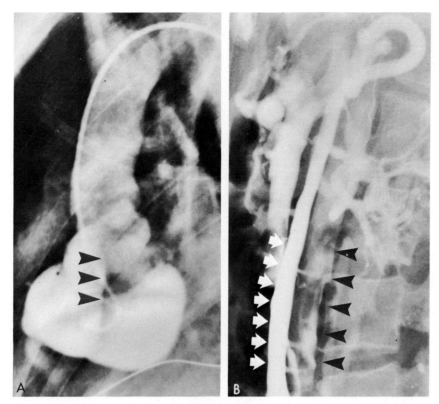

FIGURE 8–15. *A,* Cystic medial necrosis showing aortic root dissection. The junction of the true and false lumen is outlined with black arrows. *B,* Lateral aortogram of same patient as in *A,* showing double-lumen abdominal aorta, outlined with white and black arrows.

should be followed from childhood with annual echo-cardiograms to detect aortic dilation.[297] There is some evidence that β-blocker therapy initiated before the development of aortic incompetence may retard the onset of incompetence and perhaps retard aneurysmal degeneration.[298] A thoracic aortogram of a typical patient with Marfan's syndrome is seen in Figure 8–16.

Elective repair of the aortic valve and ascending aorta should be accomplished prophylactically before severe aortic insufficiency compromises left ventricular function or the ascending aorta exceeds 6 cm in diameter, at which point the risk of dissection and rupture increases.[299] Occasionally, mitral valve replacement is required. With modern surgical techniques, the life expectancy of these patients can be improved considerably, as emphasized by recent reports with low operative mortality, even in severely symptomatic patients.[300,301]

Ehlers-Danlos Syndrome

The Ehlers-Danlos syndrome refers to a group of diseases, first clearly described by von Meekeren in 1682,[302] characterized by hyperextensible skin, hypermobile joints, fragile tissues, and a bleeding diathesis primarily related to fragile vessels. At least seven different types of Ehlers-Danlos syndrome have been described, each with variable clinical signs, symptoms, and patterns of inheritance. The biochemical basis for some of the types is known and involves defects in collagen production. For further specific information regarding Ehlers-Danlos syndrome the reader is referred to standard works.[293]

The extreme fragility of tissues in many patients with Ehlers-Danlos syndrome leads to problems of surgical importance. The skin and soft tissues are easily disrupted, tend to fragment and tear with manipulation, and hold sutures and heal poorly. Wound dehiscence is common when surgery is required.[303] In addition to these significant problems incident to any surgery, a number of patients with Ehlers-Danlos syndrome are prone to arterial disorders, which may require surgical intervention. Three types of Ehlers-Danlos syndrome, types I, III, and IV, frequently have arterial complications, especially type IV. These patients produce little or no type III collagen, which is of major structural importance in vessels, viscera, and skin.[304] The result of this defect is that patients with the syndrome are prone to spontaneous rupture of major vessels, aneurysm formation, and acute aortic dissections. The difficulty in dealing with these critical problems is emphasized by reports describing vessels so friable that clamping is unsuccessful and arterial disintegration occurs with attempted simple ligation.[305]

In spite of the extreme difficulty in dealing with these friable tissues, several authors have reported successful vascular operations in patients with Ehlers-Danlos syndrome. Most authors agree that arteriography carries special risks of vessel laceration

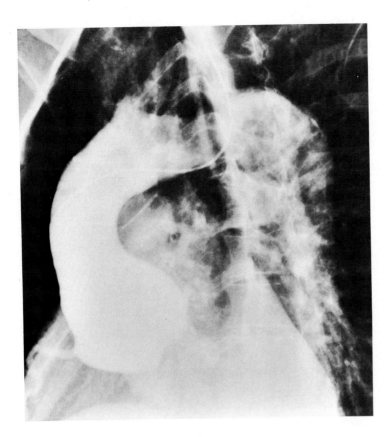

FIGURE 8–16. Thoracic aortogram of a patient with Marfan's syndrome showing massive aortic dilation and associated aortic insufficiency.

and hemorrhage in these patients and should be avoided if possible.[305–307]

Treatment of spontaneous arterial rupture in patients with Ehlers-Danlos syndrome should be nonoperative, consisting of compression and transfusion whenever possible.[305] If operation for major arterial disruption is required, the therapeutic objective should be ligation to control bleeding if this can be accomplished without tissue loss. Gentle dissection, proximal vessel control with external tourniquets or internal balloon catheters, and the use of carefully applied heavy ligatures reinforced with fine vascular sutures have been emphasized as keys to success.[305–307] Major arterial reconstruction can be accomplished in patients with Ehlers-Danlos syndrome, as emphasized by Burnett and associates, who successfully replaced an abdominal aortic aneurysm with a Dacron bifurcation graft in a 17-year-old female.[308]

Pseudoxanthoma Elasticum

Pseudoxanthoma elasticum is an inherited disorder of elastic tissue manifested clinically by loose, baggy skin with multiple creases and small yellow-orange cutaneous papules in intertriginous areas.[309] These patients also have changes in the eye (angioid streaks) and distinct vascular abnormalities.

The exact biochemical defect responsible for the syndrome is unknown. The basic pathologic change in the arteries is replacement of normal medial elastic tissue by calcium deposits. This change results in a markedly abnormal pulse contour due to loss of the elastic recoil and distensibility of vessels and may be clearly demonstrated plethysmographically.[310,311] Arterial stenoses and/or occlusions and arterial hypertension are the end results of this pathologic process. Roentgenography frequently reveals extensive arterial calcification in a young patient without obvious risk factors for atherosclerosis.[311] Arterial occlusive disease occurs at an early age, usually presenting in the third or fourth decade. Gastrointestinal hemorrhage is common and is believed to originate from the widespread arterial degeneration.[312] Hypertension is common in these patients and is usually ascribed to extensive vascular calcification, although renovascular hypertension has been reported.[313] The vascular disease in patients with pseudoxanthoma elasticum may involve the cerebral, coronary, visceral, and peripheral arteries.[275,309]

Standard techniques of vascular surgery, including autogenous vein bypass[315] and endarterectomy (J. M. Porter, G. M. Baur, and L. M. Taylor, unpublished case material, 1982), have been utilized with success in patients with pseudoxanthoma elasticum. The indications for surgery in these patients are the same as for patients with arteriosclerotic occlusive disease.

Arteria Magna Syndrome

Leriche was the first to describe patients with this peculiar condition, characterized by extreme arterial dilation, elongation, and tortuosity. He termed the condition "dolicho et mega-artere."[316,317] Since then many such patients have been recognized and the terms "arteria magna," "arteria dolicho et magna," and "arteriomegaly" have all been used to describe it.

Although the condition was initially thought to resemble a variety of arteriosclerosis, it has been reported in children,[318,319] and careful pathologic study reveals that the arterial media of these patients shows a striking loss of elastic tissue, which is believed to be responsible for the arterial changes.[320]

Angiography in patients with this syndrome reveals characteristic changes. The major changes visualized include arterial widening and tortuosity (100 per cent of patients), extremely slow arterial flow velocity (100 per cent of patients), and the existence of multiple aneurysms (66 per cent of patients).[321] A representative angiogram is seen in Figure 8–17. The slow arterial flow present in patients with this condition makes arteriography difficult. Large amounts of contrast must be used, and visualization of distal vessels may require multiple injections and special timing sequences with delayed filming.

The strong propensity for these patients to form arterial aneurysms at multiple sites results in the frequent need for surgical correction. Because of their generalized arterial dilation, standard criteria for determining size of aneurysms to be operated upon may not be useful. All patients with arteria magna

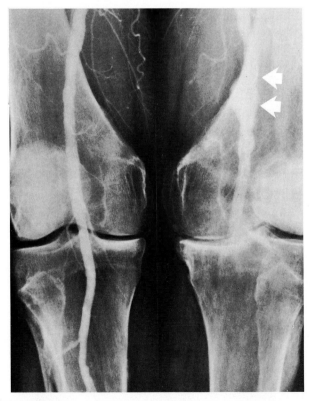

FIGURE 8–17. Arteriogram of a 68-year-old male showing very dilated popliteal arteries and a left popliteal aneurysm. This patient's arterial dilation extended throughout his body, a condition termed "arteria magna syndrome."

should have a careful examination of all pertinent sites (aorta, iliac, femoral, popliteal) together with ultrasound imaging of nonpalpable or questionable areas. These examinations should be repeated annually. Any aneurysm that reaches 2 to 2.5 times the size of the parent vessel or becomes symptomatic should be replaced. Arterial occlusions, when they occur in patients with an arteria magna syndrome, are almost always complications of aneurysmal disease, including thrombosis or embolism. The relationship of arteria magna to typical atherosclerosis is uncertain. The syndrome occurs, albeit rarely, in young people with no evidence of atherosclerosis. Clinical experience suggests that most patients in the United States with arteria magna have significant associated atherosclerosis along with the usual risk factors, such as tobacco use. In these patients, however, the atherosclerosis is typically nonocclusive and dilation predominates.

HOMOCYSTEINEMIA

Homocystinuria, an inborn error of metabolism in which homocysteine accumulates abnormally in plasma, tissues, and urine, was described in 1962.[322] Patients with this disorder suffer from multiple abnormalities, including ectopia lentis, mental retardation, rapidly progressive arteriosclerotic vascular disease, and thromboembolic disorders.[322,323] Three specific enzyme deficiencies, each of which may be responsible for homocystinuria, have been identified: (1) cystathionine synthetase deficiency,[324] (2) homocysteine methyltransferase deficiency,[325] and (3) methylene tetrahydrofolate reductase deficiency.[326] These enzymes require cofactors, including pyridoxine, folate, and cobalamin.[327–329] Regardless of the primary cause, all forms of homocystinuria in humans have been associated with premature atherosclerosis, frequently complicated by thrombosis.[323]

The arteriosclerotic lesions occurring in homocystinuria, whether resulting from cystathionine synthetase deficiency, homocysteine methyltransferase deficiency, or methylene tetrahydrofolate reductase deficiency, are typical fibrous plaques.[330–332] Microscopic evaluation reveals medial hypertrophy, elaboration of extracellular matrix and collagen, and degeneration and destruction of the elastic laminae. Lipid deposition in the plaques is characteristically absent.[330–332]

Accumulation of homocysteine leads to the production of homocysteine thiolactone by the liver, which has been implicated as the toxic substance in homocysteinemic atherogenesis.[332] In patients with homocysteinemia, homocysteine thiolactone is found in increased quantities in lipoproteins and cell membranes, altering surface charges and perhaps predisposing to cellular aggregation within the vascular lumen.[334] Homocysteine thiolactone causes platelet aggregation and release of prostaglandin metabolites in vitro.[334] Interestingly, the metabolism of homocysteine thiolactone appears abnormal in patients with arteriosclerosis without homocysteinemia.[335]

Homocysteine exists in human plasma in at least three forms: as the mixed disulfide homocysteine-cysteine; as free homocysteine, which requires dietary methionine loading for detection; and as protein-bound homocysteine.[336,337] Men have higher levels of plasma homocysteine than women, and premenopausal women have lower levels than postmenopausal women.[338,339] Increasing evidence indicates that mildly elevated levels of plasma homocysteine may be associated with symptomatic atherosclerotic disease.[340–342] Boers et al. detected a heterozygous trait they termed "homocysteinemia" in a group of 14 patients with premature atherosclerotic vascular disease.[340] The detection of elevated plasma homocysteine in high-risk groups has historically required use of a cumbersome dietary methionine load.[338] Kang et al. simplified these investigations when they demonstrated elevated levels of protein-bound homocysteine in patients with coronary artery disease without any requirements for dietary methionine loading.[343] This has become the standard clinical assay.

Our ongoing evaluation of patients with peripheral vascular disease has confirmed elevated total plasma homocysteine levels in a significant number of patients compared to age- and sex-matched controls.[342,344] Recent investigations have focused on lowering these supranormal plasma homocysteine levels through alteration of the homocysteine-methionine pathways using pharmacologic doses of the cofactors for these enzymatic pathways, specifically folic acid, pyridoxine, and vitamin B_{12}.[345] Although reduction of plasma homocysteine levels to normal has been observed with this therapy, no study to date has shown clinical benefit from homocysteine reduction. Intuitively one would expect clinical improvement once the toxic homocysteine levels have declined. Serial evaluation of the progression of peripheral vascular disease in groups randomized to treatment and nontreatment will be necessary to determine clinical effect.

HYPERVISCOSITY SYNDROMES

Multiple conditions that result in an increase in the viscosity of blood, through increase in either the formed elements or the dissolved proteins, can cause arterial or venous thromboembolism. A list of such conditions is presented in Table 8–5 with a current reference to each. In our clinical experience, hyperviscosity syndromes result in thrombosis frequently in the venous system, next most often in the small peripheral arteries (i.e., hands and fingers), and least often in the major arteries.

Treatment of these problems should be directed primarily at correction of the underlying disorders, with appropriate anticoagulation therapy as needed. Vascular surgery procedures are rarely required in these patients.

TABLE 8–5. DISORDERS RESULTING IN INCREASED BLOOD VISCOSITY, WHICH MAY RESULT IN ARTERIAL OR VENOUS THROMBOEMBOLISM

Myeloproliferative disorders
   Polycythemia rubra vera[345]
   Thrombocytosis[346]
   Leukemia[346]
Serum protein abnormalities
   Myeloma[346,347]
   Benign monoclonal gammopathy[347]
   Macroglobulinemia[347]
   Cryoglobulinemia[348]
   Tumor-produced globulins[346]
   Myeloid metaplasia[346]

NEUROFIBROMATOSIS

Neurofibromatosis has been associated with multiple vascular abnormalities, including abdominal coarctation, renal artery stenosis, aneurysm formation in multiple sites, and arteriovenous malformations.[247,350–352] No widely accepted explanation for the apparent relationship between the two conditions has been offered. An example of a large vertebral artery aneurysm arising in the area of neurofibromatosis arterial involvement is shown in Figure 8–18.

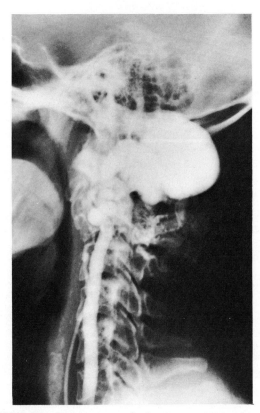

FIGURE 8–18. Enormous vertebral artery aneurysm in a patient with neurofibromatosis.

REFERENCES

1. Lie JT: Vasculitis, 1815 to 1991: Classification and diagnostic specificity. J Rheumatol *19*:83–89, 1992.
2. Savage COS: Pathogenesis of systemic vasculitis. *In* Churg A, Churg J (eds): Systemic Vasculitides. New York, Igaku-Shoin, 1991, pp 7–30.
3. Arkin A: A clinical and pathological study of periarteritis nodosa. Am J Pathol *6*:401–427, 1930.
4. Lanham JG, Elkon KB, Pusey CD, et al: Systemic vasculitis with asthma and eosinophilia: A clinical approach to Churg-Strauss syndrome. Medicine *63*:65–81, 1984.
5. Yoshikawa Y, Watanabe T: Pulmonary lesions in Wegener's granulomatosis: A clinicopathologic study of 22 autopsy cases. Hum Pathol *17*:401–410, 1986.
6. Rosen S, Falk RJ, Jennette JC: Polyarteritis nodosa, including microscopic form and renal vasculitis. *In* Churg A, Churg J (eds): Systemic Vasculitides. New York, Igaku-Shoin, 1991, pp 57–77.
7. D'Agati V, Chandler P, Nash M, et al: Idiopathic microscopic polyarteritis nodosa: Ultrastructural observations on the renal vascular and glomerular lesions. Am J Kidney Dis *7*:95–110, 1986.
8. Jennette JC, Wilkman AS, Falk RJ: Anti-neutrophil cytoplasmic antibody associated glomerulonephritis and vasculitis. Am J Pathol *35*:921–930, 1989.
9. Travers RL, Allison DJ, Brettle RP, et al: Polyarteritis nodosa: A clinical and angiographic analysis of 17 cases. Semin Arthritis Rheumatol *8*:184–199, 1979.
10. McCauley RL, Johnston MR, Fauci AS: Surgical aspects of systemic necrotizing vasculitis. Surgery *97*:104–108, 1985.
11. Selke FW, Williams GB, Donovan DL, et al: Management of intra-abdominal aneurysms associated with periarteritis nodosa. J Vasc Surg *4*:294–299, 1986.
12. Capps JH, Klein RM: Polyarteritis nodosa as a cause of perirenal and retroperitoneal hemorrhage. Radiology *94*:143–146, 1970.
13. Robins JM, Bookstein JJ: Regressing aneurysms in polyarteritis nodosa. Radiology *104*:39–42, 1972.
14. Fauci AS, Katz P, Haynes BF, et al: Cyclophosphamide therapy of severe systemic necrotizing vasculitis. N Engl J Med *301*:325–328, 1979.
15. Cohen RD, Conn DL, Ilstrup DM: Clinical features, prognosis, and response to treatment in polyarteritis. Mayo Clin Proc *55*:140–144, 1980.
16. Kawasaki T: MCLS—clinical observations of 50 cases. Jpn J Allergy *16*:178–182, 1967.
17. Kawasaki T, Kosaki F, Okawa S, Shigematsu I, Yanagawa H: A new infantile acute febrile mucocutaneous lymph node syndrome (MLNS) prevailing in Japan. Pediatrics *54*:271–276, 1974.
18. Goldsmith RW, Gribetz D, Strauss L: Mucocutaneous lymph node syndrome in the continental United States. Pediatrics *57*:431–435, 1976.
19. Feigen RD, Schleien CL: Kawasaki disease. Curr Clin Top Infect Dis *4*:30, 1983.
20. Bell DM, Morens DM, Holman RC, et al: Kawasaki syndrome in the United States. Am J Dis Child *137*:211–214, 1983.
21. Melish ME: Kawasaki syndrome (the mucocutaneous lymph node syndrome). Ann Rev Med *33*:569–585, 1982.
22. Rauch AM: Kawasaki syndrome: Critical review of U.S. epidemiology. Proceedings of the Second-International Kawasaki Disease Symposium, Kauai, Hawaii, November 30 to December 3, 1986. New York, Allan R. Liss, 1987, pp 33–44.
23. Kawasaki T: Clinical features of Kawasaki syndrome. Acta Pediatr Jpn Overseas Ed *25*:79–90, 1983.
24. Landing BH, Larson EJ: Pathological features of Kawasaki disease (mucocutaneous lymph node syndrome). Am J Cardiovasc Pathol *1*:215–229, 1987.
25. Kato H: Cardiovascular involvement in Kawasaki disease: Evaluation and natural history. Proceedings of the Second International Kawasaki Disease Symposium, Kauai, Hawaii, November 30 to December 3, 1986. New York, Allan R. Liss, 1987, pp 277–286.
26. Vargo TA, Huhta JC, Moore WH, et al: Recurrent Kawasaki disease. Pediatr Cardiol *6*:199–202, 1986.
27. Capannari TE, Daniels SR, Meyer RA, et al: Sensitivity, specificity, and predictive value of two-dimensional echocardiography in detecting coronary artery aneurysms in patients with Kawasaki disease. J Am Coll Cardiol *7*:355–360, 1986.
28. Gribetz D, Landing BH, Larson EJ: Kawasaki disease: Mucocutaneous lymph node syndrome (MCLS). *In* Churg A, Churg J (eds): Systemic Vasculitides. New York, Igaku-Shoin, 1991, pp 257–272.
29. Takahashi M, Mason W, Lewis AB: Regression of coronary aneurysms in patients with Kawasaki syndrome. Circulation *75*:387–394, 1987.
30. Kato H, Ichinose E, Yoshioka F, et al: Fate of coronary aneurysms in Kawasaki disease: Serial coronary angiography and long term follow-up study. Am J Cardiol *49*:1758–1766, 1982.
31. Inoue O, Akagi T, Ichinose E, et al: Systemic artery involvement in Kawasaki disease. Proceedings of the Third International Kawasaki Disease Symposium, Tokyo, November 29 to December 2, 1988. New York, Allan R. Liss, 1988, p 53.
32. Bierman FZ, Gersony WM: Kawasaki disease: Clinical perspective. Pediatrics *111*:789–792, 1987.
33. Koren G, Rose V, Lavi S, Rowe R: Probable efficacy of high-dose salicylates in reducing coronary involvement in Kawasaki disease. JAMA *254*:767–769, 1985.
34. Saalouke MG, Venglarcik JS III, Barker DR, et al: Rapid regression of coronary dilatation in Kawasaki disease with intravenous γ-globulin. Am Heart J *121*:905–909, 1991.
35. Kitamura S, Kawashima Y, Fujita T, et al: Aortocoronary bypass grafting in a child with coronary obstruction due to a mucocutaneous lymph node syndrome. Circulation *53*:1035–1040, 1976.
36. Suma K, Takeuchi Y, Shiroma K, et al: Early and late postoperative studies in coronary arterial lesions resulting from Kawasaki's disease. J Thorac Cardiovasc Surg *84*:224–229, 1982.
37. Suzuki A, Kamiya A, Ono Y, et al: Indication of aortocoronary bypass for coronary obstruction due to Kawasaki's disease. Heart Vessels *1*:94–100, 1985.
38. Kitamura S, Kawachi K, Oyama C, et al: Severe Kawasaki heart disease treated with an internal mammary artery graft in pediatric patients. J Thorac Cardiovasc Surg *89*:860–866, 1985.
39. Myers JL, Gleason MM, Cyren SE, Baylen BG: Surgical management of coronary insufficiency in a child with Kawasaki's disease: Use of bilateral mammary arteries. Ann Thorac Surg *46*:459–461, 1988.
40. Takeuchi Y, Gomi A, Okamura Y, et al: Coronary revascularization in a child with Kawasaki disease: Use of a right gastroepiploic artery. Ann Thorac Surg *50*:294–296, 1990.
41. Sethi S, Ott DA, Nihill M: Surgical management of the cardiovascular complications of Kawasaki's disease. Tex Heart Inst J *10*:343–348, 1983.
42. Fukushige J, Nihill M, McNamar DG: Spectrum of cardiovascular lesions in mucocutaneous lymph node syndrome: Analysis of eight cases. Am J Cardiol *45*:98–102, 1980.
43. Citron BP, Halpern M, McCarron M, et al: Necrotizing angiitis associated with drug abuse. N Engl J Med *283*:1003–1011, 1970.
44. Yu YJ, Cooper DR, Wellenstein DE: Cerebral angiitis and intracerebral hemorrhage associated with methamphetamine abuse. J Neurosurg *58*:109–111, 1983.
45. Ellertson DG, Lazarus AM, Averbach R: Patterns of acute vascular injury after intra-arterial barbiturate injection. Am J Surg *126*:813–817, 1973.

46. Maxwell TM, Olcott C, Blaisdell FW: Vascular complications of drug abuse. Arch Surg 105:875–882, 1972.
47. Lindell TD, Porter JM, Langston C: Intraarterial injection of oral medications. A complication of drug addiction. N Engl J Med 287:1132–1133, 1972.
48. Cogan DG: Syndrome of nonsyphilitic interstitial keratitis and vestibulo-auditory symptoms. Arch Ophthalmol 33:144–149, 1945.
49. Cheson BD, Bluming AZ, Alroy J: Cogan's syndrome: A systemic vasculitis. Am J Med 60:549–555, 1976.
50. LaRaja RD: Cogan syndrome associated with mesenteric vascular insufficiency. Arch Surg 111:1028–1031, 1976.
51. Behçet H: Uber rezidivierende aphthose durch ein virus verusachte Geschwure Am Mund, Am Mauge und an den Genitalien. Dermatol Ubchenschr 105:1152–1157, 1937.
52. Chajek T, Fainaru M: Behçet's disease. Report of 41 cases and a review of the literature. Medicine 54:179–182, 1975.
53. Shimutzu T, Ehrlich GE, Inaba G, Hayashi K: Behçet's disease (Behçet's syndrome). Semin Arthritis Rheum 8:223–260, 1979.
54. The Lancet Editors: Behçet's disease. Lancet 1:761–762, 1989.
55. Namba K: Behçet's disease and streptococcal infection. Abstract presented at Royal Society of Medicine International Conference on Behçet's disease, June 5–6, 1985.
56. Mizushima Y, Matsuda T, Hoshi K, Ohno S: Induction of Behçet's disease symptoms after dental treatment and streptococcal antigen skin test. J Rheumatol 15:1029–1030, 1988.
57. Sezer FN: The isolation of a virus as the cause of Behçet's disease. Am J Ophthalmol 36:301–315, 1953.
58. Sezer FN: Further investigations of the virus of Behçet's disease. Am J Ophthalmol 41:41–54, 1956.
59. Williams BD, Lehner T: Immune complexes in Behçet's syndrome and recurrent oral ulceration. Br Med J 1:1387–1389, 1977.
60. Yamana K, Kosuga K, Kinoshita H, et al: Vasculo-Behçet's disease: Immunological study of the formation of aneurysm. J Cardiovasc Surg 29:751–755, 1988.
61. Little AG, Zarins CK: Abdominal aortic aneurysm and Behçet's disease. Surgery 91:359–362, 1982.
62. Park JH, Ham MC, Bettman MA: Arterial manifestations of Behçet's disease. AJR 143:821–825, 1984.
63. Lehner T, Batchelor JR, Chailacombe SJ, Kennedy L: An immunogenetic basis for the tissue involvement in Behçet's disease. Immunology 37:895–899, 1979.
64. Dhobb M, Ammar F, Bensaid Y, et al: Arterial manifestations in Behçet's disease: Four new cases. Ann Vasc Surg 1:249–252, 1986.
65. Jenkins AM, Macpherson AS, Nolan B, et al: Peripheral aneurysms in Behçet's disease. Br J Surg 63:199–202, 1976.
66. Schwartz P, Weisbrott M, Landau M, Antebi E: Peripheral false aneurysms in Behçet's disease. Br J Surg 74:67–68, 1987.
67. Hamza M: Large artery involvement in Behçet's disease. J Rheumatol 14:554–559, 1987.
68. Mowatt AG: Gangrene in Behçet's syndrome. Br Med J 2:636–639, 1965.
69. Shimizu T: Vascular lesions of Behçet's disease. Cardioangiology 1:124–127, 1977.
70. Kingston M, Ratcliffe JR, Alltree M, et al: Aneurysm after arterial puncture in Behçet's disease. Br Med J 1:1766–1767, 1979.
71. Aoki K, Sugiura S: Immunosuppressive treatment of Behçet's disease. Med Probl Ophthalmol 16:309–312, 1976.
72. Cupps TR, Fauci AS: The Vasculitides. Philadelphia, WB Saunders Company, 1981, pp 142–202.
73. O'Duffy JD, Lehner T, Barnes CG: Summary of the Third International Conference on Behçet's Disease. J Rheumatol 10:154–158, 1983.
74. Sheps SG, McDuffie FC: Vasculitis. In Juergens JL, Spittell JA, Gairbaim JF (eds): Peripheral Vascular Disease. Philadelphia, WB Saunders Company, 1980, pp 493–553.
75. Cosgriff TM, Arnold WJ: Digital vasospasm and infarction

associated with hepatitis B antigenemia. JAMA 235:1362–1363, 1976.
76. Levo Y, Gorevic PD, Kassab HJ, et al: Association between hepatitis B virus and essential mixed cryoglobulinemia. N Engl J Med 296:1501–1504, 1977.
77. Alarcron-Segovia D: The necrotizing vasculitides—a new pathologic classification. Med Clin North Am 61:240–260, 1977.
78. Andrasch R, Bardana EJ, Porter JM: Digital ischemia and gangrene preceding renal neoplasm. Arch Intern Med 136:486–490, 1976.
79. Taylor LM, Baur GM, Porter JM: Finger gangrene caused by small artery occlusive disease. Ann Surg 193:453, 1981.
80. Baur GM, Porter JM, Bardana EJ, et al: Rapid onset of hand ischemia of unknown etiology. Ann Surg 186:184–189, 1977.
81. Porter JM, Taylor LM: Small artery disease of the upper extremity. World J Surg 07:326:333, 1983.
82. Rivers SM, Porter JM: Treatment of Raynaud's syndrome. In Bergan JJ (ed): Clinical Surgery International. Edinburgh, Churchill Livingstone, 1983.
83. Taylor LM, Rivers SP, Porter JM: Treatment of finger ischemia with Bier block reserpine. Surg Gynecol Obstet 154:39–43, 1982.
84. Porter JM, as discussed in Pardy BJ, Hoare MC, Eastcott HHG, et al: Prostaglandin E₁ in severe Raynaud's phenomenon. Surgery 92:953–965, 1982.
85. Huston KA, Hunder GG, Lie JT, et al: Temporal arteritis: A 25 year epidemiologic, clinical, and pathologic study. Ann Intern Med 88:162–167, 1978.
86. Bengtsson B, Malmvall B: Giant cell arteritis. Acta Med Scand (Suppl) 658:1–102, 1982.
87. Hollenhorst RW, Brown JR, Wagener HP, et al: Neurologic aspects of temporal arteritis. Neurology 10:490–498, 1960.
88. Hamrin B, Jonsson N, Landberg T: Arteritis in polymyalgia rheumatica. Lancet 1:397–401, 1964.
89. Austen WG, Blennerhassett JB: Giant cell aortitis causing an aneurysm of the ascending aorta and aortic regurgitation. N Engl J Med 272:80, 1965.
90. Healey LA, Wilskie KR: The Systemic Manifestations of Temporal Arteritis. New York, Grune & Stratton, 1978.
91. Klein RG, Hunder GG, Stanson AW, et al: Large artery involvement in giant cell temporal arteritis. Ann Intern Med 83:806–812, 1975.
92. Swinson DR, Goodwill CJ, Talbot IC: Giant cell arteritis presenting as subclavian artery occlusion. Postgrad Med J 52:525–529, 1976.
93. Rivers SP, Baur GM, Inahara T, et al: Arm ischemia secondary to giant cell arteritis. Am J Surg 143:554–558, 1982.
94. Lupi-Herrera E, Sanchez-Torres G, Marcustiamer J, et al: Takayasu's arteritis. Clinical study of 107 cases. Am Heart J 93:94–103, 1977.
95. Case reports of the Massachusetts General Hospital (Case 43:1978). N Engl J Med 299:1002–1008, 1978.
96. Austen WG, Shaw RS: Surgical treatment of pulseless (Takayasu's) disease. N Engl J Med 270:1228–1231, 1964.
97. McKusick VA, Harris WS, Ottesen OE, et al: Buerger's disease—a distinct clinical and pathologic entity. JAMA 181:5–12, 1962.
98. Wessler S, Ming SC, Gureuch V, et al: A critical evaluation of thromboangiitis obliterans. The case against Buerger's disease. N Engl J Med 262:1149–1160, 1960.
99. Buerger L: Thromboangiitis obliterans: A study of the vascular lesions leading to presenile spontaneous gangrene. Am J Med Sci 136:567–580, 1908.
100. Adar R, Papa MZ, Halpern Z, et al: Cellular sensitivity to collagen in thromboangiitis obliterans. N Engl J Med 308:1113–1116, 1983.
101. Lie JT: Thromboangiitis obliterans (Buerger's disease) in women. Medicine 65:65–72, 1987.
102. Ohta T, Shionaya S: Fate of ischemic limbs in Buerger's disease. Br J Surg 75:259–262, 1988.
103. Juergens JL: Thromboangiitis obliterans (Buerger's disease). In Fairbairn JF, Juergens JL, Spittell JA (eds): Allen-Barker-

Hines Peripheral Vascular Disease, 5th ed. Philadelphia, WB Saunders Company, 1980, pp 468–491.

104. Mills JL, Porter JM: Buerger's disease. *In* Cameron JL (ed): Current Surgical Therapy III. Philadelphia, BC Decker, 1989, pp 575–578.

105. Shionaya S, Ban I, Nakata Y, et al: Diagnosis, pathology, and treatment of Buerger's disease. Surgery 75:695–700, 1974.

106. McKusick VA, Harris WS: Buerger's syndrome in the Orient. Bull Johns Hopkins Hosp 109:242–248, 1961.

107. Abu-Dalu J, Giler SH, Urea I: Thromboangiitis obliterans of the iliac artery. Angiology 24:359–364, 1973.

108. Biller J, Asconape J, Challa VR, et al: A case for cerebral thromboangiitis obliterans. Stroke 12:686–689, 1981.

109. Inada K, Iwashima Y, Okada A, Matsumoto K: Nonatherosclerotic segmental arterial occlusions of the extremity. Arch Surg 108:663–667, 1974.

110. Shionaya S: What is Buerger's disease? World J Surg 7:554–557, 1983.

111. Eadie DGA, Mann CV, Smith PG: Buerger's disease: A clinical and pathological reexamination. Br J Surg 55:452–456, 1968.

112. Mills JL, Porter JM: Buerger's disease in the modern era. Am J Surg 154:123–129, 1987.

113. Rivera R: Roentgenographic diagnosis of Buerger's disease. J Cardiovasc Surg 14:40–46, 1973.

114. Szilaygi DE, DeRusso FJ, Elliot JP: Thromboangiitis obliterans. Clinico-angiographic correlations. Arch Surg 88:824–835, 1964.

115. Allen EV, Brown GE: Thromboangiitis obliterans: A clinical study of 200 cases. Ann Intern Med 1:535–549, 1928.

116. Corelli F: Buerger's disease: Cigarette smoker disease may always be cured by medical therapy alone. Uselessness of operative treatment. J Cardiovasc Surg 14:28–36, 1973.

117. Perler BA: Buerger's disease. *In* Cameron JL (ed): Current Surgical Therapy II. Philadelphia, BC Decker, 1986, pp 385–388.

118. Craven JL, Cotton RC: Hematological differences between thromboangiitis obliterans and atherosclerosis. Br J Surg 54:862–867, 1967.

119. Spittell JA: Thromboangiitis obliterans—an autoimmune disorder. N Engl J Med 308:1157–1158, 1983.

120. Simi'c L, Pirnat L: Immunological aspects of smoking in patients with thromboangiitis obliterans. Vasa 14:349–352, 1985.

121. McLoughlin FA, Helsby FR, Evans CC, et al: Association of HLA-A1 and HLA-B5 with Buerger's disease. Br Med J 2:1165–1166, 1976.

122. Ohtawa T, Juji T, Kawano N, et al: HLA antigens in thromboangiitis obliterans. JAMA 230:1128–1131, 1974.

123. Stojanovic VK, Marcovic A, Arsov V, et al: Clinical course and therapy of Buerger's disease. J Cardiovasc Surg 14:5–8, 1973.

124. Van der Stricht J, Goldstein M, Flammand JP, Belenger J: Evolution and prognosis of thromboangiitis obliterans. J Cardiovasc Surg 14:9–16, 1973.

125. Mills JL, Firedman EI, Taylor LM Jr, Porter JM: Upper extremity ischemia caused by small artery disease. Ann Surg 206:521–528, 1987.

126. Machleder HI, Wheeler E, Barber WF: Treatment of upper extremity ischemia by cervico-dorsal sympathectomy. Vasc Surg 13:399–404, 1979.

127. Nielubowicz J, Rosnowski A, Pruszynski B, et al: Natural history of Buerger's disease. J Cardiovasc Surg 21:529–540, 1980.

128. Largiader J, Schneider E, Bruner U, Bollinger A: Arterial reconstruction in Buerger's disease (thromboangiitis obliterans). Vasa 15:174–179, 1986.

129. Vollmar J: Surgical considerations on the terminology and treatment of the so-called Buerger's disease. J Cardiovasc Surg 14:37–39, 1973.

130. Cupps TR, Fauci AS: Thromboangiitis obliterans (Buerger's disease, endarteritis obliterans). *In*: The Vasculitides. Philadelphia, WB Saunders Company, 1981, pp 133–136.

131. Pardy BJ, Lewis JD, Eascott MS: Preliminary experience with prostaglandins E1 and I2 in peripheral vascular disease. Surgery 88:826–828, 1980.

132. Clifford PC, Martin MFR, Dieppe PA, et al: Prostaglandin E1 infusion for small vessel arterial ischemia. J Cardiovasc Surg 24:503–508, 1983.

133. McFadyen IJ, Housley E, MacPhersons AIS: Intra-arterial reserpine administration in Raynaud's syndrome. Arch Intern Med 132:526–528, 1973.

134. Prandoni AG, Moser M: Clinical appraisal on intraarterial priscoline therapy in the management of peripheral arterial diseases. Circulation 9:73–81, 1954.

135. Wilding RP, Flute PR: Dipyridamole in peripheral upper limb ischemia. Lancet 1:999–1000, 1974.

136. Fonkalsrud EW, Sanchez M, Zervbavel R, et al: Serial changes in arterial structure following radiation therapy. Surg Gynecol Obstet 145:395–400, 1977.

137. Benson EP: Radiation injury to large arteries. Radiology 106:195–197, 1973.

138. Budin JA, Casarella WJ, Harisiadis L: Subclavian artery occlusion following radiotherapy for carcinoma of the breast. Radiology 118:169–173, 1976.

139. McCready RA, Hyde GL, Bivins BA, et al: Radiation induced arterial injuries. Surgery 93:306–312, 1983.

140. Elerding SC, Fernandez RN, Grotta JC, et al: Carotid artery disease following external cervical irradiation. Ann Surg 194:609–615, 1981.

141. Silverberg GD, Britt RH, Goffinet DR: Radiation induced carotid artery disease. Cancer 41:130–137, 1978.

142. Rawitscher RE, Smith GW, Muller WH: Experimental canine coronary atherosclerosis. Ann Surg 177:357–361, 1973.

143. Jarrett F, Darling R, Mundth E, et al: Experience with infected aneurysms of the abdominal aorta. Arch Surg 110:1281–1286, 1975.

144. Stengel A, Wolforth C: Mycotic (bacterial) aneurysms of intravascular origin. Arch Intern Med 31:527–554, 1973.

145. Chiff MM, Soulen RL, Finestone AJ: Mycotic aneurysms—a challenge and a clue. Arch Intern Med 126:977–987, 1970.

146. Blum L, Keefer BC: Clinical entity of cryptogenic mycotic aneurysm. JAMA 188:503–508, 1964.

147. Bardin J, Collins G, Devin J, et al: Nonaneurysmal suppurative aortitis. Arch Surg 116:954, 1981.

148. Bennett DE, Cherry JK: Bacterial infection of aortic aneurysms. Am J Surg 113:321–326, 1967.

149. Malone JM, Lalka SG, McIntyre KE, Bernhard VM, Pabst TS: The necessity for long-term antibiotic therapy with positive arterial wall cultures. J Vasc Surg 8:262–267, 1988.

150. Macbeth GS, Rubin JR, MacIntyre JE Jr, et al: The relevance of arterial wall microbiology to the treatment of prosthetic graft infections: Graft infection vs. arterial infection. J Vasc Surg 1:750–756, 1984.

151. Dougherty SH, Simmons RL: Infections in bionic man: The pathobiology of infection in prosthetic devices. Parts I & II. Curr Probl Surg 19:1–314, 1982.

152. Lalka SG, Malone JM, Fisher DF Jr, Bernhard VM, Sullivan D, Stroecklemann D, Bergstrom RF: Efficacy of prophylactic antibiotics in vascular surgery: An arterial wall microbiologic and pharmacokinetic perspective. J Vasc Surg 10:501–510, 1989.

153. Bergamini TM, Bandyk DF, Govostis D, et al: Identification of *Staphylococcus epidermidis* vascular graft infections: A comparison of culture techniques. J Vasc Surg 9:665–670, 1989.

154. Wilson SE, Van Wagenen PV, Passaro E: Arterial infection. Curr Probl Surg 15(8):12–38, 1978.

155. Ernst C, Campbell H, Daugherty M, et al: Incidence and significance of intra-operative cultures during abdominal aortic aneurysm-ectomy. Ann Surg 185:626–633, 1977.

156. Mendelowitz D, Ramstedt R, Yao J, et al: Abdominal aortic salmonellosis. Surgery 85:514, 1979.

157. Zak F, Strauss L, Saphra I: Rupture of diseased large arteries in the course of enterobacterial (salmonella) infections. N Engl J Med 258:824, 1958.

158. Miller BM, Waterhouse G, Alford RH, et al: Histoplasma infections of abdominal aortic aneurysms. Ann Surg 197:57–62, 1983.

159. Benoit G, Icard P, LeBaleur A, et al: Mycotic aneurysms and renal transplantation. Urology 31:63–65, 1988.

160. Kyriakides GK, Simmons RL, Najarian JJ: Mycotic aneurysms in transplant patients. Arch Surg 111:472–475, 1976.

161. Houssin D, Ortega D, Richardson A, Ozier Y, Stephan H, Soffer M, Chapius Y: Mycotic aneurysm of the hepatic artery complicating human liver transplantation. Transplantation 46:469–472, 1988.

162. Porter LL, Houston MC, Kadir S: Mycotic aneurysm of the hepatic artery: Treatment with arterial embolization. Am J Med 65:697–672, 1979.

163. Tzakis AG, Carroll PB, Gordon RD, et al: Arterial mycotic aneurysm and rupture: A potentially fatal complication of pancreas transplantation in diabetes mellitus. Arch Surg 124:660–661, 1989.

164. Walstra BJ, Jorning PG, Koostra G, van Hoof JP, Janevski BK: Pancreas transplantation complicated by a mycotic false aneurysm: Diagnostic features. J Med Imaging 2:133–136, 1988.

165. Thomson D, Menkis A, Pflugfelder P, Kostuk W, Ahmad D, Mckenzie FN: Mycotic aortic aneurysm after heart-lung transplantation. Transplantation 47:195–197, 1989.

166. Atnip RG: Mycotic aneurysms of the suprarenal abdominal aorta: Prolonged survival after in situ aortic and visceral reconstruction. J Vasc Surg 10:635–641, 1989.

167. Mundth ED, Darling RC, Alvarado RH, et al: Surgical management of mycotic aneurysms and the complications of infection in vascular reconstructive surgery. Am J Surg 117:460–470, 1969.

168. Scher L, Brener B, Goldenkranz R, et al: Infected aneurysms of the abdominal aorta. Arch Surg 115:975, 1980.

169. Cooke PA, Ehrenfeld WK: Successful management of mycotic aortic aneurysm. Report of a case. Surgery 75:132–136, 1974.

170. Oz MC, Brener BJ, Buda JA, et al: A ten-year experience with bacterial aortitis. J Vasc Surg 10:439–449, 1989.

171. Davies OG, Thorburn JD, Powell P: Cryptic mycotic abdominal aortic aneurysms. Am J Surg 136:96–101, 1978.

172. Johansen K, Devin J: Mycotic aortic aneurysms. Arch Surg 118:583–588, 1983.

173. Yeager RA, Hobson RW, Padberg FT, Lynch TG, Chakravarty M: Vascular complications related to drug abuse. J Trauma 27:527–554, 1987.

174. Huebl HC, Read RC: Aneurysmal abscess. Minn Med 49:11–16, 1966.

175. Greelhoed GW, Joseph WL: Surgical sequelae of drug abuse. Surg Gynecol Obstet 39:749–755, 1974.

176. Feldman AJ, Berguer R: Management of an infected aneurysm of the groin secondary to drug abuse. Surg Gynecol Obstet 57:519–522, 1983.

177. Fromm SH, Lucas CE: Obturator bypass for mycotic aneurysm in the drug addict. Arch Surg 100:11–16, 1970.

178. Johnson JR, Ledgerwood AM, Lucas CE: Mycotic aneurysms. New concepts in therapy. Arch Surg 118:577–582, 1983.

179. Reddy DJ, Smith RF, Elliot JP, Haddad GK, Wanek EA: Infected femoral artery pseudoaneurysms in drug addicts: Evolution of selective vascular reconstruction. J Vasc Surg 3:718–724, 1986.

180. Reddy DJ: Treatment of drug related infected false aneurysm of the femoral artery. J Vasc Surg 8:344–345, 1988.

181. Patel KR, Sumel L, Vaus RH: Routine revascularization with resection of infected femoral pseudoaneurysms from substance abuse. J Vasc Surg 8:321–328, 1988.

182. Stanley JC, Gewertz BL, Bove EL, et al: Arterial fibrodysplasia histopathologic character and current etiologic concepts. Arch Surg 110:561–566, 1978.

183. Leadbetter WF, Burkland CE: Hypertension in unilateral renal disease. J Urol 39:611–626, 1938.

184. Descotes J, Pelissier PH, Chignier E: Dystrophy of the media with aneurysmal tendency in the abdominal aorta-iliac segments. J Cardiovasc Surg 17:413, 1976.

185. Harrington OB, Crosby VG, Nicholas L: Fibromuscular hyperplasia of the internal carotid artery. Ann Thorac Surg 9:516–524, 1970.

186. Youngberg SP, Sheps SG, Strong CG: Fibromuscular disease of the renal arteries. Med Clin North Am 61:623–641, 1977.

187. Foster JH, Maxwell MH, Franklin SS, et al: Renovascular occlusive disease: Results of operative treatment. JAMA 231:1043–1048, 1975.

188. Mahler F, Probst PN, Haertel M, et al: Lasting improvement of renovascular hypertension by trans-luminal dilatation of atherosclerotic and non-atherosclerotic renal artery stenosis. A followup study. Circulation 65:611–617, 1982.

189. Kelly TF, Morris GC: Arterial fibromuscular disease: Observations on pathogenesis and surgical management. Am J Surg 143:232–236, 1982.

190. Houston C, Rosenthal D, Lamis PA, et al: Fibromuscular dysplasia of the external iliac arteries: Surgical treatment by graduated interval dilatation technique. Surgery 85:713–715, 1979.

191. Ejrup B, Hiertonn T: Intermittent claudication. Three cases treated by free vein graft. Acta Chir Scand 108:217, 1954.

192. Richardson JD, Polk HC: Adventitial cystic disease of the popliteal artery. Arch Surg 116:478–479, 1981.

193. Flanigan DP, Burnham SJ, Goodreau JJ, et al: Summary of cases of adventitial cystic disease of the popliteal artery. Ann Surg 189:165–175, 1979.

194. Eastcott HHG: Cystic myxomatous degeneration of the popliteal artery. Br Med J 2:1270, 1963.

195. Ishikawa K, Mishima Y, Kobayashi S: Cystic adventitial disease of the popliteal artery. Angiology 12:357, 1961.

196. Stuart TP: A note on a variation in the course of the popliteal artery. J Anat Physiol 13:162, 1879.

197. Hamming JJ: Intermittent claudication at an early age, due to an anomalous course of the popliteal artery. Angiology 10:369–371, 1959.

198. Love JW, Whelan TJ: Popliteal artery entrapment syndrome. Am J Surg 109:620–624, 1965.

199. Gibson MH, Mills JG, Johnson GE, et al: Popliteal entrapment syndrome. Ann Surg 185:341–348, 1977.

200. Senior HD: The development of the arteries of the human lower extremity. Am J Anat 26:55–59, 1919.

201. Bardeen CR: Development and variation of the nerves and the musculature of the inferior extremity and of the neighboring regions of the trunk in man. Am J Anat 6:259–390, 1907.

202. Bouhoustos J, Daskalakis E: Muscular abnormalities affecting the popliteal vessels. Br J Surg 68:501–506, 1981.

203. Insua JA, Young JR, Humphries AW: Popliteal artery entrapment syndrome. Arch Surg 101:771, 1970.

204. Rich NM, Collins GJ, McDonald PT, et al: Popliteal vascular entrapment: Its increasing interest. Arch Surg 114:1377–1384, 1979.

205. Biemans RG, Van Bockel JH: Popliteal artery entrapment syndrome. Surg Gynecol Obstet 144:604–609, 1977.

206. Baker WH, Stoney RJ: Acquired popliteal entrapment syndrome. Arch Surg 105:780–781, 1972.

207. Brener BJ, Alpert J, Brief DK, et al: Iatrogenic entrapment of femoro-popliteal saphenous vein bypass grafts by the gastrocnemius muscle. Surgery 78:668–674, 1975.

208. Hall KV: Anomalous insertion of the medial gastrocnemic head, with circulatory complications. Acta Pathol Scand (Suppl) 148:53, 1961.

209. diMarzo L, Cavallaro A, Sciacca V, et al: Diagnosis of popliteal artery entrapment syndrome: The role of duplex scanning. J Vasc Surg 13:434–438, 1991.

210. Miles S, Roediger W, Cooke P, Mieny CJ: Doppler ultrasound in the diagnosis of the popliteal artery entrapment syndrome. Br J Surg 64:883–884, 1977.

211. Olson SK, Parker DG, Reul GJ: Popliteal artery entrapment: A diagnosis that may be overlooked. Tex Heart Inst J 10:305–310, 1983.

212. Collins PS, McDonald PT, Lim RC: Popliteal artery entrapment. An evolving syndrome. J Vasc Surg 10:484–490, 1989.
213. Muller N, Morris DC, Nichols DM: Popliteal artery entrapment demonstrated by CT. Radiology 151:157–158, 1984.
214. Rizzo RJ, Flinn WR, Yao JST, et al: Computed tomography for evaluation of arterial disease in the popliteal fossa. J Vasc Surg 11:112–119, 1990.
215. Fermand M, Houlle D, Fiessinger JN, et al: Entrapment of the popliteal artery: MR findings. AJR 154:425–426, 1990.
216. Darling RC, Buckley SJ, Abbot WM, Raines J: Intermittent claudication in young athletes: Popliteal artery entrapment syndrome. J Trauma 15:543–552, 1974.
217. Lee BY, La Pointe DG, Madden JL: The adductor canal syndrome. Am J Surg 123:617–620, 1972.
218. Koman M, Hardaker WT, Goldner JL: Wick cathether in evaluating and treating compartment syndromes. South Med J 73:303–309, 1981.
219. Eaton RG, Green WT: Volkmans ischemia: A volar compartment syndrome of the forearm. Clin Orthop 117:58–64, 1975.
220. Jepson PS: Ischemic contracture: Experimental study. Ann Surg 84:785, 1926.
221. Matsen FA: Compartmental Syndrome: A Unified Concept. New York, Grune & Stratton, 1980.
222. Ashton H: Critical closing pressure in human peripheral vascular beds. Clin Sci 22:79, 1962.
223. Matsen FA, Winquist RA, Krugmire RB: Diagnosis and management of compartmental syndromes. J Bone Joint Surg [Am] 62:286–291, 1980.
224. Mubarak SJ, Hargens AR: Acute compartment syndromes. Surg Clin North Am 63:539–551, 1983.
225. Russell WL, Burns RP: Acute upper and lower extremity compartment syndromes. In Bergan JJ, Yao JST (eds): Vascular Surgical Emergencies. Orlando, FL, Grune & Stratton, 1987, pp 203–217.
226. Perry MO, Shires GT III, Albert SA: Cellular changes with graded limb ischemia in reperfusion. J Vasc Surg 1:536–543, 1984.
227. Roberts JP, Perry MO, Hariri RJ, et al: Incomplete recovery of muscle cell function following partial but not complete ischemia. Circ Shock 17:253, 1985.
228. DelMaestro RF: An approach to free radicals in medicine and biology. Acta Physiol Scand 492 (Suppl):153–168, 1980.
229. Shlater M, Kane PF, Kirsh MM: Superoxide dismutase plus catalase enhance the efficacy of hypothermic cardioplegia to protect the globally ischemic, reperfused heart. J Thorac Cardiovasc Surg 83:803–809, 1982.
230. Perler BA, Tohmeh AG, Bulkley GB: Inhibition of the compartment syndrome by ablation of free radical–mediated reperfusion injury. Surgery 108:40–47, 1990.
231. McCord JM: Oxygen-derived free radicals in post-ischemic tissue injury. N Engl J Med 313:154–157, 1985.
232. Mubarak SJ, Owen CA, Hargens AR: Acute compartment syndromes: Diagnosis and treatment with the aid of the Wick catheter. J Bone Joint Surg [Am] 60:1091–1095, 1978.
233. McDermott AGP, Marble AE, Yabsley RH: Monitoring acute compartment pressures with the STIC catheter. Clin Orthop 190:192–197, 1984.
234. Matsen FA, Krugmire RB: Compartmental syndromes. Surg Gynecol Obstet 147:943–949, 1978.
235. Willey RF, Corall RJ, French EB: Noninvasive method for the measurement of anterior tibial compartment pressure. Lancet 1:595–596, 1982.
236. Auerbach N, Bowen A: Sonography of leg in posterior compartmental syndrome. AJR 136:407–408, 1981.
237. Paton DF: The anterior tibial syndrome. Practitioner 255:151–153, 1981.
238. Whitesides TE, Haney TC, Morimoto K, et al: Tissue pressure measurements as a determinant of the need of fasciotomy. Clin Orthop 113:43–49, 1975.
239. Sheridan GW, Matsen FA: An animal model of the compartmental syndrome. Clin Orthop 113:36, 1975.
240. Ashton H: Effect of inflatable plastic splints on blood flow. Br Med J 2:1427, 1966.
241. Rollins DL, Bernhard VM, Towne JB: Fasciotomy: An appraisal of controversial issues. Arch Surg 116:1474–1481, 1981.
242. Hutton M, Rhodes RS, Chapman G: The lowering of postischemic compartment pressures with mannitol. J Surg Res 32:239–242, 1982.
243. Buchbinder D, Karmody AM, Leather RP, et al: Hypertonic mannitol. Arch Surg 116:414–418, 1981.
244. Haimovici H: Metabolic complications of acute arterial occlusions. J Cardiovasc Surg 20:349–354, 1979.
245. Perry MO: Compartment syndromes and reperfusion injury. Surg Clin North Am 68(4):853–864, 1988.
246. Quain R: Partial contraction of the abdominal aorta. Trans Pathol Soc Lond 1:244, 1847.
247. Glenn F, Keefer EB, Speer DS, et al: Coarctation of the lower thoracic and abdominal aorta immediately proximal to the celiac axis. Surg Gynecol Obstet 94:561, 1952.
248. DeBakey ME, Garrett HE, Howell JF, et al: Coarctation of the abdominal aorta with renal arterial stenosis: Surgical considerations. Ann Surg 165:830, 1967.
249. Graham LM, Zelenock GB, Erlandson ED, et al: Abdominal aortic coarctation and segmental hypoplasia. Surgery 86:519, 1979.
250. Hallett JW, Brewster CD, Darling RC, et al: Coarctation of the abdominal aorta: Current options in surgical management. Ann Surg 191:430, 1980.
251. Hejhal L, Hejhal J, Firt P: Coarctation of the abdominal aorta. J Cardiovasc Surg 14:168, 1973.
252. Scott HW, Dean RH, Boerth R, et al: Coarctation of the abdominal aorta: Pathophysiologic and therapeutic considerations. Ann Surg 189:746, 1979.
253. Stanley JC, Graham LM, Whitehouse WM: Developmental occlusive disease of the abdominal aorta and the splenic and renal arteries. Am J Surg 142:190, 1981.
254. Siassi B, Glyman G, Emmonouilides GC: Hypoplasia of the abdominal aorta associated with the rubella syndrome. Am J Dis Child 120:426, 1970.
255. Robicsek F, Sanger PW, Daugherty HK: Coarctation of the abdominal aorta diagnosed by aortography. Ann Surg 162:277, 1965.
256. Sen PK, Kinore SG, Engineer SD, et al: The middle aortic syndrome. Br Heart J 25:610, 1963.
257. Lande A: Takayasu's arteritis and congenital coarctation of the descending thoracic and abdominal aorta: A critical review. Am J Roentgenol 127:277, 1976.
258. Meacham PW, Dean RH, Lawson JW, et al: Study of the renal pressor system in experimental coarctation of the abdominal aorta. Am Surg 43:771, 1977.
259. Kaufman JJ: The middle aortic syndrome: Report of a case treated by renal autotransplantation. Trans Am Assoc Genitourin Surg 64:39, 1972.
260. Robicsek F, Daugherty HK, Cook JW, et al: Coarctation of the abdominal aorta with stricture of the major vessels. Surgery 87:545, 1980.
261. Doberneck RC, Varco RL: Congenital coarctation of the abdominal aorta. Lancet 1:143, 1968.
262. Huang TT, Walma FJ, Tyson KR: Coarctation of the abdominal aorta. Am J Surg 120:598, 1970.
263. Pierce WS, Vincent WR, Fitzgerald E, et al: Coarctation of the abdominal aorta with multiple aneurysms. Ann Thorac Surg 20:687, 1975.
264. Pirker E, Schmidberger H: Die Arteria ischiadica: Eine seltene getassvariente. Fortschr Geb Roentgenstr Nuklearmed Erganzungsband 116:434, 1972.
265. Hutchinson JE, Cordiac WV, McAllister FF: The surgical management of an aneurysm of a primitive persistent sciatic artery. Ann Surg 167:277, 1968.
266. Tisnodo J, Beachley ML, Amendola MA, et al: Aneurysm of a persistent artery. Cardiovasc Radiol 2:257, 1979.
267. Cowie TN, McKellan HJ, McLean N, et al: Unilateral congenital absence of the external iliac and femoral arteries. Br J Radiol 33:520, 1960.

268. Senior HD: The development of arteries of the human lower extremity. Am J Anat 25:55, 1919.
269. Greebe J: Congenital anomalies of the iliofemoral artery. J Cardiovasc Surg 18:317, 1977.
270. Steele G, Saunders RJ, Riley J, et al: Pulsatile buttock masses: Gluteal and persistant sciatic artery aneurysms. Surgery 82:201–204, 1977.
271. Erdheim J: Medionecrosis aortae idiopathica cystica. Virchows Arch [A] 276:187–229, 1930.
272. Roberts AJ, Jaffe RB, Michaels LL, et al: Cystic medial necrosis. A correctable cause of the superior vena cava syndrome. Arch Surg 109:84, 1974.
273. Tredal SM, Carter JB, Edwards JE: Cystic medial necrosis of the pulmonary artery. Arch Pathol 97:183, 1974.
274. Tse TF, Yu DY: Unusual clinical manifestations of cystic medionecrosis: Report of a case. Am Heart J 84:794, 1972.
275. Read RC, Wolf P: Symptomatic disseminated cystic medial necrosis. N Engl J Med 271:816, 1964.
276. Tsipouras P, Borresen Al, Bamforth S, et al: Marfan syndrome: Exclusion of genetic linkage to the COLIA2 gene. Clin Genet 30:428–432, 1986.
277. Dalgleish R, Hawkins JR, Keston M: Exclusion of the alpha 2(I) and alpha 1(III) collagen genes as the mutant loci in a Marfan syndrome family. J Med Genet 24:148–151, 1987.
278. Francomano CA, Streeten EA, Meyers DA, et al: Marfan syndrome: Exclusion of genetic linkage to three major collagen genes. Am J Med Genet 29:457–462, 1988.
279. Huttunen K, Kaitila I, Savolainen A, et al: The linkage analysis with RFLP markers of elastin and type III collagen genes in Finnish Marfan families (abstr). Am J Med Genet 32:244, 1989.
280. Low FN: Microfibrils: Fine filamentous components of the tissue space. Anat Rec 142:131–137, 1962.
281. Raviola G: The fine structure of the ciliary zonule and ciliary epithelium. Invest Ophthalmol 10:851–869, 1971.
282. Gibson MA, Kumaratilake JS, Cleary EG: The protein components of the 12 nanometer microfibrils of elastic and nonelastic tissues. J Biol Chem 264:4590–4598, 1989.
283. Maddox BK, Sakai LY, Keene DR, Glanville RW: Connective tissue microfibrils. J Biol Chem 264:2181–2185, 1989.
284. Hollister DW, Godfrey MP, Keene DR, et al: Marfan syndrome: Abnormalities of the microfibrillar array detected by immunohistopathologic studies (abstr). Am J Med Genet 32:244, 1989.
285. Hollister DW, Godfrey MP, Sakai LY, et al: Immunohistologic abnormalities of the microfibrillar-fiber system in the Marfan syndrome. N Engl J Med 323:152–159, 1990.
286. Kainulainen K, Pulkkinen L, Savolainen A, et al: Location on chromosome 15 of the gene defect causing Marfan syndrome. N Engl J Med 323:935–939, 1990.
287. Dietz HC, Pyeritz RE, Hall BD, et al: The Marfan syndrome locus: Confirmation of assignment to chromosome 15 and identification of tightly linked markers at 15q15-15q21.3. Genomics 9:355–361, 1991.
288. Dietz HC, Cutting GR, Pyeritz RE, et al: Marfan syndrome caused by a recurrent de novo missense mutation in the fibrillin gene. Nature 353:337–339, 1991.
289. Lee B, Godfrey MP, Vitale E, et al: Linkage of Marfan syndrome and a phenotypically related disorder to two different fibrillin genes. Nature 353:330–334, 1991.
290. Tsipouras P, Del Mastro R, Sarfarazi M, et al: Genetic linkage of the Marfan syndrome, ectopia lentis, and congenital contractural arachnodactyly to the fibrillin genes on chromosomes 15 and 5. N Engl J Med 326:905–909, 1992.
291. Beals RK, Hecht F: Congenital contractural arachnodactyly: A heritable disorder of connective tissue. J Bone Joint Surg 53:987–993, 1971.
292. McKusick VA: The defect in Marfan syndrome. Nature 352:279–281, 1991.
293. McKusick VA: Heritable Disorders of Connective Tissue, 4th ed. St. Louis, CV Mosby, 1972, pp 61–223.
294. Roberts WC, Honig HS: The spectrum of cardiovascular disease in the Marfan syndrome: A clinico-morphologic study of 18 necropsy patients and comparison to 151 previously reported necropsy patients. Am Heart J 104:115–135, 1982.
295. Perejda AJ, Abraham PA, Carnes WH, et al: Marfan syndrome: Structural, biochemical, and mechanical studies of the aortic media. J Lab Clin Med 106:376–383, 1985.
296. Hirata K, Triposkiadis F, Sparks E, et al: The Marfan syndrome: Abnormal elastic properties. J Am Coll Cardiol 18:57–63, 1991.
297. Come PC, Bulkley BH, McKusick VA, et al: Echocardiographic recognition of silent aortic root dilatation in Marfan's syndrome. Chest 72:789, 1977.
298. Pyeritz RE: Propranolol retards aortic root dilation in the Marfan syndrome (abstr). Circulation 111:365, 1983.
299. Pyeritz RE, McKusick VA: The Marfan syndrome: Diagnosis and management. N Engl J Med 300:772, 1979.
300. Davis Z, Pluth JR, Giuliana ER: The Marfan syndrome and cardiac surgery. J Thorac Cardiovasc Surg 75:505, 1978.
301. McDonald GR, Schaff HV, Pyeritz RE, et al: Surgical management of patients with the Marfan syndrome and dilatation of the ascending aorta. J Thorac Cardiovasc Surg 81:180, 1981.
302. Van Meekeren JA: De dilatabilitate extraordinaria cutis. In: Observations Medicochirugicae. Amsterdam, 1682.
303. Beighton P, Horan FT: Surgical aspects of the Ehlers-Danlos syndrome. A survey of 100 cases. Br J Surg 56:255, 1969.
304. Pope FM, Martin FR, Lichtenstein JR, et al: Patients with Ehlers-Danlos syndrome type IV lack type III collagen. Proc Natl Acad Sci USA 72:1314, 1975.
305. Wesley JR, Mahour GH, Wooley MM: Multiple surgical problems in two patients with Ehlers-Danlos syndrome. Surgery 87:319, 1980.
306. Hunter GC, Malone JM, Moore WS: Vascular manifestations in patient with Ehlers-Danlos syndrome. Arch Surg 117:495, 1982.
307. Wright CB, Lamberth WC, Ponseti IV, et al: Successful management of popliteal arterial disruption in Ehlers-Danlos syndrome. Surgery 85:708, 1979.
308. Burnett HF, Bledsoe JH, Char F: Abdominal aortic aneurysmectomy in a 17-year-old patient with Ehlers-Danlos syndrome: Case report and review of the literature. Surgery 74:617, 1973.
309. Carlborg U, Lund EG: Pseudoxanthoma elasticum: Short summary and discussion of the general clinical and histopathologic cardiovascular findings. Acta Med Scand (Suppl) 350:56, 1959.
310. Carlborg U: Studies of circulatory disturbances, pulse wave velocity, and pressure pulses in larger arteries in cases of pseudoxanthoma elasticum and angioid streaks. Acta Med Scand (Suppl) 151:1, 1944.
311. Eddy DO, Farber EM: Pseudoxanthoma elasticum. Arch Dermatol 86:729, 1962.
312. Wahlquist ML, Fox FM, Beech AM, et al: Peripheral vascular disease as a mode of presentation of pseudoxanthoma elasticum. Aust NZ Med J 7:523, 1977.
313. Alinder I, Bostrom H: Clinical studies on a Swedish material of pseudoxanthoma elasticum. Acta Med Scand 191:273, 1972.
314. Farreras-Valenti P, Rozman C, Jurado-Gran J, et al: Touraine syndrome with systemic hypertension due to unilateral angioma: Cure of hypertension after nephrectomy. Am J Med 37:355, 1965.
315. Carter DJ, Vince FP, Woodword DAK: Arterial surgery in pseudoxanthoma elasticum. Postgrad Med J 52:291, 1976.
316. Leriche R: Dilatation pathologique des arteres es en dehors des aneurysmes vie tissulaire des arteres. Presse Med 50:641, 1942.
317. Leriche R: Dolicho et mega-artere: Dolicho et mega-verne. Presse Med 51:554, 1943.
318. Beuren AJ, Hort W, Kalbfleisch H, Muller H, Stoermer J: Dysplasia of the systemic and pulmonary arterial system with tortuosity and lengthening of the arteries. Circulation 39:109, 1969.
319. Staple TW, Friedenberg MJ, Anderson MS: Arteria magna et dolicho g leriche. Acta Radiol Diagn 4:293, 1966.

320. Randall PA, Omar MM, Rohner R, et al: Arteria magna revisited. Radiology *132*:295, 1979.
321. Thomas ML: Arteriomegaly. Br J Surg *71*:690, 1971.
322. Carson HAJ, Cusworth DC, Dent CE, et al: Homocystinuria: A new inborn error of metabolism associated with mental deficiency. Arch Dis Child *38*:425, 1963.
323. McCully KS: Homocysteine theory of atherosclerosis. Development and current status. Atherosclerosis Rev *11*:157–247, 1983.
324. Mudd SH, Finkelstein JD, Irrevere F, Laster L: Homocystinuria: An enzymatic defect. Science *143*:1443–1445, 1964.
325. Mudd SH, Levy HL, Abeles RH: A derangement in the metabolism of vitamin B-12 leading to homocystinuria, cystathionuria, and methyl malonic aciduria. Biochem Biophys Res Commun *35*:21–26, 1969.
326. Mudd SH, Uhlendorf BW, Freeman JM, et al: Homocystinuria associated with decreased methylene tetrahydrofolate reductase activity. Biochem Biophys Res Commun *46*:905–912, 1972.
327. Smolin LA, Crenshaw TD, Kurtyca D, Benevenga NJ: Homocysteine accumulation in pigs fed diets deficient in vitamin B-6 (pyridoxine). Relationship to atherosclerosis. J Nutr *133*:2022–2028, 1983.
328. Kang SS, Wong PWK, Norusis M: Homocysteine due to folate deficiency. Metabolism *36*:458–465, 1987.
329. Brattstorm L, Israelsson B, Lindgarde X, et al: Higher total plasma homocysteine in vitamin B-12 deficiency than in heterozygosity for homocystinuria due to cystathionine B-synthetase deficiency. Metabolism *37*:175–182, 1988.
330. Gibson JB, Carson NAJ, Neil DW: Pathological findings in homocystinuria. J Clin Pathol *17*:427–437, 1964.
331. McCully KS: Vascular pathology of homocysteinemia: Implications for the pathogenesis of atherosclerosis. Am J Pathol *56*:111–128, 1969.
332. Kanwar YS, Manaligod JR, Wong WK: Morphologic studies in a patient with homocystinuria due to 5,10-methylene tetrahydrofolate reductase deficiency. Pediatr Res *10*:598–609, 1976.
333. McCully KS, Ragsdale BC: Production of arteriosclerosis by homocysteinemia. Am J Pathol *61*:1–11, 1970.
334. McCully KS, Carvalho ACA: Homocysteine thiolactone, N-homocysteine thiolactonyl retinamide, and platelet aggregation. Res Commun Chem Pathol Pharmacol *6*:349–360, 1987.
335. McCully KS, Vezeridis MP: Homocysteine thiolactone in arteriosclerosis and cancer. Res Commun Chem Pathol Pharmacol *59*:107–119, 1988.
336. Refsum H, Helland S, Ueland PM: Radioenzymatic determination of homocysteine in plasma and urine. Clin Chem *31*:624–628, 1985.
337. Wilcken DEL, Gupta VJ: Cysteine-homocysteine mixed disulfide: Differing plasma concentrations in normal men and women. Clin Sci *57*:211–215, 1979.
338. Wilcken DEL, Wilcken B: The pathogenesis of coronary artery disease: A possible role for methionine metabolism. J Clin Invest *57*:1079–1082, 1976.
339. Boers GHK, Smals AGH, Trijbels FJM: Unique efficiency of methionine metabolism in premenopausal women may protect against vascular disease in the reproductive years. J Clin Invest *72*:1971–1975, 1983.
340. Boers GHK, Smals AGH, Trijbels FJM, et al: Heterozygosity for homocystinuria in premature peripheral and cerebral occlusive arterial diseases. N Engl J Med *313*:709–714, 1985.
341. Brattstrom LE, Hardebo JE, Hutberg BL: Moderate homocysteinemia—a possible risk factor for arteriosclerotic cerebrovascular disease. Stroke *15*:1012–1015, 1984.
342. Malinow MR, Kang SS, Taylor LM Jr, et al: Prevalence of hyperhomocysteinemia in patients with peripheral arterial occlusive disease. Circulation *79*:1180–1188, 1989.
343. Kang SS, Wong PWK, Cook HY, et al: Protein bound homocysteine. A possible risk factor for coronary artery disease. J Clin Invest *77*:1482–1486, 1986.
344. Harris EJ Jr, Taylor LM Jr, Malinow MR, et al: The association between elevated plasma homocysteine and symptomatic peripheral arterial disease. Surg Forum *XL*:307–309, 1989.
345. Olszewski AJ, Szostak WB, Bialkowska M, et al: Reduction of plasma lipid and homocysteine levels by pyridoxine, folate, cobalamin, choline, riboflavin, and troxerutin in atherosclerosis. Atherosclerosis *75*:1–6, 1989.
346. Fills WT, Melissinos EG: Polycythemia vera. *In* Sabiston DC (ed): Textbook of Surgery. Philadelphia, WB Saunders Company, 1977, p 146.
347. Williams WJ, Beutler E, Erslev AJ, et al: Hematology. New York, McGraw-Hill, 1977.
348. Block KJ, Maki DG: Hyperviscosity syndromes associated with immunoglobulin abnormalities. Semin Hematol *10*:113, 1973.
349. Brouet C, Clauvel J, Danon F: Biologic and clinical significance of cryoglobulins. Am J Med *57*:775, 1974.
350. Bloor K, Williams RT: Neurofibromatosis and coarctation of the abdominal aorta with renal artery involvement. Br J Surg *50*:811, 1963.
351. Mena E, Bookstein JJ, Holt JF, et al: Neurofibromatosis and renovascular hypertension in children. Am J Roentgenol Radium Ther Nucl Med *118*:39, 1973.
352. Schurch W, Messerli FH, Genest J, et al: Arterial hypertension and neurofibromatosis: Renal artery stenosis and coarctation of abdominal aorta. Conn Med Assoc J *113*:879, 1975.

REVIEW QUESTIONS

1. Arteritis is a central feature in all of the following syndromes except:

   (a) Kawasaki disease
   (b) Cogan's syndrome
   (c) Behçet's syndrome
   (d) Takayasu's disease
   (e) Gilbert's disease

2. The majority of patients with temporal arteritis are encompassed in which of the following groups?

   (a) 50 years, male, white
   (b) 50 years, females, nonwhite
   (c) 50 years, male, nonwhite
   (d) 50 years, male and female, nonwhite
   (e) 50 years, female, white

3. Optimal initial treatment for subacute upper extremity ischemia caused by temporal arteritis is:

   (a) steroids
   (b) endarterectomy
   (c) saphenous vein bypass
   (d) thrombolytic therapy
   (e) warfarin anticoagulation

4. Which of the following is of greatest benefit in the treatment of patients with Buerger's disease?

   (a) sympathectomy
   (b) oral vasodilators
   (c) arterial reconstructive surgery
   (d) warfarin anticoagulation
   (e) cessation of tobacco use

5. Which of the following organisms is most frequently cultured from primary arterial mycotic aneurysms?
   (a) *Haemophilus*
   (b) *Salmonella*
   (c) *Pseudomonas*
   (d) *Neisseria*
   (e) *Clostridium*

6. Calf claudication in a nonsmoker less than 30 years of age is most commonly caused by:
   (a) popliteal entrapment syndrome
   (b) atherosclerosis
   (c) polyarteritis nodosa
   (d) Takayasu's disease
   (e) homocystinemia

7. The early objective diagnosis of anterior compartment syndrome is best made by:
   (a) absent dorsal pedal pulse
   (b) foot drop
   (c) tense swelling
   (d) localized compartmental pain
   (e) compartment pressure greater than 40 mm Hg

8. Extensive vascular calcification in a young patient with normal parathyroid function suggests:
   (a) hyperlipidemia
   (b) Hurler's syndrome
   (c) pseudoxanthoma elasticum
   (d) Marfan's syndrome
   (e) Ehlers-Danlos syndrome

9. Abdominal coarctation is most frequently discovered during evaluation for:
   (a) claudication
   (b) blue toe syndrome
   (c) weight loss
   (d) hypertension
   (e) abdominal pain

10. Ischemic finger ulcerations most frequently result from:
    (a) digital vasospasm
    (b) accidental arterial drug injection
    (c) cold injury
    (d) hypothenar hammer syndrome
    (e) diffuse palmar and digital arterial obstruction

ANSWERS

1. e	2. e	3. a	4. e	5. b	6. a	7. e
8. c	9. d	10. e				

9
PRIMARY ARTERIAL INFECTIONS

JOE A. CATES and HUGH A. GELABERT

Although "primary" or "spontaneous" infections of the arterial tree are relatively uncommon, this clinical entity remains one of the most challenging problems in the field of vascular surgery. Despite dramatic advances in our understanding of the pathophysiology as well as improvements in both antibiotic treatment and modern surgical technique, arterial infections continue to commonly result in limb loss and/or death. This chapter focuses on the pathophysiology, diagnosis, and treatment of primary arterial infections, and reviews changing patterns in these three areas.

HISTORICAL PERSPECTIVE

Among the earliest reports of arterial infections was that offered by Paré during the 16th century. He described suture ligation and excision of vessels that had become infected following battle injuries. This early treatment subsequently became a mainstay of therapy and, in combination with the modern techniques of vessel substitution, remains as such today. Rokitansky[1] and others[2] recognized an association between arterial infection and aneurysm formation early in the 19th century. Osler, in 1885,[3] presented the first comprehensive description of this relationship. In addressing the Royal College of Physicians, he described a 30-year-old male who had succumbed with fever, chills, and pneumonia. At autopsy the patient was found to have endocarditis involving the aortic valve, as well as multiple aneurysms of the thoracic aorta. Based on carefully described pathologic findings, Osler proposed a causal relationship between infection of the aortic wall and subsequent aneurysm formation. Due to a similarity between the beaded appearance of these aneurysms and fungal vegetations, he introduced the term "mycotic aneurysm," and thus the concept of primary arterial infection.

DEFINITION

A universally accepted definition of primary arterial infection has not been well established. More-over, there continues to be confusion regarding the general classification of native arterial infections. The term mycotic aneurysm was initially introduced by Osler to signify those infected aneurysms found in association with bacterial endocarditis. Currently, the term has come to denote an infected aneurysm of any type. Additionally, the majority of published literature has focused on specific subtypes of arterial infections; namely, aneurysmal dilatation secondary to arterial infection and those resulting from infection of a traumatic pseudoaneurysm. Another problem is that there exists considerable disparity among the several definitions that have been proposed. Finally, it should be recognized that with the exception of a secondarily infected arterial aneurysm, most of these lesions are in fact infected pseudoaneurysms. Most arise by the local destruction of the arterial wall and the fibrous encapsulation of an expanding hematoma, and thus do not have the histologic components of an arterial wall. Thus, the very term mycotic aneurysm is frequently a misnomer. For the purposes of this chapter, we will utilize the following definition to describe a primary arterial infection: the direct invasion or extension of a specific pathogen into the intima, media, or adventitia of a native artery, irrespective of the preexisting state of the underlying artery or source of the pathogen. Similarly, the term mycotic aneurysm will be used to denote both true aneurysm and false aneurysm.

PATHOGENESIS

Mycotic Aneurysm

Five basic pathophysiologic mechanisms have been implicated in the genesis of arterial infections. They may broadly be grouped under the following names: mycotic aneurysm, microbial arteritis with aneurysm formation, infected aneurysm, mechanical injury with contamination, and arteritis from contiguous spread. It should be noted that the same name applies to both the pathophysiologic mechanism and the resultant aneurysm.

Osler described the first of these, the mycotic aneurysm. It was most common during the preantibiotic era, when bacterial endocarditis was far more prevalent. As described by Osler, the true mycotic aneurysm is limited to the unique clinical condition characterized by bacterial endocarditis with septic embolization from valvular vegetations. These septic emboli lodge within this arterial wall, where a suppurative infection develops. The arterial wall is destroyed by the infection, and the resultant pseudoaneurysm is recognized as a mycotic aneurysm.

As noted, considerable confusion has subsequently arisen because the term mycotic aneurysm has been applied to various types of infected aneurysms. Crane attempted to classify mycotic aneurysms into primary and secondary types.[4] He introduced the term "primary mycotic aneurysm" to refer to infected aortic aneurysms not associated with endocarditis or an infectious focus. In contrast, secondary types were those that formed as a result of precedent endocarditis. Ponfick[5] and Eppinger[6] were among the first to pathologically characterize the anatomical features of these aneurysms. Ponfick proposed that the initial insult to the arterial wall was a mechanical injury inflicted by the embolization of septic material. Eppinger, in 1887, provided further support for the theory of septic emboli by culturing the same strain of bacteria from both vegetative lesions and the wall of an aneurysm in a patient with endocarditis. He applied the term "embolomycotic" to describe the combination of infectious and embolic components that lead to the formation of mycotic aneurysms.

Microbial Arteritis with Aneurysm Formation

The second mechanism of arterial infection involves the microbial seeding of arteries during an episode of bacteremia. This mechanism is responsible for two distinct types of arterial infections that are differentiated by the state of the preexisting artery. Microbial arteritis with aneurysm formation occurs when a normal or atherosclerotic artery becomes infected and the weakened artery subsequently becomes aneurysmal. In contrast, an infected aneurysm refers to the infection of a preexisting aneurysm—most often by hematogenous microbiological seeding of the aneurysm.

In 1906, the German pathologist Weisel described distinctive pathologic changes in arterial walls that occurred during the course of an infectious disease, but which were not of embolic origin.[7] Lewis and Schrager[8] and Cathcart[9] presented case reports of infected peripheral aneurysms that developed in normal arteries of patients with osteomyelitis and typhoid fever, respectively. Despite these reports, nearly 30 years passed before consideration was given to the mechanism by which bacteremia led to arterial infection. Crane, in 1937, described an infected aneurysm that occurred in a patient with hypoplasia of the aorta, but with no associated bacterial endocarditis or other identifiable source of infection.[4] He proposed that the combination of the "force of the blood stream" and abnormal development of the aorta allowed bacteria to invade that portion of the aorta. This resulted in an arterial infection, disruption of the aortic wall, and subsequently an infected pseudoaneurysm. Revell extended the concept of aortic bacterial seeding one step further, and proposed that the route of infection was through the aortic vasa vasorum. Lastly, Hawkins and Yeager, acknowledging the resistance of arterial intima to infection, suggested that an intimal defect such as that produced by arteriosclerosis would allow bacterial localization and infection.[10]

Infected Aneurysm

Within the category of arterial infections developing from bacteremia, there exists a specific subset, which consists of those preexisting aneurysms that become secondarily infected. These lesions are referred to as infected aneurysms. The original aneurysms are most commonly atherosclerotic. However, they may also be traumatic or syphilitic in origin. The mechanism of infection is hematogenous spread of the bacteria to the aneurysm. The diseased artery becomes host to the bacterial pathogens when these lodge within the intramural thrombus and arteriosclerotic intima. While some of these infected aneurysms may proceed to rapid expansion and rupture, many appear to remain quiescent. These are often discovered in the course of incidental microbiological investigation of aneurysm contents.

Mechanical Injury with Contamination

A third means by which arterial infections occur is that of mechanical arterial injury with contaminated instruments. This type of infection can occur as an inadvertent arterial puncture with a contaminated needle in drug abuse, as an accidental contamination during radiological procedures, during placement of hemodynamic monitoring catheters, or as a result of traumatic injury. The combination of mechanical disruption of the intima along with the seeding of the arterial lesion with pathogenic bacteria leads to the formation of suppurative arteritis and destroys a portion of the arterial wall. This subsequently becomes an infected arterial pseudoaneurysm.

An alternative route of development of the traumatic arterial infection is the secondary contamination of a traumatic pseudoaneurysm. In this scenario, a pseudoaneurysm is created as a consequence of an arterial puncture. Bacterial seeding occurs as a secondary event in the course of a bacteremic episode. For reasons that are not clear, the bacterial colonization develops into an invasive infection. This in turn becomes an infected arterial pseudoaneurysm.

Arteritis from Contiguous Spread

The fourth mechanism by which arterial infections develop is spread of the infection from a contiguous focus. Contiguous infections that have been recognized as potential sources of these bacteria include lesions such as osteomyelitis, infected lymph nodes, tuberculous lymph nodes, and abscesses from narcotic injection.[11] Bacteria and, less commonly, mycobacteria or fungi invade the artery either by direct extension or via lymphatics. They subsequently produce a necrotizing invasive infection of the arterial wall with eventual destruction of the vessel wall. This process, depending on the rate of progression, leads either to pseudoaneurysm formation or free arterial rupture.

Other Forms of Arterial Infection

There are three other less common forms of infected aneurysms that are tangentially included in the above classification: syphilitic aortitis, true fungal aneurysms, and spontaneous aortoenteric fistulas. Because of significant differences in the pathogens and the pathogenesis of these lesions, they merit separate notice.

Syphilitic aneurysms represent a rarely encountered complication of advanced syphilis. These lesions occur in approximately 10 per cent of patients with the tertiary form of the disease.[12] These aneurysms commonly arise in the ascending aorta, frequently involve the aortic valve, and are secondary to treponemal invasion of the vasa vasorum. Reasons for the preference of the *Treponema* for this portion of the aorta remain unclear. Following spirochete penetration, an infiltrate develops within the vessel wall, consisting of plasma cells, epidermal cells, and giant cells. This infiltrate results in destruction of the elastic and muscular components of the tunica media, replacement of the normal wall with fibrous tissue, and dilation and subsequent formation of saccular aneurysms.

Fungal arterial infections are also extremely rare, and most often occur in patients who are immunosuppressed. Common risk factors include diabetes, immunosuppressive medications, or chronic hematologic disorders such as leukemias or lymphomas. Species most often implicated are *Histoplasma capsulatum*, *Aspergillus fumigatus*, *Candida albicans*, and *Penicillium* species. These lesions most commonly result from either colonization of a preexisting aneurysm or infection of a damaged artery.

Spontaneous aortoenteric fistulae arise as a consequence of progressive aneurysmal enlargement with gradual erosion into the adjacent gastrointestinal tract. The erosion is thought to be facilitated by the indurated, atherosclerotic artery pressing against a tethered portion of bowel. The most common location for this erosion is the third portion of the duodenum. In reviewing a series of 16,633 autopsies, Hirst and Affeldt reported the incidence of this type of fistula to be 0.05 per cent.[13] Currently, because the majority of patients diagnosed with aortic aneurysms now undergo elective operation, the incidence of these lesions is thought to be considerably lower. Patients with spontaneous aortoenteric fistulas may present with an initial or "herald" bleed. This represents the initial hemorrhage of blood into the duodenum. It may stop for a period of time and then resume in a more prolonged and dramatic manner. Clot within the aortoenteric fistula is responsible for the intermittent nature of the bleeding episodes.

ETIOLOGIC ORGANISMS

The bacteriology of primary arterial infections has undergone considerable transformation since its original description in the mid 1800s (Fig. 9–1). Brown et al.[14] and others suggest that the reason for this change is antibiotic-selective pressure leading to bacterial adaptation. Also, there has been a change in the relative incidence of pathogenic mechanisms with the more common use of invasive diagnostic modalities as well as increased illicit use of intravenous drugs. The majority of arterial infections during the preantibiotic era were true mycotic aneurysms; that is, related to bacterial endocarditis. The bacteriology of arterial infections during this period, therefore, was that of endocarditis. Stengal in 1923[15] and Revell in 1945[16] both reported that the predominant organisms were nonhemolytic streptococci, staphylococci, and pneumococci. Magilligan in a more contemporary review, subdivided 91 patients with bacterial endocarditis into two groups—those known to be intravenous drug abusers (36 patients), and those who were not (55 patients).[17] Of the first group, the most common organisms were *Staphylococcus aureus* (36 per cent), *Pseudomonas* species (16 per cent), polymicrobial organisms (15 per cent), *Streptococcus faecalis* (13 per cent), and *Streptococcus viridans* (11 per cent). Organisms in the second group (nonintravenous drug abusers) were *S. viridans* (22 per cent), *S. aureus* (20 per cent), *S. faecalis* (14 per cent), and *Staphylococcus epidermidis* (11 per cent). The declining incidence of rheumatic fever and the adoption of early, appropriate antibiotic treatment has resulted in a significant decrease of bacterial endocarditis. This in turn has resulted in a decline in the incidence of Oslerian mycotic aneurysm in the recent decades.

Concurrent with the declining incidence of mycotic aneurysms was an increase in various other types of primary arterial infections. Principal amongst these are microbial arteritis and infected aneurysms. This in part may be due to the increasing age of the population and the simultaneous increase in the prevalence of atherosclerosis. The bacteriology of these arterial infections is different from that of mycotic aneurysms. The microorganisms most commonly associated with microbial arteritis are *Salmonella*, *Staphylococcus*, and *Escherichia coli*. *Salmonella* species in

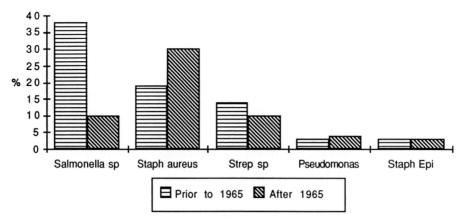

FIGURE 9–1. Organisms cultured from mycotic aneurysms. Staph aureus, *Staphylococcus aureus*; Strep, *Streptococcus*; Staph epi, *Staphylococcus epidermidis*. (From Brown SL, Busuttil RW, Baker JD, et al: Bacteriologic and surgical determinants of survival in patients with mycotic aneurysms. J Vasc Surg 1:541–547, 1984.)

particular have a striking propensity toward invasion of diseased (atherosclerotic) aortas. In selected series, the involvement of *Salmonella* has been reported to be as high as 50 per cent. The most virulent species, *S. choleraesuis* and *S. typhimurium*, account for over 60 per cent of the reported cases of *Salmonella* arteritis.[18] Less commonly reported organisms associated with microbial arteritis include fungi and anaerobic organisms. Amongst the latter, *Bacteroides fragilis* has been reported in association with supraceliac aortic aneurysms.

The bacteriology of infected aneurysms is similar to that of both mycotic aneurysms and microbial arteritis. Despite this, some variation exists between reported series. While Bennett and Cherry[19] reported a 66 per cent incidence of *Salmonella* infections, Jarrett and associates[20] described a predominance of gram-positive cocci (59 per cent), with *S. aureus* representing 41 per cent. In two prospective studies of patients undergoing aneurysmectomy, cultures obtained from both aneurysm wall and bowel bag revealed a predominance of gram-positive organisms.[20,21] Both of these series are thought to represent cases of bacterial colonization. Despite the relative infrequency of gram-negative organisms observed in Jarrett's series, the distinction between gram-negative and gram-positive cultures proved clinically important. Patients with gram-negative bacteria demonstrated a greater likelihood of aortic rupture than those with gram-positive organisms. Specifically, the rupture rate for gram-negative bacterial isolates was 84 per cent, while that of the gram-positive bacterial cultures was 10 per cent.

According to Brown and associates, the most common infected aneurysms since 1965 are those that occur as a result of mechanical arterial injury with contamination of the vessel wall.[14] The organism most frequently implicated in this type of arterial infection is *S. aureus*. It has been cultured in as many as 30 per cent of their cases. Reddy and associates, in reporting a series of infected femoral false aneurysms, made note of a 65 per cent incidence of *S. aureus*.

Cultures also demonstrated a 33 per cent rate of polymicrobial infection.[22] While arterial infections secondary to contiguous spread are most commonly bacterial, mycobacterial and fungal infections have also been noted to occur in these lesions. As with microbial arteritis, *Salmonella* is the predominating pathogen with *Staphylococcus* second in frequency (Fig. 9–2).

DISTRIBUTION OF PRIMARY ARTERIAL INFECTIONS

The anatomic distribution of primary arterial infections varies somewhat depending on the pathologic type of infection. True mycotic aneurysms, due to their embolic etiology, may occur in any artery larger than end-digital vessels. They most often involve the larger muscular and elastic arteries. Both Lewis[8] and Brown,[14] in retrospective reviews, demonstrated the most common sites of infection to be abdominal aorta, femoral, and superior mesenteric arteries (Fig. 9–3). The predisposition toward aortic involvement is thought to be related to the higher incidence of underlying atherosclerotic aneurysms in this location as compared to other anatomical sites.

Microbial arteritis with aneurysm formation occurs when a pathogen localizes at the site of an arterial lesion such as an atherosclerotic plaque. As one would anticipate, the arteries most commonly involved are the same ones that demonstrate advanced atherosclerotic changes; namely, the distal aorta, femoral, iliac, and popliteal vessels. Infected aneurysms may, in theory, occur at any site within the arterial tree where there is a preexisting aneurysm. It is curious that all series in the literature demonstrate a strong propensity toward involvement of the abdominal aorta. Involvement of this artery has been reported to occur in as many as 79 per cent of these cases. Whether this represents a tendency of the bacteria to infect aortic aneurysms, or is a study bias toward aortic aneurysms, is not clear. Certainly, aortic aneurysms

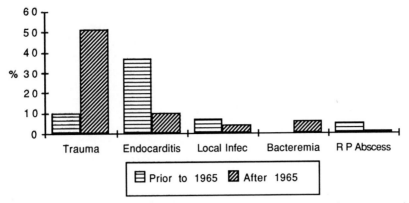

FIGURE 9–2. Etiology of mycotic aneurysms. *Local Infect,* local infection; *R P Abcess,* retroperitoneal abcess. (From Brown SL, Busuttil RW, Baker JD, et al: Bacteriologic and surgical determinants of survival in patients with mycotic aneurysms. J Vasc Surg 1:541–547, 1984.)

have been subjected to closer scrutiny than other peripheral arterial aneurysms. This may account, in part, for this reported predilection.

Arterial infections due to mechanical injury with contamination most commonly involve arteries that have minimal soft tissue coverage. There are three main etiologies: accidental drug injections, vascular access, and trauma. Since these etiologies are related to the accessibility of the arteries and their superficial locations, these infections most commonly involve the femoral or brachial arteries. These locations also have an important impact on the presentation of these lesions, since femoral and brachial arterial aneurysms are most frequently identified by virtue of the prominence, erythema, and tenderness of the aneurysm rather than by symptoms of arterial sepsis.

CLINICAL PRESENTATION

The most common clinical presentation in patients with primary arterial infection is fever, leukocytosis,

and tenderness over the affected artery. Patients may present with a wide range of signs and symptoms depending on the pathophysiology, bacteriology, and location of the infected artery or arteries. Most components of the clinical presentation may be assigned to one of two general groups: signs and symptoms resulting from infection and/or bacteremia, and signs and symptoms occurring secondary to local arterial involvement and/or aneurysm formation. Night sweats, general malaise, arthralgias, and increased fatigability in conjunction with fever and leukocytosis occur as a consequence of the recurrent bacteremias associated with primary arterial infections. These are the signs of sepsis caused by the arterial infection. In certain patients, these signs may also be attributed to the primary source of bacteremia. In patients with true mycotic aneurysms, the clinical signs and symptoms of bacterial endocarditis may be difficult to distinguish from those associated with the arterial infection. Similarly, symptoms in those patients with arterial lesions that developed by spread from a con-

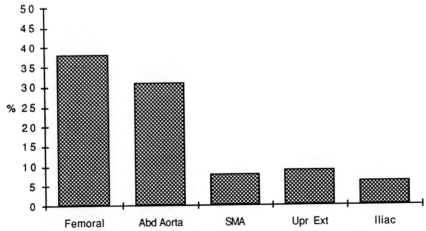

FIGURE 9–3. Distribution of mycotic aneurysms. *Abd Aorta,* abdominal aorta; *SMA,* superior mesenteric artery; *Upr Ext,* upper extremity. (From Brown SL, Busuttil RW, Baker JD, et al: Bacteriologic and surgical determinants of survival in patients with mycotic aneurysms. J Vasc Surg 1:541–547, 1984.)

tiguous suppurative source may derive from either infectious focus.

A second group of signs and symptoms occurs as a result of inflammation and aneurysmal dilatation of the infected artery. Localized tenderness is the most readily recognized symptom related to the inflammatory destruction of the arterial wall. Characteristics such as abdominal or peripheral bruits, neurological defects from nerve compression, or pulsatile masses may be included in this group.

Thrombosis and thromboembolization are common sequela of such arterial aneurysms. When they present, they elicit a host of associated symptoms such as ischemic digital or limb pain. Initially, these embolic presentations may be indistinguishable from similar events in uninfected aneurysms. If the embolic material is infected and causes a secondary arterial infection, then the mycotic nature of the lesion may be revealed. Other findings of arterial infections include petechial skin lesions and septic arthritis.

Arterial rupture is not an uncommon event in cases of infected arterial aneurysms. This presentation is identical to that with any arterial rupture. If the damaged artery is contained and supported by a capsule of fibrous connective tissue, then it may progress to form a pseudoaneurysm, and its principal symptom would be pain. If the rupture is uncontrolled, then the presentation will be that of hypotensive shock. If the rupture is in a superficial artery that erodes through the skin, then the presentation will be that of evident life-threatening hemorrhage.

The development of periarterial gas formation signals the presence of a gas-producing organisms and should be a clear signal indicating urgency in treating these patients. While this is not a very common presentation, it should be considered in any patient who presents with unexplained periaortic gas and symptoms suggestive of sepsis.

DIAGNOSTIC TESTING

The diagnosis of a primary arterial infection is based on the recognition of elements of the clinical presentation along with appropriate use of various testing modalities. The primary factor in making such a diagnosis is an acute clinical suspicion and the subsequent search for evidence to support the diagnosis of primary arterial infections. The choice and use of diagnostic testing is of singular importance in identifying and substantiating the presence of an arterial infection. Because of the potentially fulminant course of these infections and the fatal outcome of improperly managed cases, both speed and accuracy of diagnosis are crucial. The basic elements of diagnostic testing that are used in this process include bacteriologic and radiologic techniques.

Blood Cultures

The demonstration of bacterial organisms in association with an arterial lesion is central to the di-

agnosis of an arterial infection. The bacteria may be detected by either blood cultures or cultures of the arterial wall itself. Blood cultures, by virtue of their availability, are frequently among the first tests drawn in patients suspected of having a significant infection. If the patient is floridly bacteremic, the blood cultures may detect the circulating bacteria. However, several problems limit the usefulness of blood cultures. The incidence of negative blood cultures testifies to the fact that in only a fraction of symptomatic patients will the blood cultures help in the diagnosis. Many patients with arterial infections will never have positive blood cultures. In Brown's review of the UCLA experience with mycotic aneurysms, only 60 per cent of patients had positive preoperative blood cultures.[14] Finally, many blood cultures may not detect the infectious organism until several days or weeks have elapsed, limiting the test with regard to its ability to impact clinical management.

The presence of bacteria in the blood of the patient may be an important early clue to an arterial infection, but the information from such tests must be evaluated in the proper clinical context. Most bacteremic patients have an evident source of the bacteremia that should be identified and treated. Patients with positive blood cultures and no clinical evidence of a concurrent infection should be considered and examined for possible arterial pathology. The significance of a positive blood culture in an otherwise asymptomatic individual is difficult to determine without considering the patient's underlying problems and risk factors. It should also be noted that patients who are relatively asymptomatic (no systemic manifestations of sepsis) will tend to have fewer positive blood cultures. Thus, in Wakefield's study of patients undergoing clean arterial procedures, only 2 per cent of blood cultures were positive, whereas 12 per cent of arteries and 14 per cent of periarterial adipose tissues harbored bacteria. Obvious clues, such as a recently noted aneurysm or history of drug abuse, may serve to promote further investigation.

The type organism identified in blood cultures may further suggest a source of the infection. Certain pathogens are related to certain types of infections. The association between gram-negative bacteria and urinary tract infections is one example. Similarly, if a blood culture reveals *Salmonella* in a patient with an aneurysm, then an arterial infection should be seriously considered. While *Staphylococcus* is a common pathogen in arterial infections, its ubiquitous presence on skin will often confuse the diagnosis and call into question the results of the blood culture.

The importance of preoperative blood cultures is difficult to understate. They represent the earliest reliable clue to the presence of an arterial infection. Even in the event of a delayed result, when several days have passed before the blood cultures are able to identify the bacteria, the information that these tests provide may be invaluable in managing the patient.

Arterial Cultures

Arterial wall cultures may also serve to secure the diagnosis of an arterial infection. The principal drawback to arterial wall cultures is the time they require before revealing information regarding the infection. Patient management must therefore depend on other factors such as the clinical setting, the index of suspicion, the presence of prior blood culture data, and the results of angiographic studies. The patient's presentation may be important, since Wakefield discovered that tissue cultures in asymptomatic patients had significantly higher sensitivity than blood cultures. This stands in contrast to symptomatic patients in whom blood cultures tend to have a higher sensitivity than the arterial cultures.

Because clinical decisions cannot always be based on arterial culture results, the use of other techniques is often considered. Intraoperative Gram staining and frozen section of the arterial tissue are amongst these techniques. Unfortunately, these methods may not provide significant improvement in the detection of bacteria. In Brown's study, while 60 per cent of patients had positive preoperative blood cultures, only 20 per cent of intraoperative Gram stains were positive.[14] While arterial wall frozen sections have not had widespread use, they may yet prove helpful. Histologic findings of inflammation and bacterial invasion are strong evidence supporting the diagnosis of arterial infection.

In obtaining both blood and arterial wall cultures, it should be kept in mind that the type of organism may affect the yield of the tests. In Brown's study, he noted that 60 per cent of available arterial wall cultures were negative.[14] About 25 per cent of their cultures failed to detect any organism at all. Presumably these were difficult organisms to collect and culture. *Staphylococcus epidermidis* may be difficult to culture without sonicating the specimen. *Treponema pallidum* may require dark-field examination for identification. *Mycobacterium tuberculosis* is a fastidious organism and difficult to grow. These considerations should prompt a notice to the pathology lab requesting special attention as well as collection of adequate specimens.

Nuclear Imaging: Tagged White Blood Cell Scans

Nuclear imaging has become an important tool in the identification of arterial graft infections, but has not served as important a role with regard to the identification of primary arterial infections. The technique is based on the ability of various radioisotope markers to become involved in inflammatory processes. The strength of these tests is their relatively low risk to the patient, and the facility of their application. The principal drawback is that the tests may serve to detect many inflammatory lesions, not just those that are the result of an arterial infection.

The physician interpreting the results of a nuclear scan must take into account the clinical condition of the patient in order to improve the diagnostic accuracy. Although the usefulness of these tests have been debated, in the absence of recent trauma or infection, radiolabeled indium or gallium as markers may allow localization of an arterial infection.

Perhaps the most significant problem with the isotopic detection of arterial infections is that these techniques have not been widely applied to this problem. The role of these tests is not well established. As a consequence, in cases where the diagnosis of arterial infection is apparent, the tests are forsaken. When the diagnosis of an arterial infection is not established, other testing modalities are frequently used first. Those lesions that are not clearly apparent, such as intraabdominal aneurysms, are often better visualized by other forms of imaging such as angiography, computed tomography (CT), or magnetic resonance imaging (MRI). Finally, the specificity and selectivity of the nuclear imaging tests is not well established in these lesions.

Imaging: CT and MRI Scanning

The success of computerized imaging techniques such as CT and MRI scanning in identification of a primary arterial infection depends largely on the ability of these scans to resolve the characteristic anatomic features of the lesions. Because of the detailed anatomic data that these scans present, they have become very popular in the evaluation of intraabdominal vascular lesions. There are some significant limitations, however, with regard to the scans' ability to secure the diagnosis of an arterial infection.

The essential diagnostic characteristics of arterial infections include the presence of a focal defect in the wall of the aorta, the saccular shape of the aneurysms, and the edema in the tissues that accompanies the inflammatory reaction. The current reconstruction of CT images does not readily allow recognition of the diagnostic features of mycotic aneurysms. Current scanners will detect the presence of an aneurysm in the proximity of the aorta, but they frequently do not have the resolving power to detect small arterial wall defects. Additionally, current CT scanners are not able to routinely reconstruct images in the same three-dimensional manner as magnetic image scanners. It is reasonable to expect that the use of more advanced methods of computerized reconstruction and higher resolution will improve these abilities.

Magnetic resonance imaging represents an improvement over CT scanning because current computer analysis of the MRI images allows more flexible assemblage of the data and facilitates recognition of essential diagnostic characteristics. Additionally, the resolution of MRI scanners may be better than that of CT scanners. MRI scanners do not require intravascular contrast agents, which are frequently needed with CT scanners. Finally, MRI scanners are able to detect tissue differences with regard to certain molecular constituents. An advantage of MRI is its ability to detect the accumulation of water in tissues. This accumulation, tissue edema, is frequently the hallmark of an inflammatory process, and may identify an arterial infection.

Angiography

Angiography is the most widely used technique for the investigation and definition of arterial infections (Fig. 9–4). Its applications include the imaging of both central (abdominal and thoracic) and peripheral arterial lesions. Historically, it was the first method by which the characteristics of primary arterial infections—specifically, infectious aortic aneurysms—were identified. Angiography has thus served not only to identify, but also to define the characteristics of these lesions. Not surprisingly, angiography is able to surpass computerized imaging in identifying the characteristic signs of arterial infections. Additionally, angiography is clearly superior in areas such as the intestinal mesentery and the visceral vessels, where the size of the arterial lesions may be below the resolution of the computerized techniques. In the detection of aortic mycotic aneurysms, the angiogram will usually provide excellent definition of the defect in the aortic wall, the saccular pseudoaneurysm, as well as the contiguous arterial anatomy. Finally, the

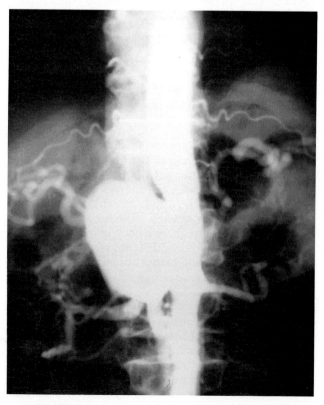

FIGURE 9–4. Angiogram of aortic mycotic aneurysm.

arteriogram will offer the best definition of the relationship between the visceral vessels and the arterial defect—an essential step in the planning of management. The strength of angiography, then, is the detection of the arterial lesions and the definition of the arterial anatomy. These two elements are essential in planning an arterial reconstruction.

The role of arteriography in the management of a peripheral arterial infection has been questioned. Since some peripheral arterial infections are managed with ligation and débridement without reconstruction, then an angiogram may not be required. On the other hand, it is important to assess the native circulation before attempting an arterial ligation. Should the limb require urgent revascularization following arterial ligation, an angiogram from before the ligation is very helpful in planning the revascularization. It should be noted that an arteriogram obtained following ligation and resection of the vessel will often be less than satisfactory. For this reason, an arteriogram of the involved vessels is required in all but emergent cases.

TIMING OF DIAGNOSIS

The diagnosis of a primary arterial infection may be made preoperatively, intraoperatively, or postoperatively. The point at which the diagnosis is made is important, since the earlier the diagnosis is made, the more readily it may be attended. Ideally, the diagnosis is made in the preoperative period. In this circumstance, plans and preparations may be made for the repair of the aneurysm and the treatment of the infection. If the diagnosis is not made until the intraoperative findings are noted, then some of the preparative measures may not be possible. Still, an alert discovery of an infected aneurysm at this stage allows for the implementation of appropriate therapy.

Should the diagnosis be made in the postoperative period, then the possibility of an undesirable outcome is increased. The arterial reconstruction will probably have been made in the bed of the infected artery, and the patient will probably not have had the benefit of prolonged intravenous antibiotics.

The point at which the diagnosis of a primary arterial infection is made is dependent upon the astute recognition of the presenting signs and symptoms. The classic combination of fever, positive blood cultures, and a tender aneurysm are not always present in a given patient. Furthermore, the symptoms of a primary arterial infection may not be evident to the casual observer. The preoperative diagnosis requires a high index of suspicion.

NATURAL HISTORY

Given the pathogenesis of a primary arterial infection—the bacterial invasion, colonization, and destruction of an artery—the sequence of events that follow this initial insult are predictable and inexorable. Destruction of the arterial wall will lead to either the development of an arterial pseudoaneurysm or a life-threatening hemorrhage. Which of these two events occurs is probably related to the rate of progression of the infection, the location of the infection, and the subsequent development of an inflammatory response. If the destruction of the arterial wall is gradual and accompanied by a vigorous inflammatory response, then the arterial infection may produce a pseudoaneurysm. If the process of the arterial infection leads rapidly to loss of the arterial integrity, then the arterial infection will lead to hemorrhage.

Complications of arterial infections include those common to all aneurysms: embolization, thrombosis, and rupture. The incidence of rupture is thought to be increased in those instances where the arterial wall is invaded by infectious pathogens. The high rupture rate is reflected in both the virulent course (rapid expansion and progression to rupture) as well as the high mortality of these lesions. For these reasons, mycotic aneurysms are urgent cases that should be repaired at the soonest possible date. One final complication that is significantly increased in cases of primary arterial infection is the rate of infection of the vascular reconstruction. Whereas the anticipated incidence of graft infection in "clean" cases is less than 1 or 2 per cent, the incidence of graft infection following remote (extraanatomic) reconstruction in cases of primary arterial infections may be as high as 15 per cent. In older series, when in situ reconstruction was performed in the face of a purulent infection and without current antibiotics, the reinfection rates approached 100 per cent.

PRINCIPLES OF MANAGEMENT

Arterial infections have the potential for causing significant morbidity and/or mortality. A low index of suspicion coupled with an aggressive diagnostic evaluation is essential to maximize the likelihood of a positive clinical outcome. Once the diagnosis has been established, early, definitive intervention must be initiated. Two elemental principles form the basis of therapy in primary arterial infections: control of sepsis, and establishment of arterial continuity.

Control of Sepsis

Antibiotic therapy and surgical débridement represent the predominant treatment modalities for the control of sepsis in arterial infections. All infected arterial tissue must be débrided. It is important that the arterial resection encompass all inflamed tissues. It should continue to the point where the arterial tissue is normal and healthy. This helps prevent subsequent recurrence of the infection and disruption of the arterial suture line.

Soft tissues adjacent to the infected artery that appear to be involved in the infection should also be débrided. Major structures such as the vena cava and ureters should be left intact. Retroperitoneal tissues that appear involved should be resected. Once all infected tissues have been removed, the wound should be thoroughly irrigated with an antibiotic solution. Ideally, the irrigating solution should contain antibiotic directed toward the suspected pathogens (as detected by preoperative blood cultures). Surgical drains are useful in situations where there is clear evidence of purulence. In the absence of an abscess or fluid collection, drains may not be required.

The use of antibiotics in an adjunctive role for the treatment of such infections represents one of the least controversial issues in the surgical literature. Broad-spectrum antibiotics should be initiated as soon as a strong clinical suspicion of arterial infection has been established. Blood cultures should be drawn prior to the initiation of antibiotics. When positive, these cultures should be used in selecting an antibiotic regimen with the highest therapeutic value and lowest side effects. Negative cultures should not preclude the institution of such broad-spectrum antibiotics in a setting where arterial infection is suspected. The use of high-dose preoperative antibiotics should be directed toward sterilizing the aneurysm and adjacent tissues in order to minimize bacteremia and local contamination during surgical manipulation of infected tissues. Preoperative antibiotic treatment, however, should not delay surgical intervention. In patients with true mycotic aneurysms, specific consideration must be given to sterilization of cardiac valvular vegetations. Antibiotics must be continued until the source of the bacteremia has been corrected either surgically or medically. Likewise, the primary source of bacteremia or local bacterial invasion must be controlled as a mainstay of therapy in all types of primary arterial infections.

The duration of antibiotic treatment remains somewhat controversial. Several authors have suggested that intravenous antibiotics be initiated prior to surgery and extended for a period of time no less than 6 weeks postoperatively.[23-25] Additionally, these authors recommend that in patients with prosthetic reconstructions, and especially those with in situ prosthetic reconstructions, that the patient be placed on a lifelong oral regimen of suppressive antibiotics. Typically, Bactrim, sulfa drugs, or a first-generation cephalosporin or penicillin are the agents of choice.

When treating primary arterial infections, surgical intervention represents the mainstay of therapy in the control of sepsis. The surgical goal is control of sepsis by means of radical débridement of all infected tissues and drainage of any purulent collections. Ideally, the infected artery and surrounding tissues should be removed in their entirety. It is important that the affected arteries should be resected to the point where normal arterial wall is encountered. In instances where collateral circulation allows, the excision may be accompanied by proximal and distal ligation and no effort to reconstruct the artery, as first described by Paré.

Important technical points include the use of monofilament suture material in ligation, and oversewing the arteries. This recommendation is based on the superiority of monofilaments over braided suture in resisting recurrent infection. Additionally, whenever possible, the resected arterial stump should be covered with a pedicle of healthy, viable tissue so as to further reduce the possibility of a recurrent infection and to accelerate the healing of the arterial segment. In the abdomen, this tissue pedicle is frequently the omentum. A flap of fascia from the prevertebral fascia and ligaments has been used to reinforce the aortic suture line. In the periphery, muscle transposition is the preferred means of obtaining tissue coverage. In the femoral region, this is most readily accomplished by rotating the head of the sartorius.

Nonoperative therapy for arterial infections in specific subsets of patients has been proposed by Kaufman[26] and others. This treatment modality, although effective in anecdotal cases, remains controversial. Future investigation will be necessary to further evaluate this unique treatment approach.

Reestablishment of Arterial Continuity

When ligation and excision of infected arteries is inadequate due to lack of collateralization, some form of arterial reconstruction must be performed to avoid tissue ischemia. This situation is most common with infections involving the visceral arteries, the aorta, and the femoral artery bifurcation. Blakemore, in 1947, was among the first to utilize a graft to replace an infected artery when he implanted a Vitallium tube. Over the subsequent 45 years, a wide range of bypass materials have been utilized, with varying success rates. These include autologous tissues such as saphenous vein and arterial homografts, as well as various synthetic materials such as polytetrafluorethylene (PTFE) and Dacron. Use of arterial homograft has been disappointing. These conduits were vulnerable to both recurrent infection as well as disruption. The resultant hemorrhage yielded a 100 per cent mortality in selected series. Autologous vein grafts are currently considered the optimal material with which to reconstruct most arterial infections. Vein grafts tend to be superior to prosthetic material in resisting recurrent infection. Furthermore, they are durable and familiar to most vascular surgeons. Prosthetic grafts have been used, and are the graft of choice in certain instances. These are subject to recurrent infection to a greater extent than autologous vein grafts. They are important in allowing reconstructions that would be difficult or dangerous with autologous tissue. Most prosthetic graft reconstructions of arterial infections are found in extraanatomic bypasses and in the rare instances of in situ reconstruction of the paravisceral aorta.

Successful management of arterial infections depends largely on the location and size of the affected artery. General principles indicate that when bypass procedures must be performed, autologous materials such as the patient's own arteries or veins harvested from clean sites should be utilized as the graft of first choice. When prosthetic grafts must be used, every attempt should be made to place them through clean planes, including extraanatomic bypass when necessary.

Infrarenal Aorta

Primary arterial infections of the infrarenal aorta invariably require excision and bypass grafting. The "gold standard" of therapy that has evolved for infections in this location combines excision and débridement of the aneurysm and adjacent tissues with extraanatomic bypass (e.g., axillofemoral bypass). In selected patients, in situ aortic graft reconstruction may be performed at a later time, once the infection has been completely eradicated. In a review of spontaneous abdominal aortic infections, Ewart and associates demonstrated a 23 to 63 per cent reoperation rate for graft infection following immediate in situ reconstruction and a 7 per cent recurrent infection rate when patients were initially treated with arterial débridement and remote reconstruction.[27]

Brown and associates, in their review of 51 cases of mycotic aneurysms, noted that the mortality of local graft reconstruction was 32 per cent, whereas the mortality of extraanatomic reconstruction was 13 per cent.[14] Still, the authors advocated in situ reconstruction on selected cases: they proposed that if no gross purulence was encountered intraoperatively, and if Gram stains were negative, in situ reconstruction utilizing prosthetic (Dacron) material could safely be performed. This approach is predicated on the recommendation that postoperative antibiotics be continued for a minimum of 6 to 8 weeks. They demonstrated a 63 per cent survival rate and a 19 per cent reinfection rate for aneurysms treated using this approach. In comparison, the rate of infection of extraanatomic bypasses following repair of mycotic aortic aneurysms has been reported to be as high as 13 per cent.

Suprarenal Aneurysms

Because of their unique anatomic characteristics, arterial infections of the paravisceral and suprarenal aorta will almost always require immediate in situ arterial reconstruction. It is nearly impossible to bypass the visceral vessels without traversing the bed of the infected paravisceral aorta. Experience gained from these repairs of suprarenal mycotic aneurysms has given credence to the concept of in situ repair with adjunctive lifelong antibiotic therapy.

When combined with débridement of grossly infected tissue and appropriate use of antibiotics, most reported series utilizing this type of reconstruction have demonstrated acceptable morbidity and mortality rates. Chan and associates have reported a series of 22 patients with mycotic aneurysms of the thoracic and abdominal aorta.[25] Of these, 13 had involvement of the paravisceral aorta. All 13 required in situ reconstruction. Twelve of the 13 survived surgery and were placed on lifelong suppressive antibiotics. None was reported to have had a clinical recurrence of the infection. In the overall series, three patients died; two of the deaths were attributable to multisystem organ failure and one to aspiration pneumonia. The authors concluded that in situ reconstruction along with surgical débridement and lifelong antibiotics offers the best chance for survival in these difficult patients. It should be noted that while this form of therapy (in situ reconstruction) is inescapable in the reconstruction of infected paravisceral aneurysms, its application to arterial infections at other sites (e.g., infrarenal aorta or femoral artery) is less well established, and should be approached with caution.

Femoral, Iliac, and Mesenteric Arterial Infections

Other anatomic locations where primary arterial infections are considered relatively common include the femoral, superior mesenteric, and celiac arteries. Attempts at ligation and excision of these vessels for the treatment of primary arterial infections may be associated with a high rate of irreversible ischemia. Currently, the patients who are at greatest risk of developing these infections are intravenous drug abusers. Because these patients have a tendency toward recidivism, they are at risk of reinfecting their arterial reconstructions. This has generated debate regarding the best treatment of these patients. The simplest approach is to ligate and resect, then observe the ligated vascular bed for signs of severe ischemia. Revascularization is performed only if severe ischemia develops. The second choice is to proceed with an autogenous reconstruction at the time of resecting the infected lesion.

The Infected Femoral Pseudoaneurysm

Infections of the vessels of the femoral region are the most common type of arterial infection. In the review by Brown and colleagues, these lesions accounted for 38 per cent of all arterial infections.[14] The most common presentation is that of an inflamed, tender, pulsatile inguinal mass. The more common complications include erosion through the skin and hemorrhage, embolization, compression of adjacent structures (femoral vein and nerve), and thrombosis. Of these, erosion and hemorrhage are the most feared complications.

The debate regarding reconstruction is of particular interest in the subset of patients with infected pseudoaneurysms of the femoral bifurcation that are the result of intravenous drug abuse. Because of the addict's tendency to re-use the femoral sites for further drug administration, the arterial reconstruction may be in jeopardy of recurrent infection. If the reconstruction required prosthetic material, then the resultant reinfection would be all the more complicated and dangerous.

Finally, the incidence of graft infection following immediate reconstruction is sufficient by itself to warrant hesitation in such reconstructions. Because of these concerns, some authors have advocated simple arterial ligation and resection of the infected tissues. The problem is that simple ligation of the femoral arteries at the level of the arterial bifurcation may have a subsequent amputation rate approaching 33 per cent.[22,28]

An alternative school of thought holds that the limbs should be reconstructed, and if these are subsequently infected, then the infection should be dealt with as necessary. In the course of these reconstructions, the infected arteries and adjacent tissues should be débrided and the reconstruction should be coursed through uninfected tissues.[29] Finally, the reconstruction should be performed with autogenous tissue if possible.

The third option is to combine both approaches so that the arterial lesion is resected and the adjacent tissues are débrided. The artery is ligated, but no reconstructions are performed in the initial setting. The limb is observed for signs of severe ischemia. If the limb appears viable with collateral perfusion alone, then no effort is made to reconstruct. If the limb appears severely ischemic, then revascularization is attempted. Femoral artery reconstruction should be carried out with either in situ saphenous vein interposition grafting or through an extraanatomic approach such as a transobturator bypass.

Infection and pseudoaneurysm of the common femoral, superficial femoral, or the profunda femoris do not appear to suffer a similar fate. These vessels stand a far better chance of tolerating simple ligation without requiring reconstruction. Reddy and colleagues have reported a very low incidence of amputation following ligation and resection without amputation in this circumstance. In a series of 39 patients with such infections, they noted an amputation rate of 5 per cent.[30] They further noted that these amputations occurred in two patients who had impaired collateral circulation from prior (contralateral) common femoral artery ligation. In the absence of these two cases, the amputation rate in this group of patients was 0 per cent.

Mesenteric Artery Infections

Mesenteric artery infections tend to present as pseudoaneurysms within the mesentery of the intestine. These lesions may be asymptomatic; however, the more common presentation is that of abdominal pain. These lesions may develop as a consequence of intravenous drug abuse. Pathophysiologically, they are considered to be the result of mycotic embolization. Because of this, it is necessary to consider both the possible source of the emboli, as well as the possibility of other embolic targets. In practical terms, this means that these patients should be screened for both cardiac vegetations and other arterial lesions. Preoperative angiography is recommended if it is possible. Postoperative angiography should be considered if a preoperative study was not obtained.

The mesenteric arterial infections tend to develop rapid expansion and intramesenteric hemorrhage. Alternatively, these aneurysms may result in thrombosis and infarction of the intestine. The management of these vessels is related to the location of the lesion, the available collateral circulation, and the presence and extent of intestinal infarction. Lesions of the proximal mesenteric arteries will frequently require reconstruction with autogenous tissues. More distally located pseudoaneurysms may frequently be managed by simple excision. If a small area of intestinal ischemia develops, then a limited bowel resection may also be necessary. In instances of extensive intestinal ischemia, a second-look celiotomy may be advisable following restoration of intestinal perfusion.

Arterial Infections of the Upper Extremity

Infections of the arteries of the upper extremities are fairly rare. Collectively they represented about 10 per cent of arterial infections in the review by Brown and colleagues.[14] Frequently these lesions are associated with trauma. Like other infections of peripheral vessels, these lesions may present in a number of ways. The most common presentation is that of an inflamed, tender, pulsatile mass. In the upper extremities, careful inspection should detect evidence of digital embolization (i.e., splinter hemorrhages and ischemic lesions).

Because of the extensive collateral blood supply to the upper extremities, infections of the arteries to the upper extremities may often be treated with simple ligation and excision. This is particularly true when the involved segment occurs between the thyrocervical trunk and subscapular artery or distal to the profunda brachia. Reconstruction, when required, should be accomplished with a saphenous vein graft or similar autogenous tissues. As with all mycotic aneurysms, preoperative and postoperative antibiotics should be given for a prolonged period of time.

CONCLUSIONS

Primary arterial infections are relatively rare. These lesions are frequently lethal. They often follow a rapidly progressive course toward expansion and rupture. Only an astute diagnosis along with the correct management will allow for improved chances of survival. The diagnosis is established by a high index of suspicion along with identification of risk factors and appropriate testing. Once identified, the management must be tailored to the organism involved, the site and severity of the infection, as well as the condition of the patient. Surgical excision is almost always necessary in the course of management. Long-term intravenous antibiotics (for 6 weeks) are also almost always required. The subsequent use of lifelong oral antibiotic suppression is strongly recommended for these patients. Optimal care may reduce the mortality of these lesions from nearly 100 per cent to less than 10 to 15 per cent.

REFERENCES

1. Rokitansky CF: Handbuch der Paathologischen Anatomic, 2 edition. 1844, p 55.
2. Koch L: Uber Aneurysma der Arteriae Mesenterichae Superioris [inaug dis]. Erlangen, 1851.
3. Osler W: The gulstonian lectures on malignant endocarditis. Br Med J 1:467, 1885.
4. Crane A: Primary multilocular mycotic aneurysm of the aorta. Arch Pathol 24:634, 1937.
5. Ponfick CE: Ueben Embolishe Aneurysmen, nebst Bermerkungen uber das acute Herzaneurysma (herzge schwur). Virchows Arch 58:528, 1873.
6. Eppinger H: Pathogenesis (Histogenesis und Aetiologie) der Aneurysman ein Schliesslich des Aneurysma equi Verminosum. Arch Klin Chir 35:404, 1887.
7. Weisel J: Die Erkrankuger Arterieller Gerfasse im Verlaufe akuter Infektionen. Z Heilk 27:269, 1906.
8. Lewis D, Schrager V: Embolomycotic aneurysms. JAMA 53:1808, 1909.
9. Cathcart R: False aneurysms of the femoral artery following typhoid fever. South Med J 2:593, 1909.
10. Hawkins J, Yeager G: Primary mycotic aneurysm. Surgery 40:747, 1956.
11. Yellin A: Ruptured mycotic aneurysm, a complication of parenteral drug abuse. Arch Surg 112:981, 1977.
12. Lande A, Beckman Y: Aortitis—pathologic, clinical and arteriographic review. Radiol Clin North Am 14:219, 1976.
13. Hirst AJ, Affeldt J: Abdominal aortic aneurysm with rupture into the duodenum: A report of eight cases. Gastroenterology 17:504, 1951.
14. Brown SL, Busuttil RW, Baker JD, et al: Bacteriologic and surgical determinants of survival in patients with mycotic aneurysms. J Vasc Surg 1:541–547, 1984.
15. Stengal A, Wolferth C: Mycotic (bacterial) aneurysms of intravascular origin. Arch Intern Med 31:527, 1923.
16. Revell S: Primary mycotic aneurysms. Ann Intern Med 22:431, 1943.
17. Magilligan D, Quinn E: Active infective endocarditis. *In* Magilligan DJ, Quinn E (eds): Endocarditis: Medical and Surgical Management. New York, Marcel Dekker, 1986, p 207.
18. Wilson S, Van Wagenen P, Passaro EJ: Arterial infection. Curr Probl Surg 15:5–89, 1978.
19. Bennett D, Cherry J: Bacterial infection of aortic aneurysms: A clinicopathological study. Am J Surg 113:321, 1967.

20. Jarrett F, Darling R, Mundth E, et al: Experience with infected aneurysms of the abdominal aorta. Arch Surg 10:1281, 1975.
21. Ernst C, Campbell H, Daugherty M, et al: Incidence and significance of intra-operative bacterial cultures during abdominal aortic aneurysmectomy. Ann Surg 185:626–633, 1977.
22. Reddy D, Smith R, Elliot JJ, et al: Infected femoral artery false aneurysms in drug addicts: Evolution of selective vascular reconstruction. J Vasc Surg 3:718, 1986.
23. Mundth E, Darling RC, Alvarado RH, et al:Surgical management of mycotic aneurysms and the complications of infections in vascular reconstructive surgery. Am J Surg 117:460, 1969.
24. Crawford E, Crawford J: Diseases of the Aorta Including an Atlas of Angiographic Pathology and Surgical Techniques. Baltimore, Williams & Wilkins, 1984.
25. Chan F, Crawford E, Coselli J, et al: In-situ prosthetic graft replacement for mycotic aneurysm of the aorta. Ann Thorac Surg 47:193–203, 1989.
26. Kaufman J, Smith R, Capel G, et al: Antibiotic therapy for arterial infection: Lessons from the successful treatment of a mycotic femoral artery aneurysm without surgical reconstruction. Ann Vasc Surg 4:592, 1990.
27. Ewart J, Burke M, Bunt T: Spontaneous abdominal aortic infections. Essentials of diagnosis and management. Am Surg 49:37–49, 1983.
28. Johnson J, Ledgerwood A, Lucas C: Mycotic aneurysms: New concepts in therapy. Arch Surg 118:577–582, 1983.
29. Patel K, Semel L, Clauss R: Routine revascularization with resection of infected femoral pseudoaneurysm from substance abuse. J Vasc Surg 8:321–328, 1988.
30. Wright D, Shepard A: Infected femoral artery aneurysm associated with drug abuse. In Stanley J, Ernst C (eds): Current Therapy in Vascular Surgery. Philadelphia, BC Decker, 1990, pp 350–353.

REVIEW QUESTIONS:

1. Mycotic aneurysms as described by Osler were the result of vegetative cardiac emboli. (true of false)

2. Arterial trauma is involved in the pathogenesis of most primary arterial infections. (true or false)

3. The most common location for infected arterial aneurysms is in the brachial arteries. (true or false)

4. Prosthetic grafts should be used to replace excised mycotic aneurysms:
   (a) if the surgical field is lavaged with antibiotics
   (b) in the upper extremities
   (c) only if absolutely necessary
   (d) in fungal arterial infections
   (e) never

5. In mycotic aneurysms of the great vessels, surgery may be avoided if large doses of antibiotics are given.
   (a) true
   (b) sometimes true
   (c) never true
   (d) only in cases of *Pseudomonas* infection

6. Since 1965 the most common organism cultured from mycotic aneurysms is:

   (a) *Salmonella* species
   (b) fungi
   (c) *Mycobacteria*
   (d) *Pseudomonas* species
   (e) *Staphylococcus aureus*

7. In the management of a mycotic pseudoaneurysm of the femoral artery, it is always necessary to revascularize the leg. (true or false)

8. In the management of a mycotic mesenteric aneurysm located in the distal arterial arcade (adjacent to the intestine), the recommended management is:
   (a) reconstruction with Dacron graft
   (b) reconstruction with PTFE graft
   (c) reconstruction with umbilical vein graft
   (d) reconstruction with vein graft
   (e) ligation and excision without reconstruction

9. Suprarenal mycotic aneurysms that involve the paravisceral aorta should never be reconstructed with in situ prosthetic material. (true or false)

10. The recommended management of infrarenal mycotic aneurysms involves the use of antibiotics, débridement of the infected tissues, and reconstruction through a remote (extraanatomic), uninfected field.

ANSWERS

1. T	2. T	3. F	4. c	5. c	6. e	7. F
8. e	9. F	10. T				

10

CONGENITAL VASCULAR MALFORMATIONS OF THE EXTREMITIES

BENJAMIN O. ANDERSON, JANETTE D. DURHAM, and
ROBERT B. RUTHERFORD

Congenital vascular malformations (CVMs) comprise a spectrum of developmental abnormalities that may involve all components of the peripheral circulation: arteries, veins, capillaries, and lymphatics. The majority of clinically significant lesions contain primarily arterial and venous elements. Pure venous anomalies are rare and are simpler to manage than venous malformations. While anomalous lymphatic elements are frequently intermixed with arteriovenous anomalies, pure lymphatic congenital lesions (i.e., lymphoceles) are infrequently seen. Understandably, therefore, the emphasis in this chapter will be on arteriovenous malformations (AVMs).

Structurally dissimilar CVMs may present in clinically similar ways. For example, enlarged or swollen legs can result from lymphatic anomalies, pure venous dysplasias, or arteriovenous malformations, and varicose veins and local signs of venous hypertension can result from either of the latter two. The different etiology obviously warrants a different therapeutic approach. Therefore, the crux of CVM management lies in the appropriate application of diagnostic tools to arrive at a precise diagnosis. This allows confident and early prognostic projections to be made and guides the selective and properly timed use of appropriate therapeutic interventions. The aims of this chapter are: (1) to describe the incidence, etiology, classification, and clinical presentation of CVMs; (2) to propose the appropriate use of a diagnostic approach that has some practical advantages over angiography alone; and (3) to discuss the relative merits of current therapeutic options with suggestions for their clinical use.

Arteriovenous malformations are that subset of CVMs that contain both arterial and venous components, but the most common and clinically important AVMs are those containing arteriovenous fistulae (AVFs) which shunt a significant amount of blood directly from artery to vein, bypassing the nutritive capillary bed. Ninety per cent of AVMs occur in the extremities, pelvis, body shell of the trunk, and shoulder girdle. The anatomic sites of involvement are shown in Table 10–1. Congenital CVMs with major AV shunting are particularly problematic because they (1) tend to enlarge with time, (2) may steal blood from the distal extremity, (3) cause continual venous hypertension, and (4) may even increase cardiovascular demand. The major focus of this chapter, therefore, will be on the diagnostic evaluation of AVMs, emphasizing the identification and quantification of arteriovenous shunt flow. This emphasis will carry over into the management strategies proposed.

INCIDENCE

Congenital vascular malformations are rare, unless one includes capillary/cavernous hemangiomas of such little consequence that medical attention for diagnosis or intervention is not sought. Thus, they account for only 1 in 10,000 hospital admissions, and with an increasingly conservative approach to therapy, even this may decrease. The literature is weighted by cases presenting for surgical evaluation or treatment. Possibly because of this, no American authors have reported experiences exceeding 100 cases. The largest personal experience with congenital AVMs, reported by Szilagyi, was 82 cases and was accumulated over 22 years, between 1952 and 1974 (approximately four new cases a year in a center known for its expertise on this subject).[1] Most vascular surgeons see far fewer cases, and the English literature, when reviewed about a decade ago by one of the authors (R.B.R.), contained barely 400 cases. Thus, the relative rarity of CVMs means that individual surgeons are unlikely

TABLE 10–1. ANATOMIC SITES OF INVOLVEMENT

Artery	Cases
Femoral	30
Iliac	20
Popliteal	8
Radial	4
Radial and ulnar	4
Anterior and posterior tibial	4
Anterior tibial	3
Posterior tibial	2
Subclavian	2
Ulnar	2
Axillary	2
Brachial	1
Total	82

to develop a meaningful personal experience with them and may also have difficulty finding reliable therapeutic recommendations in the literature.

NOMENCLATURE

The plethora of names applied over time to CVMs reflects their wide spectrum of clinical presentations, which vary from subtle, asymptomatic birthmarks or scattered varicosities to grotesquely deformed extremities and hemodynamic compromise. The long list of designations also reflects a futile attempt by earlier physicians to reduce the protean clinical manifestations into distinct entities. These names include hemangioma simplex, angioma telangiectaticum, hemangioma cavernosum, strawberry birthmark, nevus angiectoides, port-wine mark, angioma arteriole racemosum or plexiform, cirsoid aneurysm, serpentine aneurysm, congenital arteriovenous aneurysm, and congenital arteriovenous fistula. Some categories of lesions have acquired eponyms such as Klippel-Trenaunay syndrome[2] (varicose veins, enlarged limb, and a birthmark) and Parkes-Weber syndrome[3] (the same triad *with* arteriovenous fistulae). This confusing diversity in nomenclature developed because early authors did not have the modern diagnostic tools by which to demonstrate that these visibly dissimilar lesions shared common vascular components. Reid[4] and Rienhoff[5] in the 1920s were the first to suggest that CVMs result from an arrest or misdirection in development of the primitive vascular system. Pursuit of this concept, soon aided by the frequent use of angiography, eventually allowed this archaic descriptive nomenclature to be replaced by simpler terms that reflect the common congenital etiology of CVMs and the stage and location of the responsible "errors" in embryonic development. While a universally accepted nomenclature system has not yet been adopted, the one used in this chapter is based on the embryological development of the vascular system, and is expected to form the framework of the system ultimately adopted.[1,6]

EMBRYOLOGY OF ANGIOGENESIS

The vascular system first appears during the third gestational week as a network of interlacing blood spaces in the primitive mesenchyme.[7] The blood does not yet circulate in any organized fashion and no separate arterial or venous channel can yet be identified. The vascular system gradually develops by processes of vascular coalescence and cellular differentiation, culminating in the appearance of separate arterial and venous conduits. This process was described by Woollard in 1922 as a sequence which he divided into three stages.[8] During the *undifferentiated* stage (I), primitive blood lakes coalesce into more organized capillary networks. No arterial or venous conduits can yet be recognized. During the *retiform* stage (II), the capillaries formed in stage I themselves coalesce into larger plexiform structures which are the progenitors of arterial and venous channels. During the *maturation* stage (III), histologically mature vascular channels and principal arterial stems appear. The capillary network that persists beyond fetal life into adulthood may be thought of as a remnant from the original blood lakes in stage I.

CLASSIFICATION

A number of classifications have been proposed for CVMs. Malan proposed an elaborate and complete system to accommodate the numerous varieties of clinical lesions.[9] A more workable system, proposed by deTakats in the 1930s, is based on the concept that abnormal developmental events in utero determine the morphologic characteristics that become apparent ex utero.[10] The classification system proposed here, conceptually similar to that of deTakats, is based on the correlation of clinical and angiographic findings with the stages of angiogenesis and consists of the following categories: (1) cavernous or simple hemangioma; (2) microfistulous AV communications; (3) macrofistulous AV communications; and (4) anomalous development of mature vascular channels (e.g., persistent primitive sciatic artery). Purely venous or lymphatic anomalies (without arterial involvement), although thought also to be of developmental etiology, would be classified as separate categories of vascular malformations.

Cavernous or simple (capillary) hemangiomas histologically resemble the unorganized capillary network of stage I and are thought to represent an arrest in development during that stage. The term "hemangioma" means "a tumor of blood vessel origin," which, strictly speaking, is incorrect, since the majority of these vascular "tumors" are nonneoplastic. Hemangiomas presenting in infancy may be separated into two categories based on endothelial cell proliferation.[11] The first and more common lesion has a normal rate of endothelial cell turnover and is a vascular malformation with no malignant potential and thus is not literally a "hemangioma." These lesions are typically first seen at birth and grow commensurately with the child. Enlargement results from changes in blood or lymphatic pressure, collateralization, or hormonal modulation. The second category of hemangiomatous vascular lesions are characteristically hypercellular with increased cellular turnover and neoplastic proliferative capacity. This lesion is not a vascular malformation, but a true "hemangioma." Typically these appear just after birth and show rapid neonatal growth and, usually, slow involution. The latter is almost always the rule with cutaneous or subcutaneous hemangiomas. Some of the more aggressive parenchymal hemangiomas have a poor prognosis if untreated; however, recent work by White and colleagues with pulmonary hemangiomatosis reports encouraging results using recombinant interferon α-2a with clinical arrest of tumor growth.[12]

Microfistulous AV communications are a network of extensive interconnections between arteries and veins that are too small to be seen on angiography. Significant arteriovenous shunting can occur in these lesions, as inferred by secondary angiographic findings such as early venous filling, increased vascularity in the area of the mass, and dilation of the proximal supplying artery, but more commonly the hemodynamic consequences are quite modest. These lesions represent developmental arrest in angiogenesis during stage II, with the persistence of immature channels resulting from the coalescence of embryonic capillaries.

Macrofistulous AV communications contain multiple, grossly visible interconnections between arteries and veins that are apparent even on angiography. The more complex of these lesions usually have hemangiomatous, fistulous, and aneurysmal elements, which have been described as cirsoid ("varicose") or racemose ("cluster-of-grapes–like"). If superficial enough to be palpable, these lesions are characteristically warm and have a bruit or thrill because of very high AV shunt flow. This category of lesions is thought to result from arrest during stage III of angiogenesis, prior to complete vessel maturation.

Anomalous development of mature vascular channels consists of lesions containing mature but aberrant vessels such as isolated venous angiomata and arterial malformations. This category does not, strictly speaking, include lesions that cause arteriovenous shunting, indicating that they have arisen from the end of stage III after vessel maturation and loss of arteriovenous connections have occurred.

Any of the above types of CVMs can, and not infrequently do, coexist in a single lesion. In such cases, the lesion is categorized by the dominant or most serious component, the usual order being arteriovenous, arterial, venous, lymphatic, and capillary.

CLINICAL FINDINGS

Although patients with CVMs present in myriad ways, certain patterns in presentation have emerged.

In general, the age at the time of first clinical presentation for evaluation is inversely related to the severity of the lesion. Younger children present with more obvious vascular masses, limb enlargements, or huge birthmarks. Older children (and adults) more often present with subtler signs; for example, developing varicose veins, swelling, limb length discrepancies, or even aching or "heavy" sensations in the affected extremity, in addition to a previously recognized birthmark. As listed in Table 10–2, birthmarks are the most common finding in patients with congenital AVMs (70 per cent) and should be recognized as potential indicators of more serious underlying pathology.[1] Venous varicosities, the second most common finding (60 per cent), can also be associated with venous angiomas (compressible grapelike clusters of large venous spaces) or ambulatory venous hypertension from dysplastic venous segments and/or segments with absent valves. Atypical distribution and early onset distinguish them from the usual varicosities caused by saphenofemoral incompetence. *Asymmetric limb length* can result from significant regional AV shunting, by an incompletely understood mechanism, or can indicate significant osseous involvement. However, increased girth or, in fact, increased overall dimensions are also seen, sometimes to a striking degree. In the latter instance, osseous and soft tissue changes go hand in hand, but it must be remembered that "giant" hypertrophy of one limb can occur *without* an underlying CVM. In such cases, it is present at birth with little proportional change with time. *Edema*, in contradistinction, may develop with time due to underlying venous and/or lymphatic abnormalities, assuming the same characteristics as edema of those respective origins. *Ulceration* and *bleeding* are late presentations. A subcutaneously located vascular "tumor" or varix under pressure may bleed readily following minor trauma. Such focal lesions can progress to ulceration just like venous ulcers in patients with other forms of chronic venous insufficiency, but with AVMs, the venous hypertension is never totally relieved by elevation and healing may be further impaired by a

TABLE 10–2. INCIDENCE OF PHYSICAL CHANGES IN 82 AFFECTED EXTREMITIES[a]

Changes	Patients	
	No.	%
Color changes	57	69.5
Erythema	(33)	
Cyanosis	(24)	
Venous varices	49	59.7
Edema	46	56.0
Increased length	20	24.3
Deformity	9	11.0
Ulceration	8	9.8
Pulse deficit	3	3.6
Bleeding	3	3.6

[a] From Szilagyi DE, Smith RF, Elliott JP, Hageman JH: Congenital arteriovenous anomalies of the limbs. Arch Surg *111*:423–429, 1976.

degree of superimposed ischemia. Regional or distal "steal" may contribute to the latter and may result in a diminution of distal pulses.

As shown in Table 10–3, *hemangioma* rarely presents alone in those with congenital AVM. Unless huge or disfiguring, hemangiomas are usually accepted as a cosmetic problem until additional signs develop. As an isolated finding, *swelling* is more common than varicosities, while *bruit* is rarely the sole indication of an AVM. It is noteworthy that, in this experience,[1] less than one third (32 per cent) presented with a single physical finding. On the other hand, the classic triad of "birthmark, varicosities, and limb enlargement," which characterizes the syndromes of Klippel-Trenaunay (without AVFs) and Parkes-Weber (with AVFs), was seen in barely 30 per cent, with various other double or triple combinations of signs being seen in the remainder (38 per cent). Nevertheless, significant birthmarks, early-onset varicose veins, and limb asymmetry, either singly or in combination, all warrant further testing and close clinical follow-up over time.

DIAGNOSTIC METHODS

Angiography has been routinely applied in the past as the definitive study or "gold standard" for evaluating AVMs.[13] However, because of the advent of new noninvasive diagnostic techniques, angiography can now be limited, as in arterial occlusive disease, to those patients who are likely soon to undergo interventional therapy. This is not only because angiography is uncomfortable and invasive and, in children, can be technically difficult, cause arterial injury, and requires anesthesia,[14] but also because it does not regularly provide definitive information about anatomic extent (i.e., involvement of muscle, bone, and other surrounding tissues), does not identify microfistulous communications, and does not characterize venous, capillary, or lymphatic abnormalities. This latter information, plus hemodynamic assessment, can better be provided by other simpler tests, including noninvasive vascular tests, shunt quantification with labeled microspheres, and noninvasive imaging.[15]

TABLE 10–3. INCIDENCE OF DIAGNOSTIC PHYSICAL SIGNS[a]

Physical Sign	No. of Patients (N = 82)
Hemangioma, varices, bruit, swelling	17
Varices, swelling	14
Swelling	14
Hemangioma, swelling	10
Varices	9
Hemangioma, varices, bruit, swelling	8
Bruit, swelling	5
Bruit	3
Varices, bruit, swelling	2

[a] From Szilagyi DE, Smith RF, Elliott JP, Hageman JH: Congenital arteriovenous anomalies of the limbs. Arch Surg *111*:423–429, 1976.

Noninvasive Vascular Tests

For well over a decade, noninvasive vascular tests have been accepted as the initial, if not primary, means of evaluating peripheral vascular diseases. However, it is not generally appreciated that the same noninvasive methods used primarily for evaluating peripheral arterial *occlusion* can also be applied to peripheral AV *shunting*. These tests include segmental limb pressures, segmental plethysmography (or pulse volume recordings), and Doppler analog tracings or velocity waveforms.

Segmental limb pressures (SLPs) are systolic arterial pressure determinations at multiple levels along an extremity. The pattern of SLPs can be helpful in localizing peripheral AVFs. Proximal to a fistula, systolic pressure is often *increased*. Distal to a fistula, systolic pressure is usually normal but can be *decreased* secondary to a "steal" phenomenon.[16] SLPs, then, help locate peripheral AVFs by demonstrating a step-off in systolic pressure from above the fistula to below it when compared to the normal contralateral extremity (Fig. 10–1).

Pulse volume recordings (PVRs) use sensitive cuffs wrapped around the extremity at multiple levels to monitor the changing limb circumference that results from pulsatile arterial flow. This flow is increased proximal to a hemodynamically significant AVF because of lowered vascular resistance. PVR tracings illustrate this increased flow by *sharper, higher systolic peaks*. In addition, because blood flows more readily through the low-resistance fistula than through a normal capillary bed, *the normal anacrotic notch is decreased or absent* (Fig. 10–2). Distal to an AVF, PVRs are often unchanged, although again, if there is a distal "steal" there will be a discernible decrease in flow, particularly at the digital level.[16]

Doppler analog tracings or velocity waveforms (VWFs) record blood flow velocity. Because of its greater peripheral resistance, the velocity pattern in a resting extremity artery is normally triphasic, with major forward flow in early systole, some flow reversal in later systole, minor forward flow in early diastole, and negligible forward flow in late diastole. As a result of the latter, the normal VWF "rests" on (or lies close to) the zero baseline. Significant AVF flow eliminates any end-systolic flow reversal and produces significant flow all through diastole so the VWF tracing proximal to the fistula *never drops near the zero baseline* (Fig. 10–3). In fact, the degree of elevation of the velocity tracing above baseline is directly proportioned to fistula flow. The VWF is the most sensitive and least specific noninvasive vascular test for AVFs. Any physiologic or pathophysiologic change causing extremity hyperemia (e.g., exercise, warming, vasodilators, inflammation, relief from ischemia, or recent sympathectomy) can produce a similar pattern to that seen with AVF. Fortunately, in this clinical setting, most of these conditions are easily controlled or clinically ruled out.

The above tests have the advantage of being easy,

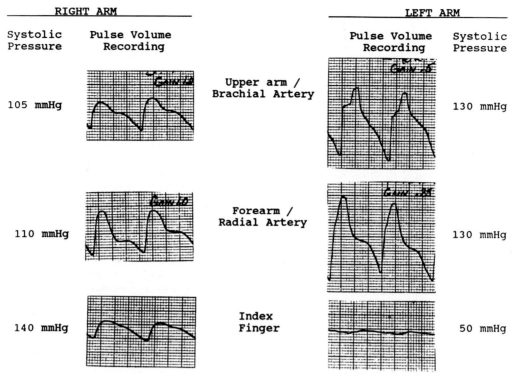

FIGURE 10–1. Systolic limb pressures (SLP) and pulse volume recording (PVR) in 13-year-old girl (C.W.) with left palm arteriovenous fistula (AVF) involving distal ulnar and palmar arch arteries. The SLPs illustrate increased systolic pressure and decreased digital pressure distal to the fistula, demonstrating pronounced steal. The PVRs illustrate sharp, high systolic peaks and slightly decreased anacrotic notches proximal to this fistula.

fast, inexpensive, and readily obtainable. When used in combination, they will detect almost any hemodynamically significant peripheral AVF flow. They are ideal for screening children with birthmarks, unilateral limb enlargement, asymmetry, and early-onset varicosities. However, they are not helpful in detecting AVFs proximal to the upper limb cuff or groin/axilla, and will miss minor or diffusely distributed microfistulas (constituting together less than 10 to 15 per cent of all extremity AVFs). Obviously, they are not necessary to make the diagnosis in the patient presenting with a discolored, mass lesion associated with local warmth, bruit, and prominent varicosities.

Labeled Microspheres

The labeled microsphere method is a minimally invasive technique which *quantitates* AV shunting in an extremity.[17,18] A bolus of ^{99m}Tc-labeled human albumin microspheres is injected *intraarterially* proximal to an AVF (e.g., in the femoral artery) and the amount of radioactivity subsequently arriving at the lungs is measured with a gamma camera. Less than 3 per cent of 25- to 35-μm microspheres will pass through a normal extremity capillary bed and on to the lungs, where essentially all of them should lodge.

To calibrate the amount passing through AVFs and to normalize for differences among patients and microsphere preparations, a second bolus of microspheres is injected *intravenously* in any peripheral vein, since 100 per cent of these microspheres should lodge in the lungs. In this way, the absolute counts measured in the patient's lungs can be converted to a percentage of AV shunting.[17,18]

The labeled microsphere method is useful both as an initial diagnostic test and to evaluate therapy. In diagnosis, labeled microspheres distinguish shunting from nonshunting CVMs (e.g., a microfistulous AVM from a pure venous anomaly). The level of shunting has prognostic value. For example, the parents of a child with a 9 per cent AV shunting lesion can be reassured that future symptomatology should be mild and easily controlled without intervention, whereas if the shunt level is 36 per cent, counseling would pursue the opposite path. In therapy, labeled microspheres measure the decrease in shunting achieved by surgery or embolization. Since AV shunting in congenital AVFs recurs with time following most therapeutic interventions,[1] labeled microspheres may be used following embolization or ablative surgery to quantify recurrence and time future interventions. The labeled microsphere method cannot be used effectively under anesthesia because all general and

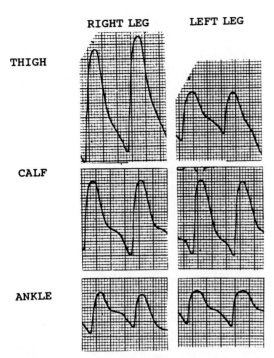

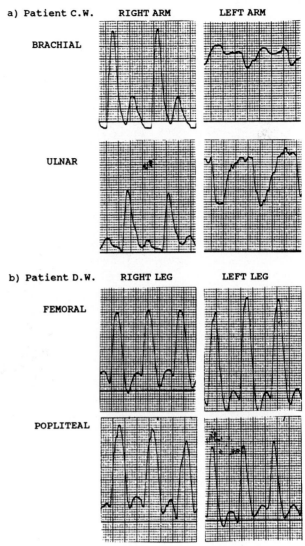

FIGURE 10–2. Pulse volume recording (PVR) in 3-year-old male (D.W.) with right thigh arteriovenous fistula (AVF). This study shows sharpened high systolic peaks and nearly absent anacrotic notches distal to the fibula. Steal is not evident in this study.

FIGURE 10–3. Doppler velocity waveforms (VWFs) from the same patients as in Figures 10–1 and 10–2. VWF from C.W. shows extreme elevation in baseline diastolic velocity consistent with large arteriovenous shunting in left arm. VWF from D.W. shows mild elevation in baseline diastolic velocity consistent with lesser arteriovenous shunting in the right leg.

regional anesthesias induce vasodilatation and AV shunting, as does any sympathetic blockade.

Noninvasive Imaging

The resectability of a CVM is determined by its anatomic location, extent, and involvement of important surrounding structures. Computerized tomography (CT) and magnetic resonance imaging (MRI) both help define anatomic involvement of vascular malformations.

CT scanning with contrast enhancement can often demonstrate muscle and bone involvement,[19–21] but highly cellular lesions, having little vascular space, may not enhance, causing an underestimation of a CVM's extent,[22] and diffuse microfistulous AVMs may not be distinguishable from primarily venous anomalies. The optimal technique for contrast infusion (bolus versus constant infusion) has not yet been determined[20,21] and may vary from lesion to lesion. The value of CT scans is also limited by the difficulty in obtaining sections in multiple orientations[23] and the inability to generate information about blood flow.

MRI is superior to CT for evaluating CVMs for several reasons: MRI needs no contrast; it differentiates muscle, bone, fat, and blood vessels,[23] and thus identifies involvement of these tissues by the vascular malformation; it generates axial, coronal, and sagittal sections readily; and it characterizes blood flow through a lesion. High- and low-flow lesions can be

distinguished.[22,24] High-flow lesions increase the risk of developing functional impairment or serious hemodynamic abnormalities in subsequent months or years. Hemorrhage into soft tissues can be observed and aged with MRI, and cellularity can be estimated. Because it accurately assesses both anatomic relationships and flow characteristics with multiplanar views, MRI is more useful than any other single test in the management of CVMs. Its major *current* drawback is cost. The potential clinical value of obtaining an MRI is illustrated in representative longitudinal and axial views (Figs. 10–5 and 10–6, respectively) obtained on a patient referred for operation with a "localized, resectable" AVM based on clinical exam and arteriography (Fig. 10–4).

Magnetic resonance angiography (MRA) has been em-

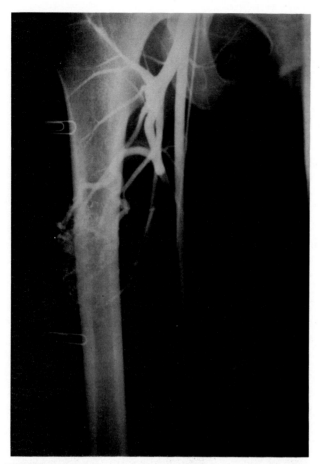

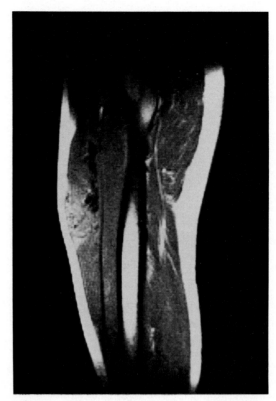

FIGURE 10–5. MRI, longitudinal view, of right thigh AVM in same patient as in Figure 10–4. A high-flow (dark) draining vein and low-flow (light) vascular spaces can be seen to involve the anterior thigh muscles.

FIGURE 10–4. Arteriogram of 19-year-old patient with right thigh CVM. The arteriogram illustrates an extensive vascular network fed by profunda femoris branches. Early venous filling was seen in later views (not shown).

ployed in the evaluation of CVMs.[25] With this technique, vascular contrast is produced noninvasively by the phase response of moving protons. Diastolic and systolic gated images produce, respectively, flow signal and flow void. The difference image is a map of pulsatile flow. Although these advances have not yet been fully developed, improvements like them will undoubtedly increase the diagnostic accuracy of magnetic resonance technology for CVMs of the extremity in the future.

RECOMMENDED DIAGNOSTIC APPROACH

There are three basic diagnostic goals in evaluating patients with congenital vascular malformations: (1) to establish the diagnosis and categorize the dominant lesion; (2) to define the lesion's anatomic extent and involvement of adjacent structures; and (3) to determine the local, regional, and, if significant, the systemic hemodynamic effects. While the first two goals are directed at defining lesion type and anatomic limits (i.e., potential resectability), the third goal helps gauge the likely *need* for intervention. Only lesions with significantly increased vascularity and arteriovenous

shunting are likely to cause significant and progressive functional impairment or affect limb dimensions. In the absence of these flow characteristics, most CVMs may be successfully managed conservatively. Even in the presence of high AV shunt flow, diffuse anatomic

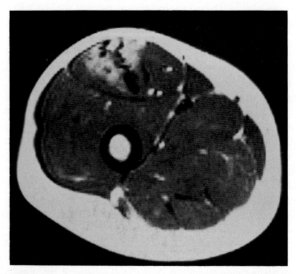

FIGURE 10–6. MRI, axial view, of right thigh AVM in same patient as in Figure 10–4. The vascular mass with high-flow (dark) vessels can be observed to involve most of the vastus medialis muscle.

involvement may preclude resectability and dictate carefully timed palliative interventions.

With this in mind, diagnostic tests should be employed in a logical sequence that helps direct management, as indicated in Figure 10–7. Noninvasive vascular tests are obtained, with VWFs for diagnosis of AVFs, and SLPs and PVRs for their localization. With clearly positive noninvasive vascular tests, we recommend an MRI to characterize anatomic extent and confirm flow characteristics. If an extensive, high-flow lesion is seen on MRI, then a macrofistulous communication is present and an arteriogram may be avoided until intervention is necessary. If a low-flow lesion is seen on MRI, than a labeled microsphere study would be useful to differentiate microfistulous communications from nonshunting lesions (i.e., venous angiomas, capillary/cavernous hemangiomas). If *arterial* noninvasive tests are entirely normal at the initial screening, *venous* Doppler studies and duplex scanning may be performed in the same vascular laboratory to identify venous dysplasias or venous angiomas. Normal venous studies then would suggest capillary/cavernous hemangioma in the patient presenting with a "birthmark" or lymphatic hypoplasia in a patient presenting with diffuse swelling, although minor venous dysplasia or angiomas are not absolutely ruled out without "closed space" venography (performed similar to a Bier block but with contrast instead of an anesthetic agent being injected).[26] Like arteriography, venography and lymphangiography should be reserved for the patient in whom intervention is required by significant functional or cosmetic problems.[27] With unequal limb length, radiographic documentation of bone age and length is indicated to predict the need for and timing of epiphyseal closure.

RECOMMENDED THERAPEUTIC APPROACH

Management of CVMs (outlined in Fig. 10–8) depends on the patient's symptoms as well as the malformation's characteristics. Many lesions are self-limiting, most lesions are incurable, and all invasive treatments have associated complications. Therefore, interventional therapy should be reserved for specific pressing indications. *Absolute indications* for treatment of symptomatic AVMs, venous malformations, and (rarely) hemangiomas include hemorrhage, ischemia from arterial steal, refractory ulceration from venous hypertension, and congestive heart failure. *Relative indications* for treatment include disabling pain, limiting claudication, functional impairment of an extremity, and significant cosmetic deformity. Unequal limb length alone is not an indication for intervention, since appropriately timed epiphyseal closure in the ipsilateral extremity yields good results.

Therapeutic options include conservative management, surgical resection, and embolotherapy. The most frequently chosen management course is conservative, using support stockings and extremity elevation to control the sequelae of venous hypertension. Although this approach fails to retard the progression of high-flow lesions, it may adequately control symptoms that might otherwise demand aggressive therapy. Primary surgical excision is appropriate only for accessible, localized lesions. If successfully excised, CVMs are cured, although lesions amenable to complete resection are rare (5 to 10 per cent). Surgical resection is made easier by prior embolization, use of pneumatic tourniquets, autotransfusion, and, occasionally, deep hypothermia. Experience has demonstrated that ligating "feeding" arteries and performing partial excisions are fruitless. The transient

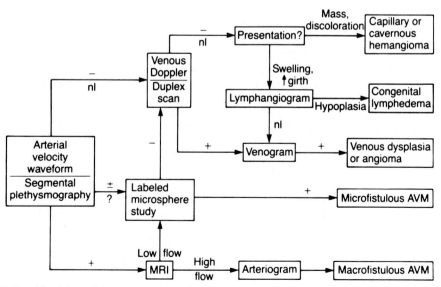

FIGURE 10–7. Algorithm of diagnostic approach to categorize peripheral CVMs. +, Positive; −, negative; *nl*, normal.

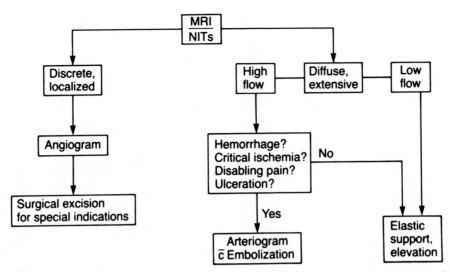

FIGURE 10–8. Algorithm shows how the use of noninvasive tests (NITs), including MRI, can help guide management of peripheral CVMs.

palliation promoted by these techniques does not justify their tendency to complicate or preclude later attempts at embolization.[1] Embolization may be employed alone or in conjunction with surgery. Preoperative embolization simplifies excision and reduces blood loss during resection of larger lesions (Fig. 10–9). If the anatomic extension of the CVM prevents complete resection, palliative embolization should be undertaken for appropriate indications, as defined above. Curative embolization has been possible in only a fraction of treated lesions; thus, embolization therapy necessitates a commitment to long-term surveillance and repeated intervention as required.

Currently, embolotherapy is performed in stages. First, an arteriogram is obtained to confirm the diagnosis, characterize the lesion, and identify the primary feeding arteries and draining veins. Selective catheterization of feeding arteries may be necessary to precisely localize AVFs. Venography may also be needed to delineate venous anomalies. Then embolization is performed, using general anesthesia to obviate pain and improve tolerance for an often lengthy procedure—this is almost always necessary in children. Multiple embolization sessions are generally required for large malformations, to limit contrast volume, anesthesia time, and excessive tissue necrosis. If a combined embolization and surgical approach is elected, then operation should be performed *immediately* following embolization before new vasculature can be recruited. Tissue edema developing 24 to 48 hours after embolization can make surgical resection difficult and tedious.

The goal of embolization therapy for AVMs is to thrombose the so-called nidus of abnormal vasculature that promotes vascular recruitment and arteriovenous shunting. Permanent nidus occlusion is desirable since, otherwise, AVMs typically recur in an almost malignant fashion. Embolization of arterial feeders proximal to the nidus only promotes colla-

teralization and prevents nidus ablation. Therefore, the embolic agents that are most appropriate for embolization include microscopic particles or liquids that can reach the nidus' small-calibre vascular bed. Ivalon (polyvinyl alcohol) particles ranging in size from 100 to 500 μm are useful for precapillary occlusion, allowing embolization of multiple arterial feeders near the nidus. Absolute ethanol and cyanoacrylate adhesives allow obliteration of the nidus itself.

Embolic material is injected only after the feeding arteries are selectively catheterized to avoid the inadvertent embolization of normal vasculature. Recent improvements in digital imaging, live subtraction fluoroscopy, and roadmapping make this possible. Multiple arteriograms may be required, making digital filming essential. Small, steerable catheter and guidewire systems allow the selective catheterization of lesions that at first glance appear inaccessible. Previous arterial ligation or embolization may prevent a *remote* percutaneous transarterial approach, in which case, surgical exposure or *direct* percutaneous puncture and catheterization may be necessary. Blood pressure cuffs, tourniquets, and intraarterial occlusion balloons are often employed to slow blood flow through dynamic lesions and control the deposition of embolic agents. With venous lesions, sequential sclerosis of abnormal veins in symptomatic areas of these typically diffuse abnormalities is feasible. Direct puncture followed by sclerosis with ethanol or Sotradecol (sodium tetradecyl sulfate) has been described.[28]

Leukocytosis, fever, and mild to moderate pain is typically observed following most embolization procedures. Limited tissue necrosis and transient sensory or motor deficits comprise minor complications that do not require specific treatment. The major complications of embolic therapy include extensive tissue necrosis necessitating skin grafting, inadvertent embolization of normal vasculature, pulmonary embolization, and permanent neurologic loss resulting from embolization of

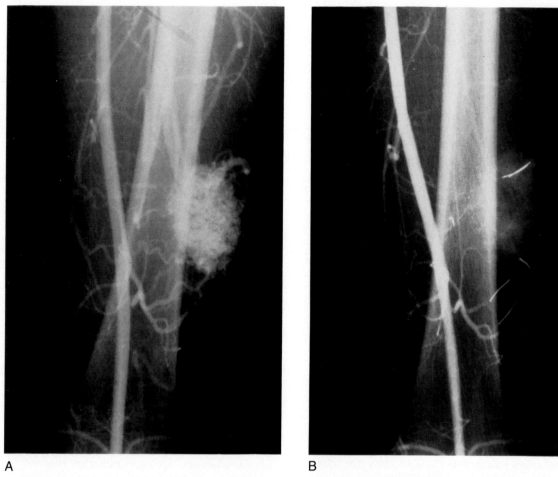

A

B

FIGURE 10–9. Arteriovenous malformation (AVM) of left thigh (*A*) before and (*B*) after embolotherapy with ethanol.

critical vasa nervosum. Although major complications occur infrequently, they emphasize the importance of careful patient selection in order to assure that the risk:benefit ratio is in favor of intervention.

Although the best embolic agent remains controversial, the overall approach, therapeutic results, and complication rates are similar among several published patient series. Rosen and colleagues, who advocate the use of cyanoacrylate adhesives, have successfully treated 47 patients with peripheral AVMs, with 79 per cent of patients benefiting from therapy.[29] Thirteen patients appeared cured at 3-year follow-up, 11 patients had residual malformations but were asymptomatic, 12 patients were improved but remained symptomatic, and nine patients either were unchanged or had worsened. Six per cent of patients suffered major complications including two patients with temporary hemiparesis and one patient with intractable hematuria. Yakes and colleagues used alcohol to treat 10 patients with CVMs, eight AVMs and two venous malformations.[30] Eight of 10 patients benefitted from treatment with two apparent cures at 1-year follow-up. They reported a 20 per cent major complication rate, including one patient who suffered a fatal pulmonary embolus 4 days postembolization and one patient who developed an L3-4 radiculopathy. Widlus and colleagues treated 16 patients with symptomatic AVMs using a combination of tissue adhesive and particles.[31] All patients were improved following treatment. Two patients required skin grafting after a procedure, but no other major complications developed.

These encouraging results support the use of palliative embolization to treat symptomatic CVMs not amenable to complete surgical resection. The combination of better vascular imaging techniques and more limited use of surgery for palliative indications (and its replacement in this setting by embolotherapy, made possible by a decade of technological refinement), now offers a more optimistic outlook for even the more challenging congenital vascular malformations.

REFERENCES

1. Szilagyi DE, Smith RF, Elliott JP, Hageman JH: Congenital arteriovenous anomalies of the limbs. Arch Surg *111*:423–429, 1976.

2. Lindenauer SM: The Klippel-Trenaunay syndrome: Varicosity, hypertrophy and hemangioma with no arteriovenous fistula. Ann Surg *162*:303–314, 1965.

3. Parkes-Weber F: Angioma formation in connection with hypertrophy of limbs or hemihypertrophy. Br J Dermatol *19*:231, 1907.

4. Reid MR: Studies on abnormal arteriovenous communications, acquired and congenital: 1. Report of a series of cases. Arch Surg *10*:601–638, 1925.

5. Rienhoff WF: Congenital arteriovenous fistula: An embryologic study with the report of a case. Johns Hopkins Hosp Bull *35*:271–284, 1924.

6. Szilagyi D, Elliott J, DeRusso F, et al: Peripheral congenital arteriovenous fistulas. Surgery *57*:61–68, 1965.

7. Moore KL: The cardiovascular system. *In*: The Developing Human: Clinically Oriented Embryology, 4th ed. Philadelphia, WB Saunders Company, 1988, pp 286–333.

8. Woollard HH: The development of the principle arterial stems in the forelimb of the pig. Cont Embryol *14*:139–154, 1922.

9. Malan E (ed): Vascular Malformations. Milan, Carlo Erba Foundation, 1974, pp 41–43.

10. DeTakats G: Vascular anomalies of the extremities. Surg Gynecol Obstet *55*:227–237, 1931.

11. Mulliken J, Glovacki J: Hemangiomas and vascular malformation in infants and children: A classification based on endothelial characteristics. Plast Reconstr Surg *69*:412–420, 1982.

12. White CW, Sondheimer HM, Crouch EC, Wilson H, Fan LL: Treatment of pulmonary hemangiomatosis with recombinant interferon α-2a. N Engl J Med *320*:1197–1200, 1989.

13. Woolley MM, Stanley P, Wesley JR: Peripherally located congenital arteriovenous fistulae in infancy and childhood. J Pediatr Surg *12*(2):165–176, 1977.

14. Rutherford RB, Pearce WH: Acute problems following diagnostic and interventional radiologic procedures. *In* Bergan JJ, Yao JST (eds): Vascular Surgery Emergencies. Orlando, FL, Grune & Stratton, 1986, pp 417–430.

15. Rutherford RB, Anderson BO: Diagnosis of congenital vascular malformations of the extremities: New perspectives. Int Angiol *9*(3):162–167, 1990.

16. Rutherford RB: Noninvasive testing in the diagnosis and assessment of arteriovenous fistula. *In* Bernstein EF (ed): Noninvasive Diagnostic Techniques in Vascular Disease, 3rd ed. St. Louis, CV Mosby Company, 1985, pp 666–679.

17. Sumner DS, Rutherford RB: Diagnostic evaluation of arteriovenous fistulas: Radionuclide assessment. *In* Rutherford RB (ed): Vascular Surgery, 3rd ed. Philadelphia, WB Saunders Company, 1989, pp 1037–1038.

18. Rutherford RB, Fleming RW, McLeod FD: Vascular diagnostic methods for evaluating patients with arteriovenous fistulas. *In* Diethrich EB (ed): Noninvasive Cardiovascular Diagnosis: Current Concepts. Baltimore, University Park Press, 1978, pp 217–230.

19. Rauch RF, Silverman PM, Korobkin M, et al: Computed tomography of benign angiomatous lesions of the extremities. J Comput Assist Tomogr *8*:1143–1146, 1984.

20. Wilson JS, Korobkin M, Genant HK, Bovill EG Jr: Computed tomography of musculoskeletal disorders. AJR *131*:55–61, 1978.

21. Bernardino ME, Jing BS, Thomas JL, Lindell MM Jr, Zornoza J: The extremity soft tissue lesion: A comparative study of ultrasound, computed tomography, and xeroradiography. Radiology *139*:53–59, 1981.

22. Pearce WH, Rutherford RB, Whitehill RA, Davis K: Nuclear magnetic resonance imaging: Its diagnostic value in patients with congenital vascular malformations of the limbs. J Vasc Surg *8*:64–70, 1988.

23. Cohen JM, Weinreb JC, Redman HC: Arteriovenous malformations of the extremities: MR imaging. Radiology *158*:475–479, 1986.

24. Mills CM, Brant-Zawadzki M, Crooks LE: Nuclear magnetic resonance: Principles of blood flow imaging. *142*:165–170, AJR 1984.

25. Meuli RA, Wedeen VJ, Geller SC, et al: MR gated subtraction angiography: Evaluation of lower extremities. Radiology *159*(2):411–418, 1986.

26. Braun SD, Moore AVJ, Mills SR, et al: Closed-system venography in the evaluation of angiodysplastic lesions of the extremities. AJR *141*(6):1307–1310, 1983.

27. O'Donnell TFJ, Edwards JM, Kinmonth JB: Lymphography in congenital mixed vascular deformities of the lower extremities. J Cardiovasc Surg (Torino) *17*(6):535–540, 1976.

28. Yakes WF, Parker SH: Diagnosis and management of vascular anomalies. *In* Castaneda-Zuniga WR, Tada-Varthy SM (eds): Interventional Radiology, 2nd ed. Philadelphia, Williams & Wilkins, 1991, pp 152–189.

29. Rosen RJ, Riles TS, Berenstein A: Congenital vascular malformations. *In* Rutherford RB (ed): Vascular Surgery, 3rd ed. WB Saunders Company, 1989, pp 1049–1061.

30. Yakes WF, Haas DK, Parker SH, et al: Symptomatic vascular malformations: Ethanol embolotherapy. Radiology *170*:1059–1066, 1989.

31. Wildus DM, Murray RR, White RI, et al: Congenital arteriovenous malformations: Tailored embolotherapy. Radiology *169*:511–516, 1988.

11

VASCULOGENIC IMPOTENCE

RALPH G. DePALMA

The past 14 years witnessed increasing information about pathogenesis, diagnosis, and treatment of impotence. In 1978 it was believed that impotence was due mainly to arterial insufficiency, and efforts were directed to direct corpus cavernosal revascularization.[1] However, beginning in 1984 the treatment emphasis changed to a variety of medical and surgical therapies.[2] Among the reasons for this evolution was the recognition that cavernosal or arteriolar abnormalities often predispose to impotence.[3] From the standpoint of the vascular surgeon, the work-up for impotence should be accurate and cost-effective; vascular reconstructive approaches should be based on specific guidelines. Mainly, vascular surgeons require information about prevention of impotence during aortoiliac reconstruction; they may also be required to evaluate the contribution of large vessel disease to vasculogenic impotence. This chapter emphasizes surgical approaches for prevention of vasculogenic impotence. Evolutionary arterial reconstructive and venoablative procedures will be discussed as well as current approaches to diagnosis and medical therapy.

PHYSIOLOGY OF ERECTION

Penile erection requires adequate arterial inflow and closure of cavernosal outflow.[4,5] Erection is controlled primarily by relaxation of the smooth muscle of the corporal bodies. These are endothelial-mediated relaxation responses[6] stimulated by neural mechanisms. Recently, the role of nitric oxide as the chemical mediator has been recognized.[8] With increased corporal arterial inflow, the emissary veins are compressed against the tunica albuginea, causing venous outflow occlusion. During full erection cavernosal artery flow virtually ceases. During the flaccid state, there is a constant venous leak and penile inflow and outflow are balanced. As the corpora do not fill when arterial inflow is insufficient, a venous leak will also be present. In the erect state intercavernous pressure increases from 10 to 15 mm Hg to levels ranging from 80 to 90 mm Hg. Higher pressures that contribute to penile rigidity are generated by perineal muscle contraction.[5]

ETIOLOGY OF IMPOTENCE

Table 11–1 summarizes general etiologic factors contributing to impotence. In modern practice more cases are now recognized as organic in origin than appreciated previously; however, in most cases of organic impotence psychogenic components are also often present. In screening 1023 impotent men from September 1983 through March 1992, 461 demonstrated some type of arterial inflow problem as judged by noninvasive criteria using penile brachial indices and pulse volume recordings. However, many impotent men exhibit other factors including diabetes, neuropathy in about 20 per cent, the need to take antihypertensive medications, and cavernosal malfunction including Peyronie's disease. Men with multiple factors contributing to impotence are not candidates for reconstruction; only about 4 to 5 percent of impotent men ultimately become candidates for vascular intervention. Furthermore, in the author's series only 15.6 per cent of the men with decreased arterial perfusion exhibited large vessel disease. Thus, when a screening sequence[8] is imposed for surgical case selection there is a sharp funnel effect so that for arterial reconstructions, for example, in a previous study, 334 men ultimately yielded only 18 operations.[9]

Table 11–2 offers an updated classification of vasculogenic impotence. Some type of small vessel, cavernosal, or arteriolar cause appears to be present in 43.3 per cent of men exhibiting abnormal penile perfusion. An additional 41.1 per cent of men with the primary complaint of impotence exhibit a combination of large and small vessel involvement as can be best ascertained by noninvasive and physical criteria. Most men presenting with the primary complaint of impotence will most likely have small vessel rather than large vessel disease.

However, in men with frank Leriche's syndrome or aortoiliac disease, impotence is an important complaint. Many men are potent prior to reconstruction

TABLE 11–1. GENERAL ETIOLOGIC FACTORS IN IMPOTENCE

Vasculogenic
Neurogenic
Endocrine
Drug-Induced
Psychogenic

for aneurysm or occlusive disease, and an accurate history of their sexual activity must be obtained. In spite of the best surgical technique to preserve sexual function, impotence can occur after reconstructions for aneurysms and occlusive disease. Importantly, the complaint of impotence has been found to be associated with undiscovered aneurysm disease in approximately 1 in 100 patients in the author's clinic. Therefore, prior to aortoiliac reconstruction, the surgeon must make careful inquiries into sexual function and probably carry out selective noninvasive measures of penile artery perfusion.[10]

HISTORY AND PHYSICAL EXAMINATION

A history of gradual erectile failure, in the absence of traumatic life events and correlated with symptoms such as claudication, suggests large vessel arteriogenic impotence. In these men, both the intensity and duration of atherosclerotic risk factors, mainly cigarette smoking, hypertension, diabetes, and hypercholesterolemia, probably contribute to atherosclerosis. This pattern signals those patients with involvement of the aorta or the iliac systems. As mentioned previously, abdominal aneurysms or ulcerative atheromatous disease can cause small penile vessel emboli. A history of perineal injuries predisposes to interruption of the cavernosal artery and these histories should be sought. The immediate onset of erectile failure following urologic, vascular, or rectal operations is an important diagnostic point. While erectile dysfunction can result from either neural or vascular interruption or both, neural interruption is more commonly associated with ejaculatory disorders. Alcohol and drug abuse contribute to erectile failure, while drugs used to treat hypertension and diabetes cause erectile failure because of their neuropathic and metabolic effects. Other hormonal disorders such as hypogonadism are less common. The author has seen one prolactinoma in the past decade.

On physical examination the major findings of aortoiliac disease are decreased femoral pulses or bruits. Sensory testing of the extremities, perineum, or glans occasionally reveals neuropathies associated with diabetic impotence. However, these abnormalities are best sought by neurovascular testing, using pudendal evoked potentials and measurement of bulbo cavernosal reflex times.[11] The prostate must be examined and nodular abnormalities investigated—the author has frequently obtained prostatic-specific antigen determinations in these men. Examination is completed by methodical palpation of the corpora cavernosa for Peyronie's plaques and estimation of testicular size. In the majority of men with the chief complaint of impotence, the physical examination is completely normal.

At this point the erectile mechanism can be tested in the clinic by intracavernous injection of 10 to 20 μg of Prostin E1.[12] Rigid erection sufficient for intercourse demonstrates adequate arterial inflow and venoocclusive mechanisms. Provided aneurysmal disease is ruled out (e.g., by sonography), cavernosal injection therapy can be selected at this point for treatment in many men.

NEUROVASCULAR TESTING

Neurovascular testing[8,10] is used primarily to select patients for further studies and as candidates for reconstructive procedures. These are also needed in deciding on the dosage of intracavernous injection of vasoactive agents—patients with neurologic deficits are often exquisitely sensitive and dosage must be reduced.

Penile brachial indices (PBI) are the ratio between systolic pressure detected by a Doppler probe placed distal to the penile cuff and systemic or brachial arm pressure. A cuff of 2.5 cm is used in an average size penis. The cuff is inflated, then deflated, and reappearance of the Doppler signals in the dorsal artery branch proximal to the corona signals reflow. Normally, this pressure approaches systemic pressure. A PBI above .75 suggests no major obstacle between the aorta and the distal measurement point. Generally, PBIs less than .6 relate to major vascular obstructions in the aortoiliac bed, while PBIs between .6 and .75 are considered abnormal. Flow can be further characterized by use of penile pulse volume recording. Penile pulse volume recording, as performed by the author, uses a pneumoplethysmographic cuff (Buffington) with a contained transducer.

This test is performed in the flaccid state. The variables recorded are the same used for those in the

TABLE 11–2. CLASSIFICATION OF VASCULOGENIC IMPOTENCE

Arterial

Large-vessel	Aorta and branches to internal iliac artery
Small-vessel	Anterior division of internal iliac artery and penile arteries
Combined	Atheroembolism from aortoiliac segment

Cavernosal

Fibrosis	Postpriapic, drug injection, idiopathic with aging
Peyronie's disease	Deformity; venous leakage
Refractory states	Hormonal, diabetic, blood pressure medication

Venous

Acquired	Various patterns; dorsal vein, crural; spongiosal
Congenital	Cavernous spongiosus leak

lower extremity. These include crest time, waveform, and the presence or absence of a dicrotic notch. This technique measures the total pulsation of all penile arteries as the cuff compresses the cavernous tissues. The measurements are taken with the cuff inflated to mean arterial pressure, calculated as diastolic pressure plus one third of systemic pulse pressure. Waveforms on a polygraph with a chart speed of 25 mm/sec and sensitivity setting in one will demonstrate in normal patients that the upstroke of the waveform is completed by 0.2 seconds, while normal waveform amplitudes vary from 5 to 6 to 30 mm in height. Waveforms can be distinctly abnormal with small vessel disease or cavernosal disorders, while PBI is normal.

These noninvasive tests help in the detection of arteriogenic impotence. However, cases of vasculogenic impotence caused by venous leak or Peyronie's disease or cavernosal fibrosis are not detected. In these instances color-flow duplex scanning after an intracavernous injection to produce erection can be useful.[10] The noninvasive tests are not completely sensitive and specific. We have found that the combination of penile brachial indices and pulse volume recording will predict an abnormal arteriogram with a sensitivity of 85 per cent and a specificity of 70 per cent. In suspected cases of venogenic impotence (i.e., normal arterial noninvasive tests), we have discovered that 12 to 15 per cent of these men demonstrate an arterial abnormality.[9] Therefore, prior to small vessel interventions, both pudendal arteriography and dynamic infusion cavernosography are recommended.

CAVERNOSOMETRY AND CAVERNOSAL ARTERY OCCLUSION PRESSURE

These invasive studies provide quantitative information about arterial inflow and venoocclusive mechanisms.[10] A calibrated pump provides flow of warm heparinized saline via 20-gauge needles inserted into the corpora. During maximum erection, intracavernous pressure at some point equilibrates with arterial inflow pressure. Flow in the deep cavernosal artery will stop. This value is called cavernosal artery occlusion pressure (CAOP). CAOP is measured using Doppler insonation at the point of full erection. It is taken as normal when greater than 90 mm Hg. A pressure gradient from brachial levels greater than 30 mm Hg suggests arterial inflow occlusion. Dynamic infusion cavernosography measures the flow to maintain erection. This value is normally taken to be 40 ml or less following intracavernous injection of a standard papaverine-phentolamine mixture. To visualize venous leaks, diluted nonionic contrast is injected. Spot filming in various obliquities identifies specific abnormal or leaking veins when cavernosography is positive. As mentioned previously, failure of erection is associated with an excess of venous leakage over inflow. Venous leakage can be due to arterial insufficiency and, as mentioned, prior to con-

templated venous ablation we recommend routine highly selective pudendal arteriography.

LARGE VESSEL RECONSTRUCTION— PREVENTION OF VASCULOGENIC IMPOTENCE

Given the usual indications for large vessel aortoiliac reconstruction (i.e., aneurysm and occlusive disease), a procedure must be selected that provides perfusion of one or both internal iliac arteries wherever possible. Embolization into the internal iliacs is avoided. The dissection must spare the neural fibers about the aorta and the iliac arteries (which are especially rich on the left side) and about the inferior mesenteric artery. In all these cases a specific history of preoperative sexual activity must be sought. If an elderly couple manifests no interest in this activity, further investigation is not needed. However, where interest exists, penile brachial indices and pulse volume recordings preoperatively will be helpful in comparing with postoperative findings. In addition, positive findings of abnormal pudendal and somatosensory evoked potentials are helpful, particularly in diabetics demonstrating preoperative neuropathy.

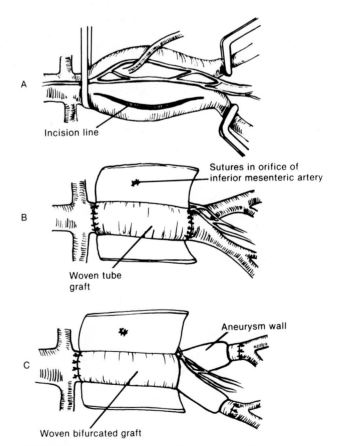

FIGURE 11–1. Inlay nerve-sparing techniques for aneurysm repair. Note incision on right side of aneurysm. (From DePalma RG: Prevention of sexual dysfunction in aortoiliac surgery. *In* Jamieson CW (ed): Current Operative Surgery. Eastborne, East Sussex, Bailliere-Tindall, 1985.)

OPERATIVE TECHNIQUES

These techniques have been described previously[13] and illustrations have been reproduced from a recent review.[14] Exposure for aortoiliac reconstruction is best accomplished by dissecting the aortoiliac segment from the right side and sparing the nerves and inferior mesenteric artery. In cases of aortoiliac aneurysm, perfusion of the internal iliac is assured by an inlay technique, illustrated in Figure 11–1. Again, the aneurysmal sac is incised well to the right, avoiding interruption of a dominant left periaortic nerve plexus. The inferior mesenteric artery is sutured from within the aneurysmal sac. Figures 11–2 and 11–3 show techniques for occlusive disease. In men with buttock claudication and impotence related to local disease in the arterial distribution of the internal iliac artery, an extraperitoneal approach with endarterectomy or bypass is a convenient procedure. This approach involves a longitudinal incision along the edge of the rectus muscle with reflection of the peritoneal medially (Fig. 11–4). In renal transplant patients, end-to-side renal artery anastomosis to the external iliac artery avoids division of an internal iliac artery.

Fredberg described sexual dysfunction in conventional aortoiliac operations.[15] In this series, 55 per cent (11/20) aneurysms were preoperatively impotent, while 95 per cent (19/20) were postoperatively impotent. For occlusive disease, 31 per cent (15/48) were preoperatively impotent and 60 per cent (29/48) were postoperatively impotent. In contrast, a series of men operated upon by the author using techniques previously described were followed for at least 3 years up to 1990. Of 125 men operated for aortoiliac disease, four became impotent as a result of emergency operations (rupture) or internal iliac aneurysms. Fifty-three men, average age 64.6, were impotent preoperatively and postoperatively; 30 men, average age 57 years (39 to 71), were potent preoperatively and postoperatively, while 39 men, average age 58.0 years

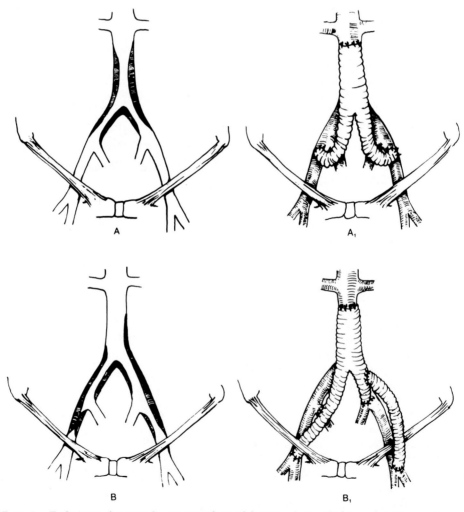

FIGURE 11–2. Techniques for aortoiliac or aortofemoral bypass: *A, A₁,* End-to-end aortic anastomosis with suprainguinal end-to-side bypass where external iliac and common femoral arteries are spared. *B, B₁,* end-to-end, aortic anastomosis with side-to-side reconstruction of right internal iliac and two limbs on left side. (From DePalma RG: Prevention of sexual dysfunction in aortoiliac surgery. *In* Jamieson CW (ed): Current Operative Surgery. Eastborne, East Sussex, Bailliere-Tindall, 1985.)

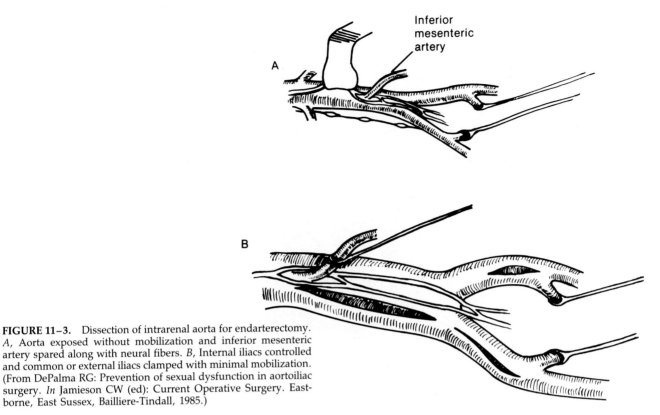

FIGURE 11–3. Dissection of intrarenal aorta for endarterectomy. *A,* Aorta exposed without mobilization and inferior mesenteric artery spared along with neural fibers. *B,* Internal iliacs controlled and common or external iliacs clamped with minimal mobilization. (From DePalma RG: Prevention of sexual dysfunction in aortoiliac surgery. *In* Jamieson CW (ed): Current Operative Surgery. Eastborne, East Sussex, Bailliere-Tindall, 1985.)

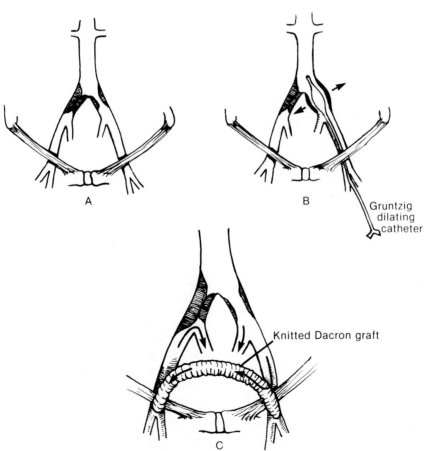

FIGURE 11–4. Femorofemoral bypass with transluminal angioplasty. (From DePalma RG: Prevention of sexual dysfunction in aortoiliac surgery. *In* Jamieson CW (ed): Current Operative Surgery. Eastborne, East Sussex, Bailliere-Tindall, 1985.)

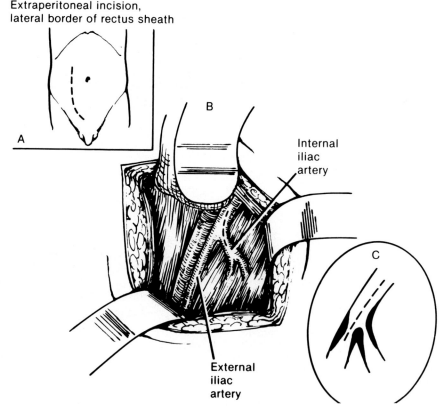

Extraperitoneal incision,
lateral border of rectus sheath

A

B

Internal
iliac
artery

C

External
iliac
artery

FIGURE 11–5.   Isolated iliac artery endarterectomy. *A,* Incision for retroperitoneal exposure. *B,* Incision for isolated plaque of internal iliac. *C,* Linear incision when external iliac artery also involved. (From DePalma RG: Prevention of sexual dysfunction in aortoiliac surgery. *In* Jamieson CW (ed): Current Operative Surgery. Eastborne, East Sussex, Bailliere-Tindall, 1985.)

(38 to 69), impotent preoperatively, regained function postoperatively. Among 125 men undergoing aortoiliac surgery, about 3 per cent were rendered impotent, commonly in emergency settings. Overall, the author was able to restore or maintain function in 54 per cent of men requiring aortoiliac surgery. The average age of men postoperatively potent was 57.5 years (range 38 to 71), while those preoperatively and postoperatively impotent averaged 64.6 years. The author has noted in his patients decreasing potency with aging that does not appear to be related to arterial occlusion per se. Schiavi et al.[16] have shown age-related decreases in nocturnal penile tumescence in frequency, duration, and degree that correlate with desire, arousal, and coital frequency. Thus, age of patient preoperatively and postoperative aging contribute to diminished sexual function. In the author's opinion this decrement in function is not linearly related to arterial inflow compromise as previously believed.

In certain men femorofemoral bypass combined with intraluminal dilation of donor external or common iliac arteries is an excellent choice (Fig. 11–5). The procedure avoids completely an aortoiliac dissection and the results can be quite durable. Objective information with pulse volume recordings before and after femorofemoral bypass correlate with improved patterns of penile plethysmography and pressures after reconstruction.[17]

Common iliac artery transluminal dilation has been found useful. Transluminal dilation of the external iliac arteries can improve penile perfusion, relieving steal via the internal iliac and gluteal arteries. While transluminal dilatation of the common iliac arteries works, the internal iliac arteries are difficult to dilate; junctional lesions at the common iliac bifurcation are best treated surgically.

SMALL VESSEL RECONSTRUCTIONS

Small vessel reconstructions were initially attempted using direct arterialization of the corpus cavernosum. These procedures failed because they induced priapism or thrombosed due to fibrosis at the anastomosis of the artery with the corpus cavernosum.[1] Two types of operations of microvascular bypasses are now used. One involves microvascular bypass into the dorsal artery and the other involves arterialization of the deep dorsal vein. The source for inflow is usually the inferior epigastric artery or in some hands a vein graft originating from the femoral artery. The author prefers the inferior epigastric artery as inflow source that is most often possible, and the direct arterial reconstruction over the deep dorsal vein arterialization.

Patient Selection

The candidate for microvascular correction of impotence must be rigorously screened. Ideally, these are young men with a history of trauma or localized disease.[18] Some exhibit diffuse distal penile lesions of unknown origin. The candidate will exhibit absence of neural, hormonal, or medication-induced causes of impotence. The author has not accepted diabetic patients for these procedures; the oldest patient selected thus far has been 61. All patients require pudendal arteriography. Appropriate candidates with communication between the dorsal and the cavernosal artery are selected using careful visualization of individual penile vessels after intracavernous injection of a small dose of papaverine to produce tumescence. As mentioned previously, a full erection masks inflow into the cavernosal artery and is not appropriate for evaluation of the penile microvasculature. The inferior epigastric artery is harvested (ligating side branches) and turned down for microvascular anastomosis to the appropriate dorsal artery.

DEEP DORSAL VEIN ARTERIALIZATION

These patients are generally younger individuals with small vessel disease whose dorsal arteries are not suitable for direct bypass. Physiology of this operation was thought to be due to reverse flow via emissary veins into the corpus cavernosum. However, the author's arteriographic observations and those of others indicate that flow is largely by the circumflex veins into the spongiosum. While results vary, this operation is said to be successful in 60 to 70 per cent of men for limited follow-up periods. Using the inferior epigastric artery, a microvascular anastomosis is done between the inferior epigastric artery and deep dorsal vein. There is one serious and specific complication of this arterialization—glans hyperperfusion. To prevent this, the anastomosis is performed proximally under the arch of the pubis and the dorsal vein is ligated proximally and distally, sparing circumflex veins, which provide outflow. When this complication does occur, further distal venous ligation or graft occlusion is urgently required.

VENOUS LIGATION

Success rates for venous ligation vary widely from 28 to 73 per cent.[8] Venous ligation implies both direct ligation and excision of the veins in cases selected by dynamic infusion cavernosography. The author has confined these procedures to excision of the dorsal vein[19] and has not approached crural veins directly. Other draining veins can be occluded using Gianturco coils inserted by the invasive radiologist. At times an introducing catheter inserted via the deep dorsal vein is useful. Yu et al. recommended routine dynamic cavernosography and cavernosometry at 3 months in all cases of venous ligation to rule out sham effect.[20] At this time additional embolization for new leaks can be done and with these combined procedures about 70 per cent of men regain erectile function or can then function with intracorporeal injections.

MEDICAL TREATMENT OF VASCULOGENIC IMPOTENCE

Multiple treatment options are summarized in Table 11–3. It is wise to try medical treatment first. As pointed out by Lue this can be done early in the work-up.[21] In particular, cessation of cigarette smoking and control of obesity are recommended, although no control study exists to support efficacy of these steps. It is also possible to alter or minimize antihypertensive treatment by weight control, exercise, or drug change. Some men improve after one or two intracavernosal injections producing artificial erection, and then resume spontaneous function. With mild arteriogenic impotence this effect can be enhanced by the addition of isoxsuprine hydrochloride 10 to 20 mg four times a day and yohimbine three times a day.

The majority of men with vasculogenic impotence are now treated medically, with self-administered intracorporeal injections or with vacuum constrictor devices.[22,23] From the standpoint of the practicing vascular surgeon, it is important to recognize the requirements for aortoiliac reconstruction that prevent or relieve impotence associated with large vessel disease. With conscientious screening and medical treatment, only 4 to 5 per cent of men become candidates for vascular surgical intervention.

TABLE 11–3.   TREATMENT OF VASCULOGENIC IMPOTENCE

Medical	Surgical
Risk-Factor Intervention	Arteriogenic
Smoking cessation	Aortoiliac and/or internal iliac
Diabetes control	reconstruction
Blood pressure medication	Dorsal artery bypass
Change	Dorsal vein arterialization
Drugs	Cavernosal or neurogenic
Isoxsuprine hydrochloride	Prostheses
Pentoxifylline	
Intracorporal injections	Cavernosal leakage
Prostaglandin E_1	Vein resection; interruption
Papaverine	Transcatheter embolization
Phentolamine	
Mixtures of above	
Miscellaneous	
Vacuum constrictor	
devices	

References

1. DePalma RG, Kedia K, Persky L: Vascular operations for preservation of sexual function. *In* Bergan JJ, Yao JST (eds): The Surgery of the Aorta and its Body Branches. New York, Grune & Stratton, 1979, pp 277–296.
2. DePalma RG, Schwab FJ: Vasculogenic impotence. *In* Young JR, Graor RA, Olin JW, Bartholomew TR (eds): Peripheral Vascular Disease. St. Louis, Mosby Year Book Publishers, 1991, pp 395–400.
3. Bookstein FJ, Valjl: The arteriolar component in impotence: A possible paradigm shift. Am J Radiol *157*:932, 1991.
4. Michal V: Arteriogenic impotence. Angiol Arch *8*:4, 1985.
5. DePalma RG: Anatomy and physiology of male sexual function. *In* Giordano JM, Trout HH III, DePalma RG (eds): The Basic Science of Vascular Surgery. Mt. Kisco, NY, Futura Publishing Company, 1988, pp 699.
6. DeTejada IS, Goldstein I, Azadzoi K, et al: Impaired neurogenic and endothelium-mediated relaxation of penile smooth muscle from diabetic men with impotence. N Engl J Med *32*:1025, 1989.
7. Rajfer J, Aronson WJ, Bush PA, Dorey FJ, Ignarro LJ: Nitric oxide as a mediator of the corpus cavernosum in response to nonadrenergic noncholinergic neurotransmission. N Engl J Med *326*:90, 1992.
8. DePalma RG, Emsellem HA, Edwards CM, et al: A screening sequence for vasculogenic impotence. J Vasc Surg *5*:228, 1987.
9. DePalma RG, Schwab FJ, Emsellem E, Massarin E, Bergsrud D, Olding MJ: Vascular interventions for impotence: Effect of screening sequence. Int J Impot Res *2* (Suppl):358, 1990.
10. DePalma RG, Schwab FJ, Emsellem HA, et al: Noninvasive assessment of impotence. Surg Clin North Am *70*:119, 1990.
11. Emsellem HA, Bergsrud DW, DePalma RG, et al: Pudendal evoked potentials in the evaluation of impotence (abstr). J Clin Neurophysiol *359*:5, 1988.
12. Stackl W, Hasun R, Marberger M: Intracavernous injection of prostaglandin E1 in impotent men. J Urol *140*:66, 1988.
13. DePalma RG, Edwards CM, Schwab FJ, Steinberg DL: Modern management of impotence associated with aortic surgery. *In* Bergen JJ, Yao JST (eds): Arterial Surgery: New Diagnostic and Operative Techniques. Orlando, FL, Grune & Stratton, 1988, pp 337–348.
14. DePalma RG: Prevention of sexual dysfunction in aortoiliac surgery. *In* Jamieson CW (ed): Current Operative Surgery: Vascular Surgery. London, Bailliere-Tindall, 1988, pp 80–96.
15. Fredberg U, Mouritzen C: Sexual dysfunction as a symptom of arteriosclerosis and as a complication to reconstruction of the aortoiliac segment. J Cardiovasc Surg *29*:149, 1988.
16. Schiavi RC, Schreiner-Engel P, Mandeli J, Schanger H, Cohen E: Healthy aging and male sexual function. Am J Psychiatry *147*:766, 1990.
17. Merchant RF Jr, DePalma RG: The effects of femoro-femoral grafts on postoperative sexual function: Correlation with penile pulse volume recordings. Surgery *90*:962, 1981.
18. Krane RJ, Goldstein I, DeTejada IS: Impotence. N Engl J Med *321*:1648, 1989.
19. DePalma RG, Schwab F, Druy EM, Miller HC, Emsellem HB: Experience in diagnosis and treatment of impotence caused by cavernosal leak syndrome. J Vasc Surg *10*:117, 1989.
20. Yu GW, Schwab FJ, Melograna FS, DePalma RG, Miller HC, Rickhdt AL: Preoperative and postoperative dynamic infusion cavernosography and cavernosometry: Objective assessment of venous ligation for impotence. J Urol *147*:618, 1992.
21. Lue TF: Impotence: A patient's goal-directed approach to treatment. World J Urol *8*:67, 1990.
22. Nadig PW, Ware TC, Blumoff R: Noninvasive device to produce and maintain an erection-like state. Urology *27*:126, 1986.
23. Witherington R: Vacuum constriction device for management of erectile impotence. J Urol *141*:320, 1989.

12

HEMODYNAMICS FOR THE VASCULAR SURGEON

R. EUGENE ZIERLER and D. EUGENE STRANDNESS, JR.

Blood flow in human arteries and veins can be described in terms of strict hemodynamic principles. While the elements of hemodynamics are derived from engineering, mathematics, and physiology, these principles also form the theoretical foundation for the surgical treatment of vascular disease.

The major mechanisms of arterial disease are obstruction of the lumen and disruption of the vessel wall. Arterial obstruction or narrowing may result from atherosclerosis, emboli, thrombi, fibromuscular dysplasia, trauma, or external compression. The clinical significance of an obstructive lesion depends on its location, severity, and duration, as well as the ability of the circulation to compensate by increasing cardiac output and developing collateral pathways. Surgical treatment requires the identification and correction of arterial lesions associated with significant hemodynamic disturbances. Disruption of the arterial wall is caused by ruptured aneurysm or trauma. The tendency of aneurysms to rupture is determined by arterial wall characteristics, intraluminal pressure, and size. In this situation, the role of surgery is to prevent rupture or to reestablish arterial continuity after rupture occurs.

On the venous side of the circulation, the major hemodynamic mechanisms of disease are obstruction and valvular incompetence. These are generally the sequelae of thrombosis in the deep venous system, and they produce venous hypertension in the circulation distal to the involved venous segment. The clinical consequences of venous hypertension are the signs and symptoms of the postthrombotic syndrome: pain, edema, subcutaneous fibrosis, pigmentation, stasis dermatitis, and ulceration. Treatment of this condition involves elevation, external compression, venous interruption, and, rarely, direct venous reconstruction.

This chapter begins with a discussion of the hemodynamic principles and wall properties that govern arterial flow. The hemodynamic alterations produced by arterial stenoses and their effect on flow patterns in human limbs are considered next. These principles are then related to the treatment of arterial obstruction. Finally, the hemodynamics of the venous system are briefly reviewed and related to the pathophysiology and treatment of venous disease.

BASIC PRINCIPLES OF ARTERIAL HEMODYNAMICS

Fluid Pressure

The pressure in a fluid system is defined as force per unit area (given in dynes per square centimeter). Intravascular arterial pressure (P) has three components: (1) the dynamic pressure produced by contraction of the heart, (2) the hydrostatic pressure, and (3) the static filling pressure. Hydrostatic pressure is determined by the specific gravity of blood and the height of the point of measurement above a specific reference level. The reference level in the human body is considered to be the right atrium. The hydrostatic pressure is given by:

$$P \text{ (hydrostatic)} = -\rho g h \qquad (1)$$

where ρ is the specific gravity of blood (approximately 1.056 g/cu cm), g is the acceleration due to gravity (980 cm/sec^2), and h is the distance in centimeters above or below the right atrium. The magnitude of hydrostatic pressure may be quite large. In a man 5 feet 8 inches tall, this pressure at ankle level is approximately 89 mm Hg.[1]

The static filling pressure represents the residual pressure that exists in the absence of arterial flow. This pressure is determined by the volume of blood and elastic properties of the vessel wall, and it is usually in the range of 5 to 10 mm Hg.

Fluid Energy

Blood flows through the arterial system in response to differences in total fluid energy. Although pressure gradients are the most obvious forces involved, other forms of energy drive the circulation.[2] Total fluid energy (*E*) can be divided into potential energy (E_p) and kinetic energy (E_k). The components of potential energy are intravascular pressure (*P*) and gravitational potential energy.

The factors contributing to intravascular pressure have already been discussed. Gravitational potential energy represents the ability of a volume of blood to do work because of its height above a specific reference level. The formula for gravitational potential energy is the same as that for hydrostatic pressure (Eq. 1) but with an opposite sign: $+\rho gh$. Since the gravitational potential energy and hydrostatic pressure usually cancel each other out and the static filling pressure is relatively low, the predominant component of potential energy is the dynamic pressure produced by cardiac contraction. Potential energy can be expressed as

$$E_p = P + (\rho gh) \qquad (2)$$

Kinetic energy represents the ability of blood to do work on the basis of its motion. It is proportional to the specific gravity of blood and the square of blood velocity (*v*), in centimeters per second:

$$E_k = \tfrac{1}{2}\rho v^2 \qquad (3)$$

By combining Eqs. 2 and 3, an expression for the total fluid energy per unit volume of blood (in ergs per cubic centimeter), can be obtained:

$$E + P + (\rho gh) + (\tfrac{1}{2}\rho v^2) \qquad (4)$$

Fluid Energy Losses

Bernoulli's Principle

When fluid flows from one point to another, its total energy (*E*) along any given streamline is constant, provided that flow is steady and there are no frictional energy losses. This is in accordance with the law of conservation of energy and constitutes Bernoulli's principle:

$$P_1 + \rho gh_1 + \tfrac{1}{2}\rho v_1^2 = P_2 + \rho gh_2 + \tfrac{1}{2}\rho v_2^2 \qquad (5)$$

This equation expresses the relationship between pressure, gravitational potential energy, and kinetic energy in an idealized fluid system. In the horizontal diverging tube shown in Figure 12–1, steady flow between point 1 and point 2 is accompanied by an increase in cross-sectional area and a decrease in flow velocity. Although the fluid moves against a pressure gradient of 2.5 mm Hg and therefore gains potential energy, the total fluid energy remains constant because of the lower velocity and a proportional loss of kinetic energy. In other words, the widening of the tube results in the conversion of kinetic energy to potential energy in the form of pressure. In a converging tube the opposite would occur; a pressure drop and increase in velocity would be noted as potential energy was converted to kinetic energy.

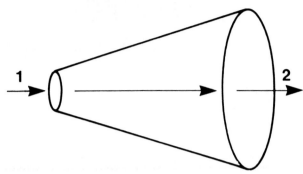

A_1=1 cm^2 A_2=16 cm^2
V_1=80 cm/sec V_2=5 cm/sec
P_1=100 mm Hg P_2=102.5 mm Hg

FIGURE 12–1. Effect of increasing cross-sectional area on pressure in a frictionless fluid system. While pressure increases, total fluid energy remains constant as a result of a decrease in velocity. (Redrawn from Sumner DS: The hemodynamics and pathophysiology of arterial disease. *In* Rutherford RB (ed): Vascular Surgery, Philadelphia, WB Saunders Company, 1977.)

The situation depicted in the preceding example is not observed in human arteries because the ideal flow conditions specified in the Bernoulli relationship are not present. The fluid energy lost in moving blood through the arterial circulation is dissipated mainly in the form of heat. When this source of energy loss is accounted for, Eq. 5 becomes

$$P_1 + \rho gh_1 + \tfrac{1}{2}\rho v_1^2$$
$$= P_2 + \rho gh_2 + \tfrac{1}{2}\rho v_2^2 + \text{heat} \qquad (6)$$

Viscous Energy Losses and Poiseuille's Law

Energy losses in flowing blood occur either as viscous losses resulting from friction or as inertial losses related to changes in the velocity or direction of flow. The term "viscosity" describes the resistance to flow that arises because of the intermolecular attractions between fluid layers. The coefficient of viscosity (η) is defined as the ratio of shear stress (τ) to shear rate (*D*):

$$\eta = \frac{\tau}{D} \qquad (7)$$

Shear stress is proportional to the energy loss due to friction between adjacent fluid layers, whereas shear rate refers to the relative velocity of adjacent fluid layers. Fluids with particularly strong intermolecular attractions offer a high resistance to flow and have high coefficients of viscosity. As an example, motor oil has a higher coefficient of viscosity than water.[3] The unit of viscosity is the "poise," which equals 1 dyne sec/sq cm. Since it is difficult to measure viscosity directly, relative viscosity is often used to relate the viscosity of a fluid to that of water. The relative viscosity of plasma is approximately 1.8, whereas for whole blood the relative viscosity is in the range of 3 to 4.

Since viscosity increases exponentially with hematocrit, the concentration of red blood cells is the most important factor affecting the viscosity of whole blood. The viscosity of plasma is determined largely by the concentration of plasma proteins. These constituents of blood are also responsible for its non-Newtonian character. In a Newtonian fluid, viscosity is independent of shear rate or flow velocity. Because blood is a suspension of cells and large protein molecules, its viscosity can vary greatly with shear rate (Fig. 12–2). Blood viscosity increases rapidly at low shear rates, but approaches a constant value at higher shear rates. In most of the arterial circulation, the prevailing shear rates place the blood viscosity on the asymptotic portion of the curve. Thus, for arteries with diameters greater than about 1 mm, human blood resembles a constant-viscosity or Newtonian fluid.

Poiseuille's law describes the viscous energy losses that occur in an idealized flow model. This law states that the pressure gradient along a tube ($P_1 - P_2$ in dynes per square centimeter) is directly proportional to the mean flow velocity ($\bar{V}$, in centimeters per second) or volume flow (Q, in cubic centimeters per second), the tube length (L, in centimeters), and the fluid viscosity (η, in poise), and inversely proportional to either the second or fourth power of the radius (r, in centimeters):

$$P_1 - P_2 = \bar{V}\frac{8L\eta}{r^2} = Q\frac{8L\eta}{\tau r^4} \qquad (8)$$

When this equation is simplified to pressure = flow × resistance, it is analogous to Ohm's law of electrical circuits.

The strict application of Poiseuille's law requires the steady, laminar flow of a Newtonian fluid in a straight, rigid, cylindrical tube. Since these conditions seldom exist in the arterial circulation, Poiseuille's law can only estimate the minimum pressure gradient or viscous energy losses that may be expected in arterial flow. Energy losses due to inertial effects often exceed viscous energy losses, particularly in the presence of arterial disease.

Inertial Energy Losses

Energy losses related to inertia (ΔE) are proportional to a constant (K), the specific gravity of blood, and the square of blood velocity:

$$\Delta E = K\tfrac{1}{2}\rho v^2 \qquad (9)$$

Since velocity is the only independent variable in this equation, inertial energy losses result from the acceleration and deceleration of pulsatile flow, variations in lumen diameter, and changes in the direction of flow at points of curvature and branching.

The combined effects of viscous and inertial energy losses are illustrated in Figure 12–3. When the pressure drop across an arterial segment is measured at varying flow rates, the experimental data fit a line with both linear (viscous) and squared (inertial) terms. The viscous energy losses predicted by Poiseuille's law are considerably less than the total energy loss actually observed.

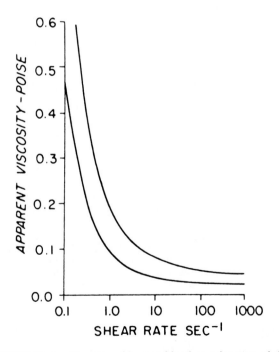

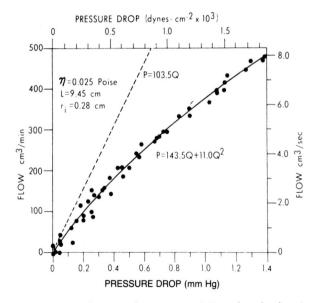

FIGURE 12–2. Viscosity of human blood as a function of shear rate. Values range between the two lines. (From Strandness DE, Sumner DS: Hemodynamics for Surgeons. New York, Grune & Stratton, 1975.)

FIGURE 12–3. Pressure drop across a 9.45-cm length of canine femoral artery at varying flow rates. The experimental data line (solid) has both linear and squared terms, corresponding to viscous and inertial energy losses. The pressure-flow curve predicted by Poiseuille's law (dashed line) depicts much lower energy losses than those actually observed. (From Sumner DS: The hemodynamics and pathophysiology of arterial disease. *In* Rutherford RB (ed): Vascular Surgery. Philadelphia, WB Saunders Company, 1977.)

Vascular Resistance

Hemodynamic resistance (R) can be defined as the ratio of the energy drop between two points along an artery ($E_1 - E_2$) to the mean blood flow (Q):

$$R = \frac{E_1 - E_2}{Q} \cong \frac{P_1 - P_2}{Q} \qquad (10)$$

If the kinetic energy term ($\frac{1}{2}\rho v^2$) is considered to be a small component of the total energy, and the artery is assumed to be horizontal so that the gravitational potential energy terms ($\rho g h$) cancel, Eq. 4 can be used to express resistance as the simple ratio of pressure drop ($P_1 - P_2$) to flow. Thus, Eq. 10 becomes a rearranged version of Poiseuille's law (Eq. 8), and the minimum resistance or viscous energy losses are given by the resistance term

$$R = \frac{8L\eta}{\pi r^4} \qquad (11)$$

The hemodynamic resistance of an arterial segment increases as the flow velocity increases, provided the lumen size remains constant (Fig. 12–4). These additional energy losses are related to inertial effects and are proportional to $\frac{1}{2}\rho v^2$.

According to Eq. 11, the predominant factor influencing hemodynamic resistance is the fourth power of the radius. The relationship between radius and pressure drop for various flow rates along a 10-cm vessel segment is shown in Figure 12–5. For a wide range of flow rates, the pressure drop is negligible until the radius is reduced to about 0.3 cm; for radii less than 0.2 cm, the pressure drop increases rapidly. These observations might explain the frequent failure of femoropopliteal autogenous vein bypass grafts less than 4 mm in diameter.[4]

The calculation of total resistance (R_t) depends on whether the component resistances ($R_1 \ldots R_n$) are arranged in series or in parallel. This is also analogous to electrical circuits.

$$R_t(\text{series}) = R_1 + R_2 + \ldots R_n \qquad (12)$$

$$\frac{1}{R_t(\text{parallel})} = \frac{1}{R_1} + \frac{1}{R_2} + \ldots \frac{1}{R_n} \qquad (13)$$

The standard physical units of hemodynamic resistance are dyne seconds per centimeter to the fifth power. A more convenient way of expressing resistance is the peripheral resistance unit (PRU), which has the dimensions of millimeters of mercury per cubic centimeter per minute. One PRU is approximately 8×10^4 dyne sec/cm⁵.

In the human circulation, approximately 90 per cent of the total vascular resistance results from flow through the arteries and capillaries, while the remaining 10 per cent results from venous flow. The arterioles and capillaries are responsible for over 60 per cent of the total resistance, whereas the large and medium-sized arteries account for only about 15 per cent.[2] Thus, the arteries that are most commonly affected by atherosclerotic occlusive disease are normally very low-resistance vessels.

Blood Flow Patterns

Laminar Flow

In the steady state conditions specified by Poiseuille's law, the flow pattern is laminar. All motion is parallel to the walls of the tube, and the fluid is arranged in a series of concentric layers or laminae like those shown in Figure 12–6. While the velocity within each lamina remains constant, the velocity is lowest adjacent to the tube wall and increases toward the center of the tube. This results in a velocity profile that is parabolic in shape (Fig. 12–7). As previously discussed, the energy expended in moving one lamina of fluid over another is proportional to viscosity.

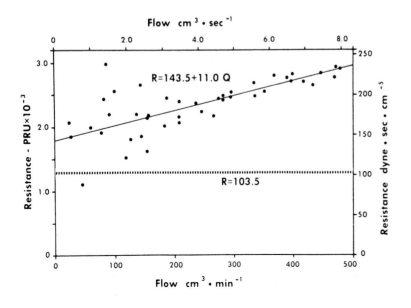

FIGURE 12–4. Resistance derived from pressure-flow curve in Figure 12–3. The resistance increases with increasing flow. Constant resistance predicted by Poiseuille's law is shown by the dotted line. (From Sumner DS: The hemodynamics and pathophysiology of arterial disease. *In* Rutherford RB (ed): Vascular Surgery. Philadelphia, WB Saunders Company, 1977.)

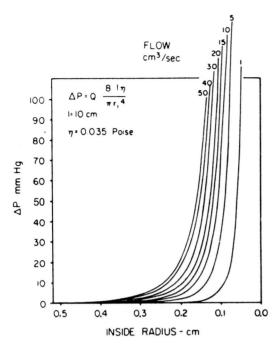

FLOW
cm³/sec

$$\Delta P = Q\ \frac{8\ l\ \eta}{\pi\ r_i^{4}}$$

l = 10 cm

η = 0.035 Poise

FIGURE 12–5. Relationship of pressure drop to inside radius of a cylindrical tube 10 cm in length at various rates of steady laminar flow. Flow rates are comparable to those in the human iliac artery. (From Strandness DE, Sumner DS: Hemodynamics for Surgeons. New York, Grune & Stratton, 1975.)

Turbulent Flow

In contrast to the linear streamlines of laminar flow, turbulence is an irregular flow state in which velocity varies rapidly with respect to space and time. These random velocity changes result in the dissipation of fluid energy as heat. The point of transition between laminar and turbulent flow depends on the tube diameter (*d*, in centimeters), the mean velocity, the specific gravity of the fluid, and the fluid viscosity. These

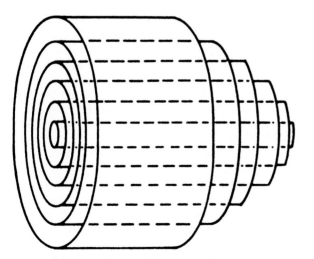

FIGURE 12–6. Concentric laminae of fluid in a cylindrical tube. Flow is from left to right. The center laminae move more rapidly than those near the periphery, and the flow profile is parabolic. (From Strandness DE, Sumner DS: Hemodynamics for Surgeons. New York, Grune & Stratton, 1975.)

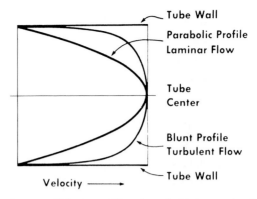

FIGURE 12–7. Velocity profiles of steady laminar and turbulent flow. Velocity is lowest adjacent to the tube wall and maximal in the center. (From Sumner DS: The hemodynamics and pathophysiology of arterial disease. *In* Rutherford RB (ed): Vascular Surgery. Philadelphia, WB Saunders Company, 1977.)

factors can be expressed as a dimensionless quantity called the Reynolds number (Re), which is the ratio of inertial forces to viscous forces acting on the fluid:

$$\mathrm{Re} = \frac{d\bar{V}\rho}{\eta} \tag{14}$$

In flowing blood at Reynolds numbers greater than 2000, inertial forces may disrupt laminar flow and produce fully developed turbulence. With values under 2000, localized flow disturbances are damped out by viscous forces. In the normal arterial circulation, Reynolds numbers are usually less than 2000, and true turbulence is unlikely to occur; however, Reynolds numbers over 2000 can be found in the ascending aorta, where small areas of turbulence develop.[3] Although turbulent flow is uncommon in normal arteries, the arterial flow pattern is often disturbed.[5] The condition of disturbed flow is an intermediate state between stable laminar flow and fully developed turbulence. It is a transient perturbation in the laminar streamlines that disappears as the flow proceeds downstream. Arterial flow may become disturbed at points of branching and curvature.

When turbulence is the result of a stenotic arterial lesion, it generally occurs immediately downstream from the stenosis and may be present only over the systolic portion of the cardiac cycle when the critical value of the Reynolds number is exceeded. Under conditions of turbulent flow, the velocity profile changes from the parabolic shape of laminar flow to a rectangular or blunt shape (Fig. 12–7). Because of the random velocity changes, energy losses are greater for a turbulent or disturbed flow state than a laminar flow state. Consequently, the linear relationship between pressure and flow expressed by Poiseuille's law cannot be applied. This deviation from Poiseuille's law in arterial flow is shown in Figure 12–3.

Boundary Layer Separation

In fluid flowing through a tube, the portion of fluid adjacent to the tube wall is referred to as the boundary layer. This layer is subject to both frictional interactions with the tube wall and viscous forces generated by the more rapidly moving fluid toward the center of the tube. When the tube geometry changes suddenly, such as at points of curvature, branching, or alteration in lumen diameter, small pressure gradients are created that cause the boundary layer to stop or reverse direction. This results in a complex, localized flow pattern known as an area of flow separation or separation zone.[6]

Areas of boundary layer separation have been observed in models of arterial anastomoses and bifurcations.[7,8] In the carotid artery bifurcation shown in Figure 12–8, the central rapid flow stream of the common carotid artery is compressed along the inner wall of the carotid bulb, producing a region of high shear stress. An area of flow separation has formed along the outer wall of the carotid bulb that includes helical flow patterns and flow reversal. The region of the carotid bulb adjacent to the separation zone is subject to relatively low shear stresses. Distal to the bulb, in the internal carotid artery, flow reattachment occurs and a more laminar flow pattern is present.

The complex flow patterns described in models of the carotid bifurcation have also been documented in human subjects by pulsed Doppler studies.[9,10] As shown in Figure 12–9, the Doppler spectral waveform obtained near the inner wall of the carotid bulb is typical of the forward, quasi-steady flow pattern found in the internal carotid artery. However, sam-

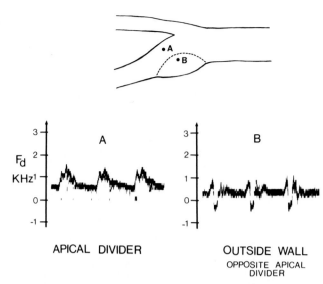

FIGURE 12–9. Flow separation in the normal carotid bulb shown by pulsed Doppler spectral analysis. The flow pattern near the apical divider (*A*) is forward throughout the cardiac cycle, but near the outside wall (*B*) the spectrum contains both forward (positive) and reverse (negative) flow components. The latter pattern indicates an area of flow separation. (Reproduced with permission of J. F. Primozich, B.S., and D. J. Phillips, Ph.D.)

pling of flow along the outer wall of the bulb demonstrates lower velocities with periods of both forward and reverse flow. These spectral characteristics are consistent with the presence of flow separation and are considered to be a normal finding, particularly in young individuals.[10] Alterations in arterial distensibility with increasing age make flow separation less prominent in older individuals.[11]

The clinical importance of boundary layer separation is that these localized flow disturbances may contribute to the formation of atherosclerotic plaques.[12] Examination of human carotid bifurcations, both at autopsy and during surgery, indicates that intimal thickening and atherosclerosis tend to occur along the outer wall of the carotid bulb, while the inner wall is relatively spared.[8] These findings suggest that atherosclerotic lesions form near areas of flow separation and low shear stress. Whether flow separation represents a true causative factor or simply promotes the development of previously existing lesions is not known.

Pulsatile Flow

In a pulsatile system, pressure and flow vary continuously with time, and the velocity profile changes throughout the cardiac cycle. The hemodynamic principles that have been discussed are based on steady flow, and they are not adequate for a precise description of pulsatile flow in the arterial circulation; however, as previously stated, they can be used to determine the minimal energy losses occurring in a specific flow system.

The complex interactions of cardiac contraction, arterial wall characteristics, and blood flow are extremely difficult to define rigorously. For example,

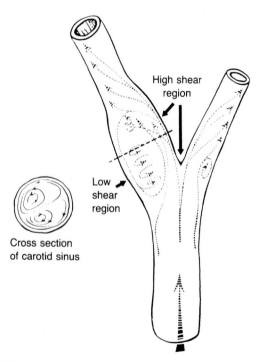

FIGURE 12–8. Carotid artery bifurcation showing an area of flow separation adjacent to the outer wall of the bulb. Rapid flow is associated with high shear stress, whereas the slower flow of the separation zone produces a region of low shear. (From Zarins CK, Giddens DP, Glagov S: Atherosclerotic plaque distribution and flow velocity profiles in the carotid bifurcation. *In* Bergan JJ, Yao JST (eds): Cerebrovascular Insufficiency. New York, Grune & Stratton, 1983.)

estimation of the inertial energy losses in pulsatile flow requires a value for the velocity term (Eq. 9); however, in pulsatile flow, velocity varies with both time and position across the flow profile. Furthermore, skewing of the velocity profile may occur as a result of curvature or branching. The resistance term of Poiseuille's law (Eq. 11) estimates viscous energy losses in steady flow, but it does not account for the inertial effects, arterial wall elasticity, and wave reflections that influence pulsatile flow. The term "vascular impedance" is used to describe the resistance or opposition offered by a peripheral vascular bed to pulsatile blood flow.[3]

Pulsatile flow appears to be important for optimum organ function. For example, when a kidney is perfused by steady flow instead of pulsatile flow a reduction in urine volume and sodium excretion occurs.[13] The critical effect of pulsatile flow is probably exerted on the microcirculation. While the exact mechanism is unknown, transcapillary exchange, arteriolar tone, and lymphatic flow are all influenced by the pulsatile nature of blood flow.

Bifurcations and Branches

The branches of the arterial system produce sudden changes in the flow pattern that are potential sources of energy loss. However, the effect of branching on the total pressure drop in normal arterial flow is relatively small. Arterial branches commonly take the form of bifurcations. Flow patterns in a bifurcation are determined mainly by the area ratio and the branch angle. The area ratio is defined as the combined area of the secondary branches divided by the area of the primary artery.

Bifurcation flow can be analyzed in terms of pressure gradient, velocity, and transmission of pulsatile energy. According to Poiseuille's law, an area ratio of 1.41 would allow the pressure gradient to remain constant along a bifurcation. If the combined area of the branches equals the area of the primary artery, then the area ratio is 1.0 and there will be no change in the velocity of flow.[14] For efficient transmission of pulsatile energy across a bifurcation the vascular impedance of the primary artery should equal that of the branches, a situation that occurs with an area ratio of 1.15 for larger arteries and 1.35 for smaller arteries.[15] Although human infants have a favorable area ratio of 1.11 at the aortic bifurcation, there is a gradual decrease in the ratio with age. In the second decade of life the average area ratio is less than 1.0, in the third decade it is less than 0.9, and by the fifth decade it drops below 0.8.[16] This decline in the area ratio of the aortic bifurcation leads to an increase in both the velocity of flow in the secondary branches and the amount of reflected pulsatile energy. For example, with an area ratio of 0.8, approximately 22 per cent of the incident pulsatile energy will be reflected in the infrarenal aorta. This mechanism may play a role in the localization of atherosclerosis and aneurysms in this arterial segment.[17]

The curvature and angulation of an arterial bifur-cation can also contribute to the development of flow disturbances. As blood flows around a curve, the high-velocity portion of the stream is subjected to the greatest centrifugal force; rapidly moving fluid in the center of the vessel tends to flow outward and be replaced by the slower fluid originally located near the arterial wall. This can result in complex helical flow patterns such as those observed in the carotid bifurcation.[9] As the angle between the secondary branches of a bifurcation is increased, the tendency to develop turbulent or disturbed flow also rises. The average angle between the human iliac arteries is 54 degrees; however, with diseased or tortuous iliac arteries this angle can approach 180 degrees.[3] In the latter situation, flow disturbances are particularly likely to develop.

Physical Properties of the Arterial Wall

Composition of the Arterial Wall

Blood vessels are viscoelastic tubes. In this context, viscosity refers to the resistance of a material to shear, and elasticity describes the tendency of a material to return to its original shape after being subjected to a deforming force. As blood proceeds from the large arteries of the thorax and abdomen to the medium-sized arteries of the extremities, the relative amount of elastic tissue in the vessel wall decreases as the amount of collagen and smooth muscle increases. At the level of the arteriole, the wall consists almost entirely of smooth muscle. Thus, the viscoelastic properties of an artery depend primarily on the elastin-collagen ratio. Elastin is the predominant component of the thoracic aorta that allows energy to be stored during cardiac systole and returned to the system in diastole. Since collagen is much less extensible than elastin, the more distal arteries, such as the brachial and femoral, do not store much of the pulsatile energy but serve mainly as conduits for blood. The function of the muscular arterioles is to control blood pressure and flow by actively altering the lumen diameter.

As the structure of the arterial wall changes, each successive branching also increases the total cross-sectional area of the arterial tree. The cross-sectional area at the arteriolar level is approximately 125 times that of the aorta; at the capillary level it has increased approximately 800 times.[3] The reduced elastin-collagen ratio and increased stiffness of the peripheral arteries result in a more rapid pulse wave velocity and a high vascular impedance. While the impedance of the thoracic aorta must be low to minimize cardiac work, the impedance of peripheral arteries should match the high arteriolar impedance to decrease the reflected components of the pulse wave.

Tangential Stress and Tension

The tangential stress (τ) within the wall of a fluid-filled cylindrical tube can be expressed as

$$\tau = P\frac{r}{\delta} \qquad (15)$$

where P is the pressure exerted by the fluid (in dynes per square centimeter), r is the internal radius (in centimeters), and δ is the thickness of the tube wall (in centimeters). Stress (τ) has the dimensions of force per unit area of tube wall (dynes per square centimeter). Thus, tangential stress is directly proportional to pressure and radius, but inversely proportional to wall thickness.

Equation 15 is similar to Laplace's law, which defines tangential tension (T) as the product of pressure and radius

$$T = Pr \qquad (16)$$

Tension is given in units of force per tube length (dynes per centimeter). The terms "stress" and "tension" have different dimensions and describe the forces acting on the tube wall in different ways. Laplace's law can be used to characterize thin-walled structures like soap bubbles; however, it is not suitable for describing the stresses in arterial walls.

Arterial Wall Properties in Specific Conditions

Aging and Atherosclerosis. Arterial walls become less distensible with age. This increase in stiffness cannot be explained on the basis of atherosclerosis alone.[3] Alterations in the elastin fibers and elastic lamellae, together with an increase in wall thickness, probably account for this increase in arterial stiffness. Changes associated with aging include fragmentation of elastic lamellae and deposition of collagen between the elastin layers. This tends to maintain the elastin fibers in the extended state. Calcium is also deposited near the elastin fibers and contributes to the increased thickness of the arterial wall.

The effects of atherosclerosis on the mechanical properties of the arterial wall are complex and difficult to distinguish from those due to aging. In the early stages, arterial distensibility may actually increase as elastin fibers are disrupted; however, as the disease progresses, fibrosis and calcification tend to make the arterial wall less distensible.

Endarterectomy. During an endarterectomy, the atherosclerotic plaque is removed along with the intima and a portion of the media, leaving behind a tube consisting of the outer media and adventitia. This reduces the wall thickness to approximately one third of its original value and should result in an increase in tangential stress according to Eq. 15. As would be expected, endarterectomy decreases the stiffness of an artery to circumferential expansion.[18] Still, the endarterectomized artery remains stiffer and less distensible than a normal artery. This indicates that the components responsible for strength and stiffness are concentrated in the outer layers of the arterial wall. It is because of this anatomic arrangement that endarterectomy is possible.

Aneurysms. When the structural components of

the arterial wall are weakened, aneurysms may form. Rupture occurs when the tangential stress within the arterial wall becomes greater than the tensile strength. Figure 12–10 shows a tube with an outside diameter of 2.0 cm and a wall thickness of 0.2 cm, dimensions similar to those of atherosclerotic aortas.[1] If the internal pressure is 150 mm Hg, the tangential wall stress will be 8.0×10^5 dyne/cm². Expansion of the tube to form a 6.0-cm diameter aneurysm results in a decrease in wall thickness to 0.06 cm. The increased radius and decreased wall thickness will increase the wall stress to 98.0×10^5 dyne/cm², assuming that the pressure remains constant. In this example, the diameter has been enlarged by a factor of 3 and the wall stress has increased by a factor of 12.

While the tensile strength of collagen is extremely high, it constitutes only about 15 per cent of the aneurysm wall.[19] Furthermore, the collagen fibers in an aneurysm are sparsely distributed and subject to fragmentation. The tendency of larger aneurysms to rupture is readily explained by the effect of increased radius on tangential stress (Eq. 15) and the degenerative changes in the arterial wall. The relationship between tangential stress and blood pressure accounts for the contribution of hypertension to the risk of rupture.

The diverging and converging geometry of aneurysms can result in complex flow patterns that include areas of boundary layer separation and flow reversal.[20] These patterns explain the frequent accumulation of clot in aneurysms that confines the flow stream to an area not much larger than the native artery. Since this clot increases the effective thickness of the vessel wall, it may reduce tangential stress and provide some protection against rupture. However, the tensile strength of clot and arterial wall

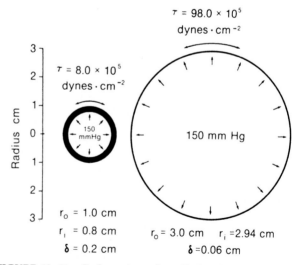

FIGURE 12–10. End-on view of a cylinder, 2 cm in diameter, that is expanded to 6 cm in diameter while wall area remains constant. τ = wall stress, δ = wall thickness, r_i = inside radius, r_o = outside radius. (From Sumner DS: The hemodynamics and pathophysiology of arterial disease. *In* Rutherford RB (ed): Vascular Surgery. Philadelphia, WB Saunders Company, 1977.)

are not the same, and the contribution of clot to the integrity of an aneurysm is impossible to predict.[3] Furthermore, the clot within an aneurysm is often not circumferential. In this situation, Eq. 15 can be applied to the wall segment without clot, and the tangential stress at that site will depend on the maximum internal radius.

Another factor to consider is that in about 55 per cent of the ruptured abdominal aortic aneurysms the site of rupture is in the posterolateral aspect of the aneurysm wall.[21] The posterior wall of the aorta is relatively fixed against the spine, and repeated flexion of the wall in that area could result in structural fatigue. This would produce a localized area of weakness that might predispose to rupture.

HEMODYNAMICS OF ARTERIAL STENOSES

Energy Losses Related to Arterial Stenoses

According to Poiseuille's law (Eq. 8), the radius of a stenotic segment will have a much greater effect on viscous energy losses than its length. Inertial energy losses, which occur at the entrance (contraction effects) and exit (expansion effects) of a stenosis, are proportional to the square of blood velocity (Eq. 9). Energy losses are also influenced by the geometry of a stenosis; a gradual tapering results in less energy loss than an irregular or abrupt change in lumen size. A converging vessel geometry tends to stabilize laminar flow and flatten the velocity profile, while a diverging vessel produces an elongated velocity profile and a less stable flow pattern. The energy lost at the exit of a stenosis may be quite significant because of the sudden expansion of the flow stream and dissipation of kinetic energy in a zone of turbulence.

The energy lost in expansion (ΔP) can be expressed in terms of the flow velocity distal to the stenosis (v), and the radii of the stenotic lumen (r_S) and the normal distal lumen (r):

$$\Delta P = k \frac{\rho}{2} v^2 \left[\left(\frac{r}{r_S} \right)^2 - 1 \right]^2 \qquad (17)$$

Figure 12–11 illustrates the energy losses related to a 1-cm long stenosis. The viscous losses are relatively small and occur within the stenotic segment. Inertial losses due to contraction and expansion are much greater. Since most of the energy loss in this example results from inertial effects, the length of the stenosis is relatively unimportant.[1]

Bruits and Poststenotic Dilation

The presence of an audible sound or bruit over an artery is usually regarded as a clinical sign of arterial disease. Stenoses or irregularities of the vessel lumen produce turbulent flow patterns that set up vibrations in the arterial wall. These vibrations generate displacement waves that radiate through the surrounding tissues and can be detected as audible sounds. Such vibrations are probably the main source of sound in the arterial system.[3]

Generally, a soft, midsystolic bruit is associated with a relatively minor lesion that does not significantly reduce flow or pressure. A bruit with a loud diastolic component suggests a stenosis severe enough to reduce flow and produce a pressure drop. Thus, the intensity and duration of a bruit serve as a rough guide to the severity of an arterial stenosis. A bruit may be absent when an artery is nearly occluded or when the flow rate is extremely low.

A dilated area distal to a stenosis is a common clinical finding. Poststenotic dilation has been observed in the thoracic aorta below coarctations, distal to arterial stenoses at the thoracic outlet, and distal to atherosclerotic lesions. The most likely explanation for this phenomenon is that arterial wall vibrations result in structural fatigue of elastin fibers. In a series of animal model studies, poststenotic dilations did not develop unless a bruit was present distal to the stenosis.[22] It appears that vibrations in the audible range may weaken elastin fibers and break down links between collagen fibers. When this occurs, the arterial wall distal to the stenosis becomes more distensible and subject to localized dilation.

Critical Arterial Stenosis

The degree of arterial narrowing required to produce a significant reduction in blood pressure or flow is called a *critical stenosis*. Because the energy losses associated with a stenosis are inversely proportional to the fourth power of the radius at that site (Eqs. 8 and 17), there is an exponential relationship between energy loss (pressure drop) and reduction in lumen size. When this relationship is illustrated graphically, the curves have a single sharp bend (Figs. 12–5 and 12–12). These observations provide theoretical support for the concept of critical stenosis.[23,24]

As previously noted, blood flow velocity is a major determinant of fluid energy losses (Eqs. 8, 9, and 17). Thus, the pressure drop across a stenosis varies with the flow rate. Because flow velocity depends on the distal hemodynamic resistance, the critical stenosis value also varies with the resistance of the runoff bed. In Figure 12–12, a system with a high flow velocity (low resistance) shows a reduction in pressure with less narrowing than a system with low flow velocity (high resistance). The higher flow velocities produce curves that are less sharply bent making the point of critical stenosis less distinct.

Another observation related to critical stenosis is that the decrease in flow is linearly related to the increase in pressure gradient as long as the peripheral resistance remains constant (Fig. 12–13).[24] In this situation, the curves for pressure drop and flow re-

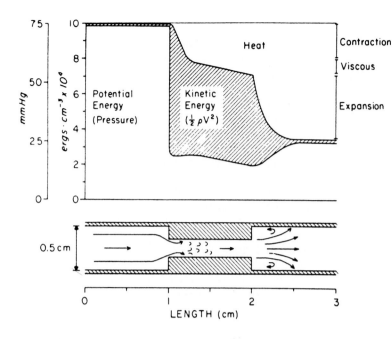

FIGURE 12–11. Energy losses resulting when blood flows steadily through a 1-cm-long stenosis. Inertial losses (contraction and expansion) are more significant than viscous losses. (From Sumner DS: The hemodynamics and pathophysiology of arterial disease. *In* Rutherford RB (ed): Vascular Surgery. Philadelphia, WB Saunders Company, 1977.)

duction are mirror images of each other, and the critical stenosis value is the same for both. Many vascular beds are able to maintain a constant level of blood flow over a wide range of perfusion pressures by the mechanism of autoregulation. This is achieved by constriction of resistance vessels in response to an increase in blood pressure and dilation of resistance vessels when blood pressure decreases. For example, autoregulation permits the brain to maintain normal flow rates down to perfusion pressures in the range of 50 to 60 mm Hg.[25]

Significant changes in pressure and flow begin to

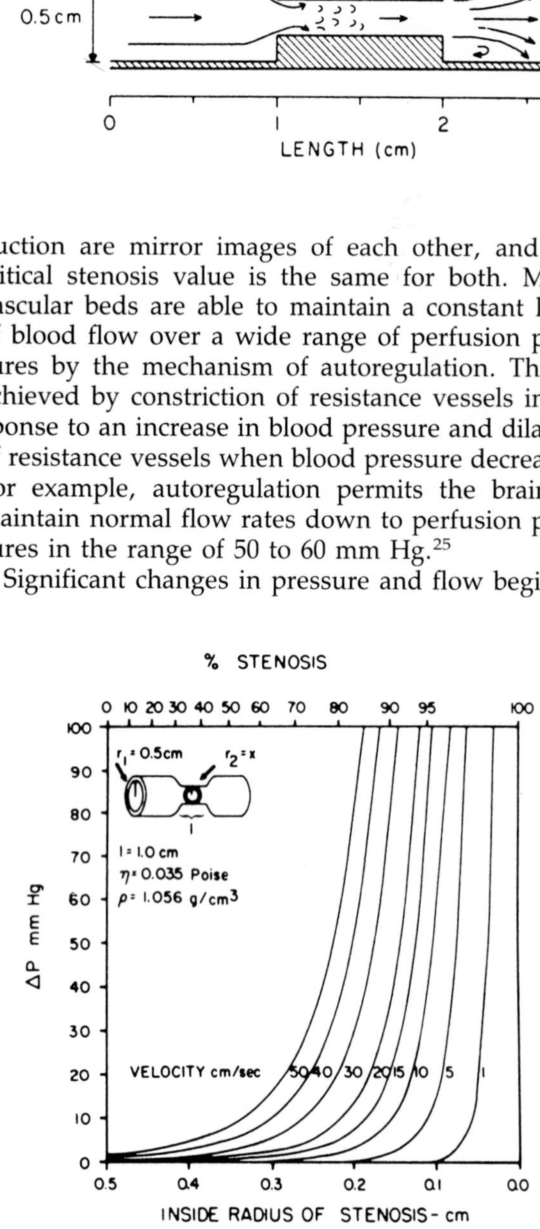

FIGURE 12–12. Relationship of pressure drop across a stenosis to the radius of the stenotic segment and the flow velocity. (From Strandness DE, Sumner DS: Hemodynamics for Surgeons. New York, Grune & Stratton, 1975.)

occur when the arterial lumen has been reduced by about 50 per cent of its diameter or 75 per cent of its cross-sectional area; however, the concept of critical stenosis is strictly valid only when the flow conditions are specified. Consequently, a stenosis that is not significant at resting flow rates may become critical when flow rates are increased by reactive hyperemia or exercise. For example, iliac stenoses that do not appear severe by arteriography may be associated with significant pressure gradients during exercise.[26] Because of the complex geometry of atherosclerotic lesions and the wide variation in arterial flow rates, it is often difficult to predict the hemodynamic significance of a lesion based on the apparent reduction in lumen size. Therefore, physiologic testing by blood pressure measurement must be used to document the clinical severity of arterial lesions.[27,28]

Effect of Stenosis Length and Multiple Stenoses

Poiseuille's law predicts that the radius of a stenosis will have a much greater effect on viscous energy losses than its length (Eq. 8). If the length of a stenosis is doubled, the viscous energy losses are also doubled; however, reducing the radius by one half increases energy losses by a factor of 16. Furthermore, inertial energy losses are independent of stenosis length and are especially prominent at the exit of a stenosis (Fig. 12–11 and Eq. 17). Since energy losses are primarily due to entrance and exit effects, separate short stenoses tend to be more significant than a single longer stenosis. It has been shown experimentally that when stenoses that are not significant individually are arranged in series, large reductions in pressure and flow can occur.[29] Thus,

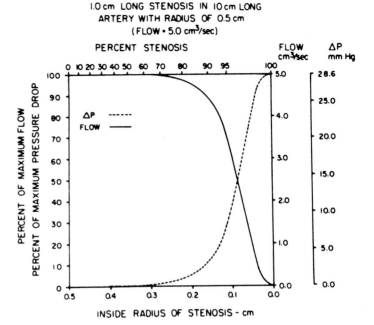

FIGURE 12–13. Effect of increasing stenosis on blood flow and pressure drop across the stenotic segment. Collateral and peripheral resistances are considered to be fixed. (From Strandness DE, Sumner DS: Hemodynamics for Surgeons. New York, Grune & Stratton, 1975.)

multiple subcritical stenoses may have the same effect as a single critical stenosis.

Based on the preceding discussion, several points can be made about stenoses in series. When two stenoses are of similar diameter, removal of one will provide only a modest increase in blood flow. If the stenoses have different diameters, removal of the least severe will have little effect while removal of the most severe will improve blood flow significantly.

These principles apply only to unbranched arterial segments such as the internal carotid. In the presence of a severe stenosis in the carotid siphon, removal of a less severe lesion at the carotid bifurcation is not likely to result in significant hemodynamic improvement. On the other hand, when the proximal lesion involves an artery that supplies a collateral bed that parallels a distal lesion, removal of the proximal lesion can be beneficial. For example, when there is an iliac stenosis and superficial femoral occlusion, removal of the iliac lesion usually improves perfusion of the lower leg by increasing flow through the profunda-geniculate collateral system.

ARTERIAL FLOW PATTERNS IN HUMAN LIMBS

Collateral Circulation

When arterial obstruction occurs, blood must pass through a network of collateral vessels to bypass the diseased segment. The functional capacity of the collateral circulation will vary according to the level and extent of occlusive lesions. As mentioned in the preceding example, the profunda-geniculate system can compensate to a large degree for an isolated super-

ficial femoral artery occlusion; however, the addition of an iliac lesion will severely limit collateral flow.

A typical hemodynamic circuit includes the diseased major artery, a parallel system of collateral vessels, and the peripheral runoff bed (Fig. 12–14). The collateral system consists of stem arteries, which are large distributing branches, a midzone of smaller intramuscular channels, and reentry vessels that join the major artery distal to the point of obstruction.[30] These vessels are preexisting pathways that enlarge when flow through the parallel major artery is reduced. The main stimuli for collateral development are an abnormal pressure gradient across the collateral system and increased velocity of flow through the midzone vessels.[31] This mechanism is consistent with the gradual improvement in collateral circulation that results from a regular exercise program in patients with lower extremity arterial occlusive disease.[32]

Collateral vessels are smaller, longer, and more numerous than the major arteries that they replace. Although considerable enlargement may occur in the midzone vessels, collateral resistance is always greater than that of the original unobstructed artery. In addition, the acute changes in collateral resistance during exercise are minimal.[33] Therefore, the resistance of a collateral system is, for practical purposes, fixed.

Distribution of Vascular Resistance and Blood Flow

Unlike collateral resistance, the resistance of a peripheral runoff bed is quite variable. The muscular arterioles are primarily responsible for regulating peripheral resistance and controlling the distribution of

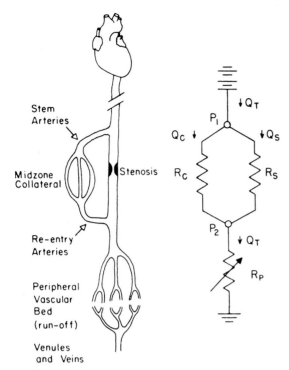

FIGURE 12–14. Major components of a hemodynamic circuit containing a stenotic artery. The analogous electrical circuit is shown on the right with the heart represented as a battery and the central veins as a ground. Flows are represented by Q_T (total), Q_C (collateral), and Q_S (stenosis). Resistances are represented by R_C (collateral), R_S (stenosis), and R_P (peripheral runoff); R_C and R_S are fixed. R_P is variable. (From Sumner DS: The hemodynamics and pathophysiology of arterial disease. *In* Rutherford RB (ed): Vascular Surgery. Philadelphia, WB Saunders Company, 1977.)

blood flow to various capillary beds. Arteriolar tone is mainly determined by the sympathetic nervous system, but it is also subject to the influence of locally produced metabolites.

When discussing blood flow in the lower limb, it is useful to separate vascular resistance into segmental and peripheral components. Segmental resistance consists of the relatively fixed parallel resistances of the major normal or diseased artery and the by-passing collateral vessels, such as the superficial femoral artery and the profunda-geniculate system. Peripheral resistance includes the highly variable resistances of the distal calf muscle arterioles and cutaneous circulation. The total vascular resistance of the limb can be estimated by adding the segmental and peripheral resistances (Eqs. 12 and 13).

Normally, the resting segmental resistance is very low and the peripheral resistance is relatively high; therefore, the pressure drop across the femoropopliteal segment is minimal. With exercise, the peripheral resistance falls and flow through the segmental arteries increases by a factor of up to 10, with little or no pressure drop.

With moderate arterial disease, such as an isolated superficial femoral artery occlusion, the segmental resistance is increased as a result of collateral flow, and an abnormal pressure drop is present across the

thigh. Because of a compensatory decrease in peripheral resistance, the total resistance of the limb and the resting blood flow often remain in the normal range.[34] During exercise, the segmental resistance remains high and fixed, while the peripheral resistance decreases further. However, the capacity of the peripheral circulation to compensate for a high segmental resistance is limited, and exercise flow is less than normal. In this situation, exercise is associated with a still larger pressure drop across the diseased arterial segment. The clinical result is calf muscle ischemia or claudication.

When arterial disease becomes severe, as in combined iliofemoral and tibioperoneal occlusive disease, the compensatory decrease in peripheral resistance may be unable to provide normal blood flow at rest. In this case, there is a marked pressure drop across the involved arterial segments and little or no increase in blood flow with exercise. Claudication will be severe, and ischemic rest pain or ulceration may develop.

These changes in the distribution of vascular resistance in the lower limb explain the alterations in blood pressure and flow observed in patients with arterial occlusive disease.

Arterial Pulses and Waveforms

The heart generates a complex pressure pulse that is modified by arterial wall properties and changes in vascular resistance as it progresses distally. Normally, the peak systolic pressure is amplified as it passes down the lower limb.[3] This is due to a progressive decrease in arterial compliance and reflections originating from the relatively high peripheral resistance. Consequently, the systolic pressure at the ankle is higher than that in the upper arm, and the ankle-arm pressure ratio is greater than 1. However, the diastolic and mean pressures gradually decrease as the blood moves distally.

When blood flows through an arterial stenosis or a high-resistance collateral bed, the distal pulse pressure is reduced to a greater extent than the mean pressure.[35] This indicates that the systolic pressure beyond a lesion is a more sensitive indicator of hemodynamic significance than the mean pressure. It is well known that palpable pedal pulses in patients with superficial femoral artery stenosis can disappear after leg exercise. This occurs when increased flow through high-resistance vessels causes a reduction in pulse pressure. The contour of the pressure pulse also reflects the presence of proximal arterial disease. These changes can be demonstrated plethysmographically and include a delayed upslope, rounded peak, and bowing of the downslope away from the baseline.[36]

Changes in the flow pulse are also useful to characterize the state of the arterial system. While the peak pressure increases, the peak of the flow pulse decreases as the periphery is approached.[3] The flow pattern in the major arteries of the leg is normally triphasic (Fig. 12–15). An initial large forward-velocity phase resulting from cardiac systole is followed by a brief phase of flow reversal in early diastole and a third smaller phase of forward flow in the late diastole. This triphasic pattern is modified by a variety of factors, including proximal arterial disease and changes in peripheral resistance. For example, body heating, which causes vasodilation and decreased resistance, will abolish the second phase of flow reversal; on exposure to cold, resistance increases and the reverse-flow phase becomes more prominent. Since a stenotic lesion is accompanied by a compensatory decrease in peripheral resistance, one of the earliest changes noted distal to a stenosis is the disappearance of the reverse-flow phase (Fig. 12–15). As a stenosis becomes more severe, the distal flow pattern becomes monophasic, with a slow rise, a rounded peak, and a gradual decline toward the baseline in diastole. The character of the flow pulse proximal to an arterial obstruction is variable and depends on the capacity of the collateral circulation. These flow patterns can be studied noninvasively using a Doppler velocity detector and strip-chart recorder.

Pressure and Flow in Normal Limbs

As the pressure pulse moves distally, the systolic pressure rises, the diastolic pressure falls, and the pulse pressure becomes wider. The fall in mean arterial pressure between the heart and ankle is normally less than 10 mm Hg. In normal individuals at rest, the ratio of ankle systolic pressure to brachial systolic pressure

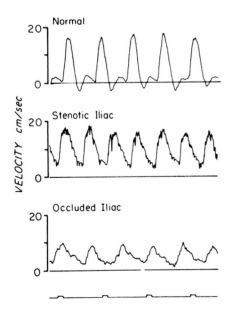

FIGURE 12–15. Velocity flow waveforms obtained with a directional Doppler velocity detector from the femoral artery of a normal subject, a patient with external iliac stenosis, and a patient with common iliac occlusion. (From Strandness DE, Sumner DS: Hemodynamics for Surgeons. New York, Grune & Stratton, 1975.)

(ankle-arm index) has a mean value of 1.11 ± 0.10.[37] Moderate exercise in normal extremities produces little or no drop in ankle systolic pressure. Strenuous effort may be associated with a drop of several millimeters of mercury; however, pressures return rapidly to resting levels after cessation of exercise.

The average blood flow in the normal human leg is in the range of 300 to 500 ml/min under resting conditions.[3] Blood flow to the muscles of the lower leg is approximately 2.0 ml/100 g/min. With moderate exercise, total leg blood flow increases by a factor of 5 to 10, and muscle blood flow rises to around 30 ml/100 g/min. During strenuous exercise, muscle blood flow may reach 70 ml/100 g/min. After cessation of exercise, blood flow decreases rapidly and returns to resting values within 1 to 5 minutes.

Pressure and Flow in Limbs with Arterial Obstruction

If an arterial lesion is hemodynamically significant at rest, there will be a measurable reduction in distal blood pressure. Generally, limbs with a lesion at one anatomic level have ankle-arm indices between 0.9 and 0.5, whereas limbs with occlusions at multiple anatomic levels have indices less than 0.5.[28] The ankle-arm index also correlates with the clinical severity of disease: in limbs with intermittent claudication, the index has a mean value of 0.59 ± 0.15; in limbs with ischemic rest pain, 0.26 ± 0.13; and in limbs with impending gangrene, 0.05 ± 0.08.[37]

Because of the increased segmental vascular resistance in limbs with arterial occlusive disease, the ankle systolic blood pressure will fall dramatically during leg exercise. As indicated in Figures 12–16, 12–17, and 12–18, the extent and duration of the pressure drop are proportional to the severity of the arterial lesions. Recovery of pressure to resting levels may require up to 30 minutes.[28]

Resting leg or calf blood flow in patients with intermittent claudication is not significantly different from values obtained in normal individuals. However, the capacity to increase limb blood flow during exercise is quite limited, and pain occurs in the muscles that have been rendered ischemic. The pain of claudication is presumably due to the accumulation of metabolic products that are removed under normal flow conditions. As the occlusive process becomes more severe, the decrease in peripheral vascular resistance can no longer compensate, and resting flow may be less than normal. When this occurs, ischemic rest pain or ulceration may appear. As shown in Figures 12–16, 12–17, and 12–18, the capacity to increase calf blood flow with exercise depends on the severity of arterial disease. With increasing degrees of disease, the hyperemia that follows exercise becomes more prolonged, and the peak calf blood flow is both decreased and delayed. In some cases, flow may fall below resting levels.[28] The ankle blood pressure returns to normal after peak flows have started to decline.

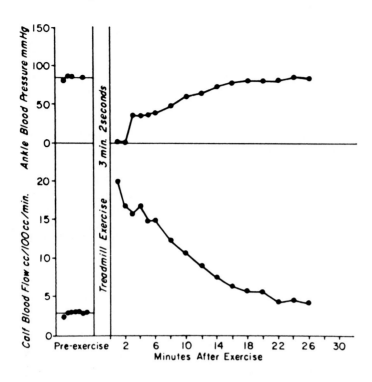

FIGURE 12–16. Preexercise and postexercise ankle blood pressure and calf blood flow in a patient with severe stenosis of the superficial femoral artery. (From Sumner DS, Strandness DE: The relationship between calf blood flow and ankle blood pressure in patients with intermittent claudication. Surgery *65*:763, 1969.)

The changes in blood pressure and flow in lower limbs with arterial occlusive disease provide the basis for noninvasive diagnostic tests. By monitoring the ankle systolic pressure before and after treadmill exercise or reactive hyperemia, two components of the physiologic response can be evaluated: (1) the magnitude of the immediate pressure drop, and (2) the time for recovery to resting pressure. The changes in both of these parameters are proportional to the severity of arterial disease.[38]

Vascular Steal

Hemodynamic arrangements in which one vascular bed draws blood away or "steals" from another

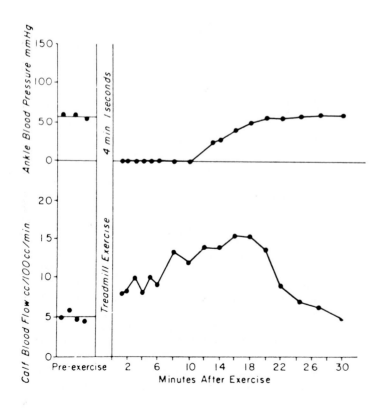

FIGURE 12–17. Preexercise and postexercise ankle blood pressure and calf blood flow in a patient with iliac stenosis and superficial femoral artery occlusion. (From Sumner DS, Strandness DE: The relationship between calf blood flow and ankle blood pressure in patients with intermittent claudication. Surgery *65*:763, 1969.)

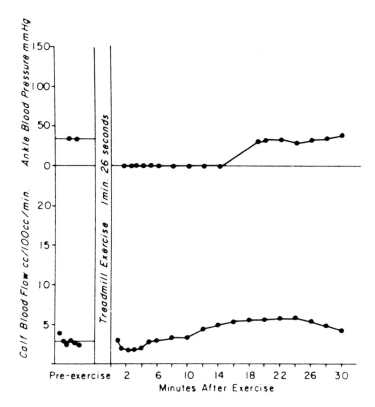

FIGURE 12–18. Preexercise and postexercise ankle blood pressure and calf blood flow in a patient with occlusion of the iliac, common femoral, and superficial femoral arteries. This patient had moderate rest pain and severe claudication. (From Sumner DS, Strandness DE: The relationship between calf blood flow and ankle blood pressure in patients with intermittent claudication. Surgery 65:763, 1969.)

can occur in a variety of situations. A vascular steal may arise when two runoff beds with different resistances must be supplied by a limited source of inflow.

Multiple Level Occlusive Disease

One example of the steal phenomenon involves a limb with lesions in both the iliac and superficial femoral arteries.[1] Between the fixed resistances of these two arterial lesions is the profunda orifice, which supplies the variable resistance of the thigh. The resistance of the distal calf runoff bed is also variable. Under resting conditions, normal leg blood flow can be maintained by a nearly maximal decrease in calf resistance and a moderate decrease in thigh resistance. This will be apparent clinically as an abnormally low ankle systolic pressure. With the increased metabolic demands of exercise, the thigh resistance can decrease further, but the calf resistance has already reached its lower limit. This results in a further pressure drop across the proximal iliac lesion, which reduces the pressure perfusing the calf. Blood flow to the calf will be decreased until the thigh resistance rises and thigh blood flow begins to fall. In this situation, the effect of exercise is to increase thigh blood flow, decrease calf blood flow, and decrease distal blood pressure. The thigh steals blood from the calf because the proximal iliac lesion restricts inflow to both runoff beds.

Subclavian Steal Syndrome

In the subclavian steal syndrome, reversal of flow in the vertebral artery is associated with subclavian artery occlusion and symptoms of brainstem ischemia.[39] When occlusion is present in the proximal subclavian artery on the left or the innominate artery on the right, the pressure at the origin of the ipsilateral vertebral artery is reduced. This can result in reversal of flow in the vertebral artery, which then serves as a source of collateral circulation to the arm. The increased demands of arm exercise tend to augment the reversed flow, and the patient may experience ischemia of the brainstem. The hemodynamic effect is more severe with innominate artery occlusion than with isolated subclavian occlusion. With innominate occlusion, the origin of the right common carotid is also subject to reduced pressure, and the patterns of collateral circulation to the arm and brain become quite complicated. Blood passing down the vertebral artery on the side of the occlusion may be recovered, in part, by the right common carotid artery; however, during arm exercise, flow in the right common carotid may be reduced.

It is important to distinguish between symptomatic and asymptomatic subclavian steal. The presence of reversed vertebral artery flow, as demonstrated by arteriography, may be a normal variant without clinical significance.[40] In true subclavian steal syndrome, there is often a definite relationship between arm exercise and symptoms of brainstem ischemia. There will also be objective evidence of decreased blood flow to the involved arm, such as a diminished radial pulse and lowered brachial blood pressure relative to the contralateral arm.[41]

Extraanatomic Bypass Grafts

When an extraanatomic bypass is performed, a single donor artery must supply several vascular beds. In the case of a femorofemoral crossover graft, one iliac is the donor artery, the leg ipsilateral to the donor artery is the donor limb, and the contralateral leg is the recipient limb. Studies of crossover grafts in animal models have shown that the immediate effect of the graft is to double the flow in the donor artery.[42,43] When an arteriovenous fistula is created in the recipient limb, graft flows may increase by a factor of 10 without any evidence of a steal from the donor limb.

These experimental observations are consistent with hemodynamic data from patients with femorofemoral grafts.[44] Improvement in the ankle-arm index on the recipient side can be achieved, even in the presence of significant occlusive disease in both the donor and recipient limbs. Although the ankle-arm index may decrease slightly on the donor side, a symptomatic steal is extremely uncommon. The most important factor contributing to vascular steal with a femorofemoral graft is stenosis of the donor iliac artery. With iliac stenosis, a steal is most likely to occur during exercise, when flow rates are increased. A mildly stenotic iliac can be used as a donor artery when high flow rates are not needed, such as in the treatment of ischemic rest pain. However, when increased flow rates are required to improve the walking distance of a patient with claudication, stenosis of the donor iliac may result in a steal from the donor limb. Occlusive disease in the arteries of the donor limb distal to the origin of the graft will not result in a steal providing that the donor iliac artery is normal.

These principles also apply to other types of extraanatomic bypass grafts, including axillary-axillary, carotid-subclavian, and axillofemoral grafts.[42,45]

HEMODYNAMIC PRINCIPLES AND THE TREATMENT OF ARTERIAL DISEASE

It should be apparent from the preceding discussion that the high fixed segmental resistance of the diseased major arteries and collaterals is responsible for decreased peripheral blood flow. Therefore, to be most effective in improving peripheral blood flow and relieving ischemic symptoms, therapy must be directed toward lowering this abnormally high segmental resistance. Since the peripheral resistance has already been lowered to compensate for the increased segmental resistance, attempts to further reduce the peripheral resistance are seldom beneficial.

While exercise therapy has been shown to improve collateral function, the degree of clinical improvement is usually modest.[32] In general, exercise therapy is best suited for patients with mild, stable claudication who are not candidates for direct intervention. Another method for improving peripheral blood flow in limbs with arterial disease is medically induced hypertension.[46] The administration of mineralocorticoid and sodium chloride raises systemic blood pressure and increases the head of pressure perfusing the diseased arterial segment. Although this technique has not been widely applied, it has been used successfully in patients with severe distal ischemia and ulceration.[46]

Direct Arterial Intervention

The most satisfactory approach to reducing the fixed segmental resistance is direct intervention by surgical or radiologic techniques. Depending on the nature of the lesions, endarterectomy, embolectomy, replacement grafting, or bypass grafting may be indicated. Percutaneous transluminal angioplasty may also be appropriate in selected cases.[47] In patients with occlusive disease involving a single anatomic level, a successful procedure should return all hemodynamic parameters to normal or near normal. This should be evident as an increase in the ankle-arm index and an improvement in the ankle pressure response to leg exercise.[48] However, since it is seldom possible to perform a perfect arterial reconstruction, it is common to detect a minor degree of residual hemodynamic impairment. When occlusions involve multiple levels, the treatment of one level should result in significant improvement, and the persisting hemodynamic abnormality will then reflect the remaining untreated disease. In such cases, the improvement is usually sufficient to increase claudication distance or relieve ischemic rest pain. The relative severity of lesions at different levels is often difficult to determine clinically; however, the basic principle is to initially treat the most proximal level of hemodynamically significant occlusive disease.

The factors required for optimal function of arterial bypass grafts can be analyzed in terms of basic hemodynamic principles. As previously noted, vessel diameter is the main determinant of hemodynamic resistance, so the diameter of a graft is considerably more important than its length. All prosthetic grafts develop a pseudointimal layer of variable thickness that further reduces the effective diameter.[3] Therefore, whenever the situation permits, a graft with a relatively large diameter should be used. Graft diameter is often limited by arterial size. In order to minimize energy losses associated with entrance and exit effects, the diameter of a graft should approximate that of the adjacent artery. When arteries of unequal size must be joined, a gradual transition is preferable. Thus, the graft should be slightly smaller than the proximal artery and slightly larger than the distal artery.

Theoretically, end-to-end anastomoses are preferable to those done end-to-side, since the end-to-end configuration eliminates energy losses due to curvature and angulation. However, these losses appear to be minimal under physiologic conditions, and in most clinical situations the anastomotic angle will be determined by technical factors. For example, reversed angulation has been used successfully in the construction of aortorenal and femorofemoral bypass grafts. Nevertheless, as a general rule, the smallest anastomotic angle that is technically feasible should be used. The width of an end-to-side anastomosis should be approximately equal to the diameter of the graft; the length of an anastomosis is less important but does serve as the main determinant of anastomotic angle. A carefully everted suture line also helps to minimize energy losses at anastomoses.

Bifurcation grafts, such as those used for aortofemoral bypass, are subject to the same general hemodynamic considerations as arterial bifurcations and branches. Most commercially available grafts have secondary limbs with diameters that are one half that of the primary tube, resulting in an area ratio of 0.5. In this configuration each of the secondary limbs has 16 times the resistance of the primary tube, and in parallel they offer 8 times the primary tube resistance. The flow velocity in the secondary limbs is doubled, and almost 50 per cent of the incident pulsatile energy is reflected at the graft bifurcation.[3] As previously discussed, the area ratio determines the hemodynamic characteristics of a bifurcation with respect to pressure gradient, flow velocity, and transmission of pulsatile energy. However, the optimal area ratio for grafts has not been established, and the geometry of bifurcation grafts has received relatively little attention. Instead, the development of prosthetic grafts has emphasized features such as graft material, porosity, and surface characteristics. In spite of their theoretical disadvantages, commercially available grafts have functioned extremely well in a variety of clinical applications.

Vasodilators

The rationale for the use of vasodilators is that they lower peripheral vascular resistance and improve limb blood flow. While this may occur in normal limbs, it is unlikely to be beneficial in limbs in which peripheral resistance is already decreased as a result of arterial disease. There is even a theoretical possibility that dilating vessels in relatively normal areas could divert blood away from the areas of ischemia. Most clinical studies of vasodilator therapy have failed to show a significant effect.[49,50] There is no conclusive evidence that vasodilators can increase flow in either collateral vessels or severely ischemic tissues. Consequently, there is no theoretical or clinical support for vasodilator therapy.

Sympathectomy

Since the purpose of sympathectomy is to reduce peripheral resistance by release of vasomotor tone, it is subject to the same general criticisms as vasodilator therapy. Because sympathectomy has little, if any, influence on collateral resistance, there is no rational basis for its use in the treatment of intermittent claudication.[51] Furthermore, exercise-induced muscle ischemia alone is a potent stimulus for peripheral vasodilation.

The use of sympathectomy for cutaneous ischemia has some physiologic basis, since the predominant effect is dilation of cutaneous arterioles. However, clinical improvement can occur only if the ischemic tissues are capable of further vasodilation, as demonstrated by reactive hyperemia testing.[36] Beneficial results have been obtained in patients with mild rest pain and superficial ischemic ulcers; patients with severe rest pain and extensive tissue loss are not likely to respond.[51] While sympathectomy has been recommended as an adjunct to arterial operations, there is little objective evidence that it improves either the early or late results of arterial reconstructive surgery.[52]

Rheologic Agents

According to Poiseuille's law, hemodynamic resistance is directly proportional to the blood viscosity (Eqs. 8 and 11). If the pressure remains constant and viscosity is reduced, flow will increase in proportion to the fall in viscosity. Procedures for lowering blood viscosity are most often used in the immediate postoperative period to increase flow through a reconstructed arterial segment.

Low-molecular-weight dextran (molecular weight 40,000) is the most commonly used agent for reducing blood viscosity. The increased peripheral blood flow observed after intravenous administration of low-molecular-weight dextran is the result of both peripheral vasodilation secondary to blood volume expansion and changes in viscosity due to hemodilution.[3] Dextran solutions also influence red cell aggregation and platelet function.[53]

An orally administered rheologic agent, pentoxifylline, has been evaluated in a multicenter clinical trial for the treatment of patients with intermittent claudication.[54] Pentoxifylline reduces blood viscosity by improving the membrane flexibility of red blood cells. The drug also has an inhibitory effect on platelet aggregation. During the clinical trial, the distance walked prior to onset of claudication increased in both the pentoxifylline and placebo groups; however, the degree of improvement was significantly greater in those receiving pentoxifylline. It was concluded that pentoxifylline is a safe and effective drug for use in patients with intermittent claudication. While this agent may provide a modest degree of functional improvement in some patients, its effect on the progression of arterial disease is unknown.

HEMODYNAMICS OF THE VENOUS SYSTEM

The structure of the vein wall is considerably different from that of the companion arteries. Some of these major differences are as follows: (1) the vein wall is much thinner, being anywhere from one third to one tenth as thick as the systemic arteries; (2) there is very little elastic tissue in the wall of the vein; (3) the venous media is almost exclusively a muscular layer; (4) venules have no media and no smooth muscle; and (5) a major part of the walls of the larger veins is composed of adventitia. An important characteristic of the veins is the presence of valves, which are essential for proper function. The distribution and number of valves correspond quite well to those regions in which the effects of gravity are greatest. They have a bicuspid structure with a fine connective tissue skeleton covered by endothelium on both surfaces. Their major function is to ensure antegrade flow and prevent reflux from the deep to the superficial veins.

From the clinical standpoint, the area of greatest interest is found below the knee. This is the most common site for the development of venous thrombosis, and it is also the region of the leg where the complications of the postthrombotic syndrome are evident. The veins of the soleus muscle are often termed the "soleal sinuses" because of their capacious size and lack of venous valves. These sinuses are the most common site for the development of venous thrombosis.

The perforating veins that normally carry blood from the superficial to the deep veins are key elements in venous function. These short channels have the following features: they penetrate the deep fascia; they contain valves; they are found predominantly below the knee; the majority are small and inconstant in location; and they vary in number from 90 to 200.[55] While not commonly thought of as such, the greater and lesser saphenous veins have all the characteristics of perforating veins. One relatively constant large perforator can be found on the medial aspect of the distal thigh, and this is one of the few that establishes a direct communication between the greater saphenous vein and the deep system of veins. A common misconception is that the perforating veins along the medial aspect of the lower leg communicate directly with the greater saphenous vein. In fact, they communicate most commonly with its major tributary, the posterior arch vein. Normally there are four relatively constant perforators that join the posterior arch vein, and when these are diseased they contribute to the pathogenesis of the postthrombotic syndrome. The region in the vicinity of the lowest two perforating veins is often referred to as the gaiter area.[55]

As will be discussed, the function of the venous wall and its associated valves becomes evident when the effects of gravity and the calf muscle pump are considered.

Normal Pressure and Flow Relationships

A major factor in venous physiology that explains the capacitance function of these vessels is that they can undergo large changes in volume with very little change in transmural pressure. This is not due to the elastic properties of the walls, but rather to the fact that they tend to collapse under the influence of a low transmural pressure. Veins are actually stiffer than arteries when compared at the same distending pressure. This results from the paucity of elastic tissue and the very prominent adventitia, which consists largely of collagen.

One of the remarkable features of the venous system is the wide range of flow rates that can be found. These can vary from high flows to nearly complete stasis. Flow rates depend on a host of complex interactive factors such as body position, level of activity, vascular fluid volume, and ambient temperature. Since it is virtually impossible to measure instantaneous venous flow in either the superficial or the deep veins, it is necessary to look at measurements of venous pressure and relate these to specific conditions or disease states.

Resting Venous Pressure

The pressures that exist in the absence of pulsatile flow are shown in Figure 12–19, which is the hydrostatic model of a 6-foot-tall "dead man." If the case of an open rigid tube is considered, pressure at the top would be zero (atmospheric). In the body, the arteries and veins can be represented as a series of parallel tubes, with the veins being collapsible and the arteries rigid. With the system filled with fluid, but not enough to entirely distend the collapsible tube (venous), the pressure in the collapsed portion of the tube is atmospheric. Pressures in the rigid tube (arterial) must be equal to those in the collapsible tube up to the zero point. Above the zero pressure point, the pressures in the rigid tube are negative, since the collapsed tube representing the veins prevents free communication between the two segments.

When we examine the pressure relationships in a living man, supine and erect, some important facts can be noted (Fig. 12–20).[56] There is a point just below the diaphragm where the pressures in the arteries and veins remain constant regardless of position. This has been termed the "hydrostatic indifferent point" (HIP). This point only changes when the subject is placed head down, and then it is located at the level of the right atrium. The zero pressure level is in the region of the right atrium, usually at the level of the fourth intercostal space. The effect of gravity is the same throughout the vascular system in the supine subject. Raising an arm above the head in the erect position does produce some dramatic changes. The arteriovenous pressure gradient in the foot remains the same (83 mm Hg), but in the hand it falls to a level of 31 mm Hg.[57]

While there is no difference in the pressure gradient across the capillaries in the feet between the supine and the standing position, some important changes do occur. On assuming the standing position there is a translocation of blood into the veins of the legs that is on the order of 500 ml.[58] There is also a marked increase in the transmural venous pressure at the foot as a result of the effect of gravity. With

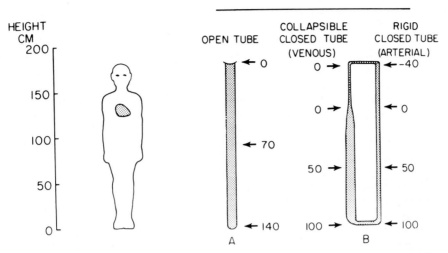

FIGURE 12–19. Hydrostatic pressures measured in the upright "dead man." *A*, The pressures in the open tube are those expected in a rigid tube of equal height. *B*, The pressures shown are those expected in a system of closed, connected parallel tubes. (From Strandness DE, Sumner DS: Hemodynamics for Surgeons. New York, Grune & Stratton, 1975.)

this increase in pressure, fluid is forced out of the capillaries into the tissues. Although some of this fluid may be picked up by the lymphatics, other factors must come into play if edema is to be prevented. The single most important element in preventing the continued accumulation of interstitial fluid is the calf muscle pump. This can dramatically lower the pressure in the veins and capillaries, thus promoting the return of interstitial fluid to the circulation.

Pressure Changes During Exercise

Features that distinguish normal subjects from patients with venous disease are best understood by examining the pressure changes that occur with leg exercise. While patients with chronic arterial disease can usually be distinguished from normal subjects under resting conditions by measurement of distal arterial blood pressure, this is not the case with venous disease. For patients with venous problems, it is only when the muscle pump is activated that the abnormality will be apparent. The calf muscle pump produces important changes in venous volume, flow rate, and flow direction. The muscle pump fulfills three useful functions: it lowers the venous pressure in the dependent limb; it reduces venous volume in the exercising limb; and it increases venous return.

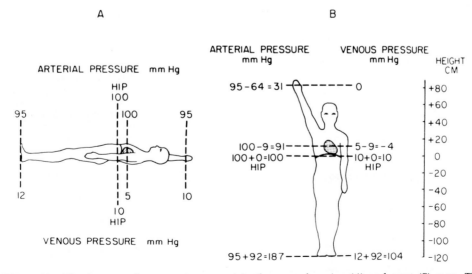

FIGURE 12–20. The intravascular pressures present in the normal supine (*A*) and erect (*B*) man. The *HIP*, (hydrostatic indifferent point) is located just below the diaphragm. (From Strandness DE, Sumner DS: Hemodynamics for Surgeons. New York, Grune & Stratton, 1975.)

With quiet standing, the venous pressure at the level of the foot remains constant, but this is dramatically altered even with a single step (Fig. 12–21). As noted in the figure, at the completion of a single step, the venous pressure is very low and requires several seconds to return to the prestep level.[59] When a normal subject walks, the venous pressure remains at a low and steady level throughout the period of exercise. Calf volume initially falls but gradually increases during exercise as the arterial inflow rises (Fig. 12–22). It is essential to understand that the observed pressure changes at the level of the foot are entirely dependent on intact and functioning venous valves in the distal limb. The calf muscle pump essentially empties the local venous system during contraction. With relaxation, the veins are nearly empty and the venous pressure is very low. These changes are vital to maintaining normal venous return and protecting the limb. As will be shown, destruction of the valves dramatically alters these changes.

Venous Flow Patterns

Flow on the venous side of the circulation is influenced by a variety of factors, including respiration, the filling pressure of the right heart, body position, the activity of the calf muscle pump, and the amount of arterial inflow. The patterns of blood flow in the femoral artery and vein are shown in Figure 12–23. Flow velocity in the normal femoral vein is lowest at peak inspiration when the intraabdominal pressure resulting from descent of the diaphragm is at its maximum. In theory, the changes in velocity of venous flow in the subclavian vein should be opposite to those in the femoral vein; that is, highest at peak inspiration when intrathoracic pressure is at its minimum.

As noted earlier, the presence of competent valves prevents reflux of blood and an increase in venous pressure. This can be shown when the pressure is suddenly increased above a competent iliofemoral valve (Fig. 12–24). A cough and a Valsalva maneuver result in a sharp increase in pressure above the valve, but not below it. There is no reflux of blood flow through the valve during either of these maneuvers.

Abnormal Pressure and Flow Relationships

The most common manifestations of abnormal venous function are primary varicose veins and the postthrombotic syndrome. Current evidence suggests that primary varicose veins are often familial in etiology. The initial abnormality in this condition appears to be incompetence of the terminal valves of the greater and lesser saphenous veins, which permits reflux of blood. With the passage of time, progressive incompetence of the other valves occurs. Dodd and Cockett also include patients with idiopathic perforator vein incompetence in the primary varicose vein group.[60] While this may be valid, it is likely that many of these incompetent perforators occur secondary to episodes of calf vein thrombosis that result in destruction of the valves.

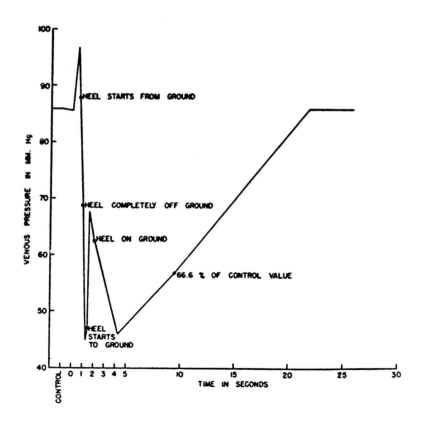

FIGURE 12–21. Changes in the mean saphenous vein pressure measured at the level of the ankle that occur with a single step. (Redrawn from Pollack AA, Wood EH: Venous pressure in the saphenous vein at the ankle in man during exercise and changes in posture. J Appl Physiol 1:649, 1949.)

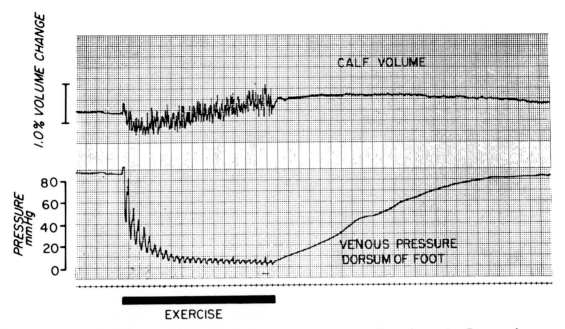

FIGURE 12–22. Normal calf volume and venous pressure response to calf muscle exercise. Pressure changes measured in a dorsal foot vein. Venous pressure falls rapidly, remains low throughout the period of exercise, and returns slowly to the baseline after calf muscle contraction ceases. (From Strandness DE, Sumner DS: Hemodynamics for Surgeons. New York, Grune & Stratton, 1975.)

The flow abnormality produced by loss of valvular competence at any level of the venous system is easily demonstrated with a Doppler ultrasonic velocity detector. The flow patterns shown in Figure 12–25 are from the greater saphenous vein of a patient with primary varicose veins. In the supine position, flow with a calf contraction (C) is antegrade with a slight and transient period of reflux during relaxation (R); however, with standing the opposite is noted, with flow being toward the foot. Walking in place illustrates clearly the rapid changes in direction that occur with each step as a result of loss of valvular competence. When the pressure in the veins on the dorsum of the foot is measured during exercise in a patient with primary varicose veins, the deviations from normal are evident (Fig. 12–26). The pressure does not fall to normally low levels, and it returns to the preexercise level much faster when walking is stopped. If a tourniquet is placed around the upper calf, this pattern will be normalized as long as the valves in the deep system are competent.

With the development of acute deep vein thrombosis, two major factors determine the long-term outcome: the location and extent of the residual venous

FIGURE 12–23. Comparison between the flow velocity patterns in the common femoral artery (*top*) and vein (*bottom*) in the supine position with normal respiration. The venous velocity patterns are dominated by the pressure changes that occur with respiration. *F*, Doppler shift frequency, which is proportional to velocity. (From Strandness DE, Sumner DS: Hemodynamics for Surgeons. New York, Grune & Stratton, 1975.)

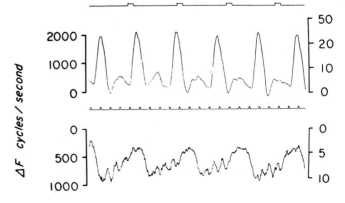

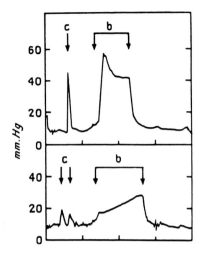

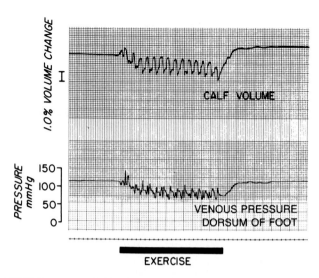

FIGURE 12–24. Effect of a cough (*c*) and a Valsalva maneuver (*b*) on the venous pressure in a patient with a competent valve at the iliofemoral level. *Upper panel,* pressure changes above the valve; *lower panel,* pressure changes below the valve. (From Ludbrook J, Beale G: Femoral venous valves in relation to varicose veins. Lancet *1*:79, 1962.)

FIGURE 12–26. Calf volume and venous pressure changes recorded from a dorsal foot vein of a patient with primary varicose veins. The pressure does not fall to the low levels seen in normal subjects, and it returns to the baseline much faster. (From Strandness DE, Sumner DS: Hemodynamics for Surgeons. New York, Grune & Stratton, 1975.)

obstruction, and the condition of the valves below the knee in the area of the calf muscle pump.[61] Since these will vary greatly from one patient to another, it is not surprising that the pressure responses would also show a wide variation. Four examples of the types of patterns that can be observed are shown in Figure 12–27. It is clear that even with primary varicose veins the pressure changes at the level of the foot are abnormal with exercise (Figs. 12–26 and 12–

27). However, patients with this very common condition generally complain of minimal edema and rarely develop ulceration. The factors that appear to be responsible for the development of the postthrombotic syndrome relate primarily to the status of the deep veins below the knee and the perforating veins. The most abnormal venous pressures and flows occur in the area where ulceration develops and are due to valvular incompetence in both the distal deep veins and their connections with the superficial venous system. With this combination, the very high pressures that can be generated by activation of the calf muscle pump result in ambulatory venous hypertension in the lower leg.

Browse and Burnand in 1978 offered a reassessment of the factors responsible for the development of the postthrombotic syndrome.[62] They recognized that the clinical condition could only occur with damage to the deep venous system and postulated that the abnormally high venous pressures led to the development of multiple new capillaries in the dermis with large pores in the venular side. As a result, there would be extravasation of large molecules such as fibrinogen and coagulation factors. These, in conjunction with tissue factors, would lead to the conversion of fibrinogen to fibrin. If this were combined with inadequate fibrinolysis, fibrin would accumulate in the tissues and produce a barrier to the diffusion of both oxygen and nutrients. The end result would be tissue anoxia and death of the skin in the affected region.

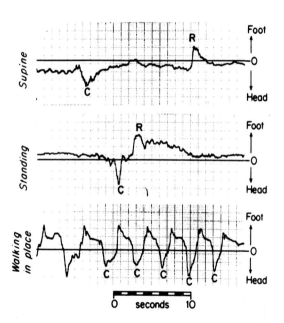

FIGURE 12–25. Venous velocity changes recorded from an incompetent greater saphenous vein in a patient with primary varicose veins. The effects of muscular contraction (*C*) and relaxation (*R*) are indicated for the supine and standing positions. The bidirectional flow that occurs with walking is also shown. (From Strandness DE, Sumner DS: Hemodynamics for Surgeons. New York, Grune & Stratton, 1975.)

Hemodynamic Principles and the Treatment of Venous Disease

In contrast to the arterial side of the circulation, there are very few direct therapeutic approaches that

Hemodynamics for the Vascular Surgeon

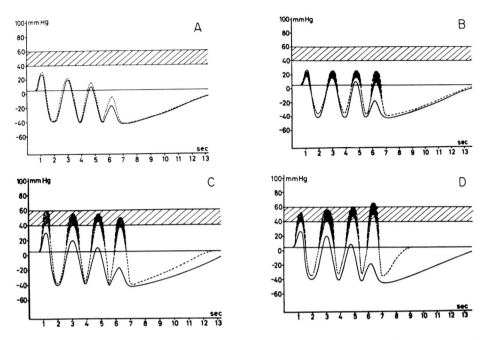

FIGURE 12–27. The pressure changes in the greater saphenous vein at the ankle during four steps. In each panel, the normal response is noted by the solid line. *A,* Primary varicose veins and no leg ulcers. *B,* Varicose veins, incompetent ankle perforators, normal deep veins, no leg ulcers. *C,* Varicose veins, incompetent ankle perforators, normal deep veins, leg ulcers present. *D,* Varicose veins, incompetent ankle perforators, abnormal deep veins, leg ulcers present. (From Arnoldi CC, Linderholm H: On the pathogenesis of the venous leg ulcer. Acta Chir Scand *134*:427, 1968.)

can correct the underlying hemodynamic abnormalities of venous disease. While obstruction of inflow to a limb is the most commonly treated arterial abnormality, mechanical interference with venous outflow is a rare cause of chronic venous insufficiency.

One exception to this observation is the patient with venous claudication. This entity is uncommon and may not be recognized. It occurs in the specific clinical setting of chronic iliofemoral venous occlusion. In most cases, the major deep veins distal to the groin are patent and competent. With vigorous exercise, the patient is unable to adequately decompress the deep venous system, and the thigh becomes tense and very painful. After the patient stops exercising, if often requires 15 to 30 minutes for the pain and tightness to disappear. It is important to recognize that this syndrome rarely occurs with ordinary exercise, and thus tends to be seen is relatively young patients who indulge in vigorous activities such as jogging, skiing, or tennis. The underlying mechanism of venous claudication involves the collateral veins that bypass the obstructed segment and have a relatively high, fixed resistance.[63] This high outflow resistance results in a marked increase in venous volume during exercise. In some circumstances it may be feasible to provide therapeutic relief by a crossover saphenous vein graft using the proximal saphenous vein from the opposite limb. This is rarely

done because the symptoms in most patients produce only minimal disability.

Other surgical procedures designed to treat chronic venous insufficiency do so by either removing the offending vein or interrupting it at some point in its course. This is done to eliminate sites of reflux and restore the pressure-flow relationship to normal. The value of this particular approach is limited because the most common site of the disease responsible for chronic venous insufficiency is the distal deep veins, an area not amenable to direct surgical intervention.

In recent years, there has been a good deal of interest in promoting valvular competence in the proximal superficial femoral vein. This has been done by a direct surgical approach through a longitudinal venotomy or by transposition of a competent venous valve.[64,65] The validity of these techniques can be questioned for the following reasons: there is no evidence to support the concept of the so-called critical valve; the alterations of pressure and flow are nearly always secondary to deep venous abnormalities in the distal limb; and proof of the effectiveness of such an approach is at present lacking.

The most common form of therapy for chronic venous insufficiency is the use of support stockings that provide external compression and thus minimize the amount of edema that occurs during ambulation.[66] The exact mechanism of compression therapy remains poorly understood. In theory, the stocking should reduce the transmural venous pressure gradient in a graduated fashion, with the highest compression pressures in the ankle area and diminishing pressures proximally up the limb. The amount of pressure exerted by a stocking depends on the elastic tension in the garment and the radius of the limb. Compression pressure should be in the range of 80 to 90 mm Hg while standing, 50 to 60 mm Hg while sitting, and 0 mm Hg in the recumbent position. This is obviously not possible with any single stocking, so a compromise must be accepted.

Elevation of the legs above the level of the heart is also a standard method for relieving the symptoms of chronic venous insufficiency. The physiologic basis for the use of elevation depends on three major effects: it reduces venous pressure by decreasing the hydrostatic component related to gravity; it promotes the reabsorption of edema fluid; and it prevents ambulatory venous hypertension. Periodic elevation and external compression therapy are essential for the treatment of chronic venous insufficiency. When strictly adhered to, a regimen of elevation and compression will minimize edema, improve skin nutrition, and avoid ulceration in the majority of patients.

CONCLUSION

The fundamental principles of hemodynamics often seem remote from the everyday clinical problems faced by the vascular surgeon. The purpose of this chapter has been to show how these mathematical and physical concepts provide the basis for a rational approach to the pathophysiology, diagnosis, and treatment of vascular disease. These principles are also important in understanding the recent advances in noninvasive diagnostic techniques that are discussed elsewhere in this book. The use of objective hemodynamic data is an essential step in the clinical evaluation of patients. This increased reliance on physiologic testing should encourage the vascular surgeon to consider the patient with vascular disease in terms of basic hemodynamic principles.

REFERENCES

1. Sumner DS: The hemodynamics and pathophysiology of arterial disease. *In* Rutherford RB (ed): Vascular Surgery. Philadelphia, WB Saunders Company, 1977, pp 25–46.
2. Burton AC: Physiology and Biophysics of the Circulation, 2nd ed. Chicago, Year Book Medical Publishers, 1972, pp 86–94.
3. Strandness DE Jr, Sumner DS: Hemodynamics for Surgeons. New York, Grune & Stratton, 1975.
4. Barnes RW: Hemodynamics for the vascular surgeon. Arch Surg 115:216–223, 1980.
5. Attinger EO: Flow patterns in vascular geometry. *In* Attinger EO (ed): Pulsatile Blood Flow. New York, McGraw-Hill, 1964, pp 179–200.
6. Gutstein WH, Schneck DJ, Marks JO: In vitro studies of local blood flow disturbance in a region of separation. J Atherosclerosis Res 8:381–388, 1968.
7. Logerfo FW, Soncrant T, Teel T, Dewey F: Boundary layer separation in models of side-to-end arterial anastomoses. Arch Surg 114:1364–1373, 1979.
8. Zarins CK, Giddens DP, Glagov S: Atherosclerotic plaque distribution and flow velocity profiles in the carotid bifurcation. *In* Bergan JJ, Yao JST (eds): Cerebrovascular Insufficiency. New York, Grune & Stratton, 1983, pp 19–30.
9. Ku DN, Giddens DP, Phillips DJ, et al: Hemodynamics of the normal human carotid bifurcation—in vitro and in vivo studies. Ultrasound Med Biol 1:13–26, 1985.
10. Phillips DJ, Greene FM Jr, Langlois Y, et al: Flow velocity patterns in the carotid bifurcations of young, presumed normal subjects. Ultrasound Med Biol 1:39–49, 1983.
11. Reneman RS, van Merode T, Hick P, et al: Flow velocity patterns in and distensibility of the carotid artery bulb in subjects of various ages. Circulation 71:500–509, 1985.
12. Fox JA, Hugh AE: Localization of atheroma: A theory based on boundary layer separation. Br Heart J 28:388–394, 1966.
13. Milnor WR: Pulsatile blood flow. N Engl J Med 287:27–34, 1972.
14. Malan E, Noseda G, Longo T: Approach to fluid dynamic problems in reconstructive vascular surgery. Surgery 66:994–1003, 1969.
15. McDonald DA: Blood Flow in Arteries, 2nd ed. London, Edward Arnold Ltd, 1974.
16. Goaling RG, Newman DL, Bowden NLR, et al: The area ratio of normal aortic junctions—aortic configuration and pulse wave reflection. Br J Radiol 44:850–853, 1971.
17. Lalleman RC, Gosling RG, Newman DL: Role of the bifurcation in atheromatosis of the abdominal aorta. Surg Gynecol Obstet 137:987–990, 1973.
18. Sumner DS, Hokanson DE, Strandness DE Jr: Arterial walls before and after endarterectomy, stress-strain characteristics and collagen-elastin content. Arch Surg 99:606–611, 1969.
19. Sumner DS, Hokanson DE, Strandness DE Jr: Stress-strain characteristics and collagen-elastin content of abdominal aortic aneurysms. Surg Gynecol Obstet 130:459–466, 1970.
20. Scherer PW: Flow in axisymmetrical glass model aneurysms. J Biomech 6:695–700, 1973.
21. Darling RC: Ruptured arteriosclerotic abdominal aortic aneurysms—a pathologic and clinical study. Am J Surg 119:397–401, 1970.
22. Roach MR: Changes in arterial distensibility as a cause of poststenotic dilatation. Am J Cardiol 12:802–815, 1963.
23. Berguer R, Hwang NHC: Critical arterial stenosis—a theoretical and experimental solution. Ann Surg 180:39–50, 1974.
24. May AG, Van de Berg L, DeWeese JA, Rob CG: Critical arterial stenosis. Surgery 54:250–259, 1963.
25. James IM, Millar RA, Purves MY: Observations on the intrinsic neural control of cerebral blood flow in the baboon. Circ Res 25:77–93, 1969.
26. Moore WS, Hall AD: Unrecognized aortoiliac stenosis—a physiologic approach to the diagnosis. Arch Surg 103:633–638, 1971.
27. Carter SA: Response of ankle systolic pressure to leg exercise in mild or questionable arterial disease. N Engl J Med 287:578–582, 1972.
28. Sumner DS, Strandness DE Jr: The relationship between calf blood flow and ankle blood pressure in patients with intermittent claudication. Surgery 65:763–771, 1969.
29. Flanigan DP, Tullis JP, Streeter VL, et al: Multiple subcritical arterial stenosis: Effect on poststenotic pressure and flow. Ann Surg 186:663–668, 1977.
30. Longland CJ: The collateral circulation of the limb. Ann R Coll Surg Engl 13:161–176, 1953.

31. John HT, Warren R: The stimulus to collateral circulation. Surgery 49:14–25, 1961.
32. Skinner JS, Strandness DE Jr: Exercise and intermittent claudication. II. Effect of physical training. Circulation 36:23–29, 1967.
33. Ludbrook J: Collateral artery resistance in the human lower limb. J Surg Res 6:423–434, 1966.
34. Sumner DS, Strandness DE Jr: The effect of exercise on resistance to blood flow in limbs with an occluded superficial femoral artery. Vasc Surg 4:229–237, 1970.
35. Keitzer WF, Fry WT, Kraft RO, et al: Hemodynamic mechanism for pulse changes seen in occlusive vascular disease. Surgery 57:163–174, 1965.
36. Strandness DE Jr, Bell JW: Peripheral vascular disease: Diagnosis and objective evaluation using a mercury strain gauge. Ann Surg (Suppl) 161:1–35, 1965.
37. Yao JST: Hemodynamic studies in peripheral arterial disease. Br J Surg 57:761–766, 1970.
38. Zierler RE, Strandness DE Jr: Doppler techniques of lower extremity arterial diagnosis. *In* Zwiebel WJ (ed): Introduction to Vascular Ultrasonography, 2nd ed. New York, Grune & Stratton, 1986, pp 305–331.
39. Reivich MH, Holling HE, Roberts B, Toole JF: Reversal of blood flow through the vertebral artery and its effect on the cerebral circulation. N Engl J Med 265:878–885, 1961.
40. Gonzales L, Weintraub RA, Wiot JF, Lewis C: Retrograde vertebral artery blood flow: A normal phenomenon. Radiology 82:211–216, 1964.
41. Kelly WA, Strandness DE Jr: The subclavian steal syndrome *In* Strandness DE Jr (ed): Collateral Circulation in Clinical Surgery. Philadelphia, WB Saunders Company, 1969, pp 570–582.
42. Ehrenfeld WK, Harris JD, Wylie EJ: Vascular "steal" phenomenon—an experimental study. Am J Surg 116:192–197, 1968.
43. Shin CS, Chaudhry AG: The hemodynamics of extraanatomic bypass grafts. Surg Gynecol Obstet 148:567–570, 1979.
44. Sumner DS, Strandness DE Jr: The hemodynamics of the femorofemoral shunt. Surg Gynecol Obstet 134:629–636, 1972.
45. Mozersky DJ, Sumner DS, Barnes RW, et al: The hemodynamics of the axillary-axillary bypass. Surg Gynecol Obstet 135:925–929, 1972.
46. Larsen DA, Lassen NA: Medical treatment of occlusive arterial disease of the legs—walking exercise and medically induced hypertension. Angiologica 6:288–301, 1969.
47. Freiman DB, Ring EJ, Oleaga JA: Transluminal angioplasty of the iliac, femoral, and popliteal arteries. Radiology 132:285–288, 1979.
48. Strandness DE Jr, Bell JW: Ankle pressure responses after reconstructive arterial surgery. Surgery 59:514–516, 1966.
49. Coffman JD, Mannick JA: Failure of vasodilator drugs in arteriosclerosis obliterans. Ann Intern Med 76:35–39, 1972.
50. Strandness DE Jr: Ineffectiveness of isoxuprine on intermittent claudication. JAMA 213:86–88, 1970.
51. Strandness DE Jr: Role of sympathectomy in the treatment of arteriosclerosis obliterans and thromboangiitis obliterans. *In* Strandness DE Jr (ed): Collateral Circulation in Clinical Surgery. Philadelphia, WB Saunders Company, 1969, pp 450–459.
52. Barnes RW, Baker WH, Shanik G: Value of concomitant sympathectomy in aortoiliac reconstruction. Arch Surg 112:1325–1330, 1977.
53. Gruber UF: Dextran and the prevention of postoperative thromboembolic complications. Surg Clin North Am 55:679–696, 1975.
54. Porter JM, Cutler BS, Lee BY, et al: Pentoxifylline efficacy in the treatment of intermittent claudication: Multicenter controlled double-blind trial with objective assessment of chronic occlusive disease patients. Am Heart J 104:66–72, 1982.
55. Strandness DE Jr, Thiele BL: Anatomy of the venous system of the lower limb. *In*: Selected Topics in Venous Disorders. New York, Futura Publishing, 1981, pp 1–26.
56. Gauer OH, Thron HL: Postural changes in the circulation. *In* Hamilton WF, Dow P (eds): Handbook of Physiology, Section 2, Circulation, Vol III. Washington, DC, American Physiological Society, 1965, pp 2409–2439.
57. Holling HE, Verel D: Circulation of the elevated forearm. Clin Sci 16:197–213, 1957.
58. Henry JP, Slaughter OL, Greiner T: A medical massage suit for continuous wear. Angiology 6:482–494, 1955.
59. Pollack AA, Wood EH: Venous pressure in the saphenous vein at the ankle in man during exercise and changes in posture. J Appl Physiol 1:649–662, 1949.
60. Dodd H, Cockett FB: The Pathology and Surgery of the Veins of the Lower Limbs. Edinburgh, Churchill Livingstone, 1976.
61. Strandness DE Jr, Langlois YE, Cramer M, et al: Long-term sequelae of acute venous thrombosis. JAMA 250:1289–1292, 1983.
62. Browse NL, Burnand KG: The postphlebitic syndrome—a new look. *In* Bergan JJ, Yao JST (eds): Venous Problems. Chicago, Year Book Medical Publishers, 1978, pp 395–404.
63. Killewich LA, Martin R, Cramer M, et al: Pathophysiology of venous claudication. J Vasc Surg 1:507–511, 1984.
64. Kistner RL: Transvenous repair of the incompetent femoral vein valve. *In* Bergan JJ, Yao JST (eds): Venous Problems. Chicago, Year Book Medical Publishers, 1975, pp 493–509.
65. Queral LA, Whitehouse WM, Flinn WR, et al: Surgical correction of chronic deep venous insufficiency by valvular transposition. Surgery 87:688–695, 1980.
66. Husni EA, Ximenes JOC, Goyette EM: Elastic support of the lower limbs in hospital patients—a critical study. JAMA 214:1456–1462, 1970.

REVIEW QUESTIONS

1. Viscous energy losses in flowing blood result from:
   (a) changes in the velocity and direction of flow
   (b) friction between adjacent layers of moving blood
   (c) turbulent flow in areas of stenosis
   (d) disturbed flow at points of branching
   (e) areas of boundary layer separation

2. Poiseuille's law states that viscous energy losses are inversely proportional to:
   (a) mean flow velocity
   (b) tube or stenosis length
   (c) blood viscosity
   (d) tube or stenosis radius
   (e) volume flow rate

3. Inertial energy losses in blood flow are related primarily to:
   (a) changes in the velocity and direction of flow
   (b) blood viscosity
   (c) the specific gravity of blood
   (d) friction between adjacent layers of moving blood
   (e) the mean blood pressure

4. The critical stenosis value for a particular artery depends on the:
   (a) length of the arterial segment
   (b) tangential wall stress
   (c) blood viscosity
   (d) compliance of the arterial wall
   (e) flow rate and peripheral vascular resistance

5. Which of the following statements about the collateral circulation is false?
   (a) collateral vessels are preexisting pathways that enlarge when the parallel major artery is occluded
   (b) the vascular resistance of the collateral bed is relatively fixed
   (c) collateral artery resistance is usually less than that of the original unobstructed parallel artery
   (d) an abnormal pressure gradient across the collateral bed may stimulate further development of collateral pathways
   (e) the midzone of the collateral bed consists of small, intramuscular vessels

6. Which of the following is not related to rupture of arterial aneurysms?
   (a) the volume flow rate through the aneurysm
   (b) the arterial blood pressure
   (c) the internal radius of the aneurysm
   (d) the tensile strength of collagen
   (e) the thickness of the aneurysm wall

7. With an extraanatomic bypass, such as a femorofemoral crossover graft, a vascular steal from the donor limb is most likely to occur when:
   (a) there is occlusive disease in both the donor and recipient limbs
   (b) there is an occlusive lesion in the donor artery
   (c) severe occlusive disease is present in the donor limb
   (d) the recipient limb has only mild occlusive disease
   (e) the donor limb is hemodynamically normal

8. The most effective approach to the treatment of an occluded major artery such as the superficial femoral is to:
   (a) perform sympathectomy to lower the collateral resistance
   (b) lower the peripheral resistance with vasodilators
   (c) improve limb perfusion by increasing systemic blood pressure
   (d) lower blood viscosity with rheologic agents
   (e) lower segmental resistance by a direct surgical approach

9. Which of the following is not a function of the calf muscle pump?
   (a) it lowers venous pressure in the dependent limb
   (b) it reduces the venous volume in the exercising limb
   (c) it improves arterial (nutritive) blood flow to the exercising muscle
   (d) it increases venous return to the right heart
   (e) it minimizes the accumulation of interstitial fluid in the distal limb

10. All of the following contribute to the pathogenesis of the postthrombotic syndrome except:
    (a) deep vein thrombosis with obstruction of the deep veins
    (b) extravasation of blood components into the subcutaneous tissues
    (c) incompetence of the venous valves in the area of the calf muscle pump
    (d) the presence of primary varicose veins
    (e) ambulatory venous hypertension

ANSWERS

1. b	2. d	3. a	4. e	5. c	6. a	7. b
8. e	9. c	10. d				

13

THE VASCULAR LABORATORY

J. DENNIS BAKER

In the early days of vascular surgery, patient assessment was based on a careful history and physical examination. Although a few clinicians used the Collins oscillometer to estimate the pulse pressure in an extremity, there was little available in terms of quantitative assessment of arterial or venous disease. Angiography provided the only objective determination of the patient's pathology. Early experience with arteriography and phlebography demonstrated some of the limitations of these techniques, especially the problem of underestimating the severity of stenotic lesions when single-plane studies were obtained. In addition, the cost, patient discomfort, and risk of complications associated with the contrast studies precluded them from routine use for screening evaluations and for subsequent follow-up.

The growing interest in more accurate differential diagnosis, localization of disease, measurement of its severity, and documentation of progression all stimulated the development of noninvasive techniques. In the 1960s investigators started working with different plethysmographic techniques for quantitating arterial occlusive disease in the leg. Modification of ultrasound equipment to measure blood flow by the Doppler shift principle represented an important step forward in instrumentation and led to rapid development of noninvasive studies. Additional techniques were designed to evaluate carotid artery disease as well as deep venous occlusion and insufficiency. This chapter describes the main diagnostic techniques used in the noninvasive laboratory and discusses their clinical application for patients with vascular disease. Understanding the merits and limitations of each method will help the clinician make the most appropriate use of these tests.

INSTRUMENTATION

Doppler Velocity Measurement Techniques

High-frequency sound waves (2 to 10 MHz) penetrate through soft tissues and are reflected by the different interfaces encountered. Reflection from a moving interface results in the reflected frequency being increased if the motion is toward the point of observation and decreased if away. The magnitude of the shift is determined by:

$$f_s = \frac{2 V f_0 \cos \phi}{C} \qquad (1)$$

where f_s is the frequency shift, V the velocity, f_0 the transmitted frequency, ϕ the angle between the ultrasound beam and the velocity vector, and C the speed of sound in tissue (1540 m/sec). For a given velocity a greater shift f_s is obtained with a higher transmitting frequency. On the other hand, tissue penetration varies inversely with probe frequency, so that the selection of frequency for a given application is a balance between depth and velocity requirements.

Continuous-wave detectors are the simplest systems. The probe has two separate crystals, one transmitting and one receiving continuously. This system detects all velocities within the intersecting paths of the sound beams. If this zone includes more than one vessel (e.g., an artery and a vein), the resulting signal will represent both velocities. Pulsed systems use a single crystal, which repeatedly transmits a short burst of sound followed by a waiting period, during which the crystal functions in a receive mode. By selecting the time and duration of the listening phase, one can define a sample volume, the portion of the vessel from which velocity is to be measured.

The shifted frequency obtained from a vessel is within the audible range, so the data can be presented to the examiner as an audio signal. Although qualitative interpretation is helpful in patient examinations, quantitative measurements provide more objective testing. Spectral analyzers can be used to determine the main frequency components obtained from a given vessel. This information is usually displayed on a sonogram, which shows the frequency content in time (Fig. 13–1).

In some applications it is necessary to have a measure of velocity rather than the raw frequency data.

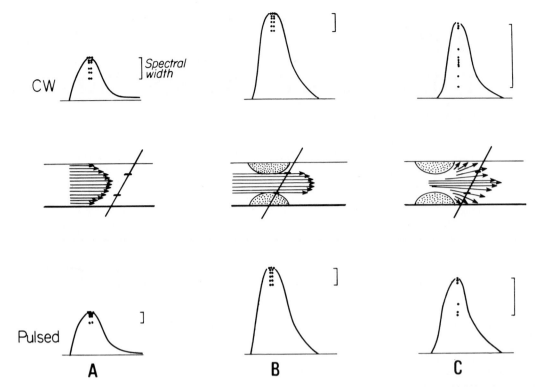

FIGURE 13–1.   Comparison of sonograms from continuous-wave (*CW*) and pulsed Doppler systems. Sonogram displays the different frequency contents detected at each point in time. CW detects all velocities across the vessel, whereas pulsed system only detects those velocity vectors within the sample volume, indicated by the marks on the ultrasound beam. *A,* Normal arterial signals. CW has more low-frequency content, since it detects flow near the walls as well as in center stream. *B,* Within stenosis there is increased peak frequency and the frequency distributions of both types of Doppler system are similar, since the sample volume encompasses the entire flow stream. *C,* Beyond stenosis peak frequency is elevated, with increased frequency distribution resulting from turbulent flow. Spectral width is greater with CW system.

If the probe angle can be measured, the velocity is estimated using the Doppler equation. The accuracy of the estimate depends greatly on the accuracy of the angle measurement. Errors are greatest when the probe is at right angles to flow and least when at low angles. Whenever possible, velocities should be measured with an angle below 60 degrees.

Duplex Scan

During the 1960s, B mode ultrasound imaging was used for visualization of soft-tissue structures. Although early devices had only crude resolution, equipment has improved to the point that clear, detailed images of vessels can be produced in real time (Fig. 13–2). In general, experience shows that where high-quality imaging is obtained the diagnostic accuracy is very high; however, in patients with advanced atherosclerosis, it is difficult to obtain optimal studies, and the diagnostic accuracies are lower. A common problem is incomplete imaging of the vessel wall as a result of calcification, which is present in varying degrees in up to half of patients studied. The interference may be limited, but in some vessels there is no visualization of substantial portions of the ar-

tery. Although calcified plaques stand out sharply in the ultrasound image, some atheromas are visualized poorly or not at all. A major source of error is that recent thrombus may have the same echo density as flowing blood, so that an occluded vessel may look normal on the ultrasound image.

In order to overcome the limitations of ultrasound imaging, the research team at the University of Washington developed the duplex scanner, combining a real-time B mode ultrasound image system with a pulsed Doppler detector.[1] The ultrasound image shows not only the vessel under study but also the location of the sample volume of the Doppler beam so that the examiner can position it to study velocity patterns at specific locations in the vessel. The device can study calcified vessels by analyzing the Doppler velocity signal distal to the areas of calcification. The evaluation of the Doppler signal from the common carotid artery and its branches is carried out using spectral analysis (Fig. 13–3). Based on the peak systolic velocity and the degree of spectral broadening, a category of stenosis is assigned to the vessel segment.

In the past 15 years there has been extensive improvement of duplex scanners both in image resolution and Doppler signal processing. The early de-

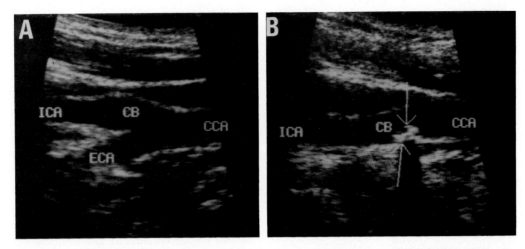

FIGURE 13–2. B mode images from carotid duplex scan. *A,* Normal bifurcation. *B,* Bifurcation with moderate plaque. Dense appearance with shadowing produced by calcium in the lesion. *CB,* carotid bulb; *CCA,* common carotid artery; *ECA,* external carotid artery; *ICA,* internal carotid artery.

vices were limited to the study of superficial vessels; however, availability of low-frequency probes (2 to 3.5 MHz) permits evaluation of abdominal vessels including the aorta, the vena cava, and the main visceral branches.

The most recent development is the color-encoded Doppler system. A linear array transducer composed of many separate elements is used to produce a grid of sample volumes encompassing the area being covered by the B mode image (Fig. 13–4). A portion of the grid is selected for color coding of velocity information. Each of the sample volumes within the area is examined sequentially. If the returning ultrasound signal has no change in phase or frequency, the amplitude information is used to create the gray-scale image at that point in the matrix. On the other hand, if there is a change in phase or frequency, the information is analyzed in terms of velocity. A color is assigned to represent the mean velocity occurring at that point in the field. Red and blue show flow toward and away from the transducer, respectively. The magnitude of the velocity is represented by the hue of the color: a dark shade indicates slow flow

and a lighter shade or white shows high flow. The aggregate of the color representation from sample volumes detecting motion produces a real-time representation of the flow patterns within vessels superimposed on the gray-scale image of the stationary tissue.

CAROTID ARTERY STUDIES

The internal carotid artery poses a unique challenge to physical examination, for it is impossible to palpate a distal pulse. It is not uncommon to find a patient whose carotid pulse in the neck is normal to palpation but who has occlusion of the internal carotid branch. This limitation stimulated development of physiological tests to assess the status of the internal carotid artery. Most of the early tests provided indirect measurement by detecting distal changes in blood flow characteristics produced by advanced stenosis. Common features of the indirect methods are that they only detect lesions that are sufficiently advanced to reduce mean blood flow, and they cannot

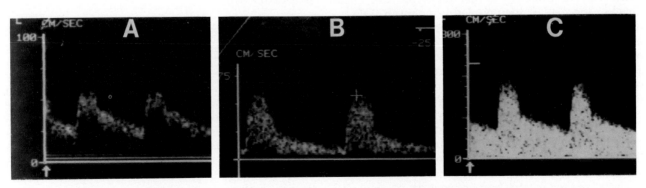

FIGURE 13–3. Doppler sonograms from carotid duplex scans. *A,* Normal study with normal spectral width. *B,* Moderate stenosis with spectral broadening but no increase in peak frequency. (Note that frequency scales are different in the three records.) *C,* Severe stenosis with high peak velocity and extensive spectral broadening.

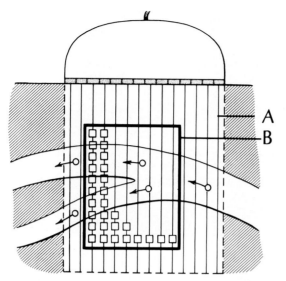

FIGURE 13–4. Color-coded duplex system. A linear array transducer is used to create a matrix of sample volumes. Gray-scale image is created within area *A*. Most examinations are carried out with color coding of velocities limited to a portion of the image (area *B*). Within this portion of the matrix ultrasound signals from sample volumes with a change in phase or frequency are interpreted as velocity data. Otherwise, the data are coded as part of the gray-scale image.

separate a tight stenosis from an occlusion, since the physiological changes in the distal bed may be indistinguishable. Later development efforts focused on direct methods, which detect changes occurring in the cervical portion of the carotid in the vicinity of the bifurcation, where the majority of the lesions occur.

Ophthalmic Artery Pressure Measurement

The internal carotid artery is not directly accessible for pressure measurements, but a flow-reducing stenosis decreases the systolic pressure in the ophthalmic branch. Ophthalmodynamometry was used for many years to detect advanced carotid stenosis indirectly by measuring differences in pressures between the two eyes. The principle of this device led Gee[2–4] to develop the ocular pneumoplethysmograph (OPG), introduced in 1974 for indirect measurement of ophthalmic artery pressure. Small suction cups (14 mm diameter) are placed on the anesthetized sclerae and are used to (1) increase the intraocular pressure by applying suction to the surface of the eye and (2) detect the arterial pulsation within the eye. Suction is applied to abolish the arterial pulsation of both eyes; as suction is reduced the systolic end-point is determined by the first arterial pulse appearing in the tracing of each eye. The suction measurements are then converted to ophthalmic artery pressure from the relationship established between these two parameters.

The test is simple to perform and is well tolerated.

Specific contraindications relate to eye pathology and include acute conjunctivitis; any history of retinal detachment, eye trauma, or surgery within the past 6 months; unstable glaucoma; and the presence of an intraocular lens prosthesis. A relative contraindication is the history of allergic reaction to local anesthetic agents; however, some patients with drug sensitivity are able to tolerate the test without the medication. Subconjunctival erythema or hematoma can occur under the contact area of the eye cup and is seen in 1 to 2 per cent of examinations. This problem is self-limited and is seen most commonly in cases where repeat determinations are required at the same sitting. A limitation of the OPG is that a systolic end-point cannot be obtained in patients with severe hypertension. In general, the ophthalmic artery pressure cannot be measured if the patient's systolic pressure is above 200 mm Hg.

Five extensive studies of clinical use of OPG have shown diagnostic accuracies of 86 to 97 per cent. All these studies use similar, but not identical, criteria for an abnormal test. Lower accuracy rates have been reported in some studies, but these use less sensitive criteria for evaluating the test results.

Although the OPG has been used most extensively for identification of internal carotid artery stenosis, the device can be used for noninvasive estimation of internal carotid artery backpressure. The ophthalmic artery pressure measurements made during external compression of the common carotid artery will reflect the collateral pressure to the ipsilateral internal carotid artery. Whenever used, the carotid compression should be applied and released slowly. If the bifurcation is palpated in an abnormally low position or if there is a carotid bruit detected low in the neck, the compression should not be carried out unless there is ultrasound scan or angiographic evidence that no substantial atherosclerotic plaque exists in the area to be compressed. Gee[2] has reported that 95 per cent of patient studies have less than 5 mm Hg difference between the carotid backpressure measured with the OPG and the direct measurements at the time of operation.

Duplex Scan

The routine examination covers as much of the common carotid artery and its branches as can be visualized with the configuration of the transducer used. Figure 13–2A shows a normal vessel; many older patients have tortuosity so that the common carotid, the bulb, and the branches cannot be visualized in a single plane, and careful scanning is required to obtain satisfactory imaging. The scan usually identifies the regions of pathology, but with advanced atherosclerosis it is often difficult to get an adequate image to permit accurate estimation of the degree of stenosis. Much of the classification of stenosis is based upon interpretation of the Doppler signal. The two branches are distinguished by the image and the velocity signals. The internal carotid has a low peripheral resistance at all times, resulting in forward flow throughout diastole, whereas the high resistance in the external carotid results in diastolic flow going to zero. Stenoses produce an increased velocity at the site of the lesion and turbulence beyond (Fig. 13–1). The turbulence is identified as spectral broadening, seen on the sonogram (Fig. 13–3). Mild stenoses may not produce a significant increase in peak systolic velocity but are identified by a moderate degree of spectral broadening. Based upon the peak systolic velocity and the degree of spectral broadening, the internal carotid artery is placed in one of six diagnostic categories, outlined in Table 13–1. Further improvement in accuracy may be obtained from using ratios of velocities in the internal carotid artery (ICA) to those in the normal portion of the common carotid artery (CCA), especially in the identification of the 80 to 99 per cent category.[5] The diagnosis of ICA occlusion must be based upon image as well as Doppler information, because the very low flow found with some "string signs" is below the threshold for velocity detection of many scanners. The stippled appearance of chronic thrombus and a small diameter of the ICA both point to occlusion. Overall, low-grade stenoses are best assessed with the image, whereas advanced lesions are best evaluated with the Doppler information.

In addition to estimating the severity of a stenosis, scanners are now being used to obtain information about the plaque itself. Most investigators have limited themselves to distinguishing between homogeneous and heterogeneous appearing plaques and describing the surface as smooth or irregular. More elaborate approaches to describing morphology are being evaluated, but no single approach has been widely adopted.

Over the past few years there has been a rapid growth in the use of duplex scanning for carotid diagnosis. Different investigators have demonstrated that the technique can be highly accurate. Studies have shown accuracies in the range of 92 to 96 per cent in the correct identification of severe stenosis.[6–8]

When these studies are analyzed in terms of correct category of stenosis, exact agreement is found in 77 to 87 per cent, with poor agreement in only 1 to 2 per cent. Of particular importance is the fact that experienced laboratories have very few errors in separating severe stenosis from occlusion.

Although the majority of work has been focused upon the carotid circulation, an increasing number of laboratories have also used duplex scanning to investigate the status of the vertebral arteries. The simplest method has been the determination of direction of flow in each vertebral; however, this limited approach only helps to identify steals. Some investigators have tried to determine the status of the origins of the vertebrals, a major site of occlusive disease in these vessels. Because of its deeper location the left vertebral takeoff is more difficult to study than the right. Ackerstaff et al. found that the status of the ostium of the vertebral could be studied satisfactorily in about 80 per cent of cases.[9] When adequate evaluation of the prevertebral portion was possible, a sensitivity of 80 per cent and a specificity of 97 per cent was achieved in the detection of diameter reductions greater than 50 per cent.

Applications

Symptomatic Patients

A large portion of transient ischemic attacks and strokes are caused by thromboembolization from ulcerations in atheromatous arterial plaques. A duplex scan may be useful for patients who are going to have an angiogram. Identification of the location and severity of lesions in the carotid system may assist in selection of the specific arteriographic technique. Occasionally the scan may demonstrate a lesion that is underestimated or missed with standard views. In recent years some centers have been using the ultrasound study as the definitive test on which to base the decision to operate. For the present time only the severe stenoses are handled in this way. Having a very experienced vascular laboratory with a validated record of high accuracy in carotid scanning is the critical element in using the duplex scan as the definitive test.

Asymptomatic Carotid Stenosis

Increasing numbers of asymptomatic patients are being referred to noninvasive vascular labs for evaluation of cervical bruits. Although some of these patients have bruits radiating from the heart or the

TABLE 13–1. CATEGORIES OF INTERNAL CAROTID ARTERY (ICA) STENOSIS DETERMINED BY DOPPLER VELOCITY CRITERIA

ICA Stenosis	ICA Velocity	Spectrum
Normal Vessel	Peak systolic velocity < 125 cm/sec	No broadening
1–19%	Peak systolic velocity < 125 cm/sec	Limited broadening in late systole
20–59%	Peak systolic velocity < 125 cm/sec	Broadening throughout systole
60–79%	Peak systolic velocity > 125 cm/sec; end-diastolic velocity < 125 cm/sec	Broadening throughout systole
80–99%	End-diastolic velocity > 125 cm/sec (severe stenoses may have very low velocity)	Broadening throughout systole
Occlusion	No ICA Doppler signal: flow to zero in CCA[a]	

[a] *CCA*, common carotid artery.

great vessels, a considerable proportion of them have bruits originating from the carotid bifurcations. Duplex scanning can provide accurate separation according to category of stenosis (Table 13–1). Patients with severe stenosis (80 to 99 per cent category) are considered at high risk of stroke and are evaluated for prophylactic carotid endarterectomy. Lesions that fall in the moderate and advanced categories (20 to 79 per cent) should have follow-up testing to detect those that progress into the high-risk group. Most people with normal vessels or early disease do not require routine follow-up.

Another indication is screening of patients with advanced atherosclerotic disease in the coronary or peripheral vessels. Due to the diffuse nature of atherosclerosis, some of these patients have occult carotid bifurcation lesions with a resulting increased risk of stroke. Screening is carried out most often in patients who are being considered for cardiac or major peripheral arterial operations, in order to detect carotid lesions that may substantially increase the risk of intraoperative and postoperative stroke. Although screening may be appropriate for patients with multiple risk factors or severe occlusive disease in other arteries, routine testing of large populations results in a low yield of stenoses in the 80 to 99 per cent category, and is not cost effective, especially if duplex scanning is used.

Postoperative Follow-up

The problem of recurrent stenosis after carotid endarterectomy has attracted increasing interest. Early studies reported as much as 5 per cent symptomatic restenosis and 8 per cent asymptomatic restenosis (as identified by noninvasive testing).[10,11] More recent studies applying life-table analysis have found 20 to 32 per cent rates for restenosis with greater than 50 per cent diameter reduction.[12,13] It has been shown that a substantial proportion of the restenoses occur early in the postoperative period. The practice of our vascular laboratory is to obtain an early postoperative study that can be used as a baseline. Follow-up evaluations are done 6 and 12 months after surgery. If the studies remain normal, noninvasive studies are repeated yearly.

LOWER EXTREMITY ARTERIAL STUDIES

Segmental Extremity Pressure Measurement

Indirect measurement of extremity pressures has been performed since the beginning of the century using a sphygmomanometer and auscultation of the Korotkoff sounds with a stethoscope. Although it is universally used for measurement of pressures in the brachial artery, its application in the lower extremity is less practical because of difficulties in listening for Korotkoff sounds in the popliteal space. The technique is certainly not applicable in the distal portions of the extremity because of the small size of the vessels involved. Investigators overcome this limitation by using a variety of plethysmographic devices. In 1950, Winsor[14] first described the clinical measurements of arterial gradients using a plethysmograph. He found that systolic pressures in the lower extremity were normally higher than those in the upper extremity. He described the blood pressure index (blood pressure of arm/blood pressure of leg), which in normal persons is above 1.0. A value below 1.0 indicates clinically significant occlusive disease proximal to the point of measurement. Likewise, a gradient between two sampling sites localizes the occlusive disease in the intervening segment. The main limitation of this method is that it detects only occlusive lesions that are sufficiently advanced to reduce the systolic pressure, so that it is not possible to detect early disease. Introduction of the Doppler velocity detector greatly simplified the indirect measurement of extremity pressures. For this application, the Doppler device is simply used to detect presence or absence of movement of blood in the artery. Measurements made by this method are very reproducible but do not provide diastolic pressure. Plethysmographic techniques are cumbersome and are not used routinely.

In clinical practice, simple screening can be carried out by measuring the pressure at the brachial arteries and at the dorsal pedal and posterior tibial arteries on each side. The ankle index (AI) is determined by dividing the ankle pressure on each side by the higher of the two brachial pressures. The resulting value reflects the severity of the occlusive disease for the entire extremity. Normally, the AI should be above 1.0, and values below 0.95 are abnormal. Figure 13–5 summarizes the general relation between AI values and clinical status. It must be emphasized that this is only a rough correlation and that patients with similar values may have substantial differences in exercise tolerance. Likewise, the index at which rest pain appears varies considerably from patient to patient, ranging from 0.30 to 0.50.

An important limitation of the indirect measurement of extremity pressure occurs in patients with abnormal stiffening of the vessel wall, most often due to heavy calcification. Such conditions occur in patients with diabetes mellitus but also can be found with other types of pathology. In these cases the systolic pressure measured reflects the cuff pressure required to collapse the vessel wall in addition to the pressure required to overcome the intraluminal pressure. In some cases it is not possible to stop the flow of blood at all. Error due to wall stiffness should be suspected whenever the AI is above 1.3 or when its value is out of proportion to the patient's clinical status. In general, a leg with normal AI should have an easily palpable ankle pulse. In some patients with stiff arteries it may be possible to obtain an accurate evaluation by measuring the toe pressure. In the normal person there is a gradient of 20 to 30 mm Hg

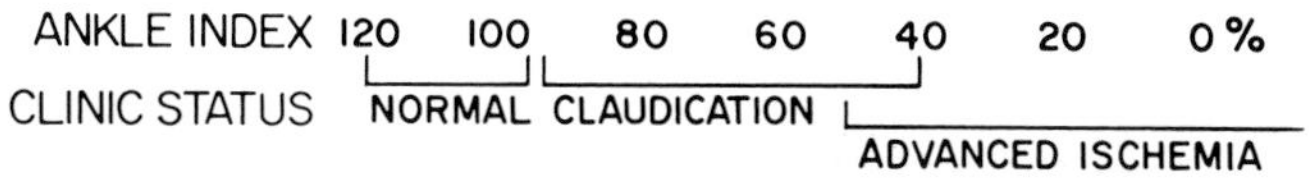

ANKLE INDEX 120   100   80   60   40   20   0 %

CLINIC STATUS   NORMAL   CLAUDICATION

ADVANCED ISCHEMIA

FIGURE 13–5. Relation of ankle index to patient symptoms.

between the ankle and the toe, so a correction must be made when toe pressures are being used.

Additional information on localization of occlusive disease can be obtained by measuring the pressures at different levels of the leg. The segmental pressure measurements are usually performed applying cuffs at the thigh, the upper calf, and immediately above the ankle artery. A standard adult-size cuff (12 cm wide) is satisfactory for calf and ankle determinations, but a thigh cuff (18 cm) should be used above the knee. (Using a narrower cuff above the knee will result in artificially high pressure measurements as a result of the size discrepancy between the cuff and the diameter of the thigh. Thigh measurements with an arm cuff will usually result in determinations that are 20 to 30 mm Hg above those obtained with the wider cuff.) A thigh pressure lower than brachial pressure indicates obstruction proximal to the location of the thigh cuff. Gradients of more than 20 mm Hg between measuring sites are diagnostic of occlusive disease in the intervening segment, and higher gradients are usually associated with more severe lesions.

An important limitation of the use of the wide cuff for thigh measurement is that it is only possible to make a single thigh measurement. As a result, it is not possible to distinguish occlusive disease above the ligament from that in the proximal portion of the superficial femoral artery, since both conditions may result in the same thigh pressure measurement. To overcome this problem some investigators have recommended using 12-cm-wide cuffs in order to obtain two separate thigh measurements. When this is done it is necessary to take into account the 20 to 30 mm Hg artifact that will result. In a study comparing the wide-cuff versus the two-narrow-cuff techniques in the same group of patients, Heintz et al.[15] reported an increased accuracy in localization of disease using the two-cuff technique. Both of the methods of thigh pressure measurement are still being used, so it is important to be aware of which method is being reported when reviewing results of patient studies. Although segmental pressures have been used extensively to detect proximal disease, diagnostic errors may occur in 25 per cent of patients. Other techniques should be used when the accurate assessment of the segmental localization is needed.

Stress Testing

Most patients with advanced arterial insufficiency are adequately evaluated by measurements at rest; however, early lesions may not produce sufficient disturbance at resting flow rates to be detected by the usual methods. An example of the problem is the patient with typical symptoms of claudication who has normal or borderline leg pressures. More accurate evaluation can be obtained by increasing the flow, thereby accentuating the hemodynamic effect of the stenosis. The simplest and most normal way to increase blood flow is to have the patient walk. The exercise produces a decrease in vascular resistance in the leg with a resulting increase in flow to the leg. With moderate levels of exercise there is no change in distal pressures in a normal extremity, but increasing the flow through a moderate stenosis causes an increased resistance at the lesion. The resulting energy loss can be detected by noninvasive tests as a pressure gradient or the attenuation of the pulse waveform.

The stress test is performed by having the patient walk on a treadmill for 5 minutes or until he is forced to stop. Most protocols use a low level of exercise (2 mph with a 10 to 12 per cent grade). This level of stress is sufficient to yield an abnormal result in most claudication patients without undue cardiac stress. Baseline arm and ankle pressures are measured with the Doppler detector. As soon as the patient stops walking he lies down on the examining table for repeat pressure measurements, which are made at 30-second intervals during the first 2 minutes and at 60-second intervals for the remainder of the examination, usually 5 to 10 minutes. The examiner always asks the patient why he stopped walking, because in some cases the limiting factor will be angina or shortness of breath rather than claudication. Identification of these limitations is an important benefit of the stress test, since it may uncover or emphasize the significance of these other conditions.

One objective measure of severity of occlusive disease is the exercise tolerance (i.e., the time the patient walks at the standardized rate). Further assessment is based on the changes in extremity pressures. Figure 13–6 shows the time-pressure relations seen in control subjects and in different categories of occlusive disease. Normal people have no significant change in ankle pressures with the modest level of exercise used for the stress test. On the other hand, patients with flow-limiting stenoses will have a drop in distal pressures as a result of vasodilation in the muscles. The amount of the drop in AI and the recovery time are both increased by greater severity of occlusive disease. Multiple lesions produce more marked depression of the recovery curve than do single lesions.

There are some situations in which treadmill exercise is not practical or does not offer the best eval-

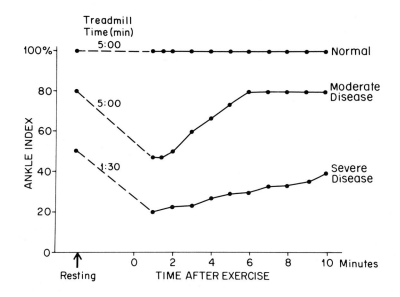

FIGURE 13–6. Changes in ankle index with exercise. The severity of the arterial stenosis is related to the exercise tolerance and the magnitude of the drop in ankle pressure and recovery time.

uation. In such cases reactive hyperemia can be used to increase blood flow in the extremities. A thigh cuff inflated above systolic pressure produces local circulatory arrest, resulting in hypoxia and local vasodilation. When the cuff is released there is a transient increase in flow, the duration of which is related to the period of ischemia and to the total blood flow to the leg. The magnitude of the pressure drop is comparable to that seen after walking but the recovery is always more rapid with reactive hyperemia. In contrast to exercise, reactive hyperemia does produce a transient pressure drop (with a rapid recovery) in normal subjects. Criteria for a normal result are: (1) lowest AI greater than 0.80 and (2) index returns to 90 per cent of baseline value within 1 minute.[16] The technique provides a useful test method for (1) patients who cannot walk on the treadmill because of disabilities, (2) full evaluation of the less involved limb in patients with marked asymmetry of their occlusive disease, and (3) people who are not willing to perform adequately on the treadmill.

Doppler Waveform Analysis

Most commercial Doppler detectors provide an analog signal that is proportional to the velocity of the blood in the vessel studied. This signal can be displayed on a screen or recorded for later analysis. The overall shape of the waveform reflects the status of the vessel proximal to the point studied (Fig. 13–7). In the lower extremity the normal velocity wave is triphasic, with reverse flow in early diastole. Proximal stenosis first eliminates the reverse flow, and with more severe lesions there is blunting of the systolic upstroke and increasing flow during diastole. Complete analysis is complicated by the fact that the waveform is also affected by the stenotic lesions below the sampling site. The simplest analysis of Doppler waveforms is the qualitative interpretation of the

curves, allowing for identification of broad categories of disease. One specific application has been the assessment of the aortoiliac segment. However, the method suffers from a high false-positive rate resulting from the fact that an attenuated wave can be caused by proximal disease, distal disease, or a combination of the two.

A quantitative analysis of the Doppler waveform was described by Gosling et al.[17] using a parameter called pulsatility index (PI), obtained by dividing the peak-to-peak frequency shift by the mean frequency shift. The effect of stenosis is defined by the sampling factor, the ratio of the distal PI to the proximal PI. Normally, the damping factor is greater than 1.0 and values below this reflect disease between the points of the two measurements. Estimation of severity of disease in the aortoiliac segment by waveform damping is not practical, since it is not normally possible to obtain a Doppler signal from the distal aorta with a continuous-wave Doppler.

Segmental Plethysmography

During systole the blood entering a limb normally causes an increase in the total volume of the extremity with a return to resting volume during diastole. This phenomenon is responsible for the pulse pressure oscillations seen with the sphygmomanometer while taking blood pressure. The total effect of the volume changes is quite small and can only be detected with the aid of sensitive devices. A variety of plethysmographic recorders have been devised using mercury strain gauge, water displacement, capacitance, and impedance systems, but the majority of these systems have proven to be impractical for routine clinical application. In the early 1970s, the pulse volume recorder (PVR), was designed specifically for peripheral arterial diagnosis. The system is based on a calibrated recording air-plethysmograph using

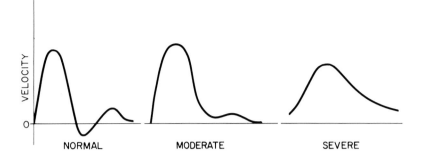

FIGURE 13–7. Doppler velocity tracings in the leg. Increasing stenosis results in elimination of reverse flow, decrease in systolic peak, and increase in flow during diastole.

standard blood pressure cuffs applied at the thigh, calf, and ankle levels. The cuffs are inflated to 65 mm Hg for the recordings in order to assure optimal contact of the cuff around the extremity. A sensitive transducer detects the small increase in pressure within the cuff resulting from the volume increase of the extremity during systole. The recorder provides a hard-copy tracing of the pulse wave, which has been demonstrated to be quite similar to arterial pressure waves measured directly.

The primary diagnosis is based on the qualitative evaluation of the PVR waveform. The tracing from each level is categorized as normal, mildly abnormal, moderately abnormal, or severely abnormal. The normal tracing has a brisk, sharp rise to the systolic peak and usually displays a prominent dicrotic notch (Fig. 13–8). Early disease is characterized by the absence of a dicrotic notch and a more gradual, prolonged downslope. Moderate disease is characterized by the rounded systolic peak. Severe occlusive disease produces a flattened wave with a slow upstroke and downstroke. The absolute amplitude measurements are of limited value from patient to patient, since substantial changes result from variations in cardiac output and vasomotor tone. Comparison of amplitudes from one side to the other in the same patient can be of value in assessing unilateral disease. In the presence of bilateral disease it can help to standardize the amplitude measurements in the lower extremities by comparing them to arm tracings, since most patients do not have major upper extremity occlusive disease. Serial PVR measurements have been shown to be reproducible in patients with stable disease, so that amplitude changes indicate progression of disease.

The PVR has received extensive application in the past 15 years. In most situations the plethysmographic studies are used in combination with segmental Doppler pressure measurements. Vascular laboratories using the PVR report that it is a useful adjunct to the routine pressure measurements. One particular advantage is the ability to accurately assess presence or absence of occlusive disease in patients with rigid arteries. In addition, the PVR has improved the detection of aortoiliac stenosis. Kempczinski[18] has reported correct identification of advanced inflow disease in 95 per cent of extremities.

Duplex Scan

In recent years there has been increasing use of the duplex scan for peripheral arteries. With appropriate scan heads, Doppler signals can be obtained from the aorta down to the tibial branches. Screening for occlusive disease can be done by comparing signals from the distal aorta and more distal sites, looking for attenuation either qualitatively or by measurement of damping factor (see earlier in chapter). A more complete assessment is obtained by examining the full length of the segment in question, looking for the increased velocity and spectral broadening produced by a stenosis. The color-coded Doppler makes tracking of the vessels and localizing of significant stenoses considerably easier than with conventional scanners. Moderate stenosis (20 to 49 per cent) produces extensive spectral broadening with local velocity increases of 30 to 100 per cent, whereas more severe stenosis is associated with velocity increases of more than 100 per cent.[19]

Scanning is being used increasingly for visceral vessels. Renal arteries of normal and transplanted kidneys as well as celiac and superior mesenteric arteries have been studied. The anterior approach to visceral branches can be made difficult by the presence of bowel gas. Flank approaches and examination

FIGURE 13–8. Pulse volume recorder tracings in the leg. Increasing stenosis results in loss of the dicrotic notch and flattening of the curve.

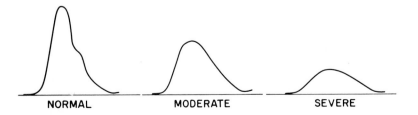

of the fasting patient increase the rate of successful studies. As with peripheral lesions the focus to date has been on distinguishing stenoses above and below 50 per cent diameter reduction.

Applications

Qualitative Assessment of Specific Vessels

Direct examination with a Doppler detector has been applied in a variety of situations. Preoperative determination of whether or not there is flow in distal vessels may help plan distal bypass operations in the calf. In the postoperative patient with no distal pulses it is often possible to detect whether a bypass graft has thrombosed. A more accurate assessment of hand circulation can be achieved by performing a modification of the Allen test, using the Doppler detector to examine flow in the palmar arch during the compression maneuvers. Patency and function of a peritoneovenous shunt (LeVeen or Denver shunt) can be determined. A sterile probe can be used intraoperatively to detect technical problems with arterial reconstructions and to assess intestinal viability.

Severity and Location of Arterial Lesions

The primary use of noninvasive tests in the patient with lower extremity problems is to obtain objective determinations to supplement the physical examination. The measurements permit reproducibility between different examiners as well as from one time to the next. In addition, the tests are valuable in measuring progression of arterial disease and assessment of arterial reconstructions. Extremity pressures and pulse plethysmographic recordings are valuable to assess severity of disease; however, duplex scanning must be used for accurate determination of level and extent of lesions. Kohler et al.[20] found a sensitivity of 89 per cent and a specificity of 90 per cent in identification of iliac stenosis greater than 50 per cent. Legemate et al.[21] used a velocity increase of 150 per cent and found a sensitivity of 92 per cent and specificity of 98 per cent. It is possible to estimate common femoral artery blood flow with duplex scan measurements, but the high variability in repeat measurements in individual patients limits the clinical usefulness of this approach.[22] Although further refinement of quantitative criteria is required, it is clear that duplex scanning can play an increasing role in evaluation of peripheral arterial insufficiency. Good results with scanning have led several groups to select patients for transluminal angioplasty.[23,24]

Resting measurements do not always provide adequate assessment; however, stress tests are only needed in a small proportion of patients. The most common indication for a stress test is the evaluation of the patient with complaints of claudication in whom resting segmental pressures are normal. Normal results rule out significant occlusive disease and point to other diagnoses such as pseudoclaudication. Ex-ercise testing may help differentiate a patient's primary limitation when he complains of a combination of symptoms, such as claudication and shortness of breath. (Arterial reconstruction will not improve the person whose primary limitation is pulmonary.)

Graft Surveillance

Because of the poor secondary patency in patients whose grafts thrombose, careful attention has been given to follow-up. For many years graft status has been monitored with pressure measurements; however, in patients with stiff tibial arteries and those with small-caliber distal grafts, other methods are required. Bandyk et al.[25] have proposed measuring velocity in the graft as an adjunctive method. Subcutaneous grafts are easily studied with a continuous-wave Doppler with a suitable signal processor, whereas anatomically placed bypasses require a duplex scanner. A peak velocity below 45 cm/sec or a drop in peak velocity of 30 cm/sec indicates a failing graft. Once there is an indication of problems with a graft, a more complete evaluation can be obtained with a duplex scan of its entire length to locate the site of stenosis. The use of graft velocity measurements continues to evolve and the optimal criteria are still being developed.

Amputation Level

There has been much interest in using noninvasive tests to predict the probability of healing major leg amputations. Barnes et al.[26] demonstrated that all patients with an AI above 70 per cent attained healing at the below-knee level, while 25 per cent of patients with lower pressures failed. From this data, it would be inappropriate to base the decision for above-knee amputation on AI results. The only finding that indicates an above-knee level is the absence of an arterial Doppler signal in the popliteal space.

VENOUS DISEASE

The correct diagnosis of venous pathology presented a challenge for many years. In contrast to arterial occlusive disease, venous pathology can be difficult to distinguish from other problems on the basis of the physical examination. In the past, diagnosis depended on phlebography, which in addition to being painful can precipitate thrombosis in a normal venous system. In the 1960s, Strandness et al.[27] and Sigel et al.[28] described using the Doppler velocity detector to identify normal and abnormal flow patterns in the veins of the leg. Along with the subsequent development of noninvasive techniques for the arterial system there was a parallel growth of venous diagnosis, initially through the application of plethysmographic techniques and more recently with duplex scanning.

Doppler Venous Examination

The flow in the veins of an extremity can be evaluated qualitatively with the Doppler detector. The patient is examined in the supine position with the head slightly elevated. The deep veins are found adjacent to the accompanying arteries. A normal vein has spontaneous flow with a phasic variation with respiration. Breath-holding or a Valsalva maneuver decreases or abolishes flow; with release there is a transient augmentation of the signal. A quick compression of the extremity distal to the probe produces a brisk augmentation, often followed by a transient decrease on release. Proximal compression decreases or abolishes the flow signal, with augmentation coming on release. Examination of a thrombosed segment of vein will show no flow, and adjacent collateral veins will have a high-pitched signal. The patent portion of the vein distal to an obstruction has a continuous flow with no respiratory variation, and the Valsalva maneuver produces no change. Limb compression may produce limited augmentation, but clearly less than in the normal vein. The vein segment proximal to an occlusion may have phasic flow similar to normal, but the compression produces little change. The Doppler examination is sensitive to alterations in venous flow patterns, and different forms of extrinsic compression can produce similar changes. Abnormal studies can result from large hematomas, massive edema, or ruptured popliteal cysts. A false-positive test can also occur with advanced pregnancy, ascites, or abdominal masses compressing the inferior vena cava.

Many groups have studied the clinical application of the Doppler venous examination by comparing the results with phlebograms. Sumner and Lambeth[29] have reviewed a large number of the published studies and found overall diagnostic accuracies ranging from 49 to 96 per cent, with a number showing accuracies above 90 per cent. Many of the errors are attributed to incomplete examination or lack of examiner experience. The greatest accuracy is obtained in the diagnosis of iliofemoral occlusions because these produce large and easily detected changes in the venous flow patterns. However, careful testing can produce satisfactory diagnosis of thrombosis below the knee, with accuracies of 84 and 86 per cent reported.[30,31]

The Doppler venous examination can also detect venous valvular insufficiency. Normally there should be no flow produced by compression proximal to the probe because the valves prevent flow toward the probe. With incompetent valves the proximal compression (or Valsalva maneuver) produces augmentation as a result of the retrograde flow. Demonstration of significant reverse flow is clear evidence for postthrombotic syndrome.

The Doppler venous examination was an important test for acute deep vein thrombosis in the leg, but it has been supplanted by quantitative and imaging techniques. Because of the simplicity of the method it still remains in use, primarily as an extension of the physical examination. An abnormal flow pattern in a patient with borderline physical findings can trigger more complete evaluation by the vascular laboratory. Simple Doppler examination is also helpful in detecting deep venous reflux in the patient with varicose veins.

Impedance Phlebography

Impedance plethysmography was developed to detect acute deep vein thrombosis by measuring volume changes in a limb by changes in electrical resistance. An increase in the volume causes a decrease in the resistance between measuring electrodes (more accurately, the electrical impedance), and conversely, a decrease in volume raises the resistance. The technique is sensitive enough to detect the small change in volume produced by the additional filling of the limb during systole. Wheeler et al.[32] developed the occlusive method of impedance phlebography (IPG), which provided a standardized method that did not require active patient participation. Two pairs of electrodes are placed on the calf to detect the volume changes in a 10-cm segment, and a blood pressure cuff is placed on the thigh. The foot of the bed is raised 15 to 20 degrees to provide rapid drainage of the veins. While making a continuous IPG recording, the thigh cuff is quickly inflated to 35 to 40 mm Hg, occluding the venous outflow. During occlusion there is an increase in the calf volume until the venous system below the cuff is maximally filled. The cuff is rapidly deflated, releasing the blood trapped in the calf veins, producing a decrease in calf volume to its baseline size.

In a normal extremity, the IPG tracing shows a steady rise, and after 45 seconds the cuff is deflated, producing a rapid fall to baseline levels, usually within 3 to 4 seconds (Fig. 13–9). In the presence of massive, acute deep vein thrombosis, the venous system is maximally filled, so there is no further increase in size when the thigh cuff is inflated and the IPG curve remains flat. With a less extensive occlusion the capacitance of the venous system is limited. The tracing will show a slow rise, often coming to a plateau in 20 to 40 seconds. Following release of the cuff, the outflow will be slow, as a result of the increased resistance of flow through collaterals. Wheeler and Anderson[33] standardized the evaluation of the IPG tracings by comparing the venous capacity (the maximum deflection during venous occlusion) to the maximum venous outflow rate (the amount the tracing drops in the first 3 seconds after cuff release). These values are plotted on a graph that separates the results into normal, borderline, and abnormal diagnostic groups.

Numerous studies have correlated the results of IPG with contrast phlebograms. Wheeler and Anderson[34] have reviewed many of the reports published in the last 8 years and found an overall ac-

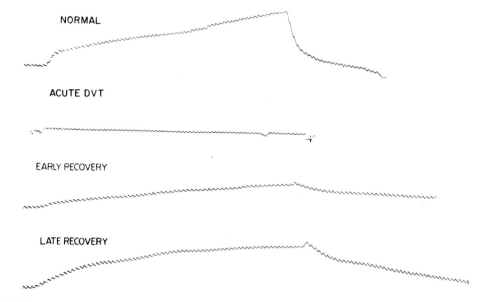

NORMAL

ACUTE DVT

EARLY PECOVERY

LATE RECOVERY

FIGURE 13–9. Impedance phlebogram tracings. Acute thrombosis produces a flat curve because the venous system is maximally distended. With less extensive thrombosis, in the recovery phases there is limited expansion (upward deflection) and slow return to baseline.

curacy of 95 per cent in the diagnosis of thrombosis at or above the popliteal vein.

Impedance phlebography is a simple and accurate technique of diagnosing acute deep vein occlusion. The method is easy to learn, perform, and interpret. It is not capable of identifying a nonocclusive thrombus or small, isolated calf thrombi, as these have no significant effect on the overall venous outflow. An important limitation is that the IPG may not detect chronic deep venous disease because in many cases lysis of clot or extensive collateral development may have reestablished normal outflow from the leg. Although IPG depends on adequate arterial inflow to fill the venous system, the IPG can be performed on most patients with arterial insufficiency; only in patients with severe rest pain (AI less than 0.25) is there a problem in obtaining a satisfactory examination.

Duplex Scan

The high resolution available with duplex scanners makes it possible to detect venous thrombosis. In this application the emphasis is upon imaging. Thrombus is seen within the vein lumen with varying degree of echogenicity (Fig. 13–10). On occasion, fresh thrombus may not appear different from flowing blood; in these instances additional assessment is obtained by compressing the vein with the probe. Normally, gentle pressure will flatten the vein completely (Fig. 13–11). The presence of partial or totally occluding thrombus prevents collapse in response to external pressure. Compression is performed in the transverse mode to assure accurate evaluation with the maneuver. When examining in the longitudinal orientation it is possible to move the ultrasound beam

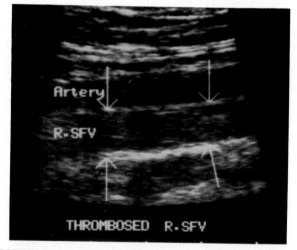

FIGURE 13–10. B mode scan of venous thrombus. Note the appearance of the vein lumen compared with the normal flow in the adjacent artery. *R-SFV*, right superficial femoral vein.

off the center of the vein so that the vein appears to collapse when it does not.

Occluded segments can also be identified by the lack of flow on Doppler examination, and examination of flow characteristics should be part of every study. Abnormalities in Doppler velocity signals either at rest or in response to augmentation maneuvers point to pathology that may not be evident with imaging. Color-coded Doppler is especially helpful in detecting partial occluding thrombi. The color scanner has also improved the examination of the tibial veins.

Most centers using duplex scanning carry out a detailed examination from the inguinal ligament to

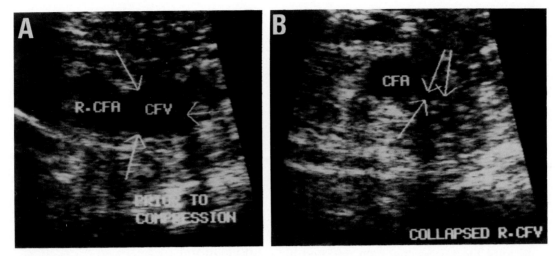

FIGURE 13–11. Transverse duplex scan. *A,* Normal appearance of vein. *B,* Complete collapse of vein in response to external compression with the probe. *R-CFA,* right common femoral artery; *R-CFV,* right common femoral vein.

the distal end of the popliteal vein. The common and superficial femoral veins are examined in the supine position with moderate leg dependency. (The deep femoral vein is usually not followed beyond its origin.) The popliteal vein is best imaged with the patient in the lateral or prone position. In addition to the deep system, superficial veins can be imaged. The greatest difficulty in many examinations is following the vein through the adductor canal. Many studies do not include tracing all the infrapopliteal branches. In some cases this is because of the fact that isolated calf thrombi are not considered important, whereas in other cases the separate branches are not sought because of the added difficulty of examination. The other problem area is the detection of thrombus in the common or external iliac veins. It is difficult to image these; therefore, one often relies on indirect evidence given by the flow signal from the common femoral vein. Proximal occlusion causes a loss of phasic variation with respiration and limited or no change with Valsalva maneuver. Vogel et al. have described using the change in common femoral vein diameter during Valsalva maneuver: increase of less than 10 per cent indicates iliofemoral thrombosis.[35]

Duplex scan of the deep leg veins for thrombus is technically difficult and requires considerable experience for accurate diagnosis. Experienced investigators have reported sensitivities and specificities on the order of 95 per cent for the diagnosis of thrombus.[35-38] Although most studies have focused on acute thrombosis, Rollins and his associates have demonstrated the same high accuracy in the identification of chronic disease as in the acute situation.[37] In addition, they had an 89 per cent accuracy in the evaluation of calf veins compared with 93 per cent for the proximal veins.

The duplex scan is also used to evaluate reflux in specific venous segments. Many laboratories perform this evaluation in a casual fashion, examining patients in the recumbent position and using manual compression to cause valve closure. Van Bemmelen and his associates have emphasized the need to examine the patient in the standing position in order to recreate the maximum stimulus for reflux.[39] In addition, they recommend using a pneumatic cuff with rapid decompression to provide the necessary reverse flow. A reverse velocity of 30 cm/sec is necessary for consistent valvular closure.[40] Manual compression produces a variable amount of reverse flow and often results in incomplete closure. In such a case slow reverse flow may occur through a normal valve, leading to an interpretation of an abnormal segment.

Venous Reflux Photoplethysmography

The venous reflux resulting from valvular insufficiency has long been recognized as the primary cause of the symptoms and complications of the post-thrombotic syndrome. The first method used to study venous hypertension was the direct measurement by insertion of a needle into a superficial foot vein with pressures determined before, during, and after walking. The response to this test is defined by the magnitude of the pressure drop during walking and the time required for the pressure to return to baseline. The main drawback of ambulatory venous pressure measurement is the need for placing a needle into a foot vein, a procedure that can be difficult or impossible in some patients with advanced postthrombotic syndrome.

Photoplethysmography (PPG) has been used to study reflux. A light in the probe shines into the superficial layers of the skin and a photoelectric detector measures the reflected light. The intensity of light reflected varies with the amount of blood in the underlying microcirculation and the device produces a pulse wave trace, which is displayed on a strip-chart recorder. The technique is sensitive enough to record the arterial pulsation in the skin. The PPG tracing varies with the venous congestion of the skin, which varies with the venous pressure in the limb. Studies made with simultaneous recording of venous pressure and PPG signals have demonstrated similar tracing configurations by the two methods.[41,42]

The test is usually performed with the patient in the sitting position. The sensor is attached with double-sided clear tape over the medial malleolus, taking care not to be directly over a superficial vein. After a short baseline tracing is obtained the patient is instructed to contract his calf five times in quick succession and then to relax the leg. The recording is continued until the tracing has fully returned to the baseline level. The recovery time is measured from the end of the calf exercise to the point at which the curve returns to baseline (Fig. 13–12). A normal recovery is over 20 seconds, with many subjects having times of 30 to 60 seconds. Times below 20 seconds indicate venous reflux, with the severity of the condition being inversely proportional to the recovery time. If an abnormal tracing is obtained, the examination is repeated with a Penrose drain tourniquet (or a narrow cuff inflated to 50 mm Hg) placed above or below the knee to exclude the effect of reflux down the superficial system insufficiency in the face of a normal deep system. Commonly, the tracing improves without being completely normal, indicating combined deep and superficial disease. In some cases of severe reflux combined with persisting iliofemoral occlusion there may be either no change or a rise in

the tracing. These findings indicate very severe disease.

PPG recording provides a simple, objective method for quantifying venous reflux. The test is easy to perform and interpret. Unlike the Doppler venous examination, which identifies the presence or absence of flow reversal at given levels, the PPG reflects the overall effect of the venous insufficiency in the leg. A limitation of the test is the possibility of having reflux in the deep system with competent valves in the perforating veins. In this situation the abnormal congestion of the deep system would not be transmitted to the skin and the PPG tracing would be normal.[43]

Applications

Acute Deep Venous Thrombosis

Clinicians have been aware of the fallibility of the physical findings in the diagnosis of acute deep vein thrombosis (DVT) of the leg, so that most of the effort in the noninvasive diagnosis of venous disease has focused on the acute occlusion. The main limitation of the IPG is the inability to detect isolated calf thrombi. Therefore, when using this test, it is advisable to repeat the test in 2 to 4 days if the initial results are negative in a patient with a suspicious clinical picture. With this approach the progression of a limited calf clot can be detected by the subsequent examination and treatment can be started.

Wheeler and Anderson[34] have reviewed the extensive experience with the IPG in his laboratory. Over a 3-year period there were 690 patients suspected of having DVT, who had negative noninvasive tests and had no phlebogram and no therapy. A small number were later suspected of having pulmonary embolization. All patients in this subgroup underwent pulmonary angiography; only one had a positive study, and the embolus was small and nonthreatening. Wheeler and Anderson have found only one anecdotal report of a fatal pulmonary embolus after a negative IPG. Two prospective studies have evaluated the clinical efficacy of managing symptomatic patients based upon IPG findings. Anticoagulation was withheld from all patients with normal IPG. Hull et al.[44] found only a single pulmonary embolus in the 645 patients followed with negative tests. Similarly, Huisman et al.[45] found a single minor embolus in 289 patients followed with negative tests. Of the patients who initially had normal IPG studies, 3 per cent in Hull et al.'s study and 6 per cent in Huisman et al.'s converted to abnormal on repeat testing.

In the past 5 years duplex scanning has become the primary modality used to diagnose acute DVT. Many institutions only perform contrast phlebograms in patients with nondiagnostic scans or where the scan cannot be done. This practice has been justified by the high accuracy achieved by different investigators.[35–38] A major advantage of the scan over IPG is the ability to identify the specific location of

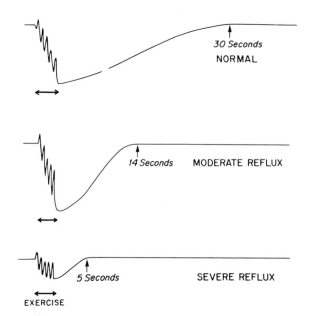

FIGURE 13–12. Photoplethysmography in evaluation of venous reflux. Incompetent valves result in recovery time below 20 seconds. Severe insufficiency causes incomplete emptying of the calf during exercise, seen as a limited downward deflection of the tracing.

disease, especially when there is thrombus at multiple levels. Another important advantage is the detection of partial-occluding thrombi, a key limitation of the IPG. In addition to confirming the initial diagnosis, scanning can be used to document change during the therapy.

Recurrent Deep Vein Thrombosis

The diagnosis of recurrent deep venous thrombosis in patients with postthrombotic syndrome presents a great challenge to clinicians. Exacerbation of symptoms may mimic the symptoms of the original thrombosis, and in many cases patients are readmitted for heparin therapy without objective evidence of recurrence. Although labeled fibrinogen is an excellent method for detecting new thrombus, this test is not available in most nuclear medicine departments. Noninvasive testing may be used to obtain objective diagnosis. In serial follow-up IPG studies Huisman et al.[46] found that 95 per cent of patients with abnormal studies after acute thrombosis reverted to normal within 12 months. Therefore, IPG can be used for subsequent diagnosis in any patient with a normal follow-up study. One of the problems is that it is not current practice to obtain follow-up IPG studies on patients with DVT.

Duplex scanning can identify residual chronic thrombus by its high echogenicity. Other characteristics include thickened vein walls, fibrosed segments of occluded veins, and valvular insufficiency with reverse flow on Doppler examination. These features allow the examiner to distinguish recent from chronic clot, unlike the contrast phlebogram, which shows all lesions as filling defects. An advantage of scanning over IPG is that a baseline follow-up study is not required prior to evaluation of possible new DVT. Although many vascular laboratories do not have experience with scanning of chronic DVT, it appears that this technique will become the best way to detect recurrence.

Venous Insufficiency

The complications of chronic stasis are usually obvious, but it may be difficult to assess the relative contributions of outflow obstruction and reflux. Although the initial conservative management is similar, further surgical treatment must be directed to the specific etiology. IPG can determine the presence of chronic high outflow resistance such as that found in the patient with persisting iliofemoral occlusion with poor collateral development. These are the people who may benefit from venous bypass operations. The Doppler exam or the PPG can determine the presence of venous reflux and whether it involves the deep or the superficial system. More recently, duplex scanning has been used to evaluate specific segments, especially in the deep system. Measurement of reverse blood velocities or flows provides a quantitative assessment not available with the simpler tests.[39,47] This information can help in the selection of procedures such as long saphenous stripping,

interruption of communicating veins, and possibly the newer methods of venous valve transfer or transposition.

Preoperative Vein Mapping

With the growing use of the greater saphenous vein for in situ bypass grafts, knowledge of the patient's specific anatomy has become more important. Using contrast phlebograms, Shah[48] and his associates demonstrated that only 65 per cent of thighs and 45 per cent of calfs had a single saphenous trunk. The rest had variants of double systems and cross-connections. Because many surgeons are concerned about the contrast phlebogram inducing acute thrombosis, there has been increasing use of preoperative duplex scanning for mapping superficial veins both in the arms and the legs.[49,50] The high resolution of the images available on contemporary machines permits satisfactory demonstration of size, course, double segments, and varicosities in most patients. These findings correlate closely with anatomy demonstrated at operation.

Screening Asymptomatic High-Risk Patients

Patients with obesity; previous venous thrombosis; and those undergoing major hip, pelvic, or intracranial operations are all at high risk of developing DVT during or shortly after surgery. Some physicians use prophylaxis against thrombosis, while others prefer to treat only if thrombosis occurs. For many years IPG has been used for screening; however, recent reports show that this and other physiologic methods are inadequate. In a study of screening of 537 patients undergoing total hip replacement, Paiement et al.[51] found that IPG had a sensitivity of only 24 per cent in detecting thigh thrombosis documented by contrast phlebogram. In a similar study Comerota et al.[52] found a 20 per cent sensitivity in the detection of asymptomatic thrombi, and he explained the poor accuracy on the high incidence of nonocclusive lesions. These recent reports show that the physiologic techniques are unsuitable for surveillance of the asymptomatic patients. As a result, increasing numbers of physicians are turning to the duplex scan for screening purposes, mainly because the technique can demonstrate nonocclusive thrombi. Recent studies of asymptomatic, high-risk patients have compared scanning and contrast venography. Although specificity has ranged from 94 to 100 per cent, sensitivity has been between 63 and 79 per cent.[53–55] The results indicate that a negative study may miss asymptomatic thrombi in a significant proportion of patients. The screening role for scanning still requires further evaluation.

CONCLUSIONS

The rapid development of noninvasive vascular laboratory techniques in recent years has increased the amount of objective data that can be accumulated about a patient. As is the case with other diagnostic modalities, it is critical to remember that the different tests should always supplement, not replace, the information gained from a careful history and physical examination. It is becoming increasingly common to find medical students or young house staff presenting patients in terms of the results of the vascular lab tests rather than describing presenting symptoms and physical findings. Another area of concern is the increasing practice of patients being sent to the noninvasive laboratory for "diagnosis of vascular condition" without having been examined. This practice results in a growing number of inappropriate tests (with the corresponding wasteful cost to the patient).

Optimal use of noninvasive test results requires an understanding of the limitations and errors of the specific examinations. The choice of tests must be based on the questions to be answered. There are some questions that cannot be answered by any of the techniques, such as the detection of small ulcers in the carotid arteries. In addition, it must be remembered that errors, both false-positives and false-negatives, occur with all diagnostic methods, so it is important to be aware of the accuracy of the tests being used. Published studies often represent the best that can be expected, and newly established laboratories often do not achieve as good results. Therefore, it is important to find out the accuracy obtained in the laboratory one is using in order to apply the noninvasive results appropriately.

REFERENCES

1. Blackshear WM, Phillips DJ, Thiele BL, et al: Detection of carotid occlusive disease by ultrasonic imaging and pulsed Doppler spectrum analysis. Surgery 86:698–706, 1979.
2. Gee W, Mehigan JT, Wylie EJ: Measurement of collateral cerebral hemispheric blood pressure by ocular pneumoplethysmography. Am J Surg 130:121, 1975.
3. Gee W: Physiologic principles of ocular pneumoplethysmography. In Bernstein EF (ed): Noninvasive Diagnostic Techniques in Vascular Disease. St. Louis, CV Mosby, 1982, pp 57–66.
4. Gee W: Carotid physiology with ocular pneumoplethysmography. Stroke 13:666–673, 1982.
5. Bluth EI, Stavros AT, Marich KW, Wetzner SM, Aufrichtig D, Baker JD: Carotid duplex sonography: A multicenter recommendation for standardized imaging and Doppler criteria. Radiographics 8:487–506, 1988.
6. Bendick PJ, Jackson VP, Becker GJ: Comparison of ultrasound scanning/Doppler with digital subtraction angiography in evaluation of carotid arterial disease. Med Instrum 17:220–222, 1983.
7. Langlois Y, Roederer GO, Chan A, et al: Evaluating carotid artery disease—The concordance between pulsed Doppler/spectrum analysis and angiography. Ultrasound Med Biol 9:51–63, 1983.
8. Londrey GL, Spadona DP, Hodgson KJ, Ramsey DE, Barkmeir LD, Sumner DS: Does color-flow imaging improve the accuracy of duplex carotid evaluation? J Vasc Surg 13:659–662, 1991.
9. Ackerstaff RGA, Grosvelt WJHM, Eikelbloom BC, Ludwig JW: Ultrasonic duplex scan of the prevertebral segment of the vertebral artery in patients with cerebral atherosclerosis. Eur J Vasc Surg 2:387–393, 1988.
10. Kremen JE, Gee W, Kaupp HA, McDonald KM: Restenosis or occlusion after carotid endarterectomy. Arch Surg 114:608–610, 1979.
11. Salvian A, Baker JD, Machleder HI, Busuttil RW, Barker WF, Moore WS: Etiology and noninvasive detection of restenosis following carotid endarterectomy. Am J Surg 146:29–34, 1983.
12. DeGroote RD, Lynch TG, Jamil Z, Hobson RW: Carotid restenosis: Long-term noninvasive follow-up after carotid endarterectomy. Stroke 18:1031–1036, 1987.
13. Healy DA, Zierler RE, Nichols SC, et al: Long-term follow-up and clinical outcome of carotid restenosis. J Vasc Surg 10:662–669, 1989.
14. Winsor T: Influence of arterial disease on the systolic blood pressure gradients of the extremity. Am J Med Sci 220:117–126, 1959.
15. Heintz SE, Bone GE, Slaymaker EE, et al: Value of arterial pressure measurements in the proximal and distal part of the thigh in arterial occlusive disease. Surg Gynecol Obstet 146:337–343, 1978.
16. Baker JD: Poststress Doppler ankle pressures. Arch Surg 113:1171, 1978.
17. Gosling RG, Dunbar G, King DH, et al: The quantitative analysis of occlusive peripheral arterial disease by nonobtrusive ultrasonic technique. Angiology 22:52–55, 1971.
18. Kempczinski RK: Segmental volume plethysmography in the diagnosis of lower extremity arterial occlusive disease. J Cardiovasc Surg 23:125–129, 1982.
19. Jager KA, Phillips DJ, Martin RL: Noninvasive mapping of lower limb lesions. Ultrasound Med Biol 11:515–521, 1987.
20. Kohler TR, Nance DR, Cramer MM, Vandenberghe N, Strandness DE: Duplex scanning for diagnosis of aortoiliac and femoropopliteal disease: A prospective study. Circulation 76:1074–1080, 1987.
21. Legemate DA, Teeuwen C, Hoeneveld H, Ackerstaff RGA, Eikelbloom BC: The potential of duplex scanning to replace aorto-iliac and femoro-popliteal angiography. Eur J Vasc Surg 3:49–54, 1989.
22. Lewis P, Psaila JV, Davies WT, McCarty K, Woodcock JP: Measurement of volume flow in the human common femoral artery using a duplex ultrasound system. Ultrasound Med Biol 12:777–784, 1986.
23. Cossman DV, Ellison JE, Wagner WH, et al: Comparison of contrast angiography to arterial mapping with color-flow duplex imaging in the lower extremities. J Vasc Surg 10:522–529, 1989.
24. Edwards JM, Coldwell DM, Goldman ML, Strandness DE: The role of duplex scanning in the selection of patients for transluminal angioplasty. J Vasc Surg 13:69–74, 1991.
25. Bandyk DF, Seabrook GR, Moldenhauer P, et al: Hemodynamics of vein graft stenosis. J Vasc Surg 8:688–695, 1988.
26. Barnes RW, Shanik GD, Slaymaker EE: An index of healing in below knee amputation: Leg blood pressure by Doppler ultra-sound. Surgery 79:13–20, 1976.
27. Strandness DE, Schultz RD, Sumner DS, Rushmer RF: Ultrasonic flow detection—a useful technique in the evaluation of peripheral vascular disease. Am J Surg 113:311–320, 1967.
28. Sigel B, Popky GL, Wagner DK, Boland JP, Mapp EM, Feigl P: A Doppler ultrasound method for diagnosing lower extremity venous disease. Surg Gynecol Obstet 127:339–350, 1968.
29. Sumner DS, Lambeth A: Reliability of Doppler ultrasound in the diagnosis of acute venous thrombosis both above and below the knee. Am J Surg 138:205–210, 1979.
30. Hull RS, Hirsh J, Carter CJ, et al: Diagnostic efficacy of impedance plethysmography for clinically suspected deep-vein

thrombosis: A randomized trial. Ann Intern Med *102*:21–28, 1985.

31. Barnes RW, Russell HE, Wu KK, Hoak JC: Accuracy of Doppler ultrasound in clinically suspected venous thrombosis of the calf. Surg Gynecol Obstet *143*:425–428, 1976.

32. Wheeler HB, O'Donnell JA, Anderson FA, Benedict K: Occlusive impedance phlebography: A diagnostic procedure for venous thrombosis and pulmonary embolism. Prog Cardiovasc Dis *17*:199–205, 1974.

33. Wheeler JB, Anderson FA: Impedance plethysmography. *In* Kempczinski RF, Yao JST (eds): Practical Noninvasive Diagnosis, 2nd ed. Chicago, Year Book Medical Publishers, 1987, pp 407–437.

34. Wheeler HB, Anderson FA: Can noninvasive tests be used as the basis for treatment of deep vein thrombosis? *In* Bernstein EF (ed): Noninvasive Diagnostic Techniques in Vascular Disease, 3rd ed. St. Louis, CV Mosby, 1985, pp 805–818.

35. Vogel P, Laing FC, Jeffrey RB, Wing VW: Deep venous thrombosis of the lower extremity: US evaluation. Radiology *163*:747–751, 1987.

36. Cronan JJ, Dorfman GS, Scola FH, Schepps B, Alexander J: Deep venous thrombosis: US assessment using venous compression. Radiology *162*:191–194, 1987.

37. Rollins DL, Semrow CM, Friedell ML, Calligaro KD, Buchbinder D: Progress in the diagnosis of deep venous thrombosis: The efficacy of real-time B-mode ultrasonic imaging. J Vasc Surg *7*:638–641, 1988.

38. Sullivan ED, Peter DJ, Cranley JJ: Real-time B-mode venous ultrasound. J Vasc Surg *1*:465–471, 1984.

39. van Bemmelen PS, Bedford G, Beach K, Strandness DE: Quantitative segmental evaluation of venous valvular reflux with duplex ultrasound scanning. J Vasc Surg *10*:425–431, 1989.

40. van Bemmelen PS, Bedford G, Beach K, Strandness DE: The mechanism of venous valve closure. Arch Surg *125*:617–619, 1990.

41. Abramowitz HB, Queral LA, Flinn WR, et al: The use of photoplethysmography in the assessment of venous insufficiency: A comparison to venous pressure measurements. Surgery *86*:434–441, 1979.

42. Nicolaides AN, Miles C: Photoplethysmography in the assessment of venous insufficiency. J Vasc Surg *5*:405–412, 1987.

43. Barnes RW, Yao JST: Photoplethysmography in chronic venous insufficiency. *In* Bernstein EF (ed): Noninvasive Diagnostic Techniques in Vascular Disease, 2nd ed. St. Louis, CV Mosby, 1982, pp 514–521.

44. Hull RS, Hirsch J, Carter CJ, et al: Diagnostic efficacy of impedance plethysmography for clinically suspected deepvein thrombosis: A randomized trial. Ann Intern Med *102*:21–28, 1985.

45. Huisman MV, Buller HR, TenCate JW, Vreeken J: Serial impedance plethysmography for suspected deep venous thrombosis in outpatients: The Amsterdam General Practitioner Study. N Engl J Med *314*:823–828, 1986.

46. Huisman MV, Buller HR, TenCate JW: Utility of impedance plethysmography in the diagnosis of recurrent deep-vein thrombosis. Arch Intern Med *148*:681–683, 1988.

47. Vasdekis SN, Clarke GH, Nicolaides AN: Quantification of venous reflux by means of duplex scanning. J Vasc Surg *10*:670–677, 1989.

48. Shah DM, Chang BB, Leopold PW, Corson JD, Leather RP, Karmody AM: The anatomy of the greater saphenous vein system. J Vasc Surg *3*:273–283, 1986.

49. Ruoff BA, Cranley JJ, Haannan LA, Aseffa N, Karkow WS, Stedje KG, Cranley RD: Real-time duplex ultrasound mapping of the greater saphenous vein before in situ infrainguinal revascularization. J Vasc Surg *6*:107–113, 1987.

50. Salles-Cunha SX, Andros G, Harris RW, Dulawa LB, Oblath RW: Preoperative noninvasive assessment of arm veins to be used as bypass grafts in the lower extremities. J Vasc Surg *3*:813–816, 1986.

51. Paiement G, Wessinger SJ, Waltman AC, Harris WH: Surveillance of deep vein thrombosis in asymptomatic total hip replacement patients: Impedance phlebography and fibrinogen scanning versus roentgenographic phlebography. Am J Surg *155*:400–404, 1988.

52. Comerota AJ, Katz ML, Grossi RJ, et al: The comparative value of noninvasive testing for diagnosis and surveillance of deep vein thrombosis. J Vasc Surg *7*:40–49, 1988.

53. Borris LC, Christiansen HM, Lassen MR, Olsen AD, Schott P: Real-time ultrasonography in the diagnosis of deep vein thrombosis in non-symptomatic high-risk patients. Eur J Vasc Surg *4*:473–475, 1990.

54. Woolson ST, McCrory DW, Walter JF, Maloney WJ, Watt JM, Cahill PD: B-mode ultrasound scanning in the detection of proximal venous thrombosis after total hip replacement. J Bone Joint Surg *72A*:983–987, 1990.

55. Mattos MA, Londrey GL, Leutz DW, et al: Color-flow duplex scanning for the surveillance and diagnosis of acute deep venous thrombosis. J Vasc Surg *15*:366–376, 1992.

BIBLIOGRAPHY

Berstein EF (ed): Noninvasive Diagnosis Techniques in Vascular Disease, 4th ed. St. Louis, CV Mosby, 1993.

Grant EC, White EM: Duplex Sonography. New York, Springer-Verlag, 1987.

Kempczinski RF, Yao JST (eds): Practical Noninvasive Vascular Diagnosis, 2nd ed. Chicago, Year Book Medical Publishers, 1987.

Salles-Cunha SX, Andros G: Atlas of Duplex Ultrasonography. Pasadena, CA, Appleton Davies, 1988.

Zwiebel WJ (ed): Introduction to Vascular Ultrasonography, 3rd ed. Philadelphia, WB Saunders Company, 1992.

REVIEW QUESTIONS

1. Measuring thigh pressures with a regular arm blood pressure cuff will result in a determination that is:

   (a) higher than the actual pressure
   (b) equal to the actual pressure
   (c) lower than the actual pressure

2. An ankle index (ankle pressure–arm pressure) of 160 per cent indicates:

   (a) normal arterial system
   (b) significant arterial insufficiency
   (c) pathologic vessel wall stiffness
   (d) arteriovenous fistula in the extremity
   (e) none of the above

3. When evaluating a patient with an exercise stress test, the severity of occlusive disease is evaluated by:

   (a) walking time
   (b) magnitude of drop in ankle index

(c) recovery time
(d) all of the above
(e) none of the above

4. Noninvasive cerebrovascular techniques are accurate for all except:
   (a) detecting advanced stenosis of the internal carotid artery
   (b) detecting internal carotid occlusion
   (c) detecting arterial ulceration
   (d) detecting abnormal turbulence in the internal carotid artery

5. For a given arterial velocity the magnitude of the Doppler shift is related to:
   (a) distance from the probe
   (b) frequency of the probe
   (c) type of system (pulse or continuous-wave)
   (d) all of the above
   (e) none of the above

6. Noninvasive evaluation of the carotid system with ocular pneumoplethysmography (OPG) is limited by the fact that:
   (a) test can only detect presence or absence of advanced stenosis
   (b) test cannot differentiate tight stenosis from occlusion

(c) both (a) and (b)
(d) neither (a) nor (b)

7. Spectral broadening of a Doppler signal is:
   (a) greatest proximal to a stenosis
   (b) greatest in the stenosis
   (c) greatest just beyond a stenosis
   (d) the same at all of the above sites

8. Asymptomatic deep venous thrombosis of the leg is best detected by:
   (a) impedance phlebography (IPG)
   (b) duplex scan
   (c) both
   (d) neither
   (e) none of the above

9. A venous reflux photoplethysmography (PPG) exam of a patient with postphlebitic syndrome will show:
   (a) increased recovery time
   (b) unchanged recovery time
   (c) decreased recovery time

10. Suitability of a superficial femoral artery for treatment with balloon dilation can be determined by:
    (a) segmental pressures
    (b) volume plethysmography
    (c) duplex scan
    (d) all the above
    (e) none of the above

ANSWERS

1. a	2. c	3. d	4. c	5. b	6. c	7. c
8. b	9. c	10. c				

14
NATURAL HISTORY AND NONOPERATIVE TREATMENT OF CHRONIC LOWER EXTREMITY ISCHEMIA

LLOYD M. TAYLOR, JR. and JOHN M. PORTER

Traditionally, vascular surgeons have practiced in the United States without a related medical subspecialty concerned with the nonoperative care of patients with vascular disease. Thus, in contrast to many other surgical specialists, vascular surgeons have been obligated to function as diagnosticians, primary caregivers, and nonoperative therapists for patients with vascular disease, in addition to their more traditional role as operative therapists. This situation is changing at present. Vascular medicine, long a recognized area of specialization in a few academic centers, has been identified by the National Institutes of Health as an area of priority in both research and clinical areas. New centers have been established, and specific training in vascular medicine is now available in a number of medical centers, with more to come. Thus, in the near future, vascular surgeons may readily turn to well-trained medical colleagues who provide primary and nonoperative care for their vascular patients. Arrival of significant numbers of clinical specialists upon the scene will require time, however, and at least for the intermediate-term future, patients with clinical vascular disease will continue to rely upon vascular surgeons for both operative and nonoperative speciality care.

The need for such care is obvious with regard to lower extremity ischemia. The population is aging rapidly. At least 10 per cent of persons over the age of 70 have claudication, as well as 1 to 2 per cent of those ages 37 to 69.[1,2] Currently about 100,000 procedures per year are performed for treatment of lower extremity ischemia.[3] Clearly most patients with lower extremity ischemia are treated nonoperatively.

In this chapter we will review the available information regarding the natural history of chronic lower extremity ischemia. Such information must obviously serve as the foundation upon which all treatment decisions are based. We will then describe our preferred approach to the nonoperative management of patients with this condition. The subjects discussed include diagnostic testing, risk factor modification, and pharmacologic therapy.

NATURAL HISTORY OF CHRONIC LOWER EXTREMITY ISCHEMIA

In the past patients with chronic lower extremity ischemia were considered in two groups, based upon an assumption of markedly different natural histories. Patients in the first group, those with intermittent claudication, were considered to have a relatively benign prognosis, with a low cumulative incidence of amputation and/or need for corrective surgery. In contrast, patients with limb-threatening ischemia (ischemic rest pain, gangrene) were thought to have a uniformly grim prognosis, with amputation the inevitable result unless the ischemia could be corrected surgically. This artificial division of patients with a single disease process into two groups, while a serviceable approach in years past, is no longer optimal. As will become apparent from the information that follows, chronic lower extremity ischemia presents a spectrum of severity, which is particularly suited to objective quantitative noninvasive evaluation. The prognosis for patients with chronic lower extremity ischemia is more closely related to the results of such objective evaluation than to any subjective description of symptoms.

Historic Studies of the Natural History of Claudication

Intermittent claudication is a clinical condition characterized by lower extremity muscular pain induced by exercise and relieved by short periods of rest. The syndrome is caused by arterial obstruction at sites proximal to the muscle bed that restrict the normal exercise-induced increase in muscle blood flow, producing ischemia. It is obvious that the significance of this symptom complex will vary widely, depending upon levels of exercise and the perception of discomfort by each individual. Studies have demonstrated that between 50 and 90 per cent of patients with intermittent claudication have never complained of this symptom to their doctors.[4,5] When questioned, patients typically responded that they considered increasing difficulty walking to be a normal consequence of aging.

Aside from the inconvenience imposed by its symptoms, intermittent claudication is of concern to both patients and physicians because of the fear of disease progression with ultimate need for amputation. Multiple large studies of claudication have established that this is an unusual outcome. The classic study of Boyd[6] is an example, in which 1440 claudicants followed prospectively for 10 years had an amputation incidence of 12.2 per cent. Similarly, in the Framingham study, 1.6 per cent of claudicants followed for a mean of 8.3 years required amputation.[7] Data from several other historic studies of the natural history of claudication are listed in Table 14–1, confirming the relatively benign prognostic implications of claudication symptoms.

This historic picture of claudication must be carefully reviewed. Although the claudication symptom complex is relatively specific, many other causes of leg pain exist. Most historic claudication studies used patient history alone as inclusion criteria and doubtless were flawed by inclusion of a variable but significant number of patients with normal arterial circulation and leg pain of other etiologies. The effect of this sampling error is that of assigning too benign a prognosis. The results of claudication studies including only patients whose arterial obstructive disease was objectively documented are reviewed in the section that follows.

Natural History of Claudication as Determined by Objective Studies

Arterial obstruction producing claudication can be objectively demonstrated by arteriography, or by noninvasive means such as measurement of ankle-arm blood pressure index. The results of studies of claudication in which abnormal results of such testing were an entry requirement are summarized in Table 14–2. These studies reveal a more somber prognosis than that described in most historic studies cited above. The report of Cronenwett et al.,[11] in which 91 male veteran patients were followed for a mean of 2.5 years, is an example of the newer objectively documented studies. In this group, 60 per cent experienced worsening during the study, and fully 22 per cent required operation to prevent amputation. Similar results were noted by Rosenbloom et al.,[12] who retrospectively reviewed 195 patients followed for up to 8 years. By life-table analysis, 24 per cent of limbs developed critical ischemia by 5 years of follow-up and 41 per cent by 8 years of follow-up.

Multiple investigators have examined the outcome of patients with claudication to identify factors associated with a higher likelihood of progression to severe ischemia. Cigarette smoking and diabetes have both been identified as such factors. Importantly, however, all studies in which arterial disease has been objectively assessed have clearly identified *severity of arterial occlusive disease at the time of initial patient encounter* as the most important risk factor for subsequent development of severe ischemia. This is true for studies in which disease was initially assessed by noninvasive means[7,11,12,14] as well as for those in which assessment was by angiography.[13]

Natural History of Limb-Threatening Ischemia

Limb-threatening ischemia occurs when arterial occlusion progresses to the point at which resting blood flow is insufficient to meet minimal metabolic requirements. The clinical manifestations of this pathophysiologic state include rest pain, ulceration, and gangrene. Ischemic rest pain is typically described as a burning, dysesthetic discomfort primarily involving the forefoot and toes. The pain is typically induced or aggravated by elevation and partially or totally relieved by dependency, presumably as a result of the increase in arterial pressure due to gravity. Ischemic ulceration occurs when minor traumatic le-

TABLE 14–1.   NATURAL HISTORY OF CLAUDICATION AS DETERMINED BY STUDIES BASING DIAGNOSIS ON PATIENT HISTORY

Author and Year	Reference Number	Number of Patients	Mean Follow-up (Years)	Stable or Improved (%)	Worse (%)	Amputated (%)
Boyd, 1960	6	1440	10	—	—	12.2
Schadt et al., 1961	8	362	9	93	7	—
Peabody et al., 1974	2	162	8.3	—	—	4.3
Begg and Richards, 1962	9	198	5	73	26	7
McAllister, 1976	10	100	6	78	22	7

TABLE 14–2. NATURAL HISTORY OF CLAUDICATION AS DETERMINED BY STUDIES BASING DIAGNOSIS ON OBJECTIVE TESTING

Author and Year	Reference Number	Number of Patients	Mean Follow-up (Years)	Stable or Improved (%)	Worse (%)	Amputated (%)
Cronenwett et al., 1984	11	91	2.5	40	60	—
Rosenbloom et al., 1988	12	195	8[a]	59	41	—
Imparato and Kim, 1975	13	104	2.5	79	21	5.8
Jonason and Ringquiest, 1985	14	224	6	78	22	—

[a]Life-table follow-up to 8 years.

sions fail to heal because of inadequate blood supply. Gangrene occurs when arterial inflow is so inadequate that spontaneous necrosis occurs in the areas with least perfusion.

It is well recognized that limb-threatening ischemia incident to acute arterial occlusion may rapidly resolve as a result of the development of collateral circulation. Traditional teaching, however, states that chronic ischemic rest pain is inevitably followed by progressive gangrene and need for amputation. Review of the available data indicates that this uniformly grim prognosis is probably inaccurate and excessively simplistic. Clearly, progressive gangrenous changes and/or continuous ischemic rest pain are unstable conditions requiring treatment. In contrast, a number of patients with advanced ischemia describe occasional episodes of rest pain relieved by dependency and maintain stable symptoms for months or years. Similarly, with care, severely ischemic ulcerations may ultimately heal without revascularization.

Rivers et al.[15] described healing of ischemic ulcers in 11 of 14 patients who received no specific therapy for their limb-threatening ischemia beyond simple wound care. This study emphasizes the uncertain natural history of limb-threatening ischemia, and emphasizes the critical need for a control group in any study purporting to show therapeutic benefit for a particular treatment method. The results of studies that included such control patients may be surprising to surgeons assuming that the existence of rest pain and/or gangrene means inevitable limb loss. A trial of prostaglandin treatment performed in 1982 randomized 22 patients with arterial ischemic ulcers. In the placebo-treated group, 40 per cent of the ulcers healed.[16] A similar study of 120 patients performed in 1984 found healing of ischemic ulcers in 49 per cent of the placebo-treated patients, over 80 per cent of whom also reported improved ischemic rest pain.[17]

Just as with intermittent claudication, objective assessment of the severity of the arterial occlusive process permits stratification of prognosis in patients with limb-threatening ischemia. The likelihood of limb loss is directly related to severity of ischemia at the time of patient presentation, with the patients having absent ankle arterial Doppler signals demonstrating a uniformly poor outcome.[18]

Long-Term Survival of Patients with Chronic Lower Extremity Ischemia

Since atherosclerosis is a systemic disease process, one may accurately predict increased incidence of coronary and cerebral vascular disease in persons with chronic lower extremity ischemia. The inevitable result of such involvement is reduced long-term survival when compared with age-matched control patients. Until recently, information regarding the incidence of atherosclerotic disease at various sites has been limited to data obtained by inquiry regarding symptoms. Recently, however, objective information regarding the incidence of associated atherosclerotic coronary and cerebral lesions, whether symptomatic or asymptomatic, has become available from two sources.

The first of these is the patient series accumulated at the Cleveland Clinic under the direction of Hertzer and colleagues. These workers obtained routine coronary angiography in 1000 consecutive patients prior to elective vascular surgery without regard to the presence or absence of symptoms of coronary disease. Coronary atherosclerosis was detected in 90 per cent of all patients scheduled for operation for lower extremity ischemia.[19] Symptomatic and/or electrocardiographic evidence of disease was present in only 47 per cent of these patients, emphasizing that a considerable portion of the coronary disease detected by angiography was asymptomatic. Importantly, fully 14 per cent of the asymptomatic patients were found to have severe surgically correctable coronary disease. A summary of data from this important study is seen in Table 14–3. Although this study demonstrates an overwhelming incidence of coronary disease, the reader must recall that this information was obtained from a patient population all of whom were sufficiently symptomatic to require peripheral vascular surgery. It seems reasonable to assume that coronary disease in these persons is more advanced than would be found in the entire group of patients with lower extremity ischemia, most of whom do not require operative treatment.

The availability of duplex scanning of the carotid arteries, a noninvasive test with accuracy approaching that achieved by cerebral angiography, has made

TABLE 14–3. INCIDENCE OF CORONARY ARTERY DISEASE (CAD) IN 1000 CONSECUTIVE PERIPHERAL DISEASE PATIENTS SCREENED BY CORONARY ANGIOGRAPHY[a]

	No Indications of Coronary Disease		Suspected Coronary Disease	
	No. of Patients	Per Cent	No. of Patients	Per Cent
Normal coronary arteries	64	14	21	4
Mild to moderate CAD	218	49	99	18
Advanced but compensated CAD	97	22	192	34
Severe correctable CAD	63	14	188	34
Severe inoperable CAD	4	1	54	10

[a]From Hertzer NR, Bevan EG, Young JR, O'Hara PJ, Ruschhaupt WF, Graor RA, DeWolfe VG, Maljovec LC: Coronary artery disease in peripheral vascular patients—a classification of 1000 coronary angiograms and results of surgical management. Ann Surg *199*:223, 1984.

it possible to screen large numbers of persons with lower extremity ischemia for carotid atherosclerosis. In one such study of preoperative patients, 52 per cent were found to have detectable carotid artery disease.[20] In our own preoperative patients, 40 per cent had carotid stenosis, one fourth of whom had stenoses of 60 per cent or greater diameter reduction (J.A. Luscombe, L.M. Taylor, Jr., and J.M. Porter, unpublished data). In the majority of patients in both these surveys, the carotid artery disease was asymptomatic.

Given the prevalence of coronary and cerebral disease referred to above, the markedly reduced long-term survival in persons with chronic lower extremity ischemia when compared to age-matched controls is hardly surprising. All studies have found such reduced survival, as can be seen from the summary of information in Table 14–4. Interestingly, the severity of the anticipated reduction in survival appears to be directly related to the severity of the lower extremity occlusive disease as assessed by objective testing, or by severity of symptoms. Thus survival after 5 years of follow-up ranges from 87 per cent in a series of patients with claudication treated nonoperatively,[32] to 80 per cent in a series of patients with claudication

treated by operation,[29] to 48 per cent in a series of patients with limb-threatening ischemia treated by operation,[30] to 12 per cent in a series of patients requiring reoperative surgery for limb-threatening ischemia.[31] Similarly, multiple studies that stratified patients according to objective parameters of severity of lower extremity ischemia have demonstrated an inverse relationship with survival. The influence on survival is especially pronounced when severe arterial involvement is present below the knee.[18,33–35]

This information leads to the inescapable conclusion that the severity of the systemic atherosclerotic disease process is accurately mirrored by the severity of localized atherosclerotic changes in the lower extremities. Thus physicians obtaining objective evaluation of patients' lower extremity complaints are at the same time obtaining a valid approximation of their survival potential, information that may be critically important to therapeutic planning. A major exception to this rule appears to exist when lower extremity arterial occlusive disease is diagnosed in young patients, in whom both the cause of the condition and the implications of its presence may be different. This important patient group is discussed in the following section.

TABLE 14–4. SURVIVAL OF PATIENTS WITH CHRONIC LOWER EXTREMITY ISCHEMIA

Author and Year	Reference Number	Number of Patients	Mean Follow-up (Years)	5-Year Survival (%)	10-Year Survival (%)	15-Year Survival (%)
Bloor, 1961	21	1476	7.0	79.0	54	—
				72.0	35	—
				60.0	20	—
Silbert and Zazeela, 1958	22	1198	12.0	94.7	71	52
Kallero, 1981	23	193	9.7	—	52	—
Schadt et al., 1961	8	362	9.0	76.0[a]	59	—
				54.0[b]	38	
Leferve et al., 1959	24	500	5.0	57.0	—	—
Hansteen et al., 1975	25	307	8–16	70.0	50	37
Crawford et al., 1981	26	949	0–25	74.0	50	30
Szilagyi et al., 1986	27	1648	0–30	70.0	64	25
Hertzer, 1981	28	256	6–11	80.0	60	—
Malone et al., 1977	29	180	0–15	80.0	43	26
Veith et al., 1981	30	551	5.0	48.0	—	—
Edwards et al., 1990	31	82	2.0	12.0	—	—

[a]Nondiabetics.
[b]Diabetics.

Natural History of Chronic Lower Extremity Ischemia in Young Persons

Most patients with atherosclerotic lower extremity occlusive disease are elderly. When symptomatic peripheral occlusive disease occurs in young persons (less than 50 years of age), identifiable conditions other than idiopathic arteriosclerosis are often present. Such conditions include familial hyperlipidemia, congenital hypercoagulable states, Buerger's disease, and inborn errors of metabolism such as homocystinemia.[36–41] Progression of disease in these patients has been especially rapid, with a high incidence of amputation noted by many investigators. In the past many authorities have recommended that invasive therapy be considered only in cases of clearly threatened limb loss, both because of a high anticipated failure rate and because of a higher than usual rate of amputation following failed reconstructions in these young patients.[42]

Interestingly, the aggressive course pursued by lower extremity occlusive disease in young persons is not paralleled by a high incidence of early death, as would be predicted from the experience with patients in the more typically atherosclerotic age groups over age 60. Several investigators have noted relatively normal life expectancy in young persons with lower extremity arterial disease, particularly when a disease process separate from atherosclerosis can be identified, such as Buerger's disease.[43,44]

EVALUATION OF THE PATIENT WITH CHRONIC LOWER EXTREMITY ISCHEMIA

Review of the preceding sections makes obvious the need for objective evaluation of lower extremity ischemia in order to make rational decisions regarding etiology, severity, and therapy. Although a great deal can be learned from the clinical assessment of the patient, there is simply no substitute for noninvasive quantitative determination of the location and severity of the arterial lesions present, information that, in all studies to date, correlates much better with prognosis than the presence or absence of any subjectively assessed clinical symptom complex. The reader should not conclude from these remarks that such an evaluation need be extensive or complex. Indeed simple palpation of peripheral pulses followed by measurement of blood pressure in all four extremities provides sufficient information for initial assessment. Addition of Doppler analog waveforms, segmental pressure indices, and the response of ankle pressure to treadmill walking provides simply (and it is hoped inexpensively) obtained information from the vascular laboratory sufficient to accurately determine the presence, severity, and location of lower extremity arterial obstructive lesions in more than 90 per cent of patients. For a more detailed description of these techniques as well as methods used for complete testing in the noninvasive vascular laboratory, the reader is referred to Chapter 13.

In addition to providing objective information concerning the state of lower extremity arterial disease at the time of patient presentation, the noninvasive vascular laboratory data provide a critical baseline against which to compare future hemodynamic assessments to permit objective evaluation of the efficacy of therapy and the progression of disease. In our opinion, the initial assessment of patients with chronic lower extremity ischemia should also include noninvasive examination of the carotid arteries, both to exclude the possibility of asymptomatic critical stenosis and to permit future documentation of progression of disease at this site.

The extent of evaluation for coronary artery disease appropriate for patients with chronic lower extremity ischemia remains controversial. Certainly the physician should obtain all previous records pertaining to coronary disease, especially those of coronary angiograms and/or nuclear cardiac scanning. Given the overwhelming incidence of coronary disease revealed by the screening studies referred to above, cogent arguments can be made for extensive coronary evaluation in most patients with symptomatic lower extremity ischemia.[19] At present, however, there is little evidence that such screening has demonstrable therapeutic benefit, both because of the limited indications for prophylactic intervention in coronary artery disease, and because of the well-documented high incidence of morbidity and mortality associated with treatment of coronary artery disease in patients with lower extremity ischemia.[45] For these reasons, our practice is to reserve extensive or invasive coronary evaluation for those patients in whom such testing is indicated by severe symptoms, or for those with asymptomatic disease in whom elective therapeutic procedures are contemplated for which an accurate assessment of cardiac risk is an important element in the decision for or against treatment.

Having obtained the information above, the surgeon can make accurate predictions regarding natural history of both the patient's lower extremity symptoms and his life expectancy and coexisting disease. With this knowledge, a decision can be made regarding operative or nonoperative treatment. A description of the specific nonoperative measures used in our clinical practice forms the basis for the remainder of this chapter.

NONOPERATIVE TREATMENT OF CHRONIC LOWER EXTREMITY ISCHEMIA

Nonoperative treatment of chronic lower extremity ischemia includes modification of risk factors known to contribute to severity of symptoms and progression of disease, modification of life habits, and drug treatment. Some of these aspects are described elsewhere in the volume and will not be further considered here. The specific topics discussed here include smoking, exercise, and drug treatment.

Smoking

Smoking tobacco has been implicated as a cause of approximately 350,000 deaths per year in the United States.[46] The monotonously consistent relationship between smoking and chronic lower extremity ischemia is well known to all physicians. Smokers are 9 times more likely to develop claudication than nonsmokers.[47] More than 90 per cent of persons with claudication and an equal number of those undergoing lower extremity amputation for ischemia are smokers.[48-50] The specific pathophysiologic mechanisms through which smoking exerts adverse chronic effects on arteries remain unknown. Multiple toxicities of the myriad components of tobacco smoke are recognized, including alterations in vascular endothelium, prostaglandin metabolism, lipid metabolism, blood viscosity, platelet function, and coagulation. A complete discussion of the effects of smoking is beyond the scope of this chapter. Several excellent comprehensive reviews are available.[51-53] Besides chronic effects, an acute effect of tobacco smoke was recognized by Aronow and associates, who demonstrated immediate decreases in treadmill walking ability after smoking, presumably caused by carbon monoxide.[54]

Complete cessation of all tobacco use is the foundation of nonoperative therapy of chronic lower extremity ischemia. The first duty of the physician must be to clearly inform the patient that the smoking addiction is the most important cause of the symptoms. Most smokers recognize only an increased risk of lung cancer. In a study by Clyne et al., only 37 per cent of patients with peripheral vascular disease recognized that their smoking was contributing to their symptoms.[55] All patients with chronic lower extremity ischemia must be told without equivocation that they must stop smoking. This advice should be repeated at every patient encounter. Such an approach produces results. In the study by Kirk and associates strong and repeated advice by physicians resulted in successful cessation of smoking by one third of patients.[56]

In our opinion physicians should adopt a positive approach in attempting to influence patients to stop smoking. Threats of refusal to continue treatment if the patient does not comply are inappropriate and indicate a lack of understanding by the physician of the nature of addiction. It is appropriate and desirable to describe in detail to the patient that cessation of smoking is associated with multiple positive benefits.

There is abundant evidence that cessation of smoking improves outcome in patients with chronic lower extremity ischemia. Quick and Cotton showed significant improvement in treadmill walking when successful abstainers were compared to patients who

continued smoking.[57] In our own practice, patients who stop smoking usually experience at least a doubling of previously recorded walking distance.

Improved patency of arterial repairs in nonsmokers has been documented by multiple authors for both aortofemoral[58,59] and femoropopliteal[60] reconstructions. Greenhalgh et al. demonstrated a direct relationship between amount of smoking (as assessed by blood carboxyhemoglobin levels) and likelihood of graft failure.[61] Similarly, a markedly reduced incidence of amputation in patients with peripheral arterial disease has been demonstrated by multiple authors. In one study by Birkenstock, 85 per cent of persons who stopped smoking had improvement in symptoms of lower extremity ischemia, compared to improvement in only 20 per cent of continued smokers.[62] Even for the patients with severe rest pain, 86 per cent of the 64 patients who stopped smoking did not require amputation, whereas only 10 per cent of those who continued to smoke avoided amputation.

Information such as this should form the basis for continued insistence by the vascular surgeon that all patients with chronic lower extremity ischemia should stop smoking. Patients should be informed of the availability of community resources, including smoking cessation clinics and professionals specializing in treatment of addiction. Prescription of nicotine gum or transdermal nicotine patches as an aid to ease the transition from smoking to abstinence is appropriate. Although nicotine has adverse effects, fewer than 5 per cent of those using the gum continue to use it for more than a short period.[63]

Exercise

Patients with intermittent claudication typically greatly reduce their walking in response to the discomfort. Severely affected persons may become near prisoners in their homes, curtailing all activities including shopping, visiting, and any walking for pleasure. Many poorly informed patients assume that the pain of claudication indicates injury and further avoid walking from fear of adverse effects. In fact, the opposite is true. It has long been known that a regular program of walking exercise results in improved symptoms of claudication in a majority of affected persons. This improvement has ranged from an 80 per cent increase in walking distance documented by one British study[64] to a 234 per cent increase in a study of 148 patients from Sweden.[65] All similar studies have shown such benefit.[66-68] Thus a recommendation for regular walking exercise forms an important part of nonoperative therapy for intermittent claudication.

The mechanism by which exercise produces an improvement in walking distance was initially thought to be through improved collateral blood supply. Numerous investigators have demonstrated that neither ankle blood pressure nor calf muscle blood flow are improved by walking exercise that results in improved walking distance.[64,69-72] At present it is believed that the improved muscle performance results from typical athletic training, which can be characterized at least in part by more efficient oxygen extraction from the limited blood supply.[73] In addition, at least one study has demonstrated improved hemorrheologic behavior of erythrocytes following regular exercise.[67]

Regardless of the mechanism involved, regular walking exercise produces results with sufficient reliability that the surgeon can recommend such treatment with confidence. In our practice sedentary persons with claudication are advised to begin walking for 1 hour each day, repeatedly approaching the point of claudication, resting until the symptoms pass, then resuming walking. The majority of patients following such instructions will experience at least a doubling in walking distance.

Overview of Cessation of Smoking and Exercise

Clearly, cessation of smoking and exercise therapy form the foundation for nonoperative treatment of chronic lower extremity ischemia. With exceptions, claudicating patients with ankle brachial pressure indices greater than 0.55 rarely require treatment beyond these measures. Unfortunately, as all physicians know, patient compliance with these recommendations for changes in basic habits and addictions is poor. Despite this, the physician should maintain a positive attitude and continue to advise compliance with basic nonoperative therapy. Most persons who successfully stop smoking do so after several stops and starts. Similar vacillations characterize those who ultimately adopt the habit of regular exercise. Encouragement by the physician positively influences this process, whereas condemnation of initial failures may interrupt it.

Pharmacologic Treatment of Chronic Lower Extremity Ischemia

In recent years a large number of pharmacologic agents have been evaluated for possible benefit in treatment of chronic lower extremity ischemia. These include hemorrheologic agents, antiplatelet drugs, and vasodilators, including calcium channel blocking agents and prostaglandins, as well as drugs intended to enhance metabolism in ischemic areas. Each of these will be discussed here.

Hemorrheologic Drugs

Increasing interest is currently being directed to the study of the characteristics of blood flow, a field termed "hemorrheology." Viscosity is an important factor affecting blood flow. The important determinants of viscosity include hematocrit, plasma protein concentration (especially fibrinogen), platelet aggregability, and blood cell deformability. Cellular deformability is especially important in the microcirculation.

Since erythrocytes are 8 to 9 μ in diameter, leukocytes are 6 to 15 μ in diameter, and typical capillaries are only 4 to 5 μ in diameter, cells must obviously deform in order to traverse the capillary bed. Other factors of importance in microcirculatory flow include white cell adhesiveness and platelet adhesiveness.

A large number of observations have documented altered hemorrheology in persons with chronic lower extremity ischemia. The first of these was the observation by multiple investigators of decreased rates of passage of blood from persons with claudication through filters of constant pore size.[74,75] Since these initial observations, multiple studies have demonstrated decreased deformability of erythrocytes and leukocytes, increased aggregation of platelets, increased adhesiveness of platelets and leukocytes, and increased whole blood viscosity in patients with chronic lower extremity ischemia when compared to normal controls.[74-82]

These consistent findings of abnormal hemorrheology in patients with chronic lower extremity ischemia have led to intense interest in development of pharmacologic agents to correct the abnormalities. Currently in the United States only one drug believed to act through hemorrheologic mechanisms, pentoxifylline, is approved for use in chronic lower extremity ischemia. Interestingly, however, multiple drugs with recognized effectiveness in treatment of chronic lower extremity ischemia previously thought to act through other mechanisms may also have significant hemorrheologic effects. These drugs include the vasodilators cyclandelate and isoxsuprine as well as the antiplatelet drug ticlopidine.

The straightforward approach to improvement in hemorrheology by hematocrit reduction was evaluated by Ernst and coauthors, who used hemodilution in 24 patients with claudication and demonstrated significant improvement in treadmill walking distance when compared to controls.[83] Although this treatment approach is obviously not practical on a large-scale, chronic basis, it does illustrate the potential for alterations in hemorrheology to produce improvement in lower extremity ischemia symptoms.

Pentoxifylline. Pentoxifylline, a theobromine derivative, was initially introduced in Germany for use as a vasodilator, an effect that the drug does not produce in man.[84] In the laboratory, pentoxifylline has been demonstrated to produce improved blood filterability, decreased plasma fibrinogen, decreased platelet aggregation, and improved white cell rheology, all of which result in a demonstrable decrease in blood viscosity,[82,85-88] leading to the conclusion that pentoxifylline acts through hemorrheologic mechanisms. In humans, treatment with pentoxifylline produces increased limb blood flow as measured by plethysmography, and increased calf muscle blood flow as measured by xenon-133 clearance.[89,90] Ehrly found increased muscle pO_2 in claudicants following pentoxifylline treatment,[91] an important observation that to date remains unconfirmed.

Clinical testing of pentoxifylline for treatment of

claudication has included 12 separate double-blind trials using treadmill walking as the end point, 11 of which were conducted in Europe, as well as a single large multicenter trial in the United States.[92] Uniformly, these trials have demonstrated significant benefit from pentoxifylline when compared with placebo.

Characteristically, the improvement in walking distance resulting from pentoxifylline treatment is modest. As can be seen from Table 14–5, fewer than half of patients experience a doubling in walking distance. In the controlled studies, patients with documented improvement in treadmill walking distance often reported on questionnaires that they perceived no benefit in their daily lives. This finding is not surprising given the frequent observation by vascular surgeons that procedures that result in improvement in claudication rather than cure are often not perceived as beneficial by patients. In our own practice the drug seems most often useful in treatment of patients with extremely limited walking distance (less than 50 meters) and relatively sedentary life-styles, for whom an incremental increase in claudication distance may allow significant activities that were previously impossible (short walk to mailbox, dining hall, etc.).

The repeatedly demonstrated improvement in microcirculatory flow resulting from pentoxifylline treatment has led to interest in use of this drug in treatment of limb-threatening ischemia. Some encouraging results have been reported in healing of ischemic ulcers.[93] We have noted improvement in the ischemic ulcers of a few patients with inoperable small artery disease.[43,94] Obviously these observations require confirmation by randomized trials.

The side effects of pentoxifylline include dizziness and gastrointestinal symptoms (nausea, vomiting, bloating), which require interruption of drug therapy in about 3 per cent of patients.

Vasodilators

Tremendous interest has been focused for years on the clinical use of vasodilating agents in obstructive arterial disease. This interest seems superficially logical, given the critical relationship of blood flow to the fourth power of vessel radius described by the Poiseuille equation, as well as the frequent clinical observation of cool, blanched distal lower extremities in claudicants, suggesting abnormal vasospasm. The many different types of vasodilators that have been evaluated for treatment of chronic lower extremity ischemia are listed in Table 14-6, grouped by their presumed mechanism of action.

Unfortunately, to date, no vasodilator has ever been proven effective in the treatment of chronic lower extremity ischemia caused by obstructive arterial disease. The assumption that vasoconstriction exists in ischemic areas has been conclusively shown to be false.[95] Similarly, to date, no vasodilator has ever been shown to increase blood flow to exercising muscle. All controlled trials evaluating vasodilators for effectiveness in chronic lower extremity ischemia have failed to show benefit,[79,95,96] and for this reason, a large majority of these drugs, as indicated in Table 14–6, have been withdrawn from the market. Available evidence indicates that this withdrawal may be premature. Some previously commonly used vasodilating agents have been recently shown to have hemorrheologic properties and may prove effective for treatment of claudication.

Despite the results of vasodilator treatment to date, interest remains high in the potential clinical application of calcium channel-blocking agents and prostaglandins to the treatment of chronic lower extremity ischemia. Several agents are currently under investigation, each of which will be briefly described.

Calcium channel agents produce vasodilation by blocking smooth muscle contraction. The drugs block the influx of calcium from the extracellular space to the cytoplasm, which is an obligate requirement for smooth muscle contraction. These agents have a well-established role in the treatment of hypertension and of vasospastic disorders, including coronary vasospasm. Several of these drugs are currently under investigation for treatment of claudication.

Prostaglandin I_2 (PGI_2; prostacyclin) is a potent vasodilator that is also a powerful inhibitor of platelet aggregation. Some controlled studies, but not all, have shown benefit from this agent in decreasing ischemic rest pain[97,98] as well as improving treadmill walking distance in claudicators.[99] Clinical use of the drug has been limited both by its extremely short half-life (minutes), requiring intravenous administration, and by the frequent occurrence of significant side effects (hypotension, dizziness). Iloprost is a stable analog of prostacyclin that can be administered orally. A controlled study of Iloprost in treatment of severe lower extremity ischemia is in progress.

Metabolic Enhancing Agents

The possibility that symptoms of chronic lower extremity ischemia might be improved by alteration of the metabolism of ischemia tissues has resulted in evaluation of a number of agents. Two of these drugs, naftidrofuryl and carnitine, are of current clinical in-

TABLE 14–5. RESULTS OF PENTOXIFYLLINE TREATMENT IN CONTROLLED TRIALS

	Total Patients Treated	Per Cent with <50% Improvement	Per Cent with 50–100% Improvement	Per Cent with >100% Improvement
Pentoxifylline	375	45	24	31
Placebo	354	76	15	9

TABLE 14–6. VASODILATORS[a]

α-Adrenergic Blocking Agent	Nitrates
Guanethidine	Nitroglycerin
Phenoxybenzamine	Nitroprusside
Prazosin	
Tolazoline	
Phentolamine	
Direct-Acting Drugs	Prostaglandins
Papaverine*	PGE₁
Isoxsuprine*	PGI₂
Cyclandelate*	Iloprost
β-Stimulating Drugs	Calcium Channel Blockers
Nylidrin	Nifedipine
	Verapamil
	Diltiazem

[a]None of these drugs is currently approved for treatment of chronic lower extremity ischemia. Those indicated by an * were previously used and have been withdrawn from the market.

terest, although at the time of this writing neither is approved for use by the U.S. Food and Drug Administration. Despite this, both agents are of importance as examples of another avenue of treatment of chronic lower extremity ischemia.

Naftidrofuryl (Praxilene) is available in Europe. This drug appears to act through stimulation of carbohydrate and fat entry into the tricarboxylic acid cycle, resulting in a net increase in adenosine triphosphate (ATP) production in ischemic areas. Controlled trials of this drug in treatment of claudication[100] and of ischemic rest pain[101] have yielded mixed results. The drug is widely prescribed, however, and U.S. physicians may often encounter its use in their patients who have traveled to Europe or Mexico.

Carnitine is a naturally occurring substance that is free from recognized toxic effects at any therapeutic dose.[102] This drug facilitates aerobic metabolism by promoting entry of pyruvate into the citric acid cycle as well as facilitating the transport of fatty acids. Each molecule of pyruvate entered into the citric acid cycle by carnitine results in the production of 30 additional molecules of ATP that would otherwise have been lost to the cell as lactate. Therefore the available oxygen provides more energy in the presence of carnitine, in theory resulting in greater work capacity for muscle.[103]

Carnitine was evaluated clinically by Brevetti et al.,[104] who gave carnitine to claudicants in a double-blind randomized trial and evaluated treadmill walking, as well as popliteal venous blood lactate levels and muscle biopsy carnitine levels. These workers demonstrated a significant increase in treadmill walking distance with carnitine as opposed to placebo. Popliteal venous lactate was decreased in the patients receiving carnitine, and muscle biopsy carnitine was increased. The results of this study, if confirmed by a U.S. multicenter trial currently underway, predict significant clinical utility for this nontoxic substance.

Antiplatelet Agents

A vast array of drugs have antiplatelet actions, including aspirin and nearly all other nonsteroidal antiinflammatory agents. Calcium channel-blocking agents and the prostaglandins PGI₂ and PGE₁ also have demonstrable antiplatelet effects. New drugs whose primary mechanism of action is through an antiplatelet effect are ticlopidine and thromboxane synthetase inhibitors.

Aspirin irreversibly acetylates the enzyme cyclooxygenase, thus blocking the formation of thromboxane A₂ and eliminating an important stimulus to platelet aggregation and release. Note that aspirin does not block platelet adhesion, nor does it affect platelet aggregation or release induced by thrombin, both of which occur independent of prostaglandin mediators.[105,106] Thromboxane synthetase inhibitors selectively block this enzyme, thus theoretically shifting arachidonic acid metabolism toward the production of PGI₂, with net vasodilation and decrease in platelet aggregation.[107] Ticlopidine appears to inhibit platelet adenosine diphosphate (ADP) receptors.[108]

At present the use of aspirin in patients with symptomatic chronic lower extremity ischemia is strongly supported by at least two groups of data. The first of these is the consistently demonstrated beneficial effect of aspirin on survival of patients with atherosclerotic disease. A recent summation metaanalysis of over 30 different studies demonstrated that aspirin reduced vascular mortality by 15 per cent and reduced nonfatal stroke and myocardial infarction by 30 per cent.[109] This clear demonstration of benefit (over 29,000 patients studied) indicates that all patients with demonstrable atherosclerotic disease should be treated with aspirin, 325 mg/day, unless contraindicated by allergy or by intolerable side effects.

Aspirin also has an apparent, although less well-demonstrated, beneficial effect on the patency of arterial repairs in the lower extremity, particularly if the repair involves the use of prosthetic graft material. The beneficial effect on patency is greatest if the aspirin therapy is started preoperatively.[110,111] At present, there is no convincing evidence that any other nonsteroidal agent has any advantage in platelet inhibition over aspirin, which has the obvious advantage of low cost.

The use of thromboxane synthetase inhibitors has been explored in patients with claudication and in ischemic rest pain, with preliminary indication of some benefit in these conditions.[112,113] Obviously the use of these drugs to treat chronic lower extremity ischemia requires evaluation by blinded trials.

Ticlopidine was recently evaluated in treatment of claudication in a 21-month double-blind trial with ankle-arm blood pressure index and treadmill walking as the evaluated parameters. At the conclusion of the study, there was a significant improvement in both parameters in the ticlopidine-treated patients. No major side effects were reported.[114] The exact mechanism of the improvement is not known, although ticlopidine has been demonstrated to reduce blood viscosity.[115]

Overview of Drug Treatment of Chronic Lower Extremity Ischemia

At present it is our firm opinion that all patients with chronic lower extremity ischemia (or any other manifestation of arteriosclerotic disease) should receive aspirin, 325 mg/day, for life. Clearly, some patients with claudication are benefited by pentoxifylline therapy and a trial of this agent in conjunction with the other nonoperative measures listed above seems appropriate. The multiplicity of other agents currently under active investigation predicts a significant role for pharmacologic treatment of chronic lower extremity ischemia in the future. The most promising of these new agents have been described above, to afford the reader familiarity when and if they become available for general use.

REFERENCES

1. Droller H, Pemberton J: Cardiovascular disease in a random sample of elderly people. Br Heart J 15:199–201, 1953.
2. Peabody CN, Kannel WB, McNamara PM: Intermittent claudication—surgical significance. Arch Surg 109:693–697, 1974.
3. Rutkow IM, Ernst CB: An analysis of vascular surgical manpower requirements and vascular surgical rates in the United States. J Vasc Surg 3:74–83, 1986.
4. Hughson WG, Munn JI, Garrod A: Intermittent claudication: Prevalence and risk factor. Br Med J 1:1379, 1978.
5. Reid DD, Brett GZ, Hamilton PJS, Jarrett RJ, Keen H, Rose G: Cardiorespiratory disease and diabetes among middle aged male civil servants. Lancet 1:469, 1974.
6. Boyd AM: The natural course of arteriosclerosis of lower extremities. Angiology 11:10–14, 1960.
7. Kannel WB, Skinner JJ, Schwarz MJ, Shurtleff D: Intermittent claudication—incidence in the Framingham study. Circulation 41:875, 1970.
8. Schadt DC, Hines EA, Juergens JL, Barleer NW: Chronic athersoclerotic occlusion of the femoral artery. JAMA 175:656–661, 1961.
9. Begg TB, Richards RL: The prognosis of intermittent claudication. Scott Med J 7:341–352, 1962.
10. McAllister FF: The fate of patients with intermittent claudication managed nonoperatively. Am J Surg 132:593–559, 1976.
11. Cronenwett JL, Warner KG, Zelenock GB, Whitehouse WM, Graham LM, Lindenhauer SM, Stanley JC: Intermittent claudication: Current results of nonoperative management. Arch Surg 119:430–436, 1984.
12. Rosenbloom MS, Flanigan DP, Schuler JJ, Meyer JP, Durham JR, Eldrup-Jorgensen J, Schwarcz TH: Risk factors affecting the natural history of claudication. Arch Surg 123:867–870, 1988.
13. Imparato AM, Kim GE: Intermittent claudication: Its natural course. Surgery 78:795–799, 1975.
14. Jonason T, Ringquiest I: Factors of prognostic importance for subsequent rest pain in patients with intermittent claudication. Acta Med Scand 218:27–33, 1985.
15. Rivers SP, Veith FJ, Ascer E, Gupta SK: Successful conservative therapy of severe limb threatening ischemia: The value of nonsympathectomy. Surgery 99:759–762, 1986.
16. Eklund AE, Eriksson G, Olsson AG: A controlled study showing significant short term effect of prostaglandin E1 in healing of ischemic ulcers of the lower limb in man. Prostaglandins Leukotrienes Med 8:265–271, 1982.
17. Schuler JJ, Flanigan DP, Holcroft JW, Ursprung JJ, Mohrland JSA, Pyke J: Efficacy of prostaglandin E1 in the treatment of lower extremity ischemic ulcers secondary to peripheral vascular occlusive disease: Results of a prospective randomized, double-blind, multicenter clinical trial. J Vasc Surg 1:160–170, 1984.
18. Felix WR Jr, Sigel B, Gunther L: The significance for morbidity and mortality of Doppler absent pedal pulses. J Vasc Surg 5:849–855, 1987.
19. Hertzer NR, Beven EG, Young JR, O'Hara PJ, Ruschhaupt WF, Graor RA, DeWolfe VG, Maljovec LC: Coronary artery disease in peripheral vascular patients—a classification of 1000 coronary angiograms and results of surgical management. Ann Surg 199:223–233, 1984.
20. Turnipseed WD, Berkhoff HA, Belzer FD: Postoperative stroke in cardiac and peripheral vascular disease. Ann Surg 192:365–368, 1980.
21. Bloor K: Natural history of arteriosclerosis of the lower extremities. Ann R Coll Surg Engl 28:36–52, 1961.
22. Silbert S, Zazeela H: Prognosis in atherosclerotic peripheral vascular disease. JAMA 166:1816–1821, 1958.
23. Kallero KS: Mortality and morbidity in patients with intermittent claudication as defined by venous occlusion plethysmography: A ten year follow-up. J Chronic Dis 34:455–462, 1981.
24. Cefevre FA, Corbaciogla C, Humphries AW, DeWolfe VG: Management of arteriosclerosis obliterans of the extremities. JAMA 170:656–661, 1959.
25. Hansteen V, Lorentsen E, Sivertssen E, Bergan F: Long term follow-up of patients with peripheral arteriosclerosis obliterans treated with arterial surgery. Acta Clin Scand 141:725–734, 1975.
26. Crawford ES, Bomberger RA, Glaeser DH, Saleh SA, Russell WL: Aortoiliac occlusive disease: Factors influencing survival and function following reconstructive operation over a twenty-five year period. Surgery 90:1055–1067, 1981.
27. Szilagyi DE, Elliott JP, Smith RF, Reddy DJ, McPharlin M: A thirty year survey of the reconstructive surgical treatment of aortoiliac occlusive disease. J Vasc Surg 3:421–436, 1986.
28. Hertzer NR: Fatal myocardial infarction following lower extremity revascularization—two hundred and seventy-three patients followed six to eleven post-operative years. Ann Surg 193:492–498, 1981.
29. Malone JM, Moore WS, Goldstone J: Life expectancy following aortofemoral grafting. Surgery 81:551–555, 1977.
30. Veith FJ, Gupta SK, Samson RH, et al: Progress in limb salvage by reconstructive arterial surgery combined with new or improved adjunctive procedures. Ann Surg 194:386–401, 1981.
31. Edwards JM, Taylor LM Jr, Porter JM: Treatment of failed lower extremity bypass grafts with new autogenous vein bypass. J Vasc Surg 11:132–145, 1990.
32. Reunanen A, Takkunen H, Aromaa A: Prevalence of intermittent claudication and its effect on mortality. Acta Med Scand 537(suppl):8–35, 1972.
33. Dormandy J, Mahir M, Ascady D, et al: Fate of the patient with chronic leg ischemia. J Cardiovasc Surg 30:50–57, 1989.
34. Kallero KS, Bergqvist D, Cederholm C, Jonsson K, Olsson PO, Takolander R: Late mortality and morbidity after arterial reconstruction: The influence of arteriosclerosis in the popliteal artery trifurcation. J Vasc Surg 2:541–546, 1985.
35. Howell MA, Colgan MP, Seeger RW, Ramsey DE, Sumner DS: Relationship of severity of lower limb peripheral vascular disease to mortality and morbidity: A six-year follow-up study. J Vasc Surg 9:691–697, 1989.
36. DeBakey ME, Crawford ES, Garrett E, Colley DA, Morris GC Jr, Abbott JP: Occlusive disease of the lower extrem-

ities in patients 16 to 37 years of age. Ann Surg *159*:873–890, 1964.

37. Nunn DB: Symptomatic peripheral arteriosclerosis of patients under age 40. Ann Surg *39*:224–228, 1973.

38. Pairolero PC, Joyce JW, Skinner CR, Hollier LH, Cherry KJ Jr: Lower limb ischemia in young adults: Prognostic implications. J Vasc Surg *1*:459–464, 1984.

39. Hallet JW Jr, Greenwood LH, Robinson JG: Lower extremity arterial disease in young adults. Ann Surg *202*:647–652, 1985.

40. Eldrup-Jorgenson J, Flanigan JP, Brace L, Sawchuk AP, Mulder SG, Anderson CP, Schuler JJ, Meyer JR, Durham JR, Schwarcz TH: Hypercoagulable states and lower limb ischemia in young adults. J Vasc Surg *9*:334–341, 1989.

41. Boers GHJ, Smals AGH, Trijbels FJM, Fowler B, Bakkeren JAJM, Schoonderwaldt HC, Kleijer WJ, Kloppenborg PWC: Heterozygosity for homocystinuria in premature peripheral and cerebral occlusive arterial disease. N Engl J Med *313*:709–715, 1985.

42. N-Hsiang Y, Hildebrand H: Results of vascular surgery in younger versus older patients. Am J Surg *157*:419–422, 1989.

43. Mills JL, Taylor LM Jr, Porter JM: Buerger's disease in the modern era. Am J Surg *154*:123–129, 1987.

44. McCready RA, Vincent AE, Schwartz RW, Hyde GL, Mattingly SS, Griffen WO: Atherosclerosis in the young: A virulent disease. Surgery *96*:863–869, 1984.

45. Yeager RL, Moneta GL: Assessing cardiac risk in vascular surgical patients: Current status. Perspect Vasc Surg *2*:18–36, 1989.

46. Pollin W: The role of the addictive process as a key step in causation of all tobacco related disease. JAMA *252*:2874, 1984.

47. Hughson WG, Munn JI, Garrod A: Intermittent claudication: Prevalence and risk factor. Br Med J *1*:1379, 1978.

48. Lithell H, Hedstrand H, Karlsson R: The smoking habits of men with intermittent claudication. Acta Med Scand *197*:473–476, 1975.

49. Eastcott HHG: Arterial Surgery, 2nd ed. London, Pitman Publishers Ltd, 1973, p 3.

50. Jurgens IL, Barker NW, Hines EA: Arteriosclerosis obliterans: A review of 520 cases with special reference to pathogenic and prognostic factors. Circulation *21*:188–194, 1960.

51. Couch NP: On the arterial consequences of smoking. J Vasc Surg *3*:807–812, 1986.

52. Fielding JE: Smoking: Health effects and control. N Engl J Med *313*:555–561, 1985.

53. Krupski WC, Rapp JH: Smoking and atherosclerosis. Perspect Vasc Surg *1*:103–134, 1989.

54. Aronow WS, Stemmer EA, Isbell MW: Effect of carbon monoxide exposure on intermittent claudication. Circulation *49*:415–417, 1974.

55. Clyne CA, Arch PJ, Carpenter D, Webster JHH, Chant ADB: Smoking, ignorance, and peripheral vascular disease. Arch Surg *117*:1062–1065, 1982.

56. Kirk CJC, Lund VJ, Woolcock NE, Greenhalgh RM: The effect of advice to stop smoking on arterial disease patients, assessed by serum thiocyanate levels. J Cardiovasc Surg *21*:568–569, 1970.

57. Quick CRG, Cotton LT: The measured effect of stopping smoking on intermittent claudication. Br J Surg *69*(suppl):524–526, 1982.

58. Robiseck F, Daugherty HK, Mullen DC, Masters TN, Narbay D, Sanger PW: The effect of continued cigarette smoking on the patency of synthetic vascular grafts in Leriche syndrome. J Thorac Cardiovasc Surg *70*:107–112, 1975.

59. Provan JL, Sojka SG, Murnaghan JJ, Jauinkalns R: The effect of cigarette smoking on the long term success rates of aortofemoral and femoropopliteal reconstructions. Surg Gynecol Obstet *165*:49–52, 1987.

60. Myers KA, King RB, Scott DF, Johnson N, Morris PJ: The effect of smoking on the late patency of arterial reconstructions in the legs. Br J Surg *65*:267–271, 1978.

61. Greenhalgh RM, Laing SP, Colap V, Cole PV, Taylor GW: Progressing atherosclerosis following revascularization. *In* Bernhard VM, Towne JB (eds): Complications in Vascular Surgery. New York, Grune & Stratton, 1980, p 39.

62. Birkenstock WE, Louw JHY, Terblanche J, Immelman EJ, Dent DM, Baker PM: Smoking and other factors affecting the conservative management of peripheral vascular disease. S Afr Med J *49*:1129–1132, 1975.

63. Hjalmarson AIM: Effect of nicotine chewing gum in smoking cessation. JAMA *252*:2835–2838, 1984.

64. Clifford PC, Davies PW, Hayne JA, Baird RN: Intermittent claudication: Is a supervised exercise class worthwhile? Br Med J *280*:1503–1505, 1980.

65. Ekroth R, Dahllof AG, Gundevall B, Holm J, Schersten T: Physical training of patients with intermittent claudication: Indications, methods, and results. Surgery *84*:640–643, 1978.

66. Skinner JS, Strandness DE Jr: Exercise and intermittent claudication. II. Effect of physical training. Circulation *36*:23–29, 1967.

67. Ruell PA, Imperial ES, Bonor FJ, et al: Intermittent claudication. The effect of physical training on walking tolerance and venous lactate concentration. Eur J Appl Physiol *52*:420–425, 1984.

68. Gallasch G, Diehm C, Dorter C, et al: The influence of physical training on blood flow properties in patients with intermittent claudication. Klin Wochenschr *63*:554–559, 1985.

69. Ekroth R, Dahllof AG, Gundevall B, Holm J, Schersten T: Physical training of patients with intermittent claudication: Indications, methods, and results. Surgery *84*:640–643, 1978.

70. Saltin B: Physical training in patients with intermittent claudication. *In* Cohen LS, Mock MB, Ringquist I (eds): Physical Conditioning and Cardiovascular Rehabilitation. New York, John Wiley & Sons, 1981, pp 181–196.

71. Sprlie D, Myhre K: Effects of physical training in intermittent claudication. Scand J Clin Lab Invest *38*:217–222, 1978.

72. Dahllot AG, Holm J, Sclersten T, Sivertsson R: Peripheral arterial insufficiency. Effect of physical training on walking tolerance, calf blood flow and blood flow resistance. Scand J Rehab Med *8*:19–26, 1976.

73. Bylund AC, Hammersten J, Holm J, et al: Enzyme activities in skeletal muscles from patients with peripheral arterial insufficiency. Eur J Clin Invest *6*:425–429, 1976.

74. Ehrly AM, Kohler HJ: Altered deformability of erythrocytes from patients with chronic occlusive arterial disease. Vasa *5*:319–322, 1976.

75. Reid JL, Dormandy JA, Barnes AJ, Lock AJ, Dormandy TL: Impaired red cell deformability in peripheral vascular disease. Lancet *1*:666–677, 1976.

76. Chesebro JH, Fuster V, Frye RL: Smoking, family history and shortened platelet survival in coronary disease patients age 50 and under. Circulation *58*(suppl II):221–226, 1978.

77. Dormandy JA, Hoare E, Colley J: Clinical hemodynamic and biochemical findings in 126 patients with intermittent claudication. Br Med J *4*:576–581, 1973.

78. Ernst E, Hammerschmidt DE, Bagge U, Matrai A, Dormandy JA: Leukocytes and the risk of ischemic disease. JAMA *257*:2318–2324, 1987.

79. Hansteen V, Lorentsen E: Vasodilator drugs in the treatment of peripheral arterial insufficiency. Acta Med Scand (suppl) *556*:9–62, 1974.

80. Janssen Pharmaceutica: Ketanserin: A Novel Serotonin S2-Receptor Blocking Agent. Investigational New Drug Brochure, 7th ed. Beerse, Belgium, Janssen Pharmaceutica, 1983.

81. Johnson G Jr, Keagy BA, Rodd DW, Gabriel DA, Lucas CL, Hardison VC: Viscous factors in peripheral tissue perfusion. J Vasc Surg *2*:530–535, 1985.

82. Matrai A, Ernst E: Pentoxifylline improves white cell rheology in claudicants. Clin Hemorrheol *5*:483–491, 1986.

83. Ernst E, Matrai A, Kollar L: Placebo-controlled double-blind

study of hemodilution in peripheral arterial disease. Lancet 1:1449–1451, 1987.

84. Baumann JC: Erweiterte Moglichkeiten zur konserviten. Behandlung arterieller. Durchblutungstor ungen. Therapiewoche 27:188–196, 1977.

85. Hess HV, Franke I, Jauch M: Medikamentos Verbesserung der flieseigenschaften des blutes. Ein wirksames Prinzip zure Behandlung von arteriellen Durchblutungss torungen. Fortschr Med 91:743–748, 1973.

86. Ehrly AM: Improvement of the flow properties of blood. A new therapeutic approach in occlusive arterial disease. Angiology 27:188–196, 1976.

87. Schubotz R: Double-blind trial of pentoxifylline in diabetics with peripheral vascular disorders. Pharmatherapeutica 1:172–179, 1976.

88. Muller R: Hemorrheology and peripheral vascular disease. A new therapeutic approach. J Med 12:209–235, 1981.

89. Accetto B: Beneficial hemorrheologic therapy of chronic peripheral arterial disorders with pentoxifylline; results of a double-blind study versus vasodilator-nylidrin. Am Heart J 113:864–869, 1982.

90. Angelkort B, Doppelfield E: Treatment of chronic arterial occlusive disease. Clinical study with a new galenic preparation of pentoxifylline. Trental 400. Pharmatherapeutica 3(suppl I):18–29, 1983.

91. Ehrly AM: Effects of orally administered pentoxifylline on muscular oxygen pressure in patients with intermittent claudication. IRCS Med Sci 10:401–402, 1982.

92. Taylor LM Jr, Porter JM: Drug treatment of claudication: Vasodilators, hemorrheologic agents, and antiserotonin drugs. J Vasc Surg 3:374–381, 1986.

93. Strano A, Davi G, Avellone G, Novo S, Pinto A: Double-blind, crossover study of the clinical efficacy and the hemorrheologic effects of pentoxifylline in patients with occlusive arterial disease of the lower limbs. Angiology 35:459–466, 1984.

94. Mills JL, Friedman EI, Taylor LM Jr, Porter JM: Upper extremity ischemia caused by small artery disease. Ann Surg 206:521–528, 1987.

95. Coffman JD: Vasodilator drugs in peripheral vascular disease. N Engl J Med 300:713–717, 1979.

96. Coffman JD, Mannick JA: Failure of vasodilator drugs in arteriosclerosis obliterans. Ann Intern Med 76:35–39, 1972.

97. Belch JJP, Drury JK, Capell H, et al: Intermittent epoprostenol (prostacyclin) infusion in patients with Raynaud's syndrome: A double-blind controlled trial. Lancet 1:313–315, 1983.

98. Hossman V, Auel H, Rucker W, et al: Prolonged infusion of prostacyclin in patients with advanced states of peripheral vascular disease: A placebo-controlled cross-over study. Klin Wochenschr 62:1108–1114, 1984.

99. Linet OI, Mohberg NR, Sinzinger H, et al: Cyclo-prostin (epoprostenol) is effective in peripheral vascular disease. Paper presented at the Cardiovascular Pharmacotherapy International Symposium 1985, Geneva, Switzerland, April 22–26, 1985.

100. Clyne CAC, Gallard RB, Fox MJ, Gustave R, Jantet GH, Jamieson CW: A controlled trial of naftidrofuryl in the treatment of intermittent claudication. Br J Surg 67:347–348, 1980.

101. Greenhalgh RM: Naftidrofuryl for ischemic rest pain: A controlled trial. Br J Surg 68:265–266, 1981.

102. Bahl JJ, Bresler RD: The pharmacology of carnitine. Annu Rev Pharmacol Toxicol 27:257–277, 1987.

103. Goa KL, Brogden RN: L-carnitine: A preliminary review of its pharmacokinetics, and its therapeutic use in ischemic heart disease and primary and secondary carnitine deficiencies in relationship to its role in fatty acid metabolism. Drugs 34:1–24, 1987.

104. Brevetti G, Chiariello M, Ferulano G, Policicchio A, Nevola E, Rossini A, Attisano T, Ambrosio G, Siliprandi N, Angelini C: Increases in walking disease treated with L-carnitine: A double-blind, cross-over study. Circulation 77:767–773, 1988.

105. Roth GJ, Majerus PW: The mechanism of the effect of aspirin on human platelets. 1. Acetylation of a particulate fraction protein. J Clin Invest 56:624–633, 1975.

106. O'Brien JR: Effects of salicylates on human platelets. Lancet 1:779–781, 1968.

107. Tonak J, Knecht H, Groitl H: Treatment of circulatory disturbances with pentoxifylline. Double-blind trial with Trental. Pharmatherapeutica 46(suppl I):126–135, 1983.

108. Lips JPM, Sixma JJ, Schiphorst ME: The effect of ticlopidine administration to humans on the binding of adenosine diphosphate to blood platelets. Thromb Res 17:19–27, 1980.

109. Antiplatelet Trialists' Collaboration: Secondary prevention of vascular disease by prolonged antiplatelet treatment. Br Med J 296:320–333, 1988.

110. Clagett GP, Genton E, Salzman EW: Antithrombotic therapy in peripheral vascular disease. Chest 95:1286–1398, 1989.

111. Clyne CAC, Archer TJ, Atuhaire LK, et al: Random control trial of a short course of aspirin and dipyridamole (Persantin) for femorodistal grafts. Br J Surg 74:246–248, 1987.

112. Ehrly AM: Influence of a thromboxane synthesis inhibitor on the muscle tissue microcirculation of patients with intermittent claudication. Br J Clin Pharm 15(suppl I):117s–118s, 1983.

113. Pupita F, Rotatori P, Frausini G: Farmacologia clinica della sostanze vasoattive: Studi sulla pentoxifyllina. Ric Clin Lab II(suppl I):293–302, 1981.

114. Balsano F, Coccheri S, Libretti A, Nenci GG, Catalano M, Fortunato G, Grasselli S, Violi F, Hellemans H, Vanhove PH: Ticlopidine in the treatment of intermittent claudication: A 21 month double-blind trial. J Lab Clin Med 114:84–91, 1989.

115. Panak E, Maffrand JP, Picard-Fraire C, Vallee E, Blanchard J, Roncucci R: Ticlopidine: A promise for the prevention and treatment of thrombosis and its complications. Haemostasis 13(suppl I):1–52, 1983.

15

PRINCIPLES OF ANGIOGRAPHY AND INTERVENTIONAL RADIOLOGY

ANTOINETTE S. GOMES

Angiography is a technique in which radiopaque contrast material is injected into vessels, permitting visualization of the vascular system. The information obtained is used to make a clinical diagnosis, to formulate a preoperative therapeutic plan, and to provide anatomic information that can reduce operative time. Conventional arteriograms can be performed on an inpatient or outpatient basis. In either case the patient should be closely monitored to avoid the risk of postangiographic complications such as bleeding at the puncture site.

Access to the vascular system is obtained using aseptic technique with percutaneous puncture of the vessel. Patients undergoing routine angiographic procedures should be mildly sedated and well hydrated.

Angiography is performed by several routes. A femoral approach with puncture of the femoral artery below the inguinal ligament is the most widely used. When the femoral vessels are occluded or the catheter cannot be introduced into the femoral artery, an axillary puncture or high brachial artery puncture can be utilized. This approach is more difficult than the femoral approach owing to the small size and mobility of the vessel. It is associated with a slightly higher risk because of the proximity of the brachial plexus and the increased difficulty of obtaining hemostasis in the soft tissues.[1] Hematoma, direct nerve trauma, and brachial nerve palsy are potential complications with this technique. The incidence of complications in experienced hands is low. When the femoral arteries are not suitable for puncture, a translumbar approach with direct puncture of the abdominal aorta is another alternative. In a small percentage of patients, periaortic bleeding may occur with a possible change in hematocrit. This technique allows good images of the abdomen and legs. It should not be used when there is an aneurysm at the level of catheter entry (T12) or (L2-3), a bleeding disorder, an aortic graft at the puncture site, or systemic hypertension.

TECHNICAL COMPLICATIONS OF ANGIOGRAPHY

The most common angiographic complication is hematoma formation at the catheter site as a result of inadequate compression of the artery or trauma to the vessel following prolonged manipulation of the catheter. This is usually self-limiting and only rarely requires operative evacuation. Loss of pulse may occur because of arterial spasm or thrombus formation.[2] If the pulse is lost during the procedure, vasodilators should be given or a pullout angiogram performed. Surgical treatment of the thrombosed vessel may be necessary. Other complications that may occur at the puncture site include arteriovenous fistulas, false aneurysms, and retroperitoneal hematoma. Subintimal dissection of a catheterized vessel may also occur. These usually heal spontaneously, but may result in occlusion of the vessel. Distal embolization of blood clot or atheromatous plaque may also occur, with the sequelae determined by the size and location of the dislodged material.

CONTRAST MEDIA

The most widely used contrast agents are sodium or methylglucamine salts of triiodo-2,4,6-benzoic acid. Substitutions in the 3,5-acetylamine components distinguish the various agents: iothalamates, diatrizoates, and metrizoates. The contrast agents are available in high, medium, and low concentrations. The osmolarity of these agents is higher than that of blood, which accounts for the sensation of heat, vasodilation, and pain that patients experience with the injection. The sodium salts are less viscous than the methylglucamine salts, but more toxic.[3,4] These contrast agents are excreted by glomerular filtration. They produce a transient decrease in renal blood flow and increased vascular resistance.[5] Contrast agents induce acute renal dysfunction in a significant proportion of patients undergoing angiography both with and without a history of previous renal disease.[6] Patients with prior renal failure, proteinuria, diabetes, and dehydration are at higher risk for renal dysfunction.[7-9] The changes that occur are usually minimal and transient but can lead to progressive anuria. Contrast-induced renal failure usually resolves spontaneously within 7 days.[9] Studies have suggested that renal dysfunction may be dose related.[10] Hydration of patients prior to angiography is recommended.[11] The administration of mannitol to patients with preexisting renal disease at the time of angiography has also been recommended.[8] Lasix administration in combination with dopamine may also have a protective effect. The effects on renal function of angiographic contrast media should be considered when extensive angiographic studies are requested and when deciding on the interval between angiography and operation.

Reactions to Contrast Media

In addition to renal dysfunction from a direct nephrotoxic effect, contrast agents may precipitate an allergic reaction. These reactions may be mild, with hives or urticaria, or they may be severe anaphylactoid reactions characterized by bradycardia, hypotension, wheezing, and shock.[12] In patients with a history of a severe previous reaction, the indications for repeat angiography should be carefully evaluated. The patient should be pretreated with steroids prior to the study and given antihistamines the day of the examination. In addition, intravenous steroids during the examination may be used. An emergency cart should be available.[13,14] Pretreatment with steroids has been found to block the recurrence of the anaphylactoid symptoms in a high percentage of patients.[13]

Newer Contrast Agents

It is clear that the hyperosmolality of the ionic contrast agents is important in many of the hemodynamic, cardiac effects and unpleasant side effects.[15] Newer agents have been developed that have lower osmolality, and a higher ratio between the number of iodine atoms and the number of dissolved particles. The agents developed are nonionic monomers (metrizamide, iopamidol, ioversol, and iohexol). Also available is a monoacidic dimer (ioxaglate); this has a high ratio of iodine atoms to number of dissolved particles but still has an ionized anion in solution. These new agents have shown reduced side effects owing to osmolality, reduced organ toxicity, and fewer adverse reactions. They cause less vascular hemodynamic change and less heat and pain after intraarterial and intravenous injections. Less damage to endothelial cells occurs and less reactivity is induced in the complement and coagulation systems. Also reduced are pulmonary complications, central nervous system (CNS) toxicity, and possibly

nephrotoxicity. The recent large prospective Katayama study demonstrated a lower overall incidence of adverse reactions in patients who received low-osmolar nonionic contrast media as compared to those who received high-osmolar ionic contrast media. In cardiac use, fewer electrocardiographic changes are seen and less ventricular fibrillation is induced.

These low-osmolar contrast agents are approved for use in angiography. Their cost, however, is high: 4 to 10 times the cost of current ionic agents. Although it would be medically beneficial to use the low-osmolality agents, their high cost has somewhat restricted their use to special groups of patients, such as those with renal insufficiency or diabetes, infants, dehydrated patients, and patients with a history of prior adverse reactions to contrast media. In these high-risk patients the advantages outweigh the increased cost.

ARCH AORTOGRAPHY

The arch aortogram is used to provide visualization of the brachiocephalic vessel origins, carotid bifurcations, and high cervical portions of the carotid arteries. It is usually performed from the femoral approach using a pigtail catheter positioned in the ascending aorta just proximal to the innominate artery. Approximately 50 ml of contrast is injected with filming in both oblique projections. Conventional film-screen subtractions of the arteriograms are then made (Fig. 15–1).

Considerable controversy has existed regarding the merits of the use of arch aortography versus selective arteriography in the evaluation of extracranial carotid disease.

Selective carotid arteriography is easily and safely performed in patients with nonocclusive vascular disease or intracerebral mass lesions. In patients studied for transient ischemic attacks (TIAs), intracranial collateral flow is delicate, and the balance may be upset by hemodynamic changes induced by the placement of catheters in vessels with high-grade stenosis. The slow clearance of contrast from vessels with high-grade stenosis leads to longer cell contact with the contrast agent. The hazards of fibrin deposition on catheters in severely obstructed vessels is increased. Surgical mortality and morbidity are significantly higher in patients operated on for extracranial disease who did not have adequate intracranial visualization. In a series from Duke University,[16] 8 per cent of 350 patients studied for extracranial disease had significant intracranial pathology. Johnsrude[16] found that 85 per cent of their patients undergoing evaluation for intracranial disease could be adequately evaluated by multiple-projection aortic arch subtraction studies alone. Other authors have observed similar findings.[17,18] The complication rate from femoral cerebral angiography with cerebrovascular occlusive disease with this approach has also been reduced.[19] If the arch study does not conform to the results of non-invasive testing, a selective injection can be per-

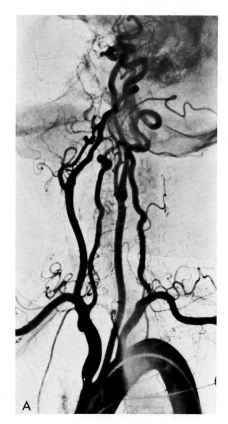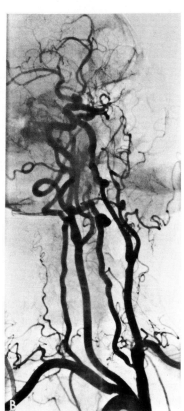

FIGURE 15–1. Subtraction films of an aortic arch study. *A,* Right posterior oblique position shows mild narrowing at the origin of the innominate artery, normal right carotid and right vertebral arteries. The left common carotid fills well. There is a smooth, nonobstructing plaque in the distal left common carotid artery. The left subclavian and left vertebral arteries are intact. *B,* On the left posterior oblique view, a plaque is seen at the origin of the right subclavian artery. The origin of the left vertebral artery has a 30 to 40 per cent narrowing. Again seen is the plaque in the distal left common carotid artery. The high cervical portions of the right and left internal carotid arteries are well seen.

formed. This offers the advantage of not having to selectively catheterize a tightly stenosed vessel. A disadvantage of the arch study is the larger volume of contrast required.

ANGIOGRAPHY OF THE EXTREMITIES

Angiography of the Lower Extremities

When visualization of the vessels of the lower extremities is desired, a femoral runoff study is obtained. The standard femoral arteriogram includes a runoff study with filling of the vessels of the legs down to the ankles. When a below-knee bypass is planned, filming to the level of the plantar arch may be necessary. A routine study also typically includes an abdominal aortogram with visualization of the aortic bifurcation. In the legs, improved visualization is obtained with reactive hyperemia induced at the time of the study. This can be accomplished using tourniquet constriction with release immediately prior to injection or with the administration of vasodilators such as papaverine. A standard runoff injection employs 75 to 85 ml of Renografin-76 (medium concentration) for visualization of the pelvis and lower legs. The abdominal injection is made with 50 ml of contrast medium for visualization of the aortic bifurcation and origins of the renal arteries. When visualization of only one leg is needed, the femoral artery on the ipsilateral side may be punctured, or the fem-

oral artery on the opposite side may be punctured and the catheter passed around the aortic bifurcation. It is important that the bifurcation of the superficial femoral and profunda femoral arteries be well visualized. If there is overlap of the vessels at this site, a significant stenosis in either the superficial femoral artery or the profunda femoral artery may be missed. It is often necessary to film the pelvis in the oblique projection with the side of interest elevated in order to open the bifurcation. In the lower leg, it is also important to avoid overlap of the tibia and fibula during positioning, because overlap of these two structures can result in poor visualization of the underlying runoff vessels. Oblique views may also be required to determine the severity of lesions in the iliac system. Visualization of the vessels in only one projection may result in a severe underestimation of the severity of the lesion. A reduction in vessel cross-sectional area of 75 per cent is considered indicative of a hemodynamically significant lesion. A 50 per cent reduction in diameter is approximately equivalent. When the hemodynamic significance of a stenosis is questioned, a pressure gradient should be measured across the lesion before and after the administration of vasodilators.[20] Gradients that are not hemodynamically significant at rest may be shown to be significant following the administration of the vasodilator. In interpreting femoral arteriograms, care must be exercised so that vessels are not presumed to be occluded when their failure to opacify is merely the result of an improper filming sequence with filming performed before arrival of the contrast bolus (Figs. 15–2, 15–3, and 15–4).

Angiography of Upper Extremities

Typical indications for angiography of the upper extremities include evaluation of atherosclerotic vascular disease or trauma, documentation of embolism, or evaluation of arteriovenous fistulae. Angiography of the upper extremities is readily performed via a percutaneous femoral artery approach. Alternatively, if the pathology is distal to the elbow, an antegrade or retrograde brachial artery puncture can be performed. Antegrade axillary punctures are employed rarely. Reactive hyperemia is used to enhance visualization of the vessels of the hand.

Specific Lesions

Atherosclerosis

In the arteries of the lower extremities, atherosclerotic changes occur most frequently in the femoral arteries, iliac arteries, the trifurcation, the popliteal arteries, and the aorta.[21] Lesions in the superficial femoral artery occur most frequently in the region of Hunter's canal. The changes may be evidenced as irregular plaques, ulceration, varying degrees of narrowing and occlusion, or areas of dilation and elongation. Patients with diabetes usually have diffuse small vessel disease with more frequent involvement below the trifurcation.

In the upper extremities, atherosclerosis involves the subclavian arteries, but rarely extends beyond them.[22] If the occlusion occurs proximal to the vertebral artery origins, a subclavian steal may occur, in which blood flow to the basilar system is decreased as blood preferentially passes retrograde down the vertebral artery into the low-pressure area of the subclavian artery distal to the stenosis. This retrograde filling of the vertebral artery is seen best on delayed films of an aortic arch injection (Fig. 15–5).

Embolism

Emboli to peripheral vessels are seen most commonly at bifurcations.[23,24] They appear radiographically as filling defects with convex margins. In acute emboli, filling of the arteries distally is usually not seen because of poor collateral formation or propagation of the thrombus. Because thrombus may form in time in the area of stagnant flow just proximal to an embolus, radiographic differentiation from thrombus can be difficult. Observations that should differentiate an embolus from a thrombus are absence of atherosclerotic changes in peripheral branches, and small collateral pathways. Thrombus superimposed on an area of stenosis may produce similar changes, but collateral pathways are usually larger and there is usually evidence of atherosclerosis distally. Emboli

may be due to clot, foreign bodies, tumor, or subacute bacterial endocarditis (SBE). Emboli most commonly originate in the left atrium. They may arise from aneurysms, atheroma, cardiac tumors, or, paradoxically, from the venous system (Fig. 15–6).

Arteritis

The most commonly seen arteritides are Buerger's disease, Takayasu's disease, and giant cell arteritis.

Buerger's Disease. Buerger's disease[25–27] involves both upper and lower extremities. It occurs primarily in young male Caucasian and Asian smokers. Migratory phlebitis is often associated. Angiographically, mural calcifications are typically absent. The lesions are segmental and symmetric and involve the distal small and medium-sized vessels with characteristically normal large proximal vessels. The angiogram typically shows absence of significant changes to suggest atheroma in large vessels. Smooth-lined vessels of even caliber are seen down to a point of abrupt occlusion. At the point of occlusion, the collateral pathways have a corkscrew, "spider-leg," or tree-root configuration around the point of focal disease. Corkscrew tortuosity of the superficial femoral and peroneal arteries may be seen. In the upper extremities, an absence of atheroma is again seen. There may be occlusion of the ulnar and/or radial arteries above the wrist, with typical collateral vessels and recanilization of the radial or ulnar arteries. The palmar arch may be attenuated or interrupted.[24]

Takayasu's Disease. This arteritis is seen more frequently in young females and most often involves the arch and brachiocephalic vessels. It can, however, involve the aorta and its branches, as well as the pulmonary arteries. It causes coarctation, occlusion, or aneurysmal dilation of the affected vessels.[28,29] The angiograms show narrowing and occlusion of the brachiocephalic vessels, particularly the subclavian arteries. Typically, long coarctations of the thoracic aorta and abdominal aorta occur with concomitant occlusion of renal and mesenteric vessels. Aneurysms of the aorta also occur (Fig. 15–7).[28]

Giant Cell Arteritis. This self-limited arteritis[30–33] usually presents in older patients with the prodrome of polymyalgia rheumatica characterized by fever, malaise, and headache. It has a predilection for medium-sized vessels of the carotid system, especially the temporal arteries, but can involve the major aortic arch branches, producing upper extremity symptoms. The femoral and popliteal arteries may also be involved. Once the patient's systemic symptoms subside, there are usually residual arterial narrowings. Angiographically, these appear as long segments of smooth arterial stenoses alternating with areas of normal or increased caliber. There is an absence of irregular plaques and ulceration. The radiographic findings may be indistinguishable from Takayasu's arteritis.

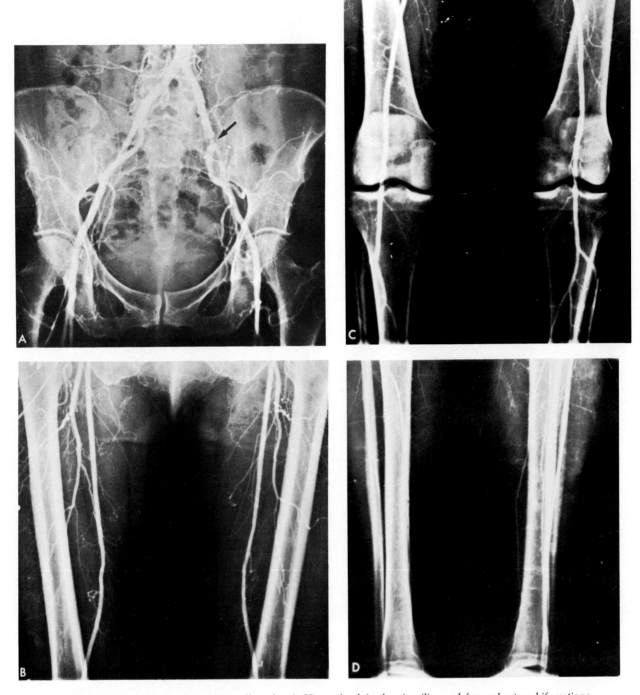

FIGURE 15–2. Typical femoral runoff study. *A,* View of pelvis showing iliac and femoral artery bifurcations. A localized stenosis is seen in the distal left common iliac artery (arrow). *B,* View of thigh showing patent right and left superficial femoral arteries. *C,* Popliteal artery and trifurcation view showing patent origin of anterior and posterior tibial and peroneal arteries. *D,* Lower leg runoff view showing normal runoff bilaterally.

Miscellaneous Causes of Occlusive Disease of Medium-Sized and Small Vessels

Medium-sized and small vessel occlusive disease may be the end result of a wide number of diseases, and frequently the diagnosis must be based on laboratory and clinical findings.[34,35] Chronic recurrent trauma to the hand can produce occlusion of digital vessels. Collagen diseases such as scleroderma can produce spasm and small vessel occlusion. Polyarteritis nodosa can present with small vessel aneurysms and occlusion. Dysproteinemias, polycythemia vera, and pseudoxanthoma elasticum can manifest with vessel occlusion, as can adverse reaction to drugs such as ergot derivatives and warfarin.[36]

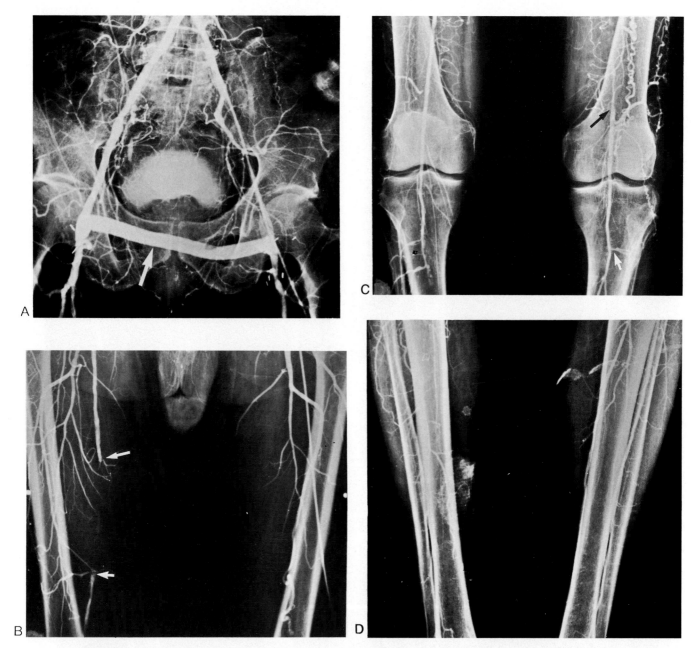

FIGURE 15–3. Runoff study. *A,* Catheter has passed via a left femoral artery puncture. Injection shows filling of the right common iliac and external iliac arteries with filling of a right femoral–to–left femoral graft (arrow). There is subsequent antegrade filling of the left profunda femoral artery. On the right, there is filling of both the profunda femoral and the superficial femoral arteries. *B,* Complete occlusion of the right superficial femoral artery midthigh (long arrow) with reconstitution at the level of the adductor hiatus (short arrow). To the left is opacification of the left profunda femoral artery with no filling of the left superficial femoral artery. *C,* Filling of the right popliteal artery with occlusion of the distal popliteal artery at the level of the posterior tibial, common peroneal trunk. The right anterior tibial artery is diffusely diseased at its origin. On the left, there is reconstitution of the popliteal artery by myriad collaterals (black arrow). The distal popliteal artery gives rise to the anterior and posterior tibial arteries. The left anterior tibial artery has a high-grade stenosis at its origin (short white arrow). The peroneal artery is patent. *D,* To the right is reconstitution of the posterior tibial artery just proximal to the ankle; the peroneal artery reconstitutes in the midcalf. The anterior tibial artery is occluded proximally. On the left, the posterior tibial and peroneal arteries fill to ankle level. The left anterior tibial has a high-grade stenosis at its origin but fills distally to the ankle.

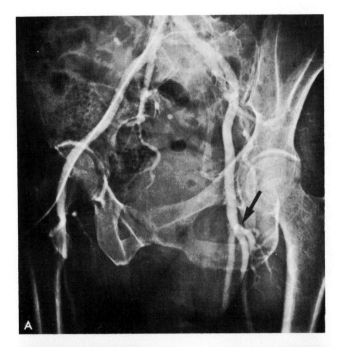

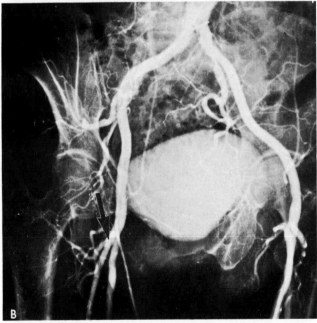

FIGURE 15–4. Oblique views of the pelvis. When the femoral bifurcations are not well visualized in the posteroanterior view, oblique views with the side of interest elevated should be performed; otherwise, hemodynamically significant bifurcation lesions may be missed. *A,* Right posterior oblique view opens up the left femoral bifurcation (arrow). *B,* Left posterior oblique view opens up right bifurcation (arrow).

Aneurysms of the Peripheral Vessels

Aneurysms of the peripheral vessels may be fusiform, saccular, mycotic, or false. They are due to a variety of causes, including atherosclerosis, medial degeneration, vasculitis, fibromuscular dysplasia, and trauma. Radiographically, the aneurysm is seen as a collection of contrast media. Laminated thrombus in the wall of the aneurysm may result in failure to diagnose the presence of aneurysms. Care should be taken to look for the presence of calcification in the wall of a vessel. In some cases, particularly popliteal artery aneurysms, ultrasonography may be necessary to determine the true size of the aneurysm (Fig. 15–8).

Congenital Arteriovenous Malformations

Congenital arteriovenous malformations may be of several types. They may be hyperdynamic, with increased small branching vessels that show early arteriovenous shunting into enlarged draining veins. They may involve small vessels or capillaries only, as in capillary hemangiomas. Angiographically, capillary hemangiomas typically show normal-sized arteries with an intense delayed capillary phase with normal or mildly dilated draining veins. Arteriovenous malformations may also involve only venous structures. These patients typically show normal arteries and capillaries. The dilated veins are seen best on venography.

Angiography of congenital arteriovenous malformations is necessary to determine the nature and full extent of the malformation, and should be performed prior to operative treatment. Angiography invariably reveals these lesions to be larger than appreciated on physical examinations. Selective injections with high volumes of contrast and rapid filming rates should be employed (Fig. 15–9).

VASCULAR TRAUMA

Vascular trauma can result from direct injury to the vessel from fracture dislocations, penetrating wounds, blunt trauma, repeated small trauma, or thermal injury. The angiographic findings in arterial trauma vary.[37–39] The most common observation is arterial spasm characterized by tapering and attenuation of the vessel with delayed flow. The vessels are usually draped and stretched in the areas of soft tissue swelling. Abrupt occlusion of the vessel may also be seen. Subintimal tears and dissections may be present. Thrombosis may occur, sometimes with distal emboli. False aneurysms may be seen as well as frank extravasation (Fig. 15–10). Arteriovenous fistulas are other sequelae. The arteriovenous fistulas characteristically show early filling of venous structures in the area of injury following an arterial injection (Fig. 15–11).

An important point that merits emphasis is that the clinical site of peripheral pulses distal to the site of trauma is not always a reliable indicator of extent of disease. The pulses may be reduced or absent when only spasm is present. Paradoxically, pulses may be good even when fairly severe trauma to the artery is present.[40,41] Because of this known disparity between the anatomic and clinical findings, angiog-

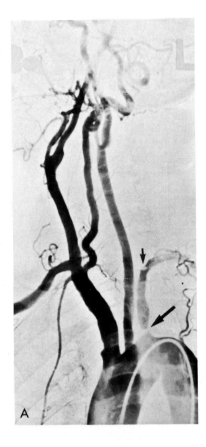 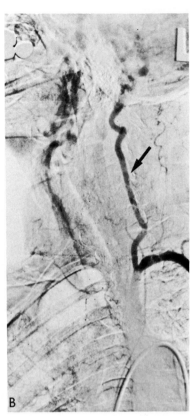

FIGURE 15–5. Subclavian steal syndrome. *A,* Aortic arch injection in the right posterior oblique position shows a patent innominate, right common carotid, and right vertebral artery. Left common carotid origin is normal. A high-grade stenosis is seen at the origin of the left subclavian artery (long arrow). At the point of expected origin of the left vertebral artery a lucency is identified (short arrow). *B,* Delayed films of the same injection show retrograde filling of the left vertebral artery (arrow) with opacification of the proximal left subclavian artery. Findings are typical for a subclavian steal syndrome.

raphy should be used early and often in cases of vascular trauma.

ABDOMINAL AORTOGRAPHY

Abdominal flush aortograms are usually performed via the femoral route. These are performed when evaluation of the abdominal aorta and its major branches is indicated. When specific information regarding organs supplied by major vessels is desired, selective arterial injections are made into the major aortic branches.

Specific Lesions

Atherosclerotic Disease

Atherosclerotic disease most commonly produces plaques, varying degrees of aortic narrowing, occlusion, and aneurysms of the aorta. Stenosis and occlusion of the aorta and its major branches occur most commonly below the renal arteries. Arteriograms will show localized or diffuse changes and eccentric or concentric narrowing. With high-grade stenoses, collateral vessels occur. When there is complete occlusion, arteriograms will demonstrate the level of occlusion and site of reconstitution if the collateral vessels are opacified (Fig. 15–12). It is important to be aware of the major collateral pathways between visceral branches of the aorta. Major collateral pathways oc-

cur between the celiac and superior mesenteric artery and inferior mesenteric artery. The arc of Bühler is a fetal remnant connecting between the celiac and superior mesenteric arteries. The middle colic branch of the superior mesenteric artery and the left colic of the inferior mesenteric artery form anastomoses when there is occlusion or stenosis. Another major collateral channel between the superior and inferior mesenteric arteries is via the marginal artery of Drummond (Figs. 15–13, 15–14, and 15–15).

Abdominal Aneurysms

Abdominal flush aortograms are commonly used to delineate the size and extent of arteriosclerotic aneurysms. The opacified lumen of the aorta does not always indicate the lumen and width of the aneurysm. The plain films obtained before the arrival of contrast must be carefully evaluated for the presence of linear calcifications. These represent calcification in the wall of the aorta. The distance between the linear calcification and the contrast-opacified aorta represents laminated thrombus in the aneurysm. The size of the aneurysm is estimated by measuring the total width of the aorta (Fig. 15–16).

Aneurysms of the hepatic and splenic artery may be identified on a flush injection or may require subselective catheterization. Splenic aneurysms appear as bulbous, dilated structures and occur more frequently than those in the hepatic artery.

Mycotic aneurysms differ in appearance from atherosclerotic aneurysms in that they characteristi-

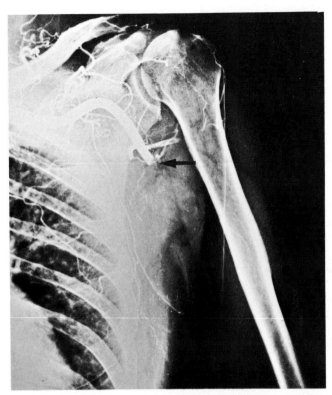

FIGURE 15–6. Embolic occlusion of proximal brachial, medial, and lateral circumflex humeral arteries. This patient experienced acute pain and loss of pulses in the left arm. Transfemoral selective left subclavian arteriogram shows abrupt termination of the brachial artery with evidence of a lucency indicative of embolus (arrow). In addition, there is a filling defect seen in the anterior humeral circumflex artery and complete occlusion of the posterior humeral circumflex. Note the absence of collateral vessels in this acute embolic occlusion.

cally are saccular or rounded in appearance. The lack of associated atherosclerotic changes and calcification aids in the diagnosis. These aneurysms have a propensity for rupture.[42]

Emboli arising from the aneurysms of the left ventricle following myocardial infarction, left atrial tumors, or aneurysms in the midaorta may embolize and produce complete occlusion of the abdominal aorta. Piercing trauma to the abdominal aorta can produce intimal damage, false aneurysms, hemorrhage, and arteriovenous fistulas.

Mesenteric Ischemia

More than 50 per cent of cases of mesenteric ischemia are due to reduced mesenteric flow from splenic vasoconstriction due to reduced cardiac output or shock.[43,44] The vessels radiographically appear intensely vasoconstricted. Multiple segmental constrictions at the origins of vessels are seen. The finer arterial vessels fill poorly. The changes may be localized or diffuse. Treatment with intra-arterial vasoconstrictors and correction of the shock are necessary to prevent irreversible bowel infarction.[45]

In other cases, bowel ischemia is due to atherosclerotic narrowing with thrombosis or emboli to ma-

jor visceral branches. Superior mesenteric artery emboli are responsible for 40 to 50 per cent of episodes of acute mesenteric ischemia. These emboli usually originate from a mural or an atrial thrombus.[46,47]

Occlusions or narrowings involving the origin of the celiac axis, superior mesenteric artery, and inferior mesenteric artery are best seen on an off-lateral view using an abdominal flush injection. Other causes of narrowing include median arcuate ligament of the diaphragm, fibromuscular dysplasia, tumors, aneurysms, or arteritis (Fig. 15–17).

Aortic Grafts

Arteriography used to evaluate the status of abdominal and peripheral grafts may reveal a variety of problems. Occlusion of the graft is the most frequently seen problem; others are the development of aneurysms in the host artery near the suture line and stenosis of host arteries at anastomotic sites. Infection or poor healing can result in disruption of the anastomosis, with rupture and retroperitoneal leaking, false aneurysm, fistula, or sinus formation (Fig. 15–18). Aortoenteric or aortocaval fistulas may occur. Angiography is useful for demonstrating these graft complications. In the aortoenteric fistula, however, the aortogram may or may not reveal the site of the fistula. Barium studies are often helpful, showing signs of a mass eroding the duodenum. Upper gastrointestinal endoscopy may identify the lesion and demonstrate the site of bleeding.[48]

In aortography of prosthetic grafts, it is preferable to avoid puncture of the graft itself because of the potential disruption of the pseudointima, introduction of infection, or induction of thombosis. In some instances, however, puncture of a graft is necessary owing to unavailability of other sites of entry. Graft puncture can be performed safely with careful technique.[49] Punctures of infected grafts, however, should be avoided.

GASTROINTESTINAL BLEEDING

Selective arteriography is useful in the detection of bleeding into the peritoneal cavity or bleeding into the gastrointestinal tract. Bleeding sites may be missed angiographically if selective injections are not employed. Bleeding sites are identified angiographically as collections of extravasated radiopaque contrast medium at the site of blood vessel disruption.[50] The bleeding may arise from lesions of the gastrointestinal tract such as ulcers, gastritis, esophageal varices, diverticuli, false aneurysms, arteriovenous malformations, hemangiomas, or tumors. Bleeding rates of 0.5 ml/min may be detected. Slow-bleeding sites are difficult to localize. Endoscopy should be performed prior to arteriography for upper gastrointestinal bleeding in order to help localize the bleeding site and thus minimize the time and volume of contrast required for the arteriogram. With slow bleeding, the success rate is low unless an anatomic defect is pres-

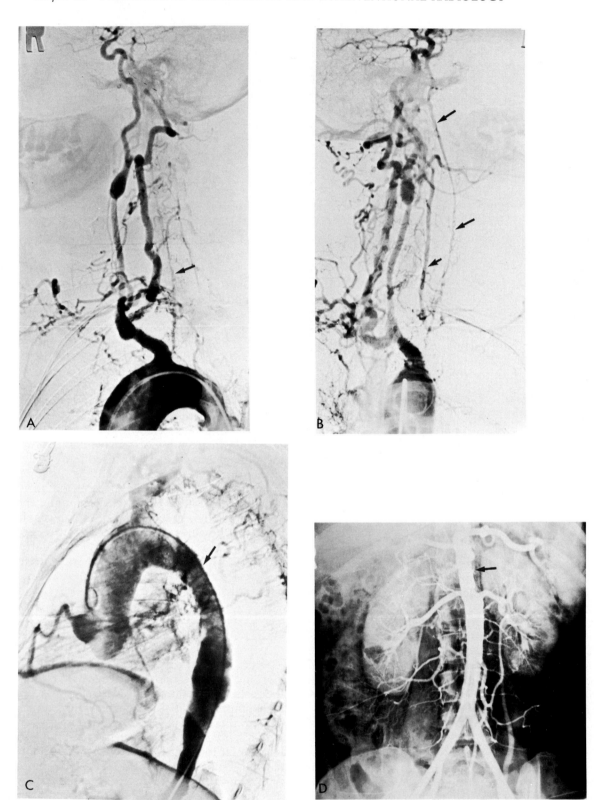

FIGURE 15–7. Takayasu's arteritis. This 28-year-old female presented with a history of a right hemiparesis at age 13. *A*, Aortic arch injection in the right posterior oblique projection shows filling of the right innominate artery, the right common carotid, and a hypertrophied left vertebral artery. There is delayed filling of the proximal portion of a narrowed threadlike left common carotid artery (arrow). The left vertebral artery does not opacify on this injection. Extensive collaterals are seen in the neck and supraclavicular region. Both subclavian arteries are occluded proximally. *B*, The left posterior oblique view again shows opacification of the right common carotid artery and right vertebral artery. This film, obtained late in the run, shows better filling of the diffusely narrowed irregular left common carotid artery (long arrows). A segment of this vessel may be recanalized (lower long

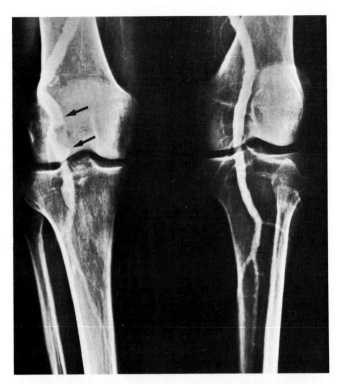

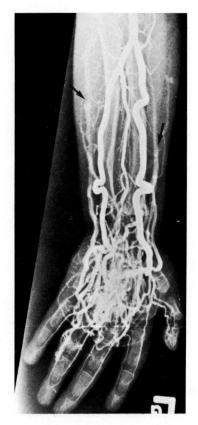

FIGURE 15–8.   Aneurysm of left popliteal artery. Runoff study shows dilation of the left popliteal artery with intraluminal filling defects consistent with thrombus (arrows). Popliteal artery aneurysms may show as areas of fusiform or saccular dilation or in the presence of laminated thrombus may show only minimal vessel irregularity. Ultrasound is a useful method for determining the true extent of the aneurysm.

FIGURE 15–9.   Congenital arteriovenous malformation. This 1.5-year-old female was noted to have a pulsatile mass on the left hand. Transfemoral left subclavian arteriogram reveals markedly dilated brachial, radial, and ulnar arteries. A dense tangle of vessels is seen projected over the metacarpals. Note the early-draining veins (arrows). This is a hyperdynamic type of arteriovenous malformation that will progressively increase in size.

ent at the bleeding site. Findings such as the presence of a large early-draining vein may indicate the site of an arteriovenous malformation. Angiodysplasia arteriographically presents as a dense stain with an early-draining vein. Tumor neovascularity or arterial encasement may help localize the site of a slow ooze. A preferable approach to the localization of slowly bleeding sites is the utilization of ⁹⁹ᵐTc sulfur colloid[51] or other ⁹⁹ᵐTc-labeled blood pool agents[52] injected intravenously. These blood pool agents collect at the site of hemorrhage as radioactive blood that can be detected using a gamma camera 2 to 40 minutes after injection. These agents can be utilized to detect active sites of bleeding in the gastrointestinal tract and are capable of detecting rates as slow as 0.1 ml/min. They are particularly useful in the diagnosis of lower gastrointestinal bleeding. The technique can serve as a direct guide to surgery or can aid in delineation of the region to be further studied angiographically.

PORTAL HYPERTENSION

Evaluation of the patient with portal hypertension may be required to demonstrate the site of gastrointestinal bleeding or to provide preoperative vascular evaluation in preparation for a shunt procedure. In the presence of portal hypertension, gastrointestinal

FIGURE 15–7.   *Continued*
arrow). There is retrograde filling of the left vertebral artery (short arrow). *C,* Injection into the thoracic aorta shows typical findings of Takayasu's aortitis, with dilation of the ascending aorta, narrowing of the upper thoracic aorta (arrow), followed by an area of dilation in the descending thoracic aorta. *D,* Abdominal aortogram again shows characteristic findings in Takayasu's aortitis, with narrowing of the abdominal aorta in the segment between celiac axis and origin of the renal arteries (arrow). The infrarenal abdominal aorta is within normal limits. Takayasu's aortitis can extend inferiorly to involve the distal aorta and common iliacs and has been reported to involve the femoral arteries.

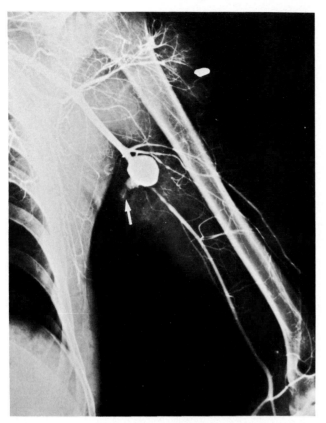

FIGURE 15–10. Posttraumatic false aneurysm with extravasation. This 34-year-old male was shot in the left shoulder. The bullet fragment is seen in the upper arm. He presented with diminished pulses distally in the left arm and decreased neurologic function in the distribution of the ulnar and median nerves. Selective left axillary artery injection shows a large false aneurysm at the site of vessel disruption. There is evidence of spasm and displacement of the circumflex humeral arteries and muscular branches of the brachial artery in the area of soft tissue swelling. Extravasation of contrast is identified (arrow).

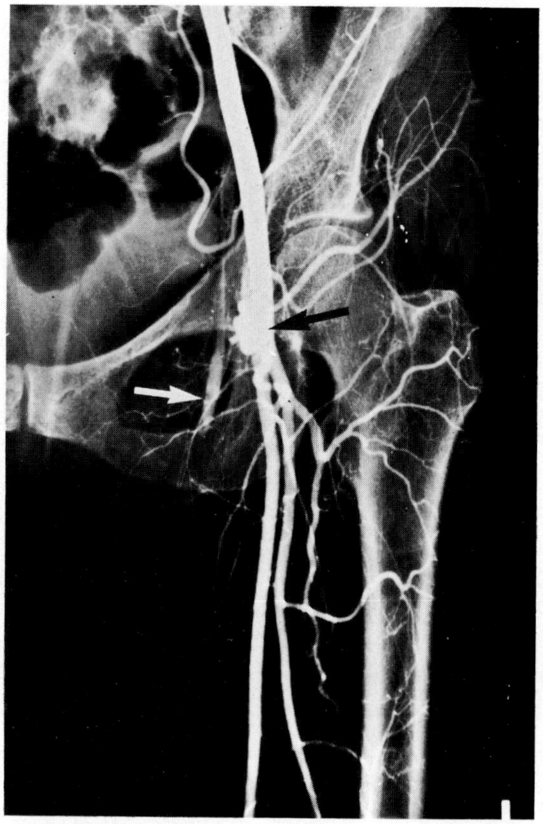

FIGURE 15–11. Posttraumatic arteriovenous fistula in left groin. This patient had undergone a left transfemoral aortogram for evaluation of hypertension. Two days later, a pulsatile mass appeared in the left groin. A continuous bruit was present. Selective right transfemoral–left external iliac arteriogram reveals a false aneurysm of the common femoral artery at the puncture site (black arrow). Fistulous communication with the femoral vein is present (white arrow).

bleeding may be from varices or other causes, such as gastritis, Mallory-Weiss tears, or ulcer disease. If selective arterial injections fail to reveal the bleeding site, the bleeding can be assumed to be from varices. Venous bleeding is almost never demonstrated angiographically, and the diagnosis of esophageal bleeding is made on angiography only indirectly by demonstrating portal hypertension and excluding other sites of bleeding.

Portal hypertension may be due to prehepatic obstruction, such as portal vein or splenic vein thrombosis. Intrahepatic obstruction is due to such entities as Laënnec's or biliary cirrhosis. Schistosomiasis causes an intrahepatic presinusoidal obstruction. Suprahepatic obstruction occurs in Budd-Chiari syndrome.

Routine angiographic evaluation of the portal system in patients with portal hypertension can be performed in several ways. Evaluation consists of measurement of the hepatic vein wedge pressure and visualization of the portal system. Hepatic vein wedge pressures are readily obtained by entry into hepatic veins using a catheter that has been passed up the

inferior vena cava and into a hepatic vein. In the wedge position, the catheter in the hepatic vein measures the pressure in the communicating sinusoids. The normal sinusoidal pressure is between 3 and 11 mm Hg. This pressure includes not only that within the sinusoids, but also the intra-abdominal pressure, which can be increased by heart failure or ascites. The true corrected sinusoidal pressure is obtained by subtracting from the wedge pressure the component of pressure transmitted from the inferior vena cava. This can be done by subtracting the wedge pressure from the pressure measured with the catheter lying free within the hepatic vein. The free hepatic vein pressure normally measures between 1 and 6 mm Hg. Therefore, the corrected sinusoidal pressure is normally 1 to 5 mm Hg. The sinusoidal pressure may be elevated owing to increased resistance at the sinusoidal or postsinusoidal level, as in cirrhosis. With mild portal hypertension, the corrected sinusoidal pressure is 6 to 10 mm Hg. Severe portal hypertension is present when the corrected sinusoidal pressure is 19 mm Hg or higher. In presinusoidal

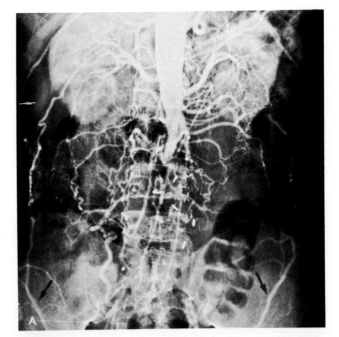

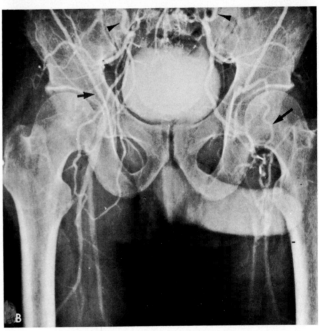

FIGURE 15–12. Collateral flow to pelvis in occlusion of the infrarenal abdominal aorta. *A,* The aorta is occluded just distal to the inferior mesenteric artery. Large lumbar arteries communicate bilaterally with the deep iliac circumflex arteries (arrows). *B,* The deep iliac circumflex artery on the right (short arrow) fills retrograde back to the common femoral artery, which then fills antegrade to give rise to the right superficial and deep femoral arteries. On the left, the deep iliac circumflex communicates with collateral branches of the left femoral circumflex (long arrow) and profunda femoral. The iliofemoral arteries (arrowheads) also fill from lumbar collaterals retrograde back to the hypogastric arteries. On the left, inferior gluteal branches of the reconstituted hypogastric artery communicate with femoral circumflex branches, which collateralize the superficial and deep femoral arteries.

obstruction or portal vein thrombosis, no pressures can be transmitted to the sinusoids, and the hepatic vein wedge pressures are usually normal or subnormal.[53–55]

At present, visualization of the portal vein is most commonly accomplished using arterial portography with injection of the celiac and superior mesenteric arteries and filming carried to the venous phase. Vasodilators such as Priscoline (Ciba) are administered intra-arterially to enhance visualization of the venous phase.[56] Adequate volumes of contrast are necessary, and filming must be sufficiently delayed. Visualization of the portal vein can be accomplished with the direct injection of contrast into the spleen, but this is associated with a risk of bleeding.[57] A percutaneous transhepatic approach can also be used, but is also associated with increased morbidity. Rarely, a transjugular vein approach is used.

Postoperative evaluation of portosystemic shunts can also be accomplished with arterial injections. Delayed films show filling of the inferior vena cava. In many instances the shunt can be directly cannulated by manipulation of the catheter passed into the inferior vena cava. Pressure gradients may be measured with this technique.

When evaluation of the hepatic veins is desired, direct injection of contrast into the hepatic veins is performed. This is indicated in the work-up of sus-

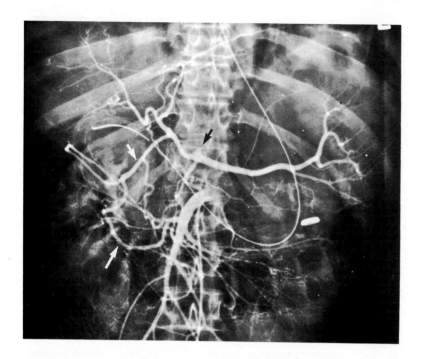

FIGURE 15–13. Collateral flow in occlusion of celiac axis. On the selective superior mesenteric artery injection there is filling of the inferior pancreatic duodenal artery (long white arrow). This artery fills retrograde to communicate with the gastroduodenal artery (short white arrow), which then fills retrograde back to the celiac trunk (short black arrow). There is filling of the splenic and hepatic arteries. This collateral pathway is important in instances in which there is occlusion of either the celiac axis or the superior mesenteric artery.

pected cases of Budd-Chiari syndrome. In this entity, the hepatic veins appear as a disorganized, spidery network.

SPLENIC ARTERIOGRAPHY

The indications for splenic arteriography have changed with the availability of other noninvasive imaging modalities. Good visualization of the spleen can be accomplished with computed tomography (CT), ultrasonography, or liver scans. CT is capable of detecting both splenic laceration and subcapsular hematomas.[58] Isotope studies lack specificity and may miss small subcapsular hematomas, but in selected cases may obviate the need for angiography. A useful algorithm[59] for splenic evaluation is CT scintigraphy or ultrasonography as the primary imaging method. If these studies are normal or diagnostic or show a diffuse infiltrative disease, no further imaging is needed. If the nature of the lesions remains uncertain, angiography is employed as the definitive diagnostic method. The algorithm is short-circuited only if there is a high suspicion of splenic trauma in the precarious patient. Even in pediatric patients, scintigraphy may be adequate as part of the effort to avoid splenectomy and preserve immunologic competency. Angiography is indicated in the evaluation of splenic artery aneurysms and the diagnosis of splenic arteriovenous fistulas.

Splenic arteriography is performed by selective splenic artery injection.

Typical Angiographic Findings

Extravasation of contrast is the diagnostic finding in splenic rupture. Mottling of the parenchymal phase is not specific and may be seen with splenic contusion in the absence of rupture. Other characteristic findings are a large avascular area with displacement of the intrasplenic branches, compression of the opacified spleen in the region of the hematoma, and clear fracture in the splenic contour. Simultaneous filling of the splenic artery and vein may be seen.[60,61]

Splenic artery aneurysms are the most common intra-abdominal aneurysms, following those in the aorta and iliac arteries. They are observed most frequently in women of childbearing age and have a high propensity for rupture. Some may be congenital, and others arteriosclerotic, in origin. They may calcify and typically appear as a large, smooth-walled, contrast-filled sac.

RENAL ARTERIOGRAPHY

Evaluation of the renal arteries is performed with a flush aortogram followed by selective arterial injections. Flush injections are utilized to identify accessory renal arteries, which can arise anywhere from the low thoracic aorta down to the iliac artery. These are also necessary for identification of collateral vessels to the kidney when flow in the renal artery is obstructed. The extrarenal collateral vessels arise from the ureteric, gonadal, adrenal, lumbar, and intercostal arteries.[62] The flush injection may provide sufficient information for diagnosis. Selective injections should be performed carefully if there is severe atherosclerotic plaqueing, because elevation of a plaque during injection can result in renal artery occlusion.

Angiographic Findings

Obstruction of the renal arteries may be due to diseases of the aorta. Atherosclerotic plaques or an-

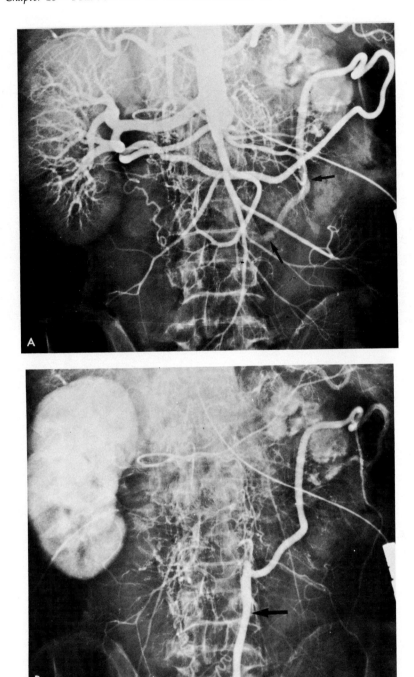

FIGURE 15–14. Collateral supply to inferior mesenteric artery. *A,* Translumbar aortogram shows complete occlusion of the abdominal aorta just distal to the takeoff of the right renal artery. The left renal artery is occluded. The left kidney is atrophic and calcified secondary to previous tuberculosis. The superior mesenteric artery is visualized. The middle colic branch is markedly hypertrophied. In the region of the splenic flexure it communicates with a hypertrophied left colic artery, which fills retrograde back to its origin from the inferior mesenteric artery (arrows). *B,* The inferior mesenteric then fills antegrade (arrow). This collateral network provides flow to the descending colon and rectum in instances when the inferior mesenteric artery is occluded.

eurysms can obstruct renal artery origins. Thrombotic occlusion of the aorta above the renal arteries and aortic dissections that extend into the renal artery can also compromise renal blood flow, as can aortitis, abdominal coarctation, and neurofibromatosis. Atherosclerotic disease of the renal arteries usually involves the proximal third of the artery, producing small plaques or complete occlusion. Atherosclerotic lesions may be eccentric or concentric and may be bilateral. Intrarenal branch stenoses also occur. They may be due to atherosclerotic disease, renal artery dysplasias, thrombosis, embolus, or arteritis. Occasionally, these may be difficult to detect on flush aortography. The parenchymal phase of the arter-

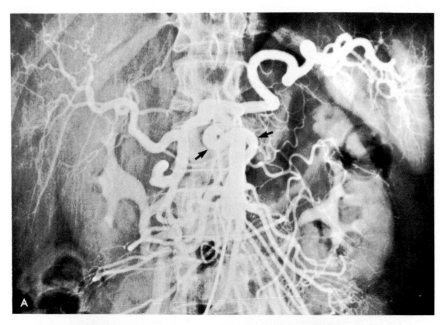

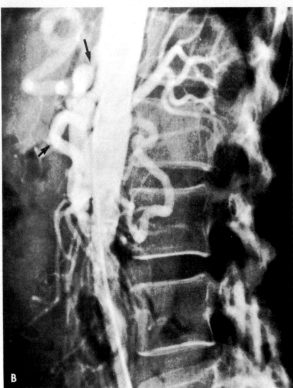

FIGURE 15–15.   Hypertrophied arc of Bühler in celiac axis stenosis. *A,* On this superior mesenteric artery injection there is retrograde filling of the gastroduodenal artery with filling back to the celiac axis, with filling of the splenic artery and hepatic artery. In addition, there is a vessel connecting the superior mesenteric artery with the celiac trunk. This ventral anastomosis represents a remnant of the tenth vitelline artery and is called the arc of Bühler (short arrows). *B,* The lateral view shows a high-grade stenosis at the origin of the celiac axis (long arrow) and the ventral position of the arc of Bühler (short arrow). The gastroduodenal artery in this patient projects posteriorly.

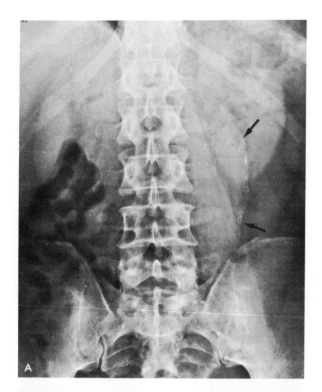

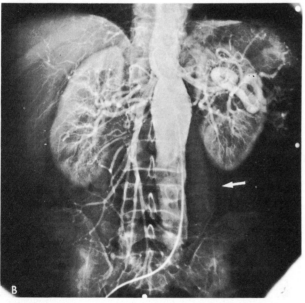

FIGURE 15–16. Abdominal aortic aneurysm. *A*, Plain films of the abdomen show calcification in the wall of the aneurysm (arrows). *B*, Flush abdominal aortogram shows an infrarenal fusiform abdominal aneurysm extending down to the iliac bifurcation. The origin of the right renal artery was seen on earlier films. The opacified channel does not indicate the true extent of the aneurysm. The calcifications indicate the width of the aneurysm (arrow). The soft tissue density between the opacified lumen and the calcified wall of the aorta represents laminated thrombus. In some instances, the calcifications may be very subtle. Abdominal aortic aneurysms can be missed on angiography if this pitfall is not considered.

iogram may show the ischemic area well. When there is a question of branch stenoses, selective arteriography with multiple views is indicated.

Fibromuscular Dysplasia

Fibromuscular dysplasia, affecting primarily young females, occurs most frequently in the middle and distal third of the main renal arteries.[63,64] The lesions are usually bilateral. Branch stenoses occur more frequently than in atherosclerotic disease.

Several types of fibromuscular dysplasia occur. They include (1) intimal fibroplasia, (2) medial fibroplasia with aneurysms, (3) medial fibromuscular hyperplasia, (4) adventitial hyperplasia, and (5) subadventitial hyperplasia.[65,66] Angiographically, they may be difficult to distinguish. The commonest type is medial fibroplasia with aneurysms. Angiographically, this typically gives a string-of-beads appearance to the renal artery. The appearance is caused by alternating areas of narrowing due to thickened segments of media partially replaced with collagen, alternating with areas of dilation where the internal elastic lamina and media are partially disrupted. Focal short stenosis or long segmental stenoses may be due to medial fibromuscular hyperplasia or intimal fibroplasia. In subadventitial perimedial fibroplasia, the segment of the vessel with the string-of-beads appearance is narrower than areas of uninvolved vessel. Tubular lesions characterized by elongated smooth concentric narrowing of the renal arteries may be due to adventitial hyperplasia. Mixed lesions can occur in the same patient. Mural aneurysms may form at the site of medial disruption, and true aneurysms may form in the region of poststenotic dilation of the renal artery. In a minority of patients, dissection of the renal artery can occur, with the dissection extending into primary or secondary renal branches.

Multiple vessels may be involved, including the carotid arteries, vertebral arteries, and splanchnic and celiac arteries (Fig. 15–19).[67]

Renal Trauma

A clinical radiologic classification has been proposed as an aid to the utilization of radiographic procedures in the diagnosis of renal trauma.[68] Minor renal injuries are those in which there has been damage to the renal parenchyma, but no extension to the renal capsule and no involvement of the pelvocalyceal system. These rarely require arteriography. The intravenous urogram in these patients usually shows a normal urinary tract, with only minimal delay in function on the affected side. Major renal injuries in which both parenchymal and capsular involvement are present usually result in damage to the collecting system. The intravenous urogram in these patients may show extravasation of contrast. Arteriography

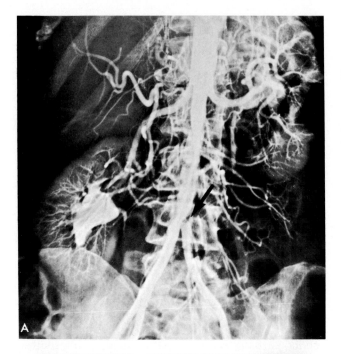

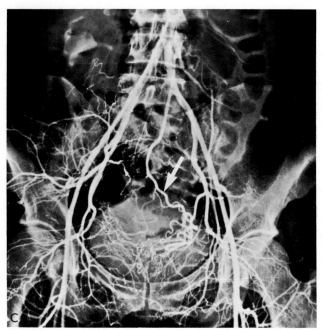

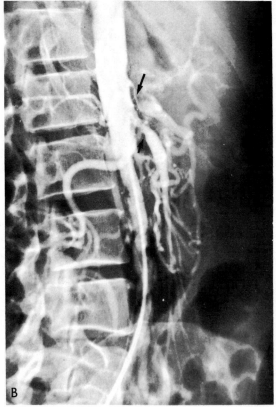

FIGURE 15–17. Abdominal angina due to superior mesenteric, celiac, and inferior mesenteric artery occlusion. This female presented with symptoms of claudication and abdominal angina. *A,* Flush aortogram shows no filling of the celiac axis. The superior mesenteric artery is patent, and there is retrograde filling of the gastroduodenal artery by way of the pancreatic arcade. There is faint opacification of the left splenic artery. There is no filling of the inferior mesenteric artery branches. In addition, a high-grade stenosis is seen at the origin of the left common iliac artery (arrow). *B,* Off-lateral view abdominal aortogram shows a tapered occlusion of the celiac axis at its origin (long arrow) and a significant stenosis at the origin of the superior mesenteric artery with poststenotic dilation (short arrow). The inferior mesenteric artery is occluded. *C,* Pelvic arteriogram shows collaterals arising from the left hypogastric artery communicating with the superior hemorrhoidal artery, which fills retrograde back to the main trunk of the inferior mesenteric artery (arrow). This collateral supply to the large bowel is jeopardized by the presence of the high-grade left common iliac stenosis.

is indicated in these patients to determine the extent of the injury and the status of the vascular anatomy. When multiple organ involvement is suspected and the patient shows no signs of impending shock, CT may be of value in the detection of early hemorrhage. Critical injuries of the kidney are those in which the renal rupture extends into the pedicle. Exsanguin-

ating hemorrhage may occur in a few minutes. The intravenous urogram is useful in determining the status of the contralateral kidney. The involved kidney is usually nonfunctioning. If the patient is sufficiently stable, arteriography will demonstrate the avulsed pedicle or laceration. There is a notable incidence of adjacent organ involvement in pedicle in-

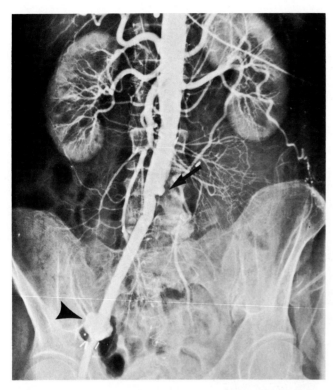

FIGURE 15–18. Aortobifemoral graft complications. Translumbar aortogram shows the left limb of the aortobifemoral graft to be completely occluded at its origin (arrow). Collaterals are seen along the left lateral aspect of the abdominal wall, which will reconstitute the left superficial and deep femoral arteries distally. The right limb of the graft is patent. A false aneurysm is seen at the distal anastomosis (arrowhead).

jury. Liver, splenic, or pancreatic damage or damage to the contralateral kidney may be present. Arteriography should encompass an evaluation of these other organs. Thrombosis of the renal artery secondary to trauma is uncommon. It usually involves the left kidney.

Renal Arteriovenous Fistulas

Renal arteriovenous fistulas may be acquired or congenital in origin.[69] Acquired traumatic fistulas are most commonly the result of percutaneous biopsy, occurring in almost 15 per cent of patients undergoing biopsy.[70] Penetrating abdominal trauma is another major cause. Arteriography is indicated and will typically show a dilated renal artery with fistulous communication to an early-draining vein. Many of these fistulas can be treated by selected transcatheter arterial occlusion rather than operation.

Renal Artery Aneurysms

Renal artery aneurysms may be congenital, traumatic, degenerative, or inflammatory in origin. They may occur in children, but are usually seen in elderly patients, except when they are a sequela of renal artery dysplasia. Hypertension is associated in 72 to 85 per cent of patients.[71] Aneurysms are saccular or fusiform, with the fusiform type seen most frequently in atherosclerotic vascular disease. Approximately 50 per cent of renal artery aneurysms have calcium in their walls. As a rule, calcified aneurysms do not tend to rupture, whereas those without calcium tend to rupture spontaneously.

RENAL DIALYSIS FISTULAS

These surgically constructed arteriovenous fistulas are usually placed in the forearm connecting the radial artery and cephalic vein. The fistulas may be externally created shunts, such as the Scribner shunt,[72] or internal fistulas.[73] The internal fistulas are end-to-side, side-to-side, or end-to-end anastomoses. Dacron prostheses, saphenous veins, or bovine carotid arteries may be interposed between the radial artery and the cephalic vein.[74] Arteriography is indicated in the evaluation of these shunts when there is evidence of shunt failure.[75,76] Problems indicative of faulty shunt function include reduction in the thrill over the shunt. Increased resistance to return during dialysis suggests stenosis or blockage in the venous limb, whereas decreased flow on withdrawing suggests obstruction in the proximal venous limb or in the artery supplying the fistula. Arteriography is used to delineate stenosis or thrombosis. These can occur in either the arterial or the venous limb of the graft. Venous stenoses may arise a considerable distance from the fistula. Pseudoaneurysms develop in the graft at venipuncture sites, and aneurysms may occur in the artery (Figs. 15–20 and 15–21).

Angiographic evaluation of the aforementioned lesions is performed by direct percutaneous puncture and injection into the shunt. Ischemia of the hand distal to the shunt may also occur. This is best evaluated with a subclavian artery injection performed via the femoral artery approach.

VENOGRAPHY

Extremities

Venography of an extremity is indicated in the evaluation of venous obstruction. The obstruction may be due to thrombosis, tumor invasion, extrinsic compression, or trauma.

Acute venous thrombosis radiographically appears as an intraluminal filling defect outlined by a rim of contrast media. As the thrombus organizes and adheres to the vessel wall, the rim is lost, and complete occlusion of the vessels occurs. Recanalized vessels have a thin, stringy appearance in which the venous valves have been obliterated. Webs may develop, and collateral vessels become prominent. Superficial varices develop.

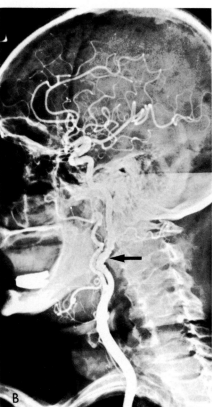
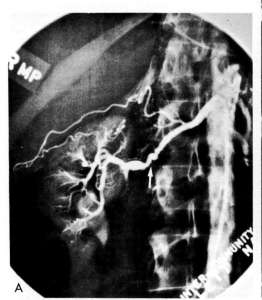

FIGURE 15–19. Fibromuscular dysplasia. *A,* The middle and distal portion of the right renal artery shows a string-of-beads appearance typical of medial fibroplasia with aneurysm (arrow). *B,* Selective left internal carotid artery injection shows typical string-of-beads appearance of fibromuscular dysplasia (medial fibroplasia with aneurysm) in the proximal portion of the left internal carotid artery (arrow).

Lower Extremity Venography

Contrast venography is the most reliable technique for the detection of deep venous thrombosis.[77–79] Color duplex flow imaging has been found to have high accuracy for detection of deep venous thrombosis above the knee. It is less accurate in the detection of thrombi below the knee. Currently it is used frequently for screening and may obviate the need for contrast venography.[80] Contrast venography is performed by introducing a 21- or 19-gauge scalp vein needle into a dorsal foot vein and injecting contrast medium. The patient should be on a radiographic tilt table at a 45- to 60-degree tilt with the extremity under study non–weight bearing. Renografin-60 (low concentration) is injected and overhead or spot films made as the contrast travels up the venous system. Studies are usually done with filming both with and without the application of tourniquets to improve filling of the deep venous system. Complications of the procedure are few, but include exacerbation of thrombophlebitis as a result of endothelial irritation from contact with the contrast medium. Phlebitis may be induced. The incidence of these complications can be reduced if the contrast is flushed from the veins with heparinized saline at the end of the study. Extravasation of contrast at the injection site may result in a skin slough.

Upper Extremity Venography

Upper extremity venography is performed with the injection of contrast introduced via a scalp vein needle positioned in an arm vein. The technique is useful for the detection of thrombus and in evaluation of patients with venous obstruction due to the thoracic outlet syndrome.

Arteriography is indicated in the work-up of the thoracic outlet syndrome in patients with diminished pulses or asymmetric cuff blood pressures in the two extremities. It is also indicated when a bruit is present in the affected extremity or when a source of peripheral emboli is sought. The arteriogram can be performed via a femoral artery approach with the catheter tip positioned in the subclavian artery. The arteriogram should be performed with the arm in a neutral position and following maneuvers that elicit symptoms.[81,82] In positive studies, the site of arterial compression will be identified. More recently, digital subtraction angiography has been used as an alternative to standard arteriography in the evaluation of these patients.

Venacavography

Superior venacavography is used primarily for the evaluation of the superior vena cava syndrome, for

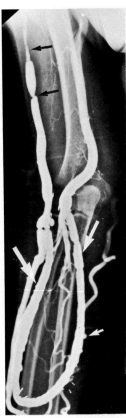

FIGURE 15–20. Bovine graft arteriovenous fistula. The "U"-shaped limb of the bovine graft is identified (long white arrows). Multiple small false aneurysms are seen at site of previous puncture for dialysis. Note the dilation of the arterial lumen (short white arrow). Arterialization of vessels is a common finding in long-standing dialysis fistulas. In the venous limb, multiple stenoses are seen in the vein (black arrows).

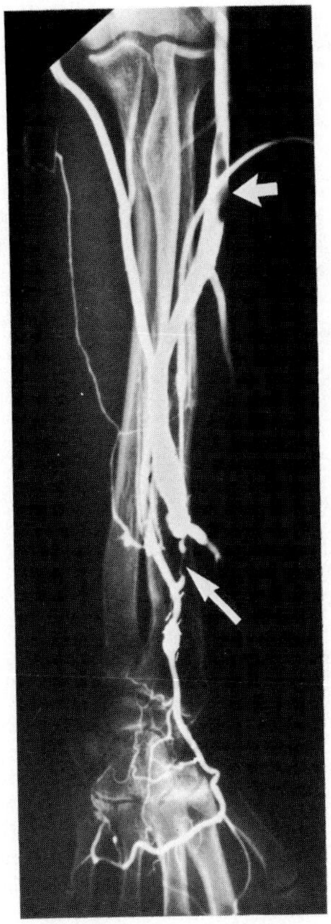

FIGURE 15–21. Dialysis arteriovenous (AV) fistula. A long, high-grade stenosis is seen in the venous limb of this dialysis AV fistula (long arrow). In addition, an intraluminal filling defect representing thrombus is seen proximally in the venous limb (short arrow). Lesions in the venous limb may arise a considerable distance from the fistula.

evaluation of mediastinal masses, and for delineation of superior vena cava anatomy in patients with suspected anomalies of pulmonary or systemic venous return.[83,84] Scalp vein needles are placed in each antecubital vein and contrast injected bilaterally. Radiographic signs of occlusion are the presence of intraluminal filling defects and collateral vessels (Fig. 15–22).

Inferior venacavography is indicated in the detection of caval obstruction. It should also be performed prior to caval umbrella placement. Caval obstruction may be secondary to thrombus, webs, or primary or secondary tumors (Figs. 15–23 and 15–24). The preferred approach is with placement of catheters in both femoral veins and simultaneous injection of contrast. Alternatively, a single catheter may be placed just at the origin of the inferior vena cava. In the presence of femoral vein occlusion, the catheter may be introduced by an antecubital vein and passed down the superior vena cava. The cava is easily visualized. If selective renal or adrenal venography is desired, selective catheterization of these vessels can be performed using either a femoral or antecubital vein approach.

DIGITAL SUBTRACTION ANGIOGRAPHY

Digital subtraction angiography (DSA) is a form of digital radiography. In digital radiography, x-ray signals are detected electronically, converted to digital form, and processed prior to being recorded and displayed. Computer subtraction techniques are utilized to remove uninteresting background information from the image so that the clinically significant details can be displayed with enhanced visibility. In DSA, the aim is to obtain visualization of the vascular system. With digital subtraction techniques and logarithmic amplification of the x-ray signal, one is able to detect and amplify small differences in density.[85–87] This permits detection of very low concentrations of iodinated contrast medium, such as those that occur in the arterial system following the intravenous injection of contrast, or on the venous phase of an arterial injection.

Although the contrast sensitivity is high in DSA, spatial resolution is less than in conventional film-screen arteriograms. As a result, the DSA images are less sharp than those obtained in the conventional arteriogram, but this is acceptable, because it is not

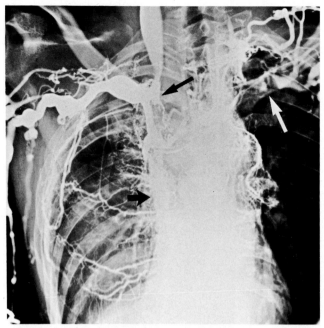

FIGURE 15–22. Superior vena cava syndrome. This 37-year-old male with carcinoma of the lung developed progressive superior vena cava syndrome. His superior venacavogram, performed by simultaneous injection into right and left antecubital veins, shows complete occlusion of the right subclavian vein (long black arrow) with reflux up the right internal jugular vein. Abundant collaterals are present. Mediastinal and intercostal collaterals are identified on the right side communicating with the azygous (short black arrow). On the left, there is thrombus with occlusion of the left subclavian vein (white arrow) and extensive collaterals to the azygous.

always necessary to have high detail in order to make a diagnosis or plan therapy.

The standard DSA unit consists of an x-ray tube, image intensifier, television camera, and image processor (computer). The subtraction technique most widely used at present is temporal subtraction, in which a mask image obtained prior to x-ray contrast arrival is stored in the computer memory. Subsequent images obtained during the arrival of the contrast bolus are obtained and then subtracted from the mask. The difference image (the opacified vessels) is displayed and stored. In instances in which motion artifact has occurred between the acquisition of the mask and the subtraction images, postprocessing of the images may then be performed. In postprocessing, a new mask is selected or the mask is shifted to partially compensate and correct for the motion artifact. The radiation dose in DSA is similar to or slightly less than that in conventional arteriography.[88]

When DSA was first developed, initial interest centered around its use for intravenous angiography. There are, however, serious limitations to the use of intravenous DSA. Motion artifacts interfere with subtraction and large volumes of contrast may be used with the multiple injections required to evaluate regions of vessel overlap. Intravenous applications are now used infrequently. Currently the most frequent application of digital techniques is with arterial injections of contrast. Arterial DSA allows arteriography using diluted contrast or reduced volumes of contrast and with reduced film costs. The availability of small French-sized, high-flow catheters makes outpatient digital arteriography feasible. Image quality with arterial DSA is superior to that with intravenous DSA, because there is less dilution of the contrast bolus and less problem with motion artifact, the injection site being closer to the structures imaged.

Arterial DSA is often used in conjunction with conventional arteriography allowing completion of the study with less contrast and fewer films. Rapid video display of images reduces angiographic study time. Arterial DSA may be used as a substitute for conventional arteriography in many situations,[89] and facilitates the performance of interventional procedures. The resolution of arterial DSA is less than that with conventional film-screen arteriography, and vessels less than 200 μ are seen better with conventional studies. Arterial DSA, however, has superior contrast detectability when compared to conventional arteriography and offers improved visualization of tumor blushes and venous structures.

FIBRINOLYTIC THERAPY

In the past few years there has been a progressive increase in the use of fibrinolytic therapy for peripheral vessel and graft thrombolysis. Streptokinase, urokinase, and recombinant human tissue-type plasminogen activator (rt-PA) are the currently available agents. All are plasminogen activators and produce lysis by stimulating the conversion of plasminogen to its active form, plasmin. Urokinase and rt-PA act directly on plasminogen to form plasmin; streptokinase must first form an activated complex with plasminogen. Urokinase and streptokinase act not only on plasminogen within the clot, but also on plasminogen throughout the circulation. Streptokinase and urokinase convert both circulating and fibrin-bound plasminogen to plasmin, the proteolytic enzyme that digests fibrin. The plasmin that is formed subsequently degrades plasma proteins, including fibrin, fribrinogen, plasminogen, and factors V and VIII. A systemic lytic state is achieved that is characterized by depletion of fibrinogen, plasminogen, and α_2-antiplasmin, prolongation of the thrombin time, and accumulation of fibrin split products, rt-PA, on the other hand, is a potent, relatively fibrin-specific thrombolytic agent.

Streptokinase was first used in man in 1959,[90] and the clinical use of urokinase soon followed.[91] Both agents were utilized in the cooperative Urokinase Pulmonary Embolism Trials in the early 1970s.[92,93] While the benefit of systemic fibrinolytic therapy was noted, it soon became apparent that systemic therapy was associated with a high incidence of hemorrhagic complications. In an effort to circumvent these hem-

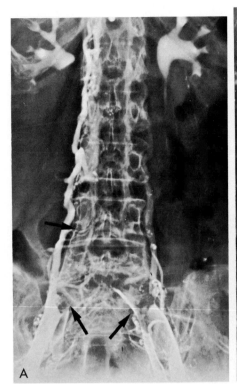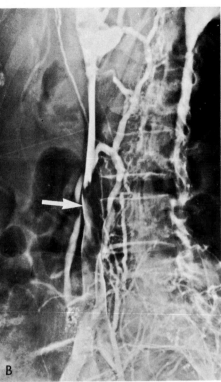

FIGURE 15–23. Thrombosis of the inferior vena cava. This patient with lymphoma was admitted with hemoptysis. During attempted pulmonary angiography, thrombosis of the inferior vena cava was identified. *A,* Shows large intraluminal thrombus in both common iliac veins and in the inferior vena cava (black arrows). There is filling of both right and left ascending lumbar veins and extensive paravertebral collaterals. *B,* Oblique view showing extent of thrombus (white arrow).

orrhagic complications, Dotter et al. proposed a "low-dose regimen"[94] with injection of the streptokinase intra-arterially through a catheter with the tip embedded in the clot. Concomitantly, renewed interest developed among cardiologists with the use of short-term (1.5 hour), high-dose intracoronary streptokinase for lysis of coronary thrombi.[95] Nonetheless, Dotter et al., in a group of 17 patients, described three in whom systemic lytic effects developed and two others in whom hemorrhagic complications occurred.[94] Hargrove et al.[96] reported their experience in 17 patients who underwent therapy with low-dose intra-arterial streptokinase for treatment of acute peripheral graft thromboses with doses of 5000 units/hour. They experienced five minor complications and one major one secondary to the fibrinolytic therapy. The five minor complications were hematomas of various sizes, and there was one major stroke. In addition, systemic fibrinolytic effects were noted in eight of nine patients in whom laboratory measurements were obtained. Subsequently, Becker et al.,[97] with 57 infusions in 50 patients, observed complete lysis of thrombus in 47 per cent. Major complications occurred in 15.7 per cent, with major bleeding occurring in 12 per cent of the infusions. Mori et al.,[98] in 50 infusions performed in 45 patients, obtained complete clot lysis in 44 per cent with a mean infusion duration of 37 hours. Major bleeding occurred in 8 per cent.

Hemorrhage, therefore, remains a serious hazard in low-dose streptokinase therapy (Fig. 15–25). Additional problems with low-dose therapy include sheathing of thrombus around the proximal portion of the catheter and distal embolization of thrombus fragments during fibrinolytic therapy. With low-dose local intraarterial fibrinolytic therapy, the catheter position must be checked at regular intervals to advance the catheter into the remaining clot. This requires repeated arteriography. At present, while using streptokinase or urokinase, there is no one laboratory test that reflects the degree of fibrinolytic therapy or the likelihood of hemorrhage.[99] However, bleeding is more likely to occur if the fibrinogen level is less than 100 mg/dl. There is a lack of correlation between embolus dissolution and changes in fibrinolytic assay and coagulation results. Because of the risk of hemorrhage and the lack of specific laboratory monitoring guidelines, contraindications to streptokinase therapy include recent ischemic CNS event, active bleeding, open wounds, coagulopathy, and recent operation (within 10 days). When heparin therapy is used concomitantly with streptokinase therapy or heparin therapy is instituted following the cessation of streptokinase infusions, extreme care should be taken and the thrombin time allowed to return to less than twice normal, or, preferably, reduced doses of heparin should be used initially. Bleeding is likely to occur

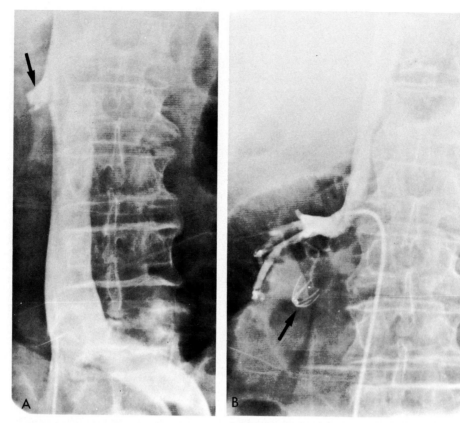

FIGURE 15–24. Misplaced Mobin-Uddin umbrella. *A,* Inferior venacavogram prior to umbrella placement shows reflux into right renal vein. Because of poor filling, the wash-in defect in the left renal vein is not identified. *B,* Selective right renal vein injection following placement of the Mobin-Uddin umbrella shows the umbrella (arrow) to reside outside the inferior vena cava. The umbrella is positioned in an aberrant double right renal vein. The point of entry into the inferior vena cava was not detected. Multiple renal veins occur more frequently on the right side.

from previous arterial puncture sites, and when lytic infusion is planned, the study should be performed from a single site of catheter entry. Results with low-dose urokinase infusions have not been markedly better than those with streptokinase.[100]

The role and dose of concomitant heparin therapy during low-dose fibrinolytic therapy is also undefined; however, its routine use with urokinase is recommended.

Allergic reactions to streptokinase may occur. Fever occurs in approximately one third of patients. The presence of antibodies to streptokinase may interfere with its action. Urokinase has not been shown to induce antibody formation, and fever occurs in only 2 to 3 per cent of patients.

Urokinase is three times more expensive than streptokinase. McNamara and Fischer[101] reported good success using a high-dose urokinase regimen starting with 4000 IU/min until lysis of a channel through the occlusion with reestablishment of antegrade flow has been accomplished, usually within 2 hours. The dose is then decreased to 1000 to 2000 IU/min until complete clot lysis has occurred. Intravenous heparin, 1000 IU/hr, is concomitantly administered and modified to maintain a partial thromboplastin time of 100

to 150 seconds. Of the 93 infusions in their series complete clot lysis occurred in 70 (75 per cent). Contrasting the cumulative average results of 155 previously reported standard low-dose streptokinase infusions with those obtained in McNamara and Fischer's 93 high-dose urokinase infusions, the high-dose urokinase regimen resulted in a higher incidence of complete clot lysis (75 per cent versus 45 per cent). A lower incidence of significant bleeding was observed (4 per cent versus 13 per cent) and the mean infusion time was shorter (18 versus 41 hours). However, longer durations of urokinase infusions, greater than 24 hours, are common. The advantages of the high-dose urokinase regime were believed to outweigh the lower cost of streptokinase. Of particular importance, there is a lower incidence of bleeding complications with urokinase.

Cragg et al.[102] recently compared high-dose and low-dose urokinase regimens in lysis of native arterial and graft occlusions. Their high-dose regimen was 250,000 IU/hr followed by 125,000 IU/hr and the low-dose was 50,000 IU/hr. The mean time to lysis was 20.8, 26.0, 16.5, and 18.2 hours for their high-dose artery, low-dose artery, high-dose graft, and low-dose graft, respectively. Respective mean infusion

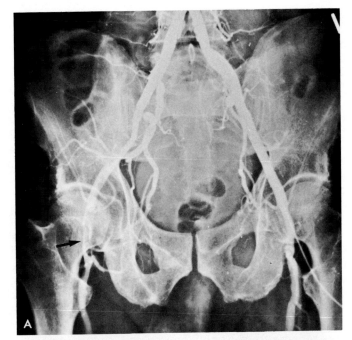

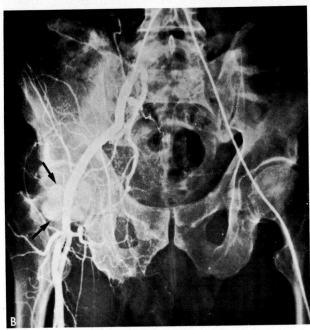

FIGURE 15–25.   Low-dose streptokinase infusion therapy. *A*, Shortly after cardiac catheterization, this patient developed claudication of the right lower extremity. A left transfemoral pelvic arteriogram shows narrowing of the right external iliac artery and intraluminal thrombus in the common femoral artery (arrow). The right superficial femoral artery was occluded. He was treated with low-dose intraarterial streptokinase for lysis of the clot for 24 hours. *B*, Following streptokinase, a selective right common iliac artery injection shows normal caliber of the external iliac artery, lysis of the thrombus in the common femoral artery, and filling of the superficial femoral artery. There is, however, also a new false aneurysm (arrows), which developed as a result of clot lysis at the previous heart catheterization site.

durations were 27.1, 35.4, 22.2, and 25.3 hours. No significant differences were noted between the high-dose and low-dose groups. Clinical success was achieved in 65 to 85 per cent of cases. The major drawback with the use of streptokinase and urokinase relates to the development of systemic effects, because the fibrinolytic agents act not only on plasminogen within the clot, but also on plasminogen throughout the circulation.

Tissue-type plasminogen activator (t-PA) is a serine protease present in most body tissues[103] and similar to the plasminogen activator produced by human vascular endothelial cells.[104] t-PA has a low affinity for circulating plasminogen, but a high affinity for fibrin. In the presence of thrombus, both t-PA and plasminogen bind to the fibrin on the surface of the clot. The proteolytic capacity of t-PA increases dramatically in the fibrin domain and fibrin-bound t-PA activates the conversion of fibrin-bound plasminogen to plasmin, which lyses the thrombus. Because plasmin production is confined primarily to the site of the clot, there is less derangement of systemic coagulation than that seen with urokinase or streptokinase. Any plasmin that enters the circulation is inactivated by α_2-antiplasmin. t-PA circulating in the blood has a low affinity for circulating plasminogen,[105] and therefore plasmin is not formed in the circulation. The half-life of t-PA in the circulation is 5 minutes. There is evidence that the fibrinolytic activity at the site of a thrombus may continue for several hours after administration is completed.[106] The currently used t-PA is produced by recombinant DNA techniques (rt-PA). Two-chain and one-chain configurations are available. Currently available rt-PA (manufacturing process G11035) is predominantly single chain but is likely converted in vivo to the two-chain form by the action of plasmin. The circulating half-life of single-chain rt-PA is on the order of 4 minutes. The contraindications to its use are similar to those of the other thrombolytic agents.

Experience with the use of rt-PA in the treatment of peripheral vascular disease is limited. Risius et al.[107] used rt-PA at a dose of 0.1 mg/kg/hr for 1 to 6 hours in 25 patients with lower extremity thromboembolic occlusions (13 thrombosed arteries, 12 thrombosed bypass grafts). The infusion catheter was inserted directly into the thrombus. Thrombolysis occurred is 23 of 25 patients (92 per cent), with time to lysis ranging from 1 to 6.5 hours (average lysis time of 3.6 hours). In 15 of 25 patients fibrinogen levels were maintained above 50 per cent of baseline. No major complications directly attributable to rt-PA infusions occurred. rt-PA infusions resulted in decreases in plasma fibrinogen, plasminogen, and α_2-antiplasmin levels and in increased plasma levels of fibrin split products. In general longer infusion times (i.e., higher total dose) resulted in a greater decrease in the aforementioned levels. The decreases noted in plasma fibrinogen, plasminogen, and α_2-antiplasmin levels indicated that a systemic lytic state does occur and is associated with varying degrees of fibrinolysis. Whether fibrinogen breakdown was a function of infusion duration or total dose infused, or both, could not be determined. Verstraete et al.[108] demonstrated that as infusion durations increase α_2-antiplasmin will be consumed and systemic fibrinogenolysis will occur. In addition, they demonstrated that a large dose infused over a short period of time results in less systemic lytic activity than a small dose infused over a long period of time.[108] Further investigation is necessary to determine if higher doses will produce more rapid thrombolysis and decrease infusion time and therefore spare fibrinogen. The current experience suggests that the fibrin specificity of rt-PA is relative. With longer infusion times, this fibrin specificity can be overcome and fibrinogenolysis can occur. Nonetheless, the rt-PA exerts less of a systemic effect than does streptokinase or urokinase.

Newer thrombolytic agents are also under development. One of these, single-chain urokinase (prourokinase), in animal studies showed greater clot selectivity than urokinase and caused only minimal fibrinogen breakdown.[109] Whether this new agent constitutes an important relatively clot-selective thrombolytic agent remains to be determined.

TRANSLUMINAL CATHETER RETRIEVAL OF FOREIGN BODIES FROM THE VASCULAR SYSTEM

The majority of foreign bodies removed from the vascular system have been retrieved from the venous system, right heart chambers, or pulmonary arteries.[110] The items most frequently retrieved are catheter fragments, broken off guidewires, and pacing catheters. From the arterial system, items removed are guidewire fragments and, more recently, Gianturco-Wallace coil occluders.[111]

Foreign body retrieval using catheter technique requires fluoroscopy and is usually accomplished through a percutaneous puncture or cutdown.[112] A sheath may sometimes be employed. Several different types of devices may be used: loop snare catheters,[113] basket retrievers,[114] hook-tip catheters,[115] or grasping forceps,[116,117] and more recently the Amplatz nitinol gooseneck snare.[118] Loop snare catheters (catheters through which a double length of guidewire is passed to make a loop) and wire catch baskets similar to Dormia baskets are the most widely used retrieval instruments. The nitinol gooseneck snare is the easiest to use. Bronchoscopic grasping forceps are of limited use owing to their lack of flexibility.[117] They usually require a cutdown to the vessel. Balloon catheters may be used percutaneously to remove items from blood vessels.[190] The removal of foreign bodies utilizing transcatheter techniques is associated with a very low complication rate and presents far less hazard than surgical removal of these items.[120]

PERCUTANEOUS TRANSLUMINAL ANGIOPLASTY

Percutaneous transluminal angioplasty (PTA) is a technique in which specially constructed catheters equipped with a balloon in their distal shaft are passed percutaneously to an area of vessel stenosis. When the catheter has been positioned at the level of stenosis, the catheter is inflated and the stenotic area dilated. The most widely used catheters are those designed by Gruntzig.[121,122] Early attempts at vessel dilation date to the mid-1960s when Dotter introduced coaxial catheters for angioplasty.[123] This system involved the passage of coaxial catheters of progressively increasing size across a stenotic area. This technique met with mixed success. This was followed by development of caged balloon catheters.[124,125] These were associated, however, with a high failure rate. The van Andel catheter, which involves the use of dilators of increasing diameter, is still used in situations in which the balloon catheters are not suitable.[126] Other balloon catheter designs are presently under development.[127] The presently available Gruntzig balloon catheters are made in various sizes. In performing angioplasty, pressure is measured on entry to the artery. The guidewire is manipulated across the lesion. A small French-sized catheter is then advanced over the guidewire across the obstruction. The wire is removed and the catheter position verified with injection of contrast. Repeat pressure recordings are then made unless the catheter obstructs the narrowed lumen. The guidewire is reintroduced and the small French-sized cathether exchanged for a balloon catheter. When the balloon is placed across the lesion, it is inflated. Postdilation pressures are recorded to evaluate for residual gradient.

Based on experimental studies, Castaneda-Zuniga et al.[128] proposed a theory for the mechanism of angioplasty. During balloon dilation, the atherosclerotic intima is ruptured and partially dehisced. This frees the media from the restraint of the atherosclerotic intima, allowing it to become overstretched with damage to the elastic properties of its elastic collagen and muscle fibers. The increased blood flow through the lesion keeps the media distended as it heals by collagen deposition. This rupture of the media results in permanent widening of the arteries.

Gruntzig balloon dilation has been used successfully in the dilation of renal arteries, the abdominal aorta, iliac arteries, and superficial femoral and profunda femoral arteries (Fig. 15–26). Improved balloon technology has allowed dilation of infrapopliteal vessels. The long-term results of PTA are still under analysis.

In PTA of the iliac arteries, the primary success rate (i.e., ability to cross the lesion and perform dilatation) is approximately 93 to 95 per cent.[129,130] Iliac PTA is best applied in patients with a short focal stenosis of the iliac arteries. It is generally not recommended for patients with diffuse iliac disease unless they are poor surgical candidates. PTA alone is also not recommended in totally occluded iliac arteries because of the high incidence of complications.[130,131] Table 15–1 summarizes the results of long-term follow-up with iliac artery PTA.

Complication rates with iliac PTA range from 2 to 4 per cent.[133,135] When compared to surgical results, Malone et al.[140] reported an immediate patency rate for aortoiliac reconstruction of 99.2 per cent for aortofemoral grafts, with a 4 per cent thrombosis rate each subsequent year. The 5-year patency rate for aortoiliac reconstruction is 91 per cent.[63] Several series have now shown that the long-term results with iliac PTA are comparable to those achieved with reconstructive surgery.[129–131,133] On the basis of these findings iliac angioplasty may be considered the sole treatment modality for limb ischemia caused by an isolated iliac lesion or for treatment of an iliac lesion prior to distal bypass surgery.[129,133]

PTA of the femoropopliteal arteries has a primary success rate of approximately 84 per cent,[122,130,141] which is lower than iliac PTA. The incidence of significant complications ranges from 4 to 6 per cent.[130,141]

The long-term patency rates after femoropopliteal PTA are summarized in Table 15–2. Johnston et al.[139] noted a lower cumulative patency rate. However, their criteria for success were excessively strict and

not always indicative of the status of the dilated segment. Multiple factors affect the outcome of PTA of the femoropopliteal arteries. Experience of the radiologist and catheter configuration have been shown to be important.[141] The success rate with femoropopliteal PTA varies with the site[141] and length of the lesion.[130,141] The success rate is higher in distal superficial femoral artery (SFA) lesions. Krepel et al.[141] obtained a success rate of 97 per cent in SFA lesions less than 3 cm long, compared to 26 per cent in lesions longer than 3 cm.

In long lesions of the femoropopliteal vessels, therefore, PTA is not recommended. The long-term results following PTA are better if the lesions are short and concentric and have a regular appearance. Results are also better when the postangioplasty morphology is near normal and the runoff is at least fair.[141]

In comparison with femoropopliteal bypass surgery, Naji et al.[147] and Mehta[148] reported a 3-year patency rate of 79.5 per cent and 77 per cent, respectively, in patients who underwent bypass surgery for claudication. In patients undergoing bypass surgery for limb salvage the 3-year patency rates were 54.1 per cent[142] and 68 per cent.[148] Spence et al.[130] contrasted these results with PTA, in which they observed a 73 per cent patency rate at 3 years in patients undergoing PTA for claudication and a 2-year patency rate of 76.1 per cent in patients undergoing PTA for limb salvage. Veith et al.[149] in their large series obtained a 66 per cent cumulative life-table limb salvage rate at 6 years for all patients having femoropopliteal-tibial artery reconstructive operations. The subset undergoing a femoropopliteal artery bypass showed a 73 per cent 6-year cumulative life-table analysis limb salvage rate.

Taylor et al.,[150] in a series of 231 patients undergoing femoropopliteal bypass, reported an operative mortality of 1.4 per cent. Thirty-one per cent underwent bypass for claudication, and 64 per cent for limb-threatening ischemia. The overall primary graft patency for all femoropopliteal grafts was 79 per cent at 5 years. The 5-year patency rate for saphenous vein bypass grafts was 85 per cent, and the 5-year patency for bypass grafts other than saphenous vein was 73 per cent. Patients undergoing a repeat bypass after a prior failed bypass had a patency rate of only 57 per cent.

The mortality and morbidity from PTA are less than the 4 per cent average mortality reported for the femoropopliteal surgery.[148] Although additional studies describing the long-term results of femoropopliteal PTA are required, the currently available long-term results in appropriately selected patients are encouraging (Table 15–2).

Experience with PTA of the infrapopliteal arteries has lagged behind that of PTA of the iliac and femoropopliteal vessels. PTA of these vessels has been considered a high-risk procedure because occlusion of a distal peripheral leg vessel might result in amputation or preclude a bypass operation. The balloon

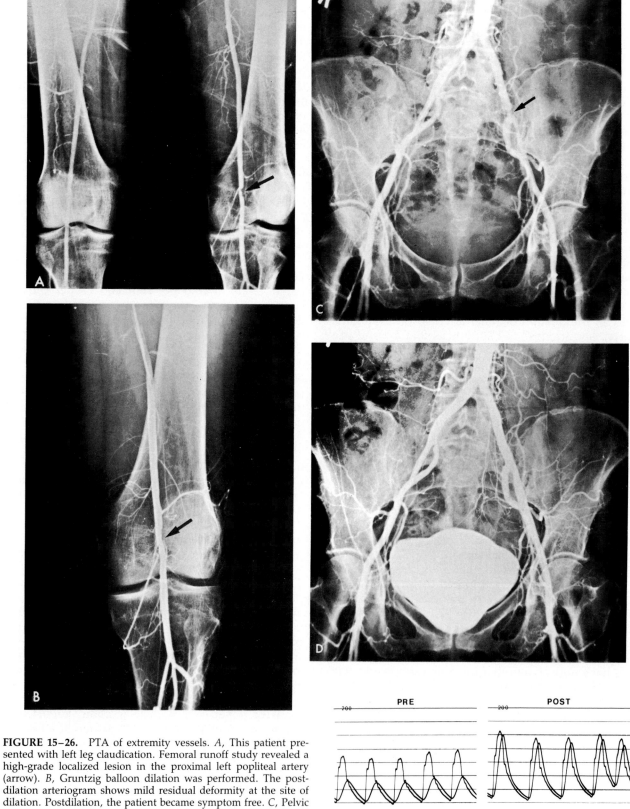

FIGURE 15–26. PTA of extremity vessels. *A,* This patient presented with left leg claudication. Femoral runoff study revealed a high-grade localized lesion in the proximal left popliteal artery (arrow). *B,* Gruntzig balloon dilation was performed. The postdilation arteriogram shows mild residual deformity at the site of dilation. Postdilation, the patient became symptom free. *C,* Pelvic arteriogram in another patient (same patient as in Fig. 15–2) shows a localized left common iliac artery stenosis (arrow). *D,* Post-PTA the stenosis is relieved. *E,* Pressure tracings measured across the iliac lesion, before and after dilation, show abolition of the gradient post-PTA.

TABLE 15–1.   ILIAC ANGIOPLASTY: RESULTS[a]

References	Published Date	No. of PTAs	Recurrences (%)	Long-Term Patency Rate (%)	Follow-up Period (mo)	Contains Life Table	Test
Gruntzig[132]	1977	36	17	83	24	yes	c
Van Andel[133]	1980	51	4	92	8–65	no	c
Spence et al.[130]	1981	148	13[b]	79	30	yes	d
Schneider et al.[134]	1982	186	12	85	60	yes	c
Johnston et al.[135]	1982	186	—	66	30	yes	
Gallino et al.[136]	1982	50	—	87	48	yes	c
Kumpe and Jones[137]	1982	65	—	82	36	yes	c
Kadir et al.[131]	1983	185	8	89	36	yes	e
Schwarten[138]	1984	58	9	89	24	no	f
Van Andel et al.[126]	1985	185	7	90	84	yes	c
Johnston et al.[139]	1987	376	—	60	60	yes	c

[a]Adapted from Van Andel GJ, Van Erp WFM, Krepel VM, Breslau PJ: Percutaneous transluminal dilation of the iliac artery: Long-term results. Radiology 156:321–323, 1985.
[b]Successfully redilated restenoses were not considered failures.
[c]At least anamnesis, physical examination, and ankle-arm index.
[d]Pulse volume recordings when indicated.
[e]Ankle-arm index in two thirds of the patients.
[f]Ankle-arm index in combination with digital subtraction angiography.

catheters initially available for PTA were not suitable for dilation of these small distal vessels. The development of small, coaxial, low-profile balloon catheters and small, atraumatic, steerable guidewires, as well as the use of pharmacologic agents such as nifedipine, nitroglycerin, and thrombolytic agents when necessary in addition to heparin are responsible for the favorable results now achievable with PTA of the infrapopliteal vessels. Also important is the use of digital arteriography, which allows rapid visualization of the runoff vessels.[152] Results of several large series are now available.[153–155] Primary success rates range from 86 to 97 per cent. Schwarten et al.,[153] in a series of 98 patients with infrapopliteal stenoses or occlusions 5 cm or less in length, reported a 1-year limb salvage rate of 89 per cent and a 2-year (37 limbs)

limbs) limb salvage rate of 86 per cent. Horvath et al.,[155] in a series of 71 patients (103 stenosed crural vessels), utilized both PTA and laser angioplasty. With life-table analysis for single-vessel runoff they obtained a cumulative patency rate of 92.5 per cent after 6 months ($n = 45$), 79.8 per cent after 1 year ($n = 27$), and 64.6 per cent after 3 years ($n = 3$). Complications have been low. Prompt clinical improvement following infrapopliteal PTA has been noted in patients in whom angioplasty restored straight line flow to the foot via at least one calf vessel narrowed by no more than 75 per cent of its diameter.[154] The success in these series demonstrates a role for infrapopliteal PTA in appropriately selected patients. These results compare favorably with surgical results at 3 years.

TABLE 15–2.   LONG-TERM RESULTS OF FEMOROPOPLITEAL ANGIOPLASTY[a]

References	Published Date	No. of PTAs	Recurrences	Patent Arteries/Follow-up Period (yr)[b] 2	3	4	5	7	Test
Gruntzig[132]	1977	184	27	65(78)[d]	—	—	—	—	e
Greenfield[142]	1980	70	6	84	—	—	—	—	e
Spence et al.[130]	1981	122	20[c]	75	70	—	—	—	f
Frieman et al.[143]	1981	88	—	67	—	—	—	—	e
Kumpe and Jones[137]	1982	50	—	56	—	—	—	—	e
Schneider et al.[134]	1982	682	162	70	—	—	68	—	e
Gallino et al.[136]	1982	200	—	62(71)[d]	—	69	—	—	e
Colapinto[144]	1983	112	—	58	55	—	—	—	e
Berkowitz et al.[145]	1983	110	30	67	63	—	—	—	e
Mahler et al.[146]	1983	252	—	71	—	—	—	—	e
Krepel et al.[141]	1985	164	38	77	70	70	70	60	e
Johnston et al.[139]	1987	253	—	53	50	44	40	—	e

[a]Adapted from Krepel VM, Van Andel GJ, Van Erp WFM, Breslau PJ: Percutaneous transluminal angioplasty of femoropopliteal artery: Initial and long-term results. Radiology 156:325–328, 1985.
[b]All results analyzed by life-table method.
[c]Successfully redilated recurrent stenoses were not considered failures.
[d]Second number is patency rate without "partial" recurrences.
[e]At least anamnesis, physical examination, and ankle-arm index.
[f]Pulse volume recordings when indicated.

The life-table primary patency rates for isolated popliteal or infrapopliteal runoff vessel surgical by-pass grafts range from 59 to 69 per cent,[149,156–158] with lower rates seen with prosthetic graft material.[156] Cumulative life-table limb salvage rates reported are 51 per cent,[149] 61 per cent,[156] and 82 per cent.[155] These results are obtained in the presence of 5-year patient survival rates ranging from 35 to 44 per cent.[156,158]

The length of hospitalization, patient costs, and discomfort are significantly less with PTA than with reconstructive surgery. The ease of dilation and the opportunity for repeat dilation are additional advantages. The performance of PTA in aortoiliac or femoropopliteal vessels does not preclude later operation. In patients with iliac disease PTA can be used in conjunction with distal surgery. There is no risk to pelvic autonomic nerves, or male sexual functioning. It can be used in obese patients and allows preservation of the saphenous vein for later cardiac or peripheral artery bypass surgery. PTA can also be used to treat inflow or outflow stenoses in patients with failing grafts.[151] Percutaneous balloon angioplasty has also been used in the treatment of venous stenoses in the subclavian veins, the inferior vena cava, and in stenosis in dialysis fistulas.

Presently available data indicate PTA has an important role in the management of patients with peripheral vascular disease.

LASER-ASSISTED BALLOON ANGIOPLASTY

Balloon angioplasty requires crossing of the vessel stenosis with a guidewire over which the balloon catheter can then be passed. In complete vascular occlusions, particularly long-segment ones, the guidewire cannot be passed and balloon angioplasty is not possible. This problem has stimulated the development of other techniques such as laser-assisted balloon angioplasty. In laser-assisted percutaneous balloon angioplasty, laser energy is used to produce a channel that can then be crossed with the guidewire. Laser light is both collimated and coherent. From the laser power source it can be transmitted over a distance through an optical fiber and focused to a highly intense light spot, allowing the focal removal of tissue. Because the channel produced by the current lasing systems is small, in most instances the laser-created channel is widened using balloon angioplasty.

A variety of laser catheters and laser sources are currently being used for peripheral percutaneous assisted balloon angioplasty. Laser sources which have been used include neodymium: yttrium-aluminum-garnet (Nd:YAG), argon, excimer, and tunable dye. Other potential sources exist. A variety of catheter designs are also being tested. Some are commercially available, others experimental.

The earliest experiments described the use of a laser source and an unmodified 600-nm optical fiber. This resulted in a high incidence of perforation and vessel spasm.[159] Attempts to minimize perforation and create larger channels led to the development of "hot tip" systems—those in which a metallic cap is applied to the tip of an optical fiber. The hot tip systems rely on mechanical tissue contact by the probe and a thermal mechanism of tissue removal (Trimedyne, Santa Ana, CA). When the fiber tip is capped there is no direct light beam exposure and, therefore, no selective absorption of argon laser wavelengths by plaque tissue.[160] Rather, the laser energy is converted to thermal energy in the metal alloy tip. The atheromatous tissue is ablated by heat radiated from the fiber tip and by the mechanical force exerted on the fiber. Argon laser energy in the aforementioned system generates catheter temperatures in the range of 130° to 400°C depending on local tissue environment. Nd:YAG laser energy has also been employed to heat the metal tip at the end of the laser probe.

Another laser source is 308-nm wavelength excimer laser energy. This laser energy is capable of vaporizing even densely calcified material such as bone. In contrast to thermal recanalization, the excimer ablates by photochemical mechanisms.[161] Ultraviolet photons possess sufficient energy to break organic bonds directly, producing photochemical desorption of constituent products.[162] This process occurs with minimal heat generation and is not dependent upon tissue water.

Although a variety of laser energy sources are available, the guidance of the laser probe through the occluded segment of vessel is a problem. If the laser probe passes subintimally into the vessel wall, dissection or perforation may occur. Perforation with a small laser probe has been reported without major significant sequelae, but passage of a balloon catheter through the same channel may lead to vessel damage and limit long-term patency.

In attempting to overcome this limitation, one laser-catheter device being tested utilizes an argon laser source that is transmitted through a 200-μ optical fiber that contains a diverting lens at its distal end to increase the diameter of the area of ablation. Directional control is enhanced by the presence of an attached centering/dilation balloon (LASTAC System, GV Medical Inc., Minneapolis, MN). A more promising approach is a laser system that has both a diagnostic laser and a treatment laser (smart laser, MCM Laboratories, Mountain View, CA). It utilizes computerized plaque detection and targeting as a feedback mechanism to reduce the risk of vessel perforation. Light from the diagnostic laser is transmitted through the optical fiber and emitted from the distal tip. This light excites fluorophores in the target tissue, resulting in fluorescent light that is transmitted back through the same optical fiber to the computerized detector, where it is analyzed, and a spectral curve is produced. If fluorescence characteristic of plaque or thrombus is found, the treatment laser is triggered and sends high-energy light down the optical fiber to ablate the diseased area. Clinical trials with this laser are underway.

Several authors have reported early results of laser therapy. Sanborn et al.[163] described 1-year follow-up results with the hot tip laser in 129 femoropopliteal lesions in 112 patients. They reported initial angiographic and clinical success in 99/127 (77 per cent) of femoropopliteal stenoses and occlusions: 21 of 22 (95 per cent) stenoses; 17 of 17 (100 per cent) short (1- to 3-cm) occlusions; 26 of 37 (70 per cent) medium-length (4- to 7-cm) occlusions; and 35 of 53 (66 per cent) long (greater than 7 cm) occlusions. There was a 4 per cent frequency of vessel perforation without clinical sequelae. The 1-year cumulative clinical patency was 77 per cent for the 99 lesions with an initial clinical success. In the 21 stenoses and 17 short occlusions, the cumulative clinical patency rates were 95 per cent and 93 per cent, respectively. In the longer occlusions (4 to 7 cm and greater than 7 cm), the clinical patency rates were 76 per cent and 58 per cent, respectively.

Similar results were obtained in a recent multicenter review of 602 cases of thermal laser-assisted balloon angioplasty with follow-up to 30 months (mean: 11.3 months). Two hundred ninety-two laser-assisted balloon angioplasties were performed for severe multifocal stenotic disease: 258 for complete occlusion, and 52 for both superficial femoral artery stenosis and occlusion. Overall, 60 per cent of initially successful procedures have remained patent, but long segment occlusions greater than 7 cm have fared poorly, with only a 25 per cent patency at 30 months.[164]

Experience with percutaneous excimer laser and excimer laser–assisted angioplasty of the lower extremities is less. However, early experience has been reported.[165] In a series of 30 patients, 28 of whom underwent laser-assisted balloon angioplasty and two of whom underwent excimer laser angioplasty alone, acute angiographic success was obtained in 24 of 31 (77 per cent) femoropopliteal stenoses and occlusions. Seven of nine (78 per cent) stenoses, six of seven (86 per cent) short (0- to 5-cm) occlusions, seven of eight (88 per cent) medium-length (6- to 10-cm) occlusions, three of four (75 per cent) long (11- to 15-cm) occlusions, and one of three (33 per cent) extreme (greater than 15 cm) occlusions were successfully treated. Inability to treat total occlusions was in each case related to inability to remain intraluminal, with consequent subintimal passage of the catheter. At a mean follow-up of 9.1 ± 3.5 months (range of 1 to 52 weeks) a restenosis rate of 29 per cent (7 of 24 patients) was observed. Three of the severe successfully treated stenotic lesions had restenosed, as did 4 of the 18 successfully treated occlusions. Of the four restenotic lesions in the original occlusion group, none was totally occlusive at the time of follow-up, and all were successfully dilated with subsequent standard balloon technique. The long-term results with 308-nm excimer laser balloon angioplasty are pending, as are long-term results with the tunable dye laser.

Currently, the long-term results of laser-assisted balloon angioplasty are unknown. It is not known at this time whether long-term patency of occluded vessel segments will be maintained following laser-assisted angioplasty. Technology is evolving, and a major question is whether the use of laser catheters that produce a larger channel will result in improved patency.

RENAL ARTERY PTA

PTA has been demonstrated to be effective in the management of renovascular hypertension due to atherosclerotic disease and to fibromuscular dysplasia.

PTA in Renal Artery Stenosis due to Atherosclerotic Disease

Sos et al.[166] described a group of 89 patients undergoing PTA. Fifty-one had atherosclerotic lesions (30 unilateral disease, and 21 bilateral disease). Follow-up extended from 4 to 40 months, with a mean of 16 months. In these patients, angioplasty was technically successful in 57 per cent of those with unilateral lesions, and in only 9.5 per cent of those with bilateral disease. Failure was primarily due to the anatomy of the lesion, with a success rate in unilateral disease of only 20 per cent (2/10) if the vessel was completely occluded or if the lesion was located at the ostium. The success rate with nonosteal, nonoccluded lesions was 75 per cent. Eighty-two per cent of patients with unilateral disease who were successfully dilated were cured or improved. Successful dilation in two patients with bilateral atheromatous disease resulted in cure.

In patients with advanced bilateral renal artery stenoses, angioplasty is rarely curative, undoubtedly because of the presence of underlying nephrosclerosis or atrophic kidneys.

PTA in Fibromuscular Disease

PTA has been demonstrated to be effective in the management of renovascular hypertension due to fibromuscular dysplasia (FMD). The success rates with PTA for FMD[167–169] with follow-up to 3 years equal the success rates of bypass surgery for FMD.[170–172] Furthermore, the morbidity, expense, length of hospital stay, and recuperation after PTA are significantly less than those of operation. Recurrence can be treated with repeat PTA, whereas reoperation after failure of bypass surgery usually necessitates nephrectomy.[170] Long-term results with percutaneous transluminal angioplasty of renal artery stenosis due to fibromuscular dysplasia have recently been reported by Tegtmeyer et al.[173] In a series of 66 patients with 85 renal artery stenoses due to fibromuscular dysplasia followed for as long as 121 months, 26 patients were cured (39 per cent), 39 (59 per cent) were improved, and one did not respond to PTA. Cumulative patency rate predicted for 10 years was 87.1 per cent.[173] As a result, PTA is the preferred initial treatment for FMD at many centers (Fig. 15–27).[167–169,173]

The complications of PTA of renal arteries include renal artery dissection, occlusion, perforation, renal infarction, hematoma, or acute tubular necrosis. In

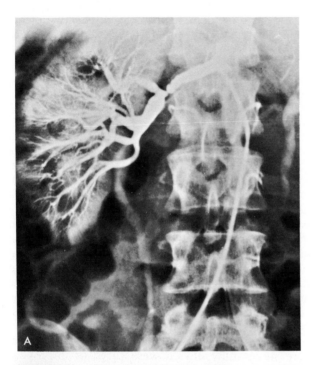

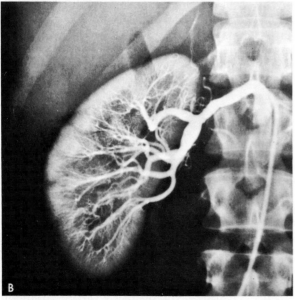

FIGURE 15–27. PTA of renal artery. *A,* Baseline arteriogram in this young hypertensive female shows typical string-of beads appearance of fibromuscular disease. *B,* Post-Gruntzig balloon dilation arteriogram shows relief of stenosis. This patient is now normotensive.

large series, the overall complication rate of PTA varies from 5.7 per cent[167] to 12.5 per cent.[168] Overall surgical results show benefit rates of 74 to 97 per cent,[170,174] with cure or improvement of hypertension expected in more than 90 per cent of young patients, particularly those with fibromuscular disease or focal atherosclerotic lesions. The similar results of surgery and angioplasty have led to the conclusion that angioplasty is the treatment of choice for uncomplicated fibromuscular disease and nonosteal unilateral atheromatous disease of the renal arteries.[163]

ANGIOGRAPHIC EMBOLIZATION THERAPY

Transcatheter embolization therapy involves the delivery of occluding agents through catheters selectively positioned in vessels. A wide variety of embolic agents are used. Some are permanent mechanical occluders, such as the Gianturco-Wallace coils,[175] detachable balloons,[176] Ivalon particles,[177] silicone,[178] and bucrylate tissue adhesives.[179] Other agents, such as autologous clot and Gelfoam, are embolic agents that are slowly absorbed by the body over a variable period of time.

A major application of embolization therapy is in the treatment of congenital arteriovenous malformations (AVMs). Congenital AVMs are difficult management problems. Surgery is of limited value,[181] being most useful in those situations in which the AVM can be totally excised. Partial removal with ligation of feeders has been shown to be ineffective owing to regrowth of collateral vessels. In those AVMs that cannot be treated by surgical excision or that require amputation, embolization therapy is a useful palliative technique.[182–184] Baseline selective arteriography should be performed in all patients with suspected congenital AVMs prior to operative or embolization therapy. Arteriography is necessary to delineate the type and extent of the AVM. These lesions are usually more extensive than suspected.

It is important that the interstices of the AVM be occluded and that the embolic agent reach the center of the AVM. Occlusion of the feeding arteries without ablation of the central portion of the AVM is equivalent to ligation of feeding vessels, which has been found to be of little use.

Permanent embolic agents are recommended for occlusion of congenital AVMs. More recently, in situations in which the AVM nidus cannot be reached directly owing to previous surgical ligation, direct percutaneous puncture of the AVM can be performed, and, using fluoroscopic guidance, the embolic agent is delivered directly into the AVM.

Most patients manifest a systemic response to embolization therapy for several days, characterized by pain, fever, and elevated muscle enzymes. Clinical symptoms respond to supportive therapy. Risks of the procedure include inadvertent distal reflux of particulate or liquid embolic agents or misplacement of the mechanical occluders, with resultant occlusion of inappropriate vessels. These mishaps may necessitate urgent operative embolectomy. Minor complications that have been reported are transient or permanent nerve injury or small areas of skin slough. With proper technique, however, the benefits of the procedure outweigh the risks, and embolization therapy may permit limb salvage. It is an effective palliative therapy, and, should new collateral feeders develop, they can be embolized.[182–184]

Transcatheter embolization is also useful in the treatment of hemorrhage. Embolization therapy has been used successfully in the control of bleeding from bronchial arteries,[185] renal bleeding,[186] splenic bleeding,[56] and gastrointestinal bleeding originating in the stomach. Massive pelvic hemorrhage following trauma or surgery or as a complication of genitourinary tumors can be effectively treated with embolic techniques. Experience has shown that any or all of the branches of the internal iliac artery can be occluded without great risk.[187,188] Embolization therapy can be performed at the time of diagnostic arteriography.

INFERIOR VENA CAVA FILTERS

The value of inferior vena cava filter placement for prophylaxis against pulmonary embolism has been recognized for many years. Initially, filter placement required a cutdown of the internal jugular vein, but in 1984 percutaneous transjugular and transfemoral placement of the Greenfield filter was described.[189] Currently, a variety of caval filters are available. In addition to improving functional performance of the filter and clot-trapping capability of the filters, an emphasis has been placed by manufacturers on the development of smaller sized introduction systems more suitable for percutaneous placement. Currently approved filters include the Greenfield stainless steel filter, the Bird's Nest and Modified Filter, the Titanium Greenfield filter, the Vena Tech filter, and the Simon nitinol filter.

The Greenfield filter has had the longest availability. It requires a large 24-Fr introducer system with a maximal diameter of 30 mm (recommended for IVC sizes of 28 mm).[190] The Greenfield filter has a reported recurrent embolism rate of 5 per cent[191,192] and a vena cava occlusion rate of 3 to 5 per cent.[191,193–196] Optimal filtration of caval blood flow results with angles less than 15 degree tilt from the vertical. The large 24-Fr size of the stainless steel Greenfield filter is a disadvantage, and there is a 10 to 24 per cent prevalence of sonographically identified femoral vein thrombus.[197] The Titanium Greenfield filter (Medi-tech, Watertown, MA) is a significantly modified design of the stainless steel Greenfield filter, which was modified to provide a smaller introduction size for percutaneous insertion. It can be delivered in a 12-Fr carrier. It has a broader base (38 mm versus 30 mm) and is recommended for caval diameters up to but not exceeding 28 mm. Initially, its use was associated with a high frequency of

vena caval perforation, but this problem has been corrected.[198]

The Bird's Nest and Modified Filter (Cook, Bloomington, IN) first tested in 1982 has the advantage of a small 12-Fr sheath size. It consists of a series of preshaped wires that assume a mesh configuration resembling a bird's nest.[199] The rate of recurrent pulmonary embolism is reported at 2.7 per cent and the rate of caval occlusion 2.9 per cent. Follow-up, however, has been largely clinical. The actual incidence of vena caval occlusion is unknown, but in a subset of 40 patients who underwent radiologic follow-up, caval occlusion was documented in 19 per cent. Because of its large size, it can be inserted in vena cavae up to 40 mm in diameter. The Vena-Tech Filter (L. G. Medical, Chasseneuil, France) is the Food and Drug Administration (FDA)–approved version of the LGM filter. Clinical follow-up shows a recurrent pulmonary embolism rate of 2 per cent, and vena caval occlusion rate of 7 per cent in 1-year follow-up.

The Simon nitinol filter (Nitinol Medical Technologies, Woburn, MA) is composed of thermal memory alloy composed of nickel and titanium. The filter wires are in straightened form at cooled temperatures (4° to 10°C) and reform to filter configuration at body temperatures.[201] The device is inserted through a 9-Fr outer sheath, and can be delivered via a transfemoral or transjugular route. Multicenter clinical trials show a symptomatic recurrent pulmonary embolism rate of 1.1 per cent and an asymptomatic pulmonary embolism rate of 0.7 per cent diagnosed by ventilation perfusion lung scan or pulmonary angiogram. The vena caval occlusion rate is 7.8 per cent (symptomatic) and 1.9 per cent (asymptomatic).[202]

The major indications for filter placement in venous thromboembolism are: (1) contraindication to anticoagulation, (2) failure of adequate anticoagulation, and (3) prophylactic placement in selected high-risk patients.

Controversy surrounds the use of prophylactic filters. Most agree that prophylactic filter placement is reasonable in patients who develop iliofemoral thrombosis while on adequate anticoagulation and in patients who have long free-floating femoral or iliac vein thrombi. Prophylaxis in other high-risk patients is the subject of much dispute. The longevity of these newer filters is not clearly known, and this should be taken into consideration when they are placed in young patients.[202]

VASCULAR STENTS

Several intraluminal vascular stents are currently in use. Currently, the two most frequently used intravascular stents are the Palmaz stent (Johnson & Johnson Interventional Systems, Warren, NJ) and the Wallstent (Medinvent, Lausanne, Switzerland; Schneider, Minneapolis, MN).

The Palmaz stent consists of a slotted, seamless, stainless steel tube of varying diameters mounted on an angioplasty balloon. The Wallstent consists of surgical grade stainless steel alloy filaments woven to form a tubular braid. It is constrained on a special delivery catheter by a membrane that is retracted during delivery. Unlike the Palmaz stent, the catheter is flexible and adapts to vessel curvature. Both stents are currently used intravascularly as an adjunct to percutaneous balloon angioplasty in cases in which relief of stenosis has not been achieved, the stenosis has recurred, or when a spontaneous or postcatheter dissection has occurred. The majority of the vascular experience has been with the deployment of stents in the iliac arteries.

Palmaz et al.[203] reported their results with 171 iliac artery stent procedures in 154 patients using the Palmaz stent. Of the 261 stents placed, 181 were placed in the iliac arteries and 80 in the external iliac arteries. Complications occurred in 18 patients (11.7 per cent). At follow-up (average: 6 months; range: 1 to 24 months) 137 patients demonstrated clinical benefit, 113 had become asymptomatic, 11 had no benefit, and 6 improved initially, but later developed new symptoms. Long-term follow-up continues.

Zollikofer et al.[204] recently reported midterm results with Wallstent placement in 31 patients. Twenty-six iliac and 15 femoropopliteal complex stenoses or occlusions with inadequate response to percutaneous transluminal angioplasty were treated. In the iliac artery group, 96 per cent of the stents were patent at a mean follow-up of 16 months (range: 6 to 30 months). In the femoropopliteal artery group, of the 11 patients available for follow-up, only six had patent stents at 7 to 26 months (mean: 20 months). Four of the six required one to three secondary interventions. Results are clearly superior with the iliac arteries and these authors recommend that placement in the femoral arteries be performed with caution.

Favorable long-term results with iliac artery stenting have been reported by Long et al.[205] using the Wallstent and the Strecker stent (Medi-Tech, Boston Scientific, Watertown, MA) in a series of 49 patients with 53 iliac artery lesions. Indications for stent deployment included recanalization of total occlusions,

15 lesions (28 per cent); dissection, 22 lesions (42 per cent); post-PTA restenosis, 11 lesions (21 per cent); and immediate post-PTA unsatisfactory results, 5 lesions (9 per cent). Mean follow-up was 15 months (range: 1 to 36 months) with follow-up angiograms in 50 vessels. Complications occurred in 14 patients (26.9 per cent). Primary patency was 85.3 per cent at 12 months and 80.9 per cent at 18 months. Secondary patency was 96.1 per cent at 12 and at 18 months. These results indicate intravascular stents have a role in the management of iliac artery lesions. Their use in other vessels is under investigation.

Transjugular Intrahepatic Portosystemic Shunts

Another important application of the intravascular stents is their use in the nonsurgical creation of intrahepatic portosystemic shunts. The nonsurgical creation of a portosystemic shunt consisting of an artificial tract between the inferior vena cava and portal vein was first accomplished in swine by Rosch et al.[206] Colapinto et al.[208] were the first to perform the technique in humans. Using a transjugular approach to puncture a portal vein branch from a hepatic vein, the artificial tract was widened by balloon dilation. Their results were limited by early and late shunt occlusion and an overall mortality of 50 per cent. Palmaz, using his stent, was able to achieve long-term shunt patency in a canine model of portal hypertension.[209]

The use of the newer vascular stents to maintain patency of the artificial tract between the hepatic vein and portal vein has resulted in improved patency of the shunts. Several series have described interim results, with reported patency at 10 months thus far.[210-212] The procedure is accompanied by a drop in portal pressure, and cessation of variceal bleeding. Early experience suggests it is a useful procedure in the management of patients with variceal bleeding due to portal hypertension or as an interim technique prior to liver transplantation.

REFERENCES

1. Molnar W, Paul DJ: Complications of axillary arteriotomies: An analysis of 1,762 consecutive studies. Radiology 104:269–276, 1972.
2. Jacobsson B, Schlossman D: Thromboembolism of the leg following percutaneous catheterization of the femoral artery for angiography: Predisposing factors. Acta Radiol Diagn 8:109–118, 1969.
3. Fischer HW: Viscosity, solubility and toxicity in the choice of an angiographic contrast medium. Angiology 16:759–763, 1965.
4. Gonzalez L, Stieritz D: Experimental evaluation of sodium methylglucamine iothalamate (MP3064): Cardiovascular responses following proximal aortic injection. Invest Radiol 2:266–271, 1967.
5. Sherwood T, Lavender J: Does renal flow rise or fall in response to diatrizoate? Invest Radiol 4:327–328, 1969.
6. Older R, Miller J, Jackson D, et al: Angiographically induced renal failure and its radiographic detection. AJR 126:1039–1045, 1976.
7. Pillay V, Robbins P, Schwartz F, et al: Acute renal failure following intravenous urography in patients with long-standing diabetes mellitus and azotemia. Radiology 95:633–636, 1970.
8. Port F, Wagoner R, Fulton R: Acute renal failure after angiography. AJR 121:544–550, 1974.
9. Talner L: Urographic contrast media in uremia. Radiol Clin North Am 10:421–432, 1972.
10. Gomes AS, Baker JD, Martin-Paredero V, et al: Acute renal dysfunction after major arteriography. AJR 145:1249–1253, 1985.
11. Eisenberg RL, Bank WO, Hedgcock MW: Renal failure after major angiography. AJR 136:859–861, 1981.

12. Pendergrass HP, Hodes PJ, Tondreau RL, et al: Further considerations of deaths and unfavorable sequelae following the administration of contrast media in urography in the United States. AJR 74:262–287, 1955.
13. Greenberger P, Patterson R, Kelly J, et al: Administration of radiographic contrast media in high risk patients. Invest Radiol 15:540–549, 1980.
14. Kelly JF, Patterson R, Lieberman P, et al: Radiographic contrast media studies in high risk patients. J Allergy Clin Immunol 62:181–184, 1978.
15. Spataro F: Newer contrast agents for urography. Radiol Clin North Am 22:365–380, 1984.
16. Johnsrude IS: Aortic arch and brachiocephalic angiography. *In* Johnsrude IS, Jackson DC (eds): A Practical Approach to Angiography. Boston, Little, Brown & Co, 1979, p 296.
17. Eisenman J, Jenkin C, Pribram H, et al: Evaluation of the cerebral circulation by arch aortography supplemented by subtraction technique. AJR 115:14–26, 1972.
18. Hoffman R, Rein B: The routine use of subtraction in aortic arch studies. Radiology 102:575–578, 1972.
19. Haas W, Fields W, North R, et al: Joint study of extracranial arterial occlusion: II. Arteriography, techniques, sites and complications. JAMA 203:159–166, 1968.
20. Castaneda WZ, Knight L, Formanek A, et al: Hemodynamic assessment of obstructive aortoiliac disease. AJR 127:559–561, 1976.
21. Haimovichi H: Patterns of arteriosclerotic lesions of the lower extremities. Arch Surg 95:918–933, 1967.
22. Crawford ES, DeBakey ME, Morris GC: Thrombo-obliterative disease of the great vessels arising from the aortic arch. J Thorac Cardiovasc Surg 43:38–53, 1962.
23. Champion HR, Gill W: Arterial embolus to the upper limb. Br J Surg 60:505–508, 1973.
24. Darling CR, Austen WG, Linton RR: Arterial embolism. Surg Gynecol Obstet 124:106–114, 1967.
25. Lambeth J, Yong N: Arteriographic findings in thromboangiitis obliterans. AJR 109:553–562, 1970.
26. McKusick VA, Harris WS, Otteson OE, et al: Buerger's disease: A distinct clinical and pathologic entity. JAMA 181:5–12, 1962.
27. Wessler S: Thromboangiitis obliterans. Fact or fancy. Circulation 23:165–167, 1961.
28. Lande A, Gross A: Total aortography in the diagnosis of Takayasu's arteritis. AJR 116:165–178, 1972.
29. Lande A, Rossi P: The value of total aortography in the diagnosis of Takayasu's arteritis. Radiology 14:287–297, 1975.
30. Hamrin B, Jonsson N, Landberg T: Involvement of large vessels in polymyalgia rheumatica. Lancet 1:1193–1196, 1965.
31. Harrison C: Giant cell or temporal arteritis: A review. Gen Clin Pathol 1:197–211, 1948.
32. Hauser WA, Ferguson RH, Holley KE, et al: Temporal arteritis in Rochester Minn 1951–1967. Mayo Clin Proc 46:597–602, 1971.
33. Hunder GG, Ward LE, Burbank MK: Giant cell arteritis producing an aortic arch syndrome. Ann Intern Med 66:578–582, 1967.
34. Benedict K, Chang W, McCready F: The hypothenar hammer syndrome. Radiology 111:57–60, 1974.
35. Laws J, Lillie J, Scott J: Arteriographic appearances in rheumatoid arthritis and other disorders. Br J Radiol 36:477–493, 1963.
36. Fagerberg S, Jorulf H, Sandberg C: Ergotism: Arterial spastic disease and recovery studied angiographically. Acta Med Scand 182:769–772, 1967.
37. Love L: Arteriography of peripheral vascular trauma. AJR 102:431–440, 1968.
38. McDonald E, Goodman P, Winestock D: Clinical indications for arteriography in trauma to the extremity: A review of 114 cases. Radiology 116:45–47, 1975.
39. Pochaczevsky R, Mufte M, LaGuerre J, et al: Arteriography of penetrating wounds of the extremities: Help or hindrance: J Can Assoc Radiol 24:354–361, 1973.

40. Lumpkin MB, Logan WD, Couves CM, et al: Arteriography as an aid in the diagnosis and localization of acute arterial injuries. Ann Surg 147:353–358, 1958.
41. Perry MO, Thal ER, Shires GT: Management of arterial injuries. Ann Surg 173:403–408, 1971.
42. Cliff MM, Soulen RL, Finestone AJ: Mycotic aneurysms—a challenge and a clue. Arch Intern Med 126:977–982, 1970.
43. Boley SJ, Sprayregen S, Siegelman SS, Veith FJ: Initial results from an aggressive roentgenological and surgical approach to acute mesenteric ischemia. Surgery 82:848–855, 1977.
44. Ottinger LW, Austen WG: A study of 136 patients with mesenteric infarction. Surg Gynecol Obstet 124:251–261, 1967.
45. Siegelman SS, Sprayregen S, Boley SJ: Angiographic diagnosis of mesenteric arterial vasoconstriction. Radiology 112:533–542, 1974.
46. Boley SJ, Feinstein R, Sammartano RJ: Superior mesenteric embolus. Paper presented at the American College of Surgeons, Atlanta, Georgia, October 1980.
47. Ottinger LW: Surgical management of acute occlusion of the superior mesenteric artery. Ann Surg 188:721–731, 1978.
48. Crummy AB: Arteriography of the patient with previous aortoiliac surgery. *In* Abrams HI (ed): Abrams Angiography Vascular and Interventional Radiology, 3rd ed. Boston, Little, Brown & Co, 1983, pp 1830–1831.
49. Wade GL, Smith DC, Mohr LL: Followup of 50 consecutive angiograms obtained utilizing puncture of prosthetic vascular grafts. Radiology 146:663–664, 1983.
50. Nusbaum M, Baum S: Radiographic demonstration of unknown sites of gastrointestinal bleeding. Surg Forum 14:374–375, 1963.
51. Alavi A, Dann RW, Baum S, et al: Scintigraphic detection of acute gastrointestinal bleeding. Radiology 124:753–756, 1977.
52. Miskowiak J, Nielsen SL, Munck O: Scintigraphic diagnosis of gastrointestinal bleeding with Tc^{99m} labeled bloodpool agents. Radiology 141:499–504, 1981.
53. Johnsrude IS: Splanchnic angiography. *In* Johnsrude IS, Jackson DC (eds): A Practical Approach to Angiography. Boston, Little, Brown & Co, 1979, pp 205–271.
54. Leevy C, Gliedman M: Practical and research value of hepatic vein catheterization. N Engl J Med 258:696–700, 1958.
55. Viamonte M Jr, Warren W, Fomon J: Liver panangiography in the assessment of portal hypertension in liver cirrhosis. Radiol Clin North Am 1:147–167, 1970.
56. Redman H: Mesenteric arterial and venous blood flow changes following selective arterial injection of vasodilators. Invest Radiol 9:193–198, 1974.
57. Leger L: Splenoportography: Diagnostic Phlebography of the Portal Venous System. Springfield, IL, Charles C. Thomas, 1966.
58. Korobkin M, Moss AA, Callen PW, et al: Computed tomography of subcapsular splenic hematoma. Clinical and experimental studies. Radiology 129:441–445, 1978.
59. Shirkhoda A, McCartney WH, Staab EV, et al: Imaging of the spleen: A proposed algorithm. AJR 135:195–198, 1980.
60. Baum S, Roy R, Finkelstein AK, Blakemore AS: Clinical application of selective celiac and superior mesenteric angiography. Radiology 84:279–294, 1965.
61. Haertel M, Ryder D: Radiologic investigation of splenic trauma. Cardiovasc Radiol 2:27–33, 1979.
62. Abrams HL, Comell SH: Patterns of collateral flow in renal ischemia. Radiology 84:1001–1012, 1965.
63. Brewster DC, Darling AC: Optimal methods of aortoiliac reconstruction. Surgery 84:739–748, 1972.
64. Palubinskas AJ, Wylie EJ: Roentgen diagnosis of fibromuscular hyperplasia of the renal arteries. Radiology 76:634–639, 1961.
65. Kincaid OW, Davis GD, Hallerman N, et al: Fibromuscular dysplasia of the renal arteries: Arteriographic features, classification and observations on natural history of the disease. AJR 104:271–282, 1968.

66. McCormack LJ, Dustan HP, Meany TF: Selected pathology of the renal artery. Semin Roentgenol 2:126–138, 1967.

67. Palubinskas AJ, Ripley H: Fibromuscular hyperplasia in extra-renal arteries. Radiology 82:451–454, 1964.

68. Wholey MH, Cooperstein LA: Renal trauma. *In* Abrams HL (ed): Abrams Angiography Vascular and Interventional Radiology, 3rd ed. Boston, Little, Brown & Co, 1983, pp 1231–1237.

69. Love L, Moncada R, Lescher AJ: Renal arteriovenous fistulae. AJR 95:364–371, 1965.

70. Ekelund L, Lindholm T: Arteriovenous fistulae following percutaneous renal biopsy. Acta Radiol Diagn (Stockh) 11:38–48, 1971.

71. Hageman JH, Smith RF, Szilagyi E, et al: Aneurysms of the renal artery. Problems of prognosis and surgical management. Surgery 84:563–572, 1978.

72. Quinton W, Dillar D, Scribner BH: Canulation of blood vessels for prolonged hemodialysis. Trans Am Soc Artif Intern Organs 6:104–113, 1960.

73. Brescia MJ, Cimino JE, Appel K, et al: Chronic hemodialysis using venipuncture and a surgically created arteriovenous fistula. N Engl J Med 275:1089–1092, 1966.

74. Butt KM, Friedman EA, Kountz SL: Angioaccess. Curr Probl Surg 13:36–38, 1976.

75. Gilula LA, Staple TW, Anderson CB, Anderson LS: Venous angiography of hemodialysis fistulas. Radiology 115:555–562, 1975.

76. O'Reilly RJ, Hansen CC, Rosental JJ: Angiography of chronic hemodialysis arteriovenous grafts. AJR 130:1105–1113, 1978.

77. Kirschner LP, Twigg H, Farkas J: Drip infusion venography. Radiology 96:413–415, 1970.

78. Rabinov K, Paulin S: Roentgen diagnosis of venous thrombosis in the leg. Arch Surg 104:134–144, 1972.

79. Thomas ML: Phlebography. Arch Surg 104:145–151, 1972.

80. Rose SC, Zwiebel WJ, Nelson BD, Priest DL, et al: Symptomatic lower extremity deep venous thrombosis: Accuracy, limitations, and role of color duplex flow imaging in diagnosis. Radiology 175:639–644, 1990.

81. Lange EK: Arteriography of thoracic outlet syndrome. *In* Abrams HI (ed): Abrams Angiography Vascular and Interventional Radiology, 3rd ed. Boston, Little, Brown & Co, 1983, pp 1001–1015.

82. Lang EK: Arteriographic diagnosis of the thoracic outlet syndrome. Radiology 84:296–302, 1965.

83. Okay N, Bryk D: Collateral pathways in occlusion of the superior vena cava and its tributaries. Radiology 92:1493–1498, 1969.

84. Steinberg I: Superior vena cava obstruction. *In* Abrams HL (ed): Angiography, 2nd ed. Boston, Little, Brown & Co, 1971, pp 625–640.

85. Kruger RA, Mistretta CA, Riederer SJ, et al: Computerized fluoroscopy in real time for noninvasive visualization of the cardiovascular system. Radiology 130:49–57, 1979.

86. Mistretta CA, Ort MG, Cameron JR, et al: Multiple images subtraction technique for enhancing low contrast periodic objects. Invest Radiol 8:43–44, 1973.

87. Ort MG, Mistretta CA, Kelcz F: An improved technique for enhancing small period contrast changes in television fluoroscopy. Opt Engl 12:169–175, 1973.

88. Buonocore E, Meany TF, Borkowski GP, et al: Digital subtraction angiography of the abdominal aorta and renal arteries. Radiology 139:281–286, 1981.

89. Brant-Zawadzki M, Gould R, Norman B, et al: Digital subtraction cerebral angiography by intra-arterial injection: Comparison with conventional angiography. AJR 140:347–353, 1983.

90. Johnson AJ, McCarty WR: The lysis of artificially induced intravascular clots in man by intravenous infusion of streptokinase. J Clin Invest 38:1627–1643, 1959.

91. Sherry S, Lindemeyer RI, Fletcher AP, et al: Studies on enhanced fibrinolytic activity in man. J Clin Invest 38:810–822, 1959.

92. The Urokinase Pulmonary Embolism Trial. A Cooperative Study. Phase I results. JAMA 214:2163–2172, 1970.

93. The Urokinase Pulmonary Embolism Trial. A National Cooperative Study. Phase II results. JAMA 229:1606–1613, 1974.

94. Dotter CT, Rosch J, Seaman AJ: Selective clot lysis with low dose streptokinase. Radiology 111:31–37, 1974.

95. Rentrop P, Blanke H, Karsch KR, et al: Selective intracoronary thrombolysis in acute myocardial infarction and unstable angina pectoris. Circulation 63:307–317, 1981.

96. Hargrove WC, Barker CF, Berkowitz HD, et al: Treatment of acute peripheral arterial and graft thromboses with low dose streptokinase. Surgery 92:981–993, 1982.

97. Becker GJ, Rabe FE, Richmond BD, et al: Low dose fibrinolytic therapy: Results and new concepts. Radiology 148:663–670, 1983.

98. Mori KW, Bookstein JJ, Heeney DJ, et al: Selective streptokinase infusion: Clinical and laboratory correlates. Radiology 148:677–682, 1983.

99. Martin M: Thrombolytic therapy in arterial thromboembolism. Prog Cardiovasc Dis 21:351–374, 1979.

100. Totty WG, Gilula LA, McClellan BL, et al: Low dose intravascular fibrinolytic therapy. Radiology 143:59–69, 1982.

101. McNamara TO, Fischer JR: Thrombolysis of peripheral arterial and graft occlusions: Improved results using high dose urokinase. AJR 144:769–775, 1985.

102. Cragg AH, Smith TP, Corson JD, et al: Two urokinase dose regimens in native arterial and graft occlusions: Initial results of a prospective, randomized clinical trial. Radiology 178:681–686, 1991.

103. Astrup T, Stage A: Isolation of a soluble fibrinolytic activator from animal tissue. Nature 170:929–930, 1952.

104. Booyse FM, Scheinbuks J, Radek J, Osikowicz G, Feder S, Quarfoot AJ: Immunological identification and comparison of plasminogen activator forms in cultured normal human endothelial cells and smooth muscle cells. Thromb Res 24:495–504, 1981.

105. Collen D, Verstraete M: Systemic thrombolytic therapy of acute myocardial infarction? Circulation 68:462–465, 1983.

106. Eisenberg PR, Sherman LA, Tiefenbrunn AJ, Ludbrook PA, Sobel BE, Jaffe AS: Sustained fibrinolysis after administration of t-PA despite its short half-life in the circulation. Thromb Haemost 57:35–40, 1987.

107. Risius B, Graor RA, Geisinger MA, Zelch MG, Lucas FV, Young JR, Grossbard EB: Recombinant human tissue-type plasminogen activator for thrombolysis in peripheral arteries and bypass grafts. Radiology 160:183–188, 1986.

108. Verstraete M, Bounameaux H, DeCock F, et al: Pharmacokinetics and systemic fibrinogenolytic effects of recombinant human tissue-type plasminogen activator (rt-PA) in humans. J Pharmacol Exp Ther 235:506–512, 1985.

109. Collen D, Stump D, van de Werf F, Jang IK, Nobuhara M, Lijnen HR: Coronary thrombolysis in dogs and intravenously administered human pro-urokinase. Circulation 72:384–388, 1985.

110. Bloomfield DA: The nonsurgical retrieval of intracardiac foreign bodies—an international survey. Cathet Cardiovasc Diagn 4:1–14, 1978.

111. Chuang VP: Non-operative retrieval of Gianturco coils from the abdominal aorta. AJR 132:996–997, 1979.

112. Dotter CT, Rosch J, Bilbao MK: Transluminal extraction of catheter and guide fragments from the heart and great vessels; 29 collected cases. AJR 111:467–472, 1971.

113. Curry JL: Recovery of detached intravascular catheter or guide wire fragments. A proposed method. AJR 105:894–896, 1969.

114. Lassers BW, Pickering D: Removal of an iatrogenic foreign body from the aorta by means of a ureteric stone catheter. Am Heart J 73:375–378, 1967.

115. Rossi P: "Hook catheter," technique for transfemoral removal of foreign body from right side of the heart. AJR 109:101–106, 1970.

116. King JF, Manley JC, Zeft HJ, et al: Nonsurgical removal of foreign body from right heart. J Thorac Cardiovasc Surg 71:785–786, 1976.

117. Millan VG: Retrieval of intravascular foreign bodies using a

modified bronchoscopic forceps. Radiology *129*:587–589, 1978.

118. Yedlicka JW Jr, Carlson JE, Hunter DW, Castaneda-Zuniga WR, Amplatz K: Nitinol gooseneck snare for removal of foreign bodies: Experimental study and clinical evaluation. Radiology *178*:691, 1991.

119. Dotter CT: Interventional radiology—review of an emerging field. Semin Roentgenol *6*:7–12, 1981.

120. Dotter CT, Keller FS, Rosch J: Transluminal catheter removal of foreign bodies from the cardiovascular system. *In* Abrams HL (ed): Abrams Angiography Vascular and Interventional Radiology, 3rd ed. Boston, Little, Brown & Co, 1983, pp 2395–2403.

121. Gruntzig A, Hopff H: Perkutane Rekanalisation chronischer arterieller Verschlusse mit einem neuen Dilatationskather: Modification der Dotter—Technik. Deutsch Med Wochenschr *99*:2502–2505, 1974.

122. Gruntzig A, Kumpe DA: Technique of percutaneous transluminal angioplasty with the Gruntzig balloon catheter. AJR *132*:547–552, 1979.

123. Dotter CT, Judkins MP: Percutaneous transluminal treatment of arteriosclerotic obstruction. Radiology *84*:631–643, 1965.

124. Dotter CT, Rosch J, Anderson JM, et al: Transluminal iliac artery dilatation: Non-surgical catheter treatment of atheromatous narrowing. JAMA *230*:117–124, 1974.

125. Portsmann W: Ein nuer Korsett-Balloon Katheter zur transluminalen Rekanalisation nach Dotter unter besonderer Berucksichtigung von obliterationend an den Beckenarterien. Radiol Diagn (Berlin) *14*:239–244, 1973.

126. van Andel GJ, van Erp WFM, Krepel VM, et al: Percutaneous transluminal dilation of the iliac artery: Long term results. Radiology *156*:321–323, 1985.

127. Fogarty TJ, Chin A, Shoor PM, et al: Adjunctive intraoperative arterial dilation. Arch Surg *116*:1391–1398, 1981.

128. Castaneda-Zuniga WR, Formanek A, Tadavarthy M, et al: The mechanism of balloon angioplasty. Radiology *135*:565–571, 1980.

129. Neiman HL, Bergan JJ, Yao JS: Hemodynamic assessment of transluminal angioplasty for lower extremity ischemia. Radiology *143*:639–643, 1982.

130. Spence RK, Frieman DB, Gatenby R, et al: Long-term results of transluminal angioplasty of the iliac and femoral arteries. Arch Surg *116*:1377–1386, 1981.

131. Kadir S, White RI, Kaufman SL, et al: Long term results of aortoiliac angioplasty. Surgery *94*:10–14, 1983.

132. Gruntzig A: Die Perkutane Transluminal Re-Kanalisation Chronischer Arterienverschlusse mit einer Neuen Dilation-Stechnik. Baden-Baden, Witzstrock, 1977.

133. van Andel GJ: Transluminal iliac angioplasty; long term results. Radiology *135*:607–611, 1980.

134. Schneider E, Gruntzig A, Bollinger A: Langzeitergebnisse nach perkutaner transluminaler Angioplastie (PTA) bei 882 Konsekutiven Patienten mit iliakalen und femorpoplitealen Obstruktionen. Vasa *11*:322–326, 1982.

135. Johnston KW, Colapinto RF, Baird RJ: Transluminal dilation. An alternative? Arch Surg *117*:1604–1610, 1982.

136. Gallino A, Mahler F, Probst P, et al: Fruh-und Spatergebnisse bei 250 perkutanen transluminalen Dilatationen an den unteren Extremitaten. Vasa *11*:319–321, 1982.

137. Kumpe DA, Jones DN: Percutaneous transluminal angioplasty; radiologic viewpoint. Appl Radiol *11*:29–40, 1982.

138. Schwarten DE: Percutaneous transluminal angioplasty of the iliac arteries: Intravenous digital subtraction angiography for followup. Radiology *150*:363–367, 1984.

139. Johnston KW, Rae H, Hogg-Johnston B, Colapinto RF, Walker PM, Baird RJ, Sniderman KW, Kalman P: 5 year results of a prospective study of percutaneous transluminal angioplasty. Ann Surg *206*:403–413, 1987.

140. Malone JW, Moore WS, Goldstein J: The natural history of bilateral aortofemoral bypass grafts for ischemia of the lower extremities. Arch Surg *110*:1300–1306, 1975.

141. Krepel VM, Van Andel GJ, Van Erp WF, et al: Percutaneous

142. Greenfield AJ: Femoral, popliteal and tibial arteries: Percutaneous transluminal angioplasty. AJR *135*:927–935, 1980.

143. Freiman DB, Spence RK, Gatenby R: Transluminal angioplasty of the iliac and femoral arteries: Follow up results without anticoagulation. Radiology *141*:347–350, 1981.

144. Colapinto RF: Long-term results of iliac and femoropopliteal angioplasty. *In* Dotter CT, Gruntzig A, Schoop W, Zietler E (eds): Percutaneous Transluminal Angioplasty. Berlin, Springer, 1983, pp 202–206.

145. Berkowitz HD, Spence RK, Frieman DB, et al: Long-term results of transluminal angioplasty of the femoral arteries. *In* Dotter CT, Gruntzig A, Schoop W, Zietler E (eds): Percutaneous Transluminal Angioplasty. Berlin, Springer, 1983, pp 207–214.

146. Mahler F, Gallino A, Probst P, et al: Factors influencing early and late follow-up results after percutaneous transluminal angioplasty of the lower limb arteries. *In* Dotter CT, Gruntzig A, Schoop W, Zietler E (eds): Percutaneous Transluminal Angioplasty. Berlin, Springer, 1983, pp 199–201.

147. Naji A, Chu J, McCombs PR, et al: Results of 100 consecutive femoropopliteal vein grafts for limb salvage. Ann Surg *188*:162–165, 1978.

148. Mehta S: A Statistical Summary of the Results of Femoropopliteal Bypass Surgery. Newark, DE, WL Gore & Assoc, Inc, 1980, pp 1–32.

149. Veith FJ, Gupta SK, Samson RH, et al: Progress in limb salvage by reconstructive arterial surgery combined with new or improved adjunctive procedures. Ann Surg *194*:386–400, 1981.

150. Taylor LM, Porter JM: Clinical and anatomic considerations for surgery in femoropopliteal disease and the results of surgery. Circulation *83*(suppl I):I-63–I-69, 1991.

151. Sanchez LA, Gupta SK, Veith FJ, Goldsmith J, Lyon RI, Wengerter KR, Panetta IF, Marin ML, Cynamon J, Berdejo G: A ten-year experience with one hundred fifty failing or threatened vein and polytetrafluoroethylene arterial bypass grafts. J Vasc Surg *14*:729–736, 1991.

152. Casarella WJ: Percutaneous transluminal angioplasty below the knee: New techniques, excellent results. Radiology *169*:271–272, 1988.

153. Schwarten DE, Cutcliff WB: Arterial occlusive disease below the knee: Treatment with percutaneous transluminal angioplasty performed with low-profile catheters and steerable guide wires. Radiology *169*:71–74, 1988.

154. Bakal CW, Sprayregen S, Scheinbaum K, Cynamon J, Veith FJ: Percutaneous transluminal angioplasty of the infrapopliteal arteries: Results in 53 patients. AJR *154*:171–174, 1990.

155. Horvath W, Oertl M, Haidinger D: Percutaneous transluminal angioplasty of crural arteries. Radiology *177*:565–569, 1990.

156. Londry GL, Ramsey DE, Hodgson KJ, Barkmeier LD, Sumner DA: Infrapopliteal bypass for severe ischemia: Comparison of autogenous vein, composite, and prosthetic grafts. J Vasc Surg *13*:631–636, 1991.

157. Taylor LM, Edwards JM, Porter JM: Present status of reversed vein bypass grafting: Five-year results of a modern series. J Vasc Surg *11*:193–206, 1990.

158. Kram HB, Gupta SK, Veith FJ, Wengerter KR, Panetta TF, Nwosisi C: Late results of two hundred seventeen femoropopliteal artery segments. J Vasc Surg *14*:386–390, 1991.

159. Ginsburg R, Wexler L, Mitchell RS, Profit D: Percutaneous transluminal angioplasty for treatment of peripheral vascular disease: Clinical experience with 16 patients. Radiology *156*:619–624, 1985.

160. Sanborn TA, Faxon DP, Haudenschild CC, Ryan TJ: Experimental angioplasty: Circumferential distribution of laser thermal injury with a laser probe. J Am Coll Cardiol *5*:934–938, 1985.

161. Garrison BJ, Srinivasan R: Microscopic model for the ablative

photodecomposition of polymers by far ultraviolet radiation (193 nm). Appl Phys Lett *44*:849–851, 1984.

162. Srinivasan R, Braren B, Dreyfus RW, Hadel L, Seeger DE: Mechanism of the ultraviolet laser ablation of polymethyl methacrylate at 193 and 248 nm: Laser induced fluorescence analysis, chemical analysis, and doping studies. J Opt Soc Am (B) *3*:785–791, 1986.

163. Sanborn TA, Cumberland DC, Greenfield AJ, Welsh CL, Guben JK: Percutaneous laser thermal angioplasty: Initial results and 1-year follow-up in 129 femoropopliteal lesions. Radiology *168*:121–125, 1988.

164. Rosenthal D, Pesa FA, Gohsegen WL, Crew JR, Moss CA, Walsky R, Pallos LL: Thermal laser assisted balloon angioplasty of the superficial femoral artery: A multicenter review of 602 cases. J Vasc Surg *14*:152–159, 1991.

165. Litvack F, Grundfest WS, Adler I, Hickey AE, et al: Percutaneous excimer-laser and excimer-laser assisted angioplasty of the lower extremities: Results of initial clinical trial. Radiology *172*:331–335, 1989.

166. Sos TG, Pickering TG, Sniderman K, et al: Beneficial effects of percutaneous transluminal renal angioplasty on blood pressure in patients with renovascular hypertension due to atheroma and fibromuscular dysplasia. Paper presented at the Eighth Annual Course on Diagnostic and Therapeutic Angiography and Interventional Radiology sponsored by the Society of Cardiovascular Radiology, Fort Lauderdale, FL, 1983.

167. Schwarten DE: Transluminal angioplasty of renal artery stenosis: 70 experiences. AJR *135*:969–974, 1980.

168. Sos TA, Sniderman KW, Pickering T, et al: Percutaneous transluminal renal angioplasty: Experience in over 100 arteries. *In* Kaltenbach M, Rentrop K (eds): Transluminal Coronary Angioplasty and Intracoronary Thrombolysis. Berlin, Springer-Verlag, 1982, pp 412–425.

169. Tegtmeyer CJ, Elson J, Glass TA, et al: Percutaneous transluminal angioplasty: The treatment of choice of renovascular hypertension due to fibromuscular dysplasia. Radiology *143*:631–637, 1982.

170. Foster JH, Maxwell MH, Franklin SS, et al: Renovascular occlusive disease: Results of operative treatment. JAMA *231*:1043–1048, 1975.

171. Kaufman JJ: Renovascular hypertension: The UCLA experience. J Urol *121*:139–144, 1979.

172. Stoney RJ, DeLuccia N, Ehrenfeld WK, et al: Aortorenal arterial autografts: Long range assessment. Arch Surg *116*:1416–1422, 1981.

173. Tegtmeyer CJ, Selby JB, Hartwell GD, Ayers C, Tegtmeyer V: Results and complications of angioplasty in fibromuscular disease. Circulation *83*(suppl 2):I-155–I-161, 1991.

174. Novick AC, Straffon RA, Steward BH, et al: Diminished operative morbidity and mortality in renal revascularization. JAMA *246*:749–753, 1981.

175. Gianturco C, Anderson JH, Wallace S: Mechanical devices for arterial occlusion. AJR *124*:428–435, 1975.

176. White RI Jr, Kaufman SL, Barth KH, et al: Embolotherapy with detachable silicone balloons: Technique and clinical results. Radiology *131*:619–627, 1979.

177. Tadavarthy SM, Moller JH, Amplatz KA: Polyvinyl alcohol (Ivalon)—a new embolic material. AJR *125*:609–616, 1975.

178. Hilal SK, Sane P, Michelson WJ, et al: The embolization of vascular malformations of the spinal cord with low viscosity silicone rubber. Neuroradiology *16*:430–433, 1978.

179. Dotter CT, Goldman ML, Rosch J: Instant selective arterial occlusion with isobutyl 2-cyanoarcylate. Radiology *114*:227–230, 1975.

180. Barth KH, Strandberg JD, White RI Jr: Long-term followup of transcatheter embolization with autologous clot, oxycel and Gelfoam in domestic swine. Invest Radiol *12*:273–280, 1977.

181. Gomes MMR, Bernatz PE: Arteriovenous fistulas: A review and 10 year experience at the Mayo Clinic. Mayo Clin Proc *45*:81–102, 1970.

182. Gomes AS, Mali WP, Oppenheim WL: Embolization therapy in the management of congenital arteriovenous malformations. Radiology *144*:41–49, 1982.

183. Kaufman SL, Kumar AAJ, Roland JMA, et al: Transcatheter embolization in the management of congenital arteriovenous malformations. Radiology *137*:21–29, 1980.

184. Olcott C IVth, Newton TH, Stoney RJ, et al: Intra-arterial embolization in the management of arteriovenous malformations. Surgery *79*:3–12, 1976.

185. Remy J, Amand A, Fardon H, et al: Treatment of hemoptysis by embolization of bronchial arteries. Radiology *122*:33–37, 1977.

186. Wallace S, Chuang VP, Swenson D: Embolization of renal carcinoma. Experience with 100 patients. Radiology *138*:563–570, 1981.

187. Higgins CB, Bookstein JJ, Davis GB, et al: Therapeutic embolization for intractable chronic bleeding. Radiology *122*:473–478, 1977.

188. Ring EJ, Athanasoulis CA, Wallman AC, et al: Arteriographic management of hemorrhage following pelvic fracture. Radiology *109*:65–70, 1973.

189. Tadavarthy SM, Castenedra-Zuniga W, Salomonowitz E, et al: Kimray-Greenfield vena cava filter: Percutaneous introduction. Radiology *151*:525–526, 1984.

190. Messmer JM, Greenfield LJ: Greenfield filters: Long-term radiographic follow-up study. Radiology *156*:613–618, 1985.

191. Greenfield LJ, Michna BA: Twelve-year clinical experience with the Greenfield vena caval filter. Surgery *104*:706–712, 1988.

192. Geisinger MA, Zelch MG, Risius B: Recurrent pulmonary emboli after Greenfield filter placement. Radiology *165*:383–384, 1987.

193. Pais S, Tobin K, Austin C, Queral L: Percutaneous insertion of Greenfield inferior vena cava filter: Experience with ninety-six patients. J Vasc Surg *8*:460–464, 1988.

194. Pais SO, Tobin KD: Percutaneous insertion of the Greenfield Filter. AJR *152*:933–938, 1989.

195. Greenfield LJ, Zocco J, Wilk J, Schroeder TM, Elkins RC: Clinical experience with the Kimray-Greenfield vena caval filter. Ann Surg *185*:692–698, 1977.

196. Wingerd M, Bernhard VM, Maddison F, Towne JB: Comparison of caval filters in the management of venous thromboembolism. Arch Surg *113*:1264–1270, 1978.

197. Mewissen MW, Erickson SJ, Foley WD, et al: Thrombosis at venous insertion sites after inferior vena caval filter placement. Radiology *173*:155–157, 1989.

198. Greenfield LJ, Cho KJ, Pais SO, Van Aman M: Preliminary clinical experience with the titanium Greenfield filter. Arch Surg *124*:657–659, 1989.

199. Roehm JOF: The Bird's nest filter: A new percutaneous transcatheter inferior vena cava filter. J Vasc Surg *1*:498–501, 1984.

200. Roehm JOF, Johnsrude IS, Barth MH, Gianturco C: The bird's nest inferior vena cava filter: Progress report. Radiology *168*:745–749, 1988.

201. Simon M, Kaplow R, Salzman E, Friedman D: A vena cava filter using thermal shape memory alloy: Experimental aspects. Radiology *125*:89–94, 1977.

202. Grassi CJ: Inferior vena caval filters: Analysis of five currently available devices. AJR *156*:813–821, 1991.

203. Palmaz JC, Garcia OJ, Schatz RA, et al: Placement of balloon expandable intraluminal stents in iliac arteries: First 171 procedures. Radiology *174*:969–975, 1990.

204. Zollikofer CL, Antonucci F, Pfyffer M, et al: Arterial stent placement with use of the Wallstent: Midterm results of clinical experience. Radiology *179*:449–456, 1991.

205. Long AI, Page PE, Raynaud AC, et al: Percutaneous iliac artery stent: Angiographic long-term follow-up. Radiology *180*:771–778, 1991.

206. Rosch J, Hanafee WN, Snow H: Transjugular portal venography and radiologic portacaval shunt: An experimental study. Radiology *92*:1112–1114, 1969.

208. Colapinto RF, Stronell RD, Birch SJ, Langer B, Blendis LM, Greig PD, Gilas T: Creation of an intrahepatic portosys-

temic shunt with a Gruentzig balloon catheter. Can Med Assoc J *126*:267–268, 1982.

209. Palmaz JC, Garcia F, Sibbitt RR, et al: Expandable intrahepatic portocaval shunt in dogs with chronic portal hypertension. AJR *147*:1251–1254, 1986.

210. Richter GM, Noeldge G, Palmaz JC, Roessle M: The transjugular intrahepatic portosystemic stent-shunt (TIPSS): Results of a pilot study. Cardiovasc Intervent Radiol *13*:200–207, 1990.

211. Zemel G, Katzen BT, Becker GJ, Benenati JF, Sallee S: Percutaneous transjugular portosystemic shunt. JAMA *266*:390–393, 1991.

212. Ring EJ, Lake JR, Roberts JP, et al: Using transjugular intrahepatic portosystemic shunts to control variceal bleeding before liver transplantation. Ann Intern Med *116*:304–309, 1992.

REVIEW QUESTIONS

1. The angiographic approach associated with the highest incidence of complications is:
   (a) femoral approach
   (b) translumbar approach
   (c) axillary approach
   (d) all are associated with equal risk

2. Which of the following statements regarding radiographic contrast media are true?
   (a) contrast agents can induce renal dysfunction in patients both with and without preexisting renal disease
   (b) contrast-induced renal failure usually resolves spontaneously within 7 days
   (c) pretreatment with steroids has been found effective in preventing severe allergic reactions to contrast in patients with a prior history of allergy to x-ray contrast medium
   (d) the incidence of contrast-induced renal dysfunction is unrelated to the volume of contrast administered
   (e) patients should be dehydrated prior to arteriography, because this will result in improved visualization of vessels

3. Takayasu's disease is characterized by which of the following?
   (a) a corkscrew or tree-root configuration of vessels at the point of vessel occlusion
   (b) involvement of the aortic arch and branch vessels with coarctation, occlusion, or aneurysmal dilation of the affected vessels
   (c) increased incidence in young males
   (d) coarctation of the abdominal aorta
   (e) aneurysmal dilation, irregularity, and occlusion of the small intrarenal branches of the renal artery

4. In the evaluation of patients with arterial trauma, which of the following statements are true?
   (a) the most common angiographic observation is spasm characterized by tapering and attenuation of vessels with delayed flow or occlusion
   (b) arteriovenous fistulas and false aneurysm may occur
   (c) the status of the peripheral pulses is a reliable indicator of the extent of vascular injury
   (d) active bleeding sites are identified as areas of extravasated contrast
   (e) arteriography should be avoided, because it can result in further vascular injury

5. In the performance of visceral arteriography, which of the following statements are correct?
   (a) mesenteric ischemia may manifest angiographically as diffuse, intense vasoconstriction of mesenteric vessels in the absence of atherosclerotic changes or embolic occlusion
   (b) in mesenteric ischemia, one observes atherosclerotic narrowing with thrombosis or emboli to major vessels
   (c) the best view for visualization for the origins of the celiac, superior mesenteric, and inferior mesenteric arteries is the anteroposterior view
   (d) major venous bleeding is easier to detect arteriographically than slow arterial bleeding
   (e) in order to visualize the portal venous system, direct portal venography with percutaneous splenic puncture or transhepatic portal vein puncture is usually necessary

6. In the radiographic evaluation of the spleen, which of the following statements are correct?
   (a) arteriography should be performed first in all cases of suspected splenic trauma
   (b) CT scans, radionuclide studies, and ultrasound are of little use in the evaluation of splenic injury
   (c) splenic artery aneurysms in females are benign and associated with a low incidence of rupture
   (d) none of the above

7. The single most characteristic finding in fibromuscular dysplasia is
   (a) complete occlusion of the renal artery
   (b) renal artery aneurysms
   (c) areas of narrowing alternating with areas of dilation in the main renal arteries
   (d) involvement of the renal artery origins
   (e) none of the above

8. Which of the following statements regarding intravenous digital angiography are true?
   (a) it is a useful technique for evaluating patients who are too uncooperative or unstable to undergo conventional selective arteriography
   (b) it provides better resolution than standard film-screen angiography
   (c) the risks of the procedure are low
   (d) it has its most useful application in evaluation of the small intracranial arteries
   (e) significantly lower volumes of x-ray contrast are used as compared to conventional arteriography

9. In which of the following patients is PTA most likely to be successful?
   (a) a 30-year-old female with fibromuscular disease of the renal arteries
   (b) an elderly patient with an atherosclerotic osteal stenosis of the renal artery
   (c) a patient with an 11-cm-long superficial femoral artery occlusion
   (d) a patient with a high-grade localized stenosis of the common iliac artery
   (e) an elderly patient with bilateral atherosclerotic renal artery stenosis

10. Which of the following statements regarding interventional angiography are accurate?

   (a) transcatheter embolization therapy is useful in the control of bleeding originating in the stomach
   (b) in the treatment of posttraumatic pelvic bleeding, embolization of both hypogastric arteries should not be performed
   (c) catheter retrieval of broken wires from the venous system is less preferable than operative removal
   (d) streptokinase and urokinase therapy are associated with a high incidence of thrombotic complications
   (e) in the treatment of congenital arteriovenous malformations, arteriography should be deferred until an attempt at surgical excision has been made

ANSWERS

1. c	2. a,b,c	3. b,d	4. a,b,d	5. a,b	6. d	7. c
8. c	9. a,d	10. a				

16

ENDOVASCULAR SURGERY

SAMUEL S. AHN

The recent development of angioscopy, balloon angioplasty, laser-assisted balloon angioplasty, mechanical atherectomy, and stents has created a new multidisciplinary field that we can aptly call endovascular surgery. This field can be defined as a diagnostic and therapeutic discipline that utilizes catheter-based systems delivered through a vascular site remote from a lesion, allowing the surgeon to treat the lesion from within the vascular system. This discipline encompasses the subspecialties of vascular surgery, interventional radiology, interventional cardiology, and biomedical engineering, and integrates the expertise of these subspecialties for the common purpose of treating peripheral arterial occlusive disease. Endovascular surgery thus provides important, less invasive adjuncts and alternatives to enhance and occasionally replace conventional vascular reconstructive procedures.

Although the concept of endovascular surgery has been known for many years, the field of endovascular surgery is relatively new. Dotter in 1969 and Gruntzig in 1974 popularized and developed transluminal balloon angioplasty to its modern form.[1,2] However, the limitations of balloon angioplasty in totally occluded lesions and the high restenosis rates soon became apparent and led to the concepts of laser vaporizing or mechanically ablating and removing obstructing plaque under direct vision. Thus emerged laser-assisted balloon angioplasty and mechanical atherectomy. The need for a guidance system subsequently led to the development of miniature vascular endoscopes and, most recently, intravascular ultrasound equipment. The disappointing early restenosis rates with lasers and mechanical devices have now focused investigators to evaluate mechanical and biological stents to prevent restenosis.

Thus, the field of endovascular surgery is still evolving, rapidly changing, and largely experimental. Other than conventional balloon angioplasty, most of the devices and techniques within this field are still unproven, and there are no formal training programs. Nevertheless, some of the limited success and the less invasive nature of these techniques have generated tremendous interest and research in this new field; and this neophyte discipline of endovascular surgery is likely to establish itself as standard medical practice in the 1990s.

The purpose of this chapter is to provide the reader with an introduction to the currently available technology and some of the preliminary clinical results of the various devices and procedures within the field of endovascular surgery—vascular endoscopy, intraoperative balloon angioplasty, laser angioplasty, atherectomy, and stents. It is beyond the scope of this chapter to cover all the developmental and research studies. For an in-depth coverage of these topics, the reader is referred to the textbook "Endovascular Surgery."[3]

VASCULAR ENDOSCOPY

Description of Equipment

Vascular endoscopy equipment consists of the following complementary parts: a flexible fiberoptic scope, a light source, an irrigation system, camera, video recorder, and monitor. Figure 16–1 shows the various components of such a system. The scope itself usually contains three separate components: the light bundle for viewing, the light bundle for illumination, and a transport channel for irrigation and/or manipulating instruments (see Fig. 16–2). Multiple vascular endoscopy systems are now commercially available and a brief description of each of these endoscopes is given in Table 16–1.

Indications

Perhaps the most useful indication for vascular endoscopy is to monitor thromboembolectomy and endarterectomy. White and others have clearly shown limitations of blind thromboendarterectomy (Table 16–2).[4–7] White and Vollmar have shown that vascular endoscopy is superior to conventional angiography for detecting residual intimal flaps following endarterectomy of the iliac artery.[4,8] Mehigan and

275

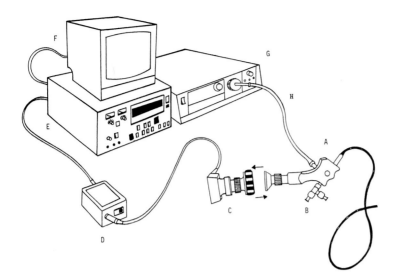

FIGURE 16–1. Components of an angioscopic system: *A*, angioscope; *B*, irrigation port; *C*, miniature camera; *D*, camera control unit; *E*, videocassette recorder; *F*, monitor; *G*, light source; *H*, light source cable. (From Hernández JJ, Quiñones-Baldrich WJ: Angioplasty: Essential, desirable, and optimal components. *In* Moore WS, Ahn SS (eds): Endovascular Surgery. Philadelphia, WB Saunders Company, 1989, pp 39–49.)

Olcott reported the potential benefits of angioscopically monitoring the completeness of carotid endarterectomy.[9]

Several investigators have also demonstrated the usefulness of vascular endoscopy to monitor the completeness of valvulotomy during in situ saphenous vein bypass grafting.[9–11] These investigators found retained valves by endoscopic examination following conventional blind valvulotomy. Matsumoto et al. also found vascular endoscopy useful for valvulotomy of nonreversed saphenous vein grafts.[12] Chin et al. recently proposed and developed an integrated angioscopy-valvulotomy system that allows valvulotomy under direct vision.[13]

Various investigators have reported a variety of other indications for vascular endoscopy, including inspection of vascular anastomosis, laser-assisted balloon angioplasty, and mechanical atherectomy.[10,14,15] Angioscopy can be useful for grabbing and retrieving organized clot, plaque, or even foreign bodies, using flexible grabbers transported through the working channel of an angioscope (Fig. 16–3).[16] Moreover, flexible biopsy-type cutters can cut residual intimal flaps under direct angioscopic view (Fig. 16–4).[16]

Technique

Vascular endoscopy is usually performed intraoperatively through an open arteriotomy. Proximal control of the inflow is obtained using a vascular clamp or a balloon catheter (Figs. 16–5 and 16–6). Distal back-bleeding can usually be controlled with irrigation injected into the scope. The endoscope may be placed directly into the artery, as shown in Figures 16–4 and 16–5, or may be placed through a standard introducer sheath with a hemostatic valve and a side-arm irrigation channel. Images can be visualized directly or recorded for later viewing. The availability of an irrigation pump or computerized digital an-

gioscopy equipment may enhance one's ability to obtain a satisfactory image, as well as avoiding fluid overload by the irrigation.

Results

White has reported residual thrombus after balloon embolectomy in almost all cases.[4] In approximately 80 per cent of 55 cases, the angioscopic findings led to further attempts at clot extraction. In our own experience at UCLA, we found residual thrombus or intimal flaps leading to altered management in 7 of 19 patients undergoing thrombectomy (S. S. Ahn, unpublished data, 1989). Grundfest et al.,[10] Mehigan and Olcott,[9] Fleisher et al.,[11] and Matsumoto et al.[12] have also reported visualization of retained valves that led to reintroduction of the valvulotome in a small but significant number of patients undergoing in situ saphenous vein bypass. Grundfest et al. have also reported anastomotic problems in 23 per cent of patients undergoing bypass procedures.[10] Olcott, however, noted very few intimal flaps or misplaced sutures in anastomotic inspections.[17] Less than 5 per cent of patients in Olcott's series required revision of the anastomosis. Our own experience at UCLA has been more consistent with Olcott's data, because we have found very few anastomotic problems following bypass surgery.

We found angioscopy beneficial to allow safe performance of mechanical atherectomy and to monitor its results (S. S. Ahn, unpublished data, 1989). Angioscopy was helpful in the placement of guidewires through the stenotic lesion and documentation of residual intimal flaps or thrombus following the procedure. Conventional angiography missed an intimal flap in one patient, and vascular endoscopy allowed placement of a guidewire in another patient in whom conventional angiographic guidance was inadequate.

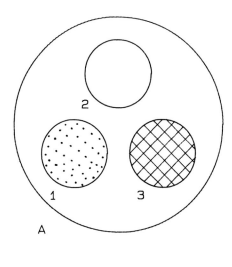

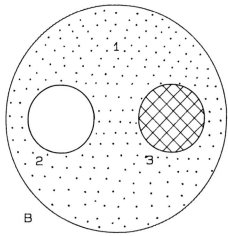

FIGURE 16–2. Light bundle patterns. *A,* A single channel (1) contains the light fibers; there are separate working/irrigation (2) and viewing (3) channels. *B,* Light fibers (1) are dispersed around the working and viewing channels (2 and 3). (From Hernández JJ, Quiñones-Baldrich WJ: Angioplasty: Essential, desirable, and optimal components. *In* Moore WS, Ahn SS (eds): Endovascular Surgery. Philadelphia, WB Saunders Company, 1989, pp 39–49.)

Limitations and Complications

Vascular endoscopy offers a direct, precise, descriptive color image of endovascular pathology, while requiring no contrast dye, no radiation, and no radiology technician. However, endoscopy is limited in its inability to visualize small runoff vessels, as well as the overall broad picture of the vascular tree. Furthermore, it is difficult to measure the percentage stenosis, unless one knows the focal length of the angioscope and the distance from the lesion to the lens. Images of a lumen visualized from a far distance may look quite small, whereas a lumen visualized close up may look quite large. Perhaps the most limiting disadvantage of angioscopy is the requirement for irrigation. Even small amounts of blood can blur or opacify the image. On the other hand, overzealous

or uncontrolled irrigation can lead to fluid overload and/or air embolus.

The irrigation pump is now available in many commercial products, and digital angioscopy is being continually refined to overcome the problem of irrigation.

Also, there is always the potential danger of injuring the vascular lumen by passing the scope into the vessel, particularly if the scope is too large for the artery. The late results of vascular endoscopy are not known, and thus potential injury-induced intimal hyperplasia cannot be completely ruled out at this time.

Finally, angioscopy may allow direct occlusion of the saphenous vein branches during in situ bypass. With further development, such a system could allow in situ saphenous vein bypass with only two incisions: one for the proximal and one for the distal anastomosis, respectively.

ENDOVASCULAR ULTRASONOGRAPHY

A whole new field of endovascular ultrasound is developing to supplement, and perhaps even replace, vascular endoscopy. Endovascular ultrasound has the advantage of not requiring any irrigation and giving more information regarding the plaque and arterial wall morphology.

The impetus for the use of endovascular ultrasonography (EU) stems from the information it provides about atherosclerotic plaque beneath the luminal surface. In 1989, using a 40-MHz ultrasound imaging device in an in vitro study, Gussenhoven et al.[18] showed that four components of atherosclerotic plaque could be distinguished by echogenicity. Lipid deposits were hyperechoic, fibromuscular tissue–casted soft echoes, fibrous tissue–elicited bright echoes, and calcification-caused bright echoes with shadowing. Soon after, Neville et al.[19] imaged 113 sheep arteries in vivo using ultrasound. The ultrasound images clearly demonstrated vessel wall architecture showing the intima, media, and adventitia as concentric layers around the echo-free lumen, thereby permitting the calculation of cross-sectional and thus the percentage stenosis. In a more recent study, Keren et al.[20] treated 18 patients for atherosclerotic vein grafts with different interventional procedures and assessed them with various imaging modalities. His in vivo study with humans revealed that EU was capable of examining transmural wall architecture, morphology of plaque subtypes, and the result of interventional procedures. Other early reports using EU in vascular surgery were favorable,[21,22] and predicted the expanded use of this technology as a guidance system for endovascular interventions. The Simpson atherectomy catheter, for example, has this technology integrated into its design to assist the surgeon in removing maximum atherosclerotic plaque without injuring the depths of the underlying media

TABLE 16–1. ANGIOSCOPY: OVERVIEW OF AVAILABLE INSTRUMENTS[a]

Manufacturer and Model	Scope		Fiberoptic System			Single Vs. Separate Unit	Channels (Irrigation Working)		Special Features
	Outer Diameter (mm)	Usable Length (cm)	Field of View	Depth (mm)	No. of Bundles (Pixels)				
Edwards LIS Inoperative (2 sizes)	2.3	80	70°	2–5	6000	Disposable separate	1.3 mm integrated		Disposable (potential lower cost)
	3.0	60	70°	2–15	6000	Disposable separate	1.5 mm integrated		
Percutaneous (2 sizes)	1.0	80	70°	2–15	6000	Reusable single	Forward flow irrigating holes		
	0.85	80	52°	2–15	2000	Reusable single	Forward flow irrigating holes		
Microvasive	6 F (2 mm)	60	90°	0.2–5	2000	Separate Visicath handle with scope; separate scope	Available: 0.6 mm, 0.9 mm		Cost-effective probe; small modular system; interchangeable probes
	8 F (2.5 mm)	60	90°	0.2–5	2000	Same as 6 F	Available: 1.1 mm		2 models (8100, 8300); 8300 available with battery pack for light source
	11 F (3.5 mm)	60	90°	0.2–5	2000	Same as 6 F	Available: 0.6 mm, 2.8 mm		Therapeutic accessories (forceps, snares, etc.)
AIS Scopecath	1.5 F (0.5 mm)	60	90°	0.2–5	2000	Single	Irrigation via coaxial catheter		Smallest diameter available for intraoperative use; coronary artery use; guidewire compatible for positioning; may use fluoroscopy for positioning
Olympus PF14	1.4	120	75°	2.1–00	32,000[b]	Single	NA	NA	Imaging only
PF22	2.2	120	75°	2.1–00	32,000	Single	NA	NA	Only scope available with steerability for acute angle vessel visualization (120° in one plane)
PF28	2.8	120	75°	2.1–00	32,000	Single	1.0 mm	NA	
Karl Storz	2.3	82	65°	1.0–00	10μ[c]	Single	0.3 mm integrated		Guidewire compatible for positioning
	3.0	82	60°	1.0–00	10μ[c]		1.2 mm integrated		In situ valvulotome; grasping and biopsy forceps for working channel
Trimedyne	2.8	105	55°	5.5–14	NA[d]	Separate optical lens and catheter	1.15 mm (additional cuff inflation channel)		

[a]From Hernández JJ, Quiñones-Baldrich WJ: Angioplasty: Essential, desirable, and optimal components. *In* Moore WS, Ahn SS (eds): Endovascular Surgery. Philadelphia, WB Saunders Company, 1989, pp 39–49.
[b]Specification as per manufacturer.
[c]Pixel number not specified.
[d]NA, not applicable.

TABLE 16–2. LIMITATIONS OF BLIND THROMBOEMBOLECTOMY[a]

Catheter injuries
 Vessel perforation
 Intimal tear or flap
 Subintimal dissection
 Rethrombosis
 Distal embolization
 Myointimal hyperplasia and arterial narrowing
Inadequate procedure
 Missed thrombus
 Adherent thrombus
 Side branch or small vessel thrombus
 Undetected atherosclerotic lesions
Absence of information
 No image
 No flow data
 No pressure measurement
Problems of angiographic control
 Time consuming
 Postprocedural monitoring only
 Requirement for equipment and technician
 Poor quality of intraoperative angiograms
 Radiation exposure to patient and staff
 Patient exposure to contrast medium
  Anaphylaxis
  Renal failure

[a]From White GF: Angioscopy to monitor arterial thromboembolectomy. *In* Moore WS, Ahn SS (eds): Endovascular Surgery. Philadelphia, WB Saunders Company, 1989, pp 55–64.

and adventitia. To date, three major applications have emerged: the diagnosis of complex arterial pathology, the guidance of intraluminal instruments, and the assessment of the outcomes of endovascular interventions.[23]

However, currently, ultrasonography is limited by the fact that the ultrasound probe must first cross the lesion and can only give a cross-section of the artery at any one point at any one time. Also, most systems are not steerable. Perhaps further developments of three-dimensional digital reproduction of the ultrasound image may overcome some of these problems. Ultrasonography has the potential to become a useful adjunct to conventional angiography, particularly in detecting posterior plaques in the iliac artery not readily visualized on conventional anteroposterior views. The ultrasound may also help de-termine the completeness of mechanical atherectomy and laser angioplasty.[24]

INTRAOPERATIVE BALLOON ANGIOPLASTY

Percutaneous balloon angioplasty is already covered in detail in another chapter in this textbook, and thus will not be covered in this chapter. This section will deal briefly with the technique of intraoperative balloon angioplasty.

Differences Between Percutaneous Balloon Angioplasty and Intraoperative Balloon Angioplasty

Intraoperative transluminal angioplasty differs from percutaneous balloon angioplasty in several ways.[25] Perhaps the most important difference is that intraoperative balloon angioplasty is used in patients with more severe and advanced peripheral vascular disease. Patients undergoing intraoperative balloon angioplasty often have multilevel and diffuse disease treated by simultaneous conventional vascular procedures in addition to the adjunctive balloon angioplasty. Percutaneous balloon angioplasty, on the other hand, is usually limited to single-level disease in patients with claudication. The second main difference is that intraoperative balloon angioplasty is performed as an adjunctive procedure in the operating room during vascular reconstruction, whereas percutaneous balloon angioplasty is a primary treatment performed in a radiology suite. Currently, the fluoroscopic equipment in most operating rooms is inferior to the equipment found in the radiology suites. Perhaps the most useful equipment in the operating room is the more modern, portable, digital C-arm units. Finally, the maintenance of sterility becomes much more important in the operating room, since the patient has an open wound. The problem of sterility becomes even more important if a synthetic graft is being implanted, such as an aortobifemoral bypass graft. Otherwise, the balloon angioplasty catheters, guidewires, and introducer sheaths are

FIGURE 16–3. Artist's conception of a flexible grabbing catheter inserted through a vascular endoscope to retrieve a piece of organized clot or plaque particle. (From Ahn SS: The use of grabbers, cutters, and shavers as an adjunct during endovascular surgery. *In* Moore WS, Ahn SS (eds): Endovascular Surgery. Philadelphia, WB Saunders Company, 1989, pp 514–517.)

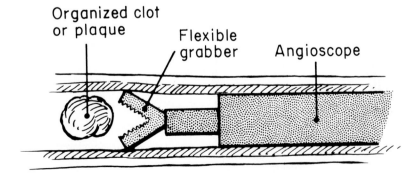

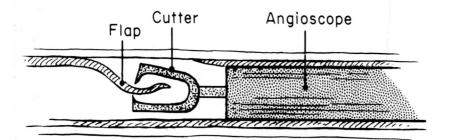

FIGURE 16–4. Artist's conception of a flexible cutter with sharp, piranha-like jaws passed through the vascular endoscope to cut an intimal flap. (From Ahn SS: The use of grabbers, cutters, and shavers as an adjunct during endovascular surgery. *In* Moore WS, Ahn SS (eds): Endovascular Surgery. Philadelphia, WB Saunders Company, 1989, pp 514–517.)

similar for both intraoperative and percutaneous balloon angioplasty.

INDICATIONS

As a general rule, most adjunctive balloon angioplasty procedures should be performed percutaneously before or after standard surgical revascularization. This applies to inflow as well as outflow lesions. Staged preoperative balloon angioplasty of an inflow lesion allows observation of the treated site to ensure that the balloon angioplasty procedure is successful before embarking upon a distal outflow bypass procedure. However, in certain situations, intraoperative balloon angioplasty may serve as an important adjunctive procedure.

Perhaps the most common indication for intra-operative balloon angioplasty is the presence of a clinically suspected, but angiographically undocumented, iliac artery stenosis or the presence of an unsuspected iliac artery stenosis in the presence of a totally occluded superficial femoral artery (Fig. 16–7). In this situation, intraoperative measurement of the femoral artery pressure, in the presence of a vasodilator, can unmask an iliac inflow lesion, which can then be treated with intraoperative balloon angioplasty as an adjunct to a femoropopliteal bypass procedure. Similarly, a balloon angioplasty of a donor iliac artery may be performed during a femorofemoral crossover bypass graft (Fig. 16–8). Furthermore, on occasion, retrograde intraoperative balloon angioplasty of a superficial femoral artery stenosis may allow the superficial femoral artery to serve as an important inflow artery to allow a shorter bypass graft distally (Fig. 16–9). This intraoperative dila-

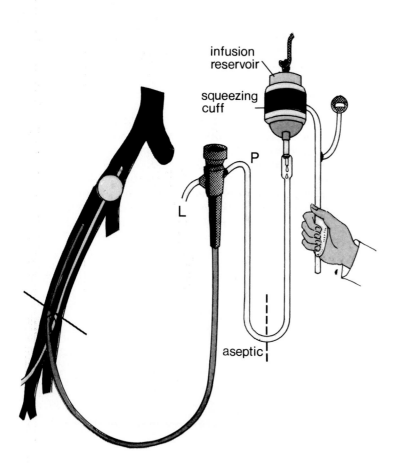

FIGURE 16–5. Principle of arterial endoscopy at the iliac level using a flexible type B endoscope introduced from a distal arteriotomy at the common femoral artery. Continuous saline perfusion is provided under controlled pressure. L, Cold light connection; P, perfusion line. (From Vollmar JF, Hutschenreiter JF: Vascular endoscopy for thromboendarterectomy. *In* Moore WS, Ahn SS (eds): Endovascular Surgery. Philadelphia, WB Saunders Company, 1989, pp 87–94.)

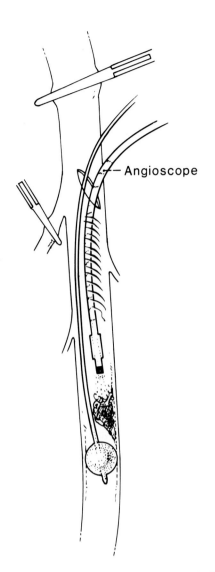

FIGURE 16–6. Standard technique of angioscopic thromboembolectomy, with a Fogarty balloon catheter inserted alongside the angioscope, allowing visualization of the thrombectomy process. (From White GH, et al: Angioscopic thromboembolectomy: Preliminary observations with a recent technique. J Vasc Surg 7:495–499, 1988.)

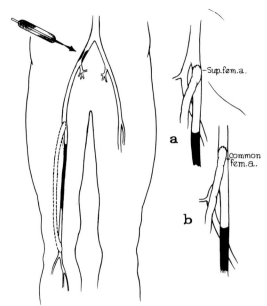

FIGURE 16–7. Iliac artery operative transluminal angioplasty (OpTA) enhances inflow to a femorodistal bypass. *a*, Graft originating from the superficial femoral artery; *b*, graft originating from the common femoral artery. (From Andros G, Harris RW, Salles-Cunha SX: Technique of intraoperative balloon angioplasty. *In* Moore WS, Ahn SS (eds): Endovascular Surgery. Philadelphia, WB Saunders Company, 1989, pp 209–222.)

tation is particularly indicated when available vein is insufficient to complete a long femoral distal bypass.

Intraoperative balloon angioplasty can also serve to augment outflow for a variety of inflow procedures to the common femoral artery, including an aortobifemoral bypass graft (Fig. 16–10), a femorofemoral bypass graft (Fig. 16–11), and a femoral endarterectomy (Fig. 16–12), in the presence of a superficial femoral artery stenosis. Similarly, improved outflow for a femoropopliteal bypass can be achieved by dilating a popliteal artery stenosis (Fig. 16–13) or a tibial artery stenosis (Fig. 16–14). Adjunctive balloon angioplasty of an obstructive popliteal or tibial artery may allow an above-knee femoropopliteal bypass, rather than a below-knee or tibial bypass.

Fogarty et al. recently reported the importance of treating underlying atherosclerotic occlusive disease following thrombectomy for acute arterial occlusion.[26] Thus, following intraoperative thrombectomy or thrombolytic therapy, the presence of residual occlusive disease, which may have incited the thrombosis in the first place, is an indication for intraoperative balloon angioplasty.

Techniques

Generally, the standard revascularization procedure is performed first, but not completed. One of the anastomotic sites is left incompletely finished to serve as the entry site for the balloon angioplasty catheters. This site is most frequently the common femoral artery. With the femoral anastomosis nearly completed, a standard introducer sheath is introduced proximally or distally, depending upon the site of the proposed dilatation. A snare is placed around the introducer sheath to prevent bleeding. The introducer sheath has a self-sealing valve that prevents blood loss during multiple passages of guidewires and catheters. The sheath also has a sidearm to allow intraoperative angiography to guide positioning of the balloon catheters and to allow completion angiograms. A standard guidewire is passed through the introducer sheath and directed past the stenotic lesion. Then an appropriately sized balloon angioplasty catheter is passed over the guidewire to the site of the obstructive lesion and balloon dilata-

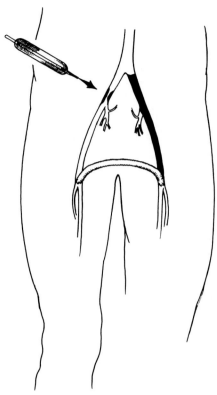

FIGURE 16–8. Iliac balloon operative transluminal angioplasty (OpTA) provides inflow to a femorofemoral bypass. (From Andros G, Harris RW, Salles-Cunha SX: Technique of intraoperative balloon angioplasty. *In* Moore WS, Ahn SS (eds): Endovascular Surgery. Philadelphia, WB Saunders Company, 1989, pp 209–222.)

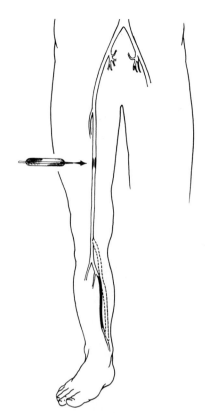

FIGURE 16–9. Adjunctive (retrograde) inflow operative transluminal angioplasty (OpTA) of the superficial femoral artery followed by distal bypass to the paramalleolar posterior tibial artery below the dilated segment (From Andros G, Harris RW, Salles-Cunha SX: Technique of intraoperative balloon angioplasty. *In* Moore WS, Ahn SS (eds): Endovascular Surgery. Philadelphia, WB Saunders Company, 1989, pp 209–222.)

tion takes place in the standard fashion. Following successful balloon angioplasty, the artery is flushed with heparin irrigation and the anastomosis is then completed.

Results

The results of intraoperative balloon angioplasty are mostly anecdotal and difficult to evaluate. The simultaneously performed intraoperative balloon angioplasty results are often intermingled with the results of sequential balloon angioplasty and vascular reconstruction. Furthermore, the more recent series have very short follow-up and the data are inherently difficult to interpret because of the difficulty of separating the effects of the balloon dilatation procedure and the standard revascularization bypass procedure. Nevertheless, there have been many anecdotal reports of success using this procedure, as summarized by Andros et al.[25]

Limitations and Complications

To quote Andros et al., "The greatest pitfalls of operative balloon angioplasty are not technical, but strategic."[25] First of all, it is important to limit the

procedure to selected cases in which the adjunctive angioplasty is indicated and not meddlesome. Failure of an iliac balloon angioplasty site can lead to permanent loss of an otherwise satisfactory femoropopliteal vein bypass. Furthermore, acute occlusion or dissection of a superficial femoral artery stenosis balloon angioplasty site can jeopardize a successful inflow bypass procedure that might otherwise have adequately revascularized the limb by an adequate profundoplasty. Second, it is important to limit the time of arterial occlusion of the balloon-dilated site. The freshly dilated site is often quite thrombogenic, with intimal flaps and dissection that may acutely thrombose in the absence of high blood flow. It is important to perform the standard bypass vascular procedure first, so that the balloon-dilated artery may be exposed to flow immediately following the balloon procedure. These pitfalls reemphasize the preference of attempting preoperative, rather than concomitant intraoperative, balloon dilatation as an adjunct to vascular bypass.

Other complications of intraoperative balloon angioplasty are similar to percutaneous balloon angioplasty: acute occlusion, distal emboli, balloon rupture, arterial rupture, and groin hematomas. On the other hand, surgically exposing the artery, using the

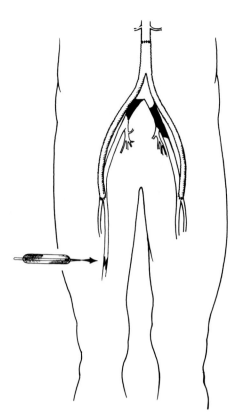

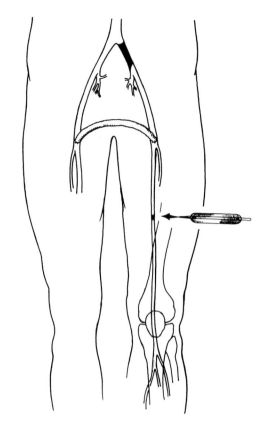

FIGURE 16–10. Operative transluminal angioplasty (OpTA) of a superficial femoral artery stenosis to increase outflow from an aortobifemoral bypass. (From Andros G, Harris RW, Salles-Cunha SX: Technique of intraoperative balloon angioplasty. *In* Moore WS, Ahn SS (eds): Endovascular Surgery. Philadelphia, WB Saunders Company, 1989, pp 209–222.)

FIGURE 16–11. Femorofemoral graft with adjunctive outflow balloon angioplasty of the superficial femoral artery on the recipient limb. (From Andros G, Harris RW, Salles-Cunha SX: Technique of intraoperative balloon angioplasty. *In* Moore WS, Ahn SS (eds): Endovascular Surgery. Philadelphia, WB Saunders Company, 1989, pp 209–222.)

open technique under controlled situations, may decrease the frequency of these complications.

Future Directions

Despite its limited indications, intraoperative balloon angioplasty is an important option with which all vascular surgeons should be familiar. Transluminal balloon angioplasty is now a well-established procedure and will likely remain so for some time. Eventually, it may well be replaced by laser or atherectomy devices. However, further refinements in these new technologies must occur before balloon angioplasty is replaced. Furthermore, improvements in guidewires, particularly the Terumo guidewire, have improved the efficacy of transluminal balloon angioplasty for tighter stenosis and even total occlusion.

The technique of transluminal balloon angioplasty requires special skills, expertise, and experience that many surgeons may not have. The surgeon should either gain the experience or, preferably, call an interventional radiology colleague into the operating room to help with the balloon dilatation procedure. A cooparative effort is most likely to lead to optimal results.

LASER ANGIOPLASTY

Basic Concepts

As of this writing, laser angioplasty is actually laser-assisted balloon angioplasty. The laser is used to recanalize a totally obstructed artery, thereby creating a pilot channel through which a guidewire and balloon angioplasty system can be delivered. The final recanalization is achieved by dilating the artery, using standard balloon angioplasty techniques.

The mechanism of laser recanalization involves several factors. The first and most widely viewed mechanism is vaporization. In actuality, very little vaporization probably takes place.[27] Vaporization occurs when rapid heating of the water content within the individual cells leads to rapid boiling and expansion, causing an explosion that disrupts the cell. This explosion produces particles that are mostly 0.3 mm in size, but occasionally as large as 1 mm in size.[28] The common denominator in this mechanism is conversion of laser light to heat and thermal energy.

The second and perhaps an equally if not more important factor is the direct mechanical effect of the laser fiber or probe. Simple pushing of the fiber probe will lead to a Dotter effect; that is, mechanical dila-

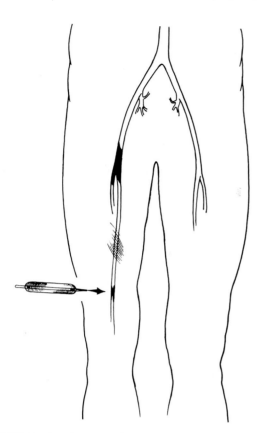

FIGURE 16–12.   Common, deep, and proximal superficial femoral artery endarterectomy with complementary intraoperative balloon angioplasty of the midsuperficial femoral artery outflow tract. (From Andros G, Harris RW, Salles-Cunha SX: Technique of intraoperative balloon angioplasty. *In* Moore WS, Ahn SS (eds): Endovascular Surgery. Philadelphia, WB Saunders Company, 1989, pp 209–222.)

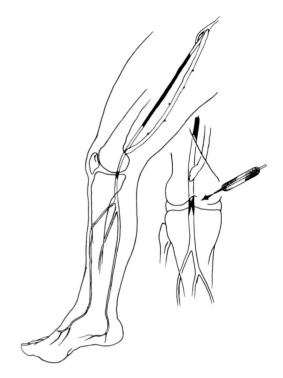

FIGURE 16–13.   Operative transluminal angioplasty (OpTA) of the midpopliteal stenosis allows a femoropopliteal bypass to terminate above the knee. (From Andros G, Harris RW, Salles-Cunha SX: Technique of intraoperative balloon angioplasty. *In* Moore WS, Ahn SS (eds): Endovascular Surgery. Philadelphia, WB Saunders Company, 1989, pp 209–222.)

tation. The laser energy may well facilitate this process in much the same way that butter or ice cream is cut easier by a heated or moist knife than by a cold, dry knife. One should note that the laser fibers and probes themselves are designed to be efficient, streamlined, tapered, probing catheters capable of recanalizing without the laser even being turned on (Figs. 16–15, 16–16, and 16–17). The excimer, or so-called cold laser, also produces a photo-decomposition reaction, leading to breakage in molecular bonds.[29]

There are now several laser systems available for laser-assisted balloon angioplasty. These include the hot thermal metal tip made by Trimedyne, HGM, Xintec; the sapphire thermal-tip laser by SLT; a direct laser fiber and balloon system by GV Medical; the multifiber coaxial system by USCI and AIS; the angioscopy-directed argon laser system by Medilase; the computer-guided dye laser made by MCM; and, the so-called nonthermal laser.

Description of Equipment

Thermal Metal Probe

The prototype of the metal thermal probe is the Trimedyne hot-tip, which is a 2.0-mm diameter, ol-

ive-shaped, metal tip that is heated by an argon continuous-wave laser (Fig. 16–15). The metal tip typically reaches 1000°C in air and 300° to 600°C in tissue, depending on the thermal conductivity of the tissue.[30] There is also a 2.5-mm diameter tip that uses continuous-wave argon and, more recently, continuous-wave neodymium: yttrium-aluminum-garnet (Nd:YAG) (Fig. 16–16). There is also a hybrid probe, or the so-called spectraprobe, which has an aperture at its tip that allows 20 per cent of the laser energy to escape directly as a laser light (Fig. 16–17). This combination gives direct laser energy recanalization followed by a thermal hot-tip that partially dilates the arterial lumen.

Optical Thermal Probes

The optical thermal probes include the sapphire tips and the quartz balls. First used in the gastrointestinal tract, the laser-heated tips have been modified for the vascular system. Artificial sapphire is a monocrystalline form of aluminum oxide, which is a physiologically neutral crystal with great mechanical strength, low thermal conductivity, and a high melting temperature (2050°C).[31] The device is round or oval in shape and acts as a divergent lens with an angle of 22 degrees and a focus of 2 mm when a 2.2-mm diameter sapphire is used. The power density is high, with maximal effect at the focus. Thus, it has been hypothesized that light energy with a short focal

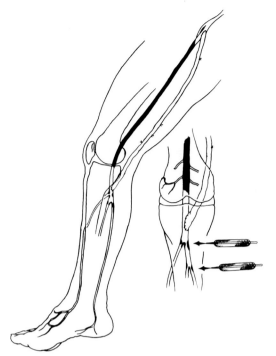

FIGURE 16–14. Femoropopliteal bypass obtaining improved outflow with infrapopliteal operative transluminal angioplasty (OpTA). (From Andros G, Harris RW, Salles-Cunha SX: Technique of intraoperative balloon angioplasty. *In* Moore WS, Ahn SS (eds): Endovascular Surgery. Philadelphia, WB Saunders Company, 1989, pp 209–222.)

length comes out directly from the sapphire tip, giving direct laser energy as well as a hot sapphire tip.

Excimer Laser

The excimer laser utilizes a halogen and a noble gas as the medium to generate laser light, and there are many types of excimer lasers, based on the type of gas used. The four most important excimer gases are argon fluoride, krypton fluoride, xenon fluoride, and xenon chloride. All of these gases produce a short-wavelength ultraviolet laser light. Perhaps the most studied system in vascular surgery is the 308-nm xenon chloride laser, which has been used with a pulse duration of 10 to 250 nsec, high energy per pulse (up to 1000 mJ/sq mm, 3.8 eV/photon), and a high-quality output beam.[32] This laser energy is delivered on a flexible quartz fiber, measuring 200 to 600 μm in diameter. There is also a multifiber, over-the-wire system using seven separate 200-μm fibers (Fig. 16–18). The laser machine itself is approximately the size of a refrigerator and is transportable.

Computer-Guided Laser

The prototype of a computer-guided system is the dual laser system made by MCM Laboratories (Mountain View, CA). This system incorporates real-time laser-excited fluorescence spectroscopic plaque recognition with subsequent pulsed-dye laser tissue ablation (Fig. 16–19).[33]

The diagnostic portion of the system consists of a shuttered 324-nm helium-cadmium laser operating at 3.0 to 5.0 mW. This low energy does not allow spectroanalysis of a characteristic fluorescent pattern intrinsically inherent to atherosclerotic plaque. A computer analyzes this spectrofluorescence pattern using algorithms that have been tested in vivo and in vitro. If the spectra pattern fits the algorithm parameters consistent with plaque, then the computer instructs a second treatment laser to activate or fire.

The treatment laser consists of a 480-nm flashlamp-excited dye laser capable of generating high energies (up to 1 joule) during short pulses (2 μsec). This cycle of the spectroanalysis of the diagnostic laser and the firing of the treatment laser is completed in approximately 100 msec and the system is operated to perform this repetitive cycle at 5 Hz or 5/sec. Both the diagnostic and treatment lasers are coupled to a single 200- or 500-μm fused silica optical fiber, and both lasers travel along the same optical pathway and are transmitted by the same common optical fiber. The laser system itself is approximately the size of a large horizontal freezer, and is transportable.

Angioscopically Guided Laser

The prototype of an angioscopy-guided laser is made by GV Medical, the so-called Medilase system. A laser fiber runs coaxially within the angioscopy catheter sheath. Ideally, the lesion is visualized using the optical fibers, and then the laser is activated under

FIGURE 16–15. The 2.0-mm diameter thermal probe (From Cumberland DC, Crew JR, Myler RK, et al: Clinical laser-assisted angioplasty using the thermal laser probe and the hybrid laser probe: Techniques, results, and indications. *In* Moore WS, Ahn SS (eds): Endovascular Surgery. Philadelphia, WB Saunders Company, 1989, pp 393–401.)

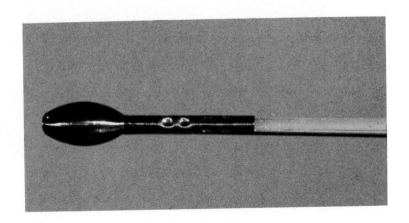

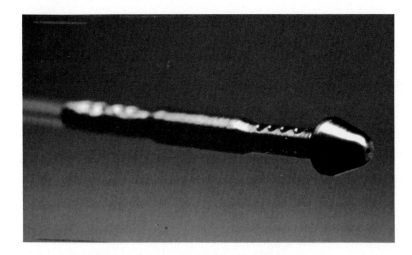

FIGURE 16–16. The 2.5-mm diameter spectraprobe. (From Cumberland DC, Crew JR, Myler RK, et al: Clinical laser-assisted angioplasty using the thermal probe and the hybrid laser probe: Techniques, results, and indications. *In* Moore WS, Ahn SS (eds): Endovascular Surgery. Philadelphia, WB Saunders Company, 1989, pp 393–401.)

direct vision. The laser fiber is eccentrically placed so that reflection of the tip allows the laser to treat more than one spot. The system utilizes a continuous-wave argon laser that is approximately the size of a small desk, and thus is easily transportable.

Indications

The indications for laser-assisted balloon angioplasty are the same as those for any other vascular procedure: limb-threatening ischemia or severe disabling claudication. The number of patients among this group who actually require laser treatment is probably quite small; those with stenotic lesions generally do not need the laser at all. Lasers are usually reserved for totally obstructive lesions, the majority of which the guidewire now can usually cross. Furthermore, the laser energy does not necessarily have to be turned on at all. The laser hot-tips are constructed in an ideal fashion to penetrate a total obstruction using simple mechanical forces. Ginsburg, for instance, found that the guidewire successfully traversed 92 per cent totally occluded arteries in 33 patients.[34] The laser probe was required only seven

times and in four of these seven cases, the laser probe was used successfully without activating the laser energy. In the remaining three patients, the laser-activated hot-tip was successful in only one case. Thus, overall, the indications for laser use are quite limited and reserved for the occasional lesion that cannot be traversed by a standard guidewire. Finally, the laser should be used in lesions that are shorter than 7 to 10 cm. Results in lesions longer than 10 cm have been quite disappointing and such lesions should be treated with conventional bypass surgery.

Techniques

Access to the artery is obtained in the standard fashion, as described previously under balloon angioplasty. The percutaneous approach is usually performed through the common femoral artery. The open approach also utilizes the common femoral, rather than the superficial femoral artery. The common femoral artery may be punctured under direct vision, or a small arteriotomy can be made to allow introduction of a no. 7- to 9-French sheath. A transverse arteriotomy is made if the patient is undergoing the laser

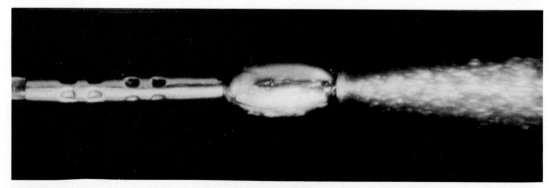

FIGURE 16–17. A 2-mm hybrid laser probe. The probe consists of a 300-μm core optical fiber with a 2-mm elliptical metal sleeve crimped onto the fiber cladding. An argon laser beam (1 watt) is seen exiting at a 15-degree angle. (From Seeger JM, Abela GS: Angioplasty using argon laser energy and fiberoptic laser probes. *In* Moore WS, Ahn SS (eds): Endovascular Surgery. Philadelphia, WB Saunders Company, 1989, pp 408–418.)

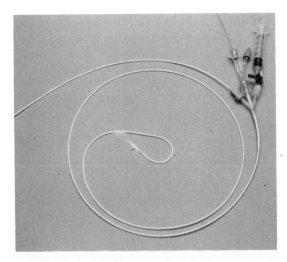

FIGURE 16–18. A multifiber excimer laser angioplasty catheter. This prototype over-the-wire catheter contains seven 200-μm fibers wrapped concentrically around an 0.018-inch movable guidewire. This prototype was used initially for recanalization of stenoses in peripheral vessels. (From Grundfest W, Litvack F, Papaioannou T, et al: Excimer laser angioplasty: From basic science to clinical trials. *In* Moore WS, Ahn SS (eds): Endovascular Surgery. Philadelphia, WB Saunders Company, 1989, pp 432–441.)

The catheter tip is carefully positioned to be as close to the center of the occlusion as possible. The laser is then activated at 5 to 10 watts, depending upon the unit used, and very gentle pressure is applied to the catheter. Care must be taken not to push the catheter too vigorously, or perforation will occur. If the fiber tip sticks to the lesion, the catheter can be released by activating the laser briefly while gently pulling back on the catheter. Serial angiograms are performed through the introducer sheath during the lasing procedure to check the progress. Although the exact relationship between the laser catheter and the arterial wall cannot be precisely identified, alignment of the distal runoff artery and the proximal segment of the artery will allow fairly accurate determination of the catheter position in relationship to the artery. After the occlusive lesion has been crossed, standard balloon angioplasty techniques are used to then enlarge the channel to its full diameter. After the procedure is completed, antiplatelet and/or anticoagulant therapy is given. We have found routine heparinization for 24 hours to be quite helpful in preventing early thrombosis. Any intraoperative thrombosis found can be treated with thrombolytic therapy intraarterially.

treatment alone, whereas a vertical arteriotomy is made if the patient is also undergoing a simultaneous vascular reconstruction. Through the introducer sheath, the laser probe or fiber is then advanced to the obstructed lesion under fluoroscopic guidance.

Results

Cumberland et al., in 1986, reported initial success in 50 of 56 cases, or 89 per cent initial success rate,

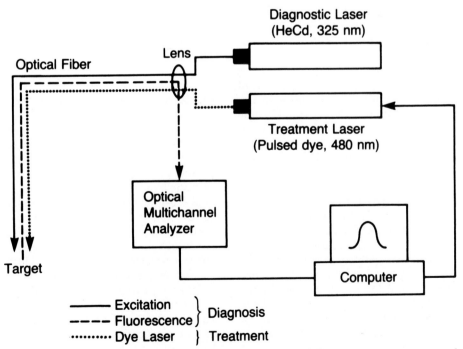

FIGURE 16–19. Dual laser system incorporating diagnostic laser-excited fluorescence spectroscopy and pulsed dye laser tissue ablation. (From Leon MD, Geschwind HJ: Fluorescence-guided laser-assisted balloon angioplasty in peripheral vascular disease. *In* Moore WS, Ahn SS (eds): Endovascular Surgery. Philadelphia, WB Saunders Company, 1989, pp 466–475.)

in their initial clinical trials using the metal thermal hot-tip.[35] These initially promising results, however, were subsequently duplicated by other investigators only in short lesions (less than 3 cm) and in stenotic lesions. In 1988, Greenfield and Sanborn subsequently reported their update results, which showed a 95 to 100 per cent success rate in stenotic lesions and total occlusions shorter than 3 cm, but only a 70 per cent initial success rate in lesions 3 to 7 cm and 67 per cent success in lesions more than 7 cm in length.[36] The long-term patency in this group of patients was similar to that of balloon angioplasty: 90 per cent 1-year patency for the stenotic lesions and lesions shorter than 3 cm, 75 per cent 1-year patency for lesions 4 to 7 cm, and less than 60 per cent 1-year patency for lesions longer than 7 cm.

More recent experiences with the thermal metal probe have been even more disappointing. Harrington et al., at the June 1989 meeting of the International Society for Cardiovascular Surgery, reported their results using the thermal hot-tip in 72 limbs with totally occluded arteries.[37] Their initial success rate was 82 per cent but, at the time of discharge, only 43 of 72 (60 per cent) of the limbs showed clinical improvement. By 4 months, only 31 of 72 limbs (43 per cent) showed continued clinical improvement. Wright et al., from the same group of investigators, reported the results of thermal hot-tip angioplasty in patients with limb salvage situations.[38] They were initially successful in only 10 of 15 cases. Within 6 months, 9 of these 10 successfully treated cases had failed, and thus, overall, 14 of 15 patients had unsuccessful results by 6 months. Perler et al. recently reported an overall success rate of only 21 of 47 (45 per cent) and found that the lesions longer than 7 cm had the worst results.[39] Their overall long-term follow-up revealed only a 30 per cent clinical success rate at 1 year.

Results using the hybrid argon laser hot-tip have been no better. Seeger et al. reported a 77 per cent initial recanalization rate, but only a 48 per cent immediate clinical success rate in 46 patients.[40] Of note is that there is a 20 per cent perforation rate. Their long-term results have not been reported to date.

Lammer and Pilger recently reported the Austrian Multi-Center Trial results using the SLT Nd:YAG sapphire contact probe in 384 patients.[41,42] Seventy per cent of the patients had claudication and the lesions were 2 to 26 cm in length of totally occluded superficial femoral artery (mean 8 cm). Their primary success rate was 81 per cent. Among the successfully treated patients, the 1-year patency was 79 per cent, the 2-year patency 73 per cent, and the 3-year patency 75 per cent. Thus, among the 384 patients initially treated with the sapphire contact probe, only 64 per cent of the patients had clinical patency at 1 year. Of note is that there was a 12 per cent dissection or perforation rate in this trial.

Lammer also reported in a previous study that the results in 250 patients were unsatisfactory in lesions longer than 15 cm.[43] Fourrier et al. reported initial success in 16 of 20 patients.[44] Failures were due to arterial wall perforation and arterial wall dissection. However, by 3-month follow-up, only 10 of the original 20 patients had continued success.

The results for excimer laser–assisted balloon angioplasty have been similar. Grundfest et al. reported initial success in seven of nine patients with stenotic lesions and 17 of 22 patients with total occlusions.[32] Subintimal dissection or perforation by the excimer laser fiber occurred in five cases. Fortunately, these complications caused no direct adverse results. Long-term follow-up revealed restenosis in 7 of 30 patients with a follow-up of 9.1 ± 3 months.

Nordstrom has recently reported initial 1-year follow-up results using the direct argon, angioscopy-guided laser, the GV Medical Medilase.[45] The initial success rate was 59 of 68 cases (87 per cent). The results in iliac arteries were 10 of 14 (71 per cent) and in the superficial femoral artery were 49 of 54 (91 per cent). Three thermal perforations occurred. Life-table analysis revealed a 1-year cumulative patency rate of 75 per cent overall; patency rates for the iliac lesions were 75 per cent, for femoropopliteal stenosis 91 per cent, and for femoropopliteal occlusion 71 per cent. These patency rates are applied to 59 of the original 68 patients who had initial success.

Geschwind et al. have the largest series, using the MCM computer-guided Smart laser (H. J. Geschwind, personal communication, 1989). The preliminary results on 53 patients showed an initial success rate of 85 per cent (45 of 53). Of these 45 patients, 42 (93 per cent) underwent subsequent successful balloon angioplasty, for an overall initial success rate of 42 of 53 (79 per cent) for the total group. There was a 9 per cent failure rate due to mechanical complications (the inability to negotiate the laser wire in the proper channel). Long-term results are not available as of this writing.

Limitations and Complications

It is interesting to note that the overall results using laser-assisted balloon angioplasty are no better than balloon angioplasty alone. Zeitler et al. in 1983 reported almost 3000 cases with very similar results for stenotic as well as total occlusive lesions.[46] Johnston et al.[47] and Sampson et al.[48] also reported very similar results using balloon angioplasty techniques alone treating occlusive as well as stenotic lesions. The similarity of results using balloon angioplasty alone versus laser-assisted balloon angioplasty is probably due to the fact that the laser angioplasty still requires final enlargement using balloon angioplasty techniques.

Laser-assisted balloon angioplasty also carries the additional complication of arterial wall perforation and/or dissection, which occurs in approximately 3 to 12 per cent of cases.[28–45] Furthermore, the usual complications of groin hematoma and/or wound infection of standard balloon angioplasty still persists. Embolic complications occur in 1 to 3 per cent of cases. Particles up to 1 mm can result from the laser vaporization, as described previously. Hard, calcified plaque is always difficult for lasers to penetrate. Calcified plaque contains hydroxyapatite, which has a melting point of 1800°C, and thus is resistant to laser thermal ablation. The excimer laser, which uses photodecompensation mechanisms, has had some success in cutting through calcified plaques. Finally, as in balloon angioplasty results, the longer lesions have poor immediate and long-term results. The best results appear to be in those lesions less than 7 cm in length.

Future Developments

Numerous laser companies are currently developing methods to enlarge the laser probe and laser beam surface coverage so that balloon angioplasty will no longer be needed. However, so far, these larger probes have caused more thermal damage and higher perforation rates and have not improved long-term patencies. Nevertheless, the trials are still early and further results are needed to evaluate the potential of laser angioplasty alone. Other investigators are looking at photodynamic therapy to enhance the specificity of laser angioplasty.[49,50] Various compounds are taken up preferentially by atherosclerotic plaque and can be selectively ablated using specific wavelengths of light. Photodynamic therapy is currently limited by delivery of the compound to the plaque in a clinically efficacious manner, while avoiding the systemic phototoxicity. Furthermore, blood products absorb the laser lights that are currently used, and thus the arterial lumen has to be cleared of blood completely prior to treatment. Moreover, there are no conclusive data that such a selective ablation will reduce the long-term restenosis rate.

Other investigators are looking at cheaper and simpler ways of heating metal tips to perform thermal angioplasty without using lasers. Radiofrequency and chemical reaction energy have been used so far.[51,52]

It is clear that current laser-assisted balloon angioplasty techniques must undergo a metamorphosis before laser angioplasty can become a routine vascular procedure.

PERIPHERAL ATHERECTOMY

Basic Concepts

Atherectomy is the selective removal of atheroma from atherosclerotic diseased arteries performed percutaneously or through a small arteriotomy remote from the disease site. Such a procedure offers three theoretical advantages over standard balloon angioplasty dilatation: (1) greater immediate success rate with less intimal dissection and occlusion; (2) wider application of endovascular technology to lesions currently not readily amenable to percutaneous balloon angioplasty (i.e., diffusely diseased vessels or

totally occluded lesions); and (3) reduction of the restonosis rate as a result of the debulking of the atheromatous mass.[53] The appeal of such theoretical benefits has led to the development and investigation of at least 12 different atherectomy devices, each with unique features that offer certain advantages and disadvantages over the other. This section will describe four atherectomy devices that have undergone preliminary clinical trials and are commercially available now or will be in the very near future. This includes the Simpson Atherocath, the Theratek Trac-Wright Catheter, the Auth Rotablator, and the Transluminal Extraction Catheter.

Simpson Atherocath

Device Description

The Simpson peripheral atherectomy catheter (Simpson Atherocath; Devices for Vascular Intervention Inc., Redwood City, CA) is a semiflexible catheter with a distal housing unit that contains a cutter, retrieval chamber, and opposing balloon (Fig. 16–20). A floppy, shapable guidewire is attached to the distal tip of this housing unit to allow the operator to advance and partially steer the catheter. Inflation of the balloon engages the longitudinal side opening of the housing unit into the atheroma. A cup-shaped cutter driven by a battery powered, hand-held motor device then slices the plaque. The plaque is then pushed into the collecting chamber in the distal tip. The cutters spin at approximately 2000 RPM. The catheters are available in nos. 7-, 8-, 9-, 10-, and 11-French sizes. The cutting windows are available in two sizes, 15 and 20 mm.

Technique

Figure 16–21 illustrates the procedure. The atherectomy catheter must first advance past the stenotic lesion. This procedure is facilitated by fluoroscopic control. The window is positioned toward the plaque by torquing the catheter appropriately under fluoroscopy. With the catheter properly positioned, the balloon is inflated to 20 to 40 PSI to push the open chamber against the arterial lesion, thereby wedging the atheroma into the window. The motor drive of the cutter is activated and the atheroma is sliced off the arterial lumen and pushed into the distal collecting chamber. Multiple passes of the cutter are taken, and the collecting chamber may be rotated to obtain full atherectomy. Multiple cuts and passages are required for complete atherectomy. Once the collecting chamber is full, the catheter is withdrawn and the atheroma slices or particles are removed from the housing. Repeat atherectomy is performed as needed to obtain complete recanalization.

Indications

The optimal lesion for Simpson atherectomy procedure is a short, discreet, eccentrically placed atheroma. Stenotic lesions are more favorable than total

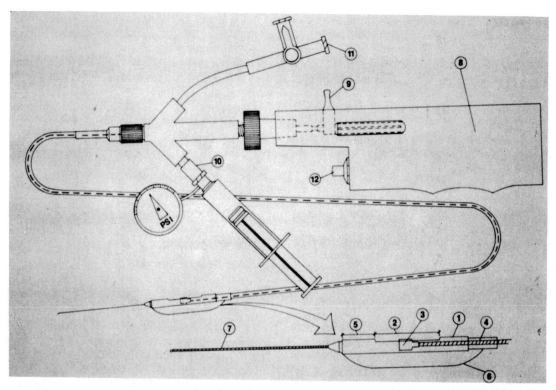

FIGURE 16–20. Atherectomy catheter system. *1,* Cylindrical housing; *2,* longitudinal opening; *3,* cutter; *4,* cutter drive cable (to motor); *5,* specimen collection area; *6,* balloon support mechanism; *7,* fixed guidewire; *8,* motor; *9,* cutter advance lever; *10,* balloon inflation port; *11,* flush port; *12,* Touhy-Borst opening for cable connector. (From Simpson JB, et al: Transluminal atherectomy for peripheral vascular disease. Am J Cardiol *61*:96G–101G, 1988.)

occlusive lesions. Concentric lesions can also be treated satisfactorily, as can short total occlusions. Ulcerative plaques are ideally suited for atherectomy. Restenotic intimal hyperplastic lesions are also quite amenable. Heavily calcified lesions may create some difficulties for the cutter, but do not pose a particular contraindication. The catheter can be used quite satisfactorily in the iliac, superficial femoral, and popliteal arteries.

Results

Simpson et al. reported their initial atherectomy experience of 136 lesions in 61 patients.[54] These investigators used the device in the superficial femoral, iliac, and popliteal arteries. Atherectomy was initially successful in 87 per cent of the patients and early failure was primarily due to the technical inability to remove adequate atheroma, leaving a residual ste-

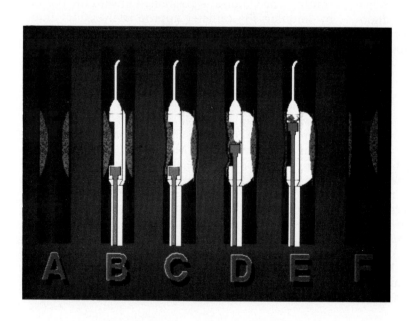

FIGURE 16–21. The atherectomy procedure. *A,* The lesion before atherectomy. *B,* Atherectomy catheter in position across the lesion. *C,* The balloon support is inflated. *D,* The cutter is advanced. *E,* The specimen is trapped in the housing. *F,* The balloon is deflated and the catheter removed. (From Hinohara T, Robertson GC, Selman MR, Simpson JB: Transluminal atherectomy: The Simpson atherectomy catheter. *In* Moore WS, Ahn SS (eds): Endovascular Surgery. Philadelphia, WB Saunders Company, 1989, pp 310–322.)

nosis of less than 50 per cent. Of the successfully treated patients, only 69 per cent had continued exercise tolerance at 6-month follow-up. Angiographic studies available in 30 of these patients revealed a restenosis rate of at least 36 per cent. The restenosis rate was greater in patients with residual stenosis greater than 30 per cent at the time of the atherectomy procedure.

Polnitz and coworkers[55] reported Simpson atherectomy procedures in 60 patients with 94 lesions (63 stenoses and 31 total occlusions) in 77 superficial femoral arteries, eight popliteal arteries, eight iliac arteries, and one anterior tibial artery. Immediate clinical success was obtained in 82 per cent (49 of 60) of the patients. Twenty-five of the successfully treated patients reached a 1-year follow-up and achieved a 72 per cent clinical patency rate; 16 per cent required repeat atherectomy, and 8 per cent required surgery for restenosis or occlusion. Six-month angiographic evaluation found restenosis in 13 (24 per cent) of 55 lesions: 3 of 13 of the concentric lesions (23 per cent), 3 of 27 of the eccentric lesions (11 per cent), and 7 of 15 of the occlusions (47 per cent).

Graor et al.[56] reported a 100 per cent and 93 per cent initial success rate in patients with lesions shorter than 5 cm and longer than 5 cm, respectively. The 12-month patency rates were 93 per cent and 83 per cent, respectively. There was a 7.1 per cent rate of major complications including one fatal myocardial infarction.

Complications

The Simpson Atherocath is a relatively safe device with few complications reported, so far. Dissection has occurred in only 3 of 61 patients and was related primarily to guidewire or introducer sheath placement or overinflation of the balloon, rather than the atherectomy procedure itself.[54] Distal embolic problems have occurred in fewer than 3 per cent of the patients. Perforations, or the need for emergency surgery, have been few to date.

Limitations

The main limitations of the Simpson Atherocath appear to be its relative ineffectiveness in long, diffusely diseased segments and long, totally occluded lesions. The time involved to atherectomize long segments can be frustrating, even to the most patient surgeon. Furthermore, restenosis rates may be significantly higher in these longer lesions. Finally, the catheters are somewhat bulky and relatively stiff to use in the tibial vessels or tortuous vessels.

Theratek Trac-Wright Atherectomy Device

Device Description

The Trac-Wright atherectomy device (Theratek Inc., Miami, FL) is also a flexible catheter with a distal cam-tip attached to a central drive shaft (Fig. 16–22). There is no coaxial leading guidewire. The cam rotates at 100,000 RPM and seeks the path of least resistance. A high-pressure water irrigating system dilates the artery, while the rotating cam pulverizes the plaque. The rotating tip appears to selectively pulverize fibrous or firm atheromatous tissue, while leaving viscoelastic tissue alone.

Technique

Atherectomy can be performed percutaneously or through a small arteriotomy in the common femoral artery. A no. 9-French introducer sheath is placed and the Kensey catheter is then slipped through the introducer sheath into the artery being treated. The catheter tip is placed directly against the obstruction under fluoroscopic guidance. Through the irrigation channel, an infusion of contrast dye, urokinase, dextran, and heparin is started with an infusion rate of 30 ml/min. The rotating cam is then activated, using an electric motor drive. The catheter is advanced diligently and slowly in a to-and-fro manner, allowing time for the rotating cam to adequately pulverize the atheroma. The catheter is advanced gradually under direct fluoroscopic control. Once the catheter has recanalized the occlusive lesion, any residual stenosis is dilated using standard balloon angioplasty techniques.

Indications

The Trac-Wright atherectomy catheter was designed particularly for totally occlusive lesions of the superficial femoral artery. By design, there is no coaxial central guidewire that must first cross the lesion. The catheter has also been touted to work expeditiously, so that long lesions can be treated as easily as short lesions.

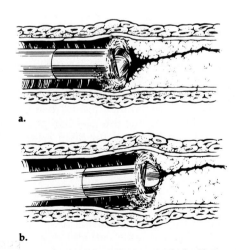

FIGURE 16–22. During recanalization with the Kensey catheter, the rotating cam seeks out the path of least resistance, tracking from a proximal arterial lumen of more normal caliber (*a*) into the narrowed lumen of the diseased segment (*b*). (From Whittemore AD: The Kensey catheter: Indications, technique, results and complications. *In* Moore WS, Ahn SS (eds): Endovascular Surgery. Philadelphia, WB Saunders Company, 1989, pp 323–326.)

Results

Whittemore reported his initial trials in 10 patients.[57] Apparently, only one patient clearly benefited from the procedure. There were two arterial wall perforations. There were no clinical peripheral embolizations.

Snyder et al. reported 23 procedures to recanalize superficial femoral artery occlusions.[58] Atherectomy was successful in 14. Eleven of these extremities underwent subsequent balloon angioplasty to enlarge the initial channel further. Perforation by the rotating cam was the main complication and occurred in 8 of 23 patients. The cumulative patency rate was recently reported to be 37 per cent at 2 years.[58]

Desbrosses et al. reported an 87 per cent (40 of 46) success rate in recanalizing femoropopliteal occlusions 2 to 24 cm long.[59] Four perforations occurred, requiring no further intervention. Failures occurred in calcified arteries. Of the successfully treated vessels, 13 per cent (5 of 40) reoccluded within 48 hours. Three patients had embolic complications postoperatively. Follow-up revealed a primary patency of 72 per cent (18 of 25) at 6 months and 70 per cent (14 of 20) at 12 months.

Complications

The main complication appears to be perforation induced by the rotating cam. Whittemore reported two perforations in 10 patients, and Snyder reported eight perforations in 23 extremities.[57,58] The catheter follows the path of least resistance, which is often away from hard calcified plaque. Although fibrous lesions are amenable to atherectomy, the hard calcified lesions, particularly at the adductor canal, have been resistant to atherectomy. Thromboembolic complications have occurred infrequently and do not appear to be a major problem.

Limitations

The main limitation of the Trac-Wright atherectomy device appears to be hard calcified plaques and perforation problems. These two factors are often related, and perforations have occurred most frequently in hard calcified plaques at the adductor canal. Because of this relatively high perforation risk, the catheter cannot be recommended for use in the iliac arteries. Furthermore, the internal damage to the artery appears to be too great for tibial arteries.

Auth Rotablator

Device Description

The Auth Rotablator (Heart Technology, Inc., Bellevue, WA) is a flexible catheter-deliverable atherectomy device with a variable-sized, football-shaped metal burr on the distal tip (Fig. 16–23). The burr is studded with multiple diamond chips (22 to 45 μ size) that function as multiple microknives. The burr comes in various sizes, ranging from 1.25 to 6.0 mm in diameter. The proper-sized burr is selected for a

given artery. The burr rotates at 100,000 to 200,000 RPM and tracks along a central guidewire. The guidewire must first traverse the lesion before rotational atherectomy can proceed. The high-speed rotation allows the diamond microchips to preferentially attack hard calcified atheroma, while leaving the surrounding elastic soft tissue of normal arterial wall intact (Fig. 16–24). The device leaves a smooth, polished intraluminal surface and no intimal flaps (Fig. 16–25). The pulverized particles are generally smaller than red blood cells and appear to pass harmlessly through the peripheral capillary circulation.[27,60,61]

Technique

Atherectomy is performed through an open arteriotomy preferentially, although percutaneous methods can be used. The percutaneous technique, however, limits the burr size to 3 mm and ultimately requires subsequent balloon angioplasty. When performing atherectomy alone, an open arteriotomy using a larger sized burr is preferred. A no. 9-, 12-, or 14-French introducer sheath is inserted into the artery through the arteriotomy. An angioscope may be inserted to document the lesion and to help with proper placement of the guidewire. Alternatively, conventional fluoroscopy can be used and is more readily available.

First, a small atraumatic guidewire is passed through the lesion, after which an exchange guide catheter is inserted. The initial guidewire is removed and then a 0.009-inch atherectomy guidewire, which is somewhat stiffer and more rigid to support the rotating burr, is passed through the lesion. The exchange guide catheter is then removed, and the burr is placed over the guidewire and then passed to the site of the obstructive lesion. Initially, a burr size half the diameter of the native artery is used; the size of the burr is progressively increased in increments of 0.5 to 1.0 mm. Atherectomy is performed gradually and slowly, recanalizing the artery by advancing the burr over the guidewire. Following atherectomy with the smallest burr, the burr is removed, leaving the guidewire in place. Then the next-sized burr is inserted and atherectomy is repeated until an adequate-sized lumen is obtained. The patient is placed on anticoagulation therapy for the first 24 hours postoperatively to prevent early thrombosis. Aspirin is then given long-term postprocedure.

Indications

The Auth Rotablator is ideally suited for hard calcified plaque, particularly in diabetics. Recanalization is achieved expeditiously in long as well as short lesions. Tibial artery lesions can be treated as well as popliteal, superficial femoral, and iliac arterial lesions. Stenotic lesions appear better suited for the Rotablator, since a central guidewire must first traverse the lesion. Total occlusions may be treated, if the guidewire can be passed initially. Eccentric plaques can be treated quite satisfactorily, since the atherectomy device preferentially attacks the calcified plaque.

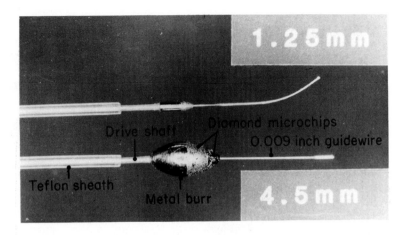

FIGURE 16–23. Rotablator atherectomy burr and guidewire. Burrs 1.25 and 4.5 mm in diameter, respectively, are shown. Note the diamond microchips embedded in the distal half of the burr. Also note the coaxial spring tip (*top*) and semirigid guidewires (*bottom*). (From Ahn SS: The Rotablator—high-speed rotary atherectomy: Indications, technique, results and complications. *In* Moore WS, Ahn SS (eds): Endovascular Surgery. Philadelphia, WB Saunders Company, 1989, pp 327–335.)

Results

The UCLA series included 41 arteries in 25 patients.[62] Limb threat was present in 56 per cent of these patients. Initial technical success was achieved in 23 of 25 patients (92 per cent) and in 39 of the 41 arterial segments (93 per cent). The in-hospital success rate was 18 of 25 (72 per cent). The primary patency rate in these 18 patients was 67 per cent at 6 months. However, at 24 months, the overall primary and secondary patency rates for the 25 patients were only 9.5 per cent and 20 per cent, respectively.

The Stanford series had 38 patients with stenoses of the superficial femoral and popliteal arteries.[63] Limb threat was present in 45 per cent. A 71 per cent (27 of 38) angiographic success rate was reported. Eighteen (47 per cent) demonstrated immediate angiographic and hemodynamic successes. Of these, 11 still were improved clinically and hemodynamically at 6 months. Six of the nine immediate angiographic successes without hemodynamic benefit required adjunctive procedures within 6 months. Of the other patients, two were lost to follow-up, and one was clinically improved but hemodynamically worse.

Complications

Combining the UCLA and Stanford data on 63 patients, complications included eight instances of peripheral emboli (one significant enough to cause thigh skin loss), seven of transient hemoglobinuria, seven wound hematomas (in six percutaneous and

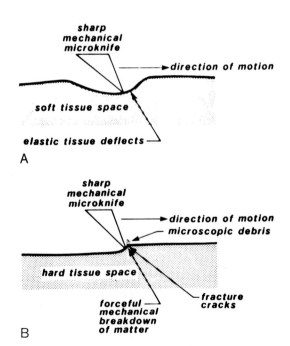

FIGURE 16–24. Differential cutting: its application in soft and hard tissue. *A,* Soft tissue is able to deflect out of the way of the microknife. *B,* Hard tissue is unable to deflect out of the way; the result is fracture and mechanical breakup of atheromatous plaque. (From Ahn SS: The Rotablator—high speed rotary atherectomy: Indications, technique, results and complications. *In* Moore WS, Ahn SS (eds): Endovascular Surgery. Philadelphia, WB Saunders Company, 1989, pp 327–335.)

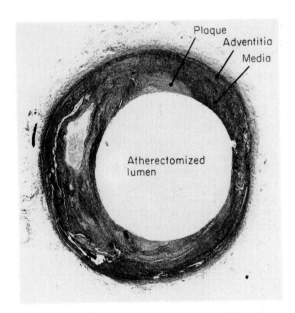

FIGURE 16–25. Photomicrographs of a successfully atherectomized artery seen in cross-section. Note the smooth, highly polished intraluminal surface denuded of intima and endothelial cells. Hematoxylin-eosin stain: original magnification × 40. (From Ahn SS: The Rotablator—high speed rotary atherectomy: Indications, technique, results and complications. *In* Moore WS, Ahn SS (eds): Endovascular Surgery. Philadelphia, WB Saunders Company, 1989, pp 327–335.)

one open procedure), five early rethromboses, three wound infections, two equipment breakages, two perforations, one intimal dissection, and three limb losses. Thromboemboli were mostly microscopic and clinically insignificant. However, a hypercoagulable patient at UCLA developed diffuse microemboli and ultimately lost her limb. Although particles are generally small, a large particle burden is a potential problem, particularly in dealing with long occluded lesions. Microscopic hemoglobinuria has occurred in several patients, particularly when the larger burs (4 mm or greater) are used. However, the effects have been clinically benign and transient. Burrs that are too large or that are advanced too rapidly are subject to entanglement and breakage.

Limitations

The Auth Rotablator is limited primarily by its inability to ablate and pulverize chronic thrombus and/or rubbery plaque.[53] These lesions preferentially deflect away from the rotating burr, which leads to suboptimal recanalization. The procedure is somewhat slowed by required multiple burrs and exchange of burrs over the guidewire. Patience is also required and care must be taken not to advance the burr too rapidly. Although particles are generally small, a large particle burden could be a potential problem. Thus, long totally occluded lesions with large particle burden resulting from atherectomy could lead to problems that have yet to be defined or identified. The device should not be used for carotid lesions, since the microemboli could lead to focal neurologic deficits and perhaps even frank, global cerebral dysfunction.

Transluminal Extraction Catheter

Device Description

The Transluminal Extraction Catheter (TEC Catheter, Inventional Technologies, Inc., San Diego, CA) is a semiflexible, torque-controlled, hollow catheter that has a rotating, cone-shaped cutter that tracks over a central guidewire (Fig. 16–26). The cone has openings on the distal tip and the catheter itself is hollow, such that the particles resulting from atherectomy can be suctioned out of the vessel and collected in a separate collecting chamber. The conical-shaped cutter itself rotates at approximately 700 RPM and leaves relatively large-sized (1-mm) particles. Suction is applied from the proximal port to suction the particles into a collecting chamber, making embolic complications unlikely. The catheter comes in nos. 5-, 7-, and 9-French sizes.

Technique

The procedure has been performed primarily percutaneously, but can be used intraoperatively as well. Because of the limited size of the TEC Catheter, standard balloon angioplasty is often required to achieve a final channel that is adequate in size. An

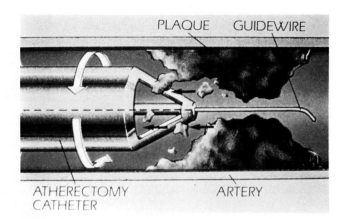

FIGURE 16–26. Artist's concept of the transluminal extraction catheter (TEC). See text for description.

appropriate-sized introducer sheath is placed into the artery in an antegrade fashion for the superficial femoral, popliteal, and tibial arteries. A guidewire is then passed through the introducer sheath and through the obstructive lesion. Once the guidewire is in place, a no. 4- or 5-French polyethylene exchange catheter is inserted. Then the initial guidewire is replaced with the TEC 0.014-inch wire. The exchange catheter is then removed and the TEC Catheter itself is then passed over the TEC guidewire until the catheter meets resistance at the obstructive lesion. The atherectomy catheter is then activated and the motor drive rotates the cutter at 700 RPM, while suction is applied. The torque tube cutter is passed freely, but gently, over the guidewire until the occluded segment has been traversed. Fluoroscopy documents the progress of the atherectomy and the final lumen. If there is significant residual stenosis, then standard balloon angioplasty is performed to dilate the artery to a final adequate size.

Indications

The indications for the TEC Catheter appear to be the same as previously described for the Simpson Atherocath.

Results

Wooley and Jarmolowski reported the initial results of 126 lesions in the first 95 patients from a multicenter trial.[64] Initial technical success was achieved in 92 per cent of the procedures. Vessels treated included superficial femoral artery (97 patients), femoropopliteal grafts (two patients), popliteal artery (14 patients), external iliac artery (eight patients), and tibial vessels (four patients). Sixty of the 95 patients had claudication. Sixty-seven of the 126 lesions (53 per cent) were treated by atherectomy alone, while the others required atherectomy plus adjunctive balloon angioplasty. Fifty patients underwent 6-month follow-up, and 16 patients underwent repeat angiography. Four of these 16 patients (25 per cent) had angiographic evidence of reocclusion. Follow-up data on the other patients were not provided in their report.

Limitations and Complications

The limitations and complications also appear to be very similar to those of the Simpson Atherocath. The specific details of the limitations and complications are not available as of this writing.

Future Developments

So far, all atherectomy devices have failed to improve the restenosis rate of standard balloon angioplasty. Despite actual removal, debulking, and even polishing of the plaque, the invariable arterial wall trauma still induces intimal hyperplasia. Until the problem of restenosis can be solved, atherectomy will be limited to those instances when balloon angioplasty may be ineffective or contraindicated. Such instances might include the presence of hard calcified lesions that are difficult to dilate, the presence of intimal flaps or dissections secondary to the balloon angioplasty itself, or ulcerative lesions that have led to thromboembolic complications.

However, if the restenosis problem can be solved, the clinical implications are enormous and the indications for atherectomy numerous. The atherectomy procedure could be performed as sole therapy to remove atherosclerotic plaque and recanalize the artery. Atherectomy could be used in conjunction with lasers to recanalize totally occluded arteries. Furthermore, atherectomy could supplement and be used as an adjunct to standard arterial revascularization. Clinical strategies using peripheral atherectomy have been outlined and illustrated already by Ahn and Moore.[65]

INTRAVASCULAR STENTS

Description of Device

The recognized problem of restenosis following transluminal angioplasty has led to a plethora of interest in intravascular stents. Several types of stents have now been described in the literature and have been used experimentally and clinically.[66-75] These include flexible, rigid, balloon-expandable, and self-expanding stents. The Palmaz stent is a balloon-expandable, rigid, stainless steel stent.[69,74] The Gianturco-Wallace stents are also metallic, rigid stents but have properties that allow for self-expansion.[67,70] The Strecker stent is balloon expandable and flexible.[72] The Wall stent is a stainless steel, flexible, self-expanding stent.[75] Most recently, there have been some experimental studies using biodegradable stents.[76]

Indications

The common denominator in all these stents is to provide a scaffold to maintain the intraluminal structure and patency of the artery. So far, stents have been used primarily in total occlusive lesions and in stenotic lesions in which balloon angioplasty gave an inadequate immediate result.[74,75] Thus, arteries that showed persistent narrowing, despite several balloon dilatation attempts, may benefit from stent placement. Another indication reported has been to prevent restenosis following a previous balloon angioplasty. Long, irregular stenotic lesions that have unfavorable results with balloon angioplasty techniques alone have also been treated with stents in order to prevent future restenosis. Stenotic lesions of the distal anastomosis of bypass grafts have been stented with some success. Stents have also been advocated to tack dissections that occur following balloon angioplasty.

Technique

So far, stent placement has been performed percutaneously as an adjunct to percutaneous balloon angioplasty. The original diameter of the vessel is estimated and bony landmarks are used to help position the stent prior to deployment. Superficial femoral arteries are usually stented with 6-mm diameter stents, whereas iliac arteries are usually treated with 8- to 10-mm stents. Multiple stents are occasionally used in a single artery, if long segments are to be treated. The balloon-expanded stents are delivered to the stenotic lesions by an introducer sheath that is advanced across the stenosis. With this protective sheath in place, the stent-balloon assembly is then advanced within the sheath to the level of the stenotic lesion. The sheath is then withdrawn, uncovering the mounted stent. Final positioning is accomplished by using bony landmarks, external metallic markers, and contrast imaging using road-mapping. The balloon is then inflated to expand the stent and the lesion simultaneously, leaving the stent mesh flush within the inner lumen. Residual irregularity or stenosis cranial or caudad to the stent is then corrected by dilating the portion of the vessel without the stent using the same balloon, or a second stent may be inserted to dilate any residual stenosis proximal or distal to the stent. After stent expansion, the balloon is deflated and withdrawn, and a completion angiogram and pressure measurements are taken.

The self-expanding stents are delivered through an introducer catheter with either a rolling membrane or a sheath covering the stent. The stent is then gradually deployed by gradual retraction of the outer membrane or sheath. It should be noted that the stents shorten during release, and thus proper placement can be somewhat inconsistent. If the catheter is only partially disengaged, then the stent can usually be pulled back but not advanced forward. Again, repeat stenting is occasionally necessary to obtain optimal results.

Routine antiplatelet use and intraoperative anticoagulation is recommended. There are some preliminary data that even suggest that long-term Coumadin postoperatively should be used to prevent early and late thrombosis.[71]

Results

Clinical results in the peripheral arteries have been limited as of this writing. Most of the experience has come from Europe using the Wall stent. Sigwart et al. reported placing 10 stents during seven procedures in six patients (four femoral and three iliac arteries).[75] Two patients had totally occluded arteries, and four patients had stenotic arteries that did not respond satisfactorily to balloon angioplasty. At 6-month follow-up, there were apparently no restenoses. Longer follow-up results are not available.

Gunther et al., also using the Wall self-expanding, flexible stent, treated 45 patients.[77] Thirty-one patients had lesions of the iliac arteries, and 14 had lesions of the superficial femoral artery. Twenty-six patients had total occlusion, and 19 patients had stenotic lesions. Thirty-seven of the patients were treated immediately after inadequate angioplasty, and the other eight patients were treated because of total occlusion or long diffuse disease. At 2- to 12-month follow-up, 40 of 45 patients had patent stents. Two patients had early thrombotic occlusions, and three patients had late intimal hyperplasia restenosis. A sixth patient subsequently developed total occlusion at 6 months. Only one of the iliac lesions had restenosis. However, 3 of 14 patients with superficial femoral artery stents had restenosis (21 per cent). Longer follow-up is not available as of this writing.

Rousseau et al., also using the Wall stent, reported 40 femoropopliteal implantations in 36 patients, with a 6-month follow-up in all patients.[71] Seventy-five per cent of the lesions were 3 to 7 cm in length, and 25 per cent exceeded 7 cm. Seventy per cent of the 40 lesions were located in the superficial femoral arteries, 16 per cent in the popliteal artery, and 14 per cent in a combination of the arteries. Seventy per cent of the lesions were stenotic lesions, and 30 per cent were total occlusions. Six patients had early thrombotic occlusions. Restenosis occurred in 10 per cent of the remaining patients. Cumulative patency rate revealed a 76 per cent 1-year patency. However, of note is that all nine patients who received postoperative Coumadin did not develop early thrombosis or late restenosis. However, Coumadin was initiated only in the last nine cases, and thus the longest follow-up is less than 1 year.

Palmaz et al. in the United States have coordinated a large multicenter trial using the rigid, metallic Palmaz stents.[74] Their initial preliminary results showed 100 per cent patency in the iliac arteries during a follow-up of 6 to 12 months. Further analysis of this study revealed a 79 per cent initial success rate of stent placement in 165 limbs of 146 patients. All 79 per cent of these patients apparently have continued clinical success at 6 months' follow-up. The Palmaz stent has not been used in the superficial femoral or popliteal artery regions so far.

Strecker et al., using the metallic tantalum filament, flexible stent reported similar good patency rates in the iliac arteries, but found several restenoses in the superficial femoral artery position.[78]

Limitations and Complications

The main complications of stent placement have been those related to percutaneous balloon angioplasty. As noted previously, there have been instances of early acute thrombosis, as well as inability to place the stents effectively. Furthermore, there has been dislodgement from the catheter delivery system, as well as misplacement of the stent requiring multiple stent placements. There have been few reported instances of stent migration and embolization. There have been vessel perforations requiring urgent surgery, as well as groin hematomas requiring blood transfusions.[68] There have been reported cases of side-branch occlusion and late thrombosis, and even distal emboli. Furthermore, accelerated intimal hyperplasia has been noted, particularly in the superficial femoral artery regions.

Future Perspectives

The preliminary results show excellent patencies of stents in the iliac artery position. However, one should note that long-term patency of balloon angioplasty in the iliac arteries is generally quite good, approaching 90 per cent patency at 1 year and 80 per cent at 3 years.[46] So far, the results in the superficial femoral and popliteal positions have been promising, but somewhat disappointing. There is no clear evidence that stents reduce the restenosis rate in the superficial femoral or popliteal artery position. Reasons for this are not clear, but it is obvious that the stents themselves may not necessarily prevent intimal hyperplasia and fibroblast overgrowth. Preliminary work using biodegradable stents is currently in progress. Nevertheless, stents have clearly shown their usefulness in certain situations, particularly to improve the early results following failed or inadequate balloon angioplasty complicated by intimal dissection or flaps. Stents also have a potential role in proximal renal artery balloon angioplasty and treatment of stricture in the distal anastomosis of a bypass graft. There has even been some preliminary work using endovascular grafts or stents to treat aortic aneurysmal disease.[79,80] Stents may also have a role in treating recurrent stenosis of arteriovenous hemodialysis access grafts.[81] Most recently, stents have been utilized successfully to perform transjugular/intrahepatic portosystemic shunt in patients with portal hypertension.[82]

CONCLUDING REMARKS

Endovascular surgery is still in its infancy and much work is needed before its full potential can be realized. The early results have been somewhat disappointing, and the initial enthusiasm has appropriately turned into more sober, realistic cautiousness. The main challenge of the future is controlling restenosis. The solution may well lie with pharmacologic manipulation and better understanding of the restenosis phenomenon. It certainly seems likely that the extensive research currently taking place will ultimately lead to significant improvement of the re-stenosis rate. If the restenosis problem is solved, then endovascular surgery will have broad applications and it will become a dominant treatment modality in peripheral vascular surgery.

The problems encountered so far should not discourage even the most pessimistic investigator. Rather, now is the time to become creative and more analytical and accelerate efforts in solving the problems currently encountered in endovascular surgery. It is imperative that vascular surgeons, in particular, continue to maintain their interest in the field and make significant contributions and shape the future course of endovascular surgery.

REFERENCES

1. Dotter CT, Jedkins MP: Transluminal treatment of atherosclerotic obstruction: Description of a new technique and preliminary report of this application. Circulation 30:645–670, 1969.
2. Gruntzig A, Hopf H: Perkutane rekanalisation chronischer arterieller Verschlusse mit einen neuen Dilationskatheter: Modifikation der Dotter-teknik. Dtsch Med Wochenschr 99:2502–2551, 1974.
3. Moore WS, Ahn SS (eds): Endovascular Surgery. Philadelphia, WB Saunders Company, 1989.
4. White GF: Angioscopy to monitor arterial thromboembolectomy. In Moore WS, Ahn SS (eds): Endovascular Surgery, Philadelphia, WB Saunders Company, 1989, pp 55–64.
5. Byrnes G, MacGowen WA: The injury potential of the Fogarty balloon catheter. J Cardiovasc Surg 75:590–593, 1975.
6. Stoney RJ, Ehrenfeld WK, Wylie EJ: Arterial rupture after insertion of a Fogarty catheter. Am J Surg 115:830–831, 1968.
7. Holm J, Schersten T: Subintimal dissection secondary to the use of the Fogarty catheter. J Cardiovasc Surg 74:684–686, 1974.
8. Vollmar JF, Hutschenreiter S: Vascular endoscopy for venous thrombectomy. In Moore WS, Ahn SS (eds): Endovascular Surgery. Philadelphia, WB Saunders Company, 1989, pp 87–94.
9. Mehigan JT, Olcott C: Video angioscopy as an alternative to intraoperative arteriography. Am J Surg 152:139–145, 1986.
10. Grundfest WS, Litvack F, Sherman T, et al: Delineation of peripheral and coronary detail by intraoperative angioscopy. Ann Surg 202:394–400, 1985.
11. Fleisher HL III, Thompson BW, McCowan TC, et al: Angioscopically monitored saphenous vein valvulotomy. J Vasc Surg 4:360–364, 1986.
12. Matsumoto H, Yang Y, Hashizume M: Direct vision valvulotomy for non-reversed vein graft. Surg Gynecol Obstet 165:181–183, 1987.
13. Chin AK, Fogarty TJ: Angioscopic preparation for saphenous vein in situ bypass grafting. In Moore WS, Ahn SS (eds): Endovascular Surgery. Philadelphia, WB Saunders Company, 1989, pp 74–81.
14. Abele GS, Seeger JM, Barbieri E, et al: Laser angioplasty with angioscopic guidance in humans. J Am Coll Cardiol 8:184–192, 1986.
15. Ahn SS, Auth D, Marcus DR, Moore WS: Removal of focal atheromatous lesions by angioscopically guided high-speed rotary atherectomy: Preliminary experimental observations. J Vasc Surg 7:292–300, 1988.
16. Ahn SS: The use of grabbers, cutters, and shavers as an adjunct during endovascular surgery. In Moore WS, Ahn SS (eds): Endovascular Surgery. Philadelphia, WB Saunders Company, 1989, pp 514–517.
17. Olcott C: Angioscopic inspection of an anastomosis: Indica-tions and techniques. In Moore WS, Ahn SS (eds): Endovascular Surgery. Philadelphia, WB Saunders Company, 1989, pp 50–55.
18. Gussenhoven EJ, Essed CE, Frietman P: Intravascular ultrasonic imaging: Histologic and echographic correlation. Eur J Vasc Surg 3:571–576, 1989.
19. Neville RF, Bartorelli AL, Sidawy AN, Almagor Y, Potkin B, Leon MB: An in vivo feasibility study of intravascular ultrasound imaging. Am J Surg 158:142–145, 1989.
20. Keren G, Douek P, Oblon C, Bonner RF, Pichard AD, Leon MB: Atherosclerotic saphenous vein grafts treated with different interventional procedures assessed by intravascular ultrasound. Am Heart J 124(1):198–206, 1992.
21. Pandian NG, Kreis A, Brockway B, et al: Ultrasound angioscopy: Real time, two dimensional, intraluminal ultrasound imaging. Am J Cardiol 62:493–494, 1988.
22. Kopchok GE, White RA, Guthrie C, et al: Intraluminal vascular ultrasound: Preliminary report of dimensional and morphologic accuracy. Ann Vasc Surg 4(3):291–296, 1990.
23. Cavaye DM, Tabbara MR, Kopchok GE, Laas TE, White RA: Three dimensional vascular ultrasound imaging. Am Surg 57:751–755, 1991.
24. Yock PG, Linker DT, Rowe MH: Clinical applications of intravascular ultrasound imaging in atherectomy. Int J Cardiac Imaging 4:117–125, 1989.
25. Andros G, Harris RW, Sales-Cunha SX: Technique of intraoperative balloon angioplasty. In Moore WS, Ahn SS (eds): Endovascular Surgery, Philadelphia, WB Saunders Company, 1989, pp 209–222.
26. Fogarty TJ, Chin AK, Olcott C, et al: Combined thrombectomy and dilatation for treatment of acute lower extremity arterial thrombosis. J Vasc Surg 10:530–534, 1989.
27. Ahn SS: In discussion of Sanborn's paper. Sanborn TA, Greenfield AJ, Gruben JK, et al: Human percutaneous and intraoperative laser thermal angioplasty: Initial clinical results as an adjunct to balloon angioplasty. J Vasc Surg 5:83–90, 1987.
28. Prevosti LG, Cook JA, Leon MB, Bonner RF: Comparison of particulate debris size from excimer and argon laser ablation. Circulation 76:410, 1987.
29. Srinivasen R: Ablation of polymers and biological tissue by ultraviolet lasers. Science 234:559–565, 1986.
30. Cumberland DC, Crew JR, Myler RK: Clinical assisted angioplasty using the thermal probe and the hybrid laser probe: Techniques, results, and indications. In Moore WS, Ahn SS (eds): Endovascular Surgery. Philadelphia, WB Saunders Company, 1989, pp 393–401.
31. Geschwind HJ: Angioplasty using the sapphire tip: Indications, technique, results, and complications. In Moore WS, Ahn SS (eds): Endovascular Surgery. Philadelphia, WB Saunders Company, 1989, pp 402–407.
32. Grundfest W, Litvack F, Papaioannou T: Excimer laser an-

gioplasty: From basic science to clinical trials. *In* Moore WS, Ahn SS (eds): Endovascular Surgery. Philadelphia, WB Saunders Company, 1989, pp 432–441.

33. Leon MD, Geschwind HJ: Fluorescence-guided laser-assisted balloon angioplasty in peripheral vascular disease. *In* Moore WS, Ahn SS (eds): Endovascular Surgery. Philadelphia, WB Saunders Company, 1989, pp 466–475.

34. Ginsburg R: Laser angioplasty as an adjunct to balloon dilatation. *In* Moore WS, Ahn SS (eds): Endovascular Surgery. Philadelphia, WB Saunders Company, 1989, pp 389–392.

35. Cumberland DC, Sanborn TA, Taylor DA, et al: Percutaneous laser thermal angioplasty: Initial clinical results with a laser probe in total peripheral artery occlusions. Lancet 1:1457–1459, 1986.

36. Greenfield et al: SCVIR, 1988, pp 41–44.

37. Harrington ME, Schwartz ME, Sanborn TA, et al: Expanded indications for laser-assisted balloon angioplasty in peripheral arterial disease. J Vasc Surg 11:146–155, 1990.

38. Wright JG, Belkin M, Greenfield AJ, et al: Laser angioplasty for limb salvage: Observations on early results. J Vasc Surg 10:29–27, 1989.

39. Perler BA, Osterman FA, White RA Jr, et al: Percutaneous laser probe femoropopliteal angioplasty: A preliminary experience. J Vasc Surg 10:351–357, 1989.

40. Seeger JM, Abela GS, Silverman SH, Jablonski SK: Initial results of laser recanalization in lower extremity laser arterial reconstruction. J Vasc Surg 9:10–17, 1989.

41. Lammer J: Paper presented at the Seventeenth International Congress of Radiology, Paris, France, July, 1989.

42. Pilger E, Lammer J, Bertuch H, et al: Na:YAG laser with sapphire tip combined with balloon angioplasty in peripheral arterial occlusions: Long-term results. Circulation 83:141–147, 1991.

43. Lammer J, Pilger E: Laser angioplasty by contact probes: Experimental and clinical experimentations. Laser Surg Med 8:328, 1988.

44. Fourrier JL, Marache P, Brunetaud JM, et al: Nouvelle methode d'angioplastie laser par saphir de contact des arteres peripheriques: Resultats preliminaires. Arch Mal Coeur 81:253–258, 1988.

45. Nordstrom LA: Argon laser assisted angioplasty: One-year follow-up results in peripheral arteries and initial coronary experience (abstr). Biotronics, *March*, 1989.

46. Zeitler E, Richter EI, Roth FJ, et al: Results of percutaneous transluminal angioplasty. Radiology 146:57–60, 1983.

47. Johnston KW, Colapinto RF, Baird RJ: Transluminal dilatation. Arch Surg 117:1604–1610, 1982.

48. Sampson RH, Sprayregen S, Veith FJ: Management of angioplasty complications, unsuccessful procedures, and early and late failures. Ann Surg 199:234–240, 1984.

49. Spears JR, Serur JR, Shopshire D, et al: Fluorescence of experimental atheromatous plaques with hematoporphyrin derivative. J Clin Invest 71:395–399, 1983.

50. Spokojny AM, Serur JR, Skelman J, Spears JR: Uptake of hematoporphyrin derivative by atheromatous plaque: Studies in human in vitro and rabbit in vivo. J Am Coll Cardiol 8:1387–1392, 1986.

51. Grundfest WS, Litvack F, Mohr F: Radiofrequency thermal angioplasty. *In* Moore WS, Ahn SS (eds): Endovascular Surgery. Philadelphia, WB Saunders Company, 1989, pp 429–431.

52. Lu DY, Leon MB, Bowman RL: Electrical thermal angioplasty: Catheter designed features in vitro tissue ablation studies and in vivo experimental findings. Am J Cardiol 60:1117–1122, 1987.

53. Ahn SS: Peripheral atherectomy. Semin Vasc Surg 2:143–154, 1989.

54. Simpson JB, Selman MR, Robertson GC, et al: Transluminal atherectomy for occlusive peripheral vascular disease. J Am Coll Cardiol 61:96–101, 1988.

55. Polinitz A, Nerlich A, Berger H, et al: Percutaneous peripheral atherectomy. J Am Coll Cardiol 15:628–688, 1990.

56. Graor R, Whitlow P: Transluminal atherectomy for occlusive

57. peripheral vascular disease. J Am Coll Cardiol 15:1551–1558, 1990.

57. Whittemore AD: The Kensey catheter: Indications, technique, results and complications. *In* Moore WS, Ahn SS (eds): Endovascular Surgery. Philadelphia, WB Saunders Company, 1989, pp 323–326.

58. Snyder SO, Wheeler JR, Gregory RT, et al: Kensey catheter: Early results with a transluminal endarterectomy tool. J Vasc Surg 8:541–543, 1988.

59. Desbrosses D, Petit H, Torres E, et al: Percutaneous atherectomy with angioplasty. Ann Vasc Surg 4:550–552, 1990.

60. Hansen DD, Auth DC, Vracko R, et al: Rotational atherectomy in atherosclerotic rabbit iliac arteries. Am Heart J 115:160–165, 1988.

61. Zacca NM, Raizner AE, Noon JP: Treatment of symptomatic peripheral atherosclerotic disease with a rotational atherectomy device. Am J Cardiol 63:77–80, 1989.

62. Ahn SS, Yeatman LR, Deutsch LS, et al: Intraoperative peripheral atherectomy: Preliminary clinical results. Ann Vasc Surg 6:272–280, 1992.

63. Jennings LJ, Mehigan JT, Ginsburg R, et al: Rotablator atherectomy: Early experience and six months' follow-up. Presented at the Western Vascular Society, Rancho Mirage, CA, January, 1991.

64. Wooley MH, Jarmolowski CR: New reperfusion devices: The Kensey catheter, the atherolytic reperfusion wire device, and the transluminal extraction catheter. Radiology 172:947–952, 1989.

65. Ahn SS, Moore WS: Lesions amenable to mechanical atherectomy: Clinical strategies. *In* Moore WS, Ahn SS (eds): Endovascular Surgery. Philadelphia, WB Saunders Company, 1989, pp 299–309.

66. Cragg AH, Lund G, Rysavy JA, Castaneda F, Castaneda-Zuniga WR, Amplatz K: Percutaneous arterial grafting. Radiology 150:45–49, 1984.

67. Duprat G Jr, Wright KC, Charnsangavej C, Wallace S, Gianturco C: Self-expanding metallic stents for small vessels: Experimental evaluation. Radiology 162:469–472, 1987.

68. Maass D, Zollikofer CL, Largiader F, Senning A: Radiological follow-up of transluminally inserted vascular endoprostheses: An experimental study using expanding spirals. Radiology 152:659–663, 1984.

69. Palmaz JC, Tio FO, Schatz RA, Alvarado R, Rees C, Garcia O: Early endothelialization of balloon-expandable stents: Experimental observations. J Intervent Radiol 3:119–124, 1988.

70. Rollins N, Wright KC, Charnsangavej C, Wallace S, Gianturco C: Self-expanding metallic stents: Preliminary evaluation in an atherosclerotic model. Radiology 163:739–742, 1987.

71. Rousseau H, Puel J, Joffre F, et al: Self-expanding endovascular prosthesis: An experimental study. Radiology 164:709–714, 1987.

72. Strecker EP, Berg G, Schneider B, Freudenberg N, Weber H, Wolf RD: A new vascular balloon-expandable prosthesis: Experimental studies and first clinical results. J Intervent Radiol 3:59–62, 1988.

73. Sutton CS, Oku T, Harasaki H, et al: Titanium-nickel intravascular endoprosthesis: A 2-year study in dogs. AJR 151:597–601, 1988.

74. Palmaz JC, Richter GM, Noeldge G, et al: Intraluminal stents in atherosclerotic iliac artery stenosis: Preliminary report of a multicenter study. Radiology 168:727–731, 1988.

75. Sigwart U, Puel J, Mirkowitch V, Joffre P, Kappenberger L: Intravascular stents to prevent occlusion and restenosis after transluminal angioplasty. N Engl J Med 316:701–706, 1987.

76. King SB III: Vascular stents in atherosclerosis. Circulation 79:460–462, 1989.

77. Gunther RW, Vorwerk D, Bohndorf K, et al: Venous stenoses in dialysis shunts: Treatment with self-expanding metallic stents. Radiology 170:401–405, 1989.

78. Strecker EP, Lierman D, Barth KH, et al: Expandable, tubular,

tantalum stents for treatment of atherosclerotic iliac and femoropopliteal occlusive disease (abstr). Biotronics, *March*: 33, 1989.

79. Mirich D, Wright KC, Wallace S: Percutaneously placed endovascular grafts for aortic aneurysms: Feasibility study. Radiology *170*:1033–1037, 1989.

80. Parodi JC, Palmaz JC, Barone HD: Transfemoral intraluminal graft implantation for abdominal aortic aneurysms. Ann Vasc Surg *5*:491, 1991.

81. Gunther RW, Vorwerk D, Bohndorf K: Iliac and femoral artery stenosis and occlusions: Treatment with intravascular stents. Radiology *172*:725–730, 1989.

82. Zemel G, Katzen BT, Becker GJ, et al: Percutaneous transjugular portosystemic shunt. JAMA *266*:390–393, 1991.

17

ROLE OF SYMPATHECTOMY IN THE MANAGEMENT OF VASCULAR DISEASE

ROBERT B. RUTHERFORD

The concept of sympathetic denervation as therapy for arterial occlusive disease was first elaborated and tested by Leriche and Jaboulay in 1913.[1] Although their experience with periarterial sympathectomy was disappointing, Adson and Brown applied the technique of sympathetic ganglionectomy in 1925 to relieve debilitating lower extremity vasospasm with better long-term results. This ushered in an era in which sympathectomy was the only alternative to amputation for severe occlusive disease. Despite technical refinements over the next 40 years, clinical results remained variable and they spawned considerable debate over the value of sympathectomy. Better understanding of extremity pain syndromes and progress in direct arterial reconstructive surgery largely eclipsed the prominent role of sympathectomy by the early 1960s. A growing body of experimental data supported the clinical impression that the beneficial effects of sympathectomy were both short lived and palliative. Current indications for upper or lower extremity sympathectomy are generally limited to patients with causalgic pain hyperhidrosis and *very selected* patients with vasospastic or distal arterial occlusive disease that is not amenable to direct surgical or drug therapy. In this chapter, the physiologic consequences, indications, techniques and results of sympathectomy will be discussed.

ANATOMIC AND PHYSIOLOGIC CONSIDERATIONS

The sympathetic nervous system is comprised of preganglionic and postganglionic neurons originating in the anteromedial columns of the thoracolumbar spinal cord. Regional sympathetic activity is the product of local reflex arcs between somatic afferent fibers and preganglionic efferent fibers. Central control of both segmental and systemic sympathetic activity is mediated through the spinothalamic tract, with important contributions from visceral nuclei in the pons and medulla. At a segmental level, pregan-glionic neurons primarily synapse with postganglionic neurons in paravertebral ganglia via white rami communicantes. A small percentage of preganglionic fibers bypass the paravertebral ganglia to form synapses in more peripherally located intermediate ganglia or cross over to innervate contralateral regions via conventional pathways.[2] Characteristically, preganglionic fibers that supply a specific region either synapse with multiple neurons in paravertebral ganglia or proceed more peripherally to synapse in intermediate ganglia, which are at a distance from their segmental source. Complete sympathetic denervation of an extremity, therefore, requires division of preganglionic fibers along their segmental origin as well as excision of their corresponding relay ganglia and intercommunicating fibers.[3] The segmental innervation levels of the upper and lower extremity as well as specific anatomic variations will be described in the sections describing dorsal and lumbar sympathectomy.

The primary functions of the sympathetic nervous system are to prevent heat loss through reduction of superficial extremity blood flow and to modify basal organ functions in preparation for the demands of "fight or flight." Only the former need to be considered here. Resting sympathetic activity primarily antagonizes the vasodilating influence of the parasympathetic nervous system on arteriolar resistance vessels, cutaneous precapillary sphincters, and capacitance venules. Local increases in sympathetic outflow cause decreased skin blood flow, pilo-erection, and sweating. Net extremity blood flow is reduced by sympathetic stimulation unless muscular activity increases perfusion by metabolic vasodilation. These vasomotor effects are mediated by the constricting influence of norepinephrine on vascular smooth muscle. Thus, the primary vascular effect of increased sympathetic tone is a large reduction in cutaneous blood flow with lesser reductions in muscular blood flow that can be overcome by metabolic vasodilation.

Complete sympathetic denervation of an extremity causes a 40 to 100 per cent increase in total resting blood flow in ischemic limb experiments.[4] The majority of this increased flow passes through cutaneous arteriovenus anastomoses with relatively modest changes in resting or exertional muscular perfusion.[5] Blood flow is redistributed more peripherally to produce the characteristic warm, pink, and dry hand or foot. Maximal vasodilation and increased extremity blood flow are noted immediately following sympathectomy. However, a progressive decline in resting vasodilation usually begins within 1 week of denervation and results in minimal augmentation of flow by 6 months.[6] Explanations for this incremental recovery of baseline sympathetic vascular tone include incomplete sympathetic denervation, regeneration of severed fibers, and vascular receptor hypersensitivity to circulating catecholamines. Biochemical examination of recovery shows that the sensitivity of *extrasynaptic* α_2 receptors to exogenous norepinephrine is increased. However, decreases in both the concentration of *synaptic* α_1 receptors and the maximal vasoconstrictive response to norepinephrine have been demonstrated.[7,8] These changes in the number and sensitivity of vascular smooth muscle α receptors seem to best explain the phenomenon of partial sympathetic tone recovery.

Despite the transient effects of sympathectomy on *resting* extremity blood flow, other effects, specifically the abolition of sweating and the vasoconstrictor response to cold, persist as long as the sympathectomy is anatomically complete.[9] Although objective assessment of symptom relief in both neuropathic and ischemic pain syndromes is difficult, aversive stimuli studies in cats have documented that sympathectomy produces enhanced tolerance of painful stimuli.[10] This pain tolerance lasts longer than the vasomotor effects of sympathectomy and may explain clinical observations of improved exercise performance in sympathectomized patients who have no objective increases in extremity blood flow.[11] Theories concerning this direct effect on pain thresholds suggest that sympathetic denervation decreases noxious stimulus perception by both decreasing tissue concentrations of norepinephrine and reducing spinal augmentation of pain stimulus transmission to cerebral centers.[12,13] This role of sympathetic denervation in modulating pain perception is the most appealing explanation for symptomatic relief.

Numerous reports of chronically ischemic extremities treated by sympathectomy alone have yielded controversial results. Both clinical and experimental studies indicate that the major circulatory effect of sympathectomy is increased distal skin blood flow. Using radioactively labeled microspheres, Cronenwett et al. claimed that most of the increased skin blood flow is shunted through arteriovenous anastomoses and does not increase nutrient capillary perfusion.[4] In contrast, Moore and Hall showed that intradermal xenon clearance, and therefore cutaneous capillary blood flow, is significantly increased

following lumbar sympathectomy.[14] Measurements of tissue oxygen concentration before and after sympathectomy suggest that tissue oxygen supply is not augmented.[15] Despite these experimental results, several uncontrolled clinical experiences suggest that sympathectomy may sufficiently improve the oxygen supply-demand balance to allow ischemic ulcer healing in 35 to 62 per cent of patients.[16–18] Unfortunately, none of these have been randomized prospective trials and healing in this 20 to 30 per cent range has been reported in the control groups of randomized trials of circulation-enhancing drugs like the prostanoids.[19]

Studies of blood flow distribution following sympathectomy have consistently shown that muscle perfusion is not improved. Using radioactively labeled microspheres, Rutherford and Valenta noted that resting and exercise blood flow to muscle remains unchanged by sympathectomy in both normal and arterial ligated extremities.[20] This lack of responsiveness has been attributed to high intrinsic myogenic tone in muscle afferent arterioles, which compensates for decreases in sympathetic tone.[21] This experimental observation is consistent with the observed ineffectiveness of sympathectomy for claudication.[22] However, relief of rest pain due to distal ischemia has been noted following sympathetic denervation in 47 to 71 per cent of patients.[16–18] This discrepancy between experimental and clinical observations requires explanation. Although relief of a causalgic component of "ischemic neuritis" has been suggested as the cause by some,[23] most feel that even small increments of improved perfusion, not measurable by clinical testing, could spell the difference in these marginal cases. Still, it is not necessary to invoke this explanation in view of the nonspecific effect of sympathectomy on pain perception. Thus, although a small fraction of patients may show improved blood flow, the majority probably obtain relief from the attenuating effects of sympathectomy on pain perception.

The influence of sympathetic denervation on resting *collateral blood flow* and vascular resistance has been studied in numerous experiments with both acute and chronic limb ischemia models. Dalessandri et al. have shown in an acute canine limb ischemia preparation that sympathectomy causes a temporary but significant increase in collateral blood flow.[24] This increase in flow around a complete arterial occlusion is thought to be caused by maximal vasodilation in collateral channels that are not fully dilated by the metabolic stimuli of acute ischemia. This phenomenon of submaximal collateral vasodilation has also been observed by Ludbrook in 30 per cent of patients with rest pain.[25] Following sympathectomy in this group, he observed an average 11 per cent decrease in collateral vascular resistance and limb salvage in 42 per cent. Although temporary, sympathectomy seems to relieve *inappropriate* vasoconstriction in the collateral blood vessels of an ischemic extremity. However, it should be emphasized that in the majority of patients with resting ischemia, regional metabolic factors dominate and cause maximal blood flow increases through existing and newly formed collateral channels.

In summary, sympathetic denervation temporarily increases blood flow to peripheral regions of the resting ischemic limb; however, much, if not most, of this flow increase is nonnutrient arteriovenous shunt flow to the cutaneous circulation. Although debatable, skin capillary perfusion may be sufficiently increased to promote healing of small or superficial ischemic ulcers in selected patients with marginally inadequate perfusion. Persistent attenuation of ischemic or neuropathic pain perception is accomplished by reduction of noxious stimulus production peripherally and pain impulse transmission centrally. This effect probably explains the subjective pain relief observed in some patients who have no objective flow improvement. Finally, increased muscular and collateral perfusion is observed in that small minority of patients who have significant limb ischemia associated with inappropriate vasoconstriction. Like its effect on sweating, the effect of sympathectomy on *abnormal* vasomotor tone is lasting. The latter is probably due to a reduction in the number and response of synaptic α receptors.

UPPER EXTREMITY SYMPATHECTOMY

Current indications for and technique of upper extremity sympathectomy are based on nearly a century of clinical experience. First used by Alexander in 1899 for epilepsy, dorsal sympathectomy has undergone multiple technical modifications to reduce its morbidity and maximize sympathetic denervation. Advice regarding the extent of ganglion resection has ranged from radical (stellate ganglion to T5) to conservative (T2 and Kuntz's nerve). Although the latter may indeed suffice for some indications, the authors' experience indicates that clinically adequate upper extremity sympathectomy is best accomplished by resection of the T2 and T3 ganglia. T4 should be included if the indication is hyperhidrosis and the axilla as well as the hand is involved. In terms of operative indications, long-term outcome analysis has shown that best results are achieved among patients with causalgia, hyperhidrosis, and vasospastic disorders complicated by digital ulceration.[26] Improved medical management of patients with Raynaud's disease has largely replaced dorsal sympathectomy as therapy for disabling digital vasospasm.[27] Patients with secondary Raynaud's phenomenon may be helped if small arteries are involved proximal to the digits, as in arterial embolism, but if the terminal digital arteries are involved, as in scleroderma, the response to sympathectomy is usually disappointing. Within this context, pertinent features of upper extremity sympathectomy will be discussed.

Anatomic Features

Proper performance of thoracic dorsal sympathectomy requires appreciation of the anatomic variations in ganglion location and innervation patterns of the upper extremity. Preganglionic neurons supplying the face, neck, and upper extremity originate at the spinal cord levels of C7 through T5. Efferents from these levels form multiple synapses in the inferior cervical, stellate, and numbered thoracic ganglia. A direct fiber tract from the T2 sympathectomy ganglion to the brachial plexus (the nerve of Kuntz) can be identified in most patients as a frequent variation in the relay chain between the spinal cord and upper extremity.[28] Other direct connections between the spinal cord and brachial plexus can be demonstrated with detailed dissection, but are too variable to list. Similar variation in interganglionic connections are present at this level of the sympathetic nervous system and thus render complete upper extremity denervation difficult if not impossible.[29] With this fact in mind, most surgeons advocate resection of T2 and T3 ganglia as well as the nerve of Kuntz and other rami contributing directly to the brachial plexus at these levels.[30] Although providing less than 15 per cent of upper extremity sympathetic innervation, the T1 and inferior portion of the stellate ganglia make significant contributions to the eyes; therefore, complete resection of these ganglia substantially increases the risk of permanent Horner's syndrome. To eliminate the potential problem of partial sympathetic denervation, Roos advocates selective division of rami from the stellate ganglion to the brachial plexus.[31] Others, including the authors, additionally resect only the lower tip, no more than the lower third of the stellate ganglion.

Operative Technique

A variety of chest, back, and axillary approaches have been used to gain exposure to the upper sympathetic ganglia. In fact, there are six distinct approaches: three anterior (supraclavicular, infraclavicular, and high anterolateral thoracotomy), one dorsal, and two axillary (through a high interspace or the bed of a resected first rib). Critical review of reported series using each technique indicates that the latter two, the axillary transthoracic (Atkins) and extrapleural axillary (Roos) approaches to the stellate and upper thoracic ganglia, have the lowest complication rates and are recommended by the authors for most cases.[31,32] Both techniques involve exposure of the posterior portion of the superior mediastinum through a transverse axillary incision. First rib resection is recommended by Roos to facilitate both extrapleural retraction of the upper lung and identification of the sympathetic connections between the brachial plexus and higher ganglia. Similar exposure is obtained using the same incision with the transthoracic approach, by entering the chest through the third intercostal space and dividing the upper mediastinal pleura (Fig. 17–1). T2 and T3 ganglionectomy is performed by metal clip interruption and division of afferent and efferent fibers after the stellate ganglion has been identified on the neck of the first rib. Separation of the ganglia from adjacent intercostal vessels is facilitated by gentle traction on the T2 ganglion and attached fibers with a right-angle clamp or nerve hook.

Transaxillary approaches are preferred because less dissection is required to fully visualize the target ganglia and the incision is cosmetically acceptable. Major disadvantages of the transthoracic approach are the pain of a rib-spreading incision and frequent need for tube thoracostomy. While preliminary first rib resection is time consuming in inexperienced hands, that time is compensated by the simple closure. Fortunately, the first rib does not need to be divided as far posteriorly as it does for thoracic outlet syndrome, and it serves as a sure landmark for the stellate ganglion lying on its inner surface near its neck.

The supraclavicular approach[33] poses the greatest risk for injury because numerous surrounding structures, including the phrenic nerve, subclavian artery, vertebral artery, thoracic duct, cupola of the lung, and brachial plexus are encountered in gaining exposure of the sympathetic ganglia (Fig. 17–2). In ad-

dition, traction and dissection from above is more likely to cause Horner's syndrome. Most painful is the posterior approach advocated by Cloward, because the extensive paraspinal muscle division, laminectomy, and rib resection are required for visualization. Common to all approaches is the risk of injury to the thoracic duct, peripheral nerve roots, azygous vein, and intercostal arteries because of their proximity to the sympathetic chain. In the authors' opinion, the overall risk of these technical complications is reduced by using the transaxillary approaches and remaining attentive to anatomic detail.

Thoracoscopic Sympathectomy

The thoracoscope is not a new idea, but the advent of new instrumentation and video systems has now made it practical for many purposes (e.g., division of pleural adhesions, lung biopsy, pleurodesis, etc.). Dorsal sympathectomy has been performed through a thoracoscope for a number of years in the United Kingdom and Australia. Early techniques use cautery to destroy the ganglion chains, but the advanced technology that laparascopic cholesystectomy and pelvic lymph node dissection has spawned has made precise excision of the upper thoracic sympathetic chain quite feasible.[34] In performing dorsal sympathectomy this way, the authors have found it to be safe and effective and *not* time consuming. After completion, a chest tube is placed in the viewing port and the two instrument parts are closed with one or two skin sutures. Chest pain is minimal and discharge on the second day is routine. This technological advance will likely impact on the willingness to apply sympathectomy for certain indications, like hyperhidrosis and Raynaud's disease, where the morbidity of operation was formerly an impediment. It should also limit the number of stellate blocks administered to causalgia or RSD patients before sympathectomy is performed. Numerous blocks will now become unnecessary and even contraindicated, since the inflammation and scarring they cause will make subsequent thoracoscopic sympathectomy difficult and dangerous, if not impossible. This approach is not feasible in those with previous thoracic operations, pulmonary infections, or diffuse pulmonary disease with severely impaired function, the latter because such patients would not tolerate a *complete* pneumothorax using a Carlen's tube.

Results of Upper Extremity Sympathectomy

Assessment of the results of upper extremity sympathectomy requires categorization according to indications for the procedure. Additional factors warranting consideration are the duration of observation and technique of sympathectomy. With these factors in mind, the most successful indication for upper extremity sympathectomy is hyperhidrosis. Although a variety of ganglionectomy combinations have been

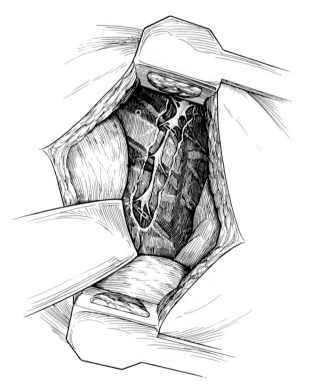

FIGURE 17–1. Transaxillary minithoracotomy through the second or third interspace provides good exposure of the upper thoracic sympathetic chain lying over the necks of the corresponding ribs. After opening the pleura, the segment of the chain from the lower tip of the stellate ganglion to T3 is resected, as shown by the dotted lines. (From Rutherford RB: A Technical Atlas of Vascular Surgery. Philadelphia, WB Saunders Company, in preparation.)

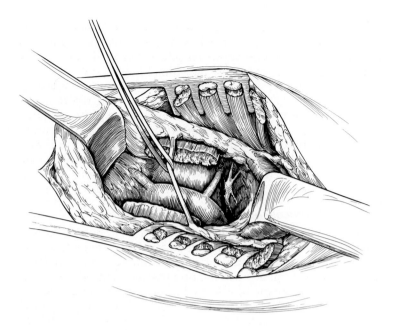

FIGURE 17–2. Through this right supraclavicular approach, the stellate ganglion is exposed just adjacent to and behind the vertebral artery, lying on the neck of the first rib. With further downward retraction, T2 and T3 can be exposed and resected with their rami and Kuntz's nerve using metal clips. (From Rutherford RB: A Technical Atlas of Vascular Surgery. Philadelphia, WB Saunders Company, in preparation.)

performed for this condition, T2, T3, and T4 ganglionectomy is sufficient. No short- or long-term failures have been reported, with maximal follow-up in one series of 7 years. Although never widely applied in North America, it remains popular in Europe.[26]

The prominent role of the sympathetic nervous system in perpetuating causalgic pain syndromes is unequivocal, despite the fact that the basic etiology of this type of posttraumatic extremity pain remains conjectural. Confident diagnosis of causalgic extremity pain requires a history of antecedent trauma, associated vasomotor dysfunction, cutaneous hypersensitivity and usually pain which is "burning" in character.[35] Consistent relief of the pain by sympathetic blockade increases that confidence immensely. Indeed, preoperative stellate ganglion blocks with local anesthetic have been advocated by Beurger and Smit and the authors, as routine, to identify patients who will most likely benefit from surgical sympathectomy.[36,49] Sham blocks to identify the "suggestive" of hysterical patients have been recommended, but the author finds using local anesthetics of different duration (e.g., Marcaine and Xylocaine) on consecutive blocks and requesting that the "blinded" patient make careful note of the duration of relief eliminates uncertainties about the validity of the response. Approximately 60 per cent of these posttraumatic pain syndromes can be managed with serial blocks, physiotherapy, mild narcotics, tricyclic antidepressants, and anticonvulsants.[37] In the remainder, T1 to T3 ganglionectomy is required. Surgical results are excellent insofar as 75 to 100 per cent of patients achieve permanent pain relief after up to 7 years of observation.[26,36–39,49]

Retrospective assessment of the success of sympathectomy in relieving symptomatic episodic vasospasm is difficult because the pathologic definition of Raynaud's disease has undergone considerable revision. Although the classical distinction between the benign "disease" and the virulent "phenomenon" is usually not made in many series, one fact is clear: the results of sympathectomy for Raynaud's disease caused by collagen vascular disease are disappointing. Characteristically, these patients suffer from progressive organic arterial disease that causes abnormal decreases in digital blood flow that are further aggravated by exposure to cold.[40] Sympathectomy initially prevents cold-induced ischemic attacks in 75 to 100 per cent of these patients. Within 2 years, however, 80 to 94 per cent of responders experience recurrent symptoms because progression of the autoimmune vascular disease further reduces resting blood flow to the digits.[26,36,41–43]

Among a small number of patients with occlusive Raynaud's disease complicated by digital ulceration, however, sympathectomy allows healing of at least 75 per cent of these lesions and prevents recurrent tissue loss even though cold-induced digital ischemia reappears.[26] Thus, sympathectomy may temporarily ameliorate symptoms and help with acute ulceration, but generally does not prevent recurrent symptoms because denervation does not affect the cause and course of the underlying vascular disease.

In contrast, occlusive Raynaud's disease caused by embolic or traumatic fibrotic lesions shows a more lasting and favorable response to sympathectomy. Abolition of cold-induced vasoconstriction in these patients reliably prevents digital ischemia because the lesions are discrete and the underlying disease is not progressive.[38,44] Similarly, Raynaud's disease caused by thrombosis or subintimal fibrosis from chronic occupational trauma also responds to sympathetic denervation and generally does not recur.[38,44–46]

Raynaud's disease resulting from abnormal digital vasoconstriction without obstructing lesions has a more benign course than the occlusive variety. Although up to 33 per cent of patients initially thought to be free of underlying disease may ultimately manifest signs of autoimmune vasculitis, true vasoconstrictive Raynaud's disease does not tend to be recurrent or associated with digital ulceration.[40,47] Treatment with α-adrenergic or calcium channel–blocking agents provides symptom relief during the acute phase of the syndrome.[27,48] Surgical sympathectomy therefore is not often indicated because medical management is sufficient and/or the symptoms are not sufficiently debilitating. Thoracoscopic sympathectomy may change this view. It is indeed unfortunate that, in this condition, surgery is least effective in those who need it the most, and vice versa. Thus clinical experience shows that sympathectomy can be justified by its overall benefit compared to risk only in patients with occlusive Raynaud's disease caused by occupation trauma, distal emboli, or autoimmune disease complicated by digital ulceration.[26,27,40,44,46]

Experience with sympathectomy in treating atherosclerotic disease of the upper extremity is limited insofar as this category accounts for only 5 to 7 per cent of dorsal sympathectomies in most large series. Although initial symptom relief or healing of ischemic ulcers is obtained in 40 to 60 per cent of patients, lasting improvement would not be expected because of the diffuse distribution of upper extremity atherosclerotic lesions.[26,27,49] An exception would be those with embolism from proximal atherosclerotic ulcerated plaques or high-grade stenoses. Among patients with preoperative arteriograms, best results are obtained in those who have primarily distal occlusive lesions. Additionally, increased digital blood flow in response to sympathetic blockade helps to identify patients likely to respond to surgical sympathectomy.[36,50] In general, however, progression of both proximal and distal occlusive disease militates against liberal use of sympathectomy for symptomatic arteriosclerotic disease of the upper extremity.

A small proportion of patients in large series of cervicothoracic sympathectomy have causalgic pain following frostbite. Such patients also commonly have vasomotor instability and a small minority may have residual organic occlusive lesions. Complete and lasting relief of symptoms following sympathectomy have been reported in essentially all such patients with these refractory afflictions of the upper extremity.[26,38] The small number of reported cases probably reflects the fact that the majority of these patients can be managed nonoperatively and have a geographic predilection. However, sympathectomy is likely to be successful because the underlying disease process is self-limited in time and discrete in distribution.

Patient Selection Criteria

The presenting symptoms of patients under consideration for upper extremity sympathectomy are usually episodic hand pain, reactive color change, or digital ulceration. Preliminary evaluation of these patients should include a disease-oriented history and examination to identify concomitant peripheral vascular disease, collagen vascular disease, antecedent trauma (isolated, occupational, or environmental), and evidence of tissue loss. Based on the presumed etiology of the pain, further testing would include serologic tests or tissue biopsy to identify collagen vascular disease as well as upper extremity and digital pressures and plethysmography to define the extent, severity, and level of occlusive disease, if present. Arteriography may be indicated to characterize both proximal and peripheral occlusive disease that is detected by segmental limb pressure measurements among those patients in whom therapeutic intervention is clearly needed.

Current Indications

Conditions most likely to permanently benefit from surgical sympathectomy are causalgia, hyperhidrosis, and Raynaud's disease caused by stable "occupational" digital thrombosis, or arterial occlusions (e.g., traumatic subintimal fibrosis, emboli). Initially favorable responses can be expected in selected patients with Raynaud's disease complicated by digital ulcerations, distal atherosclerotic peripheral vascular disease, and thromboangiitis obliterans. A trial of conservative treatment appropriate for the underlying disease is indicated for all patients. If medical measures (e.g., calcium channel blockers, cessation of smoking, etc.) fail, proper patient selection for most indications is improved by use of temporary stellate ganglion blocks to document the effectiveness of upper extremity sympathetic denervation. Among patients with vasospastic disease, abolition of cold-induced digital ischemia as monitored by digital pressures and plethysmography should be demonstrated prior to permanent sympathetic denervation. Ideally, several blocks should be done. Results indicating that sympathectomy will be efficacious are the following: (1) subjective relief of symptoms for a time period consistent with the duration of action of the local anesthetic, (2) greater than 50 per cent increase in the amplitude of the digital plethysmographic tracing as compared to baseline, and (3) abolition of the abnormally prolonged decline in the amplitude of digital plethysmographic tracings following ice-water immersion. When systematically applied, these guidelines should improve both early and late results by objectively measuring the effects of sympathetic blockade.

Complications

Injury to the adjacent neurovascular and thoracic structures may occur in a small percentage of patients undergoing thoracic dorsal sympathectomy. Horner's syndrome is the complication of sympathetic denervation that creates the most concern, but its occurrence varies directly with the extent of stellate ganglion resection. When the lower one half is resected, 3 to 36 per cent of patients experience temporary ptosis and miosis, with a 3 to 10 per cent incidence of permanent Horner's syndrome.[26,51] Even when the stellate ganglion is not completely resected, a 2 to 6 per cent incidence of permanent Horner's syndrome has been reported. It should not occur if only the lower third, or the rami connecting with it, are resected. Significant postoperative neuralgia in the face, shoulder, or chest region occurs in 20 to 40 per cent of patients.[39] The discomfort is temporary, usually lasting from 4 to 8 weeks, and requires only mild analgesics for pain relief. Unless forewarned, however, the patient may be convinced that this new discomfort outweighs the benefits of eliminating the preoperative symptoms. Significant changes in isolated pulmonary function parameters have been reported following T2 to T3 ganglionectomy by both intrapleural and extrapleural approaches. These changes consisted of a 15 to 20 per cent reduction in the total lung capacity and forced expiratory volume (in 1 second), but they resolved by the sixth postoperative month in all patients.[52] Operative mortality ranges from 0 to 4 per cent, with deaths occurring secondary to the impact of surgical stress on underlying systemic disease rather than the consequences of sympathectomy itself.

Summary

Upper dorsal sympathectomy is best performed through a transaxillary incision with intrapleural or extrapleural visualization of the stellate and upper thoracic ganglia. It may also be performed using endoscopic instruments in selected patients with reduced postoperative pain, morbidity, and hospital stay. Adequate upper extremity sympathetic denervation for most indications is achieved by resection of the T2 and T3 ganglia alone. T4 is also resected if cessation of axillary sweating is desired. The best indications for this procedure are hyperhidrosis, causalgia, and occupational or environmental digital pain syndromes. Less rewarding, but nonetheless occasionally justifiable, indications are Raynaud's disease with digital ulceration, symptomatic arteriosclerotic occlusive disease with primarily distal involvement, and those with distal thromboembolism. All patients should receive maximal appropriate medical therapy and those with vascular disease should have noninvasive definition of their digital perfusion prior to consideration of sympathectomy. Patient selection is improved by assessing symptomatic and digital perfusion responses to stellate ganglion blocks. Postoperative neuralgia and Horner's syndrome are the most common sequelae that affect patient satisfaction. The former is temporary, the latter can be minimized by restricting the extent of stellate ganglion resection.

LOWER EXTREMITY SYMPATHECTOMY

Primary indications for lumbar sympathectomy are similar to those of dorsal sympathectomy and include causalgia as well as the sequelae of distal arterial emboli and frostbite. Furthermore, a characteristic variant of causalgia following lumbar diskectomy has recently emerged as a valid indication for lumbar sympathetic denervation.[50] In terms of traditional indications, they are limited to identifying patients with "inoperable" arterial occlusive disease who can be reasonably expected to benefit. For the most part, the role of lumbar sympathectomy has become limited to threatened limbs with severe infrapopliteal occlusive disease because the limits of inoperability have been steadily reduced by newer reconstructive techniques. Its role as an adjunctive procedure to arterial reconstructions in patients with poor runoff or hypoplastic proximal or small caliber distal arteries has been supported by past experience,[53,54] but can rarely be justified if it requires a separate incision, as for infrainguinal bypass. In addition, extended use of epidural sympathetic blockade in Europe has demonstrated its utility in improving early patency of difficult infrapopliteal bypasses.[55] However, this potential role for sympathetic blockade may be more easily fulfilled by perioperative dextran 40 infusions.[56] Thus, lumbar sympathectomy has become a well-standardized technique in search of more vascular indications.

Anatomic Considerations

Sympathetic outflow to the lower extremities originates in spinal cord segments from T10 to L3. Preganglionic fibers from these segments form extensive synaptic connections in paravertebral ganglia from L1 to S3 to innervate the entire lower extremity and pelvic region. Sympathetic outflow to the lower extremity below the knee is primarily conveyed through the L2 and L3 ganglia. The remainder of the leg is supplied by ganglia from L1 to L4. Variations in the number and location of sympathetic ganglia are most common in the lumbar region, with the majority occurring at the L1, L4, and L5 levels.[57] Overall, three lumbar ganglia are most commonly found, with fusion of the L1 and L2 ganglia accounting for the reduced number.[57] Crossover fibers occur in 15 per cent of patients, with most leaving via the fourth and fifth lumbar ganglia.[58] Important structures adjacent to the lumbar ganglia are the ureter, lumbar vessels, genitofemoral nerve, aorta, and inferior vena cava. Operative injury to the inferior vena cava or its lumbar tributaries during right lumbar ganglionectomy primarily relates to their intimate association. Injuries to all adjacent structures, however, have been reported.[59]

Operative Technique

Access to the lumbar sympathetic chain is best achieved with a midabdominal oblique incision and extraperitoneal separation of the enclosed viscera from the underlying retroperitoneal structures. The ureter and gonadal vessels are reflected forward with the posterior peritoneum to expose the psoas muscle. The lumbar sympathetic chain is located medially over the transverse processes of the lumbar vertebrae, while the genitofemoral nerve lies more laterally over the midportion of the psoas (Fig. 17–3). Identification of the ganglia is facilitated by gently stroking or plucking them with the index finger and noting their characteristic "snap." Ganglion numbering is best done by distal dissection with identification of the third lumbar adjacent to a large (often crossing) lumbar vein or finding the fourth lumbar ganglion in the deepening sulcus between the iliopsoas and pelvic muscles and then proceeding upward from these ganglia. Excision of the L2 and L3 ganglia is accomplished by metal clip application and division of all encountered rami interganglionic fibers. Inspection for lumbar vein bleeding and layered closure of the abdominal wall musculature completes the procedure.

Much like upper dorsal sympathectomy, clinically adequate sympathetic denervation is usually accomplished by excision of only two ganglia, L2 and L3. More complete resection has been advocated by Imparato to reduce the possibility of incomplete denervation.[60] Inclusion of the L4 ganglion is necessary to remove crossover fibers; however, except for proximally located causalgic pain, L1 ganglionectomy seems to add little and increased the risk of ejaculatory impotence in preclimacteric males.[61]

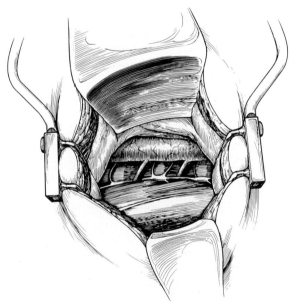

FIGURE 17–3. Retroperitoneal exposure of the right lumbar sympathetic chain from L2 to L4, lying next to the aorta of the transverse processes. The ureter has been retracted upward and the genitofemoral nerve lies laterally on the psoas muscle. As shown between L3 and L4, lumbar vessels may cross *in front of* the chain. (From Rutherford RB: A Technical Atlas of Vascular Surgery. Philadelphia, WB Saunders Company, in preparation.)

The high success rate with percutaneous sympathetic blockade using local anesthetic agents has promoted attempts to achieve extended blockade by phenol neurolysis via the same approach. Using fluoroscopic confirmation with contrast injections adjacent to the first through third lumbar vertebrae, Sanderson has shown that 80 per cent of first injections are at the desired location.[62] Second injections yielded complete lumbar sympathetic neurolysis as determined by sudomotor and foot temperature testing in 90 per cent of patients. Although their successful percutaneous neurolysis rate was only 72 per cent, Walsh et al. demonstrated that the duration of sympathectomy using 10 per cent phenol was identical to that of surgical denervation.[63] Among 31 patients with successful neurolysis, 60 per cent achieved symptomatic relief with significant increases in foot blood flow and skin temperature. Experience with phenol lumbar sympathectomy in the United States is being gained, but has not been convincing. Initial impressions are that this procedure produces less complete and less durable blockade than surgical sympathectomy. Attempts to improve this by radiofrequency heated probes with precision localization is still undergoing improvements, but to date also appears to produce less complete or less durable sympathetic denervation.[64] Further improvements in this approach may offer an alternative means of producing lasting lumbar sympathetic denervation without the morbidity (albeit now low) of a surgical procedure. However, until these techniques produce a reliably complete and lasting sympathetic denervation, they carry the disadvantage of seriously compromising the one procedure that can achieve this goal. Surgeons who have tried to perform lumbar sympathectomy through the scar and inflammatory tissue left in the wake of such attempts, including even too many lumbar anesthetic blocks, will attest to this.

Results

Although Raynaud's disease has been reported to affect the lower extremities, use of lumbar sympathectomy for this condition has been limited in published reports. Application for frostbite is more common in some climates. Comparison of sympathectomy outcomes with results of arterial reconstruction for distal occlusive disease is difficult because prospective studies have not been done and reported patient groups are not comparable. Comparisons with nonoperative treatment or other nonreconstructive procedures (e.g., prostanoids, hyperbaric oxygen, or epidural spinal cord stimulation) have not been reported but all report improvement in a minority of patients.[65] However, review of recent series allows some recommendations to be made because patient groups have been more uniformly categorized.

Ischemic Rest Pain

Critical assessment of the influence of lumbar sympathectomy on limb-threatening ischemia has previously been hampered by group variations in arteriographic extent of occlusive disease, criteria for determining operability, and magnitude of distal perfusion. Among patients with atherosclerotic arterial occlusions and thromboangiitis obliterans, primary indications for lumbar sympathectomy are limited to those who have inoperable disease complicated by rest pain or tissue loss. Experimental evidence indicates that muscular and nutrient blood flow are *not* significantly increased by sympathetic denervation of ischemic limbs. Clinical experience has shown, however, that nearly 80 per cent of patients with an ankle-brachial index greater than 0.3, no evidence of neuropathy, and limited tissue loss obtain relief of their ischemic symptoms.[66] While the criterion of an ankle-brachial index greater than 0.3 may seem arbitrary, it represents a marginal level of perfusion that might suffice to achieve limb salvage if slightly improved. Despite the known influence of sympathectomy on pain transmission that is independent of its circulatory effects, the selection criteria above define conditions in which sympathectomy seems to sufficiently improve the resting limb oxygen supply-demand ratio to prevent ischemic progression.

The primary importance of adequate arterial inflow, as determined by segmental limb pressure, was first recognized by Yao and Bergan.[67] In their retrospective review of unselected patients undergoing lumbar sympathectomy, no response was obtained in 90 per cent of limbs with an ankle-brachial index less than 0.30. Additionally, Imparato first noted the concomitant importance of intact sympathetic innervation by observing that diabetics with neuropathy rarely responded to sympathectomy.[68] He theorized that many diabetics undergo "auto-sympathectomy" secondary to associated neuropathy; therefore, surgical sympathetic denervation in such patients could not further decrease sympathetic vascular tone in the affected extremity. Indirect confirmation to this theory was provided by histologic studies showing no difference in the number of periarterial sympathetic fibers in diabetics with and without previous lumbar sympathectomy.[69]

Although seemingly self-evident, it should be emphasized that the increased blood flow requirements needed to heal deep ulcers or large areas of skin necrosis *cannot* be met by the small increases in perfusion afforded by sympathectomy. Tissue necrosis in most instances reflects a failure of both arterial inflow and local microcirculation that requires supranormal blood flow to meet the increased metabolic demands of healing. This tenet is indirectly supported by radionucleotide studies showing that small, uninfected lesions require at least a twofold increase in perfusion.[70] Large areas of tissue necrosis with infection therefore require perfusion increases that exceed the amount provided by sympathectomy alone.

Thus, lumbar sympathectomy at best restores the delicate balance between blood flow supply and demand in essentially intact but chronically ischemic limbs.

Recent series favoring use of lumbar sympathectomy for rest pain in patients with inoperable arterial disease report symptom relief in 47 to 71 per cent of unselected patients, with acute limb salvage rates of 60 to 94 per cent.[16–18,71] Best results were obtained by Perrson et al. among 37 patients who had an ankle-brachial index greater than 0.3, no evidence of neuropathy, and limited tissue necrosis; 78 per cent of this group enjoyed long-term relief of ischemic rest pain, and only 11 per cent required amputation. Worst results were noted by Fulton and Blakely among 17 unselected patients undergoing sympathectomy; only 6 per cent of this group obtained relief while 70 per cent required early amputation.[71] Although provocative, this latter older experience simply shows that disappointing results can be expected when limb-threatening ischemia is unselectively treated by sympathetic denervation.

Tissue Loss

Assessment of the results of lumbar sympathectomy for distal ischemic ulceration or gangrene is subject to the same limitations as were described for rest pain. Additionally, wound management technique is a variable requiring consideration when determining the efficacy of sympathectomy. Less impressive results than for rest pain are generally noted, with 35 to 62 per cent of patients showing complete initial healing of the ischemic lesions or arrest of gangrene progression. In addition, both early and ultimate amputation rates were higher than the rest pain group, with a range of 27 to 38 per cent.[16–18,71] Best results were again reported by Perrson et al. among 22 patients who had adequate inflow, absent neuropathy, and no evidence of subcutaneous infection; 77 per cent had ulcer healing and only 22 per cent required ultimate amputation.[66] Among patients who showed no healing, sympathectomy did not improve the amputation level required.

Adjunct for Lower Extremity Arterial Reconstruction

The role of the sympathetic nervous system in mediating vasoconstrictor responses is well known; however, assessing the adjunctive utility of sympathetic denervation with arterial reconstruction has only been studied well in patients undergoing aortofemoral bypass. When added to proximal vascular reconstruction, sympathectomy increased total extremity blood flow by a factor of 1.55, decreased vascular resistance in the foot, and reduced the incidence of early graft thrombosis.[73–75] Long-term follow-up, however, disclosed no significant difference in the need for further infrainguinal reconstructive surgery, amputation rate, or incidence of graft limb thrombosis.

European evaluation of blood flow through femoropopliteal bypass grafts in the early postoperative period shows greater flow and lower early graft thrombosis rates in limbs that are subjected to surgical or chemical sympathetic denervation.[55,76] Among patients with lumbar epidural anesthesia, Sandmann et al. implanted electromagnetic flowmeters beyond the distal popliteal anastomosis and noted consistently higher flows when compared to conventional morphine analgesia.[55] Although maximal blood flow peaked on the second postoperative day in both treatment groups, early graft thromboses were detected in the morphine control group within 4 days of operation. Similar enhancement of patency in small arterial anastomoses was noted by Casten et al. in assessing the effect of lumbar sympathectomy in an arterial trauma model.[77] Although early augmentation of graft flow seems advantageous, the chronic effects of sympathectomy on graft patency remain to be determined for infrainguinal reconstruction. The morbidity of an additional abdominal procedure, particularly a retroperitoneal dissection in a heparinized patient, seems greater than the potential benefits of high early graft patency. The use of perioperative dextran 40 infusion has been shown to increase the early patency rate of difficult distal bypasses by threefold and may prove to be more practical than sympathectomy.[56]

Current Indications

Primary indications for lumbar sympathectomy are causalgia of any cause (including frostbite), symptomatic distal arterial emboli, and selected patients with inoperable distal arterial occlusive disease. Current determinations of inoperability vary with local expertise and availability of autogenous saphenous vein for infrapopliteal bypass grafting. In the rare circumstance when such revascularization procedures are not feasible or inadvisable because of inadequate runoff or technical limitations, lumbar sympathectomy may be considered for patients with rest pain or ischemic ulceration who meet the following criteria: (1) ankle-brachial index greater than 0.3; (2) superficial tissue necrosis (confined to the forefoot or digits); (3) absent neuropathy on physical examination; (4) symptom relief or increased plethysmographic amplitude following lumbar sympathetic blockade; and (5) acceptable surgical risk for abdominal operation. Lumbar sympathectomy may also be used as an adjunct to improve early graft patency for more distal reconstructive procedures in patients with poor runoff or hypoplastic vessels, but other methods are preferable (e.g., dextran 40). The probability of the indications for sympathectomy achieving lasting benefit are summarized for both dorsal and lumbar sympathectomy in Table 17–1.

Complications

The major morbidity of lumbar sympathectomy is preventable injury to adjacent structures (lumbar veins, aorta, inferior vena cava, and ureter). Attention to

TABLE 17–1. STRATIFICATION OF INDICATIONS FOR SYMPATHECTOMY ACCORDING TO THE PROBABILITY OF ACHIEVING LASTING SYMPTOMATIC RELIEF

Indication	Dorsal Sympathectomy	Lumbar Sympathectomy
Best	Hyperhidrosis Causalgia Frostbite sequelae Raynaud's phenomenon caused by stable arterial occlusions (e.g., traumatic subintimal fibrosis, distal emboli)	Causalgia Frostbite sequelae Stable, small arterial occlusions (e.g., distal Buerger's atherosclerosis, arterial emboli) with Raynaud's or rest pain
Acceptable	Raynaud's syndrome with digital ulcerations or Distal arterial occlusions Thromboangiitis obliterans	Inoperable, Buerger's or atherosclerotic arterial occlusions with limited tissue loss Adjunctive to aortofemoral arterial reconstruction
Contraindications	Uncomplicated Raynaud's disease	Claudication Diabetes with neuropathy

detail and adequate exposure renders such injuries infrequent. Early recovery of sympathetic vascular tone ("fifth day phenomenon") and postoperative neuralgia occurs in 20 to 50 per cent of patients.[39,61] This latter syndrome is self-limited and well treated with minor analgesics, and rarely causes chronic morbidity. Similar lower extremity hyperesthetic states develop following phenol neurolysis but may last much longer. In patients with severe peripheral vascular disease, incomplete sympathectomy is difficult to distinguish clinically from progression of the underlying occlusive process. Mortality rates of 0 to 4 per cent have been reported, with cardiac and pulmonary deterioration following operation the most common cause of death. Most of the deaths were reported in earlier studies. Proper perioperative monitoring should minimize these.

Summary

Lumbar sympathectomy currently has a limited role in the treatment of limb-threatening ischemia because direct revascularization techniques yield more consistent and far better results. L2 and L3 ganglionectomy provides sufficient denervation for most indications; L4 resection is added when ablation of crossover innervation is desired. Best results are obtained when patients are selected according to threshold inflow criteria, absent neuropathy, limited or lack of tissue necrosis, and favorable response to preoperative lumbar sympathetic blockade. Lumbar sympathectomy is indicated for truly operable occlusive disease complicated by rest pain or minor tissue loss and for causalgia. The most common complications of lumbar sympathectomy are temporary neuralgia and inadequate clinical improvement. Careful selection using the suggested criteria will minimize the latter.

REFERENCES

1. Ewing M: The history of lumbar sympathectomy. Surgery *70*:791–795, 1971.
2. Simeone FA: The lumbar sympathetic. Anatomy and surgical implications. Acta Chir Belg *76*:17–16, 1977.
3. Ross JP: Surgery of the Sympathetic Nervous System. London, Bailliere, Tindall and Cox, 1958.
4. Cronenwett JL, Lindenauer SM: Hemodynamic effects of sympathectomy in ischemic canine hind limbs. Surgery *87*:417–424, 1980.
5. Cronenwett JL, Zelenock GB, Whitehouse W Jr, et al: The effect of sympathetic innervation on canine muscle and skin blood flow. Arch Surg *118*:420–424, 1983.
6. Simeone FA: Intravascular pressure, vascular tone and sympathectomy. (Presidential address, 16th Annual Meeting Society for Vascular Surgery, Chicago, IL, June 24, 1962.) Surgery *53*:1, 1963.
7. Beran RD, Tsuru H: Functional and structural changes in rabbit ear artery after sympathetic denervation. Circ Res *49*:478–485, 1981.
8. Bobik A, Anderson WP: Influence of sympathectomy on alpha 2 adrenoreceptor binding sites in canine blood vessels. Life Sci *33*:331–336, 1983.
9. Barcroft H, Swan HJC: Sympathetic Control of Human Blood Vessels. London, Edward Arnold & Co, 1952.
10. Petten CV, Roberts WJ, Rhodes DL: Behavioral test of tolerance for aversive mechanical stimuli in sympathectomized cats. Pain *15*:177–189, 1983.
11. Courbier R, Reggi M, Jansserau JM: Evaluation of effectiveness of lumbar sympathectomy by non-invasive diagnostic techniques. J Cardiovasc Surg (Torino) *20*:333–337, 1979.
12. Loh L, Nathan PW: Painful peripheral states and sympathetic blocks. J Neurol Neurosurg Psychiatry *41*:664–671, 1978.
13. Melzack R, Wall PD: Pain mechanisms: A new theory. Science *150*:971–979, 1965.
14. Moore WS, Hall AD: Effects of lumbar sympathectomy on skin capillary blood flow in arterial occlusive disease. J Surg Res *14*:151–160, 1973.
15. Perry MO, Horton J: Muscle and subcutaneous oxygen tension. Measurements by mass spectrometry after sympathectomy. Arch Surg *113*:176–178, 1978.
16. Collins GJ, Rich NM, Clagett GP, et al: Clinical results of lumbar sympathectomy. Am Surg *47*:31–35, 1981.
17. Haimovici H, Steinman C, Karson IH: Evaluation of lumbar sympathectomy. Advanced occlusive arterial disease. Arch Surg *89*:1089–1095, 1964.
18. Szilagyi DE, Smith RF, Scarpella JR, et al: Lumbar sympathectomy. Current role in the treatment of arteriosclerotic occlusive disease. Arch Surg *95*:753–761, 1967.
19. Holcroft JW, Vassar MJ: Prostaglandins and their analogues: Experience in healing ischemic ulcers. Semin Vasc Surg *4*:221–226, 1991.
20. Rutherford RB, Valenta J: Extremity blood flow and distribution: The effects of arterial occlusive, sympathectomy and exercise. Surgery *69*:332–338, 1971.
21. Lindenauer SM, Cronenwett JL: What is the place of lumbar sympathectomy? Br J Surg *69*(suppl):532–533, 1982.
22. Enjalbert A: Effect of lumbar sympathectomy on the muscles. J Cardiovasc Surg (Torino) *20*:295–300, 1979.
23. Owens JC: Indications for lumbar sympathectomy. *In* Dale WA (ed): The Management of Arterial Occlusive Disease. Chicago, Year Book Medical Publishers, Inc, 1971.
24. Dalessandri KM, Carson SN, Tillman P, et al: Effect of lumbar

sympathectomy in distal arterial obstruction. Arch Surg *228*:1157–1160, 1983.
25. Ludbrook J: Collateral arterial resistance in the human lower limbs. J Surg Res *6*:423, 1966.
26. Welch E, Geary J: Current status of thoracic dorsal sympathectomy. J Vasc Surg *1*:202–214, 1984.
27. Porter JM, Rivers SP, Anderson CJ, et al: Evaluation and management of patients with Raynaud's syndrome. Am J Surg *142*:183–187, 1981.
28. Kuntz A: Distribution of the sympathetic rami to the brachial plexus. Its relation to sympathectomy affecting the upper extremity. Arch Surg *15*:871–877, 1927.
29. Ray BS: Sympathectomy of the upper extremity. Evaluation of surgical methods. J Neurosurg *10*:624–633, 1953.
30. Roos DB: Sympathectomy for the upper extremities. *In* Rutherford RB (ed): Vascular Surgery. Philadelphia, WB Saunders Company, 1984.
31. Roos DB: Transaxillary extrapleural thoracic sympathectomy. *In* Bergen JJ, Yao JST (eds): Operative Techniques in Vascular Surgery. New York, Grune & Stratton, 1980.
32. Atkins HJB: Preaxillary approach to the stellate and upper thoracic sympathetic ganglia. Lancet *2*:1152, 1949.
33. Telford ED: The technic of sympathectomy. Br J Surg *23*:448–459, 1935.
34. Appleby TC, Edwards WHJ: Thoracoscopic dorsal sympathectomy for hyperhidrosis: Technique of choice. J Vasc Surg 1992, in press.
35. Owens JC: Causalgia. Am Surg *23*:636–640, 1957.
36. Beurger R, Smit R: Transaxillary sympathectomy (T2 to T4) for relief of vasospastic/sympathetic pain of upper extremities. Surgery *89*:764–769, 1981.
37. Thompson JE: The diagnosis and management of post-traumatic pain syndromes (causalgia). Aust NZ J Surg *49*:299–304, 1979.
38. Kirtley JA, Riddell DH, Stoney WS, et al: Cervicothoracic sympathectomy in neurovascular abnormalities of the upper extremity. Experience in 76 patients with 104 sympathectomies. Ann Surg *165*:869–879, 1967.
39. Mockus M, Rutherford RB, Rosales C: Sympathectomy for causalgia: Patient selection and long-term results. Arch Surg *122*:668–672, 1987.
40. Porter JM: Raynaud's syndrome and associated vasospastic conditions of the extremities. *In* Rutherford RB (ed): Vascular Surgery. Philadelphia, WB Saunders Company, 1984.
41. Baddely RM: The place of upper dorsal sympathectomy in the treatment of primary Raynaud's disease. Br J Surg *54*:426–443, 1965.
42. Gifford EW Jr, Hines EA Jr, Craig VM: Sympathectomy for Raynaud's phenomenon: Followup study of 70 women with Raynaud's disease and 54 women with secondary Raynaud's phenomenon. Circulation *17*:5–13, 1958.
43. Linder F, Jenal G, Assmus H: Axillary transpleural sympathectomy: Indication, technique and results. World J Surg *7*:437–439, 1983.
44. Conn J Jr, Bergan JJ, Bell JL: Hypothenar hammer syndrome: Post-traumatic digital ischemia. Surgery *68*:1122–1127, 1970.
45. Christophers AJ: Occupational aspects of Raynaud's disease: A critical historical survey. Med J Aust *2*:730–733, 1972.
46. Montorsi W, Ghringhelli C, Annoni F: Indications and results of surgical treatment in Raynaud's phenomenon. J Cardiovasc Surg (Torino) *21*:203–210, 1980.
47. Zweifler AJ, Trinkaus P: Occlusive digital artery disease in

patients with Raynaud's phenomenon. Am J Med *77*:995–1001, 1984.

48. Smith CR, Rodeffer RJ: Raynaud's phenomenon: Pathophysiologic features and treatment with calcium-channel blockers. Am J Cardiol *55*:154B–157B, 1985.

49. Welling RE, Cranley JJ, Krause RJ, et al: Obliterative arterial disease of the upper extremity. Arch Surg *116*:1593–1596, 1981.

50. Owens JG: Complications of sympathectomy. *In* Beebe HG (ed): Complications in Vascular Surgery. Philadelphia, JB Lippincott Co, 1973.

51. Romeno A, Kurchin A, Rudich R, et al: Ocular manifestations after upper dorsal sympathectomy. Ann Ophthalmol *2*:1083–1086, 1979.

52. Molno M, Shemesh E, Gordon D, et al: Pulmonary function abnormalities after upper dorsal sympathectomy. A comparison between the supraclavicular and transaxillary approaches. Chest *77*:651–655, 1980.

53. DeLaurentis DA, Friedmann P, Wolferth CC Jr, et al: Atherosclerosis and the hypoplastic aortoiliac system. Surgery *83*:27–37, 1978.

54. Satiani B, Liapis CD, Hayes JP, et al: Prospective randomized study of concomitant lumbar sympathectomy with aortoiliac reconstruction. Am J Surg *143*:755–760, 1982.

55. Sandmann W, Kremer K, Wust H, et al: Postoperative control of blood flow in arterial surgery and results of electromagnetic blood flow measurement. Thoraxchir *25*:427–434, 1977.

56. Rutherford RB, Jones DN, Bergentz SE, et al: The efficacy of dextran-40 preventing early post-operative thrombosis following difficult lower extremity bypass. J Vasc Surg *1*:765–763, 1984.

57. Yeager GH, Cowley RA: Anatomical observations on the lumbar sympathetics with evaluation of sympathectomies in organic peripheral vascular disease. Ann Surg *127*:953–967, 1948.

58. Callow AD, Simeone FA: The Grimonster Symposium on the occasion of the 50th anniversary of the first lumbar sympathectomy. Arch Surg *113*:295, 1978.

59. Rutherford RB: Complications of sympathectomy. *In* Towne JB, Bernhard VM (eds): Complications in Vascular Surgery, 2nd ed. New York, Grune & Stratton, 1984.

60. Imparato AM: Lumbar sympathectomy. Role in the treatment of occlusive arterial disease in the lower extremities. Surg Clin North Am *59*:719–735, 1979.

61. Rutherford RB: Lumbar sympathectomy: Indications and technique. *In* Rutherford RB (ed): Vascular Surgery. Philadelphia, WB Saunders Company, 1984.

62. Sanderson CJ: Chemical lumbar sympathectomy with radiologic assessment. Ann R Coll Surg Engl *63*:420–422, 1981.

63. Walsh JA, Glynn CJ, Cousins MJ, et al: Blood flow, sympathetic activity and pain relief following lumbar sympathetic blockade and surgical sympathectomy. Anesth Intensive Care *13*:18–24, 1984.

64. Noe CE, Haynsworth RF Jr: Lumbar radiofrequency sympatholysis. J Vasc Surg 1992, accepted for publication.

65. Dormandy J, Andreani D, Bell P, et al: Second European Consensus Document of Chronic Critical Ischemia. Circulation (suppl) *84*(5):IV-1–IV-26, 1991.

66. Persson AV, Anderson L, Rodberg FT Jr: Selection of patients for lumbar sympathectomy. Surg Clin North Am *65*:393–403, 1985.

67. Yao JST, Bergan JJ: Predictability of vascular reactivity relative to sympathetic ablation. Arch Surg *107*:676–681, 1973.

68. Kim GE, Igrahim IM, Imparato AM: Lumbar sympathectomy in end-stage arterial occlusive disease. Ann Surg *183*:157–160, 1976.

69. Grove JH, Bauman FG, Riles TS, et al: Effect of surgical lumbar sympathectomy on innervation of arterioles in the lower limbs of patients with diabetes. Surg Gynecol Obstet *153*:39–41, 1981.

70. Siegal ME, William GM, Giargiana FA Jr, et al: A useful objective criterion for determining the healing potential of an ischemic ulcer. J Nucl Med *21*:993–998, 1975.

71. Walker PM, Johnston KW: Predicting the success of a sympathectomy. A prospective study using discriminant function and multiple regression analysis. Surgery *87*:216–221, 1980.

72. Fulton RL, Blakely WR: Lumbar sympathectomy: A procedure of questionable value in the treatment of arteriosclerosis obliterans of the legs. Am J Surg *116*:735–744, 1968.

73. Barnes RW, Baker WH, Shanik G, et al: Value of concomitant sympathectomy in aortoiliac reconstruction. Results of a prospective, randomized study. Arch Surg *112*:1325–1330, 1977.

74. Collins GJ Jr, Rich HM, Anderson CA, et al: Acute hemodynamic effects of lumbar sympathectomy. Am J Surg *136*:714–718, 1978.

75. Shanik GD, Ford J, Hayes AC, et al: Pedal vasomotor tone following aortofemoral reconstructions: A randomized study of concomitant lumbar sympathectomy. Ann Surg *183*:136–138, 1976.

76. Faenza A, Splare R, Lapilli A, et al: Clinical results of lumbar sympathectomy alone or as a complement to direct arterial surgery. Acta Chir Belg *76*:101–107, 1977.

77. Casten DF, Sadler AH, Furman D: An experimental study of the effect of sympathectomy on patency of small blood vessel anastomoses. Surg Gynecol Obstet *115*:462–466, 1962.

REVIEW QUESTIONS

1. All of the following statements regarding the effects of sympathetic denervation are true except:
   - (a) increased extremity blood flow is primarily distributed through cutaneous arteriovenous anastomosis flow.
   - (b) partial recovery of resting vasomotor tone is mediated by increased sensitivity of extrasynaptic α_2 receptors to exogenous norepinephrine
   - (c) sympathectomy produces maximal vasodilation in an ischemic extremity 50 per cent greater than that produced by local metabolic influences
   - (d) sympathectomy is believed to enhance pain tolerance by decreasing tissue concentrations of norepinephrine and by reducing spinal transmission of impulses arising from noxious stimuli to peripheral nerves

2. Upper extremity sympathectomy produces worthwhile benefit for all of the following conditions except:
   - (a) causalgia
   - (b) hyperhidrosis
   - (c) distal emboli with Raynaud's phenomenon
   - (d) Raynaud's syndrome caused by scleroderma

3. Horner's syndrome is most likely to follow:
   - (a) resection of T2 and T3 ganglia only
   - (b) complete resection of the stellate ganglion
   - (c) resection of the lower one third of the stellate ganglion
   - (d) division of Kuntz's nerve

4. Which of the following techniques of thoracodorsal

sympathectomy poses the greatest risk of injury to the phrenic nerve?

(a) supraclavicular approach
(b) axillary transthoracic approach
(c) posterior approach
(d) axillary extrapleural approach

5. Which of the following statements concerning Raynaud's disease secondary to nonocclusive vasospasm is true?

(a) nearly all patients have recognizable signs of an associated collagen vascular disease
(b) symptom relief by surgical sympathectomy will ultimately be required by the majority
(c) up to 50 per cent of patients will develop signs of underlying collagen vascular disease within 6 months of follow-up
(d) the natural history follows a benign course with less than 50 per cent of patients manifesting the stigmata of an associated collagen vascular disease over 5 years of observation

6. Which is the most frequent complication following T2, T3, and T4 sympathetic ganglionectomy for severe hyperhidrosis?

(a) permanent Horner's syndrome
(b) postoperative neuralgia
(c) rebound vasospasm with cold sensitivity
(d) recurrent hyperhidrosis

7. Which of the following criteria should be met prior to performing a lumbar sympathectomy in a diabetic patient with toe ulceration due to inoperable infrapopliteal arterial occlusive disease?

(a) ankle-brachial index < 0.3
(b) ankle-brachial index > 0.3
(c) absent neuropathy
(d) limited tissue loss without associated infection

8. Which one of the following is not an indication for sympathectomy?

(a) Raynaud's phenomenon following emboli to small vessels supplying the hand
(b) intermittent claudication of the foot due to infrapopliteal occlusive disease
(c) rest pain in a patient with inoperable arterial occlusions
(d) postfrostbite causalgia

9. Crossover preganglionic sympathetic fibers most commonly exit the spinal axis at what level?

(a) T-10 and L1
(b) L2 and L3
(c) L4 and L5
(d) S1

10. The incidence of early postoperative thrombosis of distal bypass grafts has been demonstrably reduced by which of the following adjunctive measures?

(a) dextran 40 infusions
(b) temporary epidural block
(c) lumbar sympathectomy
(d) antiplatelet drugs

ANSWERS

1. c	2. d	3. b	4. a	5. d	6. b	7. b,c,d
8. b	9. c	10. a,c,d				

18

THROMBOLYTIC THERAPY FOR VASCULAR DISEASE

WILLIAM J. QUIÑONES-BALDRICH

The fluidity of blood postmortem is an observation that dates to the Hippocratic school in the fourth century B.C.[1] Almost 2000 years later, it was rediscovered by the Italian anatomist Malpighi.[2] In 1761, Morgagni noted that blood does not retain its liquid state after death, but frequently forms clots.[3] This is followed by partial or complete reliquification.

In 1906, Morawitz observed that postmortem blood destroyed fibrinogen and fibrin in normal blood.[4] Thus, the presence of an active fibrinolysin was postulated. The term "fibrinolysis" had been coined by Dastre in 1893 to describe the disappearance of fibrin in unclottable blood obtained from dogs subjected to repeated hemorrhage.[5] From the latter part of the 19th century until the present, intense investigation in this field has attempted to elucidate the complex and vital functions of the fibrinolytic system. Its physiology, components, activators, and inhibitors are only partially understood. The role of the fibrinolytic system from the homeostatic point of view is fully appreciated. Its potential, from the therapeutic standpoint, has emerged in the last few decades. Clearly, precise control of this system to favor resolution of a thrombotic process is in the frontier of clinical medicine. For the vascular specialist, this represents one of the most promising therapeutic modalities. Unfortunately, currently available agents lack the precise control necessary to avoid complications inherent in an overactive fibrinolytic system. Even so, in this era, thrombolytic therapy can be successfully utilized and, in some instances, is the preferential treatment.

The purpose of this chapter is to provide the reader with basic understanding of the fibrinolytic system and available agents, and offer guidelines that will help clinicians appropriately select patients who may benefit from thrombolytic therapy. Methods, dosages, complications, and new promising areas will be discussed.

THE FIBRINOLYTIC SYSTEM

The complex and intricate relationship of all components of the fibrinolytic system are not fully under-

stood. Much progress has been made in the last 5 years, mostly due to increased interest and recognition of the importance of the fibrinolytic system, both as a homeostatic system and as a therapeutic alternative. The concept of dynamic equilibrium was proposed by Astrup in 1958.[6] In a delicate balance, fibrinolysis breaks down fibrin that is continuously being deposited throughout the cardiovascular system. This is the result of limited activation of the coagulation system. This baseline fibrinolytic activity is probably under local and central control mechanisms. The feedback loop that prevents systemic fibrinolysis involves inhibitors at both the activator level and specific inhibitors of the proteolytic enzyme, plasmin.

The final common pathway in the fibrinolytic system is the conversion of the proenzyme plasminogen to the active enzyme plasmin. Plasminogen is a glycoprotein produced by the liver. Full-sized plasminogen can be divided into a heavy aminoterminal region that consists of five homologous, but distinct, triple disulfide bonded domains (kringles) fused to a lighter catalytic C-terminal domain. At least four forms occur in plasma, based on variation of the N terminus and degree of glycosylation. The two main forms are labeled Glu-plasminogen and Lys-plasminogen.[7] Glu-plasminogen contains glutamic acid and exists in high concentration in plasma. Lys-plasminogen, containing mostly lysin in the NH_2 terminal, results from limited proteolysis of the Glu form, has a shorter half-life, and is found in higher concentrations in thrombus, most likely secondary to its higher affinity for fibrin.[8] A schematic view of the fibrinolytic system is presented in Figure 18–1.

The kringle portion of plasminogen is a nonprotease, or heavy chain, consisting of five homologous domains. They exhibit a high degree of sequence homology with each other and with domains found in prothrombin, tissue plasminogen activator, urinary plasminogen activator, and factor XII. Kringle 4 shares homology with apolipoprotein A. The function of these kringles is thought to be of paramount

313

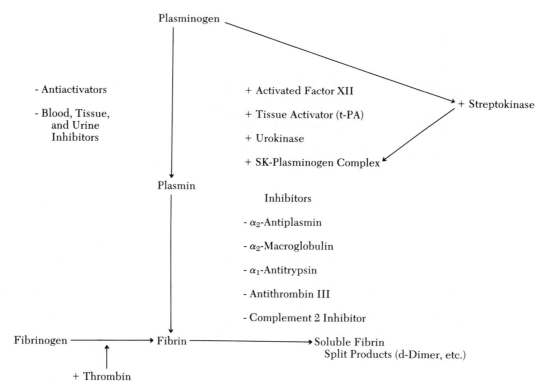

FIGURE 18-1. Simplified scheme of the fibrinolytic system with endogenous and exogenous activators.

importance in the binding of plasminogen and plasmin to fibrin, α_2-antiplasmin, and other macromolecules.[9,10] In addition, the kringle portion of plasminogen has been implicated in mediating neutrophil adherence to endothelial cells.[11] Upon binding, conformational changes occur that transform a closed structure into an open structure. Epsilon aminocaproic acid and tranexamic acid will induce this change from the closed structure to the open structure. This change renders this plasminogen far more readily cleaved to the active enzyme, plasmin, by plasminogen activators. The open conformation also binds more readily to exposed lysine residues of the fibrin's surface. Concentrations of lysine analogues, such as tranexamic acid and aminocaproic acid, that actually promote the more active open conformation of Glu-plasminogen, will also prevent its binding to fibrin, and therefore exhibit their antifibrinolytic effect.[12]

The primary substrates for the proteolytic activity of plasma in circulation are fibrinogen and fibrin. Circulating fibrinogen is comprised of three polypeptide chains known as a-alpha, b-beta, and gamma. These chains are bonded together by disulfide bonds which, in addition, are linked to a second identical chain, thus making it a dimer of trimers. Thrombin, the common pathway of the coagulation cascade, removes several amino acid peptides from the end terminus of the a-alpha chain, the b-beta chain (fibrinopeptide B), to form fibrin. As new sites are exposed, staggered polymerization is initiated.[7] Through catalysis by factor XIIIa, the domains are brought together and chemically cross-linked. Plasmin cata-

lyzes the hydrolysis of these bonds, producing peptides that can be assayed in circulation. Specifically, those produced after the cleavage of fibrinogen, consist of truncated polypeptides collectively known as X fragments. X fragments can be incorporated in both newly forming and existing thrombi, causing them to be more fragile. This has been proposed as an explanation of why fewer bleeding complications have not been observed with fibrin-specific fibrinolytic agents such as tissue-type plasminogen activator (t-PA), compared to nonspecific agents. With tissue plasminogen activator being such a potent fibrinolytic activator, the accumulation of these X fragments may make existing thrombi more susceptible to its fibrinolytic action. Several fragments are specifically produced by the action of plasmin on fibrin, as opposed to fibrinogen. Unique fragments such as d-dimers can be assayed, documenting fibrinolysis as opposed to fibrinogenolysis.[13]

Plasmin is a relatively nonspecific protease, and thus can hydrolyze many proteins found in plasma and extracellular spaces. Known targets of plasmin are factors V, VIII, and von Willebrand factor.[1] Prothrombotic activity can be shown with the initial administration of fibrinolytic agents; specifically, tissue plasminogen activator and streptokinase, which may relate to the release of fibrinopeptide A. Plasminogen can also cause the release of kinin from high molecular weight kininogen. It can also directly and indirectly activate prekalikrein, again inducing kinin formation.[14] Plasmin can also attack protein components of basement membrane, as well as other active proteases within the matrix. These include fibronectin, collagen, and laminin.[7]

Activation of factor XII by various stimuli will result in initiation of the coagulation cascade, conversion of prekalikrein to kallikrein and kinin (inflammatory response), and formation of plasmin from plasminogen. This intrinsic mechanism of activation is complemented by a second intrinsic pathway, not dependent on factor XII. The main pathway for plasminogen activation is known as the extrinsic system. Two activators are recognized in humans: urokinase-type plasminogen activator (u-PA) and t-PA. Their physiologic activity is controlled by inhibitors, mostly plasminogen activator inhibitor type 1 (PAI-1) and plasminogen activator inhibitor type 3. These inhibitors control the activity of the activators in plasma, and possibly at the cellular level. PAI-1 is synthesized in the liver and vascular endothelial cells and is normally present in trace amounts in plasma. When pharmacologic doses of these agents are administered, the inhibitor activity is suppressed. It is estimated that one third to one half of the initial pharmacologic dose of urokinase, for example, becomes inactivated shortly after administration.[11] Once plasminogen has been converted to plasmin, inhibitors of plasmin come into play. The main physiologic inhibitor of plasmin is α_2-antiplasmin. This protease inhibitor is a single-chain glycoprotein that inhibits plasminogen in two steps, a fast reversible binding step, followed by the formation of a covalent complex involving the active site of plasmin.[7] The half-life of this complex is approximately 12 hours.[16] Other inhibitors of plasmin include α_2-macroglobulin, protease nexin, and aprotinin. Protease nexin is a broad-spectrum inhibitor of serine proteinases, and inhibits, among others, trypsin, thrombin, urokinase, plasmin, and one- or two-chain tissue plasminogen activator. Once bound, these proteases are internalized via nexin receptors on the cell surface and rapidly degraded.[17] Aprotinin, also known as basic pancreatic trypsin inhibitor, has been isolated and purified and is sold under the name of Trasylol (Bayer, Germany). It is also a potent inhibitor of trypsin and kallikrein, in addition to plasmin. The use of bovine aprotinin to reduce postoperative bleeding after major surgery has been reported.[18,19] In animal models, it has been shown to serve as an antidote for bleeding induced by administration of rt-PA.[20] Since it inhibits plasmin and not the activator, it should work with other plasminogen activators.

This complex system is capable of maintaining a balanced equilibrium between clotting and lysis, such that blood fluidity is assured. It is important to recognize that although plasmin is highly selective for fibrin, it will also digest fibrinogen and other plasma proteins as well. Circulating plasmin inhibitors prevent this otherwise disordered lytic action and preclude free circulating plasmin under normal conditions. Other important biologic functions of the plasminogen-plasmin systems have now been recognized. The actions of plasminogen activators are facilitated by the presence of receptors of plasminogen, urokinase plasminogen activator, and tissue plasminogen activator on cell surfaces as well as in circulation. Expressions of these components have been observed in tissue cultures and in tissues. They are believed to be actively involved in biologic functions at the cellular level, such as embryogenesis, ovulation, neuron growth, muscle regeneration, wound healing, angiogenesis, and in tumor growth and invasion.[21] It is now postulated that tumor cell invasion (as well as cell migration) and other important biologic processes are dependent on the plasminogen-plasmin system. Endothelial cells and smooth muscle cells that take an active role in thrombosis and in atherogenesis may involve the plasminogen-plasmin system and cellular receptors in the reparative process following vascular injury. The expression seems to be modulated by a variety of cytokines including interleukin and tumor necrosis factor, hormones such as steroid, gonadotropins, and growth factors including platelet-derived growth factor.[21] Focal proteolysis, accomplished by binding of these cellular receptors as part of the plasminogen-plasmin system, allows the migrating cell to penetrate its surrounding extracellular matrix. Urokinase plasminogen activator has also been found to be a growth stimulant and mitogenic for some tumor cells.[22–24] These findings suggest that proliferation of endothelial and smooth muscle cells during vascular repair and atherogenesis induces increased expression of urokinase plasminogen activator in these cells. Both PAI-1 and PAI-2 are present on cell surfaces. Differences in distribution between urokinase plasminogen activator and its inhibitor would allow proteolysis to occur at focal points where the activator is located. The inhibitor would allow a foothold for the cell, aiding in its movement.

The synthesis and release of PAI-1 by the endothelial and hepatic cells may be under control of plasma insulin. It has been suggested that insulin stimulates synthesis and release of PAI-1 from hepatocytes, while t-PA and PAI-1 are released simultaneously from endothelial cells because of an acute-phase response to chronic vascular disease, and subsequently are rapidly inactivated by complex formation.[25] A link between lipoprotein metabolism and fibrinolytic function has been suggested by the demonstration of significant homology between the amino acid sequence of apolipoprotein A and the structure of plasminogen. Thus, a prothrombotic function by virtue of interference with the numerous physiologic functions of plasminogen has been suggested in patients with increased levels of apolipoprotein A. Apolipoprotein A has also been found to competitively inhibit the binding of plasminogen to fibrinogen and to the plasminogen receptor on endothelial cells.[26]

Plasma levels of both t-PA and PAI-1 exhibit circadian variations. t-PA activity is lowest in the early morning and highest in the afternoon. Plasma PAI activity peaks in the early morning and passes through a trough in the afternoon. Thus, overall, there is decreased fibrinolytic activity in the morning.[27-30] Differences in patterns have also been seen between men and women, suggesting a hormonal influence.[31] PAI activity has also been noted to vary secondary to diet. Caffeine-containing beverages may enhance fibrinolytic activity. On the other hand, cigarette smoking induces an acute increase in tissue plasminogen activator. This increase in tissue plasminogen activator induced by smoking may deplete normal stores and thus paradoxically decrease fibrinolytic capacity.

From the foregoing discussion, it is evident that the fibrinolytic system (plasminogen-plasmin system) plays a vital role in biologic homeostasis. In addition, an increasingly pivotal role is seen in certain disease states, ranging from atherosclerosis to carcinogenesis.

From the therapeutic standpoint, drugs capable of converting plasminogen to plasmin will achieve their lytic effect to a great extent by overwhelming circulating plasmin inhibitors and generating an abundance of plasmin (exogenous fibrinolysis). Circulating plasmin will not only produce the desired fibrinolysis, but will also proceed to digest circulating fibrinogen. A more desirable situation results in the activation of thrombus-bound plasminogen (endogenous fibrinolysis) by these agents. Thrombus-bound plasminogen is, to a certain extent, protected from circulating inhibitors, and thus proceeds with fibrin digestion much more effectively. Current investigations are concentrated in producing agents with high affinity for thrombus-bound plasminogen and little activation of the circulating zymogen. Clinical experience to date has failed to demonstrate this theoretical benefit. With better understanding of the complexity of the fibrinolytic system, it is possible that these benefits can be realized.

FIBRINOLYTIC AGENTS

Agents capable of activating the fibrinolytic system can be divided into indirect and direct activators. Indirect activators include a long list of drugs capable of increasing fibrinolytic activity in vivo without direct in vitro activity on plasminogen. The mechanism of action is variable and has not been elucidated for most of these indirect agents.

From the therapeutic standpoint, chronic enhancement of the fibrinolytic activity is attractive, although of unproven clinical value. Most indirect fibrinolytic drugs lose their effectiveness with time. Such is the case with nicotinic acid and adrenaline. Both cause an abrupt but transient increase in fibrinolytic activity by release of endothelial plasminogen activator. Thus, long-term administration is of no benefit.

Antidiuretic hormone (ADH) is capable of stimulating the fibrinolytic system at the expense of severe cardiovascular side effects. A more prolonged response without side effects has been observed with a synthetic analog of ADH, desamino-D-arginine vasopressin (DDAVP). Intranasal administration of this analog caused a plasminogen activator response with a half-life of over 6 hours.[32] The increased fibrinolytic response to DDAVP, however, seems to be clinically insignificant when compared with endothelial release of factor VIII and other important procoagulant effects, which have found clinical usefulness in managing patients with certain bleeding diatheses.

Steroids and diguanides (phenformin) are the most promising of these compounds. Stanozol, for example, is an anabolic steroid capable of producing sustained stimulation of the fibrinolytic system for periods over 5 years with daily administration.[33] In a small clinical trial, Jarret et al.[34] treated 16 patients suffering chronic recurrent thrombophlebitis with stanozol. Thirteen patients had no recurrences during short-term treatment (6 weeks). Renewed attacks were seen in five patients after discontinuation of therapy that were successfully relieved by the readministration of stanozol and phenformin.[34]

Available evidence on indirect fibrinolytic agents is mostly anecdotal. The long-term benefits of an enhanced fibrinolytic system are open to speculation. In many cases, the increased fibrinolytic activity occurs in patients whose baseline activity is depressed. In others, no clinical benefit is observed in spite of a sustained drug effect. In addition, fibrinolytic capacity may be decreased by chronic stimulation, thus rendering the system incapable of adequately responding to a thrombotic stimulus.[10] Certainly this is an area of promise that will require randomized controlled long-term studies to answer important questions on the value of chronic enhancement of fibrinolytic activity in vascular disease.

Direct Fibrinolytic Agents

Direct fibrinolytic agents are capable of converting plasminogen to plasmin both in vitro and in vivo. They do not have fibrinolytic activity by themselves, and thus require an intact enzyme system to exert their lytic action.

Streptokinase

Streptokinase is a single-chain nonenzymatic protein produced by β-hemolytic streptococci. Its discovery by Tillet and Garner in 1933 revived the interest in fibrinolysis seen in the last five decades.[35] Early clinical experience was complicated by a multitude of pyrogenic and allergic reactions. This prompted manufacturers to refine the drug, achieving the currently purified product and a marked reduction in febrile and allergic reactions.

The mechanism of action of streptokinase is complex. It initially forms an equimolar complex with plasminogen to form a plasminogen activator. Thus, it requires plasminogen as a cofactor and a substrate. The initial reaction is species specific, having excellent affinity for human and cat plasminogen, relatively poor affinity for dog and rabbit plasminogen, and no reaction with bovine proenzyme. Once the activator complex is formed, it is an excellent activator of all mammalian plasminogen. Besides converting uncomplexed plasminogen to plasmin, plasminogen within the activator complex is converted to plasmin and, during this conversion, streptokinase undergoes rapid progressive degradation.

The kinetics of these reactions have been studied in vitro. In vivo, a more complicated series of reactions will occur. Infusion of streptokinase will be followed initially by neutralization by circulating antistreptococcal antibodies. The remaining drug will then combine with circulating plasminogen to form the activator complex. This will then convert uncomplexed plasminogen to plasmin, which will either combine with any excess free streptokinase, be neutralized by circulating antiplasmins, or bind to preformed fibrin. The latter will produce the desired effect of thrombolysis. When activity is measured, however, two half-lives are detected, one at 16 and one at 83 minutes, indicating that these complex interactions have a significant impact on the concentration and activity of the drug.

From the foregoing discussion, it is evident that precise control of thrombolysis is not possible, because the dose-response relationship of streptokinase is variable from patient to patient. Initially, clinical use was guided by titers of antistreptococcal antibodies and measurement of the various components or products of the system. This proved impractical and current practice utilizes standardized dosage that will achieve the desired effect in the great majority of cases. A potential drawback of this approach is the administration of excess amounts of drug that could utilize most of the circulating plasminogen to form activator complex. This may leave inadequate amounts of zymogen to convert to plasmin. This problem of exceeding plasminogen availability may be of importance during regional, rather than systemic, administration. Some investigators have combined streptokinase with plasmin administration, with improvement in measured parameters such as plasminogen level, fibrinogen level, and potential fibrinolytic capacity.[36] Similar results are obtained by intermittent rather than continued infusion of the drug. Unfortunately, results of these noncontrolled trials have raised doubts as to the improved effectiveness of such regimens. For the average clinician, continuous infusion therapy remains the most practical method of administration.

Urokinase

Urokinase is a serine protease with direct activator activity, normally present in urine as a product of renal tubular cells. It was originally isolated by McFarlane and Pilling in 1947.[37] Urokinase is present in various molecular weight forms, with variability in its activity. Original purification was done from urine, yielding small amounts of the enzyme at a considerable cost. Current production uses human fetal kidney cell culture. This has reduced the cost considerably, making the drug available for clinical use. Urokinase is nonantigenic, and its mechanism of

action is much more direct, compared to streptokinase. Urokinase cleaves plasminogen (its only known protein substrate), by first-order reaction kinetics, to plasmin. It is relatively pH and temperature stable. The lack of circulating neutralizing antibodies and its direct mechanism of action allow for a predictable dose-response relationship. Interestingly, urokinase does not contain any lysine binding sites, and therefore does not have any fibrin-binding properties.[38] High-affinity receptors for urokinase, however, have been demonstrated in several cell types and postulated as a mechanism by which cells can invade intracellular matrix and play a role in other physiologic and pathologic processes.[39–41]

The activation of plasminogen by urokinase occurs by proteolysis of its substrate plasminogen. Once administered intravenously, urokinase is rapidly removed from circulation, mainly via hepatic clearance. It has been estimated that the half-life of urokinase in humans is on the order of 14 minutes. Urokinase will also react with other proteins, including fibrinogen. Urokinase is much more effective in cleaving the susceptible site in plasminogen when it is in the Lys form as opposed to the Glu form. The activation reaction of the latter by urokinase, however, may be enhanced by the presence of fibrin.[42]

Controversy exists as to the actual thrombolytic effect of urokinase when administered in vivo. Experimental studies have suggested exogenous fibrinolysis as the main pathway, with limited activation of plasminogen within the thrombus (endogenous fibrinolysis).[43] In vivo, however, laboratory findings in treated patients have shown a lesser fibrinogenolytic response, suggesting that plasminemia is reduced with urokinase administration when compared to streptokinase.[44] This implies a significant endogenous activity. In clinical practice, the results of urokinase therapy have paralleled those achieved with streptokinase, with a decreased incidence of bleeding complications suggested by several investigators.[45–47] Whereas major bleeding complications are seen in 15 to 20 per cent of patients treated with streptokinase, such complications have been reported in only 5 to 10 per cent of patients treated with urokinase. Thus, the benefits observed in laboratory changes and the reduced incidence of significant plasminemia with urokinase seem to translate into a decreased incidence of bleeding complication in clinical practice. Although the cost of urokinase remains high compared to streptokinase, when complications are taken into account, the cost of therapy for streptokinase and urokinase is comparable.[48]

Residual thromboplastic activity was detected in the early urokinase preparations[49] and may account for the initial hypercoagulable state reported by Kakkar and Scully.[50] Presently, this does not appear to be a clinically significant problem.

The concept of oral fibrinolytic therapy has emerged as a possibility with oral urokinase administration. Toki et al. administered 30,000 units of urokinase orally in a single capsule and demonstrated increased fibrinolytic activity in normal subjects as evidenced by shortened euglobin lysis time and raised fibrin degradation products.[51] The future of this type of intervention is open to speculation. From the peripheral vascular standpoint, chronic or perioperative administration could prove a useful adjunct.

Tissue Plasminogen Activator

Tissue plasminogen activator is a naturally occurring enzyme present in all human tissues. Its concentration is variable, with high levels detected in the uterus and moderate amounts in the heart, skeletal muscle, kidney, ovary, lung, thyroid, pituitary, and lymph nodes. Scanty amounts are found in the liver, spleen, brain, and testes.[52] It is thought to originate from vascular endothelium and, with the exception of liver and spleen, tissue concentration correlates with vascularity.

Isolation and purification of t-PA was initially hampered by inadequate sources and procedures. In 1979, Rijken et al. were successful in obtaining 1 mg of t-PA from 5 kg of human uterine tissue.[53] Recognizing the potential for this drug, investigators have concentrated on other sources.

At present, there are two main sources of t-PA. The Bowes melanoma cell line is uniquely efficient in producing large quantities of t-PA.[54] This product was subsequently proven to be identical with uterine t-PA.[55] Another source has emerged using recombinant DNA technology, with which efforts in the cloning and expression of the t-PA gene from the melanoma cell line have been successful. This product, known as rt-PA, seems as effective as melanoma t-PA, although further investigations are in progress.[56]

Tissue plasminogen activator is a direct plasminogen activator. Its main advantage is its high affinity for thrombus-bound fibrin. In addition, the presence of fibrinogen enhances its efficiency in activation of plasminogen. Two types of tissue plasminogen activator are recognized, with a commercial preparation being a mixture of both types. A single-chain form is cleaved by plasminogen to yield two-chain tissue plasminogen activator. The one- and the two-chain tissue plasminogen activator are comparable in activity, with the one-chain tissue plasminogen activator being quickly converted to the two-chain type as lysis proceeds. Most of circulating tissue plasminogen activator is in the single-chain form. Its selective action promises to produce less systemic effects, when compared to streptokinase or urokinase. The half-life of t-PA has been estimated between 4 and 7 minutes in vivo.[57] With its presumed nonantigenicity and high affinity for fibrin, t-PA is the most promising thrombolytic agent under current investigation.

When fibrin-selective agents are used for regional infusion, most of the thrombolytic effect is going to be secondary to fibrin-bound plasminogen. Recently, however, the importance of a fresh supply of plasminogen to maintain the fibrin-bound plasminogen pool has been emphasized. Experimental studies have suggested that clot lysis induced by activation of plas-

minogen is dependent on clot-associated plasminogen, which in turn depends on the concentration of plasminogen in plasma. Depletion of both will contribute to a lower frequency and rapidity of recanalization, which will be more noticeable with non–fibrin-selective agents, as compared to fibrin-selective agents, likely the result of the depletion of plasminogen that nonselective agents induce.[58]

Recent trials comparing rt-PA with streptokinase in patients with acute coronary thrombosis have failed to establish this more specific agent as a better thrombolytic agent. Systemic bleeding complications have been similar in spite of a milder homeostatic defect by laboratory evaluation in the rt-PA groups.[59] Questions regarding proper dosage to achieve effective local lysis with minimal systemic effects still exist.

Tissue plasminogen activator may also bind and be activated on platelet surfaces.[60] Due to this binding to platelet receptors, platelets can direct t-PA action on their surface, leading to rapid cleavage of glycoprotein 1B and loss of platelet binding to von Willebrand factor. This may explain why concentrations of tissue plasminogen activator achieved early in therapy may inhibit platelet aggregation.

In animal models of thrombolysis, it has been suggested that multiple bolus administration of tissue plasminogen activator has greater lytic efficacy than equal doses given as a single bolus or a continuous infusion.[61] This may have significant implications in clinical therapy where protocols requiring continuous infusion of the agent have shown a greater incidence of bleeding complications, as opposed to protocols where the drug is administered in bolus form. This may be explained by the accumulation of partially degraded fibrin (X fragments), which may increase the affinity of tissue plasminogen activator for plasminogen by about 17-fold.[7]

Limited experience is available with intraarterial t-PA administration in the treatment of peripheral arterial or graft occlusions. In 17 patients infused with rt-PA, 0.1 mg/kg/hr, all patients demonstrated thrombolysis, with 16 showing improvement clinically.[62] More important, there were no systemic complications, with a mean fibrinogen drop of 42 per cent of baseline. The infusion time was from 1 to 6 hours, compared to the usual 48 to 72 hours necessary with streptokinase. One patient died from an intracranial hemorrhage during postinfusion heparin therapy. Further clinical trials will be needed to determine the advantages, if any, of rt-PA infusion compared with urokinase infusion in the treatment of peripheral arterial occlusions.

These results suggest that t-PA is indeed fibrin selective. Systemic complications may be more related to dose and method of administration than is the case with urokinase or streptokinase. It appears that t-PA is more potent and faster than currently available agents, perhaps because of its high fibrin affinity. In this regard, t-PA may be ideally suited for intraarterial administration, because a 4- to 6-hour trial could be followed by timely surgical intervention. In addition, intraoperative use could be a welcomed adjunct to surgical embolectomy.

Investigational Fibrinolytic Agents

The ideal fibrinolytic agent should be fibrin specific, avoiding a systemic fibrinolytic state and thus digestion of other important plasma proteins such as fibrinogen. The biologic half-life of the substance should match its clinical application, with longer half-lives desirable in situations in which prolonged fibrinolytic activity is necessary. Such might be the case for treatment of acute coronary thrombosis, specifically if it can be started at the field. This might also prove beneficial in the treatment of venous thromboembolic disorders. In instances in which bleeding is a risk factor, a prolonged half-life is undesirable, because it may reduce the ability of the clinician to control the overall effect of the agent. Similarly, prolonged biologic activity of a lytic agent might be undesirable when surgical intervention may follow shortly after fibrinolytic therapy. This might be the case in peripheral vascular occlusions, in which complications and/or identification of a lesion may dictate surgical intervention. Clearly, lack of antigenicity is a desirable characteristic of any biologic agent and has been one of the main advantages of urokinase when compared to streptokinase. Investigators have concentrated on the development of agents that are fibrin specific, with some of the other characteristics taking a secondary role. Agents under current research and clinical investigations will be briefly discussed.

Anisoylated Plasminogen Streptokinase Activator Complex

Derivatives of streptokinase have been produced that change not only its biologic activity, but the duration of such activity. By chemically modulating the streptokinase molecule, greater degrees of clot specificity can be achieved.

P-anisoylated human plasminogen streptokinase activator complex (APSAC) is the most frequently used derivative of streptokinase. It is an acylated complex of streptokinase with human Lys-plasminogen. Acylation of the catalytic site of the plasminogen molecule delays the formation of the active fibrinolytic enzyme plasmin, but leaves the lysine binding sites necessary to bind the complex to fibrin. Acylation also prevents activation of circulating plasminogen by streptokinase. Deacylation of the molecule leads to activation of the streptokinase moiety. A certain amount of the complex will be bound to fibrin at the time of deacylation, but most of it will circulate in the inactive form. Thus, a larger percentage of the drug acts through endogenous fibrinolysis. Neutralizing antiplasmins will rapidly deactivate that small percentage of the drug that is deacylated in circulating plasma.[63]

APSAC has been found in vitro to have a potency 10 times that of streptokinase. This increased activity is partially dependent on fibrin binding and the deacylation process. The half-life in vitro has been estimated to be around 105 minutes in human plasma. In patients with acute myocardial infarction, this prolonged half-life is desirable. Its fibrin selectivity is a welcome improvement over streptokinase. Side effects have been reported with APSAC that are shared with the parent drug, streptokinase. Antistreptococcal antibodies have a significant inhibitory effect on APSAC, and these antibodies will form in patients treated with APSAC and be detectable in their plasma even 3 months following treatment. Therefore, retreatment with streptokinase or APSAC should be delayed for at least 6 months. At present, there is no experience reported with the regional infusion of APSAC in peripheral vascular disease. Intracoronary administration has used infusions of 5 to 30 units within 4 to 6 hours of the onset of symptoms of myocardial infarction. The prolonged half-life of APSAC may be a disadvantage for regional infusion, specifically in peripheral vascular surgery, when the possibility of having to proceed with surgical intervention shortly after fibrinolytic infusion is present. In patients with myocardial infarction, however, prolongation of the fibrinolytic activity is desirable, because it may lead to treatment with a single-dose administration at the field.

Plasmin B-Chain Streptokinase Complex

Another streptokinase derivative that has shown promise is the plasmin b-chain streptokinase complex. Streptokinase activator complexes may be prepared from different forms of plasminogen and its derivatives. Plasmin b-chain is the smallest derivative that retains enzymatic activity. The half-life of this preparation is estimated at a little over 4.5 hours, which is significantly prolonged compared with streptokinase. Using thromboelastography and whole blood, its efficiency in lysing fibrin is four times that of streptokinase. Using the fibrin plate assay, however, its activity falls somewhere between that of streptokinase and urokinase.[64]

The b-chain streptokinase complex has certain advantages over streptokinase, because it has a longer half-life, higher affinity for plasminogen, and decreased antigenicity and is not inhibited by plasma inhibitors. Nevertheless, its advantages over other currently available fibrinolytic agents, such as urokinase or t-PA, await clinical trials. No experience to date has been reported with its use in peripheral vascular occlusions.

Pro-Urokinase

Urokinase is present in various molecular weight forms and its activity is variable in nature. Pro-urokinase, or single-chain urokinase plasminogen activator (SCUPA), is a single-chain form of urokinase of about 55,000 daltons that was isolated by Husain et al. in 1979.[65] It has superior fibrin specificity and lytic efficacy compared to urokinase. Pro-urokinase is highly effective in the conversion of Lys-plasminogen to plasmin. In contrast, it has little or no activity in the conversion of Glu-plasminogen to plasmin. Since Lys-plasminogen is present in high concentrations in thrombus, this gives pro-urokinase fibrin-specific properties. In addition, plasminogen that is absorbed in thrombus changes its configuration to a pseudo–Lys-plasminogen, which is also attacked by pro-urokinase, converting it to Lys-plasmin. Circulating pro-urokinase is very stable in plasma because of its resistance to plasma inhibitors and ionized calcium.[66]

The fibrin specificities of t-PA and pro-urokinase appear to rely on differing mechanisms. Whereas t-PA is fibrin clot binding, the fibrin-selective properties of pro-urokinase are thought to be secondary to its preference for activation of Lys-plasminogen or Lys-like plasminogen substrate found in thrombus. This effect prolongs its plasma half-life, which has been estimated to be several days.[67] Such a prolonged half-life will have theoretical advantages in clinical situations in which prolonged activity is desired. In peripheral arterial occlusions, however, should the regional infusion fail to produce the desired result so that the patient must go to the operating room shortly following discontinuation of the infusion, this prolonged effect may be undesirable. At this time, there is no reported experience with such use.

Immunofibrinolysis

In an attempt to develop fibrin-specific agents, monoclonal antifibrin antibodies have been bonded to urokinase or streptokinase, rendering these agents fibrin selective. These monoclonal antibodies do not appear to cross-react with fibrinogen, and thus show marked increase in in vitro fibrinolysis compared with unmodified activator.[68] The clinical applicability of these agents remains to be determined. They may significantly alter the current approach to the management of thrombotic disease. Nevertheless, repeat therapy would require different monoclonal antibodies to avoid adverse immunologic reactions.

Summary

Most of the available clinical experience to date has been with streptokinase, urokinase, and, most recently, t-PA. The effectiveness and complication rates of each of these agents are discussed thoroughly under the specific sections dealing with the various clinical entities. Based on the experience to date, streptokinase seems to be a less desirable agent for use in peripheral vascular thrombosis, likely related to its complex mechanism of action, which translates into difficulty with dosage and complications in the clinical area.

Although fibrin selectivity has theoretical advantages, the experience so far has failed to demonstrate a significant benefit of such selectivity in the various protocols in which these drugs have been tested. Specifically, the rate of bleeding complications with t-PA has been no different than that seen with streptokinase when used in the treatment of acute myocardial infarction. In fact, a slight increased incidence of intracranial bleeding was seen with this fibrin-selective agent. This may be due to its marked potency, compared to other agents currently available. Regional administration of these agents may realize the true benefit of their selective property. In addition to the proper method of infusion (systemic versus regional), dosage may play an important role in realizing the clinical benefits of a fibrin-specific agent.

SYSTEMIC THROMBOLYTIC THERAPY

This section will discuss systemic thrombolytic therapy for venous and peripheral arterial disease. Treatment of acute coronary thrombosis is specifically omitted.

Although systemic thrombolytic therapy has been used for peripheral arterial occlusions, results have been disappointing, with bleeding complications outweighing benefits obtained. Thus, systemic therapy is reserved for venous thromboembolic diseases. Local intraarterial administration avoids some of the systemic complications, and is utilized for peripheral arterial and graft occlusion. Patient selection is probably the most important factor in obtaining good results with either modality (Table 18–1).

Patient Selection

During the course of systemic thrombolytic therapy, a systemic lytic state is achieved that is capable of lysing fibrin wherever it has been deposited throughout the body. Thus, hemostatic plugs will be as vulnerable as the clot or thrombus for which therapy has been initiated. Selection of patients for systemic lytic therapy is based on the presence of an appropriate documented indication (see below) and careful evaluation for the presence of contraindications.

Contraindications to systemic therapy are listed in Table 18–2. Absolute contraindications are active internal bleeding and recent (within 2 months) cerebrovascular accident or other intracranial pathology. Relative major contraindications include recent (less than 10 days) major surgery, trauma, obstetric delivery, organ biopsy, or puncture of a noncompressible vessel; recent gastrointestinal bleed; and severe hypertension. Relative minor contraindications (Table 18–2) carry a higher risk of complications, but the benefits of therapy may still outweigh the hazards. Peripheral embolization from a central source is a potential hazard of systemic lytic therapy. Therefore, valvular heart disease, atrial fibrillation, or previous history of emboli are relative contraindications to systemic lytic therapy. The presence of a mural thrombus is a relative contraindication to fibrinolytic therapy. The potential for peripheral embolization due to a fragmented mural thrombus may lead to dev-

TABLE 18–1. FIBRINOLYTIC AGENTS

	Streptokinase	Urokinase	Tissue Plasminogen Activator
Source	β-Hemolytic streptococcus (nonenzymatic protein)	Fetal renal cell culture (enzyme)	Recombinant DNA technology (enzyme)
Mechanism	Streptokinase-plasminogen complex	Direct plasminogen activator	Direct plasminogen activator
Metabolism	Liver	Liver	Liver
Advantages	Low cost	Direct activator; no allergic reaction	Fibrin-selective direct activator; no allergic reaction
Disadvantages	Affected by antistreptococcus A,B; allergic reactions; complex mechanism of action	High cost	High cost
Systemic dosage	250,000 units intravenously 30 minutes loading; 100,000 units intravenously/hr	2000 units/lb intravenously 10 minutes loading; 2000 units/lb intravenously/hr	50 mg intravenously over 2 hr; may repeat 30–50 mg intravenously over 4–6 hr
Regional dosage	Low dose: 5000–10,000 units/hr High dose: 30,000–60,000 units/hr	30,000–50,000 units/hr 2000–4000 units/min for 1–2 hr, then 1000–2000 units/min	0.1 unit/kg/hr

astating consequences. In patients with a demonstrable left heart thrombus by echocardiography, we would preferentially consider alternative forms of treatment. It must be recognized, however, that lysis of ventricular thrombi with urokinase has been reported with success.[69] Severe liver disease will affect the metabolism of the drug, thus making the response unpredictable. During pregnancy, a systemic lytic state may precipate abruptio or may lead to hypofibrinogenemia in the fetus, with an increased risk of bleeding. Streptokinase is specifically contraindicated in patients with known allergy, previous therapy within 6 months, or recent streptococcal infection.

One of the most devastating complications of fibrinolytic therapy is intracranial hemorrhage. The incidence of this complication is on the order of 1 per cent of treated patients in trials for acute myocardial infarction. The median time between the onset of clinical signs and the start of thrombolytic therapy ranges from 3 to 36 hours, with a mean of 16 hours. Mortality is high for this complication, with an estimated mortality of 66 per cent. Factors predictive of intracranial hemorrhage by multivariate logistic regression analysis include oral anticoagulation prior to admission, body weight less than 70 kg, and age greater than 65 years old. A small but significant increased incidence of intracranial bleeding has been observed with tissue plasminogen activator, compared to streptokinase or urokinase.[70] An increased incidence of intracerebral hemorrhage has been observed in patients receiving higher doses of t-PA. In the Thrombosis in Myocardial Infarction (TIMI) trial,[71] 1.3 per cent of patients receiving 150 mg of tissue plasminogen activator suffered an intracerebral hemorrhage, as opposed to 0.4 per cent of patients receiving 100 mg of the drug. Interestingly, in the TIMI-II trial, patients who received immediate β-blockade as part of their regimen had no incidence of intracerebral hemorrhage when given 100 mg of tissue plasminogen activator, as compared to 0.5 per cent in the group that did not receive β-blockade. This was not true, however, for the individuals treated with 150 mg of tissue plasminogen activator. The mechanism by which β-blockers may protect against intracerebral bleeding is not established.[72]

TABLE 18–2. CONTRAINDICATIONS TO SYSTEMIC LYTIC THERAPY

Absolute
  Active internal bleeding
  Recent (< 2 mo) cerebrovascular accident
  Intracranial pathology
Relative Major
  Recent (< 10 days) major surgery, obstetric delivery, or organ biopsy
  Active peptic ulcer or GI pathology
  Recent major trauma
  Uncontrolled hypertension
Relative Minor
  Minor surgery or trauma
  Recent cardiopulmonary resuscitation
  High likelihood of left heart thrombus (i.e., atrial fibrillation with mitral valve disease)
  Bacterial endocarditis
  Hemostatic defects (i.e., renal or liver disease)
  Pregnancy
  Diabetic hemorrhagic retinopathy
Streptokinase
  Known allergy
  Recent streptococcal infection
  Previous therapy within 6 months

Indications

Pulmonary Embolism

In 1968, a cooperative controlled randomized study to evaluate the use of urokinase in pulmonary embolism was initiated.[73] By 1970, 160 patients were entered and assigned to one of two therapeutic arms. Pulmonary angiography was performed on all patients before and after therapy, with lung scans repeated at 3, 6, and 12 months. The minimal eligibility was occlusion of at least one segmental pulmonary artery on angiography. Excluded from the trial were patients who had had recent operations, or those with contraindications to heparin or thrombolytic therapy. Seventy-eight patients received anticoagulants alone (heparin 75 units/lb loading dose, 10 units/lb/hr for 12 hours and 82 received urokinase 2000 units/lb/hr for 12 hours). Following the 12-hour infusion, all patients received heparin for a minimum of 5 days to maintain a prolonged bleeding time.

The randomization produced reasonably good balance between the treatment groups. Urokinase therapy resulted in a significantly accelerated resolution of pulmonary emboli at 24 hours, as shown by pulmonary arteriograms, lung scans, and right-sided pressures. No significant differences in mortality or recurrence rate were observed. Patients receiving urokinase tended to respond better if they were younger (less than 50 years), the embolus was recent (less than 48 hours old), or the embolus was large, especially if shock was present.

Bleeding complications were significant in both groups (heparin 27 per cent, urokinase 45 per cent). This high complication rate is likely the result of demands in the protocol for multiple, frequent invasive procedures, including cutdowns performed for pulmonary angiography. The study group concluded that further studies were indicated before specific therapeutic recommendations could be made.

In 1974, the second phase of this cooperative study was reported.[74] This study followed the same guidelines as phase I, comparing 12 hours of urokinase therapy with 24 hours of urokinase therapy and 24 hours of streptokinase therapy. A group treated with heparin alone was not included, because the protocol was almost identical to that in the phase I trial, which showed urokinase to be superior to heparin in clot resolution. Fifty-seven patients were given urokinase (2000 units/lb loading dose, 2000 units/lb/hr for 24 hours), and 61 patients received the same regimen for 12 hours. Fifty-eight patients received streptokinase (250,000 units loading dose, 100,000 units/hr for 24 hours).

As expected, the drop in plasminogen during therapy was steeper for patients receiving streptokinase, but otherwise the lytic effect was similar. Patients receiving 12 hours of urokinase infusion had a result nearly equivalent to those in the phase I trial receiving urokinase. No benefit was seen from 24 hours of urokinase over the 12-hour infusion. In patients with massive embolism, the greatest improvement was seen with 24-hour urokinase infusion, although the differences were not statistically significant. Streptokinase and urokinase yielded similar results, with small differences favoring urokinase. The study group concluded that all three regimens were more effective in accelerating resolution of pulmonary thromboemboli than heparin alone.

One of the major problems with the use of thrombolytic therapy for pulmonary embolism is that patients with pulmonary emboli usually have major contraindications for thrombolytic therapy. Such is the case with the occurrence of pulmonary embolism

in the postoperative patient. Recently, an experience with 13 patients treated for angiographically proven pulmonary embolism within 14 days of surgery was reported.[75] The protocol utilized consisted of 2200 units/kg of body weight of urokinase injected directly into the clot through a catheter positioned in the pulmonary artery. A continuous infusion at the same dosage was then maintained for up to 24 hours, with the simultaneous administration of heparin at 500 units/hr. Fibrinogen level was maintained at less than 0.2 gm/dl. No deaths or bleeding complications were seen, with complete lysis achieved in all patients. This selective therapy for pulmonary embolism may be appropriate for patients in the early postoperative period who suffer a major life-threatening pulmonary embolus.

The long-term results of patients randomized to the Urokinase Pulmonary Embolism Trial (UPET) study, suggests the clinical importance of resolution of the obstructive process in the pulmonary circulation. Several patients from this study were reexamined at 7 years after the original pulmonary embolus. Those assigned initially to thrombolysis had significantly higher pulmonary capillary blood volumes and preservation of the normal pulmonary vasculature response to exercise at 7 years. In contrast, patients who had been treated with anticoagulants alone demonstrated a lower pulmonary capillary blood volume at 1 year and markedly abnormal increase in pulmonary artery pressure and pulmonary vascular resistance when undergoing exercise testing during right heart catheterization.[76] These data suggest that initial management with thrombolysis can offer improved quality of life demonstrable years after the event.

More recently, rt-PA has been evaluated in the treatment of acute massive pulmonary embolism. In a multicenter trial, the intravenous administration of rt-PA was compared with intrapulmonary administration in 34 patients with massive pulmonary emboli.[77] All patients were systemically anticoagulated with heparin. Fifty milligrams of rt-PA were given over 2 hours, either intravenously or intrapulmonary, with an additional 22 patients receiving 50 mg over the subsequent 5 hours. No difference was noted between the intrapulmonary group and the intravenous administration group, and 7-hour administration was superior to a single infusion of 50 mg over 2 hours. In all groups, up to 38 per cent resolution of the angiographically determined embolism occurred. A decline in the pulmonary arterial pressure was documented in all groups. Fibrinogen levels dropped significantly, with bleeding complications limited to puncture or operative sites, and in only four patients were blood transfusions required.[77]

In a separate trial, 36 patients with angiographically documented pulmonary emboli received 50 mg of rt-PA over 2 hours, followed by repeat arteriography and, if necessary, an additional 40 mg over 4 hours of rt-PA.[78] Thirty-four of 36 patients had angiographic evidence of clot lysis, with marked improvement in 24 of the 36. Two bleeding complications occurred, one related to a pelvic tumor and the other 8 days following coronary artery bypass surgery. Again, significant improvement in the clinical condition of these patients was documented.[78]

A randomized controlled trial of recombinant tissue plasminogen activator versus urokinase in the treatment of acute pulmonary embolism was reported in 1988. Forty-five patients were randomized to rt-PA 100 mg over 2 hours versus urokinase at systemic doses. At 2 hours, 82 per cent of rt-PA patients had complete lysis, as opposed to 48 per cent of patients receiving urokinase. Eight of 23 urokinase patients required premature termination of the infusion because of bleeding complications. There was no difference in plasma fibrinogen level or improvement in lung scans between the two groups.[79]

In 1980, the NIH Consensus Development Conference[80] concluded that thrombolytic therapy results in greater improvement and normalization of the hemodynamic responses to pulmonary emboli than is observed with heparin alone. Lytic therapy may prevent permanent damage to the pulmonary vascular bed by lysing emboli and restoring pulmonary circulation to normal. The conference report also stated that although the incidence of bleeding complications in the above trials was high, recent clinical experience suggested an incidence of around 5 per cent, certainly within an acceptable range.

In current clinical practice, thrombolytic therapy should be considered in all patients with an established diagnosis of pulmonary embolism, any evidence (clinical or monitoring) of hemodynamic compromise, and no absolute contraindication to systemic lytic therapy. This excludes small pulmonary emboli with which, after the initial episode, the patient remains clinically stable. In the latter situation, the benefits of thrombolytic therapy over heparin alone are not clear.

It is important that the diagnosis of pulmonary emboli be well documented. We prefer pulmonary angiography, because it remains the "gold standard." If hemodynamic instability precludes obtaining pretreatment angiography, an alternative is to proceed with lytic therapy, which usually results in marked improvement within the hour. Angiography is then obtained to decide whether to continue therapy. If the angiogram confirms the diagnosis, the drug is continued for 12 to 24 hours, assessing hemodynamic response, and depending on the presence or absence of complications and/or risk factors. Therapy beyond 24 hours does not seem to offer any benefit.

Under these guidelines, patients who are candidates for pulmonary embolectomy should have a trial of lytic therapy. Pulmonary embolectomy is then reserved for patients who fail or have an absolute contraindication to thrombolytic therapy.

Deep Vein Thrombosis

The goal of therapy for deep vein thrombosis is the prevention of pulmonary embolism and of long-

term sequelae characterized by the postphlebitic syndrome. Anticoagulation has been highly effective in achieving the former, but ineffective in preventing valvular damage and, as a consequence, avoiding the postphlebitic syndrome. The incidence of such long-term complications can be as high as 90 per cent.[81]

Several well-controlled randomized prospective studies have compared systemic lytic therapy with conventional heparin therapy in the treatment of deep vein thrombosis.[82–86] All concluded that dissolution of deep vein thrombi with lytic therapy is faster and more complete than that observed with heparin alone. On the average, complete lysis was seen in 35 per cent of patients, compared to 4 per cent of those treated with heparin alone. At 3 to 6 months follow-up, valve function was preserved in 7 per cent of heparin-treated patients, compared to 50 per cent of patients treated with thrombolytic agents. The incidence of pulmonary embolism was similar for both regimens, with no difference in mortality. Bleeding complications averaged 4 per cent and 17 per cent for heparin and lytic therapy, respectively. In one study, phlebography at a mean of 7 months following treatment suggested an improved outcome for patients treated with fibrinolytic agents. Normal venograms were found in 40 per cent of streptokinase-treated patients, compared to 8 per cent of those who had received heparin. Clinical symptoms were related to therapeutic results and previous thrombosis. Longer follow-up was reported by Arnesen et al.,[87] who phlebographically evaluated 35 patients at a mean observation period of 6.5 years after randomly receiving streptokinase or heparin. Only seven patients had phlebographically normal veins, and all were in the streptokinase group. On clinical examination, 76 per cent of patients in the streptokinase group had normal legs, compared to 33 per cent of patients in the heparin group.[87] Contrasting results have been reported from a small prospective study in which 24 patients with major proximal deep vein thrombosis treated with heparin were compared to 25 patients similarly afflicted, treated with streptokinase.[88] After 2.5 years of follow-up, no major benefit was seen regarding hemodynamic status, as measured by foot volumetry, between the two groups. The authors questioned the validity of treatment with lytic therapy, given its inherent higher complication rate. In all of these studies, thrombi older than 3 to 5 days were less likely to respond.

Clinical experience with the use of t-PA in the treatment of deep vein thrombosis is limited. A randomized trial of rt-PA for the treatment of proximal deep vein thrombosis was carried out by Turpie et al.[89] Twenty patients with proximal deep vein thrombosis were randomized to intravenous rt-PA (0.5 mg/kg) or placebo over 4 hours, following initiation of a therapeutic dose of intravenous heparin. Patients were randomized to rt-PA (0.5 mg/kg) of saline over 1 hour, if repeat venography within 72 hours did not show complete lysis. Five of 10 patients treated with this protocol of rt-PA showed partial or complete lysis, compared with 1 of 10 patients treated with heparin. A systemic lytic effect was demonstrated by a drop in plasma fibrinogen and α_2-antiplasmin concentration with positive fibrin degradation split products and elevated euglobulin lysis time. Thus, modest effectiveness was seen in this study, similar to that achieved by urokinase or streptokinase. Long-term follow-up in these patients is not available. Three other randomized trials have shown similar results.[90-92]

It is reasonable to conclude that systemic thrombolytic therapy for deep vein thrombosis is as effective as heparin in preventing pulmonary embolic complications, with the added advantage of faster acute resolution in a significant number of patients. From the available studies, it appears that elimination of the obstructive component of deep vein thrombosis is better achieved with lytic therapy. Whether preservation of valve function is achieved by this more aggressive form of therapy remains uncertain. Clearly, with longer follow-up, more patients develop incompetent valves. This may result from minor valve damage progressing with time to a clinically significant problem. Nevertheless, it is difficult to ignore the significant improvement in the obstructive component of deep vein thrombosis, considering that the combination of obstruction and valvular incompetence will likely result in the most severe forms of postphlebitis syndrome. In view of this, should lytic therapy be offered to all patients with deep vein thrombosis? Clearly, the answer is no. When therapy started beyond 5 days following the onset of symptoms, effectiveness is significantly decreased. The incidence of deep vein thrombosis is highest in postoperative patients, women during pregnancy or after childbirth, trauma victims, or following cerebrovascular accidents or spinal injury. Lytic therapy is contraindicated in these instances, as well as in septic thrombophlebitis. Prior episodes of thrombophlebitis are likely to have destroyed delicate vein valves, and thus the benefits of lytic therapy in recurrent attacks is uncertain. If clinical evidence of valve competence is present, an attempt to prevent further damage from a recurrent attack and resolve the obstructive component is a reasonable goal. In addition, lytic therapy seems to offer an advantage in more proximal thrombosis (i.e., popliteal vein or higher), and thus treatment of isolated calf thrombi with lytic therapy is of questionable value.

From the foregoing discussion, it is evident that the impact of lytic therapy in deep vein thrombosis will be limited. However, patients suffering their first episode, with no contraindication, who present within 5 days of the onset of symptoms, will likely benefit from systemic lytic therapy. As with pulmonary embolism, documentation of the diagnosis is essential before initiating thrombolytic therapy for deep vein thrombosis. It is our practice to obtain a venogram prior to lytic therapy. Repeat venography to assess the result is not necessary, although it is very helpful in instances in which clinical response is uncertain.

Noninvasive studies are useful during therapy when an adequate clinical response is observed. The duration of therapy is guided by these studies but usually is no less than 3 days, unless complications require earlier discontinuation of the drug. Therapy beyond 5 days is rarely indicated and suggests resistance to lytic therapy. When using streptokinase, if no improvement is seen within the first 24 to 48 hours or a lytic state (see later in this section) is not documented within this time, switching to urokinase is recommended.

Phlegmasia cerulea presents with massive iliofemoral thrombosis with limb-threatening venous outflow occlusion. The results of venous thrombectomy have been variable traditionally, with a significant incidence of rethrombosis and mortality, although more recent experience has been encouraging.[93,94] Lytic therapy offers an important advantage over surgical thrombectomy; multiple peripheral thrombi not accessible to the catheter may be dissolved. In addition, a general anesthetic, frequently required for venous thrombectomy, is avoided. Although the experience with thrombolytic therapy in this entity is limited, of 14 reported cases, 13 were judged as having achieved excellent results with no mortality.[82,95-97] No long-term results are available.

Axillary Vein Thrombosis

Axillary vein thrombosis (effort thrombosis) usually occurs in young individuals and its sudden clinical manifestations lead the patient to seek early medical attention. This makes this entity ideally suited for thrombolytic therapy. Anticoagulation rarely leads to resolution and merely arrests the process, allowing for collateral drainage and amelioration of symptoms. The latter frequently leads to some degree of disability. Catheter-induced axillary subclavian vein thrombosis usually has a more gradual presentation, with slow progressive occlusion allowing for collateral venous drainage. The clinical presentation will aid in deciding whether or not to offer lytic therapy to a patient with catheter-induced axillosubclavian vein thrombosis. When symptoms have developed rapidly over the course of a few days, there is a good probability that the thrombotic material will be sensitive to lytic agents. A combination of infusion through the catheter and in the ipsilateral peripheral vein seems most effective. However, if symptoms have developed over weeks or months, they will tend to be milder in nature and less responsive to fibrinolytic agents. This is likely a result of organization of the thrombotic material.

Both forms of axillary thrombosis have been successfully managed with lytic therapy[98-100] (Fig. 18-2). Either systemic or local low-dose infusion appears to be effective.[98] Local infusion requires that the catheter be lodged in thrombus, otherwise venous collaterals will decrease its effectiveness. A systemic lytic state is avoided in the majority of patients treated by local infusion.

Once complete resolution of the clot is achieved,

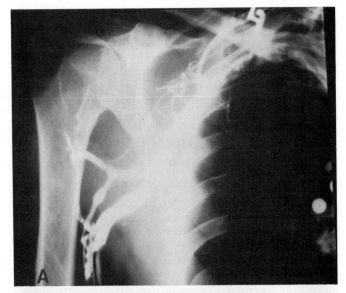

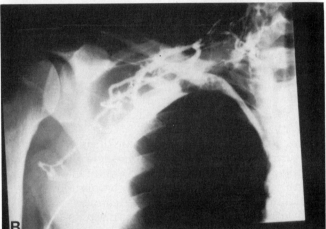

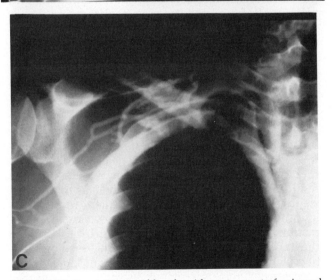

FIGURE 18–2. A 28-year-old male with acute onset of pain and swelling in the right upper extremity. *A,* Ascending venogram confirms axillary vein thrombosis. Low-dose streptokinase infusion (10,000 units/hr) initiated. *B,* Twenty-four hours later, intraluminal thrombus is seen, with patency of the system. *C,* Forty-eight hours later, there is complete resolution of the occlusion.

repeat venography with the extremity in abduction and external rotation is recommended. If an underlying thoracic outlet compression is identified, surgical correction should be advised. If a stenosis of the vein is identified, balloon dilatation has been successful to avoid rethrombosis.[98]

Superior Vena Cava Thrombosis

Superior vena cava thrombosis is frequently the result of neoplastic, traumatic, or infectious processes in the mediastinum. In these instances, external compression or inflammation precludes successful resolution of the process with lytic agents. Thrombosis secondary to an indwelling catheter is usually a slow process, allowing for organization and fibrotic replacement of the clot. It is unlikely that this will respond to lytic therapy; surgical decompression may be an option in these patients. On the other hand, patients who develop rapidly progressive symptoms may respond to lytic therapy by dissolution of the most recently formed clot, which is likely to be sensitive to lysis.

In about 4 per cent of cases, thrombosis is termed "idiopathic." Successful resolution of idiopathic vena cava thrombosis has been reported with systemic thrombolytic therapy.[101]

Method

The goal of systemic administration of fibrinolytic agents is to establish a systemic lytic state. Once the diagnosis is documented by objective means and the patient deemed a suitable candidate for lytic therapy, informed consent should be obtained. Prior to infusion, fibrinogen level, thrombin time, prothrombin time (PT), partial thromboplastin time (PTT), hematocrit, and platelet count is obtained. If heparin has been given, it is discontinued. The agent is given intravenously. If streptokinase is chosen, 250,000 units are given over 30 minutes. This will achieve a lytic state in 90 per cent of the patients. A continuous infusion of 100,000 units/hr is then commenced and continued for the duration of therapy. We routinely administer 100 mg of hydrocortisone prior to streptokinase therapy, because it may prevent or ameliorate some of the allergic reactions. If urokinase is chosen, a loading dose of 2000 units/lb is given over 10 minutes, followed by a continuous infusion of 2000 units/lb/hr for the duration of therapy. Alternatively, 50 mg of rt-PA may be given over 2 hours. If a pulmonary artery catheter is present, the drug may be administered through the atrial port of the catheter. This is preferable to administration through the distal port of the catheter, which may be located in a branch of the pulmonary artery unrelated to the location of the occlusion. Thus, either peripheral vein administration or atrial administration through the proximal port of a Swan-Ganz catheter is preferable. As an alternative, the catheter used for pulmonary angiography may be lodged within the thrombus for regional infusion. High-dose regional therapy could then be utilized (see section on "Native Vessel Occlusion" later in this chapter). Invasive procedures are to be avoided, intramuscular injections are contraindicated, and bed rest is essential during therapy. Arterial blood gases are obtained only when necessary—from the wrist and followed by at least 20 minutes of compression of the artery.

Three to four hours after commencing infusion, thrombin time (or PTT, if thrombin time is not available), fibrinogen level, and fibrin degradation product measures are obtained. A lytic state is documented by a prolonged thrombin time (twice normal) and positive fibrin degradation products. Hematocrit is followed every 6 hours, with the other parameters measured on a daily basis. A drop in fibrinogen is expected and, in the absence of bleeding complications, is well tolerated. If a lytic state is not seen after the initial 4 hours, the hourly doses are increased. Conversely, if streptokinase is used, changing to urokinase may be beneficial.

Following completion of therapy (see "Indications," earlier in this section), the patient should receive anticoagulants. Usually 2 to 3 hours after discontinuation of the lytic agent, heparin can be initiated at appropriate hourly dose without a loading dose. This is followed by warfarin in the conventional manner.

Complications

Bleeding is the most frequent and important complication of systemic lytic therapy. The incidence of major bleeding (requiring transfusions or discontinuation of the drug), as reported in the literature, varies from 7 per cent[102] to as high as 45 per cent.[73] It averages about 15 per cent and correlates with the number and type of invasive procedures during therapy. Duration of therapy also seems to influence the incidence of bleeding.

Two broad categories of bleeding are observed. Superficial bleeding, seen at invasive sites, is frequently controlled with pressure. Avoidance of unnecessary procedures and preservation of an intact vascular system are the best preventive measures. Internal bleeding, usually seen in the gastrointestinal tract or the intracranial space, is frequently the result of poor patient selection. Internal bleeding should be suspected by unexplained drops in hematocrit. As a rule, any change in the neurologic status of a patient receiving fibrinolytic therapy is considered a complication of therapy, until proven otherwise. The infusion is discontinued immediately and appropriate diagnostic and therapeutic measures instituted.

Superficial bleeding, which is controlled by local measures, can be tolerated in the final stages of therapy. Its occurrence early in the infusion, or any significant bleeding requiring transfusion, should lead to discontinuation of therapy. The hemostatic defect is corrected by the administration of fresh-frozen plasma or cryoprecipitate. These two components are rich in fibrinogen and usually result in resolution of the lytic state. Epsilon aminocaproic acid administration (plasmin inhibitor) is rarely recommended and carries a significant risk of aggravating the process for which lytic therapy was instituted. Increasing the dose of streptokinase to decrease its proteolytic effect is scientifically correct, but unnecessary. It is interesting to note that bleeding tends to occur in the lag period between termination of lytic therapy and anticoagulant administration.[54,103] Thus, heparin administration should be delayed until the thrombin time or PTT is less than twice normal, and initiated without a loading dose.

Laboratory parameters correlate poorly with the risk of bleeding. On the other hand, extremely low fibrinogen levels (less than 20 per cent of baseline) in the presence of an otherwise minor bleeding complication does increase the chances of continued bleeding, requiring cessation of therapy. An alternative is to temporarily discontinue the drug, administer fresh-frozen plasma or cryoprecipitate, and restart the infusion several hours later.

Allergic reactions are not infrequent with streptokinase, although most are minor febrile episodes of no clinical consequence. Serious allergic reactions are extremely rare with the current preparations, and the few reported have responded well to conventional therapy.[80]

Pulmonary embolism can occur during treatment for deep vein thrombosis. The incidence appears to be similar to that seen with conventional heparin therapy. In the absence of other complications, continuation of lytic therapy is the treatment of choice. If recurrent emboli are observed, discontinuation of the fibrinolytic agent, heparin administration, and placement of a caval filter may be life saving.

INTRAARTERIAL THROMBOLYTIC THERAPY

The management of acute arterial and graft occlusions by the intraarterial local administration of fibrinolytic agents has emerged as an occasional alternative and, frequently, an adjunct to surgical therapy in a selected group of patients. The exact role of lytic therapy in this setting is unclear because, to date, no randomized study has compared this approach with standard surgical intervention. Excellent results with low morbidity and mortality are now possible with modern vascular techniques. It is difficult to estimate the impact of intraarterial lytic therapy based on cases in which surgical management has traditionally been successful.

Emerging from the reported experience are a series of guidelines that have helped define the role of intraarterial lytic therapy. Unquestionably, patient selection is the most important factor in achieving good results with this nonoperative approach. As we gain experience in manipulating the fibrinolytic system, perhaps improvements in areas in which surgical results are poor will follow.

Patient Selection

As a rule, intraarterial fibrinolytic therapy should be considered when the surgical alternative carries a high morbidity or mortality, or when the surgical approach has traditionally yielded poor results. In patients with previous multiple vascular reconstructions, lytic therapy may offer an alternative to an otherwise difficult and unpredictable surgical intervention. In some cases, it may facilitate such an undertaking, thus serving as a true adjunct to surgical therapy.

In the early experience of intraarterial fibrinolytic therapy, low doses of the agent were administered close to the thrombus so as to minimize systemic effects. With a low-dose regimen, dissolution of intraarterial thrombi is a slow, gradual process, requiring anywhere between 12 and 72 hours or longer to resolve. In patients in whom this method is chosen, the viability of the ischemic tissues should be assured. Otherwise, they are better managed surgically, where prompt revascularization can be accomplished. Candidates for intraarterial lytic therapy must be able to tolerate ischemia for the duration of the infusion. With a high-dose regimen, however, frequently restoration of forward flow can be achieved in a matter of 2 to 6 hours, and thus the decision whether or not to continue fibrinolytic infusion can be made in a timely fashion.

Absolute and relative contraindications to intraarterial fibrinolytic therapy are listed in Table 18–3. Approximately 50 per cent of patients receiving low-dose intraarterial infusion of lytic drugs will develop a systemic lytic state. Thus, patients with active internal bleeding, recent cerebrovascular accidents

TABLE 18–3.   CONTRAINDICATIONS TO INTRAARTERIAL FIBRINOLYTIC THERAPY

Absolute
  Intolerable ischemia
  Active internal bleeding
  Cerebrovascular accident within 3 months
  Intracranial pathology
Relative
  Recent major surgery or trauma
  Minor GI bleeding
  Severe hypertension
  Valvular heart disease
  Atrial fibrillation
  Endocarditis
  Coagulation disorders
  Pregnancy
  Minor surgery
  Severe liver disease
  Axillofemoral graft OR knitted Dacron graft
Streptokinase
  Known allergy
  Recent streptococcal infection
  Previous therapy within 6 months

(within 2 months), or intracranial pathology are not candidates for any form of fibrinolytic therapy.

Relative contraindications represent risk factors associated with a higher incidence of complications. Recent major surgery or trauma will increase significantly the risk of bleeding in the presence of a systemic lytic state. Individualized judgment is required, but the presence of relative contraindications should not detract the clinician from utilizing regional lytic therapy if significant benefit is anticipated. These contraindications have been discussed under "Systemic Lytic Therapy" earlier in this chapter.

Several cases of embolization to the ipsilateral extremity have been reported during intraarterial lytic therapy for occluded axillofemoral grafts.[104] The length of these grafts makes them unsuitable for lytic therapy, and thus surgical thrombectomy remains the therapy of choice. Dissolution of the fibrin layer that seals Dacron prostheses can occur with systemic absorption of the drug, leading to oozing through these porous prostheses. Discontinuation of therapy usually results in stabilization of the hematoma by the surrounding capsule.

Indications

Thrombosis Following Percutaneous Angioplasty

Percutaneous angioplasty is now frequently performed in this country for stenotic arterial lesions in the iliac and femoral systems. Thrombosis following balloon angioplasty is relatively infrequent, but when it occurs local thrombolytic therapy is highly effective in restoring patency. The onset of the occlusion is known and is usually within 24 hours of the dilatation; thus the thrombotic material is fresh and highly sensitive to fibrinolysis. The underlying stenosis has been relieved by the angioplasty and when thrombosis occurs immediately, it is a simple matter to change catheters so that proximal infusion is promptly initiated.

Over 80 per cent of post–balloon dilatation thrombosis cases can be successfully treated with intraarterial lytic therapy.[105–107] The duration of therapy is short, because the infusion is started early and the thrombotic material is fresh. Thus, thrombectomy of a friable, recently dilated artery can be avoided. If dilatation of an iliac lesion was performed through an ipsilateral puncture, there is risk of bleeding and pseudoaneurysm formation (Fig. 18–3). If patency was restored by the infusion, repair of the pseudoaneurysm has been simplified to closure of the puncture site without embolectomy.

Native Vessel Occlusion

Acute occlusion of a native artery can be the result of thrombosis secondary to an underlying stenosis, or embolization from a central source. In selecting the patients for intraarterial lytic therapy, it is important to attempt to delineate the mechanism of

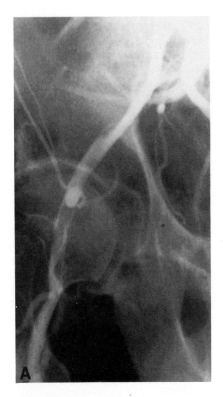

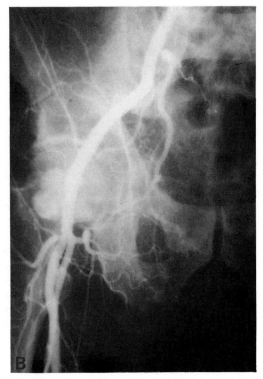

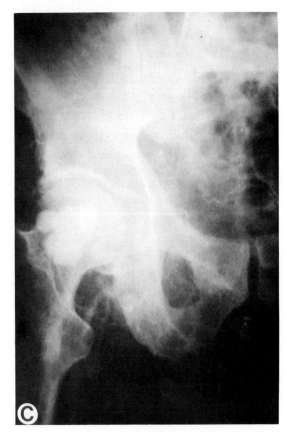

FIGURE 18–3. A 63-year-old male undergoing balloon angioplasty of a right external iliac stenosis. *A,* Postprocedural angiogram shows thrombosis of the dilated segment. *B,* After 12 hours of low-dose (5000 units/hr) intraarterial streptokinase, there is complete resolution of the thrombus. *C,* A pseudoaneurysm is evident on angiography. Repair was limited to suture closure of perforation without the need for thrombectomy.

occlusion. Lytic therapy appears to be more effective when applied to peripheral embolization.[104] Whereas 50 to 60 per cent of thrombotic occlusions will resolve with thrombolytic therapy, around 80 per cent of embolic occlusions will be effectively lysed. On the other hand, the surgical management of proximal lower extremity emboli by transfemoral embolectomy is highly successful, with low morbidity and mortality. In addition, some investigators have noted that emboli secondary to atrial fibrillation may have well-organized components and thus be resistant to fibrinolysis.[108] For these reasons, we prefer surgical embolectomy for proximal (iliac, femoral) emboli secondary to atrial fibrillation. If the embolus is secondary to a recent myocardial infarction (where the surgical risk is increased and the embolus is usually fresh clot), intraarterial fibrinolytic therapy should be considered. It must be kept in mind that the presence of mural thrombus in the ventricle, usually secondary to a recent myocardial infarction, is a relative contraindication to lytic therapy. Although the absence of such findings on echocardiography does not absolutely exclude the possibility, their presence, as demonstrated by an echocardiogram, should raise the level of concern in consideration for lytic therapy.

The management of multiple distal embolization must be individualized, depending on the viability of the extremity and the surgical risk. Intraarterial lytic therapy is a reasonable option in these patients when the extremity is viable and the anticipated surgical reconstruction difficult. If the ischemia is not well tolerated, we proceed with popliteal exploration, thrombectomy and, on occasion, intraoperative lytic therapy (see later in this section).

The use of local fibrinolytic therapy for thrombotic arterial occlusions should be based on the anticipated difficulty, morbidity, and mortality of the surgical alternative. The success rate of fibrinolytic therapy alone in thrombotic occlusion is variable. In 25 patients with atherosclerotic occlusion, Risius et al. succeeded in treating 13 (52 per cent); of these, only four required no further therapy, three had successful percutaneous transluminal angioplasty, and the remaining six required surgery or distal amputations.[109] In 40 patients with thrombotic occlusions treated by Katzen et al. with intraarterial lytic therapy, 32 (80 per cent) were considered successful.[106] No mention is made of other interventions in this group. Successful lysis was achieved by Graor et al. in 25 (56 per cent) of 45 patients with thrombotic arterial occlusions.[105] Eighteen of these 25 patients required secondary procedures. Seventy-eight per cent of patients whose thrombi were less than 30 days old were successfully lysed, compared to 37 per cent of patients with older occlusions. This trend has been observed by others and suggests an important consideration in patient selection.

Careful analysis of the reported series will reveal that although the lytic infusion may reestablish patency, additional procedures are often required. If surgical management becomes necessary, frequently this

has been simplified because better preoperative planning is possible. Thus, if the ischemia is well tolerated, the anticipated surgical intervention complex, the occlusion fairly recent (within 2 weeks), and the patient at significant increased surgical risk, thrombolytic therapy seems justified. From the reported experience, long-term results will depend mainly on whether or not a correctable lesion is identified and on the location of the occlusion. Larger vessel occlusions resolved by intraarterial lytic therapy tend to do better, with an expected patency at 2 years of 60 per cent. Superficial femoral and popliteal occlusions similarly treated, on the other hand, have a lower long-term patency of about 30 per cent at 2 years.[110] If a correctable lesion is identified and appropriately treated, long-term results are significantly improved. If no causative lesion is identified, patencies as low as 20 per cent at 2 years have been reported.[111]

There are specific instances in which surgical intervention has traditionally achieved poor results. Emboli or thrombosis of the popliteal artery with distal clot propagation or multiple tibial embolization carries a risk of amputation of 40 per cent, in spite of prompt surgical embolectomy.[3,112,113] In patients with a viable extremity at presentation, in whom no major runoff vessels are seen on angiography, a trial of local fibrinolytic therapy may improve these results. Surgical correction of the underlying lesion (stenosis or aneurysm) can be performed in a timely fashion. When severe ischemia precludes lytic therapy, we prefer to proceed with popliteal exploration and embolectomy. Intraoperative intraarterial infusion of lytic agents in an attempt to lyse clot inaccessible to the embolectomy catheter may improve results of embolectomy alone.

Thrombosis or embolization to the renal arteries is a promising area in which thrombolytic therapy may offer significant advantages over surgical intervention (Fig. 18–4). As a complication of myocardial infarction, an embolus to the renal artery carries an inordinate risk with surgical intervention. Capsular collaterals frequently maintain viability of the renal parenchyma to allow sufficient time for success with thrombolytic therapy. The material is sensitive to lysis and the length of the occlusion is short. The reported experience is limited but has been highly successful.[106,114] If a stenosis is uncovered during infusion, percutaneous dilatation or elective surgical repair may be undertaken, as deemed appropriate.

Acute mesenteric artery occlusion has been successfully treated by local intraarterial streptokinase infusion.[115] In contrast to the kidneys, the bowel is exquisitely sensitive to ischemia and reperfusion. It is difficult to assess clinically the tolerance to ischemia on presentation and during therapy. We have attempted lytic therapy in four patients with emboli to the mesenteric circulation as a complication of an acute myocardial infarction. Two patients required laparotomy and bowel resection. In one, no further revascularization was necessary. The other necessitated embolectomy and second-look laparotomy. The

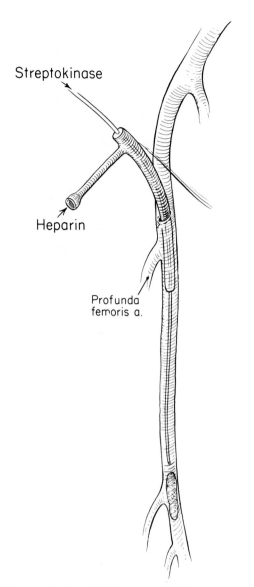

Streptokinase

Heparin

Profunda femoris a.

FIGURE 18–4. Preferred delivery method for intraarterial lytic therapy for distal lower extremity occlusions. Low-dose heparin is infused through the coaxial system to avoid upstream thrombus.

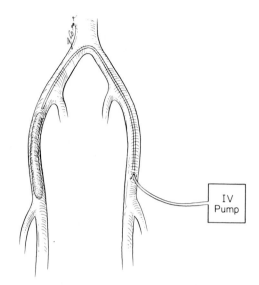

IV Pump

FIGURE 18–5. Preferred method of intraarterial lytic therapy for proximal (iliac, common femoral) occlusions. If possible, the catheter tip should be within the thrombus.

third patient had complete resolution of symptoms, avoiding laparotomy altogether (Fig. 18–5). The fourth patient required laparotomy without bowel resection or need for revascularization. The latter case underscores the difficulty in clinical follow-up during this type of nonoperative approach. If lytic therapy is elected for acute mesenteric ischemia, any deterioration in the overall clinical status, persistent acidosis, and/or sepsis should mandate emergency exploration. Otherwise, frequent angiographic assessment, as often as every 6 hours, is advisable. Failure to show progress during these intervals should trigger early, rather than delayed, exploration.

Acute Graft Occlusion

Acute occlusion of an arterial graft frequently leads to recurrent symptoms and, on occasion, limb-threatening ischemia. Thrombectomy, with or without re-

vision, achieves excellent results in prosthetic grafts and variable results in autogenous vein grafts.[116] The latter frequently require extensive revision and replacement. Intraarterial thrombolytic therapy, on the other hand, has been highly unsuccessful in resolving prosthetic graft occlusions. Of 25 prosthetic graft occlusions treated with local lytic therapy by Sussman et al., only six were successful, five of which required surgical correction of the offending lesion.[104] In the 17 failures, amputation followed in 12 patients. In the experience reported by Van Breda et al., of 19 patients with 20 prosthetic graft occlusions, only four patients were managed nonoperatively, two of whom required percutaneous transluminal angioplasty.[113] In spite of this, lytic therapy was considered beneficial, because it allowed elective surgery in 12 patients and improvement in the surgical risk in an additional two patients. An adjunctive role for lytic therapy was proposed. Although achieving successful lysis in 7 of 10 polytetrafluoroethylene (PTFE) grafts with thrombolytic therapy, Graor et al. noted that surgical revision was required in most of these patients.[105] In view of the excellent results obtained with surgical thrombectomy, one must seriously question the value of thrombolytic therapy in the management of prosthetic graft occlusions.

The results obtained with lytic therapy in the management of occluded autogenous grafts have been somewhat more gratifying. In the experience of Perler et al., occluded vein grafts were more susceptible to lytic therapy than PTFE grafts.[117] This experience is shared by others.[118] Graor et al., however, observed a similar response between PTFE and vein grafts, reporting a 75 per cent success rate in vein grafts occluded for less than 14 days.[105] Taking into account the variable results with surgical thrombectomy in the management of occluded autologous grafts, a trial of lytic therapy, when the event has been recent, is an attractive alternative. In our experience, however, long saphenous vein grafts to tibial vessels in the lower third of the leg or ankle appear to be less responsive to lytic therapy. This may have to do with limited supplies of plasminogen in these very-low-flow grafts. Nevertheless, even in unsuccessful attempts, at operation it is not unusual to find liquified, thickened blood in the graft, thus minimizing the need for mechanical thrombectomy. The operation may actually be limited to removal of the most distal occlusive material and revision of an identified lesion. Retrieving an occluded vein graft in these circumstances is possible with minimal mechanical trauma to the endothelium.

We take into account several factors when deciding whether or not to use lytic therapy for an occluded graft. Certainly, surgical risk must be assessed. Infrequently, surgery is avoided altogether. If delaying surgical intervention allows for improvement of the overall risk, lytic therapy should be considered. If little improvement is expected, it is preferable to proceed with thrombectomy in a timely fashion. When dealing with a prosthetic graft occlusion, thrombectomy remains the therapy of choice. In patients in whom multiple previous reconstructions make a surgical approach less desirable, a trial of lytic therapy is a reasonable option, realizing that the chances of success without eventual surgical correction are low. The management of an occluded vein graft differs, in that the results of surgical thrombectomy are less predictable. Thus, if the ischemia is well tolerated, a trial of lytic therapy may help restore patency of the vein graft. Correction of the causative lesion may then be undertaken without the need for thrombectomy of the graft. This approach is a welcome option in the management of occluded vein bypasses.

Hemodialysis Access

Thrombosed arteriovenous fistulas can be successfully managed by intragraft administration of fibrinolytic agents. Usually the diagnosis is established early, as the patient notices the absence of a thrill, and thus the thrombotic material is very sensitive to lysis. Administration is by direct puncture, because there are no collaterals to dilute the effect of the agent. It is usually best to lace the intragraft thrombus with the lytic agent, and then proceed with high-dose intragraft administration. Of 46 arteriovenous fistulas, Graor et al. were successful in treating 40 (87 per cent); both PTFE and vein fistulas were equally responsive.[105] Thrombi older than 4 days were less susceptible to lysis (29 per cent). Unfortunately, most patients required surgical revision of the venous anastomosis, and thus lytic therapy served as a temporizing intervention. In some patients, however, this would allow for better preoperative preparation and elective, rather than urgent, operation.

Acute Stroke

Rapid resolution of embolic material causing acute stroke has theoretical advantages that may lead to improved clinical recovery. There is considerable interest in the use of fibrin-selective thrombolytic agents in the treatment of acute stroke secondary to thromboembolic events. Thrombolytic therapy has been used in the past with extremely unfavorable outcome in the presence of an acute stroke. Nevertheless, with newer available agents and better understanding of their mechanism of action, there has been a resurgence, with promising early clinical results, of the use of lytic agents after an acute stroke.

Eight clinical trials have evaluated the results of intravenous infusion of fibrinolytic agents in patients after a completed stroke.[119-126] Although clinical improvement was seen in some, no clinical benefit could be documented in others. In addition, the incidence of intracerebral hemorrhage was significant and, therefore, supported the general impression that thrombolytic therapy is contraindicated in patients with an acute stroke.

Most recently, local intraarterial infusion of streptokinase or urokinase in patients with angiographically demonstrable acute arterial thrombotic occlusions in the carotid or vertebrobasilar territories has been reported.[127-129] Two prospective studies have evaluated the possible benefits of intraarterial fibrinolytic therapy in acute stroke. No improvement was seen in the absence of reperfusion. Nevertheless, complete recanalization was achieved in 75 per cent of patients, two thirds of whom improved clinically. Hemorrhagic transformation of a bland infarct was seen by serial computed tomography scan in 20 per cent of patients, none of whom deteriorated clinically. This percentage of change from a bland to a hemorrhagic infarct is similar to patients treated with other forms of therapy.

Intravenous infusion of rt-PA has been suggested as potentially beneficial. Four preliminary studies of various protocols are ongoing. Until results of these trials are available, treatment of an acute stroke with thrombolytic therapy should be considered only in patients subject to appropriate protocols designed to evaluate its safety and efficacy.

Method

Consideration for thrombolytic therapy should begin prior to the initial angiographic needle puncture. The approach is chosen so as to maximize access to the occlusion and minimize morbidity. Arterial punctures distal to the presumed occlusion are avoided. Sites where bleeding may cause serious morbidity (axillary, translumbar) are avoided. When the suspected occlusion is at a superficial femoral artery or below (strong femoral pulse), we prefer an antegrade ipsilateral puncture (Fig. 18–6). When the suspected occlusion is at the femoral level or above, a contralateral puncture with passage of the catheter around the aortic bifurcation is preferred (Fig. 18–7). Infusions in the upper extremities or aortic branches are carried out through a transfemoral approach. End-

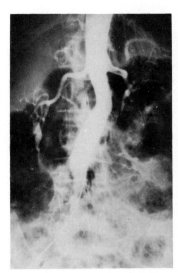 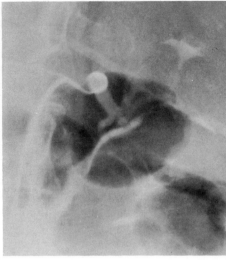 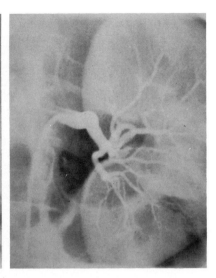

FIGURE 18–6. *Left*, Aortogram showing left renal artery embolus. *Center*, After 1 hour of high-dose intraarterial urokinase there is partial clearing and improved perfusion to left kidney. *Right*, Complete clearance of embolus after 3 hours of high-dose intraarterial urokinase.

hold catheters are used for infusion, with the tip into the thrombus. If this is not possible, there should be no large branches between the catheter tip and the occlusion. When the infusion is at the popliteal level or below, small (3-Fr) catheters are used through a coaxial system to prevent upstream clot formation (Fig. 18–8). A flush heparin infusion is maintained through the coaxial catheter.

The dosage chosen will partly depend on the length and volume of thrombus and the location and clinical importance of the vascular territory. Small-volume, short thrombi in important territories (i.e., renal) are better treated with high-dose infusions aimed at rapid fibrinolysis. Excellent results have been reported using high-dose urokinase (4000 units/min, followed after initial recanalization with 1000 to 2000 units/min).[130] These authors recommend creation of a channel into the thrombus with the angiographic guidewire. In fact, passage of the guidewire through the occlusion is a prognostic indicator as to the response to fibrinolytic infusion. Failure to pass the guidewire through the occlusion implies either plaque or well-organized thrombus, which may be resistant to fibrinolysis. On the other hand, easy passage of the guidewire through the occlusion not only establishes a channel in which the fibrinolytic agent will have the opportunity to concentrate, but implies soft, lysable thrombi. Lacing the thrombus with 50,000 units of urokinase, so that the agent is distributed within the thrombus itself, and then retrieval of the catheter for infusion, is frequently practiced and seems effective. When prolonged infusion is deemed necessary because of the amount of thrombus, then switching to a low-dose regimen (streptokinase 5000 to 10,000 units/hr; urokinase 30,000 to 50,000 units/hr) is appropriate, with angiography carried out within 12 to 16 hours to assess progress. From the accumulated experience, it appears that bleeding complications

correlate most with duration of therapy, rather than total dosage of the agent. Thus, high-dose, short-term infusions are better tolerated than long-term, low-dose infusions. Therefore, it is preferable to infuse higher doses of the agent if the duration of therapy can be shortened.

Duration of the infusion is guided by periodic angiographic and clinical monitoring, but should rarely exceed 96 hours. When high-dose infusion is used, it is best to keep the patient in the radiology suite and repeat angiography as often as every 30 minutes. For low-dose infusion, the patient is monitored in an intensive care unit and angiography is repeated daily or sooner, depending on the clinical response.

Before initiating therapy, baseline fibrinogen, thrombin time, PTT, and fibrin degradation product measurements are obtained. These are repeated 12 hours after commencing the infusion and then daily. It is expected that fibrinogen level will drop and fibrin degradation products will become positive. Prolongation of the PTT or thrombin time suggests a systemic lytic state and will occur in about 50 per cent of patients. Although specific parameters do not correlate with the risk of bleeding, the presence of the systemic lytic state does increase such risk. If good progress is being made by the infusion, a low fibrinogen value (less than 50 per cent of baseline) or evidence of a lytic state in the absence of bleeding complications is tolerated and therapy is continued. In the absence of a systemic lytic state, when little progress is evident, the dosage is increased and the result reassessed. Therapy should be discontinued if there is no improvement in any 24-hour interval, persistent or worsening ischemia, or a major bleeding complication.

The administration of heparin during regional thrombolytic therapy remains controversial. Clearly, in patients with profound ischemia, found to have

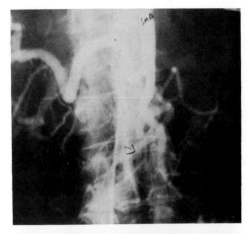

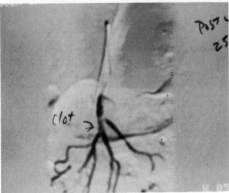

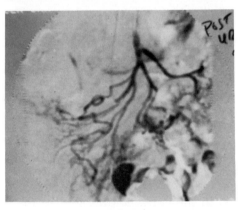

FIGURE 18–7. *Top,* Selective superior mesenteric artery angiogram showing occlusion of distal tree. *Center,* Partial clearing of embolus after 250,000 units of intraarterial urokinase (over 1 hour). *Bottom,* Complete resolution of superior mesenteric artery occlusion after 2 hours (500,000 units) of urokinase intraarterial therapy.

very low flow in the extremity, and instances where pericatheter thrombus formation would be significant (such as when 3 to 4 cm of the catheter is into a vessel with low or no flow), concomitant heparin administration should be strongly considered. Heparin administration may also be useful in increasing thrombolysis and minimizing the adverse consequences of a potential episode of distal clot migration or embolization. Heparin therapy, however, may increase the incidence and severity of pericatheter bleeding during lytic therapy and may increase the risk of distant bleeding.

Heparin administration is usually through a continuous infusion to maintain a prolonged PTT at 1.5 to 2.0 times control. A bolus infusion prior to initiation of continuous therapy is used where there is acute severe ischemia, or when low-flow states are identified in the ipsilateral system or around the catheter. When using a coaxial system, a lower dose of heparin may be administered through the larger catheter, usually at 500 units/hr. It is important that the PTT not exceed 60 seconds at the time of catheter and sheath removal. Heparin may then be restarted without a bolus.

When emergency surgery is required, the lytic agent is discontinued and fresh-frozen plasma administered if the fibrinogen level is below 100 mg/dl. The half-life of these agents is very short, and thus usually not a problem in this setting.

Complications

As with any form of lytic therapy, bleeding is the most feared and frequent complication of low-dose fibrinolytic therapy. The risk of major bleeding (requiring cessation of therapy and/or blood transfusions) ranges from 5 to 15 per cent when appropriate precautions are observed.[105,130] Bleeding is usually related to systemic effects of the drug, and management has been discussed under "Systemic Lytic Therapy" earlier in this chapter.

Considering that high-risk patients may be preferentially treated by this nonsurgical approach, the incidence of bleeding with intraarterial lytic therapy must be considered. The most recent experience seems to indicate that the risk of bleeding correlates more with duration than actual total dosage. It is therefore preferable to utilize higher dose protocols, especially in circumstances in which a short occlusion is being treated. Although specific coagulation parameters do not correlate with the risk of bleeding, the presence of a systemic lytic state increases this risk. It is important to document whether systemic effects of the drug are present, because it helps determine the most appropriate course of action. This is heralded by a 50 per cent drop in fibrinogen from baseline, a prolongation of the thrombin time to two times normal (or higher), or both. If significant progress is being made, continuation of therapy is warranted, in spite of systemic fibrinolysis. If, on the other hand, no significant improvement is noted within the last interval, reassessment should be made, weighing the risks and benefits of the alternatives.

Treatment of hemorrhagic complications depend on the severity and the progress made during lytic therapy. A small amount of oozing around the catheter entry site, without hematoma formation during the final stages of the infusion, can be controlled locally, keeping the patient under close observation until therapy is completed. The same situation in the early stages of the infusion, when more than 12 to 24 hours of therapy are anticipated, should lead to

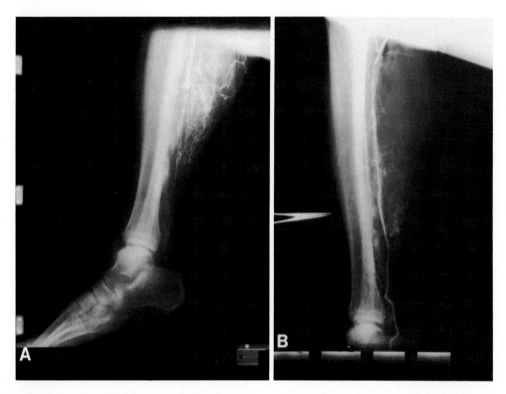

FIGURE 18–8. *A,* Intraoperative completion angiogram after popliteal embolectomy. Note absence of runoff vessels to the foot. *B,* Repeat angiogram after intraoperative infusion (streptokinase 60,000 units, heparin 1000 units) over 30 minutes through the same catheter used for angiography. Note remarkable improvement in runoff.

discontinuation of the drug. Development of a significant hematoma or bleeding at a remote site warrants cessation of therapy. Fibrinogen should be replaced by the administration of fibrinogen-rich components, such as cryoprecipitate or fresh-frozen plasma. This usually suffices, because the half-life of both urokinase and streptokinase is short.

Distal embolization occurs more frequently than is clinically appreciated. Continuation of therapy is preferable, with perhaps a temporary increase in the hourly dose. When severe ischemia is seen as the result of distal emboli, discontinuation of lytic therapy with prompt surgical embolectomy is indicated.

Several cases of embolization to the ipsilateral extremity have been reported during intraarterial lytic therapy for occlusion of axillofemoral grafts.[104] The length of these graft makes them unsuitable for lytic therapy, and thus surgical thrombectomy remains the therapy of choice.

Allergic reactions to streptokinase have been discussed under "Systemic Lytic Therapy." Routine administration of 100 mg of intravenous hydrocortisone may prevent some of these reactions and is recommended.

Pseudoaneurysm formation is rare, but may occur secondary to bleeding from an arterial puncture site. Surgical repair is recommended.

Intracranial bleeding is a recognized complication of any form of lytic therapy. Any change in the neurologic status of the patient during therapy should be viewed as related to the fibrinolytic agent until proven otherwise. Bleeding from unrecognized intracranial pathology must be ruled out. Lytic therapy should be discontinued while evaluation is proceeding. The incidence of intracranial bleeding appears to be increased in patients that have been on oral anticoagulants prior to therapy, patients weighing less than 70 kg, and patients older than 65 years old.[70]

Fatal pulmonary emboli have been reported during intraarterial fibrinolytic therapy.[107] A possible mechanism for this complication implies decreased venous circulation in the ischemic extremity, with clot formation, partial lysis, and eventual pulmonary embolization. This is a rare occurrence. Treatment options include cessation of lytic therapy with heparinization or switching to systemic intravenous lytic therapy. If the latter is chosen, leaving the intraarterial catheter in place may decrease the risk of bleeding through the arterial puncture site.

Conversion of an ischemic myocardial infarction into a hemorrhagic infarct as a complication of fibrinolytic therapy has been reported.[107] The relationship between lytic therapy and the few reported cases is unclear. Deterioration of cardiac function in the presence of an acute myocardial infarction during fibrinolytic therapy should lead the clinician to consider this possibility. Therapy should be discontinued until the etiology of the cardiac decompensation is determined.

INTRAOPERATIVE THROMBOLYTIC THERAPY

Approximately 30 per cent of lower extremity embolectomies are incomplete, with remaining intravascular defects demonstrable by completion angiography.[131] Experimental studies suggest that the true incidence may be as high as 80 per cent.[132] The idea of removing the bulk of thrombus surgically and lysing any remaining defects is attractive from the therapeutic standpoint. Alternatives include reembolectomy with the balloon catheter,[133] irrigation in an attempt to flush the residual clot,[134] passage of Dormia catheters,[135] and distal exploration. All these will further injure the endothelium, and thus increase its thrombogenicity. Certain endovascular procedures, such as endoscopy, atherectomy, or dilatations, may also temporarily increase the thrombogenicity of these vessels, leading to early thrombosis. Further mechanical manipulation is likely to result in further injury, and thus unlikely to solve the problem. For these reasons, controlled chemical intraoperative fibrinolysis may be a welcome alternative in the treatment of these complications. When dealing with delayed intervention in the presence of a thrombotic process, propagation of clot into the branches of the arterial tree may be most difficult to retrieve. Once these clots lose their integrity with the parent thrombus, enzymatic dissolution may be the only alternative.

Bleeding complications secondary to intraarterial fibrinolytic therapy are the result of prolonged infusions necessary to lyse extensive thrombus. The potential for intraoperative or perioperative lytic therapy was suggested by several investigators.[136–138] Common to all these observations was the lack of bleeding complications. There are several advantages in the intraoperative use of lytic agents, when compared to the percutaneous method. First, the bulk of the thrombus has been surgically removed, and thus there is a decrease in the amount of lysis required. Second, a higher concentration of the agent, with control of inflow and, therefore, circulation time, can be accomplished. Finally, infusion within the thrombus or adjacent to it is theoretically unnecessary, and repeat embolectomy with reassessment of the intervention can be done with repeated infusions, as necessary.

In 1985, we reported our initial experience with five patients in whom intraoperative infusions of 20,000 to 100,000 units of streptokinase was successful in restoring adequate circulation to limbs still threatened after embolectomy.[139] We have now extended this experience to 23 infusions in 22 patients.[140] In 17 of these patients, both preinfusion and postinfusion arteriograms were available and demonstrated improvement following lytic therapy in 13 (76 per cent). Only one of these reconstructions rethrombosed in the postoperative period. In the four patients without angiographic improvement, all four suffered rethrombosis. Thus, it appears that prein-fusion and postinfusion arteriography has prognostic significance, implying that failure to improve after intraoperative infusion of the lytic agent suggests a high likelihood of failure and, therefore, alternative methods of reconstruction need to be considered at the time of surgery.

Bleeding is the most feared complication of intraoperative lytic therapy. In our experience, of 23 lytic infusions carried out intraoperatively, five hematomas occurred. All of these, however, occurred in patients who were fully heparinized postoperatively. Among 12 patients who were not heparinized after surgery, there were no bleeding complications. Thus, bleeding after intraoperative lytic therapy is secondary to aggressive antithrombotic and anticoagulation regimens, rather than the lytic therapy itself.

Clinical experience to date is summarized in Table 18–4. Four additional clinical series have been reported since our initial report.[103,141–143] Cohen et al. performed 13 infusions by bolus of 25,000 to 250,000 units of streptokinase.[103] Sixty-one per cent of the infusions were successful. Five bleeding complications occurred, one of them resulting in death secondary to retroperitoneal bleeding during aortoiliac reconstruction. This suggests that caution should be exercised with intraoperative use of lytic agents during major abdominal or retroperitoneal surgery. Norem et al. reported their experience with 19 infusions of 50,000 to 200,000 units of streptokinase by bolus injection.[142] They followed the infusion by repeat embolectomy and were able to retrieve additional thrombus in each instance. Two wound hematomas occurred in the postoperative period. Heparin was maintained following surgery at low doses (200 to 500 units/hr). With this regimen, bleeding complications appeared to have been minimized.

Our preferred technique for intraoperative infusion of fibrinolytic agents consists of a drip infusion of the agent without occlusion of the inflow. Recent experimental evidence suggests that maintenance of blood flow in the system during administration of fibrinolytic agents enhances their effectiveness. This can be accomplished by insertion of a cannula distal to the arteriotomy after repair of the latter. We prefer urokinase, 250,000 units dissolved in 100 ml of saline, delivered over 30 minutes. On the basis of our original experimental study, we continue to recommend the addition of heparin to the infusate at 1 to 4 units/ml.[132] Preinfusion and postinfusion arteriography are recommended to document the effectiveness of the agent. Failure to show improvement in the postinfusion angiogram would suggest a high likelihood of failure and consideration of alternative management. More recently, the use of an isolated limb perfusion with an extracorporeal pump has shown promise in further enhancing the effectiveness of the lytic agent.[144]

Urokinase appears to be a safer agent for intraoperative use. Allergic reactions are not seen. The mechanism of action is direct and the risk of plasminogen depletion, as may occur with streptokinase, is eliminated. The best method and the appropriate

TABLE 18–4.   RESULTS OF INTRAOPERATIVE REGIONAL FIBRINOLYTIC THERAPY

Reference	No. of Cases	Drug Dose and Method[a]	Per cent Successful	Complications	Remarks
Cohen et al.[103]	13	SK: 25,000–250,000 units by bolus	61	5 rethromboses; 5 bleeding complications; 1 death after retroperitoneal surgery	2 renal infusions, 1 partly successful; death related to retroperitoneal bleeding
Norem et al.[142]	19	SK: 50,000–200,000 units by bolus	100	2 wound hematomas	All patients underwent repeat embolectomy; postoperative heparin in low doses (200–500 units/hr).
Parent et al.[143]	28	SK: 50,000–150,000 units by bolus UK: 35,000–150,000 units by bolus	88	Bleeding 11%; compartment syndrome 21%; 2 deaths	Deaths not related to lytic therapy; 2 bleeding complications in 2 patients after retroperitoneal surgery
Comerota et al.[141]	38	SK: Max 50,000 units UK: Max 150,000 units by bolus 2 patients; isolated limb—UK: 1,000,000 units	74	1 wound hematoma; 5 deaths	Deaths not related to lytic agent
Quiñones-Baldrich et al.[139]	23	SK: 60,000–100,000 units UK: 250,000–375,000 units plus heparin 1–4 units/ml Gravity infusion over 30 min	74	6 rethromboses; 5 wound hematomas	All wound hematomas in patients fully heparinized postoperatively

[a]SK, streptokinase; UK, urokinase.

dosage, however, have not been determined. The logistical advantages of bolus infusion are obvious. Nevertheless, a slow infusion has the theoretical advantage of providing a constant amount of the drug, while plasminogen is being supplied by collateral circulation. Bolus infusion, although achieving a high concentration of the agent rapidly, is likely to be washed out, and thus the effect may be very short lived. These considerations, however, remain controversial, because no study to date has evaluated these issues.

The high selectivity for fibrin of t-PA and the positive early results with relatively short-term infusion suggest that this is a promising agent for intraoperative use. To date, there are no reports of intraoperative use of t-PA.

In summary, we do not hesitate to proceed with an intraoperative fibrinolytic infusion when faced with either residual thrombus inaccessible to the balloon catheter, or persistent ischemia after restoration of flow. Although the best method of delivery and most appropriate dosage have not been fully determined, reported clinical experience has allowed guidelines that permit the clinician to obtain the benefits of fibrinolytic infusion in these difficult cases with both safety and efficacy.

REFERENCES

1. Gross R: Fibrinolyse und thrombolyse. Panorama *September*: 4, 1962.
2. Malpighi M: De polypo cordis. Opera Omnia, part 2. Ludg Batav, 1687, p 311.
3. Morgagni JB: De Sedivus et Causis Morborum per Anatomen Indagatis, 2nd ed. 1761. Translated by Alexander B: The Seats and Causes of Diseases Investigated by Anatomy, vol 3, book 4. London, Millar, 1769.
4. Morawitz P: Ner einige postmortale blutveranderugen beitr zur chem Physiol Patho. Braunschweig 8:1, 1906.
5. Dastre A: Fibrinolyse dans le sang. Arch Physiol Norn Path 5:661, 1893.
6. Astrup T: The haemostatic balance. Thromb Diath Haemost 2:347, 1958.
7. Henkin J, Marcotte P, Yang H: The plasminogen-plasmin system. Prog Cardiovasc Dis 34(2):135–164, 1991.
8. Kwaan HC: Hematologic aspects of thrombolytic therapy. *In* Comerota AJ (ed): Thrombolytic Therapy. Orlando, FL, Grune & Stratton, 1988.
9. Sugiyama N, Iwamoto M, Abiko A: Effects of kringles de-

rived from human plasminogen on fibrinolysis in vitro. Thromb Res *47*:459–468, 1987.

10. Wiman B, Lijnen HR, Collen D: On the specific interaction between the lysine-binding sites in plasminogen and complementary sites in α_2-antiplasmin and in fibrinogen. Biochim Biophys Acta *579*:142–154, 1979.

11. Lo SK, Ryan TJ, Gilboa N, et al: Role of catalytic and lysine-binding sites in plasmin-induced neutrophil adherence to endothelium. J Clin Invest *84*:793–801, 1989.

12. Thorsen S: Differences in the binding to fibrin of native plasminogen and plasminogen modified by proteolytic degradation influence of ω-aminocarboxylic acids. Biochim Biophys Acta *393*:55–65, 1975.

13. Rylatt DB, Blake LE, Cottis DA, et al: An immunoassay for human d-dimer using monoclonal antibodies. Thromb Res *31*:767, 1983.

14. Burrowes CE: Activation of human prekallikrein by plasmin. Fed Proc *30*:451, 1971.

15. Powell JR, Castellino FJ: Amino acid sequence analysis of the asparagine-288 region of the carbohydrate variants of human plasminogen. Biochemistry *22*:923–927, 1983.

16. Collen D, Wiman B: Turnover of antiplasmin, the fast-acting plasmin inhibitor of plasma. Blood *53*:313–324, 1979.

17. Low DA, Baker JB, Koonce WC: Released protease nexin regulates cellular binding, internalization, and degradation of serine proteases. Proc Natl Acad Sci USA *78*:2340–2344, 1981.

18. Royston D: Review paper: The serine antiprotease aprotinin (Trasylol™): A novel approach to reducing postoperative bleeding. Blood Coag Fibrin *1*:55–69, 1990.

19. Verstraete M: Clinical applications of inhibitors of fibrinolysis. Drugs *29*:236–261, 1985.

20. Clozel JP, Banken L, Roux S: Aprotinin: An antidote for recombinant tissue-type plasminogen activator (rt-PA) active in vivo. J Am Coll Cardiol *16*:507–510, 1990.

21. Kwaan HC: The biologic role of components of the plasminogen-plasmin system. Prog Cardiovasc Dis *34(5)*:309–316, 1992.

22. Kirchheimer JC, Wojta J, Christ G, et al: Proliferation of a human epidermal tumor cell line stimulated by urokinase. FASEB J *1*:125–218, 1987.

23. Kirchheimer JC, Wojta J, Christ G, et al: Mitogenic effect of urokinase on malignant and unaffected adjacent human renal cells. Carcinogenesis *9*:2121–2123, 1988.

24. Rabbani SA, Desjardins J, Bell AW, et al: An aminoterminal fragment of urokinase isolated from a prostate cancer cell line (PC-3) is mitogenic for osteoblast-like cells. Biochem Biophys *173*:1058–1064, 1990.

25. Juhan-Vague I, Alessi MC, Joly P, et al: Plasma plasminogen activator inhibitor-1 in angina pectoris. Influence of plasma insulin and acute-phase response. Arteriosclerosis *9*:362–367, 1989.

26. Wiman B, Hamsten A: Impaired fibrinolysis and risk of thromboembolism. Prog Cardiovasc Dis *34(3)*:179–192, 1991.

27. Andreotti F, Davies GJ, Hackett DR, et al: Major circadian fluctuations in fibrinolytic factors and possible relevance to time of onset of myocardial infarction, sudden cardiac death and stroke. Am J Cardiol *62*:635–637, 1988.

28. Grimaudo V, Hauert J, Bachmann F, et al: Diurnal variation of the fibrinolytic system. Thromb Haemost *59*:495–499, 1988.

29. Angleton P, Chandler WL, Schmer G: Diurnal variation of tissue-type plasminogen activator and its rapid inhibition. Circulation *79*:101–106, 1989.

30. Chandler WL, Trimble SL, Loo S-C, Mornin D: Effect of PAI-1 levels on the molar concentrations of active tissue plasminogen activator (t-PA) and t-PA/PAI-1 complex in plasma. Blood *76*:930–937, 1990.

31. Urano T, Sumiyoshi K, Nakamura M, et al: Fluctuation of tPA and PAI-1 antigen levels in plasma: Difference in their fluctuation patterns between male and female. J Thromb Res *60*:55–62, 1990.

32. Mannucci PM, Rota L: Plasminogen activator response after

DDAVP: A clinical fibromycological study. Thromb Res *20*:69, 1980.

33. Walker ID, Davidson JF: Long term fibrinolytic enhancement with anabolic steroid therapy: A five year study. In Davidson JF, Rowan RM, Samama MM, Desnoyers PC (eds): Progress in Chemical Fibrinolysis and Thrombolysis, vol 3. New York, Raven Press, 1978, pp 491–500.

34. Jarrett PEM, Moreland M, Browse NL: Idiopathic recurrent superficial thrombophlebitis: Treatment with fibrinolytic enhancement. Br Med J *1*:933, 1977.

35. Tillett WS, Garner RL: The fibrinolytic activity of hemolytic streptococci. J Exp Med *58*:485, 1933.

36. Kakkar VV, Sagar S, Lewis M: Treatment of deep vein thrombosis with intermittent streptokinase and plasminogen infusion. Lancet *2*:674, 1975.

37. MacFarlane RG, Pilling J: Fibrinolytic activity of normal urine. Nature *159*:779, 1947.

38. Lijnen HR, Zamarron C, Blaber M, et al: Activation of plasminogen by pro-urokinase. I. mechanism. J Biol Chem *261*:1253–1258, 1986.

39. Barnathan ES, Kuo A, Rosenfeld L, et al: Interaction of single-chain urokinase-type plasminogen activator with human endothelial cells. J Biol Chem *265*:2865–2872, 1990.

40. Behrendt N, Ronne E, Plough M, et al: The human receptor for urokinase plasminogen activator. NH_2-terminal amino acid sequence and glycosylation variants. J Biol Chem *265*:6453–6460, 1990.

41. Nykjaer A, Petersen CM, Christensen EI, et al: Urokinase receptors in human monocytes. Biochim Biophys Acta *1052*:399–407, 1990.

42. Watahiki Y, Takeda Y, Takeda A: Kinetic analyses of the activation of Glu-plasminogen by urokinase in the presence of fibrin, fibrinogen or its degradation products. Thromb Res *46*:9–18, 1987.

43. Feissinger JN, Aiach M, Capron L, et al: Effect of local urokinase on arterial occlusion of lower limbs. Thromb Haemost *45*:230, 1981.

44. McNicol GP, Gale SB, Douglas AS: In vitro and in vivo studies of a preparation of urokinase. Br Med J *1*:909, 1963.

45. Belkin M, Belkin B, Bucknam CA, Straub JJ, Lowe R: Intraarterial fibrinolytic therapy: Efficacy of streptokinase versus urokinase. Arch Surg *121*:769, 1986.

46. Tennant SN, Dixon J, Venable TC, et al: Intracoronary thrombolysis in patients with acute myocardial infarction: Comparison of the efficacy of urokinase versus streptokinase. Circulation *69*:756, 1984.

47. Van Breda A, Katzen BT, Deutsch AS: Urokinase versus streptokinase in local thrombolysis. Radiology *165*:109, 1987.

48. Graor RA, Young JR, Risius B, Ruschhaupt WF: Comparison of cost effectiveness of streptokinase and urokinase in the treatment of deep vein thrombosis. Ann Vasc Surg *1*:524, 1987.

49. Fletcher AP, Alkjaersig N, Sherry S, et al: The development of urokinase as a thrombolytic agent. Maintenance of a sustained thrombolytic state in man by intravenous infusion. J Lab Clin Med *65*:713, 1965.

50. Kakkar VV, Scully MF: Thrombolytic therapy. Br Med Bull *34*:191, 1978.

51. Toki N, Sumi H, Sasaki K, et al: Oral administration of high molecular weight urokinase in human subjects and in an experimental dog model. In Davidson JF, Nilsson IM, Astedt B (eds): Progress in Fibrinolysis, vol 5. Edinburgh, Churchill Livingstone, 1981.

52. Albrechtsen OK: The fibrinolytic agents in saline extracts of human tissues. Scand J Clin Lab Invest *10*:91, 1958.

53. Rijken DC, Wijngaards G, Zaal-DeJong M, et al: Purification and partial characterization of plasminogen activator from human uterine tissue. Biochim Biophys Acta *580*:140, 1979.

54. Collen D: Human tissue type plasminogen activator: From the laboratory to the bedside (editorial). Circulation *72*:18, 1985.

55. Rijken DC, Collen D: Purification and characterization of

the plasminogen activator secreted by human melanoma cells in culture. J Biol Chem 156:7035, 1981.

56. Collen D, Stassen JM, Marafine BJ Jr, et al: Biological properties of human tissue type plasminogen activator obtained by expression of recombinant DNA in mammalian cells. J Pharmacol Exp Ther 231:146, 1984.

57. Sherry S: Tissue plasminogen activator (t-PA): Will it fulfill its promise. N Engl J Med 313:1014, 1985.

59. TIMI Study Group: The Thrombolysis in Myocardial Infarction (TIMI) Trial. Phase I findings. N Engl J Med 312:932, 1985.

60. Gao S, Morser J, McLean K, et al: Differential effect of platelets on plasminogen activation by tissue plasminogen activator, urokinase, and streptokinase. Thromb Res 58:421–433, 1990.

61. Klabunde RE, Burke SE, Henkin J: Enhanced lytic efficacy of multiple bolus injections of tissue plasminogen activator in dogs. Thromb Res 58:511–517, 1990.

62. Graor RA, Risius B, Young JR, et al: Peripheral artery and bypass graft thrombolysis with recombinant human tissue type plasminogen activator. Circulation 72(suppl III):III-15, 1985.

63. Monk JP, Heel RC: Anisoylated plasminogen streptokinase activator complex (APSAC): A review of its mechanism of action, clinical pharmacology, and therapeutic use in acute myocardial infarction. Drugs 34:25–49, 1987.

64. Summaria L: The plasmin b-chain streptokinase complex. In Comerota AJ (ed): Thrombolytic Therapy. Orlando, FL, Grune & Stratton, 1988.

65. Husain SS, Gurewich V, Lipinski B: Purification and partial characterization of a single chain, high molecular weight form of urokinase from human urine. Arch Biochem Biophys 220:31, 1983.

66. Pannell R, Gurewich V: Pro-urokinase: A study of its stability in plasma and of a mechanism for its selective fibrinolytic effect. Blood 67:1215–1223, 1986.

67. Gurewich V, Pannell R, Louie S, et al: Effective and fibrin specific clot lysis by a zymogen precursor form of urokinase (pro-urokinase): A study in vitro and two animal species. J Clin Invest 73:1731, 1984.

68. Bode C, Matsueda G, Haber E: Targeted thrombolysis with a fibrin specific antibody urokinase conjugate. Circulation 72:111–192, 1985.

69. Kremer P, Fiebig R, Tilsner V, Bleifiel W, Mathey DG: Lysis of left ventricular thrombi with urokinase. Circulation 72:112, 1985.

71. Gore JM, Sloan M, Price TR, et al: Intracranial hemorrhage, cerebral infarction, and subdural hematoma after acute myocardial infarction and thrombolytic therapy in the thrombolysis in myocardial infarction study: Thrombolysis in Myocardial Infarction (TIMI), Phase II, pilot and clinical trial. Circulation 83:448–459, 1991.

72. Gore JM: Prevention of severe neurologic events in the thrombolytic era. Chest 100(suppl 4):124S–130S, 1992.

73. National Heart and Lung Institute Cooperative Study Group: Urokinase Pulmonary Embolism Trial: Phase I results. JAMA 214:2163, 1970.

74. National Heart and Lung Institute Cooperative Study Group: Urokinase-Streptokinase Embolism Trial: Phase II results. JAMA 229:1606, 1974.

75. Molina JE, Hunter DW, Yedlicka JW, Cerra FB: Thrombolytic therapy for postoperative pulmonary embolism. Am J Surg 163:375–381, 1992.

76. Sharma GVRK, Folland ED, McIntyre KM, et al: Longterm hemodynamic benefit of thrombolytic therapy in pulmonary embolic disease (abstract). J Am Coll Cardiol 15:65A, 1990.

77. Verstraete M, Miller AH, Bounameaux H, et al: Intravenous and intrapulmonary recombinant tissue type plasminogen activator in the treatment of acute massive pulmonary embolism. Circulation 77:353, 1988.

78. Goldhaber SZ, Markis JE, Meyerovitz MF, et al: Acute pulmonary embolism treated with tissue plasminogen activator. Lancet 2:886, 1986.

79. Goldhaber SZ, Kessler CM, Heit J, et al: A randomized controlled trial of recombinant tissue plasminogen activator versus urokinase in the treatment of acute pulmonary embolism. Lancet 2:293–298, 1988.

80. NIH Consensus Development Conference: Thrombolytic therapy in treatment. Br Med J 1:1585, 1980.

81. Berni GA, Bandyk DF, Zierler RE, et al: Streptokinase treatment of acute arterial occlusion. Ann Surg 198:185, 1983.

82. Arnesen H, Heilo A, Jakobson E: A prospective study of streptokinase and heparin in the treatment of deep vein thrombosis. Acta Med Scand 203:457, 1978.

83. Kakkar VV, Flanc C, Howe CT: Treatment of deep vein thrombosis. A trial of aspirin, streptokinase, and arvin. Br Med J 1:806, 1969.

84. Marder VJ, Soulen RL, Atichartakarn V, et al: Quantitative venographic assessment of deep vein thrombosis in the evaluation of streptokinase and heparin therapy. J Lab Clin Med 89:1018, 1977.

85. Porter JM, Seaman AJ, Common HH, et al: Comparison of heparin and streptokinase in the treatment of venous thrombosis. Am Surg 41:511, 1975.

86. Tsapogas MJ, Peabody RA, Wu KT, et al: Controlled study of thrombolytic therapy in deep vein thrombosis. Surgery 74:873, 1973.

87. Arnesen H, Hoiseth A, Ly B: Streptokinase or heparin in the treatment of deep vein thrombosis: Follow-up results of a prospective study. Acta Med Scand 211:65, 1982.

88. Kakkar VV, Lorenz D: Hemodynamic and clinical assessment after therapy for deep vein thrombosis: A prospective study. Am J Surg 140:54, 1985.

89. Turpie GG, Jay RM, Carter CJ, Hirsh J: A randomized trial of recombinant tissue plasminogen activator for the treatment of proximal deep vein thrombosis (abstract). Circulation 72:193, 1985.

90. Verhaeghe R, Besse P, Bounameaux H, et al: Multi-center pilot study of the efficacy and safety of systemic rt-PA administration in the treatment of deep vein thrombosis of the lower extremities and/or pelvis. Thromb Res 55:5–11, 1989.

91. Goldhaber SZ, Meyerovitz MF, Green D, et al: Randomized controlled trial of tissue plasminogen activator in proximal deep venous thrombosis. Am J Med 88:235–240, 1990.

92. Marder VJ, Grenner B, Totterman S, et al: Comparison of dosage schedules of rt-PA in the treatment of proximal deep vein thrombosis. J Lab Clin Med (in press).

93. Alemany J, Marsal T: Early and late results in the surgical treatment of phlegmasia cerulea dolens. Vasc Surg July/Aug:271, 1987.

94. Shionoya S, Yamada I, Sakurai T, Ohta T, Matsubara J: Thrombectomy for acute deep vein thrombosis: Prevention of postthrombotic syndrome. J Cardiovasc Surg 30:484, 1989.

95. Elliot MS, Immelman EJ, Jeffrey P, et al: The role of thrombolytic therapy in the management of phlegmasia cerulea dolens. Br J Surg 66:422, 1979.

96. Paquet KJ, Popov S, Egli H: Richtlinien und ergebnissi der konsequenten fibrinolytischen therapie der phlegmasia caerulea dolens. Dtsch Med Wochenschr 16:903, 1970.

97. Roberts WM: Some clinical problems in patients undergoing thrombolytic therapy. S Afr Med J 50:243, 1976.

98. Druy EM, Trout HH, Giordano JM, et al: Lytic therapy in the treatment of axillary and subclavian vein thrombosis. J Vasc Surg 2:821, 1985.

99. Rubenstein M, Greger WP: Successful streptokinase therapy for catheter induced subclavian vein in thrombosis. Arch Intern Med 140:1370, 1980.

100. Wilson JJ, Lesk D, Newman H: Subclavian-axillary vein thrombosis: Successful treatment with streptokinase. Can Med Assoc J 130:891, 1984.

101. Herrera JL, Wilis SM, Williams TH: Successful streptokinase therapy of acute idiopathic superior vena cava thrombosis. Am Heart J 102:1063, 1981.

102. Elliot MS, Immelman EJ, Jeffrey P, et al: A comparative randomized trial of heparin vs streptokinase in the treat-

ment of acute proximal venous thrombosis. An interim report of a prospective trial. Br J Surg 66:838, 1979.

103. Cohen LH, Kaplan M, Bernhard VM: Intraoperative streptokinase: An adjunct to mechanical thrombectomy in the management of acute ischemia. Arch Surg 121:708, 1986.

104. Sussman B, Dardik H, Ibrahim IM, et al: Improved patient selection for enzymatic lysis of peripheral arterial and graft occlusions. Am J Surg 148:244, 1984.

105. Graor RA, Risius B, Denny KM, et al: Local thrombolysis in the treatment of thrombosed arteries, bypassed grafts, and arteriovenous fistulas. J Vasc Surg 2:406, 1985.

106. Katzen BT, Edwards KC, Albert AS, et al: Low dose direct fibrinolysis in peripheral vascular disease. J Vasc Surg 1:718, 1984.

107. Sicard GA, Schier JJ, Totty WG, et al: Thrombolytic therapy for acute arterial occlusion. J Vasc Surg 2:65, 1985.

108. Taylor LM, Porter JM, Bauer GM, et al: Intraarterial streptokinase infusion for acute popliteal and tibial arterial occlusion. Am J Surg 147:583, 1984.

109. Risius B, Zelch MG, Graor RA, et al: Catheter directed low dose streptokinase infusion: A preliminary experience. Radiology 150:349, 1984.

110. McNamara TO, Bomberger RA: Factors affecting initial and six months patency following high dose intraarterial urokinase thrombolysis. Am J Surg 152:709, 1986.

111. Gardiner GA, Harrington DP, Koltun W, Whittemore A, Mannick JA, Levin DC: Salvage of occluded arterial bypass grafts by means of thrombolyses. J Vasc Surg 9:426, 1989.

112. Porter JM, Taylor LM: Current status of thrombolytic therapy. J Vasc Surg 2:239, 1985.

113. Van Breda A, Robinson JC, Feldman L, et al: Local thrombolysis in the treatment of arterial graft occlusions. Vasc Surg 1:103, 1984.

114. Cronan JJ, Dorfman GS: Low dose thrombolysis: A non-operative approach to renal artery occlusion. J Urol 130:757, 1983.

115. Pillari G, Doscher W, Fierstein J, et al: Low dose streptokinase in the treatment of celiac and superior mesenteric artery occlusion. Arch Surg 118:1340, 1983.

116. Hargrove WC, Berkowitz HD, Freiman DB, et al: Recanalization of totally occluded femoral popliteal vein grafts with low dose streptokinase infusion. Surgery 92:890, 1982.

117. Perler BA, White RI, Ernst CB, et al: Low dose thrombolytic therapy for infrainguinal graft occlusions: An idea whose time has passed? J Vasc Surg 2:799, 1985.

118. Hargrove WC, Berkowitz HD, Freiman DB, et al: Treatment of acute peripheral arterial and graft thrombosis with low dose streptokinase. Surgery 92:981, 1982.

119. Abe T, Kazawa M, Naito I: Clinical evaluation for efficacy of tissue culture urokinase (TCUK) on cerebral thrombosis by means of multicenter double-blind study. Blood Vessels 12:321–341, 1981.

120. Abe T, Kazawa M, Naito I: Clinical effect of urokinase (60,000 units/day) on cerebral infarction—comparative study by means of multiple center double-blind test. Blood Vessels 12:342–358, 1981.

121. Clarke RL, Cliffton EE: The treatment of cerebrovascular thrombosis and embolism with fibrinolytic agents. Am J Cardiol 30:546–551, 1960.

122. Fletcher AP, Alkjaersig N, Lewis M, Tuelvski V, Davies A, Brooks JE, Mardin WB, Landau WM, Raichle ME: A pilot study of urokinase therapy in cerebral infarction. Stroke 7:135–142, 1976.

123. Herndon RM, Nelson JN, Johnson JF, Meyer JS: Thrombolytic treatment in cerebrovascular thrombosis. *In* MacMillan RL, Mustart JF (eds): Anticoagulants and Fibrinolysins. Philadelphia, Lea & Febiger, 1961, pp 154–164.

124. Matsuo O, Kosugi T, Mihara H, Ohki Y, Matsuo T: Retrospective study on the efficacy of using urokinase therapy. Nippon Ketsueki Gakkai Zasshi 42:684–688, 1979.

125. Meyer JS, Gilroy J, Barnhardt ME, Johnson JF: Therapeutic thrombolysis in cerebral thromboembolism: Randomized evaluation of intravenous streptokinase. *In* Millikan CH, Siekert RG, Whisnant JP (eds): Cerebral Vascular Diseases, Fourth Princeton Conference. New York, Grune & Stratton, 1965, pp 200–213.

126. Meyer JS, Herndon RM, Gotoh F, Tazaki Y, Nelson JN, Johnson JF: Therapeutic thrombolysis. *In* Cerebral Vascular Diseases, Third Princeton Conference. New York, Grune & Stratton, 1961, pp 160–177.

127. Zeumer H, Ringelstein EV, Hassel M, Poeck K: Lokale Fibrinolysetherapie bei subtotaler Stenose der A. Cerebri Media. Dtsch Med Wochenschr 108:1103–1105, 1983.

128. Zeumer H, Hundgen R, Ferbert A, Ringelstein EB: Local intraarterial fibrinolytic therapy in inaccessible internal carotid occlusion. Neuroradiology 26:315–317, 1984.

129. Zeumer H, Hacke W, Kolmann HL, Poeck K: Lokale Fibrinolyse bei Basilaris-thrombose. Dtsch Med Wochenschr 107:728–731, 1982.

130. McNamara TO, Fischer JR: Thrombolysis of peripheral arterial and graft occlusions: Improved results using high dose urokinase. AJR 144:769, 1985.

131. Plecha FR, Pories WJ: Intraoperative angiography in the immediate assessment of arterial reconstruction. Arch Surg 105:802, 1972.

132. Quiñones-Baldrich WJ, Ziomek S, Henderson T, et al: Intraoperative fibrinolytic therapy: Experimental evaluation. J Vasc Surg 4:229, 1986.

133. Satiani B, Gross WS, Evans WE: Improved limb salvage after arterial embolectomy. Ann Surg 118:153–157, 1978.

134. Green RM, DeWeese JA, Rob CG: Arterial embolectomy before and after the Fogarty catheter. Surgery 77:24–33, 1975.

135. Greep JM, Aleman PJ, Jarrett F, Bast TJ: A combined technique for peripheral arterial embolectomy. Arch Surg 105:869–874, 1972.

136. Chaise LS, Comerota AJ, Soulen RL, et al: Selective intraarterial streptokinase therapy in the immediate postoperative period. JAMA 247:2397, 1982.

137. Feissinger JN, Vayssiarirat M, Juillet Y, et al: Local urokinase in arterial thromboembolism. Angiology 31:715, 1980.

138. Tsapogas MJ: The role of fibrinolysis in the treatment of arterial thrombosis. Experimental and clinical aspects. Ann R Coll Surg Engl 24:293, 1964.

139. Quiñones-Baldrich WJ, Zierler RE, Hiatt JC: Intraoperative fibrinolytic therapy: An adjunct to catheter thromboembolectomy. J Vasc Surg 2:319, 1985.

140. Quiñones-Baldrich WJ, Baker JD, Busuttil RW, Machleder HI, Moore WS: Intraoperative infusion of lytic drugs for thrombotic complications of revascularization. J Vasc Surg 10:408, 1989.

141. Comerota AJ, White JV, Grosh JD: Intraoperative intraarterial thrombolytic therapy for salvage of limbs in patients with distal arterial thrombosis. Surg Gynecol Obstet 160:283, 1989.

142. Norem RF, Short DH, Kerstein MD: Role of intraoperative fibrinolytic therapy in acute arterial occlusion. Surg Gynecol Obstet 167:87–91, 1988.

143. Parent III FN, Bernhard VM, Pabst TS, McIntyre KE, Hunter GC, Malone JM: Fibrinolytic treatment of residual thrombus after catheter embolectomy for severe lower limb ischemia. J Vasc Surg 9:153, 1989.

144. Quiñones-Baldrich WJ, Colburn MD, Gelabert HA, Barcliff LT, Moore WS: Isolated limb perfusion with extracorporeal pump increases effectiveness of lysis by urokinase. J Surg Res 1993 (submitted).

REVIEW QUESTIONS

1. Streptokinase and urokinase have the following similarities:
    1. both are bacterial products
    2. both are enzymes
    3. both are highly fibrin specific
    4. both are direct fibrinolytic agents
    (a) 1,2,3
    (b) 1,3
    (c) 2,4
    (d) 4 only
    (e) none of the above

2. Increasing the dose of streptokinase to decrease its lytic effect:
    (a) is indicated when bleeding occurs during therapy
    (b) is a predictable response
    (c) is scientifically correct but unnecessary
    (d) increases the risk of bleeding
    (e) none of the above

3. Tissue plasminogen activator:
    (a) is a nonenzymatic protein
    (b) has fibrinolytic activity in plasminogen-free media
    (c) is highly antigenic
    (d) is mainly an exogenous fibrinolytic activator
    (e) none of the above

4. A patient with deep vein thrombosis of the femoral system:
    1. is a candidate for lytic therapy if the thrombosis is recent and is the first episode
    2. may be treated with low-dose local lytic therapy
    3. has about a 50 to 60 per cent chance of failure to clear completely with lytic therapy
    4. is at higher risk of pulmonary embolism with lytic therapy than with heparin
    (a) 1,2,3
    (b) 1,3
    (c) 2,4
    (d) 4 only
    (e) none of the above

5. Intraarterial lytic therapy
    (a) is initiated with a loading dose
    (b) is highly effective in graft thrombosis
    (c) is highly effective in postdilatation thrombosis
    (d) can be safely administered in patients after a stroke

    (e) usually avoids a systemic lytic state

6. The dose of urokinase is:
    (a) guided by plasminogen levels
    (b) 2000 units/kg/hr without a loading dose
    (c) 2000 units/kg/hr with a loading dose of 2000 units/kg over 10 minutes
    (d) 2000 units/lb/hr
    (e) none of the above

7. Pulmonary emboli:
    (a) may be a complication of lytic therapy
    (b) requires at least 72 hours of systemic lytic therapy to completely resolve
    (c) can be effectively treated by streptokinase, 2000 units/kg/hr
    (d) should always be treated with systemic thrombolytic therapy
    (e) none of the above

8. Complications of thrombolytic therapy are:
    (a) due to the antigenicity of the agent
    (b) due to plasminemia
    (c) reduced by avoidance of invasive procedures
    (d) sometimes treated by increasing the dose
    (e) all of the above

9. Intraoperative thrombolytic therapy:
    1. is contraindicated because bleeding results from systemic absorption
    2. may improve the results of incomplete thrombectomy
    3. is done by intravenous administration of the agent
    4. should include heparin in the infusate
    (a) 1,2,3
    (b) 1,3
    (c) 2,4
    (d) 4 only
    (e) none of the above

10. Streptokinase administration
    (a) results in a drop in plasminogen
    (b) is contraindicated in patients who have received streptokinase anytime in the past
    (c) is more effective than urokinase when given intraarterially
    (d) results in a predictable lytic response
    (e) none of the above

ANSWERS

1. d	2. c	3. e	4. b	5. c	6. d	7. a
8. e	9. c	10. a				

19

EVALUATION OF CARDIAC RISK IN THE PATIENT WITH VASCULAR DISEASE

ANTHONY D. WHITTEMORE, MAGRUDER C. DONALDSON, and JOHN A. MANNICK

Successful arterial reconstruction in patients with atherosclerotic cardiovascular disease requires initial recognition and subsequent management of the underlying systemic disease process. The increased prevalence of concurrent manifestations of atherosclerosis in vascular surgical patients has been repeatedly documented in the literature. The Framingham Study represents one of the earliest reports that demonstrated that claudicators harbor a significantly higher incidence of coronary artery disease, as well as cerebrovascular and hypertensive disease, when compared with a nonclaudicating population.[1] Approximately 50 per cent of patients undergoing a variety of peripheral vascular procedures have clinically overt cardiac disease, and an additional 20 per cent have clinically silent but highly significant myocardial ischemia.[2-5] Routine coronary angiography carried out in one of the larger reported series documented a 31 per cent incidence of severe but surgically correctable coronary disease in patients with aortic aneurysms.[3] Similar findings were demonstrated in 26 per cent of patients with cerebrovascular disease and 21 per cent of those with lower limb ischemia. It is also clear that myocardial infarction remains the most common source of perioperative morbidity and mortality following a variety of arterial reconstructions.[4,5] Cardiac morbidity has been most extensively studied in patients undergoing aneurysm repair because the initially compromised myocardium is maximally stressed by aortic clamping, declamping, and attendant fluid shifts. The marked reduction in operative mortality from the initial 20 per cent rate noted in the early 1960s to the current mortality figure, consistently less than 5 per cent, is undoubtedly multifactorial.[4-8] Vast improvements in our understanding of hemodynamics, perioperative fluid administration, monitoring techniques, anesthetic management, cardiologic support, autotransfusion, and management of sepsis have all contributed to the current excellent results (Table 19–1). The primary cause of postoperative death in the vascular surgical population, however, remains cardiac. Further reduction in mortality figures, if realistically achievable at all, will require the identification of high-risk groups and appropriate alterations in management according to more specific stratification. To this end, a plethora of clinical risk parameters and laboratory procedures have emerged with which to evaluate a patient's cardiac status in an effort to minimize the considerable morbidity associated with impaired myocardial performance in patients undergoing vascular reconstruction.

CLINICAL RISK PARAMETERS

Coronary Artery Disease

While patients with angina pectoris are at higher risk for postoperative cardiac complications than those without, clinically overt angina has not been shown to be an independent predictor of postoperative cardiac complications distinct from other clinical manifestations of impaired cardiac function.[9] The significant clinical parameters available from history, physical, and routine electrocardiogram (ECG) that are of predictive value for postoperative myocardial infarction consist of age greater than 70 years, mitral insufficiency, ventricular ectopy in excess of five beats per minute, poorly controlled congestive failure, and recent antecedent myocardial infarction.[9] The evaluation and management of patients with angina, however, remains highly controversial. This controversy is founded in the recent marked reduction in postoperative incidence of cardiac events and from (1) differing methods of patient selection, (2) variable

TABLE 19–1. OPERATIVE MORTALITY RATE FOR REPAIR OF INTACT ABDOMINAL AORTIC ANEURYSMS[a]

Year	Authors	Number of Patients	30-Day Operative Mortality Rate (%)
1980	Whittemore et al.[45]	110	0
1981	Crawford et al.[60]	140	1.4
1981	Brown et al.[61]	422	2.4
1983	Hertzer[28]	206	3.4
1985	Ruby et al.[18]	227	1.3
1989	Johnston et al.[62]	666	4.8
1990	Golden et al.[29]	500	1.6

[a]Data from Golden MA, Whittemore AD, Donaldson MC, Mannick JA: Selective evaluation and management of coronary artery disease in patients undergoing repair of abdominal aortic aneurysms. Ann Surg 212:415–423, 1990.

criteria used to define postoperative myocardial infarction (50 per cent of which are entirely silent), and (3) evidence that preliminary coronary bypass reduces the number of postoperative cardiac events following noncardiac surgery.[5–10] There is little argument that patients with unstable, crescendo, or nocturnal angina require urgent coronary angiography and appropriate therapy as indicated. This course is dictated with or without contemplated vascular surgery, and in the event that such patients warrant emergent attention to an expanding abdominal aortic aneurysm or critical limb ischemia, simultaneous procedures directed toward both critical issues have been successfully carried out.[5] On the other end of the spectrum of coronary disease, as many as 20 per cent of our vascular surgical population harbor clinically silent but significant coronary artery disease, yet major vascular procedures may be undertaken without inordinate risk of postoperative cardiac events, utilizing modern principles of management.[4,5] The results of this policy are illustrated in Table 19–1, which represents the cardiac morbidity associated with 500 aneurysm repairs using our clinical method of risk stratification. The most controversial patients with ischemic heart disease remain those with chronic stable angina as defined by New York Heart Association Class II, who sustain the highest risk for cardiac events in our experience. It is primarily toward this group that current efforts at risk stratification are directed.

The single most significant predictor for postoperative cardiac complications is a recent myocardial infarction. Several reports from the early 1970s documented postoperative mortality rates ranging from 50 to 80 per cent resulting from postoperative reinfarction, and those operated upon within 3 months of a myocardial infarction sustained a risk of reinfarction or cardiac death approaching 30 per cent. Noncardiac procedures carried out 3 to 6 months following infarction were associated with a 15 per cent incidence of recurrent infarction, and after 6 months the reinfarction rate finally stabilized at 5 per cent.[9–14] Contrary to earlier reports, there appears to be no significant difference in risk imposed by transmural as compared with subendocardial infarctions.[10] Improvements in the perioperative management of these patients, however, have reduced the reinfarction rate to less than 10 per cent within 3 months

following infarction and less than 5 per cent for those undergoing noncardiac procedures between 3 and 6 months.[15,16] While further improvements have been made in management of patients who have sustained an infarction in the immediate postoperative period, it is prudent to delay elective vascular reconstruction for 3 to 6 months following antecedent myocardial infarction in an effort to minimize cardiac morbidity.[17] Emergent situations requiring immediate vascular reconstruction may be carried out but will require maximal intensive monitoring and management to reduce the added associated risk.

Congestive Heart Failure

Patients with severe congestive heart failure, clinically evident by a third heart sound or significant jugular venous distention, incur a 25 to 30 per cent risk of pulmonary edema, in sharp contrast to a 2 per cent incidence without a prior history of congestive failure.[9,18] The incidence of cardiogenic pulmonary edema correlates with the functional classification as outlined by the New York Heart Association. Of critical importance, however, is that the perioperative mortality rate correlates with the degree of congestive failure present at the time of operation, rather than with the severity of failure by history. Satisfactory preoperative control of poorly compensated congestive heart failure has therefore resulted in a substantial reduction in the overall risk of cardiac morbidity and mortality. Maximal therapy may require the use of vigorous diuresis with fluid restriction, which is invariably associated with some degree of intravascular hypovolemia. It is advisable, therefore, to allow sufficient time for reequilibration prior to surgery in order that vasodilatation associated with anesthesia is better tolerated. Conversely, under urgent circumstances, judicious diuresis should be utilized to control the failure and anesthetic technique adjusted to minimize sudden vasodilatation.

Arrhythmia

Significant risk for perioperative cardiac morbidity has been repeatedly associated with preoperative arrhythmia, particularly with frequent premature ventricular contractions.[9,10] The ischemic or congestive complications in this group, however, relate primarily to the underlying coronary artery or myocardial disease rather than to the arrhythmia itself.[19] Prophylactic pharmacologic control of the arrhythmia is usually unnecessary unless it results in ischemic changes or deterioration of myocardial function. For instance, intravenous antiarrhythmic agents would be appropriate perioperatively for patients with a history of ventricular tachyarrhythmia associated with hypotension. In most instances, however, the chronic antiarrhythmic regimen should be continued through the morning of surgery and subsequent perioperative therapy dictated by the hemodynamic significance of the specific arrhythmia.

Of particular concern is the patient with complete heart block who is at increased risk for cardiac morbidity in excess of that imposed by their underlying myocardial disease.[20] These individuals are less able to augment cardiac output in response to peripheral vasodilatation or myocardial depression induced by anesthetic agents, or successfully compensate for a wide variation in peripheral resistance and left ventricular filling pressure, particularly during major aortic surgery. Individuals with chronic heart block then should probably be provided with a pacemaker prior to surgery.

The management of patients with chronic bifascicular block has been controversial. While there is little evidence that such individuals will progress to complete heart block during the perioperative period, a significant number of patients will indeed progress during evolution of an acute myocardial infarction.[9] Appropriate monitoring usually identifies such individuals prior to sudden hemodynamic decompensation and appropriate pacing instituted as necessary. Since approximately 5 per cent of patients with established bifascicular block will develop complete heart block on an annual basis, unexplained syncope by history in these individuals might warrant the insertion of a pacing wire. Even with pacemaker backup, however, these individuals remain at increased risk for perioperative myocardial events primarily from their underlying myocardial disease rather than from the specific conduction defect.

Valvular Disease

Cardiac morbidity associated with valvular disease also reflects the degree of resultant myocardial decompensation. Asymptomatic patients, and those with a mild degree of functional limitation (New York Heart Association Class II), require no particular preoperative therapy beyond routine antibiotic prophylaxis for endocarditis. Patients with critical stenosis and significant physical limitations, however, are at substantial risk for sudden decompensation and death.[22,23] Preoperative cardiac catheterization should therefore be carried out in those patients with aortic valve stenosis associated with angina, syncopal episodes, or significant congestive failure.[24] Preliminary aortic valve replacement should be seriously considered for critical aortic stenosis, and intensive hemodynamic perioperative monitoring employed in those with symptomatic but noncritical lesions. Similar principles should apply to patients with mitral stenosis. Valvular insufficiency resulting in significant aortic or mitral regurgitation also increases the risk for postoperative cardiac morbidity associated with severe congestive failure. Valve replacement is not usually necessary unless failure cannot be adequately controlled.

Optimal management of patients with prosthetic valves who require chronic anticoagulation has not been firmly established. A significant increase in the number of thromboembolic events has not been documented when anticoagulants are withheld during the immediate perioperative period.[25,26] While chronic anticoagulation is usually withheld to minimize the incidence of hemorrhagic complications in patients undergoing noncardiac surgery, most bleeding can be ultimately controlled while the sequelae of a single thromboembolic event may be irrevocable. It is therefore not unreasonable to consider some form of anticoagulation during the preoperative period, especially in those patients with prosthetic valves known to be particularly thrombogenic. Chronic anticoagulation with warfarin is therefore discontinued approximately 3 days prior to surgery, during which time the patient should be heparinized. Intravenous dextran is often utilized during the immediate postoperative period to provide some coverage until heparin therapy or oral anticoagulation can be reinstituted safely.

CLINICAL RISK ASSESSMENT

Scoring Systems

Initial attempts to stratify risk using clinical criteria focused upon the independent parameters of prior myocardial infarction, angina, congestive heart failure, arrhythmia, and valvular disease. Several clinical scoring systems have since been developed in an attempt to provide multivariate assessment of cardiac risk.[9,27-30] One of the earliest and perhaps most rigorous of such systems is the Goldman Cardiac Risk Index, which documented the particularly ominous predictive value of poorly controlled congestive heart failure and recent myocardial infarction as previously mentioned.[9] A variety of clinical parameters were assigned a relative value based upon the association with postoperative myocardial events observed in retrospective analysis of surgical patients (Table 19-2). Goldman then developed a cardiac risk index derived from the total point score number of independent variables and relative points. As might be anticipated, patients in risk classes III and IV with the highest number of points sustained the higher incidence of postoperative cardiac complications (Table

TABLE 19–2. COMPUTATION OF MULTIFACTORIAL INDEX SCORE TO ESTIMATE CARDIAC RISK IN NONCARDIAC SURGERY[a]

Factors	Points
S$_3$ gallop or jugular venous distention on preoperative physical examination	11
Transmural or subendocardial myocardial infarction in the previous 6 months	10
Premature ventricular beats, more than 5/min documented at any time	7
Rhythm other than sinus or presence of premature atrial contractions on last preoperative electrocardiogram	7
Age over 70 years	5
Emergency operation	4
Intrathoracic, intraperitoneal, or aortic site of surgery	3
Evidence for important valvular aortic stenosis	3
Poor general medical condition[b]	3

[a]Data from Goldman L: Cardiac risks and complications of noncardiac surgery. Ann Surg *198*:780–791, 1983.
[b]As evidenced by electrolyte abnormalities (potassium, < 3.0 mEq/L; HCO$_3$, < 20 mEq/L); renal insufficiency (blood urea nitrogen, > 50 mg/dl; creatinine, > 3.0 mg/dl); abnormal blood gases (pO$_2$, aspartate transaminase or signs on physical examination of chronic liver disease); or any condition that has caused the patient to be chronically bedridden.

TABLE 19–3. INCIDENCE OF CARDIAC COMPLICATIONS FOLLOWING NONCARDIAC SURGERY IN 1001 PATIENTS CLASSIFIED ACCORDING TO RISK INDEX[a]

Risk Class	Index Points	Fatal (%)	Nonfatal (%)
I	0–5	0.7	0.2
II	6–12	5	2
III	13–25	11	2
IV	26	2	56

[a]Data from Goldman L: Cardiac risks and complications of noncardiac surgery. Ann Surg *198*:780–791, 1983.

19–3). Although proven reliable in some series, the index does not accurately reflect current management of even the most severe manifestations of coronary artery disease as demonstrated recently by Rivers, who found that patients in risk index class IV sustained a 33 per cent incidence of cardiac complications, significantly lower than the 78 per cent that would have been predicted utilizing the Goldman Cardiac Risk Index.[17] None of Rivers' patients, however, underwent surgery of the magnitude required for aortic reconstruction. A variety of additional clinical scoring systems have been devised including Dripps-ASA Score,[27] Cooperman's Equation,[30] Detsky Modified Risk Index,[28] and Eagle's Clinical Markers.[29] These clinical indicators have not proven convincingly accurate as demonstrated by Lette and associates, who found none of the systems of reliable predictive value.[31] Most of the data used to derive these systems were obtained retrospectively, and have become outdated by the dramatic advances in medical and anesthetic management of the impaired myocardium, and none account for silent ischemia.

Ejection Fraction

The ejection fraction derived by multigated radionuclide ventriculography has also proven of equivocal predictive value.[32–36] While Pasternack recently documented a 17 per cent incidence of postoperative myocardial infarction in patients undergoing aneurysm repair with an ejection fraction below 40 per cent,[33] significantly greater than the 3.4 per cent incidence found in patients with an ejection fraction in excess of 40 per cent, most recent reports attest to the lack of specificity for this derived parameter. This

is not surprising, since the ejection fraction is an estimate of the efficiency of ventricular function at a single point in time and therefore may not reflect the severity of associated ischemic coronary artery disease.

Exercise Stress Tests

The exercise tolerance test has been widely utilized to provoke evidence of myocardial ischemia but is subject to several limitations with respect to vascular surgical patients.[37–41] Approximately one third of such patients cannot successfully complete the standard examination, which has been proven a useful predictor only when patients achieve 85 per cent of their predicted maximal heart rate (PMHR).[37–39] As many as 70 per cent of patients cannot achieve their PMHR. Furthermore, results do not necessarily correlate with the relative severity of coronary atherosclerosis subsequently documented on arteriography, particularly in patients without a significant prior cardiac history.[39–41] In a large proportion of vascular surgical patients the exercise tolerance test provides equivocal results and cannot be relied upon for accurate stratification of patients most likely to benefit from coronary arteriography.

Coronary Angiography

The uncertainties with regard to the predictive value of clinical scoring systems, ejection fraction, and exercise stress tests in patients with coronary artery disease prompted some institutions to adopt a policy of routine coronary angiography.[3,42] Patients subsequently determined to harbor severe surgically reconstructable disease, such as left main or severe triple-vessel atherosclerosis, would then undergo preliminary coronary artery bypass prior to vascular reconstruction. Hertzer and associates documented severe but operable coronary disease in 25 per cent of 1000 consecutive angiograms carried out in vascular surgical patients.[3] As many as 20 per cent of such individuals had no significant history of myocardial ischemia. Subsequent coronary artery bypass in nearly 25 per cent of the entire group was associated with a 5.3 per cent operative mortality rate prior to the planned vascular reconstruction. While it is true that only one of those who survived the coronary bypass died from the subsequent vascular procedure, routine preliminary coronary arteriography for patients with stable angina is probably not justified, since the mortality associated with catheterization and subsequent bypass may be significantly greater than the risks of the same complications occurring from the anticipated noncardiac procedure alone.[3,40,43] Additional means are necessary to substratify the group of patients with stable angina who will benefit from more vigorous evaluation. Coronary angiography is usually reserved at present for those patients whose risk for myocardial ischemia is determined by other parameters.

Thallium Scan

A variety of thallium imaging techniques have been developed during the past 10 years and have demonstrated potential for identifying those patients most likely to benefit by initial cardiac intervention.[44,45] Following an initial dose of radioactive thallium chloride, the relative distribution of thallium can be documented with a gamma scintillation camera. A normally perfused segment of myocardium will demonstrate homogeneous distribution. In contrast, areas of myocardial ischemia or scar appear as initial defects (Fig. 19–1). A second image taken 3 to 4 hours later may demonstrate redistribution within an area that initially appeared as a defect, compatible with viable but relatively ischemic myocardium (Fig. 19–2). A persistent defect suggests antecedent infarction. Both exercise and intravenous dipyridamole in conjunction with thallium imaging are equally effective in inducing relative vasodilatation and increased blood flow to normally perfused myocardium, which, in turn, provide increased uptake and more rapid clearance of thallium. Regions of myocardium supplied by significantly stenotic vessels, however, show relatively decreased or delayed thallium uptake enhancing overall sensitivity. As is the case with treadmill exercise tolerance tests, a large proportion of vascular patients cannot satisfactorily sustain the exercise required for successful imaging. The dipyridamole-thallium scan has therefore become most widely used. Intravenous adenosine has a more rapid onset of action than dipyridamole, but is associated with a higher incidence of adverse reactions and its use remains primarily investigational.[46] As recently summarized by Yaeger, dipyridamole-thallium scanning has proven a sensitive and specific predictor for angiographically significant coronary disease and perioperative cardiac events associated with vascular surgery, including both myocardial infarction and cardiac death.[47] More specifically, redistribution of initial defects appears more predictive for perioperative events than fixed defects. In contrast, fixed defects are more ominous with respect to long-term survival. The dipyridamole-thallium scan is not,

however, uniformly reliable, since persistent defects determined as "fixed" at 3 hours may redistribute on further delayed gamma scan. Second, there is a significant gray zone in distinguishing persistent defects from minimal redistribution on scans or following reinjection of thallium.[48] The fact that some defects initially perceived as "fixed" but subsequently proven to reflect viable myocardium by delayed scans or by reinjection may account for the unanticipated higher incidence of cardiac complications in patients with fixed deficits reported in some recent series.[49]

Recent experience suggests that dipyridamole-thallium imaging combined with appropriate clinical parameters may be useful in identifying those patients most likely to benefit from preliminary treatment of coronary artery disease.[50–52] Several authors have addressed the issue of quantitative differences in thallium redistribution. While Eagle and Cambria recommend invasive cardiac evaluation in those patients with multiple redistribution defects,[50,52] Lette has developed a means of quantifying multiple redistribution defects that is perhaps even more precise.[51] In a relatively small group of 125 patients undergoing elective vascular surgery, quantitative indices were developed using data derived from dipyridamole-thallium scans. The myocardium was divided into six anatomic regions and the degree of reversibility scaled from 0 to 3. The number of segments affected and the degree of reversibility in each of the six anatomic regions are added to provide a "Summed Reversibility Index" (SRI). An SRI greater than 4 placed patients at high risk for postoperative cardiac events; 85 per cent of such individuals so classified sustained postoperative events in spite of intensive postoperative monitoring and antianginal medication. In contrast, only 5 per cent of patients classified as intermediate risk (SRI less than 4) sustained cardiac events. Although prior attempts to correlate the extent of reversibility with cardiac risk have provided equivocal results, this particular method of quantitation proved reliable in this study. While it is true that this study's end points were limited to cardiac death and infarction (and results may have been different if expanded to include all cardiac events), these two end points do seem the most significant. This study supports the contention that patients of intermediate risk with a limited number of reversible deficits can undergo surgery with minimal morbidity, while those in the high-risk group with multiple redistribution zones may require more aggressive coronary evaluation.

Ambulatory Holter Monitoring

Ambulatory Holter monitoring seems a relatively simple and inexpensive means of documenting myocardial ischemia.[53–55] Our prospective study of 176 patients undergoing a variety of vascular reconstructions demonstrated its potential in defining a group of patients at highest risk for postoperative cardiac

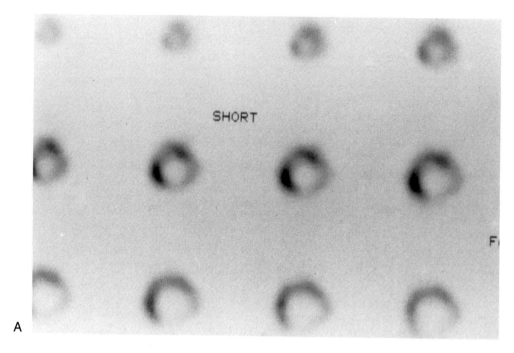

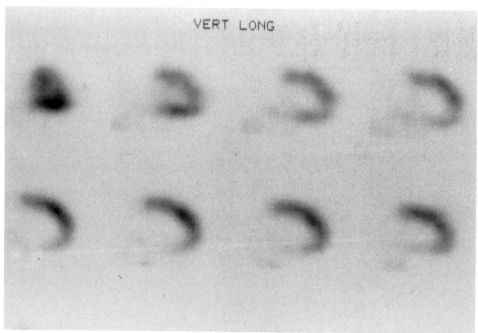

FIGURE 19–1. Initial images of myocardium following intravenous injection of dipyridamole and radioactive thallium demonstrate perfusion defects of inferior and lateral segments on short axis (*A*) and inferior segment on vertical axis (*B*).

events.[53] All but one of these events occurred in patients with positive ambulatory Holter evidence for myocardial ischemia. It is of considerable interest that all but one were entirely clinically silent. These results were similar to those reported by Pasternack, who found that 75 per cent of his patients demonstrated silent ischemic changes.[54] Mangano has also proven a significant correlation between preoperative ambulatory Holter changes and postoperative events in univariate analysis, but postoperative ischemic changes proved more highly predictive in multivariate analysis.[55] Although further investigation is ongoing, perhaps some combination of ambulatory Holter monitoring and quantitative dipyridamole-thallium scans will allow us to inexpensively and noninvasively determine those patients at highest risk for cardiac ischemia and therefore most likely to benefit from invasive coronary evaluation and treatment.

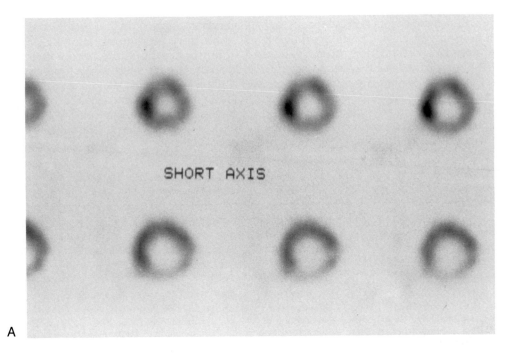

A

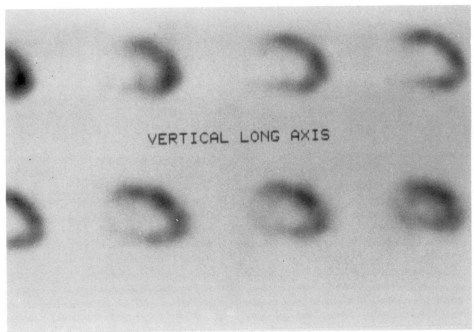

B

FIGURE 19–2. Delayed image subsequently demonstrates reperfusion of the inferior and lateral segments, suggestive of myocardium at risk for ischemia.

CONCLUSION

It has been repeatedly documented in the recent literature that patients without clinically overt coronary disease can undergo major vascular reconstructive procedures safely without further evaluation and with perhaps an irreducible minimum of postoperative cardiac fatalities.[5,50–52,56–59] In contrast, patients with severe coronary disease manifest by unstable angina, ischemic congestive failure, or recent myocardial infarction will probably benefit from invasive cardiac evaluation and either preliminary coronary intervention or an alternate vascular procedure of lesser magnitude.[5,59] Should indications for vascular reconstruction be urgent or emergent, simultaneous coronary reconstruction may well reduce the increased risk of cardiac morbidity associated with urgent procedures.[5,58] What remains uncertain is the best course of action for patients with clinically evident but stable coronary disease. Clinical scoring systems and most noninvasive laboratory methods have proven unreliable predictors of myocardial ischemic events.[50,52,60] Perhaps a more precise method of substratification of this group of patients lies in quantification of redistribution zones on dipyridamole-thallium scans as an initial screening device.[51,52] Quantitative dipyridamole-thallium scan utilizing a summed reversibility index in conjunction with preoperative ambulatory monitoring may well allow us to expeditiously identify those patients with the highest degree of susceptibility to postoperative myocardial ischemia and cardiac fatality. While the overall minimal mortality currently associated with most vascular reconstructions may represent an irreducible minimum, the persistently higher rate observed in patients with overt coronary disease justifies further effort.

REFERENCES

1. Kannel WB, Skinner JJ Jr, Schwartz MJ, et al: Intermittent claudication: Incidence in the Framingham Study. Circulation 41:857, 1970.
2. Hertzer NR, Young JR, Kramer JR, et al: Routine coronary angiography prior to elective aortic reconstruction: Results of selective myocardial revascularization in patients with peripheral vascular disease. Arch Surg 114:1336–1344, 1979.
3. Hertzer NR, Beven EG, Young JR, et al: Coronary artery disease in peripheral vascular patients. A classification of 1000 coronary angiograms and results of surgical management. Ann Surg 199:223–233, 1984.
4. Brown OW, Hollier LH, Pairolero PC, et al: Abdominal aortic aneurysm and coronary artery disease: A reassessment. Arch Surg 116:1484–1488, 1981.
5. Golden MA, Whittemore AD, Donaldson MC, Mannick JA: Selective evaluation and management of coronary artery disease in patients undergoing repair of abdominal aortic aneurysms. Ann Surg 212:415–423, 1990.
6. DeBakey ME, Crawford ES, Cooley DA, et al: Aneurysm of the abdominal aorta: Analysis of results of graft replacement therapy one to eleven years after operation. Ann Surg 160:622–639, 1964.
7. Voorhees AB Jr, McAllister FF: Long-term results following resection of arteriosclerotic abdominal aortic aneurysms. Surg Gynecol Obstet 117:355–358, 1963.
8. Szilagyi DE, Smith RF, DeRusso FJ, et al: Contribution of abdominal aortic aneurysmectomy to prolongation of life. Ann Surg 164:678–697, 1966.
9. Goldman L, Caldera DL, Nussman SR, et al: Multifactorial index of cardiac risk in noncardiac surgical procedures. N Engl J Med 297:845–850, 1977.
10. Goldman L, Caldera DL, Southwick FS, et al: Cardiac risk factors and complications in noncardiac surgery. Medicine 57:357, 1978.
11. Tarhan S, Moffitt EA, Taylor WF, et al: Myocardial infarction after general anesthesia. JAMA 220:1451, 1972.
12. Rose SD, Corman LC, Mason DT: Cardiac risk factors in patients undergoing noncardiac surgery. Med Clin North Am 63:1271, 1979.
13. Portal RW: Elective surgery after myocardial infarction. Br Med J 284:843, 1982.
14. Steen PA, Tinker JH, Tarhan S: Myocardial reinfarction after anesthesia and surgery. JAMA 239:2566, 1978.
15. Wells PH, Kaplan JA: Optimal management of patients with ischemic heart disease for non-cardiac surgery by complementary anesthesiologist and cardiologist interaction. Am Heart J 102:1029, 1981.
16. Rao TLK, El-Etr AA: Myocardial reinfarction following anesthesia in patients with recent infarction. Anesth Analg 60:271, 1981.
17. Rivers SP, Scher LA, Gupta SK, Veith FJ: Safety of peripheral vascular surgery after recent acute myocardial infarction. J Vasc Surg 11:70–76, 1990.
18. Goldman L: Cardiac risks and complications of noncardiac surgery. Ann Surg 198:780–791, 1983.
19. Schulze RA Jr, Rouleau J, Rigo P, et al: Ventricular arrhythmias in the late hospital phase of acute myocardial infarction: Relation to left ventricular function detected by gated cardiac blood pool scanning. Circulation 52:1006, 1975.
20. Lyons C: Cardiac arrhythmias as a predictable surgical risk. Surgery 35:292, 1954.
21. Wolf MA, Braunwald E: General anesthesia and noncardiac surgery in patients with heart disease. In Braunwald E (ed): Heart Disease. Philadelphia, WB Saunders Company, 1980.
22. Skinner JF, Pearce ML: Surgical risk in the cardiac patient. J Chronic Dis 17:54, 1964.
23. Chambers DA: Anesthesia for the patient with acquired valvular heart disease. In Kaplan JA (ed): Cardiac Anesthesia. New York, Grune & Stratton, 1979, p 197.
24. Perlroth MG, Hultgren HN: The cardiac patient and general surgery. JAMA 232:1279, 1975.
25. Tinker JH, Tarhan S: Discontinuing anticoagulant therapy in surgical patients with cardiac valve prostheses. JAMA 239:738, 1978.
26. Katholi RE, Nolan SP, McGuire LB: Living with prosthetic heart valves. Subsequent noncardiac operations and the risk of thromboembolism or hemorrhage. Am Heart J 92:162, 1976.
27. Dripps RD, Lamont A, Eckenhoff JE: The role of anesthesia in surgical mortality. JAMA 178:261–266, 1961.
28. Detsky AS, Abrams HB, Forbath N, et al: Cardiac assessment of patients undergoing noncardiac surgery; a multifactorial risk index. Arch Intern Med 146:2131–2134, 1986.
29. Eagle KA, Singer DE, Brewster DC, et al: Dipyridamole-thallium scanning in patients undergoing vascular surgery. JAMA 257:2185–2189, 1987.
30. Cooperman M, Pflug B, Martin EW Jr, Evans WE: Cardiovascular risk factors in patients with peripheral vascular disease. Surgery 84:505–509, 1978.
31. Lette J, Waters D, Lassande J, et al: Postoperative myocardial infarction and cardiac death. Ann Surg 211:84–90, 1990.
32. Pasternack PF, Imparato AM, Bear G, et al: The value of radionuclide angiography as a predictor of perioperative myocardial infarction in patients undergoing abdominal aortic aneurysm resection. J Vasc Surg 1:320–325, 1984.
33. Pasternack PF, Imparato AM, Riles TS, et al: The value of the radionuclide angiogram in the prediction of perioperative myocardial infarction in patient undergoing lower extremity revascularization procedures. Circulation 72:13–17, 1985.
34. Kazmers A, Cerqueira MD, Zierler RE: The role of preoperative radionuclide ejection fraction in direct abdominal aortic aneurysm repair. J Vasc Surg 8:128–136, 1988.
35. McCann RL, Wolfe WG: Resection of abdominal aortic aneurysm in patients with low ejection fractions. J Vasc Surg 10:240–244, 1989.
36. Franco CD, Goldsmith J, Veith FJ, et al: Resting gated pool ejection fraction a poor predictor of perioperative myocardial infarction in patients undergoing vascular surgery for infrainguinal bypass grafting. J Vasc Surg 10:656–661, 1989.
37. Cutler BS, Wheeler HB, Paraskos JA, Cardullo PA: Applicability and interpretation of electrocardiographic stress testing in patients with peripheral vascular disease. Am J Surg 141:501–506, 1981.

38. Arous EJ, Baum PL, Cutler BS: The ischemic exercise test in patients with peripheral vascular disease. Implications for management. Arch Surg *119*:780–783, 1984.

39. McPhail N, Calvin JE, Shariatmadar A, et al: The use of preoperative exercise testing to predict cardiac complications after arterial reconstruction. J Vasc Surg *7*:60–68, 1988.

40. Goldman L: Cardiac risks and complications of noncardiac surgery. Ann Intern Med *98*:504, 1983.

41. Gage AA, Bhayana JN, Balu V, et al: Assessment of cardiac risk in surgical patients. Arch Surg *112*:1488–1492, 1977.

42. Hertzer NR, Young JR, Drawer JR, et al: Routine coronary angiography prior to elective aortic reconstruction; results of a selective myocardial revascularization in patients with peripheral vascular disease. Arch Surg *114*:1336–1344, 1979.

43. Kennedy JW, Kaiser GC, Fisher LD, et al: Clinical and angiographic predictors of operative mortality from the collaborative study in coronary artery surgery. Circulation *63*:793–801, 1981.

44. Boucher CA, Brewster DC, Darling RC, et al: Determination of cardiac risk by dipyridamole-thallium imaging before peripheral vascular surgery. N Engl J Med *312*:389–394, 1985.

45. Cutler BS, Leppo JA: Dipyridamole-thallium 201 scintigraphy to detect coronary artery disease before abdominal aortic surgery. J Vasc Surg *5*:91, 1987.

46. Medical Letter: New ways to scan the myocardium. Med Lett *33*:87, 1991.

47. Yeager RA: Basic data related to cardiac testing and cardiac risk associated with vascular surgery. Ann Surg *4*:193–197, 1990.

48. Dilsizian V, Rocco TP, Freedman NMT, Leon MB, Bonow RO: Enhanced detection of ischemic but viable myocardium by the reinjection of thallium after stress-redistribution imaging. N Engl J Med *323*:141–146, 1990.

49. McEnroe CS, O'Donnell TF, Yeager A, Konstam M, Mackey WC: Comparison of ejection fraction and Goldman risk factor analysis to dipyridamole-thallium 102 studies in the evaluation of cardiac morbidity after aortic aneurysm surgery. J Vasc Surg *11*:497–504, 1990.

50. Eagle KA, Coley CM, Newell JB, Brewster DC, et al: Combining clinical and thallium data optimizes preoperative assessment of cardiac risk before major vascular surgery. Ann Intern Med *110*:859–866, 1989.

51. Lette J, Waters D, Lassonde J, Rene P, et al: Multivariate clinical models and quantitative dipyridamole-thallium imaging to predict cardiac morbidity and death after vascular reconstruction. J Vasc Surg *14*:158–169, 1991.

52. Cambria RP, Brewster DC, Abbott WM, et al: The impact of selective use of dipyridamole-thallium scans and surgical factors on the current morbidity of aortic surgery. J Vasc Surg *15*:43–51, 1992.

53. Raby KE, Goldman L, Creager MA, et al: Correlation between preoperative ischemia and major cardiac events after peripheral vascular surgery. N Engl J Med *321*:1296–1300, 1989.

54. Pasternack PF, Grossi EA, Baumann FG, et al: The value of silent myocardial ischemia monitoring in the prediction of perioperative myocardial infarction in patients undergoing peripheral vascular surgery. J Vasc Surg *10*:617–625, 1989.

55. Mangano DT, Browner WS, Hollenberg M, London MJ, Tubau JF, Tateo IM: Association of perioperative myocardial ischemia with cardiac morbidity and mortality in men undergoing noncardiac surgery. N Engl J Med *323*:1781–1788, 1990.

56. Perry MO, Calcagno D: Abdominal aortic aneurysm surgery; the basic evaluation of cardiac risk. Ann Surg *208*:738–742, 1988.

57. Mackey WC, O'Donnell TF Jr, Callow AD: Cardiac risk in patients undergoing carotid endarterectomy: Impact on perioperative and long-term mortality. J Vasc Surg *11*:226–234, 1990.

58. Taylor LM Jr, Yeager RA, Moneta GL, McConnell DB, Porter JM: The incidence of perioperative myocardial infarction in general vascular surgery. J Vasc Surg *15*:52–61, 1992.

59. Hollier LH: Cardiac evaluation in patients with vascular disease. Overview: A practical approach. J Vasc Surg *15*:726–729, 1992.

60. Bunt TJ: The role of a defined protocol for cardiac risk assessment in decreasing perioperative myocardial infarction in vascular surgery. J Vasc Surg *15*:626–634, 1992.

20

ANTIBIOTIC PROPHYLAXIS OF VASCULAR GRAFT INFECTION

MICHAEL M. LAW and HUGH A. GELABERT

Although infections of implanted vascular prostheses are relatively uncommon, when they do occur they are associated with significant morbidity and mortality. Complications of graft infection include pseudoaneurysm, anastamotic disruption, hemorrhage, fistula formation, and sepsis. Infection of a vascular graft almost always requires partial or complete graft removal, which is associated with a high incidence of amputation. Vascular graft infection leads to the patient's demise in one fourth to one half of cases in contemporary series. These dire consequences have prompted a continually expanding area of laboratory and clinical investigation into the role of antibiotics in the prevention of vascular graft infection. The widespread use of prophylactic antibiotics in vascular surgery has significantly altered the microbiology and clinical presentation of graft infections. New insights have been gained into the pathogenesis of this process. Alternative methods of antibiotic delivery have been developed in animal models. This chapter will present the bacteriology and current understanding of the pathogenesis of graft infection, an historic overview of the development of antibiotic prophylaxis in vascular surgery, current recommendations for prophylaxis, and new directions in antibiotic delivery.

CLINICAL SIGNIFICANCE OF GRAFT INFECTION

The reported incidence of infection following the placement of vascular prostheses ranges from 1 to 6 per cent. This relatively low rate of infection has remained stable over time, despite improvements in technique and the introduction of routine preoperative antibiotic prophylaxis. Two early series from Hoffert et al. in 1965 and Fry and Lindenauer in 1967 reported graft infection rates of 6.0 per cent (12 of 201) and 1.34 per cent (12 of 890), respectively.[1,2] In 1972, Szilagyi and colleagues reported a large series of 3397 cases in which the graft infection rate was

1.9 per cent.[3] More contemporary reports detail similar findings. Lorentzen et al.'s series from 1985 described graft infections in 62 of 2411 patients, a rate of 2.6 per cent.[4] While the overall incidence of infection has not changed significantly, the use of antibiotic prophylaxis has clearly changed the clinical presentation of most vascular graft infections. Suppurative infections presenting in the first few weeks following graft implantation have given way to more insidious, low-grade, chronic infections.[5,6]

Infection in prosthetic grafts remains an issue of critical importance in vascular surgery, despite its infrequent occurrence, because of the potentially catastrophic consequences. Reported mortality rates (Table 20–1) from graft infection in early series range from 25 to 75 per cent.[1,3,5,7–10] Mortality has been greatest for proximal grafts, with almost uniform lethality reported in aortic stump sepsis.[2,3,8,11] Despite attempts at improving mortality in aortic graft infection through staged extraanatomic bypass, graft removal, and reconstruction, mortality rates remain relatively high at 24 to 43 per cent.[12–16] Peripheral graft infections are generally associated with lower mortality rates. Modified approaches to the management of peripheral graft infection, including radical wound débridement and graft preservation when possible, have resulted in mortality rates as low as 6 per cent.[17] Amputation rates are similar for survivors of aortic and peripheral graft infections, and these rates have not improved significantly over time. Early series report amputation rates (among survivors) ranging from 22.5 to 43 per cent[3,9,18]; more contemporary series report rates of 24 to 27 per cent.[12,13,17] There is some evidence that amputation rates following aortic graft infections can be decreased by initial revascularization using extraanatomic bypass followed by immediate[15] or staged[14,15] removal of the infected graft.

PRINCIPLES OF ANTIBIOTIC PROPHYLAXIS

The goal of prophylactic antibiotic therapy is to prevent postoperative infection at the site of surgery

350

TABLE 20–1.   INFLUENCE OF GRAFT SITE ON INCIDENCE AND OUTCOME OF GRAFT INFECTION

Author	Year	Type of Graft	No. of Patients	Graft Infection Rate[a]	Amputation Rate[b]	Mortality Rate
Hoffert et al.[1]	1965	Aortoiliac	84	0%	NA	NA
		Aortofemoral	30	0%	NA	NA
		Iliofemoropopliteal	83	13%	75%	25%
Szilagyi et al.[3]	1972	Aortoiliac	418	0.7%	0%	66%
		Aortofemoral	1244	1.6%	21%	53%
		Iliofemoropopliteal	270	3.0%	40%	7%
Bouhoutsos et al.[49]	1974	Aortoiliac/aortofemoral	412	1.5%	0%	50%
		Iliofemoropopliteal	108	7.4%	25%	0%
Liekweg & Greenfield[9]	1977	Aortoiliac	NR	NR	3%	58%
		Aortofemoral	NR	NR	11%	47%
		Iliofemoropopliteal	NR	NR	30%	13%
Yashar et al.[10]	1978	Aortoiliac	300	1.0%	0%	33%
		Aortofemoral	210	2.9%	33%	50%
		Iliofemoropopliteal	65	4.6%	67%	0%
Casali[134]	1980	Aortoiliac	NR	NR	0%	50%
		Aortofemoral	NR	NR	25%	67%
		Iliofemoropopliteal	NR	NR	33%	33%
Lorentzen et al.[4]	1985	Aortoiliac	515	0%	NA	NA
		Aortofemoral	1497	3%	22%	29%
		Iliofemoropopliteal	489	3.50%	53%	18%
Edwards et al.[44]	1987	Aortic/aortoiliac	769	0%	NA	NA
		Aortofemoral	1060	0.47%	20%	40%
		Iliofemoropopliteal	583	2.90%	12%	18%

[a]Primary graft infections only; excludes aortoenteric fistulae.
[b]Amputation rate among survivors. NR, not reported; NA, not applicable.

when there is a high probability of significant bacterial wound contamination. The decision to use antibiotic prophylaxis must be based on a consideration of this potential benefit versus the likelihood of adverse consequences such as bacterial superinfection, the emergence of resistant organisms, and allergic or hypersensitivity reactions. Even with strict adherence to aseptic technique, there is no such thing as a "sterile" surgical wound. Prophylactic antibiotics, however, have been proven to be of no benefit in "clean" surgical procedures, where bacterial contamination generally consists of a small inoculum of skin flora that poses a minimal risk of postoperative infection. "Clean-contaminated" procedures that violate colonized or potentially colonized organ systems such as the respiratory, gastrointestinal, biliary, and urinary tracts are clear indications for antibiotic prophylaxis, as proven by prospective clinical trials.[19,20] Prophylaxis is also beneficial in procedures that clearly involve marked bacterial contamination, such as those involving traumatic wounds, spillage from unprepared bowel, and so forth.

Once a surgical wound has become contaminated, the likelihood of subsequent infection depends on several factors: the size of the bacterial inoculum, the infectivity and invasiveness of the organism(s) present, and the integrity of host defenses. The latter is of particular importance in patients undergoing vascular surgery. Factors that may adversely affect the host immune response include old age, inadequate blood supply, the stress of surgery and anesthesia,

renal insufficiency, and diabetes. Clearly, many of these factors apply to patients who require vascular reconstruction. Other factors that may impair the immune response or increase the risk of infection include shock, medical debility, immunodeficiency syndromes, administration of steroids and chemotherapeutic agents, preexisting infection, and obesity.

Perhaps the most important indication for antibiotic prophylaxis in vascular reconstructive surgery is the use of prosthetic materials. Foreign materials provide a protective substrate for bacterial colonization and proliferation. The presence of a foreign body in a surgical wound has been demonstrated to markedly increase the risk of postoperative infection. Long before the advent of routine antibiotic prophylaxis it was demonstrated experimentally that the presence of a foreign body increases the infectivity of *Staphylococcus aureus* 10,000-fold.[21] In light of the potentially catastrophic consequences of vascular graft infection, prophylactic antibiotics are recommended in most patients undergoing revascularization procedures, particularly when prosthetic materials are employed.

The ideal prophylactic antibiotic for surgical procedures should be (1) bactericidal for the most common pathogens causing postoperative infection, (2) adequately concentrated in serum and at the site of surgery, (3) present in adequate concentrations throughout the surgical procedure, (4) nontoxic to the patient, and (5) of cost reasonable to justify its routine use. The timing of antibiotic administration is critical, as it has been demonstrated that antibiotics administered intraoperatively and postoperatively are significantly less effective than those administered 30 minutes prior to incision time.[20,22,23] The intraoperative antibiotic concentration that is required to prevent the subsequent development of graft infection has not been determined. It is not known whether levels of antibiotic deemed acceptable for the treatment of active infections are appropriate for the indication of surgical prophylaxis. Many investigators have used the minimal inhibitory concentration (MIC) as an index of antibiotic efficacy, yet there is evidence that sub-MIC concentrations may be adequate in prophylaxis.[24] It appears that antibiotic concentration in the arterial walls is of paramount importance, as serum concentrations may not correlate well with activity in vascular tissue.[25,26] It is also clear that in long operative procedures, antibiotics should be readministered to maintain adequate serum and tissue levels for the duration of the procedure, and this may require more frequent dosing than is recommended for routine therapeutic use.[27–29]

Whether or not to continue the administration of prophylactic antibiotics into the postoperative period is a controversial issue, as antibiotics administered beyond the time of surgery have been demonstrated in some studies to provide no additional benefit and theoretically increase the likelihood of the emergence of resistant strains.[30,31] In 1984, Hassellgren and colleagues reported a randomized, double-blind study of a 1-day course of cefuroxime prophylaxis versus a 3-day course versus placebo. Wound infection rates were significantly lower in the antibiotic-treated groups, and extension of prophylaxis for 3 days provided no additional benefit.[32] It is common practice in many centers, however, to continue prophylaxis as long as a potential source of bacteremia exists, such as a bladder catheter, endotracheal tube, arterial line, or intravenous line.[33]

The route of antibiotic administration influences serum and tissue concentrations. Intramuscular administration of prophylactic antibiotics is undesirable, as this route produces lower, less reliable serum and tissue concentrations. Prophylactic antibiotics are usually administered systemically, although there is experimental and clinical evidence to suggest that local irrigation is effective in vascular surgery. In 1970, DiGiglia and colleagues reported experimental results with kanamycin-bacitracin wound irrigation in a canine model of intraoperative graft infection.[34] Femoral arteriotomies were patched with Dacron grafts and contaminated with 8 million *S. aureus*; after 30 minutes the wounds were irrigated with antibiotic solution or saline in blinded fashion. A third group received no irrigation. At 1 week following surgery, graft disruption and abscess formation was noted in the nonirrigated group, all saline-irrigated grafts were found to have gross infection with leakage and pseudoaneurysm formation, and all antibiotic-irrigated grafts were patent and intact with no gross evidence of infection. The latter, however, were culture-positive

for *S. aureus*. The antibiotic irrigation protocol was repeated with wound exploration and graft harvesting at 6 weeks, and at this time all grafts were grossly normal and culture-negative. The investigators postulated that the infecting dose of organisms was too large to be completely cleared within 1 week.

In 1976, Lord et al. reported retrospective data regarding intraoperative antibiotic wound lavage that suggested that this route of prophylaxis was effective in vascular reconstructive surgery.[35] The authors reported that the institution of antibiotic lavage (neomycin or kanamycin-cephalothin) reduced the incidence of early and late postoperative infections from 1.5 per cent (6 of 400) to 0.23 per cent (1 of 434). No parenteral antibiotics were administered to either group of patients. Pitt and colleagues have reported a prospective, randomized, blinded study of cephradine administered topically, intravenously, and by both routes to patients undergoing peripheral vascular reconstruction.[36] Infections were significantly reduced in all three groups compared to untreated controls, and no significant differences were noted between the three routes of administration. The authors concluded that both routes of administration were effective in preventing infection, and that there was no advantage in using a combination of topical and systemic antibiotics. There is also evidence that markedly higher tissue levels of antibiotic in the surgical wound may be achieved with topical than with intravenous administration.[37,38] Topical administration provides the theoretical advantage of attaining high antibiotic levels within the hematoma and dead space of a wound, where infection is most likely to develop, yet has the theoretical disadvantage of affording little protection against bacteremic seeding of vascular grafts.

As the vast majority of vascular graft infections are caused by a few specific bacteria, broad-spectrum antibiotic prophylaxis is unnecessary. Selecting an antibiotic with the narrowest spectrum of activity that includes the most common pathogens involved in graft infection will limit the emergence of resistant organisms. When possible, antibiotics that are the principal line of therapy in difficult infections (such as vancomycin in the treatment of *S. epidermidis* infections) should be reserved for that indication and not used in prophylaxis.

BACTERIOLOGY OF GRAFT INFECTION

Gram-positive cocci, the predominant flora of the skin and dermal appendages, are the organisms most often responsible for vascular graft infections. Although the bacteriology of graft infection varies somewhat by anatomic site, when all sites are considered together, approximately 60 to 65 per cent of reported cases are currently due to gram-positive organisms. The remaining 35 to 40 per cent are largely due to gram-negative rods, which account for approximately half of all infections in intraabdominal (aortic, aortoiliac) grafts. While *S. aureus* has historically been the most frequently cultured pathogen, the introduction of routine antibiotic prophylaxis along with improved culture techniques has led to the emergence of *S. epidermidis* and other coagulase-negative staphylococci as the most frequent cause of vascular graft infection (Table 20–2). The most commonly cultured gram-negative rod is *Escherichia coli*, followed by *Proteus*, *Pseudomonas*, and *Klebsiella*.

Clinical Presentation

Vascular graft infections due to *S. aureus* typically reflect the organism's virulence and invasiveness, and are characterized by early onset, suppuration, and often systemic toxicity. Extracellular enzymes such as catalase, coagulase, hyaluronidase, and proteinases destroy tissue and produce a marked inflammatory response. In contrast, *S. epidermidis* infections are generally indolent, lingering processes that present months to years postoperatively, and are characterized by serous perigraft fluid collections and chronic draining sinuses. Signs of systemic sepsis are extremely unusual. Many strains of *S. epidermidis* produce an exopolysaccharide "slime" that forms an adherent perigraft biofilm. This extracellular matrix effectively sequesters the organism from the bloodstream and tissue fluids and thus prevents adequate antibiotic penetration, and also makes culture of the organism more difficult. Slime-producing organisms are only reliably cultured from the broth culture of the graft itself, and this often requires sonication to liberate organisms from graft materials.[39] Bergamini and colleagues have reported that surface biofilm disruption and the use of a soy broth culture medium can increase the recovery rate of *S. epidermidis* to 83 per cent, in comparison to a 30 per cent recovery rate with standard blood agar media.[40] Until recently, such culture techniques have not been routinely employed, and it is therefore likely that many *S. epidermidis* infections have been reported as "culture-negative" infections.

Most gram-negative organisms are of intermediate virulence in producing vascular graft infections. They are currently a frequent cause of early graft infections, particularly in aortic prostheses. Gram-negative infections generally present in a manner similar to that of *S. aureus*, with suppuration and abscess formation. Some gram-negative infections are characterized by a necrotizing process that involves vascular wall invasion, pseudoaneurysmal degeneration, and graft disruption. This is particularly true for *Pseudomonas*, which has become notorious for the severity and mortality of pseudomonal graft infections. This observation has been demonstrated experimentally by Geary and colleagues, who in a canine model inoculated saphenous vein and polytetrafluoroethylene (PTFE) femoral artery bypass grafts intraoperatively with *S. epidermidis*, *P. aeruginosa*, or saline.[41] Grafts were excised 7 to 10 days postoperatively and examined. In the *S. epidermidis* group, graft cultures were negative (using routine culture techniques) in all cases, although 8 of 10 grafts demonstrated bacteria and neutrophils on histologic examination. There were no graft or anastamotic disruptions. In contrast, *P. aeruginosa* was recovered from all grafts infected with that organism, and marked inflammation with microabscesses was noted histologically. Additionally, three of five PTFE grafts and five of five vein grafts were disrupted. In a 1991 report on clinical experience with aortic graft infections by Quiñones-Baldrich and colleagues, three of seven patients (43 per cent) who died postoperatively had *Pseudomonas* infections, compared to 16 per cent of those who survived the initial period.[42]

The Changing Bacterial Spectrum of Graft Infection

In early reports from the 1960s and 1970s, *S. aureus* was identified as the predominant pathogen in vascular graft infections. A series of 198 aortofemoropopliteal grafts from Hoffert et al. in 1965 reported that *S. aureus* was cultured in 67 per cent (8 of 12) of

TABLE 20–2.   EFFECT OF ANTIBIOTIC PROPHYLAXIS ON THE MICROBIOLOGY OF GRAFT INFECTION

Author	Year	Type of Graft	Prophylactic Antibiotics	Cultured Organisms[a]				Culture-Negative
				S. aureus	*S. epidermidis*	*E. coli*	Other GNRs	
Hoffert et al.[1]	1965	Aortic & distal	No	67%	17%	8%	25%	17%
Fry & Lindenauer[2]	1966	Aortic	No	67%	0%	25%	8%	8%
Goldstone & Moore[5]	1974	Aortic & distal	*b*	41%	26%	15%	11%	7%
Liekweg & Greenfield[9]	1977	Aortic & distal	No	50%	4%	13%	18%	Not reported
Bandyk et al.[6]	1980	Aortofemoral	Yes	10%	60%	13%	23%	10%
Yeager et al.[13]	1985	Aortic & distal	Yes	0%	50%	0%	0%	33%
			Yes	14%	14%	0%	29%	43%
Quiñones-Baldrich et al.[42]	1991	Aortic	Yes	13%	21%	18%	45%	21%

[a]Expressed as per cent of cases from which each organism was cultured. GNR, gram-negative rods.
[b]Prophylaxis administered in 10 of 27 cases of graft infection.

cases.[1] A series of 890 aortic grafts from Fry and Lindenauer in 1966 also reported that *S. aureus* was cultured in 67 per cent (8 of 12) of cases.[2] Similarly, in 1967 Smith reported on nine cases of femoropopliteal graft infection, eight of which were due to *S. aureus*.[43] In 1977, Liekweg and Greenfield reviewed the 178 published cases of vascular graft infection reported between 1959 and 1974.[9] *Staphylococcus aureus* was responsible for 50 per cent of cases, followed by gram-negative rods (30.5 per cent) and *Streptococcus* (8.5 per cent). Only 3.6 per cent of cases were due to *S. epidermidis*.

A report from Goldstone and Moore in 1974 was one of the first to highlight the impact of antibiotic prophylaxis on the presentation and bacteriology of graft infection.[5] These investigators retrospectively reviewed the incidence of graft infection at their institution both before and after the initiation of routine antibiotic prophylaxis. The aortofemoropopliteal graft infection rate for the years 1959 to 1966, prior to the institution of antibiotic prophylaxis, was 4.1 per cent (9 of 222). From 1966 to 1973, during which time prophylaxis was administered, the graft infection rate was 1.5 per cent (5 of 344). Of all staphylococcal infections treated at that institution between 1959 and 1973, 14 of 18 occurred prior to the routine use of prophylactic antibiotics. The authors also divided the series into early (presenting up to 3.5 months postoperatively) and late (presenting later than 3.5 months postoperatively) infections. Seventy per cent (9 of 13) of early infections were due to *S. aureus*, while 50 per cent (7 of 14) of late infections were due to *S. epidermidis*.

Other reviews of graft infection since the advent of routine antibiotic prophylaxis demonstrate an increasing incidence of late infections due to fastidious organisms such as *S. epidermidis* and other coagulase-negative staphylococci. A review by Bandyk and colleagues of 30 patients treated for aortofemoral graft infections from 1972 to 1982 revealed that 60 per cent were due to *S. epidermidis*.[6] This group also examined how the time of presentation influenced the microbiology of graft infection by dividing their series into early (less than 4 months) and late (greater than 4 months) infection. There were only five early infections, four of which were due to gram-negative rods. Late infections were much more common, totalling 25, and 15 (60 per cent) of these were due to *S. epidermidis*. In 1985, Yeager and associates reported a 9-year experience in which they managed 14 aortic and 11 peripheral graft infections.[13] While peripheral graft infections presented an average of 8 months following surgery, aortic graft infections presented an average of 5 years postoperatively. Of five primarily infected aortic grafts (not graft-enteric fistulae or erosions) with positive cultures, four were due to *S. epidermidis*. A wide range of organisms were cultured from peripheral grafts, including coagulase-positive and -negative staphylococci, gram-negative rods, anaerobic streptococci, and diphtheroids.

Edwards et al. have reported on 24 infections from a series of 2614 aortofemoropopliteal grafts over a 10-year period from 1975 to 1986, in which the most common pathogen (29 per cent) was *S. aureus*.[44] The authors note, however, that in only 7 of 24 cases were prophylactic antibiotics administered according to the departmental protocol; thus, this series may be more representative of the preantibiotic era. This observation is supported by the fact that 63 per cent of these infections presented within 3 months of implantation. Additionally, cultures were negative in 21 per cent of patients, suggesting that the presence of fastidious organisms such as *S. epidermidis* may have been underestimated. In 1991, Quiñones-Baldrich and Moore reported an 18-year experience (1970 to 1988) with 45 aortic graft infections.[42] Culture results were available for 38 of 45 patients. Gram-negative organisms were cultured from 24 of 38 (63 per cent) patients, most commonly *Pseudomonas* (21 per cent) and *E. coli* (18 per cent). Gram-positive cocci were cultured from 21 of 38 (55 per cent) patients, most frequently *S. epidermidis* (21 per cent). Of note is the fact that cultures grew multiple organisms in 39 per cent of cases, and that there were eight (21 per cent) negative cultures, again suggesting that the incidence of infection due to fastidious organisms may have been underestimated.

PATHOGENESIS OF GRAFT INFECTION

A great deal of debate has surrounded the issue of how vascular prostheses become infected. There are a multitude of possible preoperative, perioperative, and postoperative sources of bacterial contamination. The two principal routes of graft infection are direct contamination, from contact with bacteria present in the surgical wound; and hematogenous or lymphatogenous seeding of graft material by blood- or lymph-borne organisms, which may occur in the immediate postoperative period but which may also represent a potential source of remote infection. It is generally accepted that most graft infections are caused by direct intraoperative contamination of the prosthesis. Potential sources of infecting organisms include the patient's skin, breaks in aseptic technique, adjacent active infections, transudation of bowel flora into the peritoneal space, and the diseased arterial tree itself, which may become colonized with pathogenic bacteria.

Skin Flora

The normal flora of the patient's own skin is probably the most important source of bacteria, as it is impossible to sterilize the skin even with appropriately timed shaving and antiseptic scrubs. It is clear that the nature of preoperative skin preparation influences subsequent infection rates. Kaiser et al. have noted a significantly higher rate of infection with a hexachlorophene-ethanol surgical scrub compared to povidone-iodine.[45] Hexachlorophene alone appears to be more effective than when used in combination with ethanol.[46] In a prospective study, Cruse has demonstrated that preoperative hexachlorophene showering can be effective in reducing wound infection rates, and that overzealous shaving may actually increase the risk of infection.[47]

While bacteria are present in essentially all surgical wounds, the presence of a foreign body such as vascular graft material may make normally inconsequential concentrations of bacteria much more significant. Wooster and colleagues studied intraoperative contamination of vascular grafts in 73 consecutive revascularization procedures, 78 per cent of which were elective.[48] Skin cultures prior to antiseptic scrubbing were uniformly positive, and of these, 80 per cent grew *S. epidermidis*. In the first 30 patients, graft cultures taken after preclotting were positive for the same organism as found on the patient's skin preoperatively in 35 per cent of cases. This number rose to 56 per cent for cultures taken after the final anastamosis. For the next 43 patients, the surgical team changed gloves prior to preclotting the graft. This reduced the number of positive cultures taken after preclotting to 25 per cent, and those taken after the final anastamosis to 35 per cent. The use of adhesive skin barriers did not influence graft contamination. Clinical graft infection developed in only one patient during the 18-month follow-up period. This study demonstrates the fact that vascular grafts routinely become contaminated with skin organisms intraoperatively, and also suggests that careful attention to aseptic technique can significantly influence the extent to which this happens.

The presence of a groin incision appears to have special significance in the development of vascular graft infections. It has long been recognized that grafts involving an inguinal wound have a higher incidence of infection than those which avoid this region.[3,5,49] In a series of 664 aortoiliofemoral reconstructions, Jamieson and colleagues reported that the presence of a groin incision increased the risk of graft infection three and a half times, and that the presence of a groin complication such as a seroma or hematoma increased the risk of infection ninefold over patients without groin complications.[8] Yashar et al. have reported a series of 15 graft infections in which five (33 per cent) of the patients had groin hematomas.[10] In Lorentzen et al.'s series of 2411 consecutive arterial reconstructions with prosthetic grafts, 62 patients (2.6 per cent) developed graft infections, and all of these occurred in patients with groin incisions.[4] The highest incidence of infection was in patients who underwent aortobifemoral grafting for abdominal aortic aneurysms (5.9 per cent), while there were no infections in 425 patients who underwent aortoiliac bypass for aneurysms (213) and occlusive atherosclerosis (212). Kaiser and colleagues, however, reported a lower incidence of infection in groin wounds (0.6 per cent) than in abdominal (4.9 per cent) or leg (3.1 per cent) wounds in a prospective study of antibiotic prophy-

laxis.[45] The authors attribute their findings to an emphasis at their institution on meticulous care of the groin. Bouhoutsos et al. have suggested that the incidence of infection in aortofemoral reconstruction can be significantly reduced when the distal anastamosis is placed above the inguinal ligament,[49] while others have noted no difference in infection rates for anastamoses on either side of this landmark.[5]

Gastrointestinal Flora

The gastrointestinal tract is a potential source of contamination during aortic reconstruction. Manipulation of the gut may lead to edema of the bowel wall, localized ischemia, and transudation of bacteria into the bloodstream or peritoneal cavity. Cultures of intestinal bag fluid have been reported by some investigators to yield enteric bacteria,[9] while others have found mainly skin organisms such as coagulase-negative staphylococci.[50] In a report on 179 bowel-bag cultures from abdominal aortic reconstructions, Scobie and colleagues found positive cultures in 14 per cent of patients.[51] *Staphylococcus epidermidis* was the single most common organism isolated ($n = 11$), while enteric flora were cultured in 12. None of these patients, however, developed graft infection. Russell et al. found only 3 of 119 bag cultures to be positive in a similar series, and also reported no instances of graft infection.[52]

Likewise, there are conflicting reports concerning the significance of concomitant gastrointestinal surgery in the development of vascular graft infection. In separate series, DeBakey et al.,[53] Stoll,[54] and Hardy et al.[55] have reported a total of 670 patients who underwent aortic graft placement and simultaneous gastrointestinal procedures, with no episodes of graft infection, leading these authors to suggest that such coincident procedures can be safely undertaken. It is notable that most of these cases predated the routine use of preoperative antibiotic prophylaxis. Other investigators, however, have described the development of graft infection in patients undergoing simultaneous appendectomy,[5] cholecystectomy and gastrostomy,[56] and anterior colon resection[49]; these authors argue for a more cautious approach.

Arterial Colonization

It is increasingly clear that the native arterial tree does not necessarily represent a sterile environment. The presence of pathogenic bacteria in previously unoperated vascular tissues, particularly coagulase-negative staphylococci, has been widely documented (Table 20–3). Lalka et al. have postulated that transient bacteremias resulting from breaks in the skin or mucous membranes may lead to arterial colonization.[26] Bacterial contamination of vascular prostheses may, therefore, be inevitable in some cases. It is not yet clear, however, to what extent the presence of

TABLE 20–3. POSITIVE ARTERIAL WALL CULTURES: INCIDENCE AND SIGNIFICANCE[a]

Author	Year	Culture Source	% of Positive Cultures	Associated with Subsequent Infection	Frequency of *S. epidermidis* Among Positive Cultures
Ernst et al.[50]	1977	Aortic aneurysms	15%	Yes	53%
Scobie et al.[51]	1979	Aortic aneurysms	23%	No	71%
Macbeth et al.[58]	1984	Femoropopliteal specimens	43%	Yes	71%
McAuley et al.[60]	1984	Aortic thrombus	14%	No	NR
Buckels et al.[57]	1985	Aortic aneurysms	8%	Yes	30%
Durham et al.[59]	1987	Aortofemoropopliteal specimens	44%	Yes	56%
Schwartz et al.[61]	1987	Aortic aneurysms	10%	No	54%
Ilgenfritz & Jordan[62]	1988	Aortic aneurysms & ASD	20%	No	55%
Brandimarte et al.[63]	1989	Aortic aneurysms	31%	No	NR
Wakefield et al.[64]	1990	Aortofemoropopliteal specimens	12%	No	60%

[a]ASD, atherosclerotic disease; NR, not reported.

positive arterial wall cultures influences the likelihood of subsequent graft infection.

Ernst et al.'s 1977 report of abdominal aortic aneurysmal wall cultures was one of the first to highlight the presence of pathogenic organisms in the native aorta.[50] The overall incidence of positive cultures was 15 per cent, and cultures were more likely to be positive when atherosclerotic disease was more advanced. Nine per cent of asymptomatic aneurysms were culture-positive, compared to 13 per cent of symptomatic and 35 per cent of ruptured aneurysms. *Staphylococcus epidermidis* was the most frequently isolated organism. Among survivors followed for at least 6 months, the late graft sepsis rate was 10 per cent in the culture-positive group versus 2 per cent in the culture-negative group. The authors recommended organism-specific antibiotic therapy when cultures of aneurysm contents are positive. In a similar report, Buckels et al. described an 8 per cent (22 of 275) incidence of positive cultures from aortic aneurysm contents, with positive cultures more likely in advanced disease.[57] The incidence of graft sepsis was 32 per cent (7 of 22) in patients with positive cultures, compared to 2.4 per cent (6 of 253) in the culture-negative group. This group also recommended prolonged organism-specific antibiotic therapy in patients with positive cultures. In 1984, Macbeth and colleagues reported on cultures of arterial wall specimens from 88 clean, elective lower extremity revascularization procedures.[58] Control cultures were taken from adjacent adipose or lymphatic tissue. While all control cultures were negative, arterial wall cultures were positive in 43 per cent (38 of 88) of cases. Seventy-one per cent (27 of 38) of these grew *S. epidermidis*. The authors described three graft infections in 335 cases (0.9 per cent infection rate), all of which had positive arterial wall cultures. Also included in this report was a retrospective review of 22 cases of graft infection for which arterial and graft culture data were available. Fifty-seven per cent (8 of 14) patients with positive arterial cultures had suture line disrup-

tion, while there were no disruptions in the culture-negative group.

Durham and colleagues have also published results that suggest an association between positive arterial wall cultures and subsequent infection.[59] In 1987, this group reported a series of 172 patients undergoing vascular reconstruction with a 44 per cent (75 of 172) incidence of positive arterial wall cultures; of these, *S. epidermidis* was responsible for 56 per cent. There were six infections (3.5 per cent) over 18 months of follow-up, and all of these patients had prior positive arterial cultures. No patients with negative arterial cultures developed graft infection. The incidence of positive cultures was essentially equivalent for primary and secondary procedures, at 43 and 45 per cent, respectively. Notably, five of the six graft infections were in patients undergoing secondary reconstruction procedures. The risk of subsequent graft infection in patients with positive cultures was estimated at 10.5 per cent, compared to 1.3 per cent for patients with negative cultures. The greatest risk for graft infection appeared to be in patients with positive arterial wall cultures undergoing reoperation. These studies suggest that the presence of bacteria in the native vessel may have a distinct association with the subsequent development of graft infection, and that postoperative antibiotic therapy directed at the cultured organisms may be indicated to prevent the development of clinical infection.

Other investigators, however, have reported conflicted findings. Scobie and colleagues have described a 23 per cent (7 of 31) incidence of positive abdominal aortic wall cultures in patients undergoing reconstruction for aneurysmal disease, but no association with the subsequent development of graft infection.[51] McAuley et al. have reported a 14 per cent (9 of 64) incidence of positive cultures in aortic thrombus at elective aneurysm resection, with no graft infections developing at a mean follow-up interval of 25 months.[60] Eight of 10 organisms cultured were sensitive to the prophylactic antibiotic administered (cefazolin or cephalexin), and these patients received only the routine 48-hour course of prophylaxis with no further therapy. Schwartz et al. found 10.4 per cent (22 of 211) of aortic aneurysm contents to be culture-positive, most commonly with *S. epidermidis* (54 per cent), but found no correlation between positive cultures and subsequent infection.[61] Ilgenfritz and Jordan have reported a 19.6 per cent (11 of 56) incidence of positive aortic aneurysm wall and atheroma cultures, with 55 per cent due to *S. epidermidis* and no graft infections over a mean follow-up interval of 24.5 months.[62] Brandimarte et al. found a 31 per cent (28 of 90) incidence of positive cultures in aortic aneurysm wall and contents, but no association with subsequent infection.[63]

Wakefield and colleagues have recently reported a study in which cultures were taken of native artery, adjacent adipose tissue, and blood in 84 patients undergoing 75 primary and 9 secondary arterial reconstructions.[64] Twelve per cent of arterial and 14 per cent of adipose tissue cultures were positive, whereas only 2 per cent of blood cultures were positive. Coagulase-negative staphylococci accounted for 60 per cent of positive arterial samples, 79 per cent of positive adipose tissue samples, and both positive blood cultures. Over a follow-up period of 1 to 29 months (mean: 15 months), there was no clinical evidence of graft infection. However, as most of the positive cultures were of *S. epidermidis*, a longer follow-up period will be required to determine the true impact of positive arterial wall cultures on the subsequent development of vascular graft infection. It remains unclear why a certain subpopulation of vascular surgery patients have arterial colonization prior to surgical intervention; also unclear is the significance of this finding in terms of subsequent infection. Although vessels with essentially normal architecture may harbor bacteria, colonization appears to be more likely in vessels with more advanced atherosclerotic disease. Colonization may therefore represent a cofactor in the development of graft infection, along with impaired host defense and technical complications at surgery.[26]

Hematogenous and Lymphatogenous Seeding

The possibility of hematogenous seeding of vascular prostheses as a source of graft infection is an actively debated issue. There are anecdotal reports in the literature of patients with urinary tract infection,[4,5] abdominal sepsis,[5,10,51] and other infections[3] that have developed a vascular graft infection with the identical organism. It is clear from well-established laboratory models of graft infection that intraoperative or immediate postoperative intravenous infusion of bacteria will result in clinical graft infection in almost all cases.[65–67] Relatively large inoculums of bacteria have been used in the majority of such experiments, on the order of 1 to 10 million organisms.

Colburn and colleagues have recently demonstrated that much smaller concentrations of bacteria, as little as 100 organisms, will reliably produce clinical graft infection in a canine model.[68]

It appears from these animal studies that different bacteria have variable affinities for different graft materials, and vice versa. Slime-producing coagulase-negative staphylococci have been found to have the highest affinity for prosthetic materials, followed by other staphylococci and then gram-negative rods.[69] PTFE is significantly more resistant to bacterial adherence than Dacron,[69,70] and this observation has led to the suggestion that PTFE is the graft material of choice in revision surgery, particularly for infected grafts. There is evidence, however, that development of a "pseudointima" occurs more rapidly with Dacron graft material, which may serve to protect the graft from hematogenous seeding.[71,72] The extent to which a pseudointimal lining protects a graft from infection is unclear. In animal models, resistance to hematogenous infection has been found to correlate with the degree of pseudointima formation.[71,73] It rarely exceeds more than 10 mm beyond an anastamosis in humans, however, which may leave large segments of graft vulnerable to infection.[74] As it is impossible to know the true incidence of the transient phenomenon of bacteremia in vascular surgery patients, it remains difficult to determine the actual impact of bacteremia on the subsequent development of graft infection.

It has been hypothesized that an open wound in the distal lower extremities may seed graft material by vascular or lymphatic routes. Hoffert and colleagues have reported a series of twelve prosthetic graft infections in which 75 per cent of patients (9 of 12) had an open, infected lesion on the distal lower extremity at the time of graft implantation, and seven of these were on the ipsilateral side.[1] In Liekweg and Greenfield's series, 20 of 60 (33 per cent) of inguinal infections occurred proximal to open foot infections.[9] Lorentzen et al., in a report of 62 graft infections, described four patients who had distal ulcers containing the same organism that was cultured from the infected graft.[4] Bunt and Mohr have described the presence of bacteria cultured from a distally infected extremity in the inguinal lymph nodes of two patients undergoing lower extremity revascularization; both patients developed graft infection.[75]

Bouhoutsos et al., however, noted no increase in the incidence of femoropopliteal graft infection in patients with infected foot lesions.[49] In a prospective study of 124 aortofemoropopliteal reconstructions, Robbs et al. noted that positive cultures of groin lymph nodes (as well as aortic clot and atheroma) did not predispose patients to postoperative infection. There were no significant differences in wound or graft sepsis rates between patients with or without infected lower extremity lesions.[76] In Edwards et al.'s series from 1987, three patients with graft infections had preoperative cultures taken of distal ulcers, and in only one case was the graft infection identical.[44]

Herbst et al. have also found no association between the presence of ischemic ulcers and subsequent infection.[33] It is worth noting that while some large series report the presence of distal lower extremity ulcers or gangrene in 20 to 50 per cent of patients, rates of graft infection remain in the range of 2 to 3 per cent.

Other Local and Systemic Factors

Prior vascular surgery has been implicated as a risk factor for vascular graft infection. Dense scar tissue, increased bleeding, and lymphatic leak may all contribute to this phenomenon. Goldstone and Moore noted that 45 per cent (12 of 27) of patients with graft infections had undergone one or more revisions of their original graft prior to the development of infection in the same region.[5] In 8 of these 12 patients, the infection was in the groin. In Edwards et al.'s series, 50 per cent (9 of 18) of patients had undergone a previous vascular surgery at the site of the graft infection.[44] Similarly, a report from Reilly and colleagues described a history of multiple previous vascular procedures at the site of graft infection in 40 per cent of cases. Johnson et al. found that prior vascular procedures were not a significant risk factor for graft infection; however, only 12 of 135 patients in this series had prior operations at the site of infection.[77]

There also is evidence that uninfected prostheses have a high incidence of bacterial colonization at explantation. Kaebnick et al. have reported culture results of 45 grafts that were revised for thrombosis (26) or anastomotic aneurysm (21), none of which had signs of infection.[78] Bacteria were isolated from 90 per cent (19 of 21) of grafts associated with anastamotic aneurysms and 69 per cent (18 of 26) of thrombosed grafts. *Staphylococcus epidermidis* was the most commonly isolated organism and accounted for 69 per cent of the isolates. Slime-producing strains were recovered from 87 per cent of the grafts with anastamotic aneurysm, compared with 33 per cent of thrombosed grafts. No patient developed graft infection following graft replacement, despite the high incidence of colonization. This study highlights the fact that organisms of low virulence, such as *S. epidermidis*, can colonize vascular grafts without evoking the typical signs of graft infection, and suggests that colonization or subclinical infection may be associated with the complications of thrombosis and the development of anastamotic aneurysm.

The immunologic status of patients with vascular disease may also impact the development of graft infection. Systemic disease, malnutrition, and medical debility may suppress the host response to invading microorganisms. Kwaan and colleagues have reported on 12 patients with advanced, fulminating graft infections, all of which had critical deficiencies in immune status as measured by serum albumin, hemoglobin, immunoglobulin, and lymphocyte assays, and by response to standard skin test antigens.[79] Eight of 12 patients who received total parenteral nutrition had significant enhancement of immune response and accelerated recovery from the graft infection. Of the four patients who did not receive nutritional support, two had a prolonged convalescence and two subsequently died from complications of graft infection.

ANTIBIOTIC PROPHYLAXIS: EXPERIMENTAL INVESTIGATIONS

The suggestion that prophylactic antibiotic therapy may be effective in the prevention of surgical infections was first made over 40 years ago.[80] In the early to mid-1950s a number of authors contended that the perioperative, systemic administration of antibiotics could in some cases prevent infections in procedures where there was a clear source of bacterial contamination, in instances of diminished host resistance to infection, and in vascular reconstructive procedures that involved the implantation of a foreign body.[81–84] In the early 1960s, Alexander and colleagues demonstrated the efficacy of penicillin prophylaxis in experimental wound infections.[85,86]

One of the first laboratory investigations into the utility of prophylactic antibiotics in vascular surgery was published by Lindenauer and colleagues in 1967.[7] Their investigation was prompted by a review of 12 cases of infected Teflon aortic prostheses in which the mortality rate was 75 per cent. In a canine model, surgical wounds were contaminated with 10,000 to 100,000 *S. aureus* following femoral arteriotomy, which was closed primarily with a Teflon patch graft or with a vein patch. A fourth group received sham operation alone. Antibiotic prophylaxis consisted of intramuscular procaine penicillin, 20,000 units/kg, every 12 hours beginning 24 hours prior to surgery and lasting for 3 days postoperatively. Control animals received no antibiotics. Arteries were cultured on the fourth postoperative day. Among control animals, the infection rate was 94 per cent (eight of nine shams, three of three arteriotomies, three of three Teflon patches, three of three vein patches). In animals treated with penicillin, the infection rate was 0 per cent (15 shams, five arteriotomies, five Teflon patches, five vein patches). The authors, therefore, demonstrated that perioperative systemic antibiotic therapy could sterilize a highly contaminated wound, even in the presence of a foreign body.

Moore and colleagues subsequently tested the utility of antibiotic prophylaxis in a canine model of hematogenous aortic graft contamination.[87] Thirty minutes prior to laparotomy, dogs were infused intravenously with 10 million *S. aureus* and then underwent placement of a Dacron infrarenal aortic graft. The experimental group received an intravenous dose of cephalothin (25 mg/kg), which was started just prior to the skin incision and continued for 30 minutes after the procedure. The animals then received

20 mg/kg of cephalothin (intramuscular) three times a day for 5 days. Control animals received similar administrations of a placebo in blinded fashion. Animals were sacrificed and grafts removed for culture at 3 weeks. Seventy-two per cent (18 of 25) of control grafts had positive cultures, compared to 24 per cent (6 of 25) of animals that received perioperative cephalothin. The investigators concluded that prophylactic antibiotics are of value in preventing infection after vascular prosthetic graft placement.

While the period of antibiotic administration in these studies was considerably more prolonged compared to today's current standards of routine prophylaxis in vascular surgery, the infecting dose of organisms was also quite large. The results clearly indicated that perioperative, systemic antibiotic therapy was capable of greatly reducing the development of infection following intraoperative bacterial contamination. This early experimental work in the prophylaxis of graft infections soon generated a large number of clinical reviews and prospective clinical investigations.

ANTIBIOTIC PROPHYLAXIS: CLINICAL INVESTIGATIONS

The relative infrequency with which vascular graft infection occurs presents some difficulties in assessing the clinical efficacy of prophylactic regimens. Large numbers of patients must be accumulated to provide a subpopulation with graft infection that is adequate for statistical evaluation. Additionally, graft infection may present at a time quite remote from graft implantation, thus prolonged follow-up is required to determine the true benefit of prophylaxis. Ethical issues may also arise, since the complication of graft infection is associated with a high degree of morbidity and mortality. This may preclude placebo-controlled studies now that antibiotic prophylaxis is almost universally accepted; it may also bring prospective studies to a premature close when trends suggest that a particular prophylactic regimen is superior to another (or to placebo), even if numbers are too small to prove statistical significance. Nevertheless, a large body of clinical investigation has accumulated over the past two decades that attempts to resolve the issue of the utility of antibiotic prophylaxis in vascular surgery.

Early Experience

Up until the mid-1970s, the use of antibiotics in vascular reconstruction with synthetic materials was largely based on personal observations and preferences. Although experimental evidence suggested that prophylactic antibiotics were of benefit, to date there had been no randomized clinical trials designed to resolve the issue. A conservative philosophy prevailed, as expressed by Szilagyi and colleagues, that until clinical trials proved the efficacy of prophylactic

antibiotics, their administration should be reserved for highly specific circumstances: the presence of an infected lower extremity ulcer or wound, gross intraoperative contamination of the graft (e.g., bowel perforation, obvious breaks in aseptic technique), cases of ruptured abdominal aortic aneurysm, and so forth.[3] Arguments against the routine use of antibiotics included the fact that no single agent could cover the entire spectrum of organisms responsible for graft infections, the rationale that an unnecessary drug may be a harmful drug (hypersensitivity reactions, drug toxicity), and the possibility that prophylactic antibiotics may only temporary suppress rather than prevent graft infection. It is notable that in Szilagyi et al.'s series from 1972, the graft infection rate among 2145 cases in which prophylactic antibiotics were not administered was 1.5 per cent.[3] Fry and Lindenauer had reported an incidence of 1.34 per cent in 890 cases where no antibiotics were used.[2] These infection rates were comparable to, and often lower than, those reported in series where prophylactic antibiotics were used.[8] Noting the preponderance of *S. aureus* in vascular graft infections, however, particularly in cases involving an inguinal incision, Szilagyi et al. suggested a clinical trial of an antibiotic directed at this organism in reconstructions that required an inguinal anastamosis.

In order to follow-up on experimental findings at their institution, in 1974 Goldstone and Moore published a review of the San Francisco VA Hospital experience with vascular prosthetic infection.[5] This series of 566 aortofemoropopliteal reconstructions was divided into two time periods: the years 1959 to 1965, during which time antibiotics were administered postoperatively only; and the years 1966 to 1973, in which prophylaxis included preoperative, intraoperative, and postoperative antibiotics. The incidence of graft infection in the former group was 4.1 per cent (9 of 222), compared to 1.5 per cent (5 of 344) in the latter. Although the investigators conceded that greater experience and skill may have contributed to the lower incidence of infection, they maintained that the major factor responsible was the more appropriate use of antibiotics in the second group of patients. The following year Perdue reported a similar retrospective review, which suggested that the institution of routine antibiotic prophylaxis reduced the incidence of wound infections and other nosocomial infections in patients undergoing major arterial reconstructive procedures.[88]

Prospective Trials

The first large prospective, randomized, blinded clinical study of antibiotic prophylaxis in vascular reconstructive surgery was published by Kaiser and colleagues in 1978.[45] Four hundred sixty-two patients undergoing aortofemoropopliteal reconstruction were randomized to receive either 1 gm of cefazolin or a saline placebo by the following protocol: an "on-call" preoperative dose, followed by three additional doses at 6-hour intervals. There were no graft infections among 225 patients who received cefazolin, compared to 4 (1.7 per cent) among 237 placebo recipients (Table 20–4). When superficial skin infections and subcutaneous skin infections were considered in the analysis (Szilagyi class I and II), the overall infection rates were 0.9 per cent in the cefazolin group and 6.8 per cent in the placebo group. There were no infections in either group among 103 patients undergoing brachiocephalic reconstruction. The mean length of follow-up after graft implantation was not reported. As no adverse drug reactions were encountered and cefazolin resistance did not emerge, the authors strongly recommended a short course of cefazolin prophylaxis in aortofemoropopliteal reconstructive surgery.

As mentioned previously, there is experimental and clinical evidence that topical antibiotic prophylaxis may be effective in preventing graft infection.[34,35] In 1980, Pitt and colleagues presented results of a controlled study of cephadrine prophylaxis in vascular procedures involving a groin incision that compared topical, systemic, and topical plus systemic administration.[36] Of 205 patients, 52 had prosthetic grafts placed, while the remainder received vein grafts. Infection rates were equivalent between these two groups. The protocol for topical administration was 1 gm in 25 ml saline instilled in the wound prior to closure; for systemic administration patients received 1 gm intravenously 1 hour prior to surgery and every 6 hours thereafter for a total of four doses. The combination-treatment group received both protocols, while controls received no antibiotics. Wound infection rates were 0 per cent for topical administration alone and systemic administration alone, 5.9 per cent for patients receiving both, and 24.5 per cent for controls. A differentiation between graft (Szilagyi class III) and isolated wound (Szilagyi class I and II) infections was not made. Minimum follow-up was 4 weeks, but mean length of follow-up was not indicated. Patients in whom synthetic graft material was used did not experience a higher incidence of wound infection. The authors concluded that topical and systemic prophylaxis were equally efficacious, and that

combined prophylaxis was unnecessary. The follow-up interval in this study, however, is not long enough to make conclusive statements.

The benefit of a short course of systemic cephalosporin prophylaxis in vascular reconstructive surgery was subsequently confirmed in a number of other prospective, randomized trials. In 1983, Salzmann and colleagues reported a trial of cefuroxime (a second-generation agent) and later cefotaxime (a third-generation agent) versus placebo in 300 patients undergoing aortofemoropopliteal reconstruction.[89] The investigators changed the prophylaxis regimen from cefuroxime to cefotaxime midway through the study, as the latter was found to be more effective in vitro against the most common graft infection pathogens at that institution. Adverse drug reactions did not occur, and the emergence of antibiotic resistance was not observed. Graft infection rates were 2.4 per cent for the placebo group and 0.8 per cent for the prophylaxis group. The incidence of wound infection was 15.1 per cent in the placebo group and 3.0 per cent in the prophylaxis group. No differences in infection rates were noted between the two antibiotics, and the authors concluded that either agent could be used effectively in the prophylaxis of postoperative infection.

In an effort to help settle the issue of how long a course of antibiotic prophylaxis was necessary, that same year Hasselgren and colleagues presented data from a trial of 1- and 3-day courses of cefuroxime versus placebo in lower extremity arterial reconstruction.[32] There was only one graft infection in this small cohort of 110 patients, and this occurred in the placebo group. The rates for wound infections were 16.7 per cent for patients receiving placebo, compared to 3.8 per cent in the 1-day and 4.3 per cent in the 3-day prophylaxis groups. No adverse reactions were noted and cefuroxime resistance did not emerge in the treatment groups. The investigators recommended that prophylactic antibiotic therapy be limited to a short-term course.

Bennion and colleagues have examined the utility of antibiotic prophylaxis in patients with chronic renal insufficiency undergoing placement of a prosthetic arteriovenous shunt for hemodialysis.[90] Patients were randomized to receive cefamandole or placebo just prior to placement of a PTFE graft, followed by two subsequent doses. The wound infection rate for the cefamandole group was 10.5 per cent (2 of 19), with one graft (Szilagyi class III) infection. The wound infection rate in the placebo group was 42.1 per cent (8 of 19), with three graft infections. This high rate of infection is not uncommon in renal failure patients, and the study emphasizes the importance of perioperative antibiotic prophylaxis.

Robbs et al. have reported a trial of cloxacillin plus gentamicin versus cefotaxime in infrainguinal arterial reconstruction.[76] This group had adopted a 48-hour course of cloxacillin plus gentamycin as their routine prophylaxis due to the predominance of *S. aureus* and gram-negative infections at their institution, and in-

TABLE 20–4. WOUND INFECTIONS AMONG PATIENTS RECEIVING CEFAZOLIN OR PLACEBO PROPHYLAXIS[9]

Prophylaxis	No. of Infections	No. of Patients	% Infected	No. of Infections by Category		
				Class I	Class II	Class III
Cefazolin	2	225	0.9%*	0	2	0
Placebo	16	237	6.8%*	4	8	4
Total	18	462	3.9%			

[a]From Kaiser AB, Clayson KR, Mulherin JL Jr, et al: Antibiotic prophylaxis in vascular surgery. Ann Surg *188*:283–289, 1978.
[b]Difference is significant at *p* < .001. Brachiocephalic procedures are not included.

itiated this trial to determine if a shorter 24-hour course of a broad-spectrum agent such as cefotaxime would be as effective. Length of follow-up ranged from 6 to 20 months. The wound infection and graft infection rates for patients receiving cloxacillin plus gentamicin were 5.4 per cent (7 of 129 wounds) and 1.5 per cent (1 of 63 grafts), respectively. The rates for patients receiving cefotaxime were 6.2 per cent (8 of 127 wounds) and 3.3 per cent (2 of 61 grafts). The differences were not statistically significant. The authors concluded that the multiagent 2-day regimen conferred no advantage over the shorter, single-agent regimen.

Comparisons of Antibiotic Regimens

As it has become evident that a short course of a cephalosporin antibiotic is the ideal prophylaxis for vascular reconstructive procedures, several recent studies have focused on whether the most widely used cephalosporin, cefazolin, is the most desirable choice. A large number of graft infections, particularly in abdominal grafts, are due to gram-negative rods. A theoretical disadvantage of first-generation cephalosporins such as cefazolin is the fact they are more vulnerable to gram-negative β-lactamase than second- and third-generation agents. Gram-negative activity is thus limited to *E. coli*, *Proteus*, and *Klebsiella*, and many hospital-acquired strains of these organisms are cefazolin-resistant. It has also been demonstrated that other cephalosporins such as the second-generation agent cefamandole have greater in vitro activities against coagulase-negative staphylococci, which have been found to colonize the native arterial wall in a large number of patients. It is clear from previous studies by Salzmann,[89] Hasselgren,[32] and Robbs[76] that second- and third-generation cephalosporins may be used effectively in vascular surgery prophylaxis.

In 1989, Lalka and colleagues examined this issue in a prospective study of arterial wall microbiology and antibiotic penetration.[26] Forty-seven patients undergoing aortofemoropopliteal reconstruction were randomized to receive perioperative cefazolin or cefamandole, 1 gm every 6 hours for nine doses. Serial samples of serum, subcutaneous fat, thrombus, atheroma, and arterial wall were obtained for culture and assay of drug levels by high-performance liquid chromatography (HPLC). Serum and tissue levels of cefazolin were significantly higher than those of cefamandole at almost all timepoints. Positive arterial wall cultures were obtained in 41.4 per cent of patients, and 68.8 per cent of bacterial isolates were coagulase-negative staphylococci (half of these were slime producers). The arterial wall concentration of both antibiotics at times fell below the geometric mean MIC for all organisms combined, but this occurred significantly more often with cefamandole. The conclusion was drawn that both antibiotics needed to be administered in larger doses (cefazolin 1.5 gm every 4 hours, cefamandole 2 gm every 3 hours), and that the antibiotics were essentially equal in efficacy if administered appropriately. The investigators corroborated the findings of Mutch and colleagues that serum antibiotic levels did not correlate well with aortic tissue concentrations of bioactive antibiotic,[25] and suggested that arterial tissue levels rather than serum levels should be a standard for comparison of antibiotic efficacy.

Edwards and colleagues have recently reported a prospective trial of cefazolin versus the more β-lactamase–stable second-generation cephalosporin cefuroxime in patients undergoing aortic and peripheral vascular reconstruction.[29] Prior studies had suggested that some failures of cefazolin prophylaxis were due to the susceptibility of this agent to staphylococcal β-lactamase, and that other cephalosporins may provide better protection than cefazolin in cardiac surgery.[91–93] Antibiotics were administered just prior to surgery, redosed intraoperatively, and continued every 6 hours postoperatively for 24 hours. Dosage and administration schedules were based on a prior pharmacokinetic study. The mean follow-up interval was not reported. The infection rate (Szilagyi class II or III) for the cefazolin group was 1 per cent (3 of 287), versus 2.6 per cent (7 of 272) in the cefuroxime group. This difference was not statistically significant. *Staphylococcus aureus* was the responsible organism in two cefazolin and five cefuroxime patients, and in vitro analysis of these isolates demonstrated greater susceptibility to cefazolin. Additionally, cefuroxime exhibited lower trough concentrations than cefazolin, and length of the operative procedure was found to be a risk factor for infection only in the cefuroxime group. The investigators concluded that cefazolin provides better perioperative prophylaxis, despite its lower resistance to β-lactamase, due to its greater antistaphylococcal potency and superior pharmacokinetic profile. Data from this and other studies[45] suggests that intraoperative redosing of cefazolin in prolonged procedures should be more frequent than in routine therapeutic administration (i.e., every 4 rather than every 6 hours) in order to maintain antibiotic levels significantly greater than the MIC for bacteria commonly implicated in graft infection.

CURRENT STATUS OF ANTIBIOTIC PROPHYLAXIS

Antibiotic Selection

Cefazolin is currently the antibiotic of choice in routine vascular surgery prophylaxis. It is relatively inexpensive, has negligible toxicity, a low incidence of severe allergic reactions, and is active against many of the bacteria commonly implicated in graft infection (Tables 20–5 and 20–6). Its pharmacokinetic profile is ideal for this indication, with reliably high peak serum concentrations and a long half-life of elimi-

TABLE 20–5.   ANTIBACTERIAL SPECTRUM OF SELECTED ANTIBIOTICS[a]

	Antibacterial Activity (MIC-90[b] in μg/ml)				
Antibiotic	*S. aureus*	*S. epidermidis*	*E. coli*	*Klebsiella*	*Pseudomonas*
Cefazolin	1	0.8	5	6	R
Cephalothin	1	0.5	5	32	R
Cefamandole	1	2	4	8	R
Cefuroxime	2	1	4	R	R
Cefotaxime	2	8	0.25	0.25	>32
Vancomycin	1	3	R	R	R
Penicillin V	P'ase(+): >25	0.02[c]	R	R	R
	P'ase(−): 0.03				
Oxacillin	0.25	0.2[c]	R	R	R
Gentamicin	0.6[c]	2[c]	4	1	2
Ciprofloxacin	0.5	0.25	0.03	0.125	0.5
Rifampin	0.015	0.015	16	32	64

[a]From Mandell RGD (ed): Principles and Practices of Infectious Diseases, 3rd ed. New York, Churchill Livingstone, 1990.
[b]MIC-90, minimum inhibitory concentration for 90 per cent of strains. MIC > 64 μg/ml considered resistant. Values are approximate and may vary between institutions.
[c]Many strains resistant.

nation compared to other cephalosporins.[29,94] It penetrates arterial tissue well, with drug concentrations exceeding the MIC of common graft infection pathogens in most instances.[26] Cefazolin is active against *S. aureus* (including penicillinase-producing strains), some strains of *S. epidermidis*, and the more commonly encountered gram-negative rods: *E. coli*, *Proteus*, and *Klebsiella*. Most other gram-negative rods are resistant, including indole-positive *Proteus* (*P. vulgaris*). Cephalothin, the other first-generation agent in common clinical use, is somewhat more resistant to staphylococcal β-lactamase, yet is less active against gram-negatives. More importantly, it is cleared from plasma four to five times as rapidly as cefazolin.[94]

Later generation cephalosporins have greater gram-negative activity and the potential benefit of increased resistance to staphylococcal β-lactamase; however, in vitro and in vivo activity against gram-positive cocci is reduced. Many investigators have tailored their choice of antibiotic to the predominant organisms responsible for graft infection at their particular institution. Cefamandole,[26] cefuroxime,[33] and cefotaxime[75] have all been used effectively as prophylactic agents in prospective trials. However, cefamandole has fallen out of favor for routine use due to an association with hypoprothrombinemia and bleeding, particularly in elderly patients and those with renal insufficiency. Cefuroxime has been shown to have antistaphylococcal potency and pharmacokinetic properties inferior to those of cefazolin.[29] The third-generation agents such as cefotaxime have broad anti–gram-negative activity, but are generally less active against staphylococci. As well, the later generation cephalosporins are in most instances significantly more expensive than first-generation agents. Cefazolin, therefore, remains the antibiotic of choice, except in specific instances where in vitro testing has revealed that another agent more adequately covers the principal pathogens of graft infection.

A potential disadvantage with cefazolin prophylaxis is the inconsistent activity of this agent against the organism that is currently responsible for the greatest number of graft infections, *S. epidermidis*. It has been shown that during hospitalization, patients acquire multiple resistant strains of this bacterium.[95,96] Up to 75 per cent of *S. epidermidis* isolates at some institutions are now cefazolin-resistant. Vancomycin is highly active against both *S. epidermidis* and *S. aureus*; resistance among these organisms is rarely encountered. Vancomycin, however, provides no gram-negative coverage. It is the drug of choice for prophylaxis in patients with a history of anaphylaxis to β-lactam antibiotics, often in combination with an aminoglycoside in procedures where there is significant risk of gram-negative infection, such as aortic reconstruction. Vancomycin is also considered the antibiotic of choice for the prophylaxis of prosthetic hemodialysis access grafts, and for patients known to be colonized with methicillin-resistant *S. aureus*. It is excreted primarily by glomerular filtration and therefore persists in high serum concentrations in

TABLE 20–6.   COST COMPARISON OF SELECTED ANTIBIOTICS

Antibiotic	Usual Dose[a]	Cost per Dose[b]	Cost per Day[c]
Cefazolin	1 gm Q 8 hr	$5.80	$32.40
Cephalothin	1 gm Q 4 hr	$2.93	$47.58
Cefamandole	1 gm Q 6 hr	$9.28	$57.12
Cefuroxime	750 mg Q 8 hr	$6.76	$35.28
Cefotaxime	1 gm Q 8 hr	$11.18	$48.54
Vancomycin	500 mg Q 6 hr	$20.04	$100.16
Penicillin V	1 million units Q 4 hr	$1.33	$37.98
Oxacillin	1 gm Q 6 hr	$5.85	$43.40
Gentamicin	80 mg Q 8 hr	$2.15	$21.45
Ciprofloxacin	400 mg Q 12 hr	$28.81	$67.62
Rifampin	600 mg Q 12 hr	$69.72	$149.44

[a]Dosages given are standard therapeutic doses for purposes of comparison. Appropriate prophylactic doses may be more frequent for some antibiotics, particularly for intraoperative administration.
[b]Source: 1992 Drug Topics Red Book. For agents available in generic form, cost is based on average wholesale price/dose.
[c]Cost per day based on price per dose, frequency of administration, and an average hospital cost per administration of $5.00.

patients with end-stage renal disease. As the incidence of graft infection is relatively low, and *S. epidermidis* infections are generally low-grade and indolent, cefazolin is currently considered to be adequate prophylaxis, with vancomycin reserved for the treatment of established *S. epidermidis* graft infections.

The broad antibacterial spectrum, excellent tissue penetration, and low toxicity of the fluoroquinolones make them potentially ideal agents for the prophylaxis of surgical infections. Limited data are available concerning the use of fluoroquinolones for this indication; however, there are reports of efficacy equal or superior to that of cephalosporin antibiotics in the prophylaxis of colorectal,[97,98] biliary,[99,100] and urologic surgery.[101–103] Auger et al. have reported a randomized study of pefloxacin (a nalidixic acid analogue) and cefazolin in patients undergoing cardiac surgery.[104] Of 111 patients, 14 receiving pefloxacin developed bacterial colonization at culture sites compared to 11 in the cefazolin group. One patient who received cefazolin developed mediastinitis from a cefazolin-resistant strain of *S. epidermidis*. As yet there are no published clinical trials of a fluoroquinolone versus a cephalosporin in the prophylaxis of peripheral vascular surgery procedures.

While rifampin is not in common clinical use in vascular surgery prophylaxis, its extremely high antistaphylococcal activity has generated a great deal of investigational interest in recent years. In 1982, Rutledge et al. reported that a preoperative intramuscular injection of rifampin was superior to cefazolin administered in the same fashion in a canine model of intraoperative graft infection.[105] Following the placement of PTFE carotid arterial grafts, 1000 *S. aureus* organisms sensitive to both antibiotics were injected over the grafts. The grafts were removed after 5 days and cultured. Only 2 of 12 grafts were infected in the rifampin-treated group, compared to 7 of 12 in the cefazolin-treated group and 7 of 7 untreated controls. Wakefield and colleagues have reported similar findings in a canine model of intraoperative aortic graft contamination.[106] Rifampin, however, provides relatively poor gram-negative coverage, and the parenteral form of this agent is at this time significantly more expensive than the cephalosporins. The clinical efficacy of parenteral rifampin in vascular surgery prophylaxis remains to be proven.

Administration

Prophylactic antibiotics are administered just prior to surgery and redosed intraoperatively during long procedures. Pharmacokinetic studies suggest that prophylactic antibiotics should be administered more frequently and in higher doses during surgery than is recommended for routine therapeutic indications (e.g., cefazolin 1.5 gm every 4 hours).[27–29] Prophylaxis is usually continued postoperatively for up to 24 hours, and possibly longer when the theoretical risk exists of postoperative bacteremia from indwelling venous catheters, arterial lines, bladder catheters, endotracheal tubes, and so forth. The advantage of continuing coverage beyond the operating room, however, has not been clearly demonstrated. In the absence of these risk factors there is clearly no advantage in extending antibiotic prophylaxis for longer than 24 hours.

Regimens of prophylaxis should be tailored to the type of vascular reconstruction that is undertaken. Cefazolin prophylaxis is recommended in all procedures involving the placement of prosthetic materials. It is probably not necessary in "clean" vascular procedures of the neck and upper extremities that do not involve the use of synthetic grafts. In contrast, the marked colonization and favorable bacterial environment of the lower abdomen and groin necessitate the use of antibiotic prophylaxis in all aortofemoropopliteal vascular procedures. The risk of gram-negative infection in aortic reconstruction may necessitate the addition of an aminoglycoside, particularly in institutions with a high degree of cefazolin resistance among gram-negative isolates. Alternatively, a second- or third-generation cephalosporin with broader anti–gram-negative activity may be substituted, as this obviates the risk of aminoglycoside-associated nephrotoxicity.

Cephalosporins should be avoided in patients with a history of anaphylaxis to β-lactam antibiotics. Patients with a history of minor allergic reactions to penicillin antibiotics may be given a cephalosporin test dose to determine if cross-reactivity is present. Reduced dosing of cefazolin and most other cephalosporins is recommended in renal insufficiency, based on the calculated creatinine clearance.

There is evidence that remote bacteremia may be implicated in vascular graft infection. Accordingly, oral prophylaxis for procedures that are highly associated with bacteremia such as tooth extraction, cystoscopy, and colonoscopy is recommended. Wooster and colleagues have demonstrated an incidence of bacteremia in 200 vascular surgery patients undergoing cystoscopy of 64 per cent among inpatients and 8 per cent in outpatients.[107] A wide variety of gram-positive cocci and gram-negative rods were identified, with multiple organisms in 22 per cent. The authors recommend antibiotic prophylaxis in these patients based on precystoscopy cultures. For procedures such as tooth extraction and colonoscopy in which preliminary cultures are not feasible, prophylaxis must be tailored to the most common normal flora of the traumatized site. Penicillins are appropriate choices for major dental procedures, while broader gram-negative and anaerobic coverage may be warranted in colonoscopy. It should be emphasized, however, that the true risk of graft infection following procedures associated with bacteremia is unclear, and there is currently no consensus of opinion on the role of antibiotic prophylaxis in this setting.

FUTURE DIRECTIONS

The desire to concentrate antibiotics at the site of potential infection has logically led to efforts to incorporate antibiotics into vascular prostheses. This method of delivery would also avoid the potential complications and expense of systemic antibiotic administration. The development of antibiotic-treated vascular grafts began over 20 years ago and has involved almost the entire spectrum of antibiotic agents in common clinical use. In recent years it has become one of the most rapidly growing areas of experimental investigation in vascular surgery.

One of the first studies involving the treatment of vascular graft material with antibiotics prior to implantation involved the first-generation cephalosporin, cephalothin (Keflin). In 1970, Richardson et al. reported that Dacron graft material soaked in cefazolin was infection resistant compared to saline-soaked controls.[108] Pieces of graft were implanted in subcutaneous pouches in guinea pigs that had been contaminated with *S. aureus* or *E. coli*, removed at 8 days, and cultured. Although the antibiotics were not bonded to the graft, and the model did not represent an actual vascular surgical procedure, the results did suggest that antibiotics concentrated at the site of surgery could be effective in limiting the deleterious consequences of intraoperative graft contamination.

It has become clear that antibiotics must be bonded to graft materials in order to prevent rapid elution and loss of antibacterial activity. The method of bonding employed must be tailored to the chemical nature of individual antibiotic agents. Greco, Harvey, Jagpal, and colleagues have pioneered the use of cationic surfactant agents such as benzylalkonium to bond anionic penicillin antibiotics to vascular graft materials.[109–112] Grafts so treated have been tested extensively in a canine model of intraoperative contamination of infrarenal aortic grafts, and were found to be highly effective in preventing (and treating) graft infection.[113–117] Benvenisty, Modak, and colleagues have employed silver in the bonding of antibiotics to vascular grafts.[118,119] Silver was found to provide two distinct advantages: it has inherent antibacterial activity, and it provides an ionic silver-antibiotic complex that is stable for weeks rather than hours or days. Penicillin and fluoroquinolone antibiotics have been bonded to graft materials in this manner and used successfully in animal models of intraoperative graft contamination.[120]

Although the cephalosporins have become the agents of choice for perioperative prophylaxis in vascular surgery, there are surprisingly few reports in the recent literature of the experimental bonding of cephalosporin antibiotics to vascular graft materials. Sobinsky and Flanagan have reported that PTFE grafts bonded with cefoxitin by glycosaminoglycan-keratin were successful in preventing infection in a canine model of intraoperative graft contamination.[121] Cephalosporins, like penicillins, are anionic in nature, and can be bonded to graft materials using cationic surfactants. Greco and colleagues reported that PTFE grafts bonded with cefoxitin using tridodecylmethyl-ammonium chloride (TDMAC) retained antibiotic activity in vivo for greater than 10 days when implanted in rat muscle pouches, and that these grafts were capable of absorbing significant amounts of systemically administered antibiotic after implantation.[122] TDMAC, however, was found to be highly thrombogenic and thus unfavorable for vascular bypass grafts.[116]

Aminoglycosides have also been used to create an infection-resistant graft. Moore and colleagues have reported that velour grafts with collagen-bound amikacin were effective in reducing infection rates in a canine model of aortic graft contamination.[65] Shenk et al. have reported similar success with a tobramycin-cyanoacrylate "glue" applied to PTFE grafts.[123] While many or most gram-positive organisms are aminoglycoside resistant, new agents with increased gram-positive activity are currently in development. Haverich and colleagues have reported the topical application of the gentamicin derivative EMD 46/217, a long-acting and poorly soluble aminoglycoside with a spectrum of activity that includes *S. aureus* and *S. epidermidis*, to Dacron prostheses using a fibrin sealant.[124]

The bacterial spectrum and pharmacologic properties of rifampin have stimulated a great deal of investigational interest into the use of this antibiotic in vascular surgery prophylaxis. Its high level of activity against *S. epidermidis* and *S. aureus* at MICs generally less than 0.008 μg/ml make it a potentially ideal antibiotic for this indication. Tissue penetration of rifampin is excellent, with concentrations in some viscera exceeding serum levels. It possesses the unusual property among antibiotics of being lipid soluble, and is therefore able to freely penetrate the cell membrane and attack intracellular organisms. Many staphylococci that are phagocytized by neutrophils remain viable and are protected from antibiotics that do not adequately penetrate the cell membrane. It has been suggested that rifampin may therefore be of value in the eradication of intracellular staphylococci that are present in leukocyte collections.[125,126] It has also been demonstrated that brief exposure to rifampin, but not cefazolin or vancomycin, can decrease the ability of *S. epidermidis* to adhere to velour-knitted Dacron.[127]

As mentioned previously, rifampin administered systemically has been shown to be superior to cefazolin in an animal model of intraoperative *S. aureus* graft contamination. The vast majority of laboratory investigation into the use of rifampin as a prophylactic agent in vascular surgery, however, has focused on the incorporation of rifampin into graft materials to produce an infection-resistant vascular prosthesis. As it has the ability to inhibit the growth of bacteria at such minute concentrations, a rifampin-bonded vascular graft might retain antibacterial activity for much longer periods of time than grafts bonded with antibiotics that have higher MICs. Additionally, its relative insolubility in water results in a much slower elution from graft materials when passively absorbed.

Powell and colleagues have reported the passive incorporation of rifampin into Dacron grafts by adding it to the blood used for preclotting.[128] These grafts were superior to cefazolin- and saline-preclotted grafts in a canine model of perioperative aortic graft contamination, although the grafts did not retain any antibiotic activity at 3 weeks.[129] Rifampin has also been passively bonded to graft materials using protein sealants. Avramovic and Fletcher have reported in vitro and in vivo success with this method.[130,131] Strachan and colleagues have recently described using such grafts clinically in four patients at high risk for postoperative infection.[132]

Chervu and colleagues have attempted to circumvent the problem of rapid elution of rifampin by using minimally cross-linked type I collagen to bind antibiotics to Dacron graft material. In an in vitro elution experiment, this group demonstrated that collagen-bonded rifampin grafts had an average duration of activity against *S. aureus* of over 22 days, compared to 2 days or less for grafts bonded with amikacin or chloramphenicol in the same manner.[133] Grafts preclotted with rifampin-containing blood had an average duration of antibiotic activity of less than 6 days. Having shown that collagen bonding can provide a sustained-release system for rifampin, the investigators then tested these grafts in a canine model of postoperative hematogenous graft infection.[67] Four groups of six dogs, each with its own group of control grafts treated with collagen alone, had aortic grafts implanted that were contaminated hematogenously with 120 million *S. aureus* at 2, 7, 10, or 12 days following surgery. Grafts were harvested 3 weeks after contamination. Of those contaminated at 2 and 7 days, none of the experimental grafts were infected, versus four of six and five of six of their controls, respectively. In the 10-day group one of six experimental grafts and only two of six controls were infected; in the 12-day group two of six experimental grafts and one of six controls were infected. The investigators conclude that grafts treated in this manner are infection resistant for 7 days following implantation, and suggest that accelerated healing of the collagen graft surface may protect against delayed bacterial seeding.

SUMMARY

Although it is not clear whether prophylactic antibiotic therapy has lowered the incidence of vascular graft infection, it has significantly changed the bacteriology and presentation of this problem. Infections due to more fastidious, less invasive organisms such as *S. epidermidis* now predominate; these infections present later and are associated with low-grade in-

flammation and chronic draining sinuses rather than abscess formation and tissue destruction.

Most graft infections appear to arise from direct intraoperative contamination of graft materials by pathogenic organisms. Hematogenous and lymphatogenous contamination may be responsible for some infections. It is clear that the native arterial tree is colonized by bacteria in a large number of cases, most commonly by *S. epidermidis*. The role of arterial colonization in the pathogenesis of graft infection has not been conclusively determined.

Most prospective studies of antibiotic prophylaxis have found that wound and/or graft infection rates are lower in patients receiving antibiotics compared to those receiving placebo. Prophylactic antibiotics are administered systemically by intravenous infusion. While there is evidence that irrigation of the surgical wound with an antibiotic solution is equally effective, systemic administration is less cumbersome and may be more cost-effective. Delivery of antibiotics by bonding to graft materials is currently under investigation, with promising results in animal models.

Cefazolin is the current antibiotic of choice in the prophylaxis of vascular reconstructive surgery. Its antibacterial spectrum, pharmacokinetic profile, low cost, and negligible toxicity make it an ideal agent for this indication. A potential drawback with the use of cefazolin is the relatively high degree of resistance currently found among hospital-acquired strains of *S. epidermidis*. Other cephalosporins may be found more appropriate for prophylaxis based on in vitro susceptibility testing at individual institutions. For hemodialysis access procedures, a single dose of vancomycin should be administered preoperatively.

Systemic antibiotic prophylaxis is recommended for all vascular procedures involving the placement of prosthetic materials. Prophylaxis is not required for clean procedures of the brachiocephalic arterial system that employ autogenous grafts. All reconstructions of the aortofemoropopliteal system mandate antibiotic prophylaxis regardless of the nature of the graft. Where there is a high degree of cefazolin resistance among gram-negative rods, an aminoglycoside may be added for aortic reconstructions. Alternately, a later-generation cephalosporin with broader gram-negative activity may be substituted.

Antibiotics should be started 30 minutes prior to incision and readministered during surgery more frequently than is suggested for "therapeutic" indications. Cefazolin should be readministered every 4 hours following the initial dose until the wound is closed, and then every 6 hours postoperatively for a total of 24 hours. There is no proven benefit from extending prophylaxis beyond this interval; however, it has been suggested that prophylaxis should continue until all sources of bacteremia have been removed, such as intravenous and arterial lines, bladder catheters, and endotracheal tubes.

REFERENCES

1. Hoffert P, Gensler S, Haimovichi H: Infection complicating arterial grafts. Arch Surg *90*:427–435, 1965.
2. Fry WJ, Lindenauer SM: Infection complicating the use of plastic arterial implants. Arch Surg *94*:600–609, 1967.
3. Szilagyi DE, Smith RF, Elliott JP, et al: Infection in arterial reconstruction with synthetic grafts. Ann Surg *176*:321–323, 1972.
4. Lorentzen JE, Nielsen OM, Arendrup H: Vascular graft infection: An analysis of sixty-two graft infections in 2411 consecutively implanted synthetic vascular grafts. Surgery *98*:81–86, 1985.
5. Goldstone J, Moore WS: Infection in vascular prostheses: Clinical manifestations and surgical management. Am J Surg *128*:225–233, 1974.
6. Bandyk D, Berni G, Thiele B, et al: Aortofemoral graft infection due to *Staphylococcus epidermidis*. Arch Surg *119*:102–108, 1984.
7. Lindenauer S, Fry W, Schaub G, et al: The use of antibiotics in the prevention of vascular graft infections. Surgery *62*:487–492, 1967.
8. Jamieson G, DeWeese J, Rob C: Infected arterial grafts. Ann Surg *181*:850–852, 1975.
9. Liekweg WG, Greenfield LJ: Vascular prosthetic infections: Collected experience and results of treatment. Surgery *81*:335–342, 1977.
10. Yashar J, Weyman A, Burnard R, et al: Survival and limb salvage in patients with infected arterial prostheses. Am J Surg *135*:499–504, 1978.
11. Buchbinder D, Leather R, Shah D, et al: Pathologic interactions between prosthetic aortic grafts and the gastrointestinal tract. Am J Surg *140*:192–196, 1980.
12. Reilly LM, Altman H, Lusby RJ, et al: Late results following surgical management of vascular graft infection. J Vasc Surg *1*:36–44, 1984.
13. Yeager R, McConnell D, Sasaki T, et al: Aortic and peripheral prosthetic graft infection: Differential management and causes of mortality. Am J Surg *150*:36–41, 1985.
14. O'Hara PJ, Hertzer NR, Beven EG, et al: Surgical management of infected abdominal aortic grafts: Review of a 25-year experience. J Vasc Surg *3*:725–731, 1986.
15. Reilly L, Stoney R, Goldstone J, et al: Improved management of aortic graft infection: The influence of operation sequence and staging. J Vasc Surg *5*:421–431, 1987.
16. Edwards MJ, Richardson D, Klamer TW: Management of aortic prosthetic infections. Am J Surg *155*:327–330, 1988.
17. Samson RH, Veith FJ, Janko GS, et al: A modified classification and approach to the management of infections involving peripheral arterial prosthetic grafts. J Vasc Surg *8*:147–153, 1988.
18. Conn J, Hardy J, Chavez C, et al: Infected arterial grafts. Ann Surg *171*:704–712, 1970.
19. Bernard H, Cole W: The prophylaxis of surgical infection: The effect of prophylactic antimicrobial drugs on the incidence of infection following potentially contaminated operations. Surgery *56*:151–157, 1964.
20. Polk HJ, Lopez-Mayor JF: Postoperative wound infection: A prospective study of determinant factors and prevention. Surgery *66*:97–103, 1969.
21. Elek S, Conen P: The virulence of *Staphylococcus pyogenes* for man. A study of the problems of wound infection. Br J Exp Pathol *38*:573–586, 1957.
22. Burke J: The effective period of preventive antibiotic action in experimental incisions and dermal lesions. Surgery *50*:161–168, 1961.
23. Stone H, Hooper A, Kolb L, et al: Antibiotic prophylaxis in gastric, biliary and colonic surgery. Ann Surg *184*:443–452, 1976.
24. Zak O, Kradolfer F: Effects of subminimal inhibitory concentrations of antibiotics in experimental infections. Rev Infect Dis *1*:862–879, 1979.
25. Mutch D, Richards G, Brown R, et al: Bioactive antibiotic levels in the human aorta. Surgery *92*:1068–1071, 1982.
26. Lalka S, Malone J, Fisher D, et al: Efficacy of prophylactic antibiotics in vascular surgery: An arterial wall microbiologic and pharmacokinetic perspective. J Vasc Surg *10*:501–510, 1989.
27. Kaiser A: Zero infection rate: An achievable irreducible minimum in clean surgery? Infect Control *7*:107–109, 1986.
28. Guglielmo B, Salazar T, Rodondi L, et al: Altered pharmacokinetics of antibiotics during vascular surgery. Am J Surg *157*:410–412, 1989.
29. Edwards W, Kaiser A, Kernodle D, et al: Cefuroxime versus cefazolin as prophylaxis in vascular surgery. J Vasc Surg *15*:35–42, 1992.
30. Stone H, Haney B, Kolb L: Prophylactic and preventive antibiotic therapy. Ann Surg *189*:691–699, 1979.
31. Mårtensson G, Norgren L, Ribbe E: Infektionsproblematik hos karlopererade patienter. Svensk Kirurgi *42*:125–131, 1984.
32. Hasselgren P, Ivarsson L, Risberg B, et al: Effects of prophylactic antibiotics in vascular surgery. Ann Surg *200*:86–92, 1984.
33. Herbst A, Kamme C, Norgren L, et al: Infections and antibiotic prophylaxis in reconstructive vascular surgery. Br J Vasc Surg *3*:303–307, 1989.
34. DiGiglia J, Leonard G, Ochsner J: Local irrigation with an antibiotic solution in the prevention of infection in vascular prostheses. Surgery *67*:836–840, 1970.
35. Lord J, Ross G, Daliana M: Intraoperative antibiotic wound lavage. Ann Surg *185*:634–638, 1977.
36. Pitt H, Postier R, MacGowan W, et al: Prophylactic antibiotics in vascular surgery. Ann Surg *192*:356–364, 1980.
37. Alexander J, Alexander N: The influence of route administration on wound fluid concentration of prophylactic antibiotics. J Trauma *16*:488–495, 1976.
38. Halasz N: Wound infection and topical antibiotics: The surgeon's dilemma. Arch Surg *112*:1240–1244, 1977.
39. Tollefson D, Bandyk D, Kaebnick H, et al: Surface biofilm disruption: Enhanced recovery of microorganisms from vascular prostheses. Arch Surg *122*:38–43, 1987.
40. Bergamini T, Bandyk D, Govostis D, et al: Identification of *Staphylococcus epidermidis* vascular graft infections: A comparison of culture techniques. J Vasc Surg *9*:665–670, 1989.
41. Geary K, Tomkiewicz Z, Harrison H, et al: Differential effects of a gram-negative and a gram-positive infection on autogenous and prosthetic grafts. J Vasc Surg *11*:339–347, 1990.
42. Quiñones-Baldrich WJ, Hernandez JJ, Moore WS: Long-term results following surgical management of aortic graft infection. Arch Surg *126*:507–511, 1991.
43. Smith R, Lowry K, Perdue G: Management of the infected arterial prosthesis in the lower extremity. Am Surg *33*:711–714, 1967.
44. Edwards W, Martin R, Jenkins J, et al: Primary graft infections. J Vasc Surg *6*:235–239.
45. Kaiser A, Clayson K, Mulherin J: Antibiotic prophylaxis in vascular surgery. Ann Surg *188*:283–289, 1978.
46. Close A, Stengel B, Love H: Preoperative skin preparation with povidone-iodine. Am J Surg *108*:398–401, 1964.
47. Cruse P: A five-year prospective study of 23,649 surgical wounds. Arch Surg *107*:206–210, 1973.
48. Wooster D, Louch R, Kradjen S: Intraoperative bacterial contamination of vascular grafts: A prospective study. Can J Surg *28*:407–409, 1985.
49. Bouhoutsos J, Chavatsas D, Martin P, et al: Infected synthetic arterial grafts. Br J Surg *61*:108–111, 1974.
50. Ernst C, Campbell H, Daugherty M, et al: Incidence and significance of intraoperative bacterial cultures during abdominal aortic aneurysmectomy. Ann Surg *185*:626–633, 1977.
51. Scobie K, McPhail N, Barber G, et al: Bacteriologic monitoring in abdominal aortic surgery. Can J Surg *22*:368–371, 1979.
52. Russell H, Barnes R, Baker W: Sterility of intestinal tran-

sudate during aortic reconstructive procedures. Arch Surg *110*:402–404, 1975.

53. DeBakey M, Ochsner J, Cooley D: Associated intraabdominal lesions encountered during resection of aortic aneurysms: Surgical considerations. Dis Colon Rectum *3*:485–489, 1960.

54. Stoll W: Surgery for intraabdominal lesions associated with resection of aortic aneurysms. Wis Med J *65*:89–90, 1966.

55. Hardy J, Tompkins W, Chavez C, et al: Combining intraabdominal arterial grafting with gastrointestinal or biliary tract procedure. Am J Surg *126*:598–600, 1973.

56. Becker R, Blundell P: Infected aortic bifurcation grafts: Experience with 14 patients. Surgery *80*:544–549, 1976.

57. Buckels J, Fielding J, Black J, et al: Significance of positive bacterial cultures from aortic aneurysm contents. Br J Surg *72*:440–442, 1985.

58. Macbeth G, Rubin J, McIntyre K, et al: The relevance of arterial wall microbiology to the treatment of prosthetic graft infections: Graft infection vs arterial infection. J Vasc Surg *1*:750–756, 1984.

59. Durham J, Malone J, Bernhard V: The impact of multiple operations on the importance of arterial wall cultures. J Vasc Surg *5*:160–169, 1987.

60. McAuley C, Steed D, Webster M: Bacterial presence in aortic thrombus at elective aneurysm resection: Is it clinically significant? Am J Surg *147*:322–324, 1984.

61. Schwartz J, Powell T, Burnham S, et al: Culture of abdominal aortic aneurysm contents, an additional series. Arch Surg *122*:777–780, 1987.

62. Ilgenfritz F, Jordan F: Microbiological monitoring of aortic aneurysm wall and contents during aneurysmectomy. Arch Surg *123*:506–508, 1988.

63. Brandimarte C, Santini C, Venditti M, et al: Clinical significance of intraoperative cultures of aneurysm walls and contents in elective abdominal aortic aneurysmectomy. Eur J Epidemiol *5*:521–525, 1989.

64. Wakefield T, Pierson C, Schaberg D, et al: Artery, periarterial adipose tissue, and blood microbiology during vascular reconstructive surgery: Perioperative and early postoperative observations. J Vasc Surg *11*:624–628, 1990.

65. Moore WS, Chvapil M, Sieffert G, et al: Development of an infection resistant vascular prosthesis. Arch Surg *116*:1403–1407, 1981.

66. White J, Benvenisty A, Reemtsma K, et al: Simple methods for direct antibiotic protection of synthetic vascular grafts. J Vasc Surg *1*:372–380, 1984.

67. Chervu A, Moore WS, Gelabert HA, et al: Prevention of graft infection by use of prostheses bonded with a rifampin/collagen release system. J Vasc Surg *14*:521–525, 1991.

68. Colburn MD, Moore WS, Gelabert HA, et al: Use of an antibiotic-bonded graft for in-situ reconstruction following prosthetic graft infections. J Vasc Surg *16*:651–660, 1992.

69. Schmitt D, Bandyk D, Pequet A, et al: Bacterial adherence to vascular prostheses. J Vasc Surg *3*:732–740, 1986.

70. Rosenman J, Pearce W, Kempczinski R: Bacterial adherence to vascular grafts after in vitro bacteremia. J Surg Res *28*:648–655, 1985.

71. Malone JM, Moore WS, Campagna G, et al: Bacteremic infectability of vascular grafts: The influence of pseudointimal integrity and duration of graft infection. Surgery *78*:211–216, 1975.

72. Moore WS, Malone JM, Keown K: Prosthetic arterial graft material. Influence on neointimal healing and bacteremic infectibility. Arch Surg *115*:1379–1383, 1980.

73. Roon A, Malone J, Moore W, et al: Bacteremic infectibility: A function of vascular graft material and design. J Surg Res *22*:489–498, 1977.

74. Berger K, Sauvage L, Rao A: Healing of arterial prostheses in man: Its incompleteness. Ann Surg *175*:118–127, 1972.

75. Bunt TJ, Mohr J: Incidence of positive inguinal lymph node cultures during peripheral revascularization. Am J Surg *50*:522–523, 1984.

76. Robbs J, Reddy E, Ray R: Antibiotic prophylaxis in aortic and peripheral arterial surgery in the presence of infected extremity lesions. Drugs *35*(suppl 2):141–150, 1988.

77. Johnson JA, Cogbill TH, Strutt PJ, et al: Wound complications after infrainguinal bypass. Classification, predisposing factors, and management. Arch Surg *123*:859–862, 1988.

78. Kaebnick H, Bandyk D, Bergamini T, et al: The microbiology of explanted vascular prostheses. Surgery *102*:756–761, 1987.

79. Kwaan J, Dahl R, Connolly J: Immunocompetence in patients with prosthetic graft infection. J Vasc Surg *1*:45–49, 1984.

80. Pulaski E, Schaeffer J: The background of antibiotic therapy in surgical infections. Surg Gynecol Obstet *93*:1–6, 1951.

81. Altemeier W, Culbertson W, Vetto M: Prophylactic antibiotic therapy. Arch Surg *71*:2–6, 1955.

82. Altemeier W, Culbertson W, Sherman R, et al: Critical reevaluation of antibiotic therapy in surgery. JAMA *157*:305–309, 1955.

83. Pulaski E: Discriminate antibiotic prophylaxis in elective surgery. Surg Gynecol Obstet *108*:385–388, 1959.

84. Linton R: The appropriate use of antibiotics in clean surgery. Surg Gynecol Obstet *112*:218–220, 1961.

85. Alexander J, McGloin J, Altemeier W: Penicillin prophylaxis in experimental wound infections. Surg Forum *11*:299–300, 1960.

86. Alexander J, Altemeier W: Penicillin prophylaxis of experimental staphylococcal wound infection. Surg Gynecol Obstet *120*:243–254, 1965.

87. Moore W, Rosson C, Hall A: Effect of prophylactic antibiotics in preventing bacteremic infection in vascular prostheses. Surgery *69*:825–828, 1971.

88. Perdue G: Antibiotics as an aid in the prevention of infections after peripheral arterial surgery. Am Surg *41*:296–300, 1975.

89. Salzmann G: Perioperative infection prophylaxis in vascular surgery: A randomized prospective study. Thorac Cardiovasc Surg *31*:239–242, 1983.

90. Bennion R, Hiatt J, Williams R, et al: A randomized prospective study of perioperative microbial prophylaxis for vascular surgery. J Cardiovasc Surg *26*:270–274, 1985.

91. Slama T, Sklar S, Misinski J, et al: Randomized comparison of cefamandole, cefazolin, and cefuroxime in open-heart surgery. Antimicrob Agents Chemother *29*:744–747, 1986.

92. Kaiser A, Petracek M, Lea J IV: Efficacy of cefazolin, cefamandole, and gentamicin as prophylactic agents in vascular surgery. Ann Surg *206*:791–797, 1987.

93. Kernodle D, Classen D, Burke J, et al: Failure of cephalosporins to prevent surgical wound infections. JAMA *263*:961–966, 1990.

94. Mandell G, Sande M: Penicillins, cephalosporins and other beta-lactam antibiotics. *In* Gilman A, Rall T, Nies A, Taylor P (eds): The Pharmacologic Basis of Therapeutics. Elmsford, NY, Pergamon Press, 1990, pp 1065–1097.

95. Archer G, Tenenbaum M: Antibiotic-resistant *Staphylococcus epidermidis* in patients undergoing cardiac surgery. Antimicrob Agents Chemother *17*:269–272, 1980.

96. Levy M, Schmitt D, Edmiston C, et al: Sequential analysis of staphylococcal colonization of body surfaces of patients undergoing vascular surgery. J Clin Microbiol *28*:664–669, 1990.

97. Offer C, Weuta H, Bodner E: Efficacy of perioperative prophylaxis with ciprofloxacin or cefazolin in colorectal surgery. Infection *16*(suppl 1):S46–S47, 1988.

98. Cooreman F, Ghyselen J, Penninckx F: Pefloxacin vs. cefuroxime for prophylaxis of infections after elective colorectal surgery. Rev Infect Dis *11*(suppl 5):S1301, 1989.

99. Kujath P: Brief report: Antibiotic prophylaxis in biliary tract surgery: Ciprofloxacin vs. ceftriaxone. Am J Med *87*(suppl 5A):255S–257S, 1989.

100. Cooreman F: Pefloxacin vs. cefazolin as single-dose prophylaxis in elective biliary tract surgery. Rev Infect Dis *11*(suppl 5):S1300, 1989.

101. Gombert M, DuBouchet L, Aulicino T, et al: Brief report:

Intravenous ciprofloxacin versus cefotaxime prophylaxis during transurethral surgery. Am J Med *87*(suppl 5A):250S–251S, 1989.

102. Cox C: Comparison of intravenous ciprofloxacin and intravenous cefotaxime for antimicrobial prophylaxis in transurethral surgery. Am J Med *87*(suppl 5A):252S–254S, 1989.

103. Christensen M, Nielsen K, Knes J, et al: Brief report: Single-dose preoperative prophylaxis in transurethral surgery. Ciprofloxacin versus cefotaxime. Am J Med *87*(suppl 5A):258S–260S, 1989.

104. Auger P, Leclerc Y, Pelletier L, et al: Efficacy and safety of pefloxacin vs. cefazolin as prophylaxis in elective cardiovascular surgery. Rev Infect Dis *11*(suppl 5):S1302–S1303, 1989.

105. Rutledge R, Baker V, Shertz R, et al: Rifampin and cefazolin as prophylactic agents. Arch Surg *117*:1164–1165, 1982.

106. Wakefield T, Schaberg D, Pierson C, et al: Treatment of established prosthetic vascular graft infection with antibiotics preferentially concentrated in leucocytes. Surgery *102*:8–14, 1987.

107. Wooster D, Krajden S: Selection of antibiotic coverage in vascular patients undergoing cystoscopy. J Cardiovasc Surg *31*:469–473, 1990.

108. Richardson RL, Pate JW, Wolf RY, et al: The outcome of antibiotic-soaked arterial grafts in guinea pig wounds contaminated with *E. coli* or *S. aureus*. J Thorac Cardiovasc Surg *59*:635–637, 1970.

109. Henry R, Harvey R, Greco R: Antibiotic bonding to a polytetrafluoroethylene (PTFE) surface. Assoc Acad Surg *13*:30–34, 1979.

110. Jagpal R, Greco R: Studies on a graphite-benzalkonium-oxacillin surface. Am Surg *45*:774–779, 1979.

111. Henry PD, Bentley KI: Suppression of atherogenesis in cholesterol-fed rabbits treated with nifedipine. J Clin Invest *68*:1366–1369, 1981.

112. Prahlad A, Harvey R, Greco R: Diffusion of antibiotics from a polytetraethylene-benzalkonium surface. Am Surg *47*:515–518, 1981.

113. Greco R, Harvey R, Henry R, et al: Prevention of graft infection by antibiotic bonding. Surg Forum *31*:29–30, 1980.

114. Greco RS, Harvey RA: The role of antibiotic bonding in the prevention of vascular prosthetic infections. Ann Surg *195*:168–171, 1982.

115. Greco RS, Harvey RA, Smilow PC, et al: Prevention of vascular prosthetic infection by a benzalkonium-oxacillin bonded polytetrafluoroethylene graft. Surg Gynecol Obstet *155*:28–32, 1982.

116. Greco R, Trooskin S, Donetz A, et al: The application of antibiotic bonding to the treatment of established vascular prosthetic infection. Arch Surg *120*:71–75, 1985.

117. Shue WB, Worosilo SC, Donetz AP, et al: Prevention of vascular prosthetic infection with an antibiotic-bonded Dacron graft. J Vasc Surg *8*:600–605, 1988.

118. Modak S, Sampath L, Fox C, et al: A new method for the direct incorporation of antibiotic in prosthetic vascular grafts. Surg Gynecol Obstet *164*:143–147, 1987.

119. Benvenisty A, Tannembaum G, Ahlnorn T, et al: Control of prosthetic bacterial infection: Evaluation of an easily incorporated, tightly bound, silver antibiotic PTFE grant. J Surg Res *44*:1–7, 1988.

120. Kinney E, Bandyk D, Seabrook G, et al: Antibiotic-bonded PTFE vascular grafts: The effect of silver antibiotic on bioactivity following implantation. J Surg Res *50*:430–435, 1991.

121. Sobinsky KR, Flanigan DP: Antibiotic binding to polytetrafluoroethylene via glucosaminoglycan-keratin luminal coating. Surgery *100*:629–634, 1986.

122. Greco RS, Harvey RA: The biochemical bonding of cefoxitin to a microporous polytetrafluoroethylene surface. J Surg Res *36*:237–243, 1984.

123. Shenk JS, Ney AL, Tsukayama DT, et al: Tobramycin-adhesive in preventing and treating PTFE vascular graft infections. J Surg Res *47*:487–492, 1989.

124. Haverich A, Hirt S, Karck M, et al: Prevention of graft infection by bonding of gentamycin to Dacron prostheses. J Vasc Surg *15*:187–193, 1992.

125. Mandell G, Vest T: Killing of intraleukocyte *Staphylococcus aureus* by rifampin: In vitro and in vivo studies. J Infect Dis *125*:486–490, 1972.

126. Simon G, Smith R, Sande M: Emergence of rifampin-resistant strains of *Staphylococcus aureus* during combination therapy with vancomycin and rifampin: A report of two cases. Rev Infect Dis *5*(suppl 3):507–511, 1983.

127. Schmitt D, Edmiston C, Krepel C, et al: Impact of postantibiotic effect on bacterial adherence to vascular prostheses. J Surg Res *48*:373–378, 1990.

128. Powell T, Burnham S, Johnson GJ: A passive system using rifampin to create an infection-resistant vascular prosthesis. Surgery *94*:765–769, 1983.

129. McDougal E, Burnham S, Johnson GJ: Rifampin protection against experimental graft sepsis. J Vasc Surg *4*:5–7, 1986.

130. Avramovic J, Fletcher J: Rifampicin impregnation of a protein-sealed Dacron graft: An infection resistant prosthetic vascular graft. Aust NZ J Surg *61*:436–440, 1991.

131. Avramovic J, Fletcher JP: Prevention of prosthetic vascular graft infection by rifampicin impregnation of a protein-sealed Dacron graft in combination with parenteral cephalosporin. J Cardiovasc Surg *33*:70–74, 1992.

132. Strachan C, Newsom S, Ashton T: The clinical use of an antibiotic-bonded graft. Eur J Vasc Surg *5*:627–632, 1991.

133. Chervu A, Moore WS, Chvapil M, et al: Efficacy and duration of antistaphylococcal activity comparing three antibiotics bonded to Dacron vascular grafts with a collagen release system. J Vasc Surg *13*:897–901, 1991.

134. Casali RE, Tucker WE, Thompson BW, et al: Infected prosthetic grafts. Arch Surg *115*:577–580, 1980.

REVIEW QUESTIONS

1. What is the average reported incidence of prosthetic graft infection?

   (a) 1 to 6 per cent
   (b) 6 to 10 per cent
   (c) 10 to 15 per cent
   (d) greater than 15 per cent
   (e) 0 to 1 per cent

2. Antibiotic prophylaxis in carotid endarterectomy should be administered:

   (a) always
   (b) never
   (c) if a synthetic prosthetic graft is to be used
   (d) if vein grafts are to be used
   (e) if there is a contralateral stenosis

3. The study by Dr. Pitt and colleagues revealed that intravenous antibiotics were much more effective than antibiotic irrigation. True or false?

4. The rate of positive aortic aneurysm wall cultures is:

   (a) 0 to 5 per cent
   (b) 10 to 25 per cent
   (c) 50 per cent
   (d) 50 to 60 per cent
   (e) none of the above

5. Risk factors for prosthetic graft infection include which of the following?
   (a) multiple reoperations
   (b) inguinal incisions
   (c) open, infected wounds on the extremities
   (d) prior graft infections
   (e) positive arterial wall cultures

6. Prophylactic antibiotics should initially be administered:
   (a) just before the start of the operation
   (b) during the operation, if the operation lasts beyond the antibiotic half-life
   (c) the day before the operation
   (d) the day after the operation if the patient has invasive lines (CVP, arterial cannula, Swan-Ganz catheter, Foley catheter)
   (e) the day after the operation if the patient has no invasive lines

7. Avenues of infection include which of the following:
   (a) the skin
   (b) the arterial wall
   (c) open wounds on the distal limb
   (d) intestinal transudate accumulated during an aortic bypass
   (e) the Foley catheter

8. The principles of selecting a prophylactic antibiotic include:
   (a) an agent with good activity against the expected pathogens
   (b) an agent with low toxicity
   (c) an agent that is relatively inexpensive
   (d) an agent reserved for difficult infections
   (e) company has good promotional materials

9. Which is the most common organism found in prosthetic graft infections?
   (a) *Proteus* species
   (b) *Escherichia coli*
   (c) *Staphylococcus aureus*
   (d) *Streptococcus viridans*
   (e) *Staphylococcus epidermidis*

10. The ideal antibiotic regimen for prophylaxis in routine vascular surgery is:
    (a) triple-antibiotic coverage
    (b) first-generation cephalosporin
    (c) second-generation cephalosporin
    (d) third-generation cephalosporin
    (e) chloramphenicol

ANSWERS

1. a 2. c 3. false 4. b 5. a,b,c,d,e 6. a,b,d 7. a,b,c,d,e
8. a,b,c 9. e 10. b

21

BIOLOGIC AND SYNTHETIC VASCULAR GRAFTS

JAMES C. STANLEY, S. MARTIN LINDENAUER, LINDA M. GRAHAM,
GERALD B. ZELENOCK, THOMAS W. WAKEFIELD, and
JACK L. CRONENWETT

Extraordinary achievements in vascular surgery must, in part, be attributed to the availability of biologic and synthetic prostheses to reconstruct diseased arteries and veins. Although autografts, homografts, allografts, and synthetic conduits have all enabled individuals to undergo limb-, organ-, and life-saving operations, the ideal vascular substitute has yet to be developed. Large-diameter synthetic grafts function quite well in high-flow situations such as with aortic reconstructive surgery. Autogenous vein grafts function well in small-vessel reconstructions. However, small-caliber grafts in general perform less well than large-diameter prostheses, and considerable contemporary research is directed at finding more suitable small-diameter prostheses for clinical use. Major recurring problems compromising the function of vascular grafts include thrombogenicity of surfaces, deterioration of biologic grafts, and infectivity of synthetic prostheses. The ideal vascular prostheses should be biocompatible, nonthrombogenic, physically durable while mimicking the elastic compliance properties of the vessel within which it is implanted, resistant to infection, and technically easy for the surgeon to implant. Our current understanding of biologic vascular prostheses (venous autografts, arterial autografts, allografts, xenografts) and synthetic vascular prostheses (fabric grafts, expanded polytetrafluoroethylene grafts), as well as a number of less often encountered alternative grafts, is considerable. This chapter is not all inclusive, but should provide a basic understanding of the common vascular prostheses used in treating patients with vascular disease.

VENOUS AUTOGRAFTS

Carrel and Guthrie clearly established the usefulness of autogenous vein transplants into the arterial circulation in experimental studies published in 1906.[1] It has been more than 40 years since the first reported successful reconstruction using saphenous vein for arteriosclerotic femoropopliteal disease,[2] and more than 25 years since similar achievements in treating coronary artery disease.[3] Autogenous saphenous vein as the conduit of choice for reconstructive surgery of small and medium-sized arteries has been widely acknowledged, and its use in the lower extremity as a reversed conduit[4,5] or in situ graft,[6,7] remains the standard by which other biologic and synthetic prostheses are judged.

Normal Vein: Anatomic Considerations

The greater saphenous vein is a subcutaneous vessel that lies close to the deep fascia within the thigh, and is more superficial within the leg. The main trunk of this vessel is formed by the confluence of the medial marginal and internal malleolar veins. As the greater saphenous vein traverses the thigh, two major tributaries, the posteromedial and anterolateral veins, merge with the main trunk of this vessel. The greater saphenous vein is a single trunk in the thigh in 65 per cent of cases, and is a single vessel at the calf level in 45 per cent of patients.[8]

The greater saphenous vein averages 60 cm in length in adult males. The precise incidence of veins too small for use in most vascular reconstructions is ill defined, but probably approaches 5 to 10 per cent. In this regard, intraoperative measurement of vein diameter may be more accurate than venographic assessments. In one study the average size of the saphenous vein was 5.5 mm following gentle distention at the time of operation, in contrast to an average diameter of 3.4 mm when the same vessels were assessed by preoperative venography.[9] In another study the diameter of the vein, as assessed by venography, was frequently underestimated, being at least 1.1 mm narrower in 80 per cent of cases.[8]

The greater saphenous vein contains approximately 8 to 12 bicuspid valves, consisting of intima with a central supporting core of connective tissue. There are nearly 1.5 times as many valves below the knee as above the knee. The most functionally important valve is located within a centimeter of the saphenofemoral junction.

Normal greater saphenous vein luminal surfaces consist of a monolayer of endothelium lying over a very thin accumulation of connective tissue within the intima (Figs. 21–1 and 21–2). The media is usually composed of an inner layer of longitudinally oriented smooth muscle cells, with a larger mass of circumferentially arranged smooth muscle cells in its outermost region. The adventitia consists of a loose arrangement of collagen fibers and elastic tissue. Not all veins procured for vascular surgical procedures are normal. In fact, intimal fibrosis and medial thickening with increased connective tissue is a common finding among veins being used in bypass operations.[10]

Vasa vasorum responsible for nourishment of the outer portion of the vein are located within the ad-

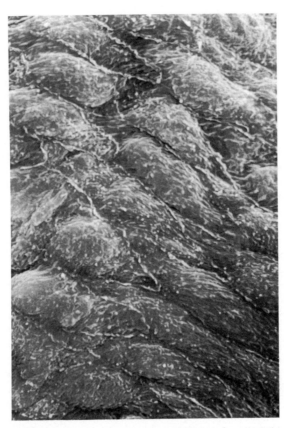

FIGURE 21–2. Normal vein lumen, exhibiting characteristic endothelial cell surface (SEM, ×30).

ventitia. Extensive communicating networks of these nutrient vessels with simple loops penetrating deep into the media have been observed in normal veins of young individuals.[11] In older-aged patients, attenuation of the adventitial communications between the vasa vasorum occur, and the simple afferent-efferent loops within the media develop into complex and more superficial networks connecting neighboring vasal loops. Such differences in nutrient blood supply may cause greater mural ischemia and subsequent aneurysmal dilation with vasa vasorum disruption during transplantation of vein segments in younger patients.

The lesser saphenous vein is sometimes used as an arterial substitute. This vein contains approximately 6 to 12 valves, and is appreciably thinner walled than the greater saphenous vein. In certain clinical settings, use of the cephalic or basilic veins may provide an acceptable alternative to synthetic grafts in small artery reconstructive procedures when other conduits are unavailable.[12,13] The cephalic vein has an average length of almost 50 cm.[14]

Vein Graft Alterations Following Arterial Implantation

Distinct morphologic and histologic changes are common within autogenous vein grafts used as ar-

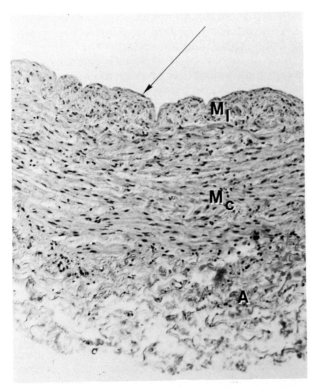

FIGURE 21–1. Normal human saphenous vein. Intimal structures (*arrow*) include a monolayer of endothelium and almost indiscernible, scant subendothelial connective tissue. Medial structures composed of an inner region of longitudinally arranged smooth muscle (M_l) and an outer region of circumferentially oriented smooth muscle (M_c). Adventitial structures appear as a loose collection of connective tissue (*a*) with occasional vasa vasorum. (Cross-section, original magnification ×120, hematoxylin and eosin stain). (From Stanley JC, Burkel WE, Lindenauer SM, Bartlett RH, Turcotte JG: Biologic and Synthetic Vascular Prostheses. New York, Grune & Stratton, 1982.)

terial substitutes.[15] These changes, often referred to as "arterialization," are perhaps erroneously considered to assist the venous conduit in adapting to the high-pressure and high-flow environment of the arterial circulation. Two specific forms of intimal thickening accompany such an event. The first is a proliferative response encompassing an overgrowth of cellular elements within the subendothelial tissue. The second is the result of fibrin layering on the graft surface, and appears to be the sequela of successive films of fibrin clot becoming organized in areas of unusually low or turbulent flow. Both of these dysplastic lesions may produce focal stenoses, as well as diffuse narrowings of the entire conduit.

Although some degree of intimal thickening is inevitable, the extent and rapidity with which it progresses is variable. In a review of lower extremity vein conduits, advanced lesions of this type were documented in 8 per cent of 260 grafts.[16] In the case of coronary artery reconstructions, this form of intimal proliferation has been alleged to account for 15 to 30 per cent of occluded grafts during the first postoperative year. Although this may be a common cause of late coronary artery bypass graft occlusions,[17] some consider it to be nonprogressive and a rare cause of such failures.[18]

The dominant pathologic feature in these lesions, like those occurring with other grafts, appears related to the presence of myofibroblasts, also referred to as myointimacytes.[19,20] The highly secretory phase exhibited by these modified smooth muscle cells may be initiated by luminal surface mitogens, such as platelet-derived growth factor that is released as platelets adhere to the deendothelialized intima. Other initiating factors may relate to local hemodynamic alterations, from circumferential distention and altered tangential stresses, from too rapid as well as too low velocity blood flow.[21-23] Smoking may be an important factor in vein graft failure,[24,25] perhaps by enhancing surface thrombotic events that contribute to underlying vessel wall proliferative phenomena. Although clinically unproven,[26] agents that lessen surface thrombosis and platelet aggregation might influence the late development of these dysplastic changes in certain cases.

Use of nonreversed in situ saphenous vein bypasses for lower extremity revascularizations has led to recognition of certain vein graft alterations unique to this particular procedure.[27] Valvulotome injury may cause obvious vessel disruption and compromise of in situ vein grafts. This may occur early as an intimal flap or late as a fibrodysplastic stenosis. Incomplete valve ablation causing early graft failure is uncommon, affecting less than 2 per cent of these conduits.[6] Malalignment of the vein, especially at the level of the knee, represents an infrequent but recognized extrinsic cause of early in situ graft failure. Intrinsic causes of graft failure account for nearly two thirds of late in situ bypass stenoses. Nearly 10 to 20 per cent of in situ veins used in lower extremity reconstructions followed for more than 5 years will develop narrowings in the body of the graft, similar to those affecting reversed conduits.[6,27]

Other specific etiologies of vein graft stenoses are known to exist. Clamp trauma causes progressive focal narrowings, manifest by transmural fibrosis and periadventitial scar tissue formation. Although uncommon in coronary artery reconstructive surgery, and relatively rare in renal reconstructive procedures, this type of traumatic stenosis has been documented in approximately 4 per cent of extremity vein grafts.[16]

Another type of vein graft stenosis has been associated with suture narrowings secondary to injudicious ligature of venous branches. This lesion appears as a focal, "hourglass" deformity and has been noted in 3 per cent of vein grafts placed in the femoropopliteal position.[152]

Occasional vein graft stenoses arise from preexisting fibrotic valves that fail to lie flat along the graft wall. These lesions appear arteriographically as focal, "conelike" narrowings. Valve cusps are often evident in immediate postoperative arteriograms, although progression to subsequent stenosis is rare. It has been generally accepted that this type of stenosis relates specifically to valve fibrosis or trapped microthrombi in the vicinity of the valve. However, experimental evidence supports the concept that stenoses may actually represent diaphragmlike strictures distal to the valve, in the form of fibroproliferative lesions affecting both medial and subendothelial regions.[28] Prevention of valve-related stenoses is controversial. Although some individuals advocate routine valvulotomy before implantation of reversed saphenous vein grafts, this is not standard clinical practice.

In general, the venous circulation is resistant to arteriosclerosis. Veins used as arterial substitutes do not maintain the same immunity to this disease. Since the first clinical description of arteriosclerosis affecting a vein graft,[29] this event has been recognized with increasing frequency and is indistinguishable from arteriosclerotic disease of the arterial circulation.[30]

The collective incidence of coronary artery vein graft arteriosclerosis was 7 per cent, with similar lesions affecting femoropopliteal vein grafts in approximately 15 per cent of cases, and comparable stenotic lesions developing in 2 per cent of aortorenal grafts.[31] Arteriosclerotic stenoses occur in nearly 8 per cent of femoropopliteal grafts, being recognized in one series at an average interval of 45 months postoperatively.[16] Progression to total occlusion may occur gradually, or be associated with acute thrombotic events in diffusely diseased grafts that appear almost aneurysmal in character.[32]

Hypercholesterolemia and hyperlipidemia are potential contributing factors in the genesis of vein graft arteriosclerosis. It is generally accepted that severe arteriosclerosis develops in vein grafts of hypercholesterolemic animals. In many patients with coronary artery bypass grafts, development of arteriosclerotic lesions appears related to elevated plasma lipid levels, although not all patients with hyperlipoproteinemia develop this complication.[24,33,34] In contrast to the apparent association of lipids with atherosclerosis affecting coronary artery grafts, Szilagyi et al. were unable to document differences in the incidence of abnormal total lipids, cholesterol and triglyceride levels, cigarette smoking, or diabetes in patients developing arteriosclerotic changes in femoropopliteal vein grafts, when compared to individuals not exhibiting this graft complication.[16] Others have noted a similar lack of an association between graft failure and lipid abnormalities.[25]

The incidence of nonarteriosclerotic aneurysmal changes within autogenous vein grafts varies with graft location. In a study of 260 femoropopliteal grafts, no aneurysms were found to be unassociated with arteriosclerosis.[16] However, in aortorenal grafts nonarteriosclerotic mural changes leading to development of aneurysmal dilation are well recognized. Nearly a third of veins placed in the aortorenal circulation undergo early nonprogressive expansion, and a 5 per cent incidence of frank aneurysmal degeneration of aortorenal vein grafts has been documented.[35] In pediatric-aged patients the incidence of aneurysmal degeneration of aortorenal vein grafts is much greater, developing in at least 20 per cent of these younger patients.[36] This is in distinct contrast to a 1.5 per cent incidence of aneurysmal aortorenal grafts in adults. Graft preparation techniques may cause structural injury to the vein wall and contribute to aneurysm formation. However, there has been no evidence that careful procurement of veins has had any lessening of the incidence of aneurysmal changes in pediatric patients. A more plausible explanation for aneurysms in this age group relates to the fact that veins from infants and children appear subject to greater initial ischemic injury when transplanted into the arterial circulation than occurs with adult veins, perhaps because of their tenuous vasa vasoral blood supply.

Arteriosclerotic injury of a vein wall may also cause subsequent aneurysmal changes. Such a process may be diffuse or it may involve isolated segments of the vein as an irregularly dilated sac. Many characteristics of these lesions are similar to arteriosclerotic aneurysmosis affecting medium-sized muscular arteries. Some of these aneurysms continue to dilate, being composed of nothing more than a fibrous sac with little cellular tissue, while others remain relatively stable accumulating arteriosclerotic debris. Thrombosis or distal embolization is a common sequela of the latter. In most instances arteriosclerotic vein graft aneurysms evolve over many years.[37] The incidence of these aneurysms has been noted to be 3.8 per cent among vein grafts placed in the lower extremity in one series,[16] and 12.5 per cent in a small number of grafts followed for 10 or more years in another report.[38]

The admonitions of Carrel and Guthrie to be gentle in dissecting veins for arterial reconstructions deserves continued emphasis. The technique of vein harvesting is of importance in contemporary practice.[39] Extensive or injudicious dissections of veins disrupts vasa vasorum, an event that is not only deleterious to the endothelial cell lining,[40] but also may be associated with subsequent acute and chronic mural abnormalities.[19,41] Cautious dissection of veins for in situ bypass is one of the best examples of the benefits of careful vein handling. Such may allow preservation of the vein's endothelial cell lining, which with its greater capacity for producing prostacyclin[42] may account for the lesser frequency of early thrombotic events accompanying in situ conduits when compared to reversed saphenous vein bypasses.

Distention of the veins using a hand-held syringe can easily generate intraluminal pressures of 700 mm Hg with complete destruction of the surface endothelium.[43] Distention pressures of 50 to 500 mm Hg are known to cause lesser diminutions in luminal fibrinolytic activity than occur with pressures of 700 mm Hg.[44] In this regard normal veins often require pressures in excess of 300 mm Hg to overcome spasm,[43] whereas those treated with smooth muscle relaxants such as papaverine may be fully distended at much lower pressures, thus lessening the risk of endothelial cell injury. Prevention of venospasm is a clear benefit of exposing veins to papaverine prior to and at the time of their excision.[45-47] Concentrations of papaverine for preoperative perivenous infiltration or intraoperative intraluminal infusions range from 0.05 to 0.6 mg/ml. Long-term studies will be necessary to establish the efficacy of preparing veins in this manner. Similarly, optimal storage solutions in which veins are maintained prior to implantation have been not adequately defined. Clearly, osmolality should approach that of blood. The latter is rarely a problem except when using "ice-slush," where osmolalities of the melting solution may rise to twice normal in the liquid portion of the medium. Heparinized blood is considered by many to be the most appropriate solution for short-term storage,[48] despite the potential for microthrombi to become deposited along luminal surfaces of some conduits. The temperature of this or other storage media is best when maintained in the neighborhood of 4°C. However, cold solutions used for initial irrigations can stimulate vein contractions, and warmer temperatures during this stage of vein preparation may be more appropriate. Although long-term data are not available to establish the superiority of any one vein graft preparation technique, it is imperative to undertake vein procurement in a careful manner.

ARTERIAL AUTOGRAFTS

The optimal substitute for a diseased artery may be the arterial autograft.[49] Unfortunately, limited availability of suitable arteries for this purpose has restricted the widespread utilization of such conduits. The most commonly used arterial autograft has been the internal iliac vessel, primarily in renal reconstructive surgery.[50-53] The radial artery and splenic artery, when used as free interposition grafts, have not afforded the same degree of clinical success as has the iliac artery. This may relate, in part, to intrinsic disease affecting the splenic vessel, and the small caliber of the radial artery. Use of arterial autografts with their origins left intact for organ revascularization, such as for internal mammary–coronary artery bypass, or splenic artery–renal artery bypass, has an appropriate place in select instances.

One of the important advantages of using autologous artery relates to maintenance of the vessel's intrinsic blood supply during the early implantation period. Vasa vasorum of medium-sized muscular arteries usually originate from small branches, and if these are undisturbed the vessel will keep its own blood supply intact as it is transplanted. The latter is not true when undertaking vein transplantation where a significant period of mural ischemia occurs prior to graft neovascularization. Although the incidence of mural thinning and aneurysmal degeneration may be less in reconstructions using autologous artery compared to autologous vein, this complication can affect arterial grafts. Long-term clinical studies are needed to establish the importance of late changes in arterial autografts.

Use of arteriosclerotic arteries after endarterectomy for bypass conduits or patch grafts is an important technical adjunct. This may be especially true in performing certain select reconstructions where contaminated fields preclude use of synthetic grafts.

HUMAN AORTIC, ARTERIAL, AND VENOUS ALLOGRAFTS

Use of fresh or preserved vessel segments from human cadaver donors was generally accepted in the early years of vascular surgery. This was particularly true in the case of aortic reconstructions. The first successful thoracic coarctation repair,[54] aortic aneurysmectomy,[55] and bypass for aortic occlusion[56] utilized aortic allografts. Aortic segments were easily sterilized by irradiation, and could be preserved by freezing, as well as by storage in either a vacuum or in β-propriolactone. Major drawbacks of allografts included their thrombogenicity and late degenerative changes with extensive calcification as well as aneurysmal rupture causing catastrophic hemorrhage.[57,58] Evolution of satisfactory large-caliber fabric grafts led to abandonment of these conduits in clinical practice.

Thromboses following implantation of small-caliber allografts caused this type of arterial substitute to be avoided in earlier practice, although approximately 30 per cent of those used in extremity reconstructions exhibited long-term patency.[59] The antigenic nature of these allografts undoubtedly contributed to their failure as an acceptable vascular graft. More recently, cryopreserved saphenous vein allografts have been reported to be useful when autogenous vein is unavailable.[60,61] In most such circumstances these conduits serve in an interim capacity, with their eventual replacement being necessary because of thrombosis, fibrosis, or aneurysmal degeneration.

UMBILICAL VEIN ALLOGRAFTS

Umbilical cord veins have been used as arterial grafts for more than 30 years. Initially, inadequate preservation and poor physical characteristics of these conduits led to unsatisfactory results and their abandonment in the early 1960s.[62,63] As vascular surgical techniques improved and bypass procedures were more widely performed, the search for alternative graft materials intensified and interest in umbilical vein was rekindled. This resulted in a commercially available graft that was used with increasing frequency in the past.[64,65]

Preparation of these conduits has been relatively well standardized. Umbilical cords, collected in delivery rooms, are individually cleaned, stripped, and refrigerated. Cords of acceptable quality are placed on mandrils and tanned for extended periods in a buffered 1 per cent glutaraldehyde solution. The resultant collagen cross-linking yields a stable, relatively nonantigenic conduit. Grafts then are subjected to multiple ethanol extractions to remove excess Wharton's gel and soluble proteins. A Dacron mesh tube is placed around the graft (Fig. 21–3A). Burst pressures for umbilical veins are near 1000 mg Hg, and are clearly in excess of strength requirements for clinical use. Human umbilical vein grafts are considerably more compliant when implanted than either expanded polytetrafluoroethylene (PTFE) or Dacron, but unfortunately, compliance falls rapidly after implantation.[66]

Because of the unique characteristics of human umbilical vein grafts, a number of specific operative techniques must be followed to achieve acceptable results.[67] If grafts are handled roughly or if clamps are applied, intimal fracture and extensive mural dissection with subsequent thrombosis may occur. Variable thicknesses of the graft wall may present technical difficulties to the inexperienced surgeon. Intimal inclusion in the anastomotic suture line is critical, but tedious with thicker portions of the graft. More recently, attempts have been made to make the graft wall thinner and easier to handle. The graft's synthetic mesh also must be included in the anastomotic suture line. Because of the Dacron mesh surrounding the umbilical vein, tunneling of the graft in a standard fashion may be difficult, and these conduits are often best passed through a metallic or plastic tube to avoid excessive friction and potential fracture of the relatively rigid graft within the flexible mesh. Umbilical vein grafts are generally used in lower extremity revascularizations when suitable autogenous vein is unavailable. Although applied to other vascular reconstructions, such as axillofemoral, aortorenal, aortocoronary, and carotid-subclavian reconstructions, there does not appear to be a clear

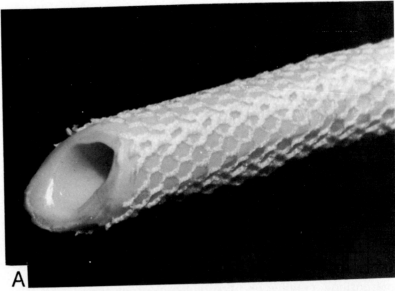

FIGURE 21–3. Human umbilical vein graft with surrounding Dacron mesh, prior to implantation (*A*) and aneurysmal segment 5 years postimplantation (*B*).

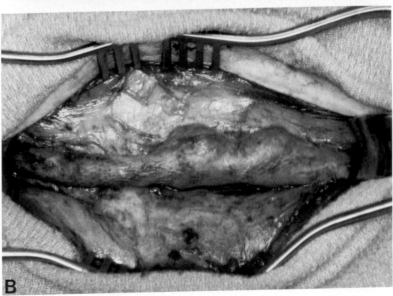

advantage of umbilical vein over other grafts in these instances.

One of the most carefully documented clinical series using glutaraldehyde-tanned umbilical vein grafts is that of Dardik et al., which included 453 femoropopliteal, 231 femorotibial, 158 femoroperoneal, 39 bypasses to the popliteal trifurcation, and 26 sequential grafts.[67] Approximately 95 per cent of the procedures were performed for gangrene, pregangrene, rest pain, or nonhealing ulcers. One-year patency rates for femoropopliteal, femorotibial, and femoroperoneal bypasses were 79 per cent, 58 per cent, and 58 per cent, respectively. Five-year patency rates for the same bypasses were 53 per cent, 26 per cent, and 28 per cent, respectively. Others have reported quite acceptable results with these conduits, but their outcomes are not as good as reported in the former experience.[68,69] A prospective randomized trial documented better patency of above-knee femoropopliteal bypasses when using umbilical vein grafts compared to expanded PTFE grafts.[70]

Complications associated with the utilization of this graft material are similar to those associated with other conduits.[71] Management of thromboses depends on multiple factors, including the time at which an occlusion occurs following implantation, the mechanism of thrombosis, and the extent of thrombosis. Late graft closures present more difficult problems. Technically, operative dissection of these grafts may be extremely difficult, particularly in the area of anastomoses. Because of the delicate nature of the grafts, thrombectomy must be performed with extreme care. Graft replacement may be necessary. Infection represents the most severe complication of using umbilical vein, and invariably necessitates graft removal. Bacteria have been demonstrated in 26 per cent of clinically noninfected grafts among a group of 80 umbilical vein conduits removed for biologic and structural studies,[72] an incidence of bacterial presence similar to that noted in clinically noninfected arteries removed during clean vascular reconstructive procedures.

Aneurysm formation in these grafts is common[67,71,73–75] (Fig. 23–3B). In several studies, aneurysmal changes affected 40 to 56 per cent of grafts, including diffuse dilations in 21 to 34 per cent of these conduits.[67,68] Deterioration of human umbilical vein grafts usually occurs after long periods of implantation. This is usually observed after 5 years' implantation and is readily detected by means of duplex imaging.[75,76] Polyester mesh, currently used to externally reinforce these prostheses, appears to provide inadequate support, and caution should be used in preferential placement of this type conduit in individuals other than those with limited life expectancies.[74,75] Fortunately, for those patients developing aneurysmal grafts, segmental resections with interposition grafting or total replacement of the prostheses is often successful.[68]

XENOGRAFTS

Interest in untreated arterial xenografts began in the early 1950s, but such grafts were discarded because of their uniformly poor performance. Development of a modified bovine carotid artery xenograft was undertaken by enzymatically removing the immunoreactive tissue, mainly smooth muscle, and leaving a relatively nonantigenic insoluble collagenous framework behind.[77] Xenograft vessels were first treated with the enzyme ficin to remove all parenchymatous proteins. The resultant soft collagen tube was then tanned over a mandril with dialdehyde starch to cross-link collagen. Carotid arteries of the adult cow became the vessel most commonly prepared in this manner, since they could be easily obtained in appropriate lengths, had very few branches complicating the preparation, and contained considerable amounts of collagen.

Utilization of these xenografts rapidly increased for both iliac artery and femoropopliteal bypasses in the 1960s and 1970s. However, after several years in the femoropopliteal position, aneurysms of the graft developed in 3 to 6 per cent of patients.[78,79] In general, patency rates resembled those with fabric prostheses, being 40 to 50 per cent at 5 years for above-knee femoropopliteal bypasses. Infection rates of 3 to 7 per cent were significantly higher than those observed with other conduits.[80] By the late 1970s utilization of this graft was limited primarily to angioaccess. These grafts appear to work well in high-flow arteriovenous fistulas, with reported patency rates of up to 87 per cent.[79] In the last several years, new forms of bovine xenografts have become available, including some with a coarse Dacron mesh net support, similar to that employed in human umbilical vein grafts. Long-term results involving these newer preparations are not available at the present time,

but in at least one study aneurysmal changes were noted in over 42 per cent of grafts 4 years following their implantation.[81]

An alternative to the dialdehyde starch–prepared bovine xenografts has been a carboxylated collagen, glutaraldehyde-tanned graft. A recent report on these "negatively charged glutaraldehyde-tanned grafts" was relatively encouraging,[82] although studies of greater numbers of patients will be necessary to define the exact role of these conduits in clinical practice. A recent variation of this type graft has involved the treatment of donor arteries with detergents to extract their cellular contents, yielding an acellular matrix consisting of the arterial skeleton of collagen and elastin, including a basement membrane.[83] While these grafts do not stimulate immune rejection and have exhibited favorable early patency in laboratory investigations, long-term studies are required to ensure lack of degeneration and sustained patency.

DACRON AND TEFLON FABRIC GRAFTS

Major advances in peripheral vascular surgery followed the dramatic experimental demonstration by Voorhees, Jaretzki, and Blakemore in 1952 that a fabric graft, in their case Vinyon N cloth, could be successfully placed into the arterial circulation.[84] A considerable body of knowledge and much clinical experience concerning fabric grafts has accumulated since then.

The usefulness of fabric vascular grafts is influenced more by the way in which the material is fabricated than by the fabric's innate biologic reactivity. Similarly, the recipient's thrombogenic potential may be more relevant to early graft occlusions than the prosthesis itself.[85] This is not to totally discount the basic material itself. For example, Nylon, Ivalon, and Orlon lose significant tensile strength after implantation, whereas Dacron (polyethylene terephthalate) and Teflon (PTFE) are essentially unchanged in tensile strength even after long periods of implantation.[86] Teflon is slightly less reactive than Dacron. This may be undesirable, however, because of less tissue bonding, and repelling of fibroblastic invasion.[87] Because of these properties, woven Teflon has been considered by some to be an unacceptable prosthetic fabric.[88] Although the synthetic fabric should not produce an excessive fibroproliferative response, a certain amount of tissue reaction may facilitate graft incorporation by the ingrowth of fibroblasts.

Fabrication

Three different kinds of yarn are utilized in the manufacture of prosthetic fabrics: (1) monofilament yarn such as nylon; (2) multifilament yarn, which contains many small continuous filaments such as Dacron and Teflon; and (3) staple yarn, which consists of short lengths of filaments spun together to form a continuous thread, such as cotton or wool.

Most multifilament yarns are texturized with spiral and coil-spring shapes within individual filaments. This produces elasticity, softness, and better handling qualities. Yarn may be fabricated in one of three ways: weaving, knitting, or braiding.

Woven fabric threads are interlaced in a simple over-and-under pattern (Fig. 21–4), both in the warp string (lengthwise on the loom) and the fill or woof (running crosswise, at right angles to the warp). Woven materials, in general, have no stretch in either the warp, in the fill, or on the diagonal bias. Furthermore, permissible looseness of the weave is limited, since a loosely woven cloth tends to fray and the yarn tends to slide and gather.

Knitted fabrics employ threads that are looped to form a continuous interconnecting chain (Fig. 21–5). Knitted fabrics have a certain amount of stretch in both length and width, but most occurs along the bias. The closer the knit, the less stretch in all directions. Knitted materials are the most versatile of fabricated grafts regarding degrees of porosity.

Braided fabrics are no longer utilized, since they require heavier yarn, tend to be bulky, and are not porous. Both woven or braided fabrics may require heat-sealing to prevent fraying of their cut edges.

Velour is a fiber variant in which loops of yarn extend upward at right angles to the fabric surface and impart a plush, velvety texture (Fig. 21–6). By varying the yarn and number of loopings, the porosity and thickness of the surface pile can be easily altered.[89] A great deal of elasticity may also be imparted to these grafts. Velour finishes may be on the internal, external, or both surfaces of graft materials. Velour grafts provide a superior matrix to fibrin for more efficient preclotting, thus providing the potential for a more porous material. Velour fabrics enhance physical binding of tissue to the fabric, since the loops of yarn extend into the fibrous tissue layer.[90]

It is seemingly important for grafts to be minimally porous at implantation but to have modest porosity for later biologic healing. Desirable fabrications include those that combine the maximum tolerable porosity with the best handling qualities. Woven, relatively nonporous materials are best suited for the thoracic aorta, and are utilized by some to repair ruptured infrarenal aneurysms. Knitted fabrics have been more widely used for most other applications, especially elective aortic reconstructions. The upper limit of graft porosity before preclotting is in the neighborhood of 7000 ml/sq cm/min, whereas from a healing perspective, grafts with a porosity of 10,000 ml/sq cm/min would be nearly perfect.[87] These figures seem inordinately high, because implantation of a graft with a porosity of 4000 ml/sq cm/min may cause bleeding that is very difficult to control even with careful preclotting. Most knitted grafts used in clinical practice have porosities in the range of 1200 to 1900 ml/sq cm/min.

Porous fabricated vascular prostheses may be rendered impervious by their coating or impregnation with albumin or collagen. These grafts need no preclotting and blood loss is less with their use.[91,92] Nevertheless, it is noteworthy that a recent prospective randomized study did not confirm this supposition.[93] Commercially available grafts prepared in this manner retain the favorable handling characteristics of knitted prostheses. Early thrombogenicity may be lessened by such graft coatings,[94] and as the protein is resorbed tissue ingrowth occurs. There are clear data that collagen-impregnated grafts do not increase platelet activation or fibrin formation.[95] Minimal differences in healing exist between grafts coated with collagen compared to those coated with albumin.[96] Collagen impregnated grafts implanted for up to 9 months in the thoracic and infrarenal aortas of animals exhibit improved initial capsular adherence, as well as greater areas of surface neoendothelialization and more capsular vasa vasorum.[97,98] These grafts have been used clinically in the descending thoracic, thor-

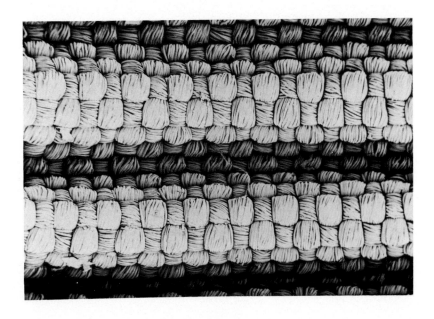

FIGURE 21–4. Woven Dacron-crimped graft with interlaced network of over-and-under threads (SEM, ×30).

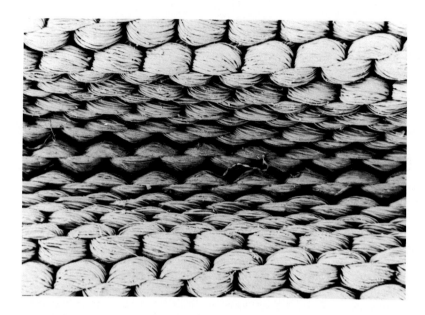

FIGURE 21–5. Knitted Dacron-crimped graft with looped threads forming a continuous chain network (SEM, ×30).

acoabdominal, and infrarenal aortic positions with no graft-related complications.[99,100] Although 40 per cent of patients with collagen-coated Dacron grafts have been observed to have increased antibodies for both graft collagen and bovine type I collagen, no severe reactions were noted among these individuals.[101] Fibrin glue and albumin may also be applied intraoperatively to porous fabricated grafts to render them impervious when hemostasis is otherwise unlikely, such as in the patient who is already anticoagulated.[102]

Prostheses are often crimped to impart elasticity and maintain shape during bending, although most of this elasticity is lost with stretching during implantation. The primary advantage of crimping lies in providing a circular tube to facilitate the technical creation of an anastomosis. Crimping has a number of disadvantages. It increases the thickness of graft

material and reduces the effective internal diameter of the prosthesis. Crimping should be narrow and shallow if it is required to provide flexibility and resistance to collapsing. Crimped prostheses may not cause difficulty in the aorta, but may pose problems when used for small arterial replacement. The adverse effects of crimping on surface thrombogenicity have prompted some to abandon crimping, and utilize external support by means of polypropylene rings or coils to create dimensional stability and avoid kinking with angulation.[103,104]

Healing of Fabric Prostheses

Shortly after implantation of any fabric graft, a fibrin layer forms on the inner surface at the interface

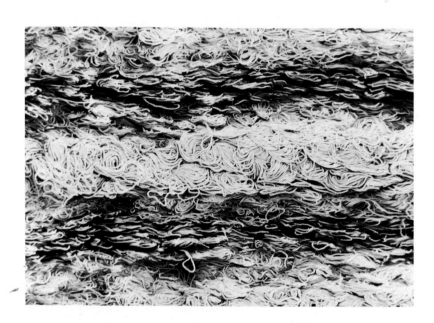

FIGURE 21–6. Knitted velour–crimped graft with loops of Dacron extending upward from surface giving it a velvety texture (SEM, ×30).

with the bloodstream. This layer usually is 1 mm or less in thickness. It does not lead to thrombosis and graft occlusion in high-flow, large caliber prostheses. However, in small prostheses, especially in low-flow environments, the fibrin layer invariably increases in thickness and often contributes to occlusion of fabric prostheses less than 5 mm in diameter. The next stage of healing is fibrous tissue encapsulation and the organization of the graft's inner lining. The inner fibrous layer may arise from cells originating from the severed ends of the host artery, from multipotential cells that are deposited from the bloodstream, or from the surrounding external tissues that grow through the interstices of the prosthesis to its inner surface. Ingrowth from the host vessel is limited in extent, and will never completely cover a prosthesis more than 4 cm in length. The most important mechanism by which inner lining organization occurs is ingrowth of fibroblasts through the interstices of the graft. Organization of the inner lining becomes apparent within days and may be quite striking within a few weeks in suitably porous grafts. Progressively longer durations of implantation produce even more organization (Fig. 21–7). Capillaries in the form of vasa vasorum traverse graft interstices to nourish the inner lining. When the porosity of the prosthesis is low, tissue ingrowth will be impeded, and organization of the inner lining is delayed.

Stability of inner and outer capsules is, in part, dependent upon the amount of fibrous tissue ingrowth through the interstices of grafts. When bonding of the outer capsule is decreased, there is a tendency for serum to accumulate around the graft, which prevents tissue ingrowth and results in subsequent inner lining degeneration. More porous grafts result in better inner capsule bonding.[87,105,106] Dacron and Teflon of comparable fabrication and porosity exhibit similar biologic fates regarding bonding.

Clinical Applications

The fabric graft is the most common conduit used for aortic replacement. Relatively nonporous woven materials are best utilized for thoracic aortic procedures because of the need to limit blood loss, which would be excessive if more porous materials are used. Woven materials should also be utilized in patients who might require immediate "full-dosage" anticoagulation postoperatively because of associated disease, or in patients with known significant coagulation defects. Woven materials also have been advocated by some for repair of all ruptured abdominal aortic aneurysms, and indeed are used routinely by some surgeons for elective aortic reconstructive procedures.

Porous knitted materials function quite satisfactorily in aortoaortic, aortoiliac, aortofemoral, axillofemoral, and femorofemoral locations. Fabric prostheses are felt by some to be suitable for above-knee femoropopliteal reconstructions. Fabric femoropopliteal grafts with the distal anastomosis below the knee should be employed only in special circumstances, because of their limited patency.

Fabric prostheses should never be implanted in contaminated or potentially contaminated locations, because of the risk of catastrophic graft infection. In nonelective circumstances, arterial reconstruction through an infected field should be avoided, in preference to reconstruction by another route. In elective circumstances, arterial reconstructive procedures in the face of active infection should always be deferred.

Care in handling fabric prostheses is essential. Clamping of vascular grafts, even with "atraumatic" vascular clamps, may crush or fracture the prosthesis. Use of rubber and plastic-shod clamps, or hydrostatic clamps, will lessen graft damage.

Most large prostheses placed in the aortoiliofemoral area function well (85 to 96 per cent long-term

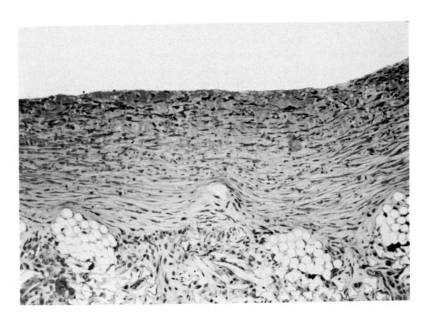

FIGURE 21–7. Inner capsule of chronically implanted knitted Dacron graft (longitudinal section, original magnification ×300, methylene blue-basic fuchsin stain).

patency), with an inner lining composed only of fibrin or unlined graft material exposed to flowing blood.[107,108] Similarly, good patency at 5 years (50 to 70 per cent) has been noted by some authors with the use of fabric prosthesis in the femoropopliteal location when the distal anastomosis is restricted to an above-knee location. Fabric prostheses also function well in the axillobifemoral location, with 5-year patency rates of 70 to 75 per cent, which are less than patency rates for aortofemoral bypass grafts but still quite acceptable, particularly in poor-risk patients. In carefully selected cases of unilateral iliac disease, femorofemoral bypass with a fabric prosthesis also yields very good patency rates at 5 years (80 to 85 per cent). Intraluminal sutureless prostheses have been used in treating aneurysms and dissections of the descending and thoracoabdominal aorta with modest success.[109–111] The recent introduction of endovascular means of introducing intraluminal grafts has great potential, although considerable testing will be required to define its exact clinical role.[112]

Complications

Fabric materials that are elastic at implantation soon become encased and ingrown by fibrous tissue, causing the loss of any preexisting elasticity. Loss of elasticity and the resultant compliance mismatch has been implicated as a cause of endothelial injury and anastomotic intimal hyperplasia, that may account, in part, for long-term failures of many prostheses.[113–117] Differences in graft construction (i.e., knitted versus woven design) do not appear to affect surface platelet adherence in chronically implanted grafts.[118] Atherosclerotic changes may occur in prosthetic linings following long-term implantation, although the role of such in fabricated graft failures has not been determined.[119]

Structural failures can affect fabric prostheses, in the form of friability, inability to hold sutures, rents in the wall, prosthetic aneurysm formation, and both early and late dilation.[120,121] Considering the enormous number of fabric prostheses inserted during the past three and a half decades, clinically overt structural failures have occurred in an exceedingly small percentage of the total implants. Defective grafts have been described in all types of fabric prostheses including Dacron and Teflon of knitted, woven, and velour construction.[122] Structural failures may reflect degenerative changes in the yarn, but more commonly seem related to mechanical failures in fabrication. In this regard, Dacron graft diameters, in one study, measured postoperatively at 33 months, revealed a 15 per cent increase in normotensive patients and a 20.8 per cent increase in hypertensive patients, findings similar to in vitro testing by manufacturers and others.[123,124] In a follow-up of an earlier report, aortic bifurcation grafts studied a mean of 175 months postimplantation exhibited greater degrees of dilation, averging increases of 67 per cent in the aortic

portion, 77 per cent in the right limb, and 54 per cent in the left limb.[125] In contrast, Dacron double-velour grafts were dilated an average of 23 per cent in another study, and little dilation occurred after 12 months implantation.[126] A modest amount of dilation, up to 20 per cent, is probably unavoidable, and should not be viewed as a major graft complication. This should be considered, however, in selecting the appropriate size of a fabric prosthesis, particularly in the hypertensive patient.

Perigraft seroma formation has been noted to affect approximately 0.008 per cent of fabricated Dacron graft implants.[127] A similar incidence of this complication has been observed with expanded PTFE conduits. The clinical presentation of such a seroma is often difficult to differentiate from a subacute graft infection.[128] Although immunologic reactions have been suggested to cause this complication, it is more likely due to inadequate adherence and ingrowth of fibroblasts to the graft substrate. Total removal of the primary graft and replacement with a conduit of a different synthetic material is successful in more than 90 per cent of patients experiencing this complication.[129]

Infection affects approximately 2 per cent of synthetic graft implantations despite careful aseptic surgical technique and administration of perioperative antibiotics. Grafts may become infected by direct inoculation with microbes during the operative procedure, as well as by hematogenous seeding from transient bacteremias months after implantation. The latter type of infection may be less likely to occur after the graft has developed a pseudointimal lining.[130] Important advances have been made toward bonding of antibiotics into prostheses as a means of lessening their infectivity. Three general concepts exist regarding application of antibacterial agents to grafts, including: (1) submersion or soaking of prostheses in agents having a high affinity for the graft material, (2) addition of antibacterial substances to blood used to preclot porous grafts, and (3) special graft preparation with materials that enhance the binding and slow the release of entrapped antibacterial agents.

Many contemporary drugs are anionic and thus amenable to easy bonding. A variety of antibiotics, including nafcillin, cefazolin, and cefamandole may be attached to grafts by their addition to preclot blood. These antibiotics are quickly bound to proteins, becoming adherent to fibrinogen, fibrin, and other plasma components, where they remain bound during the first few days following graft implantation. Canine studies using an analogue of silver-nalidixic acid, pefloxacin, have documented significant antibiotic activity in grafts subjected to continual washing for nearly 3 weeks.[131] The basis for using silver complexes relates to the strong affinity for silver to bind to Dacron. The former studies led to the bonding of silver-norfloxacin to an albumin-impregnated Dacron grafts in dogs, with evidence of inhibited bacterial proliferation 7 days following direct graft contamination with *Staphylococcus aureus* organisms.[132] The same investigators documented inhibitory levels of antibiotics in PTFE grafts impregnated with a silver-oxacillin complex, 7 days after their implantation in a canine model.[133] Binding agents were not used in the latter study. In another canine study, non-covalent bonding of benzalkonium chloride and oxacillin to expanded PTFE grafts also reduced infection following direct contamination with *S. aureus* organisms.[134]

An important development regarding infection-resistant prostheses involves the addition of antibiotics to collagen applied to Dacron grafts.[135] Gradual release of amikacin entrapped in such a collagen film has provided a high degree of protection against hematogenously induced *S. aureus* graft infections over a 3-week time period.[136] In a similar model, rifampin bonding provided early protection from graft infection.[137] Others have documented antibiotic effectiveness following direct contamination of Dacron grafts prepared with gentamycin and a fibrin sealant, and implanted in the aorta of a porcine model.[138]

Clinical application of antibiotic bonding to vascular prostheses will require extensive trials to establish its efficacy because of the relatively low incidence of graft infection. Nevertheless, research efforts on this subject are most important because of the potential catastrophic complications attending infected vascular grafts.

Anaphylactoid reactions to fabricated Dacron prostheses have been recently described.[139] Although such must be exceedingly rare, if in the presence of vasodilation and disseminated intravascular coagulation such is suspected following graft implantation, the inciting graft should be immediately removed and replaced with a graft of a different material.

EXPANDED TEFLON GRAFTS

Expanded Teflon (ePTFE) was produced for industrial purposes. ePTFE is a nontextile material unique among vascular grafts. It is highly electronegative, and thus hydrophobic, being a polymer of carbon and fluorine. Production of these grafts entails mechanical stretching, which results in a series of solid nodes of ePTFE with interconnecting small fibrils (Figs. 21–8 and 21–9). The pore size, or fibril lengths, can be controlled in the manufacturing process. Following a number of animal trials with grafts of various pore sizes, the internodal distance in most commercially available ePTFE grafts was set in the 12.5- to 30-μm range. Initial clinical trials demonstrated aneurysmal dilatation of certain ePTFE grafts,[140] resulting in a modification of the grafts with addition of an outer thin skin of solid PTFE, thickened walls, or application of an external support coil.

Clinical Applications

ePTFE grafts have been used extensively for extraanatomic and angioaccess applications, as well as for femoropopliteal reconstruction. In many centers ePTFE, shortly after its introduction, became the prosthetic material of choice for carotid-subclavian, axilloaxillary, axillofemoral, and femorofemoral bypasses.[141–146] Although the patency rates of extra-anatomic bypasses with Dacron or ePTFE are not significantly different,[147,148] ePTFE has the advantage of being impervious to blood without preclotting, relatively resistant to kinking and external pressure, and easy to declot. Many have confirmed the usefulness of ePTFE in angioaccess. Several series have compared bovine heterografts and ePTFE used for angioaccess,[149–152] with ePTFE exhibiting good long-term patency rates as well as reasonable resistance to infection. ePTFE has the added advantage of ease of revision and repair following thrombosis, infection, or pseudoaneurysm formation.[153–155] In cardiac surgery, ePTFE has found particular use in correction of certain congenital defects. This has been particularly true in repairs of atretic aortic lesions and creation of systemic-to-pulmonary shunts, where a 98 per cent patency of such reconstructions has been reported.[156] Inferior vena caval reconstructions with ePTFE actually perform better than spiral saphenous vein conduits.[157] Finally, ePTFE is useful for patch angioplasty in locations such as the aorta and the carotid or femoral arteries.

Certain early reports of ePTFE grafts in the femoropopliteal position suggested relatively acceptable patency rates.[158–160] However, with increasing follow-up, diminished patency of ePTFE grafts compared to autogenous vein grafts was confirmed.[79,145,161–163] Recently several randomized prospective trials of autogenous saphenous vein and ePTFE grafts established the poorer long-term patency of ePTFE grafts in the femoropopliteal position compared to autogenous saphenous vein.[164,165] One study revealed parallel patencies between these two types of grafts in the femoropopliteal position either above or below the knee for up to 2.5 years of follow-up.[166] Patencies in the same group of patients by 4 years at the above-knee femoropopliteal level were 61 per cent for vein and 38 per cent for ePTFE, and at the below-knee level were 76 per cent for vein and 54 per cent for ePTFE.[165] A similar study documented 5-year patencies of 70 per cent for vein and 37 per cent for ePTFE femoropopliteal grafts.[164] No distinct advantages regarding patency have been noted when externally supported (ringed) ePTFE grafts were placed in the femoropopliteal position.[167]

The difference in patency between ePTFE grafts and autogenous saphenous vein grafts in infrainguinal reconstruction increases with more distal anastomoses and in extremities with poor runoff. Thus, in a randomized trial of grafts carried to infrapopliteal arteries as femorotibial or femoroperoneal bypasses, the difference between autogenous saphenous vein and ePTFE was obvious, with patencies at 4 years being 49 per cent for vein versus 12 per cent for ePTFE.[165] Patency of ePTFE grafts may be improved with the use of antithrombotic agents such as dextran or warfarin.[69,168] Thirty-seven per cent 4-year cumulative patency has

FIGURE 21–8. Expanded PTFE graft with rather homogenous appearing surface (SEM, ×30).

been reported for infragenicular ePTFE grafts in patients maintained on warfarin postoperatively.[168] The discrepancy between low in vitro thrombogenicity and poor in vivo patency of these grafts may relate to development of an inner capsule that isolates the polymer from blood flow. That these and other polymers carry a significant risk of subsequent degeneration and aneurysmal development is a debatable topic.[169]

A bifurcated aortic ePTFE graft with a narrower flow divider than currently used in bifurcated aortic textile prostheses was recently introduced into clinical practice. In a retrospective study, patients receiving bifurcated aortic ePTFE grafts required less transfused blood and had a lower frequency of anastomotic aneurysms, late graft revisions, and amputations when compared to patients receiving knitted Dacron grafts.[170] However, the 4-year cumulative

patency for the ePTFE and Dacron grafts were not significantly different. Other retrospective studies have not documented marked advantages of these conduits.[171] In fact, in a prospective study, advantages regarding improved patency of ePTFE aortic grafts compared to Dacron grafts were not forthcoming.[172] Platelet adherence and release products in the early postoperative period appear to be less in ePTFE aortic grafts compared to Dacron aortic grafts.[173] The true value of ePTFE grafts in aortic reconstructive surgery will be better defined as results of additional prospective randomized trials become available.

Complications

ePTFE grafts, like other synthetic prostheses, may exhibit early thromboses. Since failures are not al-

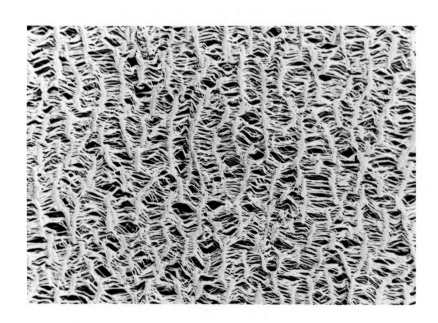

FIGURE 21–9. Expanded PTFE graft surface at higher magnification (SEM, ×300) revealing circumferentially oriented nodes of PTFE fabric interconnected by smaller fibrils of this material.

ways related to an easily defined anatomic reason, aggressive treatment of these early occlusions is clearly justified.[174,175] Late thromboses are a distinctly different aspect of this problem. Although one group has suggested that the most common cause of late failures is progression of distal arteriosclerotic disease,[176] late graft thromboses are often due to pseudointimal hyperplasia at the anastomosis.[177] Whether anastomotic pseudointimal hyperplasia is more marked in ePTFE grafts or is just more readily identified because of the ease of thrombectomy of ePTFE compared to other prosthetic grafts is not clear. Recently, more attention has been directed to the role of antiplatelet drugs in improving patency and decreasing the development of pseudointimal hyperplasia, although the clinical efficacy of this treatment remains undefined. Isolated reports of atheromatous changes in ePTFE grafts have also appeared.[178,179]

Endothelial Cell Seeding of Vascular Grafts

Seeding of prosthetic grafts with autologous endothelium and subsequent proliferation of these cells as a luminal monolayer has been well documented in experimental animal studies using both fabricated Dacron and ePTFE conduits. Widespread implantation of endothelial cells under these circumstances facilitates their replication and migration by lessening the chances of early contact inhibition.

The earliest reported method of removing endothelium for seeding involved mechanical débridement of cells,[180] but this proved cumbersome, relatively inefficient, and produced an unacceptable mixture of smooth muscle as well as endothelial cells. The latter may have contributed to the rather poor results reported in grafts seeded with mechanically derived cells in humans.[181] Derivations of cells using enzymes such as collagenase produce consistent harvests of 80 to 100 per cent of donor vessel endothelium, with clear evidence that these cells are viable and populate the linings of seeded grafts in dogs within 2 to 4 weeks.[182,183] In most of the earlier investigations, cells were affixed to implanted grafts by adding them to autologous blood used for preclotting the prostheses. Under ideal circumstances the vein surface required for effective seeding is approximately 7.5 per cent of the graft surface being endothelialized. However, given the inefficiency of contemporary preclot seeding techniques the surface area necessary to adequately seed a graft is more likely to approach 15 per cent that of the conduit being seeded. Less porous grafts, such as those made of ePTFE, are probably better substrates for seeding, in that fewer cells may be needed to bring about complete endothelial surfacing, and late proliferation of inner capsule subendothelial tissue may be less because of limited ingrowth of cells having origins external to the graft.

Although seeded endothelial cells are known to proliferate on synthetic vascular prostheses, there is a considerable lag phase in the growth of these cells to confluence. This lag may be lessened with "sodding" techniques using large quantities of microvasculature endothelium from adipose tissue, but this methodology may not provide a pure enough population of endothelial cells for clinical use.[184-187] Cultivation of enzymatically derived endothelium may provide large enough numbers of cells to provide high-density seedings, but this requires considerable time for the growth of these cells, and carries an increased potential for bacterial contamination during their processing. A second issue regarding cell growth relates to the fact that a greater initial attachment of cells to grafts prepared with various proteins may retard their later spread. Impregnation of graft surfaces with such agents as fibronectin, collagen, and laminin will certainly increase early cell attachment, but this introduces additional variables, in that preparation of these surfaces are difficult to standardize. Application of specific endothelial cell growth factors, on the other hand, may be useful in increasing the growth of seeded endothelium.

Endothelial cell–seeded synthetic grafts may perform better than conventional grafts because they have luminal surfaces functionally similar to those of native vessels. The prostacyclin-generating capacity of seeded grafts greatly exceeds that of unseeded conduits, and platelet survival returns to normal as seeded grafts become endothelialized.[188] The relevance of these physiologic findings was underscored by earlier experimental studies documenting improved patency of small-caliber endothelial cell–seeded grafts.[189,190]

The first documentation that endothelial cell seeding produced a luminal lining of endothelium in humans was reported in 1985.[191] Five preliminary clinical reports on endothelial cell seeding of vascular grafts deserve attention. The first, by Ortenwall and Risberg and their colleagues, described nine patients who had implantation of fabricated Dacron aortic bifurcation grafts.[192] These conduits had one limb seeded with a very low density of endothelium, 440 cells applied per square centimeter. Such a seeding density is much lower than most investigators use and would not necessarily be expected to be efficacious. Nevertheless, as early as 1 month postoperatively, platelet accumulation was less on the seeded limb compared to the unseeded opposite limb, implying that an antiplatelet effect was occurring. The second study, also by Ortenwall and his colleagues, documented reduced ePTFE surface thrombogenicity over a 6-month follow-up on random halves of 23 lower extremity grafts seeded with endothelial cells compared to unseeded portions of the graft.[193] The third study was that of Herring and his colleagues, in which 17 seeded ePTFE grafts placed in the femoropopliteal position were compared to 14 unseeded grafts.[194] Three-month patency rates in these groups were 93 and 84 per cent, respectively. However, at 1 year the seeded conduits exhibited an 81 per cent patency, which was significantly better than the 31 per cent patency observed in unseeded grafts. Difficulties in interpreting these data as being supportive of endothelial cell seeding technology exist, in that a greater number of more distal reconstructions were undertaken in the unseeded grafts, and the poor patency of unseeded grafts is less than would usually be expected with bypasses in these positions. In the fourth study, Zilla and his colleagues from Vienna reported on 18 patients undergoing placement of ePTFE distal femoropopliteal reconstructions.[195] In their short 14-week study, differences in platelet survival and plasma thromboxane levels both favored the seeding of conduits, although their observations were not substantiated statistically. In a fifth study, also from the Vienna group,[196] ePTFE grafts in the crural position of 13 patients performed much better than unseeded ePTFE grafts placed in 13 other patients.[196] This prospective, but nonrandomized, study in patients undergoing repeat lower extremity reconstructions is strongly supportive of this technology. Nevertheless, extensive studies are still required to clearly define the clinical utility of this technology.

ALTERNATIVE GRAFTS

A number of other vascular substitutes deserve brief comment. In most instances they represent conduits studied in the laboratory or limited clinical settings, with their relevance to contemporary practice being unknown.

Synthetic Materials

The inherent thrombogenicity and low compliance of Dacron and ePTFE prostheses have led to studies of different chemical and physical graft designs. Various polyurethanes, such as copolyetherurethane-urea are significantly less thrombogenic and more compliant when studied in vitro.[197] Reduced thrombogenicity of these conduits is related to preferential absorption of albumin rather than gamma globulin or fibrinogen, and to the microsurface characteristics of the polymer itself.[198] Unfortunately, most in vivo animal studies of polyurethane prostheses have not demonstrated better patency rates than those accompanying placement of conventional grafts.[199] The discrepancy between low in vitro thrombogenicity and poor in vivo patency of these grafts may relate to development of an inner capsule that isolates the polymer from blood flow. That these and other polymers carry a significant risk of subsequent degeneration and aneurysmal development is a continuing concern.[169]

Altering the surface composition of conventional Dacron grafts is another strategy to reduce thrombogenicity. A negative electrical charge on the graft surface can be created by carbon coating or bioelectric polyurethane.[200–202] While theoretically attractive in repelling cellular elements, these alterations in the experimental setting have not significantly improved graft patency. Recent technology has allowed the application of a very thin polymer film on Dacron grafts using tetrafluoroethylene gas and a radiofrequency glow discharge technique.[203] Although many bonding strategies appear to be theoretically efficacious, it remains to be established whether they will substantially improve patency rates of small-diameter prosthetic grafts.

Other modifications have been introduced to enhance graft patency. Electrostatic spinning of polyurethane elastomer has been used to create a microporous polymer.[204] To a similar end, replamineform grafts are formed using sea urchin spine as a cast to create unique microporous conduits from polyurethane or silicon.[205,206] It has not been demonstrated, however, that a different microporous lattice offers significant advantages over conventional microporous ePTFE.

Biologic Materials

Initial attempts to produce artificial but autogenous biologic grafts involved creation of fibrocollagen tubes as a reaction to mandrils placed in the subcutaneous tissue.[199] Fibrocollagenous conduits produced in this manner have been implanted in both animals and humans, often with associated fabric meshwork to provide structural integrity.[207] Unfortunately, even the most popular of these grafts, those using the Sparks mandril, were associated with unacceptable long-term patency, aneurysmal degeneration, and dissolution in the presence of infection.[208] Recently, glutaraldehyde-tanned mandril-generated collagen grafts have been shown to be better than ePTFE grafts when placed in the vena caval circulation of pigs.[209] It is possible that similar conduits will find a place in venous reconstructive surgery.

Bioresorbable grafts have recently been introduced in which prosthetic materials are resorbed over time and replaced by autologous cellular elements and matrix. One study involved grafts of polyglactin and polydioxanone inserted in rabbits in which subsequent generation of tissue conduits about these materials consisted of myofibroblasts and collagen beneath an endothelial-like surface.[210] Similar results have been observed with biodegradable grafts made of polyurethane and poly-1-lactic acid placed in rat aortas.[211] Although concerns remain about the long-term strength and aneurysmal formation with this type conduit, the incorporation of bioresorbable polyesters capable of slowing down the disintegration of the primary polymer may reduce such problems.[212] Considerable research is currently focused on developing a biologic graft using cell culture technology.[213]

REFERENCES

1. Carrel A, Guthrie CC: Uniterminal and biterminal venous transplantations. Surg Gynecol Obstet 2:266–286, 1906.
2. Kunlin J: Le traitement de l'arterite obliterante par la greffe veineuse. Arch Mal Coeur 42:371–372, 1949.
3. Garrett HE, Dennis EW, DeBakey ME: Aortocoronary bypass with saphenous vein graft. Seven year follow-up. JAMA 223:792–794, 1973.
4. Taylor LM, Edwards JM, Porter J: Present status of reversed vein bypass grafting: Five-year results of a modern series. J Vasc Surg 11:193–206, 1990.
5. Taylor LM Jr, Phinney ES, Porter JM: Present status of reversed vein bypass for lower extremity revascularization. J Vasc Surg 3:288–297, 1986.
6. Bergamini TM, Towne JB, Bandyk DF, et al: Experience with in situ saphenous vein bypasses during 1981 to 1989: Determinant factors of long-term patency. J Vasc Surg 13:137–149, 1991.
7. Leather RP, Shah DM, Corson JD, et al: Instrumental evolution of the valve incision method of in situ bypass. J Vasc Surg 1:113–123, 1984.
8. Shah DM, Chang BB, Leopold PW, et al: The anatomy of the greater saphenous venous system. J Vasc Surg 3:273–283, 1986.
9. Veith FJ, Moss CM, Sprayregen S, et al: Preoperative saphenous venography in arterial reconstructive surgery of the lower extremity. Surgery 85:253–256, 1979.
10. Milroy CM, Scott DJ, Beard JD, et al: Histological appearances of the long saphenous vein. J Pathol 159:311–316, 1989.
11. Short RHD: The vasa vasorum of the femoral vein. J Path Bact 50:419–430, 1940.
12. Clayson KR, Edwards WH, Allen TR, et al: Arm veins for peripheral arterial reconstruction. Arch Surg 111:1276–1280, 1976.
13. Harris RW, Andros G, Dulawa LB, et al: Successful long-term limb salvage using cephalic vein bypass grafts. Ann Surg 200:785–792, 1984.
14. Kakkar VV: The cephalic vein as a peripheral vascular graft. Surg Gynecol Obstet 128:551–556, 1969.
15. Fuchs JCA, Mitchener JS III, Hagen P-O: Postoperative changes in autologous vein grafts. Ann Surg 188:1–15, 1978.
16. Szilagyi DE, Elliot JP, Hageman JH, et al: Biologic fate of autogenous vein implants as arterial substitutes: Clinical, angiographic and histopathologic observations in femoropopliteal operations for atherosclerosis. Ann Surg 178:232–246, 1973.
17. Spray TL, Roberts WC: Fundamentals of clinical cardiology: Changes in saphenous veins used as aortocoronary bypass grafts. Am Heart J 94:500–516, 1977.
18. Lawrie GM, Lie JT, Morris GC, et al: Vein graft patency and intimal proliferation after aortocoronary bypass: Early and long-term angiopathologic correlations. Am J Cardiol 38:856–862, 1976.
19. Sottiurai VS, Stanley JC, Fry WJ: Ultrastructure of human and transplanted canine veins. Effects of different preparation media. Surgery 93:28–38, 1983.
20. Sottiurai VS, Yao JST, Flinn WR, et al: Intimal hyperplasia and neointima: An ultrastructural analysis of thrombosed grafts in humans. Surgery 93:809–817, 1983.
21. Dobrin PB, Littooy FN, Endean ED: Mechanical factors predisposing to intimal hyperplasia and medial thickening in autogenous vein grafts. Surgery 105:393–400, 1989.
22. Imparato AM, Bracco A, Kim GE, et al: Intimal and neointimal fibrous proliferation causing failure of arterial reconstructions. Surgery 70:1007–1017, 1972.
23. Zwolak RM, Adams MC, Clowes AW: Kinetics of vein graft hyperplasia: Association with tangential stress. J Vasc Surg 5:126–136, 1987.
24. Solymoss BC, Nadeau P, Millette D, et al: Late thrombosis of saphenous vein coronary bypass grafts related to risk factors. Circulation 78(suppl I):I-140–I-143, 1988.
25. Wiseman S, Kenchington G, Dain R, et al: Influence of smoking and plasma factors on patency of femoropopliteal vein grafts. Br Med J 299:643–646, 1989.
26. McCollum, C, Alexander C, Dip N, et al: Antiplatelet drugs in femoropopliteal vein bypasses: A multicenter trial. J Vasc Surg 13:150–162, 1991.
27. Donaldson MC, Mannick JA, Whittemore AD: Causes of primary graft failure after in situ saphenous vein bypass grafting. J Vasc Surg 15:113–120, 1992.
28. Bosher LP, Deck JD, Thubrikar M, et al: Role of the venous valve in late segmental occlusion of vein grafts. J Surg Res 26:437–446, 1979.
29. Ejrup B, Hiertonn, T, Moberg A: Atheromatous changes in autogenous venous grafts. Functional and anatomic aspects. Case Report. Acta Chir Scand 121:211–218, 1961.
30. Walton KW, Slaney G, Ashton F: Arteriosclerosis in vascular grafts for peripheral vascular disease. Part 1. Autogenous vein grafts. Atherosclerosis 54:49–64, 1985.
31. De Palma RG: Atherosclerosis in vascular grafts. Atherosclerosis Rev 6:147–177, 1979.
32. Beebe HG, Clark WF, DeWeese JA: Atherosclerotic change occurring in an autogenous vein arterial graft. Arch Surg 101:85–88, 1970.
33. Barboriak JJ, Batayias GE, Pintar K, et al: Pathological changes in surgically removed aorotocoronary vein grafts. Ann Thorac Surg 21:524–527, 1976.
34. Lie JT, Lawrie GM, Morris GC Jr: Aortocoronary bypass saphenous vein graft arteriosclerosis. Anatomic study of 99 vein grafts from normal and hyperlipoproteinemic patients up to 75 months postoperatively. Am J Cardiol 40:906–914, 1977.
35. Stanley JC, Ernst CB, Fry WJ: Fate of 100 aortorenal vein grafts: Characteristics of late graft expansion, aneurysmal dilation, and stenosis. Surgery 74:931–944, 1973.
36. Stanley JC, Fry WJ: Pediatric renal artery occlusive disease and renovascular hypertension. Etiology, diagnosis and operative treatment. Arch Surg 116:669–676, 1981.
37. DeLaRocha AG, Peixoto RS, Baird RJ: Arteriosclerosis and aneurysm formation in a saphenous vein graft. Br J Surg 60:72–73, 1973.
38. DeWeese JA, Rob CG: Autogenous venous grafts ten years later. Surgery 82:775–784, 1977.
39. Adcock OT, Adcock GLD, Wheeler JR, Gregory RT, Snyder SO, Gayle RG: Optimal techniques for harvesting and preparation of reversed autogenous vein grafts for use as arterial substitutes: A review. Surgery 96:886–894, 1984.
40. Corson JD, Leather RP, Balko A, et al: Relationship between vasa vasorum and blood flow to vein bypass endothelial morphology. Arch Surg 120:386–388, 1985.
41. Glas-Greenwalt P, Alton BC, Astrup T: Localization of tissue plasminogen activator in relation to morphologic changes in human saphenous veins used as coronary artery bypass autografts. Ann Surg 181:431–441, 1975.
42. Bush HL Jr, Graber JN, Jakubowski JA, et al: Favorable balance of prostacyclin and thromboxane A2 improves early patency of human in situ vein grafts. J Vasc Surg 1:149–159, 1984.
43. Bonchek LI: Prevention of endothelial damage during preparation of saphenous veins for bypass grafting. J Thorac Cardiovasc Surg 79:911–915, 1980.
44. Malone JM, Gervin AS, Kischer CW, et al: Venous fibrinolytic activity and histologic features with distension. Surg Forum 29:479–480, 1978.
45. Baumann FG, Catinella FP, Cunningham NJ Jr, et al: Vein contraction and smooth muscle cell extensions as causes of endothelial damage during graft preparation. Ann Surg 100:199–211, 1981.
46. Cunningham JN, Oatinella FP, Baumann FG, et al: Proposed mechanism for early vein graft thrombosis. Surg Forum 31:239–241, 1981.
47. LoGerfo FW, Quist WC, Crawshaw HM, et al: An improved

technique for preservation of endothelial morphology in vein grafts. Surgery 90:1015–1024, 1981.

48. Stanley JC, Sottiurai V, Fry RE, et al: Comparative evaluation of vein graft preparation media: Electron and light microscopic studies. J Surg Res 18:235–246, 1975.

49. Wylie EJ: Vascular replacement with arterial autografts. Surgery 57:14–21, 1965.

50. Ehrenfeld WK, Stoney RJ, Wylie EJ: Autogenous Arterial Grafts. *In* Stanley JC (ed): Biologic and Synthetic Vascular Prostheses. New York, Grune & Stratton, 1982, pp 291–309.

51. Novick AC, Stewart BK, Straffon RA: Autogenous arterial grafts in the treatment of renal artery stenosis. J Urol 118:919–922, 1977.

52. Stoney RJ, DeLuccia N, Ehrenfeld WK, et al: Aortorenal arterial autografts. Long-term assessment. Arch Surg 116:1416–1422, 1981.

53. Stoney RJ, Wylie EJ: Arterial autografts. Surgery 67:18–25, 1980.

54. Gross RE, Hierwitt ES, Bill AH Jr, et al: Preliminary observations on the use of human arterial grafts in the treatment of certain cardiovascular defects. N Engl J Med 239:578–579, 1948.

55. Dubost C, Allerg M, Deconomos N: Resection of an aneurysm of the abdominal aorta—re-establishment of the continuity by a preserved human arterial graft, with result after five months. Arch Surg 64:405–408, 1952.

56. Oudot J, Beaconsfield P: Thrombosis of aortic bifurcation treated by resection and homograft replacement. Report of five cases. Arch Surg 66:365–374, 1953.

57. Deterling RA, Clauss RH: Long-term fate of aortic arterial homografts. J Cardiovasc Surg 11:35–43, 1970.

58. Szilagyi DE, McDonald RT, Smith RF, et al: Biologic fate of human arterial homografts. Arch Surg 75:506–529, 1957.

59. Ochsner JL, Lawson JD, Eskind SJ, et al: Homologous veins as an arterial substitute: Long-term results. J Vasc Surg 1:306–313, 1984.

60. Fujitani RM, Bassiouny HS, Gewertz BL, et al: Cryopreserved saphenous vein allogenic homografts: An alternative conduit in lower extremity arterial reconstruction in infected fields. J Vasc Surg 15:519–526, 1992.

61. Sellke FW, Meng RL, Rossi NP: Cryopreserved saphenous vein homografts for femoral-distal vascular reconstruction. J Cardiovasc Surg 31:838–342, 1989.

62. Nasbeth DC, Wilson JT, Tan B, et al: Fetal arterial heterografts. Arch Surg 81:929–933, 1960.

63. Young NK, Eiseman B: The experimental use of heterogenous umbilical vein grafts as aortic substitutes. Singapore Med J 3:52–57, 1962.

64. Dardik H, Baier RE, Meenaghan M, et al: Morphologic and biophysical assessment of long-term human umbilical cord vein implants used as vascular conduits. Surg Gynecol Obstet 154:17–26, 1982.

65. Dardik H, Ibrahim IM, Dardik I: Modified and unmodified umbilical vein allograft and xenografts employed as arterial substitutes: A morphologic assessment. Surg Forum 26:286–287, 1975.

66. Weinberg SL, Cipolleti GB, Turner RJ: Human umbilical vein grafts: Physical evaluation criteria. *In* Stanley JC (ed): Biologic and Synthetic Vascular Prostheses. New York, Grune & Stratton, 1982, pp 433–444.

67. Dardik H, Miller N, Dardik A, et al: A decade of experience with the glutaraldehyde-tanned human umbilical cord vein graft for revascularization of the lower limb. J Vasc Surg 7:336–346, 1988.

68. Cranley JJ, Karkow WS, Hafner CD, et al: Aneurysmal dilation in umbilical vein grafts. *In* Bergan JJ, Yao JST (eds): Reoperative Arterial Surgery. New York, Grune & Stratton, 1986, pp 343–358.

69. Rutherford RB, Jones DN, Bergentz SE, et al: Factors affecting the patency of infrainguinal bypass. J Vasc Surg 8:236–246, 1988.

70. Aalders GJ, van Vroonhoven TJ, Lobach HJ, et al: PTFE versus human umbilical vein in above knee femoro-

popliteal bypass. Early results of a randomized clinical trial. J Cardiovasc Surg 29:186–190, 1988.

71. Dardik H: Reoperative surgery for complications following femorodistal bypass with umbilical vein grafts. *In* Bergan JJ, Yao JST (eds): Reoperative Arterial Surgery. New York, Grune & Stratton, 1986, pp 331–342.

72. Julien S, Gill F, Guidoin R, et al: Biologic and structural evaluation of 80 surgically excised human umbilical vein grafts. Can J Surg 32:101–107, 1989.

73. Boontje AH: Aneurysm formation in human umbilical vein grafts used as arterial substitutes. J Vasc Surg 2:524–529, 1985.

74. Dardik H, Ibrahim IM, Sussman B, et al: Biodegradation and aneurysm formation in umbilical vein grafts. Observations and a realistic strategy. Ann Surg 199:61–68, 1984.

75. Sommeling CA, Buth J, Jakimowicz JJ: Long-term behavior of modified human umbilical vein grafts; late aneurysmal degeneration established by colour-duplex scanning. Eur J Vasc Surg 4:89–94, 1990.

76. Nevelsteen A, Smet G, Wilms G, et al: Intravenous digital subtraction angiography and duplex scanning in the detection of late human umbilical vein degeneration. Br J Surg 75:668–670, 1988.

77. Rosenberg N, Gaughran ERL, Henderson J, et al: The use of segmental arterial implants prepared by enzymatic modification of heterologous blood vessels. Surg Forum 6:242, 1956.

78. Dale WA, Lewis MR: Further experiences with bovine arterial grafts. Surgery 80:711–721, 1976.

79. Rosenberg N, Thompson JE, Keshishian JM, et al: The modified bovine arterial graft. Arch Surg 111:222–226, 1976.

80. Rosenberg N: Dialdehyde starch-tanned bovine heterografts. *In* Stanley JC (ed): Biologic and Synthetic Vascular Prostheses. New York, Grune & Stratton, 1982, pp 423–432.

81. Schroder A, Imig H, Peiper U, et al: Results of a bovine collagen vascular graft (Solcograft-P) in infra-inguinal positions. Eur J Vasc Surg 2:315–321, 1988.

82. Sawyer PN, Fitzgerald J, Kaplitt MJ, et al: Ten year experience with the negatively charged glutaraldehyde-tanned vascular graft in peripheral vascular surgery. Initial multicenter trial. Am J Surg 154:533–537, 1987.

83. Malone JM, Brendel K, Duhamel RC, et al: Detergent-extracted small-diameter vascular prostheses. J Vasc Surg 1:181–191, 1984.

84. Voorhees AB Jr, Jaretzki A III, Blakemore AH: The use of tubes constructed from Vinyon "N" cloth in bridging arterial defects. Ann Surg 135:332–336, 1952.

85. Kaplan S, Marcoe KF, Sauvage LR, et al: The effect of predetermined thrombotic potential of the recipient on small-caliber graft performance. J Vasc Surg 3:311–321, 1986.

86. Creech O Jr, Deterling RA Jr, Edwards WS, et al: Vascular prostheses. Report of Committee for study of vascular prostheses for the Society of Vascular Surgery. Surgery 41:62–80, 1957.

87. Wesolowski SA, Dennis C: Fundamentals of Vascular Grafting. New York, McGraw-Hill, 1963.

88. Boyd DP, Midell AI: Woven Teflon aortic grafts: An unsatisfactory prosthesis. Vasc Surg 5:148–153, 1971.

89. Lindenauer SM, Weber TR, Miller TA, et al: Velour vascular prosthesis. Trans Am Soc Artif Intern Organs 20:314–319, 1974.

90. Sauvage LR, Berger K, Wood SJ, et al: An external velour surface for porous arterial prostheses. Surgery 70:940–953, 1971.

91. Branchereau A, Rudondy P, Gournier JP, et al: The albumin-coated knitted Dacron aortic prosthesis: A clinical study. Ann Vasc Surg 4:138–142, 1990.

92. Freischlag JA, Moore WS: Clinical experience with a collagen-impregnated knitted Dacron vascular graft. Ann Vasc Surg 4:449–454, 1990.

93. De Mol Van, Otterloo JCA, Van Bockel JH, Ponfoort ED, et al: Randomized study on the effect of collagen impregnation of knitted Dacron velour aortoiliac prostheses on

blood loss during aortic reconstruction. Br J Surg *78*:288–292, 1991.

94. Kottke-Marchant K, Anderson JM, Umemura Y, et al: Effect of albumin coating on the in vitro compatibility of Dacron arterial prostheses. Biomaterials *110*:147–155, 1989.

95. De Mol Van, Otterloo JC, Van Bockel JH, Ponfoort ED, et al: Systemic effects of collagen-impregnated aortoiliac Dacron vascular prostheses on platelet activation and fibrin formation. J Vasc Surg *14*:59–66, 1991.

96. McGee GS, Shuman TA, Atkinson JB, et al: Long-term assessment of a damp-stored, albumin-coated, knitted vascular graft. Am Surg *55*:174–176, 1989.

97. Noishiki Y, Chvapil M: Healing pattern of collagen-impregnated and preclotted vascular grafts in dogs. Vasc Surg *21*:401–411, 1987.

98. Quiñones-Baldrich WJ, Moore WS, Ziomek S, et al: Development of a "leak-proof," knitted Dacron vascular prosthesis. J Vasc Surg *3*:895–903, 1986.

99. Reigel MM, Hollier LH, Pairolero PC, et al: Early experience with a new collagen-impregnated aortic graft. Am Surg *54*:134–136, 1988.

100. Stegmann TH, Haverich A, Borst HG: Clinical experience with a new collagen-coated Dacron double-velour prosthesis. Thorac Cardiovasc Surg *34*:54–56, 1986.

101. Norgren L, Holtas S, Persson G, et al: Immune response to collagen impregnated Dacron double velour grafts for aortic and aorto-femoral reconstructions. Eur J Vasc Surg *4*:379–384, 1990.

102. Rumisek JD, Wade CE, Brooks DE, et al: Heat-denatured albumin-coated Dacron vascular grafts. Physical characteristics and in vivo performance. J Vasc Surg *4*:136–143, 1986.

103. Kenney DA, Berger K, Walker MW, et al: Experimental comparison of the thrombogenicity of fibrin and PTFE flow surfaces. Ann Surg *191*:355–361, 1980.

104. Kenney DA, Sauvage LR, Wood SJ, et al: Comparison of noncrimped, externally supported (EXS) and crimped, nonsupported Dacron prostheses for axillofemoral and above-knee femoropopliteal bypass. Surgery *92*:931–946, 1982.

105. Fry WJ, DeWeese MS, Kraft RO, et al: Importance of porosity in arterial prostheses. Arch Surg *88*:836–842, 1964.

106. Wesolowski SA, Fries CC, Karlson KE, et al: Porosity: Primary determinant of ultimate fate of synthetic vascular grafts. Surgery *50*:91–96, 1961.

107. Crawford ES, DeBakey ME, Cooley DA, et al: Use of crimped, knitted, Dacron grafts in patients with occlusive disease of the aorta and of the iliac, femoral, and popliteal arteries. *In* Wesolowski SA, Dennis C (eds): Fundamentals of Vascular Grafting. New York, McGraw-Hill, 1963, pp 356–364.

108. Szilagyi DE, Smith RF, Elliott JP, et al: Long-term behavior of a Dacron arterial substitute. Ann Surg *162*:453–477, 1965.

109. Berger RL, Karlson KJ, Dunton RF, et al: Replacement of the thoracic aorta with intraluminal sutureless prosthesis. Ann Thorac Surg *53*:920–927, 1992.

110. Oz MC, Ashton RC, McNicholas KW, et al: Sutureless ring graft replacement of ascending aorta and aortic arch. Ann Thorac Surg *50*:74–79, 1990.

111. Oz MC, Ashton RC Jr, Singh MK, et al: Twelve-year experience with intraluminal sutureless ringed graft replacement of the descending thoracic and thoracoabdominal aorta. J Vasc Surg *11*:331–338, 1990.

112. Parodi JC, Palmaz JC, Barone HD: Transfemoral intraluminal graft implantation for abdominal aortic aneurysms. Ann Vasc Surg *5*:491–499, 1991.

113. Abbott WM, Megerman J, Hasson JE, et al: Effect of compliance mismatch on vascular graft patency. J Vasc Surg *5*:376–382, 1987.

114. Clarke RE, Apostolou S, Kardes JL: Mismatch of mechanical properties as a cause of arterial prostheses thrombosis. Surg Forum *27*:208–210, 1976.

115. DeWeese JA: Anastomotic intimal hyperplasia. *In* Sawyer PN, Kaplitt MJ (eds): Vascular Grafts. New York, Appleton-Century-Crofts, 1982, pp 147–152.

116. Edwards WS: Arterial grafts, past, present and future. Arch Surg *113*:1225–1233, 1978.

117. Kinley CE, Marble AE: Compliance: A continuing problem with vascular grafts. J Cardiovasc Surg *21*:163–170, 1980.

118. Robicsek F, Duncan GD, Daugherty HK, et al: "Half and half" woven and knitted Dacron grafts in the aortoiliac and aortofemoral positions: Seven and one-half years follow-up. Ann Vasc Surg *5*:315–319, 1991.

119. Walton KW, Slaney G, Ashton F: Atherosclerosis in vascular grafts for peripheral vascular disease. Part 2. Synthetic arterial prostheses. Atherosclerosis *61*:155–167, 1986.

120. Blumenberg RM, Gelfand ML: The failure of knitted Dacron as an arterial prosthesis. Surgery *81*:493–496, 1977.

121. Ottinger LW, Darling RC, Wirthlin LS, et al: Failure of ultralightweight knitted Dacron grafts in arterial reconstruction. Arch Surg *111*:146–149, 1976.

122. Trippestad A: Dilation and rupture of Dacron arterial grafts. Acta Chir Scand [suppl] *529*:77–79, 1985.

123. Kim GE, Imparato AM, Nathan I, et al: Dilation of synthetic grafts and functional aneurysms. Arch Surg *114*:1296–1303, 1979.

124. Nunn DB, Freeman MH, Hudgins PC: Postoperative alterations in size of Dacron aortic grafts. An ultrasonic evaluation. Ann Surg *189*:741–745, 1979.

125. Nunn DB, Carter MM, Donohue MT, et al: Postoperative dilation of knitted Dacron aortic bifurcation graft. J Vasc Surg *12*:291–297, 1990.

126. Blumenberg RM, Gelfand ML, Barton EA, et al: Clinical significance of aortic graft dilation. J Vasc Surg *14*:175–180, 1991.

127. Paes E, Vollmar JF, Mohr W, et al: Perigraft reaction: Incompatibility of synthetic vascular grafts? New aspects on clinical manifestation, pathogenesis, and therapy. World J Surg *12*:750–755, 1988.

128. De Clerck LS, Houthooft D, Vermeylen J, et al: Delayed reaction to a Dacron velour bypass graft. J Cardiovasc Surg *31*:124–126, 1990.

129. Blumenberg RM, Gelfand ML, Dale WA: Perigraft seromas complicating arterial grafts. Surgery *97*:194–204, 1985.

130. Malone JM, Moore WS, Campagna G, et al: Bacteremic infectability of vascular grafts: The influence of pseudointimal integrity and duration of graft function. Surgery *78*:211–216, 1975.

131. White JV, Benvenisty AI, Reemtsma K, et al: Simple methods for direct antibiotic protection of synthetic vascular grafts. J Vasc Surg *1*:372–380, 1984.

132. Benvenisty AI, Modak S, Ahlborn TN, et al: Prevention of vascular prosthetic infection with silver-containing antibiotics using model of direct bacterial contamination. Surg Forum *36*:433–434, 1985.

133. Benvenisty AI, Tannenbaum G, Ahlborn TN, et al: Control of prosthetic bacterial infection: Evaluation of an easily incorporated, tightly bound, silver antibiotic PTFE graft. J Surg Res *44*:1–7, 1988.

134. Greco RS, Harvey RA, Smilow PC, et al: Prevention of vascular prosthetic infection by a benzalkonium-oxacillin bonded polytetrafluoroethylene graft. Surg Gynecol Obstet *155*:28–32, 1982.

135. Chervu A, Moore WS, Chvapil M, et al: Efficacy and duration of antistaphylococcal activity comparing three antibiotics bonded to Dacron vascular grafts with a collagen release system. J Vasc Surg *13*:897–901, 1991.

136. Moore WS, Chvapil M, Sieffert G, et al: Development of an infection-resistant vascular prosthesis. Arch Surg *110*:1403–1407, 1981.

137. Chervu A, Moore WS, Gelabert HA, et al: Prevention of graft infection by use of prostheses bonded with a rifampin/collagen release system. J Vasc Surg *14*:521–525, 1991.

138. Haverich A, Hirt S, Karck M, et al: Prevention of graft infection by bonding of gentamycin to Dacron prostheses. J Vasc Surg *15*:187–193, 1992.

139. Roizen MF, Rodgers GM, Valone FH, et al: Anaphylactoid

reactions to vascular graft material presenting with vasodilation and subsequent disseminated intravascular coagulation. Anesthesiology 71:331–338, 1989.

140. Campbell CD, Brooks DH, Webster MW, et al: Aneurysm formation in expanded polytetrafluoroethylene prostheses. Surgery 79:491–493, 1976.

141. Campbell CD, Brooks DH, Siewers RD, et al: Extraanatomic bypass with expanded polytetrafluoroethylene. Surg Gynecol Obstet 148:525–530, 1979.

142. Chang JB: Current status of extraanatomic bypasses. Am J Surg 152:202–205, 1986.

143. Connolly JE, Kwaan JHM, Brownell D, et al: Newer developments of extraanatomic bypass. Surg Gynecol Obstet 158:415–418, 1984.

144. Fletcher JP, Little JM, Loewenthal J, et al: Initial experience with polytetrafluoroethylene for extraanatomic bypass. Am J Surg 139:696–699, 1980.

145. Haimov M, Giron F, Jacobson JH II: The expanded polytetrafluoroethylene graft. Three years' experience with 362 grafts. Arch Surg 114:673–677, 1979.

146. Veith FJ, Moss CM, Daly V, et al: New approaches to limb salvage by extended extraanatomic bypasses and prosthetic reconstructions to foot arteries. Surgery 84:764–774, 1978.

147. Burrell MJ, Wheeler JR, Gregory RT, et al: Axillofemoral bypass. A ten-year review. Ann Surg 195:796–799, 1982.

148. Donaldson MC, Louras JC, Buckman CA: Axillofemoral bypass: A tool with a limited role. J Vasc Surg 3:757–763, 1986.

149. Anderson CB, Sicard GA, Etheredge EE: Bovine carotid artery and expanded polytetrafluoroethylene grafts for hemodialysis vascular access. J Surg Res 29:184–188, 1980.

150. Bone GE, Pomajzl MJ: Prospective comparison of polytetrafluoroethylene and bovine grafts for dialysis. J Surg Res 29:223–227, 1980.

151. Butler HG III, Baker LD Jr, Johnson JM: Vascular access for chronic hemodialysis: Polytetrafluoroethylene (PTFE) versus bovine heterograft. Am J Surg 134:791–793, 1977.

152. Tellis VA, Kohlberg WI, Bhat DJ, et al: Expanded polytetrafluoroethylene graft fistula for chronic hemodialysis. Ann Surg 189:101–105, 1979.

153. Hurt AV, Batello-Cruz M, Skipper BJ, et al: Bovine carotid artery heterografts versus polytetrafluoroethylene grafts. A prospective, randomized study. Am J Surg 146:844–847, 1983.

154. Palder SB, Kirkman RL, Whittemore AD, et al: Vascular access for hemodialysis. Patency rates and results of revision. Ann Surg 202:235–239, 1985.

155. Raju S: PTFE grafts for hemodialysis access. Techniques for insertion and management of complications. Ann Surg 206:666–673, 1987.

156. Donahoo JS, Gardne TJ, Kahka K, et al: Systemic pulmonary shunts in neonates and infants using microporous expanded polytetrafluoroethylene: Immediate and late results. Ann Thorac Surg 30:145–150, 1980.

157. Gloviczki P, Pairolero PC, Cherry KJ, et al: Reconstruction of the vena cava and of its primary tributaries: A preliminary report. J Vasc Surg 11:373–381, 1990.

158. Bergan JJ, Yao JST, Flinn WR, et al: Prosthetic grafts for the treatment of lower limb ischaemia: Present status. Br J Surg 69(suppl):534–537, 1982.

159. Graham LM, Bergan JJ: Expanded polytetrafluoroethylene vascular grafts: Clinical and experimental observations. *In* Stanley JC (ed): Biologic and Synthetic Vascular Prostheses. New York, Grune & Stratton, 1982, pp 563–586.

160. Quiñones-Baldrich WJ, Martin-Paredero V, Baker JD, et al: Polytetrafluoroethylene grafts as first-choice arterial substitute in femoropopliteal revascularization. Arch Surg 119:1238–1243, 1984.

161. Cranley JJ, Hafner CD: Revascularization of the femoropopliteal arteries using saphenous vein, polytetrafluoroethylene, and umbilical vein grafts. Arch Surg 177:1543–1550, 1982.

162. Hallett JW Jr, Brewster DC, Darling RC: The limitations of polytetrafluoroethylene in the reconstruction of femoropopliteal and tibial arteries. Surg Gynecol Obstet 152:819–821, 1981.

163. Hobson RW II, O'Donnell JA, Jamil Z, et al: Below-knee bypass for limb salvage. Comparison of autogenous saphenous vein, polytetrafluoroethylene, and composite Dacron-autogenous vein grafts. Arch Surg 115:833–837, 1980.

164. Tilanus HW, Obertop H, Van Urk H: Saphenous vein or PTFE for femoropopliteal bypass. A prospective randomized trial. Ann Surg 202:780–782, 1985.

165. Veith FJ, Gupta SK, Ascer E, et al: Six-year prospective multicenter randomized comparison of autologous saphenous vein and expanded polytetrafluoroethylene grafts in infrainguinal arterial reconstructions. J Vasc Surg 3:104–114, 1986.

166. Bergan JJ, Veith FJ, Bernhard VM, et al: Randomization of autogenous vein and polytetrafluoroethylene grafts in femoral-distal reconstruction. Surgery 92:921–930, 1982.

167. Gupta SK, Veith FJ, Kram HB, et al: Prospective, randomized comparison of ringed and nonringed polytetrafluoroethylene femoropopliteal bypass grafts: A preliminary report. J Vasc Surg 13:163–172, 1991.

168. Flinn WR, Rohrer MJ, Yao JST, et al: Improved long-term patency of infragenicular polytetrafluoroethylene grafts. J Vasc Surg 7:685–690, 1988.

169. Yeager A, Callow AD: New graft materials and current approaches to an acceptable small diameter vascular graft. Trans Am Soc Artif Intern Organs 34:88–94, 1988.

170. Cintora I, Pearce DE, Cannon JA: A clinical study of aortobifemoral bypass using two inherently different graft types. Ann Surg 208:625–630, 1988.

171. Corson JD, Reinhardt R, Von Grondell A, et al: Clinical and experimental evaluation of aortic polytetrafluoroethylene grafts for aneurysm replacement. Arch Surg 123:453–457, 1988.

172. Polterauer P, Prager M, Holzenbein T: Dacron versus polytetrafluoroethylene for Y-aortic bifurcation grafts: A six-year prospective study. Surgery 111:626–633, 1992.

173. Wakefield TW, Shulkin BL, Fellows EP, et al: Platelet reactivity in human aortic grafts: A prospective, randomized midterm study of platelet adherence and release products in Dacron and polytetrafluoroethylene conduits. J Vasc Surg 9:234–243, 1989.

174. Flinn WR, Flanigan DP, Verta MJ Jr, et al: Sequential femorotibial bypass for severe limb ischemia. Surgery 88:357–365, 1980.

175. Veith FJ, Gupta S, Daly V: Management of early and late thrombosis of expanded polytetrafluoroethylene (PTFE) femoropopliteal bypass grafts: Favorable prognosis with appropriate reoperation. Surgery 87:581–587, 1980.

176. O'Donnell TF Jr, Mackey W, McCullough JL Jr, et al: Correlation of operative findings with angiographic and noninvasive hemodynamic factors associated with failure of polytetrafluoroethylene grafts. J Vasc Surg 1:136–148, 1984.

177. Sladen JG, Maxwell TM: Experience with 130 polytetrafluoroethylene grafts. Am J Surg 141:546–548, 1981.

178. Carson SN, Hunter G, French S, et al: Occurrence of occlusive intimal changes in an expanded polytetrafluoroethylene graft. J Cardiovasc Surg 21:503–508, 1980.

179. Selman SH, Rhodes RS, Anderson JM, et al: Atheromatous changes in expanded polytetrafluoroethylene grafts. Surgery 87:630–637, 1980.

180. Herring M, Gardner A, Glover J: A single-stage technique for seeding vascular grafts with autogenous endothelium. Surgery 84:498–504, 1978.

181. Herring MB, Gardner A, Glover J: Seeding human arterial prostheses with mechanically derived endothelium. The detrimental effect of smoking. J Vasc Surg 1:279–289, 1984.

182. Graham LM, Burkel WE, Ford JW, et al: Immediate seeding of enzymatically derived endothelium in Dacron vascular grafts. Arch Surg 115:1289–1294, 1980.

183. Graham LM, Burkel WE, Ford JW, et al: Expanded polytetrafluoroethylene vascular prostheses seeded with en-

zymatically derived and cultured canine endothelial cells. Surgery *91*:550–559, 1982.

184. Jarrell BE, Williams SK, Stokes G, et al: Use of freshly isolated capillary endothelial cells for the immediate establishment of a monolayer on a vascular graft at surgery. Surgery *100*:392–399, 1986.

185. Rupnick MA, Hubbard FA, Pratt K, et al: Endothelialization of vascular prosthetic surfaces after seeding or sodding with human microvascular endothelial cells. J Vasc Surg *9*:788–795, 1989.

186. Sterpetti AV, Hunter WJ, Schultz RD, et al: Seeding with endothelial cells derived from the microvessels of the omentum and from the jugular vein: A comparative study. J Vasc Surg *7*:677–684, 1988.

187. Williams SK, Jarrell BE, Rose DG, et al: Human microvessel endothelial cell isolation and vascular graft sodding in the operating room. Ann Vasc Surg *3*:146–152, 1989.

188. Clagett GP, Burkel WE, Sharefkin JB, et al: Platelet reactivity in vivo in dogs with arterial prostheses seeded with endothelial cells. Circulation *69*:632–639, 1984.

189. Allen BT, Long JA, Welch MJ, et al: Influence of endothelial cell seeding on platelet deposition and patency in small-diameter Dacron arterial grafts. J Vasc Surg *1*:224–233, 1984.

190. Stanley JC, Burkel WE, Ford JW, et al: Enhanced patency of small-diameter, externally supported Dacron iliofemoral grafts seeded with endothelial cells. Surgery *92*:994–1005, 1982.

191. Herring M, Baughman S, Glover J: Endothelium develops on seeded human arterial prosthesis: A brief clinical note. J Vasc Surg *2*:727–730, 1985.

192. Ortenwall P, Wadenvick H, Kutti J, et al: Reduction in deposition of indium-111-labeled platelets after autologous endothelial cell seeding of Dacron aortic bifurcation grafts in humans: A preliminary study. J Vasc Surg *6*:17–25, 1987.

193. Ortenwall P, Wadenvick H, Risberg B: Reduced platelet deposition on seeded versus unseeded segments of expanded polytetrafluoroethylene grafts: Clinical observations after a 6-month follow-up. J Vasc Surg *10*:374–380, 1989.

194. Herring MB, Compton RS, LeGrand DR, et al: Endothelial seeding of polytetrafluoroethylene popliteal bypass. A preliminary report. J Vasc Surg *6*:114–118, 1987.

195. Zilla P, Fasol R, Deutsch M, et al: Endothelial cell seeding of polytetrafluoroethylene vascular grafts in humans: A preliminary report. J Vasc Surg *6*:535–541, 1987.

196. Magometschnigg H, Kadletz M, Vodrazka M, et al: Prospective clinical study with in vitro endothelial cell lining of expanded polytetrafluoroethylene grafts in crural repeat reconstruction. J Vasc Surg *15*:527–535, 1992.

197. Lyman DJ, Albo D, Jackson R, et al: Development of small

198. Lyman DJ, Metcalf LC, Albo D, et al: The effect of chemical structure and surface properties on synthetic polymers on the coagulation of blood. III. In vivo adsorption of proteins on polymer surfaces. Trans Am Soc Artif Intern Organs *20*:474–479, 1974.

199. Cronenwett JL, Zelenock GB: Alternative small arterial grafts. *In* Stanley JC (ed): Biologic and Synthetic Vascular Prostheses. New York, Grune & Stratton, 1982, pp 595–620.

200. Haubold A: Carbon in prosthetics. Ann NY Acad Sci *283*:383–395, 1977.

201. Sharp WV, Teague PC, Richenbacher WE: Thrombogenic potential of Dacron grafts after prior exposure to whole blood, plasma, or albumin. Trans Am Soc Artif Intern Organs *25*:275–279, 1979.

202. Sharp WV, Teague PC, Scott DL: Thromboresistance of pyrolytic carbon grafts. Trans Am Soc Artif Intern Organs *24*:223–228, 1978.

203. Garfinkle AM, Hoffman AS, Ratner BD, et al: Improved patency in small diameter Dacron vascular grafts after a tetrafluoroethylene glow discharge treatment. Trans Second World Congress Biomaterials *7*:337, 1987.

204. Annis D, Bornat A, Edwards RO, et al: An elastomeric vascular prosthesis. Trans Am Soc Artif Intern Organs *24*:209–214, 1978.

205. White RA, Klein SR, Shors EC: Preservation of compliance in a small diameter microporous, silicon rubber vascular prosthesis. J Cardiovasc Surg *28*:485–490, 1987.

206. White RA, White EW, Hanson EL, et al: Preliminary report: Evaluation of tissue ingrowth into experimental replamineform vascular prostheses. Surgery *79*:229–232, 1976.

207. Hallin RW, Sweetman WR: The Sparks mandril graft. Am J Surg *132*:221–223, 1976.

208. Parsonnet V, Tiro AC, Brief DK, et al: The fibrocollagenous tube as a small arterial prosthesis. *In* Dardik H (ed): Graft Materials in Vascular Surgery. Miami, Symposia Specialists, 1978, pp 249–262.

209. Ratto GB, Romano P, Truini M, et al: Glutaraldehyde-tanned mandril-grown grafts as venous substitutes. J Thorac Cardiovasc Surg *102*:440–447, 1991.

210. Greisler HP, Endean ED, Klosak JJ, et al: Polyglactin 910/polydioxanone biocomponent totally resorable vascular prostheses. J Vasc Surg *7*:697–705, 1988.

211. van der Lei B, Wildevuur CRH, Dijk F, et al: Sequential studies of arterial wall regeneration in microporous, compliant, biodegradable small-caliber vascular grafts in rats. J Thorac Cardiovasc Surg *93*:695–707, 1987.

212. Galletti PM, Aebischer P, Sasken HF, et al: Experience with fully bioresorbable aortic grafts in the dog. Surgery *103*:231–241, 1988.

213. Weinberg CB, Bell E: A blood vessel model constructed from collagen and cultured vascular cells. Science *231*:397–400, 1986.

REVIEW QUESTIONS

1. The greater saphenous vein is which one of the following?
   (a) formed by the confluence of the lateral marginal and external malleolar veins
   (b) a single trunk in the thigh in approximately 65 per cent of patients
   (c) nearly 40 cm in length in the adult male
   (d) contains more valves in the thigh than below the knee
   (e) too narrow for use in vascular reconstructions in 15 to 20 per cent of cases

2. All but which one of the following statements regarding vein graft alterations following arterial implantation are correct?
   (a) intimal thickening may follow an overgrowth of cellular elements within subendothelial tissue and fibrin layering on the surface
   (b) dysplastic lesions range from focal stenoses to diffuse narrowings of the entire graft
   (c) advanced intimal fibroplastic lesions have been noted in slightly less than 40 per cent of lower extremity vein conduits
   (d) excessive clamp trauma typically causes a focal stenosis
   (e) aneurysmal aortorenal vein grafts are more likely to develop in children than adults

3. Advantages of arterial autographs include which one of the following?

   (a) radial, splenic, and internal iliac arteries can be used as free interposition grafts with comparable clinical results

   (b) an intrinsic arterial wall blood supply that remains intact during transplantation

   (c) absolute absence of aneurysmal changes in transplanted grafts

   (d) widespread availability of suitable arterial autografts

4. Experimental and clinical experience with umbilical vein allografts reveals which one of the following?

   (a) umbilical vein grafts may be handled similar to fabric prostheses

   (b) their increased compliance persists long after implantation

   (c) aneurysmal deterioration affects nearly 50 per cent of these grafts in long-term follow-up

   (d) five-year femoropopliteal bypass patency rates are approximately 20 per cent

   (e) thrombectomy is easily performed for late thromboses in these grafts

5. The one best choice of graft material among the following is:

   (a) braided material for aortorenal bypass

   (b) knitted material for aortobifemoral bypass in a patient requiring hemodialysis

   (c) expanded PTFE for a below-knee femoropopliteal bypass

   (d) woven material for a descending thoracic aortic replacement

   (e) knitted velour material in a contaminated groin wound

6. Expanded PTFE grafts are which one of the following?

   (a) highly electronegative

   (b) comparable to saphenous vein in the femorotibial position

   (c) prone to aneurysmal dilation

   (d) very prone to infection compared to heterografts when used for angioacess

   (e) made of Teflon textile material

7. Modified bovine xenografts are which one of the following?

   (a) exhibit patency rates comparable to autogenous saphenous veins for femorotibial revascularization procedures

   (b) develop aneurysms in 80 per cent of femoropopliteal bypass grafts

   (c) commonly used for femoropopliteal bypasses

   (d) acceptable conduits for angioaccess

   (e) exhibit patency rates twice as good as with fabric grafts for femoropopliteal revascularization procedures

8. All but which one of the following is true concerning fabric prostheses?

   (a) often associated with implantation bleeding when porosity exceeds 4000 ml/sq cm/min

   (b) usefulness relates more to fabrication than particular type of material

   (c) when woven have little stretch in the warp, fill, or on the bias

   (d) may have added elasticity imparted by crimping

   (e) exhibit greater healing and incorporation when tightly woven

9. Characteristics of an ideal vascular prosthesis are best typified by which one of the following?

   (a) biocompatible with a nonthrombogenic surface

   (b) physically durable

   (c) resistant to infection

   (d) technically easy to implant

   (e) all of the above

10. All but which one of the following statements about vascular grafts are true?

   (a) autogenous saphenous vein is preferred over expanded PTFE or umbilical vein allografts for most arterial reconstructions in the lower extremity

   (b) thrombogenicity of luminal surfaces limits the usefulness of many small-caliber grafts

   (c) the ideal vascular prosthesis has yet to be developed

   (d) fibrocollagenous tubes as vascular conduits offer excellent long-term patency rates

   (e) degenerative changes often compromise the function of biologic grafts

ANSWERS

1. b	2. c	3. b	4. c	5. d	6. a	7. d
8. e	9. e	10. d				

22

THORACOABDOMINAL AORTIC ANEURYSMS

LARRY H. HOLLIER, ROBERT J. MARINO, and FRANCIS J. KAZMIER

Thoracoabdominal aortic aneurysms continue to present a dramatic challenge to the vascular surgeon. Since surgical repair involves the vasculature of multiple organ systems, the potential for major morbidity is great and the risk of operative mortality is high. Despite this, careful preoperative evaluation of the patient, identification of specific risk factors, methodical operative technique, and diligent perioperative management can allow successful thoracoabdominal aneurysm repair with acceptable morbidity and mortality.

NATURAL HISTORY

Thoracoabdominal aortic aneurysms, like infrarenal aortic aneurysms, represent degenerative structural changes within the muscular, elastic, and collagen components of the aortic wall. Simple mechanical stress factors will generally assure that progressive enlargement of the aneurysm will occur over time. Extrapolation of Laplace's law suggests that the tension on the wall of the aorta is progressively increased in direct relationship to the diameter of the aorta; thus, the larger an aneurysm, the greater the tension on the aortic wall at a given systemic pressure.

In a series reported by Crawford and DeNatale,[1] 94 patients who did not undergo aneurysm repair had a 2-year survival rate of only 24 per cent. Half of the deaths were due to aneurysm rupture. In those patients in whom the etiology of the thoracoabdominal aneurysm was dissection, 69 per cent of the deaths were due to rupture, whereas 46 per cent of the deaths were from rupture if the etiology of the aneurysm was atherosclerosis. The overall 5-year survival was 19 per cent. These data are similar to that reported by Bickerstaff et al.,[2] wherein we noted a 2-year actuarial survival rate of 28.7 per cent in patients with untreated thoracic and thoracoabdominal aneurysms. The 5-year survival of unoperated dissecting aneurysms was 7 per cent, and was 19.2 per cent for those with nondissecting aneurysms. Here

also, rupture was a major cause of death. In contrast, the expected survival of patients following repair of thoracic and thoracoabdominal aneurysms is quite good. Crawford et al. reported a 70 per cent 2-year survival and 59 per cent 5-year survival among 605 patients who underwent thoracoabdominal aneurysm repair.[3]

Although neither of these studies was able to stratify risk of rupture in relation to aneurysm size, the overall rates suggest that thoracic and thoracoabdominal aneurysms pose a greater risk of rupture than abdominal aortic aneurysms and thus an aggressive approach should be taken toward repair of these aneurysms.

DIAGNOSIS

Except for intermittent or chronic back pain (a common complaint in the elderly) thoracic and thoracoabdominal aneurysms are usually asymptomatic until the time of rupture, although some patients will report a significant worsening of back pain in the days or weeks prior to rupture; this may be due to rapid expansion of the aneurysm, localized intramural dissection, or contained perforation of the aneurysm. In a previous review of 101 patients undergoing repair of thoracoabdominal aortic aneurysm, we noted 18 per cent required emergency operation for frank or impending rupture.[4]

In most asymptomatic patients, diagnosis of thoracoabdominal aortic aneurysm is suggested on a routine chest roentgenogram (Fig. 22–1). This finding may then prompt further diagnostic evaluation (unfortunately, a thoracoabdominal aneurysm evident on a plain film is frequently misinterpreted as "tortuosity"). Although ultrasound provides satisfactory evaluation of lower abdominal aortic pathology, it is less accurate in evaluating the suprarenal aorta and is of no value in assessing the thoracic aorta.

Computed tomography is an excellent technique

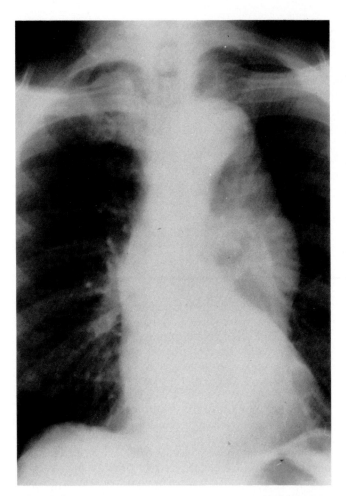

FIGURE 22–1. Chest x-ray demonstrating prominent parasternal mass in the left chest due to a large thoracoabdominal aneurysm.

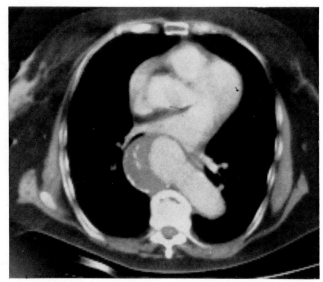

FIGURE 22–2. Computed tomographic scan of the distal thoracic aorta as it courses medially in the lower chest. Note the large amount of thrombus present at the site of aneurysmal expansion.

for evaluating thoracoabdominal aortic aneurysms, since it allows accurate delineation of aortic pathology, including extent of aneurysmal changes, relationship of the visceral vessels, and the location and amount of thrombus present within the aneurysm (Fig. 22–2). Magnetic resonance imaging is also an accurate noninvasive means of visualizing thoracoabdominal aortic aneurysm pathology, although it is somewhat more expensive than computed tomography (Fig. 22–3).

Angiography is less accurate in determining the actual size of aneurysms, since laminated thrombus in the aneurysm may result in incorrect interpretation of aortic size based on the diameter of the column of contrast material in the aortic lumen. However, in patients with thoracoabdominal aortic aneurysm angiography is usually recommended to aid in evaluating the patency of the visceral vessels (Fig. 22–4).

PREOPERATIVE EVALUATION

Patients with thoracoabdominal aortic aneurysms are generally elderly and share the various physical disorders commonly associated with age and ather-

osclerosis. Table 22–1 lists the associated risk factors and their relative prevalence among 101 patients with thoracoabdominal aortic aneurysms we previously reported.[4] To minimize the risk of operative repair it is helpful to routinely evaluate these common problems as well as any others suggested by history or physical examination.

Preoperative evaluation of a patient being considered for thoracoabdominal aortic aneurysm repair usually includes: complete blood count, chest x-ray, urinalysis, serum chemistry profile (including liver enzymes and electrolytes), platelet count, prothrombin time, partial thromboplastin time, arterial blood gases, stress electrocardiogram or cardiac function test such as dipyridamole-thallium scan, carotid duplex scan, computed tomographic scan of chest and abdomen, and visceral aortography. If the arterial blood gases are abnormal or if the patient has findings of chronic pulmonary disease, pulmonary function tests may be performed. If the patient has significant angina or if the electrocardiogram or cardiac function study suggests significant coronary artery stenosis, coronary angiography is performed; if critical coronary artery lesions are identified, they are often treated with balloon angioplasty or coronary bypass prior to repair of the thoracoabdominal aortic aneurysm. If carotid ultrasound discloses carotid stenosis of greater than 70 per cent, carotid endarterectomy is generally performed before aneurysm repair.

Patients who are to undergo thoracoabdominal aortic aneurysm repair are brought into the hospital 1 or more days prior to surgery for pulmonary preparation, including use of antibiotics and bronchodilators, preoperative hydration, and mechanical bowel preparation. Cephalosporin antibiotics are started the day prior to operation. If the patient has an elevation of creatinine that occurs after angiography, the opera-

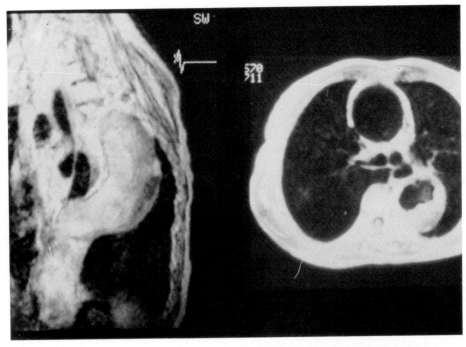

FIGURE 22–3. Magnetic resonance image of patient with type I thoracoabdominal aneurysm.

tion is usually delayed for 1 or 2 weeks to allow renal function to improve and the creatinine level to return to baseline.

OPERATIVE TECHNIQUE

When the patient is taken to the operating room, the participation of a skilled anesthesiologist is critical. A double-lumen endotracheal tube is bronchoscopically inserted to facilitate complete collapse of the left lung during exposure of the descending thoracic aorta. Monitoring lines include a Swan-Ganz catheter, a radial artery line for blood pressure monitoring and sampling of arterial blood gases, and an intrathecal catheter for drainage of cerebrospinal fluid (CSF) and continuous monitoring of spinal fluid pressure, both intraoperatively and postoperatively.[5,6] The

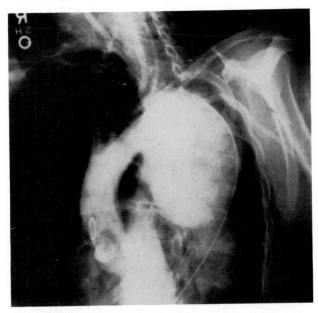

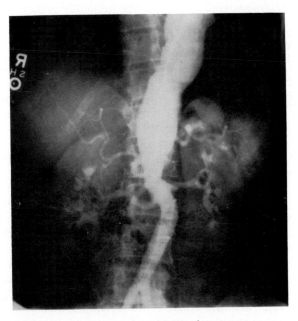

FIGURE 22–4. Angiography of patient with type I thoracoabdominal aortic aneurysm showing large upper thoracic aneurysm, a tapering aneurysm down to the level of the visceral vessels, and a normal infrarenal aorta with no renal artery stenosis.

TABLE 22–1.   RISK FACTORS

Risk Factor	Incidence (%)
Coronary artery disease	67
Strokes/transient ischemic attacks	12
Chronic lung disease	42
Renal insufficiency	38
Diabetes mellitus	6
Smoking history	90

intrathecal catheter is also used to administer 0.1 to 0.3 mg preservative-free morphine sulfate for postoperative analgesia. Two large-bore central venous catheters are placed for infusion of blood via the Haemonetics rapid infusion system. In those patients who have impaired cardiac reserve, use of transesophageal two-dimensional echocardiography is also helpful in the determination of end-diastolic ventricular volume and early detection of ischemia.

The patient is positioned in the right lateral decubitus position on an air-controlled "bean bag" and the hips are allowed to fall into a more supine position. The air is then evacuated from the "bean bag," holding the patient stable in the desired position. The thoracoabdominal incision is then made in the fourth or fifth intercostal space for a type I or high type II thoracoabdominal aortic aneurysm or in the seventh to ninth interspace for a type III or a type IV thoracoabdominal aortic aneurysm.[6]

The abdominal incision is then carried down the midline or paramedian area from a high intercostal incision or is made obliquely across the abdomen from a low intercostal incision. If necessary for added exposure, the rib above and below the incision can be transected posteriorly to allow a broader operative field and one rib may even be excised if necessary on some extensive aneurysms. We generally will try to avoid separate incisions in different interspaces, since this makes intercostal reimplantation more difficult.

The abdominal dissection is continued in an extraperitoneal plane. Small rents that might occur in the peritoneum during the course of the dissection are repaired with Prolene suture and felt pledgets. The dissection is continued down through the diaphragm in a circumferential fashion, with marking sutures of different color alternated along the incision to facilitate closure of the diaphragm at the completion of the procedure. The crus of the diaphragm is divided to the left of the aorta and the aorta is exposed along its entire length, including a segment of normal aorta both above and below the aneurysm. The visceral vessels are identified but no attempt is made to encircle or obtain specific control of them.

One thousand units of heparin are injected intraarterially through the aortic wall but systemic heparinization is otherwise not used. The distal aortic clamp is placed first; the proximal aortic clamp is then placed and the occluded segment of aneurysm is opened vertically. The left renal artery is then cannulated and the kidney is perfused with cold Collins solution. If

an area of segmental narrowing is noted along the course of the aneurysm, the distal clamp may be placed initially at this intermediate level rather than opening the entire aneurysm at once. A graft of appropriate diameter is selected and is sutured to the proximal normal aorta with running sutures of 0 Prolene on a V-7 needle. If intercostal arteries are evident near the area of the anastomosis, the edge of the graft is excised posteriorly and the proximal anastomosis is performed obliquely so that the anastomosis includes these intercostal arteries within a posterior tongue of aortic wall. After completion of this anastomosis, the proximal clamp is moved onto the graft and flow is restored to these proximal intercostal arteries. A segment of posterior graft wall is then excised and additional intercostal arteries are reimplanted into the graft in a side-to-side fashion. We try to revascularize as many pairs of intercostal arteries as is technically feasible. Occasionally, in extensive aneurysms, this may require two separate aortic wall cuffs when multiple intercostals are to be reimplanted (Fig. 22–5). In some patients with extensive difficult aneurysms we may proceed directly to visceral revascularization (to minimize risk of pre-

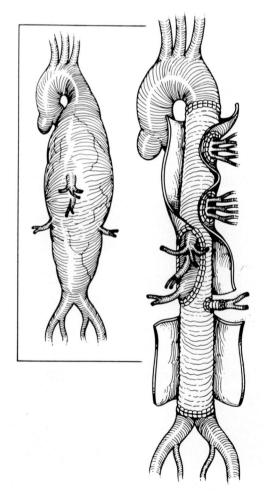

FIGURE 22–5.   Illustration of multicuff reimplantation technique for repair of extensive type II thoracoabdominal aortic aneurysm.

cipitating disseminated intravascular coagulation due to prolonged visceral ischemia[8]) and then revascularize the intercostal arteries by means of separate grafts (Fig. 22–6). After completion of intercostal reimplantation, the clamp on the graft is moved distal to this area and flow is instituted through the additional intercostal vessels. The visceral vessels are then reimplanted into the graft after excising a portion of graft wall of appropriate size. As a general rule, an attempt is made to reimplant the celiac, superior mesenteric, and renal arteries in a single cuff. In some patients this may be more safely performed in two cuffs, with the celiac, superior mesenteric, and right renal arteries in one cuff and the left renal artery in the other. Flow is then slowly restored to the visceral vessels while the distal aortic anastomosis is being completed.

At each step of sequential unclamping of the aorta, particularly when restoring flow to the visceral vessels and the lower extremities, the clamp should be opened slowly while the anesthesiologist provides rapid infusion of blood and crystalloid. This is especially important, since declamping hypotension can be particularly dramatic at this point. Additional administration of sodium bicarbonate is necessary, as well as is pharmacologic cardiac support.

After completion of revascularization, the sac of the aneurysm is closed tightly over the entire length of the graft with running suture of 3-0 or 0 Prolene. This is done primarily to achieve tamponade of any continued oozing that may occur from the graft, anastomotic sites, or aneurysm wall. If the aneurysm sac is of insufficient extent to fully cover the graft, we use a segment of Gore-Tex membrane to fill in this gap and to thus provide complete coverage of the graft (Fig. 22–7). In some cases of continued ooze from the interstices of the graft, we have injected fibrin glue into the closed sac of the aneurysm sur-

rounding the graft to stop this troublesome bleeding. At this point in the procedure, after restoration of flow, the anesthesiologist will routinely give 4 units of fresh-frozen plasma and 10 units of platelets. A thromboelastogram is then performed and additional component therapy is given as necessary to return the thromboelastogram to normal. It is not uncommon to see fibrinolysis occur at this stage of the procedure. If so, an infusion of Amicar is started and may be continued for 12 to 24 hours postoperatively.

The diaphragm is repaired with interrupted mattress sutures of 2-0 Ethibond and two chest tubes are brought out through stab incisions in the left mid-axillary line. Ordinarily, no subdiaphragmatic drains are used. The chest and abdomen are closed in layers in standard fashion and the patient is sent to the intensive care unit under close observation.

In the immediate postoperative period, the patient is continued on low-dose dopamine (2.5 mg/kg/min) and lactated Ringer's solution is given to replace urine output on a deciliter-for-deciliter basis. The patient is maintained on a respirator with no attempt being made to wean him until the following day. Blood pressure is closely regulated and maintained at the patent's normal preoperative level. Arterial blood gases, cardiac indices, coagulation studies, and serum electrolytes are monitored frequently and maintained within his preoperative normal ranges.

Maintenance fluid is decreased daily from the initial rate of 125 ml/hr in the immediate postoperative period down to 60 ml/hr by the third postoperative day. Urine replacement is stopped after the first 12 to 24 hours. By the third postoperative day the patient will generally start to mobilize fluid rapidly from the interstitial space and furosemide may be given at this point to minimize pulmonary congestion. The patient is carefully weaned from the respirator starting the day after surgery and extubated when gases

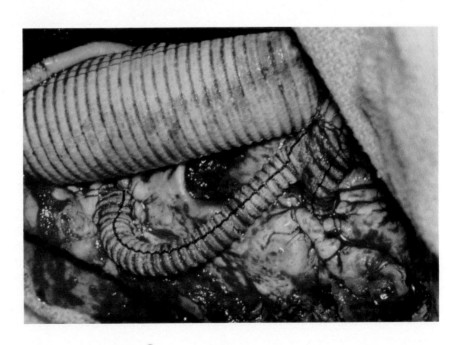

FIGURE 22–6. Operative photograph showing bifurcation graft used to revascularize multiple sets of intercostal arteries.

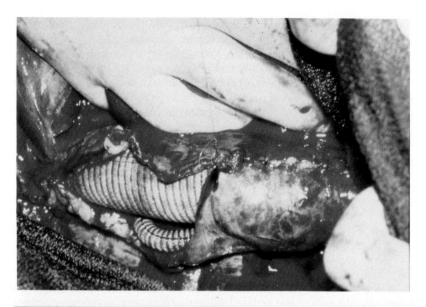

A

B

FIGURE 22–7. Operative photograph demonstrating use of Gore-Tex membrane to provide complete coverage of a thoracoabdominal graft.

are able to be maintained without support. Chest tubes are generally removed between the second and fifth postoperative day.

COMPLICATIONS

It is commonly recognized that the extensive operation required to repair thoracoabdominal aneurysms is associated with significant morbidity and mortality. Table 22–2 lists the major complications and Table 22–3 the minor complications that occurred in 83 elective thoracoabdominal aneurysm repairs that we previously reported.[4] As evident from this table, morbidity and mortality were significant. Nonetheless, in a subset of these patients who underwent elective repair under a standardized protocol, the mortality rate was reduced to 1.8 per cent, need

TABLE 22–2. MAJOR COMPLICATIONS

Complication	Incidence (%)
Death	9.6
Myocardial infarction	7.2
Dialysis	2.4
Paralysis/paresis	6.0
Pulmonary insufficiency	33.7
Cerebrovascular accident	4.8

for dialysis to 0 per cent, and the risk of myocardial infarction to 1.8 per cent.[4] A standardized protocol, however, did not reduce the incidence of pulmonary insufficiency, postoperative elevation of creatinine, or neurologic deficit. It should be noted, however, that during the time of this study adjunctive measures to prevent paraplegia, such as CSF drainage,

TABLE 22–3. MINOR COMPLICATIONS

Complication	Incidence (%)
Arrhythmia	36.1
Subendocardial myocardial infarction	8.4
Creatinine elevation without dialysis	15.7
Splenectomy	19.3
Hemorrhage	7.2
Distal emboli or thrombosis	6.0
Wound complication	12.0
Pneumonia	15.7
Urinary tract infection	14.5
Reoperation	25.3

cooling, intravenous high-dose Pentothal, etc., were not employed. Since the routine use of these adjunctive measures, paraplegia has been dramatically reduced.[15]

Pulmonary insufficiency, or prolonged need for ventilatory support, is the most common complication and to this date remains an unsolved problem.[4] Since many of these patients do have chronic obstructive pulmonary disease and a long history of smoking, this is readily understandable. Nonetheless, the occurrence of prolonged postoperative respiratory insufficiency puts the patient at an increased risk of pneumonia and other complications. This problem does not seem to be affected by the type of diaphragmatic incision used (radial versus circumferential) nor by the type of abdominal dissection (transperitoneal versus extraperitoneal). Nonetheless, meticulous attention to pulmonary toilet, serial blood gas determinations, and gradual weaning of the patient from the respirator usually allow successful extubation of the patient despite prolonged ventilatory support. More recently, we have found the use of transcutaneous oxygen monitoring to be particularly helpful in following the minute-by-minute course of these patients.

Although the patient undergoing repair of thoracoabdominal aortic aneurysm is at significant risk of developing some complication, it is important to realize that in our previous report on 101 thoracoabdominal aneurysm repairs, 41 per cent of the patients tolerated thoracoabdominal aneurysm repair without any complications and were discharged from the hospital in less than 2 weeks.[4] Currently, a patient undergoing repair of a thoracoabdominal aneurysm who suffers no complication is generally able to be discharged from the hospital in approximately 7 to 10 days.

PREVENTION OF COMPLICATIONS

Renal failure is obviously one of the major concerns following repair of thoracoabdominal aortic aneurysms. It appears that the two major determinants of postoperative renal failure are length of renal ischemia time and extent of preoperative renal dysfunction. Crawford's data clearly demonstrated these

to be the major etiologic factors that result in need for dialysis after thoracoabdominal aortic aneurysm repair.[3,7] In our experience, renal perfusion using cold Collins solution has appeared to be beneficial, especially in those patients who have preexisting renal dysfunction.

It would also seem beneficial to restore normal blood flow as rapidly as possible. However, it would seem prudent to minimize preoperative renal dysfunction by avoiding operation immediately after angiography and by providing adequate preoperative hydration. Hydration can be accomplished most safely by using a Swan-Ganz catheter and obtaining serial cardiac indices to determine the degree of volume load needed to maximize cardiac output. Obviously, this also is greatly advantageous in minimizing intraoperative cardiac dysfunction.

During operation, adequate crystalloid is given initially to maintain optimum left atrial filling pressures. We usually also give 25 gm of mannitol shortly after making the skin incision; furosemide 20 mg is given intravenously about 30 minutes prior to aortic cross-clamping. This places the kidneys in a diuretic state and minimizes the secondary renal tubular damage that can occur after ischemia. Despite these measures, however, preexisting dysfunction may still worsen and result in the need for dialysis, although it is rare for renal failure to occur if the patient had normal renal function preoperatively.

Myocardial infarction, left ventricular failure, ventricular arrhythmias, and cardiac arrest can be seen as a consequence of thoracic aortic cross-clamping. Thoracic aortic occlusion can cause increased left ventricular afterload and increased end-diastolic pressure; this can markedly decrease endocardial perfusion and result in dysfunction or infarction. Afterload can be decreased by the use of nitroprusside, nitroglycerin, heparin-bonded shunts, and femorofemoral or atriofemoral bypass. Use of any of these techniques is associated with some risks, but they are effective in reducing afterload. Femorofemoral bypass requires heparinization and is associated with increased hemorrhagic complications, and atriofemoral bypass has the risk of air embolization. Insertion of shunts can provide adequate, although limited, off-loading of the left ventricle but is sometimes complicated by aortic disruption and bleeding from the cannulation sites. Nitroprusside and nitroglycerin provide effective vasodilatation but do not ensure perfusion of the lower extremities and are thus more often associated with declamping hypotension. This latter problem can be minimized by the use of the rapid infusion pump and gradual release of the aortic clamp. Close cooperation between the surgeon and anesthesiologist is critical at this time.

Hemorrhage is a worrisome problem associated with the extensive revascularization required in repair of thoracoabdominal aortic aneurysm. Bleeding can occur not only from the sites of operative dissection and from the anastomotic suture lines, but disseminated intravascular coagulation (DIC) can occur and result in diffuse bleeding from the interstices of the graft and from the entire operative field. Experimental work by ourselves and by others[8,9] has shown that DIC can be induced by prolonged clamping of the visceral arteries, specifically the superior mesenteric artery. This provides the surgeon with added stimulus to accomplish revascularization rapidly and to promptly restore visceral blood flow. The new coated or impregnated grafts may prove to be especially beneficial in those cases in which DIC may occur; fibrin glue is sometimes useful in controlling bleeding through the graft interstices and through needle holes. After completion of the repair and restoration of flow, we routinely plan to give at least 4 units of fresh-frozen plasma and 10 units of platelets. Coagulation is evaluated by the thromboelastogram and additional coagulation components are given as needed.

Paraplegia remains an unsolved problem. Multiple techniques have been utilized over the past 15 years in attempts to prevent spinal cord injury, but no one technique has proven sufficient. Shunts and bypass techniques have been shown to be effective in reducing the incidence of paraplegia following repair of thoracic aortic aneurysms when prolonged aortic clamping was necessary[10,11]; however, they have not prevented paraplegia when used for repair of extensive thoracoabdominal aortic aneurysms.[12] Spinal cord monitoring (somatosensory-evoked potentials and motor-evoked potentials) is feasible but does not, in itself, prevent paraplegia; it merely allows one to know when neurologic injury is occurring.[13] Selective preoperative intercostal angiography has been done in an attempt to identify the arteria magna and/or predominant blood supply to the anterior spinal artery; this has allowed selective revascularization of the dominant intercostal artery but has not reduced the incidence of paraplegia.[14] More recently, we have been using CSF drainage to improve spinal cord perfusion; this has proven effective in our hands, although we, as well as other centers, have still had neurologic deficits occur.[5,15]

At the present time, our attempts to prevent paraplegia consists of a multifaceted approach: reducing cord metabolism, increasing spinal cord perfusion pressure, and reducing the effects of reperfusion hyperemia (Fig. 22–8). Spinal cord metabolism is presumably similar to that of the brain. Barbiturates have been demonstrated to reduce neuronal metabolism and decrease injury following incomplete ischemia of the brain, and cooling has shown a similar protective effect.[16–21] Recently, we have documented the effectiveness of both Pentothal and cooling in reducing the incidence of paraplegia in the rabbit spinal cord ischemia model.[21] During the early operative stages of the thoracoabdominal aortic aneurysm repair, we do not attempt to warm the patient nor do we warm the intravenous fluids. This allows the patient's temperature to drift down slightly, usually to around 32° to 34°C, reducing metabolism of the cord by approximately 20 per cent.[19,20] In addition, we give a large bolus of barbiturate, 20 mg/kg of Pentothal, intravenously about 15 minutes prior to cross-clamping the thoracic aorta. After revascularization is completed and the aorta is unclamped, the patient is warmed rapidly by warming the operating room and all intravenous fluids and blood administered. These efforts, we believe, allow prolongation of the safe clamp time, allowing time for more complete revascularization of the intercostal arteries.

Spinal cord perfusion pressure can be increased by shunts, bypass, CSF drainage, and elevation of proximal aortic pressure.[5,6] In most cases, we rely simply on CSF drainage and monitoring and use nitroprusside infusion to maintain the proximal aortic systolic pressure 20 per cent above preoperative levels, or about 140 to 160 mm Hg systolic pressure. During the time of aortic occlusion, CSF pressure is monitored continuously and additional CSF is withdrawn as necessary to keep the CSF pressure below 10 mm Hg. Postoperatively, CSF monitoring is continued for about 3 days.

The most effective method of reducing reperfusion injury is to prevent the initial ischemia of the cord. As much as possible, this is accomplished by the techniques described above. However, theoretically the additional use of free-radical scavengers would seem advantageous when ischemia does occur, and experimental use of superoxide dismutase has shown some promise in this regard, although it is not yet available for human use.[22] At the present time we use intravenous steroids, 30 mg/kg of Solu-Medrol, and 100 mg of hydrocortisone phosphate, given at the start of the operation, plus 12.5 gm intravenous mannitol (a mildly effective free-radical scavenger) just prior to declamping. We have not yet documented the effectiveness of steroids and mannitol in reducing reperfusion injury and postoperative cord edema, although experimental studies suggest they may be beneficial.[17,22]

RESULTS

In a personal series of 150 cases undergoing repair of nondissecting thoracoabdominal aortic aneurysms, the intraoperative mortality has been 3.3 per cent and the overall 30-day mortality is 10 per cent. The overall incidence of neurologic deficit (paraplegia/paraparesis) was 4.0 per cent.[15] Since the routine use of CSF drainage, no patient has awakened with a spinal cord deficit, although three patients developed late-onset paraparesis. One of these patients did not have intercostal reimplantation because of technical difficulties; she developed paresis on the fifth day after operation but is now able to walk, although she still has a persisting deficit. Another patient sustained an intraoperative cardiac arrest due to transient hyperkalemia, was successfully resuscitated, and awoke with no neurologic difficulties; around noon on the day after operation he developed paraparesis and immediately underwent drainage of an additional 40

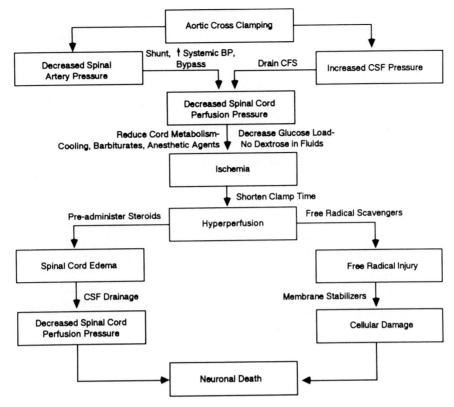

FIGURE 22–8. Schematic diagram of neurologic injury cascade precipitated by aortic clamping during thoracoabdominal aortic aneurysm repair. Potential methods of decreasing injury are depicted for each stage.

dl of CSF; within 8 hours his deficit was fully resolved and he had no further difficulty; he was discharged from the hospital, ambulatory, on the 10th postoperative day.

Since instituting our multimodality adjunctive protocol in 1989, we have repaired 42 thoracoabdominal aneurysms, including 20 type I and type II aneurysms. In these patients, we have had no occurrence of paraplegia or paraparesis.

It is obvious that these numbers are relatively small and do not allow definitive determination of the effectiveness of adjunctive techniques in the repair of thoracoabdominal aortic aneurysm. Nonetheless, it does appear that thoracoabdominal aortic aneurysms can be repaired with increasing safety. This should encourage surgeons to undertake earlier intervention in these patients.

CONCLUSION

It is evident that thoracoabdominal aortic aneurysms are being diagnosed with increasing frequency and vascular surgeons are being called upon to provide surgical correction. Although repair of diffuse aneurysms presents the spectre of formidable complications, careful preoperative evaluation, standardized operative technique, and meticulous postoperative care can result in satisfactory repair of thoracoabdominal aortic aneurysms with acceptable morbidity and mortality.

REFERENCES

1. Crawford ES, DeNatale RW: Thoracoabdominal aortic aneurysm: Observation regarding the natural course of the disease. J Vasc Surg 3:578–582, 1986.
2. Bickerstaff LK, Pairolero PC, Hollier LH, et al: Thoracic aortic aneurysms: A population-based study. Surgery 92:1103–1108, 1982.
3. Crawford ES, Crawford JL, Safi HJ, et al: Thoracoabdominal aortic aneurysms: Preoperative and intraoperative factors determining immediate and long-term results of operations in 605 patients. J Vasc Surg 3:389–404, 1986.
4. Hollier LH, Symmonds JB, Pairolero PC, et al: Thoracoab-

dominal aortic aneurysm repair: Analysis of postoperative morbidity. Arch Surg 123:871–875, 1988.
5. McCullough JL, Hollier LH, Nugent M: Paraplegia after thoracic aorta occlusion: Influence of cerebrospinal fluid drainage: Experimental and early clinical results. J Vasc Surg 7:153–160, 1988.
6. Hollier LH: Technical modifications in the repair of thoracoabdominal aortic aneurysms. *In* Greenhalgh RM (ed): Vascular Surgical Techniques, 2nd ed. London, WB Saunders Company, 1989, pp 144–151.
7. Svensson LG, Coselli JS, Safi HJ, et al: Appraisal of adjuncts

to prevent acute renal failure after surgery on the thoracic or thoracoabdominal aorta. J Vasc Surg 10:230–239, 1989.

8. Cohen JR, Angus L, Asher A, et al: Disseminated intravascular coagulation as a result of supraceliac clamping: Implications for thoracoabdominal aortic aneurysm repair. Ann Vasc Surg 5:552–557, 1987.

9. Cohen JR, Schroder W, Leal J, et al: Mesenteric shunting during thoracoabdominal aortic clamping to prevent disseminated intravascular coagulation in dogs. Ann Vasc Surg 2:261–267, 1988.

10. Livesay JJ, Cooley DA, Ventimiglia RA, et al: Surgical experience in descending thoracic aneurysmectomy with and without adjuncts to avoid ischemia. Ann Thorac Surg 39:37–46, 1985.

11. Jex RK, Schaff HV, Piehler JM, et al: Early and late results following repair of dissection of the descending thoracic aorta. J Vasc Surg 3:226–237, 1986.

12. Crawford ES, Walker HS, Saleh SA, et al: Graft replacement of aneurysm in descending thoracic aorta: Results without bypass or shunting. Surgery 89:73–85, 1981.

13. Cunningham JN Jr, Laschinger MD, Merkin HA, et al: Measurement of spinal cord ischemia during operations upon the thoracic aorta. Ann Surg 196:285–296, 1982.

14. Kieffer E, Richard T, Chiras J, et al: Preoperative spinal cord arteriography in aneurysmal disease of the descending thoracic and thoracoabdominal aorta: Preliminary results in 45 patients. Ann Vasc Surg 3:34–46, 1989.

15. Hollier LH, Money SR, Naslund TC, et al: The risk of spinal cord dysfunction in 150 consecutive patients undergoing thoracoabdominal aortic replacement. Am J Surg (accepted for publication).

16. Stein PA, Mitchenfelder JD: Cerebral protection with barbiturates: Relation to anesthetic effect. Stroke 9:140–142, 1978.

17. Hollier LH: Protecting the brain and spinal cord. J Vasc Surg 5:524–528, 1987.

18. Arnfred I, Secher O: Anoxia and barbiturates: Tolerance to anoxia in mice influenced by barbiturates. Arch Int Pharmacodyn Ther 139:67–74, 1962.

19. Vacanti FX, Ames A III: Mild hypothermia and magnesium protect against irreversible damage during CNS ischemia. Stroke 15:695–698, 1984.

20. Coles JG, Wilson GJ, Sima AF, et al: Intraoperative management of thoracic aortic aneurysm, experimental evaluation of perfusion cooling of the spinal cord. J Thorac Cardiovasc Surg 85:292–299, 1983.

21. Naslund TC, Hollier LH, Money SR, et al: Protecting the ischemic spinal cord during aortic clamping: The influence of anesthetics and hypothermia. Ann Surg 212(5):409–416, 1992.

22. Coles JG, Ahmed SN, Mehta HU, et al: Role of free radical scavengers in protection of spinal cord during ischemia. Ann Thorac Surg 41:551–556, 1986.

REVIEW QUESTIONS

1. The 2-year life expectancy of a patient with unoperated thoracoabdominal aortic aneurysm is:
   (a) 5 per cent
   (b) 24 per cent
   (c) 67 per cent
   (d) 81 per cent

2. The most accurate modality for diagnosis of thoracoabdominal aortic aneurysm is:
   (a) physical exam
   (b) ultrasound
   (c) computed tomography
   (d) angiography

3. The most frequent complication associated with repair of thoracoabdominal aortic aneurysm is:
   (a) myocardial infarction
   (b) paraplegia
   (c) prolonged ventilator dependence
   (d) disseminated intravascular coagulation

4. The major determinant of postoperative renal dysfunction following thoracoabdominal aortic aneurysm repair is:

   (a) preoperative renal dysfunction
   (b) intraoperative bleeding
   (c) prolonged aortic clamp time
   (d) use of shunts or bypass

5. Early restoration of visceral flow during thoracoabdominal aortic aneurysm repair:
   (a) reduces left ventricular afterload
   (b) reduces risk of DIC
   (c) reduces declamping hypotension
   (d) all of the above

6. Routine intercostal artery reimplantation will prevent paraplegia. True or false?

7. CSF drainage will prevent paraplegia. True or false?

8. Routine use of heparin-bonded shunts will prevent paraplegia. True or false?

9. Reducing the metabolic rate of the spinal cord may reduce neurologic injury associated with thoracoabdominal aortic aneurysm repair. True or false?

10. Avoiding use of heparin during thoracoabdominal aortic aneurysm repair will prevent hemorrhagic complications. True or false?

ANSWERS

| 1. b | 2. c | 3. c | 4. a | 5. d | 6. false | 7. false |
| 8. false | 9. true | 10. false | | | | |

23

ANEURYSMS OF THE AORTA AND ILIAC ARTERIES

JERRY GOLDSTONE

Aneurysms of the abdominal aorta are a common condition. The incidence of this entity has been estimated at between 30 and 66 per 1000 persons and in the last three decades it has tripled. Unfortunately, the age-specific death rate from ruptured aneurysms has also increased. The increasing incidence has been noted in the United States as well as other Western countries and appears to be real and not merely a reflection of the increasing age of the population and improved diagnostic methods.[1-4] The incidence and prevalence vary depending upon the population studied, being lowest in unselected groups and higher in patient groups with other atherosclerotic lesions (Table 23–1).[5-10] For example, in community screening programs, the prevalence in males 65 to 74 years old ranges from 2.7 to 3.4 per cent, while in elderly hypertensive men and women, the prevalence has been found to be from 10.7 to 12 per cent.[11,12]

Abdominal aortic aneurysms have a propensity for sudden rupture and death. Approximately 15,000 deaths per year are due to abdominal aortic aneurysm, making this the 13th leading cause of death in the United States. The importance of this condition is obvious. The only way to reduce the death rate is to identify and treat these lesions before they rupture.

There is disagreement as to what constitutes an aneurysm. The ad hoc committee on reporting standards of the Society for Vascular Surgery (SVS) and the International Society for Cardiovascular Surgery (ISCVS) (North American Chapter) has recently suggested defining an *aneurysm* as a permanent localized dilation of an artery with increase in diameter of greater than 50 per cent (1.5 times) its normal diameter.[13] The normal value for an artery depends on several factors, including age, sex, and blood pressure. The normal sizes of the aorta in males and females are listed in Table 23–2.[14] Diffuse dilatation of an artery with increased diameter of more than 50 per cent of normal is termed *ectasia*, while *arteriomegaly* represents diffuse enlargement of an artery

but not large enough to meet the criteria for aneurysm.[15] In some patients with abdominal aortic aneurysms, the entire aortoiliofemoral arterial tree is arteriomegalic or ectatic. Thus, an aorta of any given diameter might be merely dilated or an aneurysm depending on the size of the normal aorta above the dilated segment.

Aneurysms of the infrarenal aorta are by far the most common arterial aneurysms encountered in clinical practice. Men are affected more than women by a ratio of 4:1.[8] Other aneurysms frequently are present in patients with aortic aneurysms, including common or internal iliac aneurysms (41 per cent) and femoropopliteal aneurysms in about 15 per cent of patients. Conversely, popliteal aneurysms are markers of abdominal aortic aneurysms. Aortic aneurysms can be found in about 8 per cent of patients who present with a unilateral popliteal aneurysm, but in over one third of patients who have bilateral popliteal aneurysms. In at least one group of patients with carotid atherosclerosis, there was a 10 per cent incidence of abdominal aortic aneurysm, and in another group of patients with tortuous internal carotid arteries a 40 per cent incidence of aortic aneurysms was found.[16,17]

Cigarette smoking also correlates with the presence of aortic aneurysms, there being an 8:1 preponderance of aneurysms in smokers compared with nonsmokers. Hypertension is another common accompanying factor, found in up to 40 per cent of patients with aortic aneurysms.

ETIOLOGY/PATHOGENESIS OF AORTIC ANEURYSMS

There are several causes of true abdominal aortic aneurysm, including cystic medial necrosis, dissection, Ehlers-Danlos syndrome, and syphilis. Most, however, are associated with atherosclerosis and this has traditionally been considered as the usual etiology. In the past several years, the etiology of aortic

TABLE 23–1. INCIDENCE OF ABDOMINAL AORTIC ANEURYSMS

Autopsy	1.5%
Unselected patients screened by ultrasound	3.2%
Selected patients with CAD[a]	5.0%
Selected patients with PVD[b]	10.0%
Patients with femoral or popliteal aneurysms	53.0%

[a]CAD, coronary artery disease.
[b]PVD, peripheral vascular disease.

aneurysms has been actively investigated, and the new information obtained has indicated the participation of another factor or factors in addition to atherosclerosis.[18] One observation casting doubt upon atherosclerosis as the sole cause of aortic aneurysms is that most patients with aneurysmal disease do not have occlusive vascular disease involving the aorto-iliofemoral segments.[19,20] It has been estimated that no more than about 25 per cent of aortic aneurysms are associated with significant occlusive disease.[21] Also, induction of aneurysms in animals fed an atherogenic diet has not been predictable, although regression of experimental atheromata has led to aneurysm formation in monkeys.

Biochemical studies have shown decreased quantities of both elastin and collagen in the wall of aneurysms.[22-25] This has been correlated with the histopathological features of a thin, dilated wall with replacement and fragmentation of the elastin in the media by a much thinner layer of collagen. This thinned wall usually contains calcium as well as atherosclerotic lesions, rendering the wall brittle. Laminated thrombus lines the lumen concentrically, resulting in a nearly normal flow channel (Figs. 23–1 through 23–3). Elongation of aneurysms occurs as they enlarge, causing them to become bowed and tortuous.[20] It is believed that it is the weakening and fragmentation of the elastic lamellas (elastin) that permits vessels to lengthen excessively and become tortuous. Thus, failure of elastin to provide sufficient retractive force in the circumferential as well as in the longitudinal direction allows for the increased diameter and length, respectively, of aneurysms.

Mature elastin and collagen are the major structural components responsible for the integrity of the aortic wall. Collagen makes up about 25 per cent of the wall of an atherosclerotic aorta, but only 6 to 18 per cent of an aneurysmal aortic wall. In addition, the fragmentation of the elastin and the overall thinning of the wall contribute to its weakening.[20] The large loss of elastin is one of the most consistent biochemical and histochemical findings in human aortic an-

eurysms.[26] These well-established histologic features have prompted a search for nonatherogenic mechanisms that disrupt collagen and elastin in the aortic wall. Several investigators have found excessive collagenase activity in the wall of aneurysmal aortas, and others have found increased elastase activity. Increased activity of other matrix proteases in aneurysmal aortic tissue has also been reported, as has an increased leukocyte-derived elastase in the blood of smokers with aneurysms. Deficiencies in antiproteases, such as tissue inhibitor of metalloprotease (TIMP) and α_1-antitrypsin have also been described. The latter is one of the most important natural antagonists to elastase. This may explain the association of aortic aneurysm rupture and chronic obstructive pulmonary disease (emphysema patients with reduced α_1-antitrypsin levels).[27]

Although not all of the studies of this type are conclusive, many investigators are accepting an imbalance between aortic wall proteases and antiproteases as an important fact about human abdominal aortic aneurysms.

There is also considerable evidence that there is a genetic susceptibility to aortic aneurysm formation.[28] Several investigators have discovered genetically linked enzyme deficiencies that are associated with aneurysms in experimental animals. For example, Tilson and coworkers have shown that a deficiency in the copper-containing enzyme lysyl oxidase is the cause of aortic aneurysms in a strain of mice.[29,30] Lysyl oxidase is important in collagen and elastin cross-linking. Furthermore, this enzyme defect is sex chromosome linked. In addition, several reports of familial clustering of abdominal aneurysms support the notion of a genetic predisposition to this disease.[31-34] Approximately 20 per cent of patients with abdominal aneurysms have a first-order relative with the same condition.[33] The age- and sex-adjusted increased risk is 11.6 times according to one report. Male siblings are at particularly high risk. The genetic pattern of increased susceptibility has not been worked out. Available evidence supports both X chromosome–linked and autosomal dominant patterns of inheritance.

Hemodynamic (mechanical) factors may also play a role in aneurysm development. The abdominal aorta is subjected to large pulsatile stresses as a result of its tapering geometry, relatively increased stiffness, and the reflected pressure waves from the peripheral vessels. Reductions in the number of elastic lamellae and the virtual lack of vasa vasorum in the media of the distal abdominal aorta may also be factors favoring aneurysmal formation in this segment of the ar-

TABLE 23–2. NORMAL DIAMETER OF HUMAN AORTA[a]

	Eleventh Rib	Suprarenal	Infrarenal	Bifurcation
Male	26.9 ± 3.9	23.9 ± 3.9	21.4 ± 3.6	18.7 ± 3.3
Female	24.4 ± 3.4	21.6 ± 3.1	18.7 ± 3.3	17.5 ± 2.5

[a]All measurement in millimeters, plus or minus standard error. Data from Steinberg et al.[14]

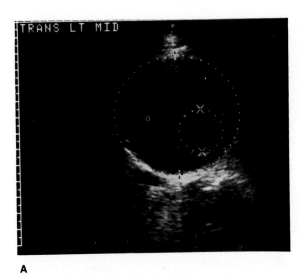

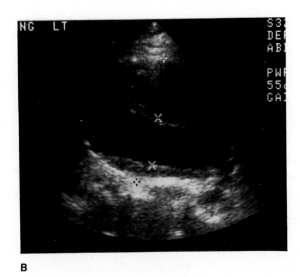

FIGURE 23–1. *A,* B mode ultrasound scan showing large aortic aneurysm measuring 74.7 mm in diameter and mural thrombus creating smaller lumen (26.4 mm) (transverse view). *B,* B mode ultrasound scan in same patient showing large aortic aneurysm, mural thrombus, and nearly normal flow channel (longitudinal view).

terial tree by making the aorta structurally less well adapted to handle the increased hemodynamic stresses that occur there.[21]

For the present time, it is probably more accurate to consider the etiology of aortic aneurysms to be multifactorial and to refer to these aneurysms as degenerative rather than atherosclerotic. They account for more than 90 per cent of abdominal aortic aneurysms.

Once an aneurysm develops, regardless of the cause, its enlargement is governed by physical principles, especially Laplace's law. This law describes the relationship between the tangential stress (T) tending to disrupt the wall of a sphere and the radius (R) and transmural pressure (P): T = PR. Thus, for a given transmural pressure, the wall tension is proportional to the radius. Once dilation of the aorta

has started, Laplace's law explains why aortic enlargement is enhanced. It also explains why large aneurysms are more prone to rupture than small ones and why hypertension is an important risk factor for rupture. Using Laplace's law, tripling the aortic radius from 2 to 6 cm results in a 12-fold increase in wall tension, and when this tension exceeds the tensile strength of the collagen in the aortic wall, disruption occurs.

CLINICAL MANIFESTATIONS

From 70 to 75 per cent of all infrarenal abdominal aortic aneurysms are asymptomatic when first discovered.[35] Most often they are discovered during a

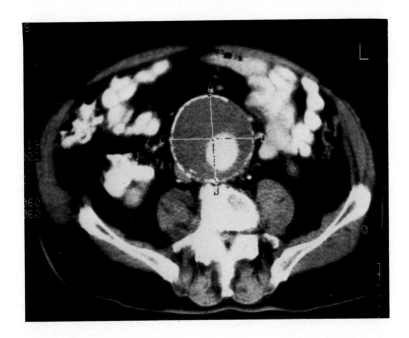

FIGURE 23–2. CT scan of abdomen showing large calcified abdominal aortic aneurysm (82.7 mm in diameter).

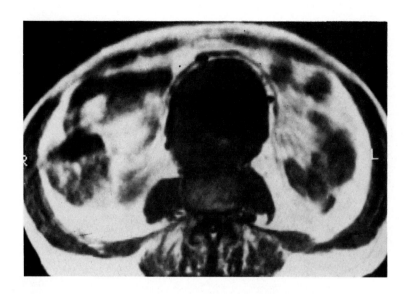

FIGURE 23–3.   Magnetic resonance image of large abdominal aortic aneurysm showing eccentric mural thrombus and flow channel.

routine physical examination or during a radiographic study performed for some other reason (i.e., upper gastrointestinal series, barium enema, intravenous pyelogram, lumbosacral spine x-rays, or abdominal computed tomography or ultrasound examination). Occasionally, an aneurysm will be first detected during the conduct of an unrelated abdominal operation.

Abdominal aortic aneurysms may cause symptoms as a result of rupture or expansion, pressure on adjacent structures, embolization, dissection, or thrombosis.[35,36] Compression of adjacent bowel can cause early satiety, and even nausea and vomiting. This fact often leads to delays in diagnosis. Virtually any type of abdominal, flank, or back pain can be due to an aneurysm and abdominal or back pain is the most common symptom and can be elicited in up to one third of patients. Large aneurysms can actually erode the spine and cause severe back pain in the absence of rupture.

The abrupt onset of severe pain in the back, flank, or abdomen is characteristic of aneurysmal *rupture* or *expansion.* It is not certain why pain is produced by an expanding but unruptured (intact) aneurysm. The best explanation is sudden stretching of the layers of the aortic wall with pressure on adjacent somatic sensory nerves. In most surgical series, symptomatic but unruptured aneurysms make up from 6 to nearly 40 per cent of cases (average of five series totaling 311 patients: 13.7 per cent).

Ruptured aneurysms comprise between 20 and 25 per cent of most series. The nature of symptoms as well as their time course vary depending upon the nature of the rupture.[37–39] Small tears of the aneurysmal sac may result in a small leak that at least temporarily seals with minimal blood loss. This is usually followed within a few hours by frank rupture, which produces a catastrophic medical emergency. The rupture most frequently occurs through the posterolateral aortic wall into the retroperitoneal space and less commonly through the anterior wall into the free peritoneal cavity. The incidence of this latter type of rupture is higher than indicated in most surgical series because most of these patients die before reaching the hospital. Rarely, an abdominal aortic aneurysm will rupture into the inferior vena cava or one of the iliac veins, producing an aortcaval (or aortoiliac) fistula, or into the gastrointestinal tract, producing a primary aortoenteric fistula.

The classic clinical manifestations of ruptured aortic aneurysm consist of mid- or diffuse abdominal pain, shock, and a pulsatile abdominal mass. The pain may be more prominent in the back or flank, or it may radiate into the groin or thigh. The severity of the shock varies from mild to profound and the duration of symptoms may vary from a few minutes to more than 24 hours. Although aneurysm rupture is usually an acute catastrophic event, it can be contained for prolonged periods. These chronic ruptures have masqueraded as radicular compression, symptomatic inguinal hernia, femoral neuropathy, and even obstructive jaundice. It is thought that chronic contained ruptures eventually progress to free rupture, and they should therefore be treated surgically on an urgent basis.[40]

The pain of expanding but intact aneurysms may closely mimic that of a ruptured one. The pain tends to be severe, constant, and unaffected by position. Hypotension and shock, however, do not usually occur in the absence of rupture. The degree of hypotension depends on the amount of blood lost from the aneurysm.

The diverse and nonspecific nature of the pain caused by expanding and leaking aneurysms all too often leads to errors in diagnosis, delays in finally establishing the correct diagnosis, and catastrophic rupture in the midst of a diagnostic procedure. Occasionally, a patient with a contained rupture will arrive in the emergency room complaining of angina pectoris, from blood loss and reflex tachycardia, and will be rapidly transported to a coronary care unit without the abdominal examination that would identify the true cause of the chest pain. Most diagnostic errors such as this are due to failure to palpate the expansile, pulsatile epigastric mass.

DIAGNOSTIC METHODS

Except in thin patients, an abdominal aortic aneurysm has to be about 5 cm in diameter to be detectable on a routine physical examination. The reported accuracy in establishing the correct diagnosis of abdominal aortic aneurysm by physical examination alone ranges between 30 and 90 per cent. Even when the aneurysm is detected, determination of its size by palpation is imprecise. Obesity, ascites, and uncooperativeness on the part of the patient impair aneurysmal detection by physical examination. On the other hand, tumors or cystic lesions adjacent to the aorta, unusual aortic tortuosity, and excessive lumbar lordosis all can lead to an erroneous diagnosis of an abdominal aortic aneurysm when it is not present. The expansile nature of a pulsatile mass is a key element in deciding whether or not it is an aneurysm.

Although physical examination will detect most large aneurysms, more objective methods are available to measure size and identify smaller aneurysms. Sizing is especially important, since it often determines management decisions. The oldest objective method for accomplishing this purpose is the plain abdominal and lateral spine x-ray, which identify aneurysms by a fine rim of calcium representing the aortic wall (Fig. 23–4). Enough calcium is in the aortic wall to make the diagnosis of aneurysm in from 67 to 75 per cent of cases, but accurate determination of maximal aortic size is possible in only about two thirds of these (Fig. 23–4). Therefore, a negative or inadequate plain film cannot be relied upon to exclude the diagnosis of aortic aneurysm.

Aortography

The limitations of aortography for the diagnosis and evaluation of aortic aneurysms, like plain film roentgenograms, are well known. Because the nearly always present mural thrombus tends to reduce the aneurysmal lumen size towards normal, aortography is not a reliable method to determine the diameter of an aneurysm or even to establish its presence. With better imaging methods now routinely available, aortography should not be used as a diagnostic method for abdominal aortic aneurysms. It is, however, useful in the preoperative evaluation of patients with aneurysms.[41,42] It can define the extent of an aneurysm, especially suprarenal and iliac involvement, and also the associated arterial lesions involving renal and visceral vessels, as well as distal occlusive lesions (Table 23–3). Although many of these associated lesions are readily detectable and manageable intraoperatively, some surgeons believe that preoperative identification of such lesions is useful in planning operative strategy and they therefore recommend routine preoperative aortography. It must be emphasized that aortography used in this way is not a diagnostic study used to determine presence or size of an abdominal aneurysm.

There are risks associated with aortography, including potential renal toxicity from the large contrast volumes that are sometimes required to adequately fill a large aneurysm and the branch vessels. In addition, manipulation of a retrograde catheter through the laminated mural thrombus risks distal embolization, and there is always the possibility of local complications at the arterial puncture site through which the angiographic catheter is introduced. The use of digital subtraction angiographic techniques has lessened but not eliminated these risks. Although there seems to be a trend favoring more frequent use of aortography in patients with abdominal aortic aneurysm, until convincing data are available, it seems prudent to perform aortography selectively in this group of patients for the following indications[43]: (1) clinical suspicion of visceral ischemia, (2) occlusive iliofemoral vascular lesions, (3) severe hypertension or impaired renal function in a patient in whom a concomitant renal artery stenosis would be repaired if discovered, (4) suspicion of presence of a horseshoe kidney, (5) suspicion of suprarenal or thoracoabdominal aneurysm, and (6) the presence of femoral or popliteal aneurysms.

Imaging Modalities for Abdominal Aortic Aneurysms

Several imaging modalities are now widely available for establishing the presence of an aortic aneurysm and accurately determining its size.[44] These include ultrasound, computed tomography (CT), and magnetic resonance imaging (MRI).

Real-time, *B mode ultrasound* is available in most hospitals. It employs no ionizing radiation, provides structural detail of vessel walls and atherosclerotic plaques, and can accurately measure aneurysm size in longitudinal as well as cross-sectional directions (three-dimensional) (Fig. 23–1). When compared to intraoperative measurements, ultrasonic measurements are accurate to within ±3 mm. Many studies have documented the ability of B mode ultrasound to establish the diagnosis and accurately determine the size of abdominal and peripheral aneurysms.[45–47] Ultrasonography has not been as useful for imaging the thoracic or suprarenal aorta because of the overlying air-containing lung. Similarly, it has been less reliable in defining the relationship between abdominal aortic aneurysms and the renal arteries. Although use of a transesophageal ultrasound transducer can largely avoid this problem, this is not practical for routine evaluation of abdominal aortic disease. Because ultrasound can obtain images in longitudinal, transverse, and oblique

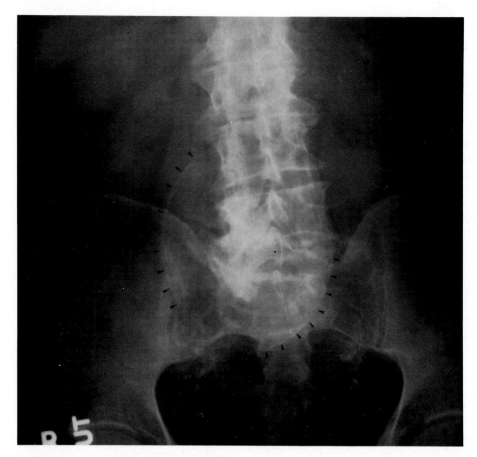

FIGURE 23–4.   Plain abdominal x-ray showing large aortic aneurysm with calcified rim (*arrowheads*).

projections, it can be especially helpful in differentiating a tortuous aorta from an aneurysm.

Ultrasound requires considerable technician skill in order to obtain a satisfactory image, and interpretation can sometimes be difficult. The images are also impaired by obesity, intestinal gas, or barium in the bowel. The overlying bowel gas often interferes with evaluation of the iliac arteries. The major advantages of ultrasound are its wide availability, its freedom from pain or other known side effects, its lack of ionizing radiation, its relatively low cost, and its ability to image vessels in longitudinal as well as cross-sectional planes. The studies can be performed quickly. In addition, the portability of ultrasound machines is advantageous for the emergency room evaluation of suspected ruptured aneurysms. These factors make ultrasound the modality of choice for the initial evaluation of pulsatile abdominal or peripheral masses and for follow-up surveillance of aneurysms to determine increase in size.

Computed tomography employs ionizing radiation to obtain cross-sectional images of the aorta and other body structures. A new format, spiral CT, is now being introduced which provides 3-D reconstructions of the aortic and branch vessel images. CT images provide reliable information about the size of the entire aorta, including the thoracic aorta, so the extent as well as the size of an aneurysm can be accurately measured. Modern CT scanners possess sufficient spatial resolution to allow identification of celiac, superior mesenteric, renal, and iliac arteries and their relationship to the aneurysm as well as adjacent organs. Major venous structures, including anomalies, can also be identified by CT.[47] The administration of intravenous contrast allows CT to evaluate the size of the aortic lumen, the amount and location of mural thrombus, and, in the presence of dissection, differentiation of the true from the false lumen (Fig. 23–2). Contrast-enhanced CT scans are also useful for assessing the retroperitoneum and can identify retroperitoneal hematoma (aneurysmal rupture) and the periaortic fibrosis associated with inflammatory aneurysms.[48–51]

CT images are degraded by patient motion and the presence of metallic surgical clips. CT scanning requires more time and is more expensive than ultrasound and only provides images in one (transverse) plane, but it gives more information about other abdominal and retroperitoneal structures than ultrasound. One of the most helpful uses of CT is to define the relationship of an aneurysm to the renal artery origins. Depending upon the thickness of each CT slice and the distance between slices, this is not always accurate, especially when there is buckling of

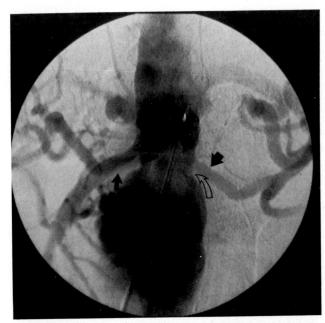

FIGURE 23–5. Digital subtraction aortogram of large juxtarenal aneurysm. This angled view allows identification of short infrarenal neck (*open arrow*) and origins of both renal arteries (*dark arrows*).

the aorta to the extent that the superior border of the aneurysm ascends anterior to the aorta. Overall, CT scans are currently the most useful imaging method for evaluation of the abdominal aorta. Most physicians have learned how to interpret the images correctly, and the images exhibit superior anatomical detail when compared to ultrasound.

Magnetic resonance imaging is the newest imaging modality available for evaluation of aortic aneurysms[49,52] (Fig. 23–3). It employs radiofrequency energy and a strong magnetic field to produce images in longitudinal, transverse, and coronal planes. Because the instruments are very expensive, they are not as widely available as ultrasound or CT and interpretation of the images requires considerable experience and skill. The spatial resolution at present is somewhat limited (about 0.8 mm) and the presence of metallic surgical clips, cardiac pacemakers, and monitoring equipment make MRI impossible to perform. Also, these studies are more expensive than either CT or ultrasound. Nevertheless, MRI images

clearly distinguish arteries and veins from viscera and other surrounding tissue. MRI of aortic aneurysms has excellent agreement with ultrasound and CT images in determining aortic diameter, and MRI is better at demonstrating involvement of branch vessels. This is especially true for the renal arteries, and some authors have reported visualization of the renal arteries in over 90 per cent of cases.[49] Other advantages of MRI over CT are the lack of ionizing radiation, its ability to obtain multiplane images, and the relatively large field of image. In addition, it is not necessary to use toxic contrast agents for MRI scans in order to achieve intravascular enhancement; however, paramagnetic contrast agents, such as gadolinium, are now available.

Newer advances in signal acquisition and computer programs now allow for MRI instruments to quantitate blood flow and construct images that look like conventional angiograms (MR angiography [MRA]).[44] When these techniques become routinely available, MR may become the only imaging method necessary for most patients with aortic disease of any type.

Objective documentation of the size should probably be accomplished with one of these imaging modalities in all patients with suspected abdominal aortic aneurysm prior to performing an elective aneurysm operation. Each method can measure the diameter accurately. An initial scan can be used for comparison with subsequent scans to determine aneurysmal enlargement. For routine situations, ultrasound is probably the method of choice because of its widespread availability, lower cost, and lack of ionizing radiation. When there is suspicion of suprarenal or thoracoabdominal aortic involvement or dissection, MRI or CT is preferable.

For symptomatic aneurysms, MRI and CT also have advantages over ultrasound because of their better ability to identify contained rupture. CT and MRI probably have equally superior capability to demonstrate unexpected features such as venous anomalies, perianeurysmal fibrosis, and horseshoe kidney, although the ureters are not easily identified by MRI.

RISK OF ANEURYSM RUPTURE

As noted earlier, the majority of abdominal aortic aneurysms are now discovered in asymptomatic pa-

TABLE 23–3.   ANGIOGRAPHICALLY DETECTED LESIONS ASSOCIATED WITH ABDOMINAL AORTIC ANEURYSMS[a]

Findings	Total Patients	Number	Percentage
Suprarenal extension	680	46	6.7
Renal stenosis/occlusion	763	138	18.0
Accessory/multiple renal artery	680	92	13.5
Celiac/superior mesenteric artery stenosis	628	87	13.8
Iliofemoropopliteal stenosis/occlusion	680	298	43.5
Iliofemoropopliteal aneurysm	680	243	34.2

[a]Collected data from Rich et al.[41] and Gaspar.[43]

tients or during an evaluation for an unrelated problem. They are being discovered at a smaller size than when the original studies on their natural history were first published by Estes, Wright, Szilagyi, and others.[53–55] Even though aneurysms can cause symptoms and serious consequences from thrombosis and distal embolization, rupture is the most important risk, and it has been established that the size of an aneurysm is the most important factor that determines the risk of rupture. In general, the risk of rupture correlates directly with size: the larger the aneurysm the greater the risk of rupture. For example, the **yearly** risk of rupture for abdominal aortic aneurysms[5,27,56,57] between 5.0 and 5.7 cm in size is 6.6 per cent, and increases to 19 per cent for aneurysms over 7.0 cm in diameter.[5,57,58] Calculated as 5-year rupture rates, these figures become 33, 0, and 95 per cent, respectively. The steepness of a curve plotting this type of data increases sharply at a diameter of about 6 cm, and this led to earlier recommendations to defer elective aneurysm repair until an aneurysm reached this size. More contemporary data, obtained from objective imaging studies, indicate that aneurysm rupture risk begins to increase at a diameter of 5.0 cm, and the recently published practice guidelines of the SVS-ISCVS have adopted this size as the important surgical decision point. However, even this value should not be used as a rigid cutoff point for recommending an elective aneurysm operation. Smaller aneurysms can and occasionally do rupture. Autopsy studies have shown that 23.4 per cent of aneurysms 4.1 to 5.0 cm rupture, and the same is true for up to 10 per cent of aneurysms less than 4 cm in diameter.[5] Data such as these have led surgeons to recommend operation for almost all aortic aneurysms in good-risk patients.

There is little debate about the appropriateness of elective aneurysm surgery for patients with large aneurysms (those greater than 6 cm in diameter) because of the high risk of rupture and associated mortality when rupture occurs. Several recent reports have questioned the need to operate on small asymptomatic aneurysms.[59–62] The population-based data from Rochester, Minnesota showed a mean enlargement rate for aneurysms less than 5.0 cm diameter of only 0.32 cm/year, and after 5 years of observation no aneurysm less than 5.0 cm ruptured. Rupture occurred in 25 per cent of patients whose aneurysm measured 5.0 cm or more, and the authors recommended elective repair of aneurysms 5 cm or more in diameter. This recommendation is in agreement with the SVS-ISCVS practice guidelines noted above. Cronenwett et al. have shown that chronic obstructive pulmonary disease and systolic hypertension were predictors of increased risk of rupture of small abdominal aneurysms.[27] In a subsequent study, they found that the rate of enlargement of small aneurysms was unpredictable but that either increased systolic or decreased diastolic pressure (i.e., increased pulse pressure) was associated with an increased rate of aneurysm expansion.[63] In this study, there was considerable variability in the rate of aneurysm enlarge-

ment even though the average rate of expansion was 0.4 cm/year in anteroposterior dimensions and 0.5 cm/year in lateral dimensions. Other studies have shown that aneurysms are frequently elliptical rather than round and that aneurysmal expansion is initially more rapid in the lateral direction. It is interesting to recall that aneurysms most frequently rupture in the lateral wall.

In a review of four series, including their own, Cronenwett et al. described the outcome of 378 patients with small aortic aneurysms initially treated nonoperatively.[63] After an average follow-up of 31 months, 27 per cent of the patients were alive with intact aneurysm, 29 per cent had died of other causes, 39 per cent had had elective aneurysm operations because their aneurysm diameter reached 5 to 6 cm, and 4 per cent suffered aneurysm rupture or acute expansion leading to emergency operation. Overall, there was a mean 5-year survival of 54 per cent in these patients. It appears, therefore, that patients can be carefully observed using serial ultrasound measurements until an aneurysm size of 5 cm is reached. The 4 to 6 per cent per year rupture rate of aneurysms smaller than this is similar to the 5 per cent operative mortality reported in this collective experience and appears to support this approach, although several authors have reported essentially zero mortality for small aneurysms operated upon during the very recent past.[65–68]

It must be emphasized that while the risk of aneurysm rupture correlates with aneurysm size, and the average rate of aneurysmal enlargement is known (0.4 to 0.5 cm/year), it is impossible to predict when a small aneurysm will rupture in any given patient.[69] The harmlessness of the small, asymptomatic abdominal aortic aneurysm is deceptive. The mere presence of an aortic aneurysm is more important than its diameter as an indication for surgical treatment.[71]

RISK OF SURGICAL TREATMENT

The natural history of untreated abdominal aortic aneurysms is well documented. Since the first successful surgical resection and graft replacement of an infrarenal aortic aneurysm was reported in 1952, there have been a large number of publications documenting the operative and long-term survival following surgical treatment. There has been a steady improvement in operative results for elective operations. Several large, contemporary series have reported operative mortality rates of between 0.9 and 5 per cent for university medical centers and only slightly higher rates for community hospitals[65–74] (Table 23–4).

Operative mortality in this range (5 per cent or less) justifies elective repair, even for small aneurysms.[87] Most of the details, even in elective operations, occur in so-called high-risk patients. Chronological age is not as important as physiological age in assessing operative risk, so patients should not be denied elective operation based solely on age.[88] Even octogenarians can undergo elective aneurysm sur-

TABLE 23–4.   OPERATIVE MORTALITY AND LATE SURVIVAL OF ELECTIVE SURGICAL TREATMENT OF AAA[a]

Author/Year	No. of Patients	Age (Years)[b]	Mortality (%)[c]	5-Year Survival (%)[d]
Vasko et al., 1963[75]	136	—	10.0	39.0[e]
Cannon et al., 1963[76]	66	65	15.0	50.0[e]
Voorhees & McAllister, 1963[77]	170	65	18.0	53.0
DeBakey et al., 1964[73]	1,332	—	7.0	58.0
Levy et al., 1966[78]	100	64	17.0	34.0
Szilagyi et al., 1966[55]	401	—	15.0	49.0
May et al., 1968[79]	135	—	13.0	49.0
Baker & Roberts, 1970[80]	240	63	9.0	54.0
Stokes & Butcher, 1973[81]	87	—	3.0	60.0
Hicks et al., 1975[82]	225	67	8.0	60.0
O'Donnell et al., 1976[83]	63	82	5.0	70.0
Whittemore et al., 1980[68]	110	68	0.0	84.0
Crawford et al., 1981[84]	860	66	5.0	63.0
Reigal et al., 1987[85]	499	76	3.0	66.0
Bernstein et al., 1988[86]	123	71	1.0	72.0

[a] Abdominal aortic aneurysm.
[b] Mean.
[c] Operative mortality.
[d] Cumulative.
[e] Actual.

gery with low morbidity and mortality rates.[74] Most vascular surgeons have successfully treated ruptured aneurysms in patients previously rejected for elective operation because they were "too old."

The major risks for elective abdominal aortic aneurysm resection are similar to those for other major intraabdominal operations, and include adequacy of cardiopulmonary and renal function. High-risk patients are those with unstable angina or angina at rest, cardiac ejection fraction less than 25 to 30 per cent, congestive heart failure, serum creatinine greater than 3 mg/dl, and pulmonary disease manifest by room air pO_2 of less than 50 mm Hg and/or elevated pCO_2. A substantial percentage of these high-risk patients will die of ruptured aneurysm and not from the diseases that led to their categorization as high risk. With intensive perioperative monitoring and support, aneurysm resection has been carried out even in these high-risk patients with operative mortality of less than 6 per cent by Hollier et al. and others.[68,70,81] Thus, large abdominal aneurysms should be considered for elective treatment even in high-risk patients if the appropriate support facilities are available.

In spite of the fact that the incidence of aneurysm rupture has decreased as a result of aggressive elective resection programs, a substantial percentage (50) of patients whose aneurysms rupture die before reaching a medical facility.[1,8] Another 24 per cent arrive at a hospital alive but die before a definitive operation can be performed. Thus, operative mortality figures underestimate the true significance of aneurysmal rupture. The overall mortality from ruptured aneurysms, as reported in two community-based studies, ranges from 74 to more than 90 per cent.

The operative results for ruptured aneurysms are not nearly as favorable and have not generally improved as much over the years, as have the results of elective aneurysm operations.[37,89–92] Although there are a few series with better results, overall, nearly 50 per cent of patients die after being operated upon for rupture. The nature of the rupture influences the results. Less than 10 per cent of patients presenting in shock with free intraperitoneal rupture survive. In contrast, stable patients with small contained leaks have a better than 80 per cent survival rate.

The factors contributing to failure in the treatment of ruptured abdominal aortic aneurysm have been reviewed by Hiatt and associates.[89] The four most important were failure to perform elective aneurysmectomy in patients with known aneurysms; errors in diagnosing rupture when it occurred, leading to delay in operation; technical errors committed during the operation (all venous injuries); and undue delays in induction of anesthesia. These are all realistically preventable. Other series have also attempted to identify factors leading to death after aortic aneurysm rupture. Repeatedly, delays in performing the surgery and the total volume of blood transfused are found to be important. Discrepancies in operative mortality between various reports are due in part to failure to properly categorize patients and instead considering all forms of rupture together. Many of these series also fail to separate patients with unruptured but symptomatic aneurysms who undergo emergency operations. The operative morbidity and mortality for this group is intermediate between elective, asymptomatic patients and those with frank rupture, averaging 16 to 19 per cent.[27,66] It has been postulated that the reason for this increased mortality is the omission of thorough preoperative evaluation and preparation necessitated by the emergency operation.

LATE SURVIVAL

In the foregoing pages, it has been shown that the commonest cause of death among patients with abdominal aortic aneurysm is rupture and that elective surgical repair of aneurysms prevents rupture and is associated with excellent survival rates. The next questions that must be answered are: What is the long-term outlook for survivors? Is life prolonged by aneurysmectomy? Several long-term studies using life-table methods have been published revealing 5-year survival rates ranging from 49 to 84 per cent (averaging 61 per cent) (Table 23–4).[93–96] Although these data are far better than the survival of patients not undergoing operation, they do not equal the survival expected for the normal age-matched population. For example, Johnson et al. reported a 50 per cent survival of 7.4 years for patients surviving operative treatment for abdominal aneurysm, whereas the figure for the United States general population was 15.7 years and that for North Carolina was 14.5 years.[94] These authors could not identify any influence of age on operative mortality, although it affected late mortality, as one would expect. Most of the excess mortality can be attributed to coronary artery disease. This has led some centers to pursue an aggressive coronary evaluation and treatment protocol prior to elective aortic aneurysm operations.[97] Several large surveys have shown that the safety of vascular surgical procedures in patients who have had previous coronary revascularization is comparable to that of patients with no evidence of ischemic cardiac disease, but this has not been evaluated by randomized clinical trials.[98–102]

ASSESSMENT OF CARDIAC RISK

Approximately 30 to 40 per cent of patients with aortic aneurysms have no clinically evident coronary artery disease (e.g., no angina pectoris, no history of myocardial infarction, normal electrocardiogram [ECG], normal exercise stress test).

There is a high prevalence (50 per cent) of angiographically documented severe coronary artery disease in patients in whom coronary disease is clinically suspected (about 50 per cent of the total).[97,102] The prevalence is still 20 per cent in patients in whom the traditional clinical indicators of coronary disease are absent. Coronary artery disease is responsible for at least 50 to 60 per cent of all perioperative and late deaths following operations on the abdominal aorta.[103,104] The incidence of fatal myocardial infarction following elective abdominal aortic aneurysm surgery has been reported to be as high as 4.7 per cent, and nonfatal infarction occurs in up to 16 per cent of patients. It is possible to identify the high-risk cardiac patient using clinical assessment, exercise stress testing, radionuclide angiography (multiple gated scan), echocardiography, dipyridamole-thallium scanning, continuous portable electrocardiographic Holter monitoring, and coronary angiography.[103,105,106] Clinical factors predictive of increased risk for postoperative cardiac complications include a history of previous myocardial infarction, congestive failure, angina pectoris, abnormal preoperative ECG, diabetes mellitus, and advanced age.[105] Dipyridamole-thallium myocardial scanning has replaced exercise stress testing for these elderly patients in many hospitals. It identifies areas of myocardium that are reversibly ischemic and is quite sensitive for identifying patients likely to have a perioperative cardiac complication, but unfortunately its specificity is relatively low.[107,108] Determination of left ventricular ejection fraction by radionuclide angiography identifies patients with poor ventricular function. Although ejection fraction less than 30 per cent has been associated with increased cardiac complications in some series, it does not predict postoperative myocardial infarction or death. Continuous portable ECG monitoring of vascular surgical patients for silent ischemia associated with ST-T segment changes has been shown to correlate with postoperative myocardial infarction in some series, but additional studies are needed to verify the value of this technique. Routine preoperative screening of all aortic aneurysm patients with coronary angiography is not feasible or prudent, even though Hertzer has reported a nearly fivefold increase in operative mortality (5.1 per cent) in aneurysm patients with suspected coronary disease, compared to those with no (1.1 per cent mortality) or corrected (0.44 per cent mortality) coronary artery disease.[97,98] Late survival was also better in the groups with no or corrected coronary artery disease. In spite of these data, no single means exists to accurately predict perioperative risk after aortic aneurysmorrhaphy, but this is an area of intensive current research.

Each of the modalities discussed above has its own usefulness as well as limitations. Older patients with congestive heart failure, active angina pectoris, previous myocardial infarction, or markedly abnormal noninvasive cardiac studies deserve thorough cardiac evaluation before elective aortic aneurysm surgery. Younger patients without overt cardiac disease and with a normal ECG probably do not need this type of evaluation. The difficult decisions are in patients that fall between these two extremes (about 50 per cent of the total), in whom unexpected coronary events still occur.[109] Since the ultimate objective of a cardiac evaluation is to identify and correct dangerous coronary artery lesions, the results of the subsequent interventions (i.e., coronary artery bypass grafting, percutaneous transluminal angioplasty) in the appropriate hospital must be considered and balanced against the relatively low myocardial infarction rates that can be achieved in patients who do not undergo coronary revascularization. Overall, preliminary myocardial revascularization prior to aortic aneurysm repair should be necessary in only about 10 per cent of patients.

INDICATIONS FOR ABDOMINAL AORTIC ANEURYSM REPAIR

The objectives of surgical treatment of abdominal aortic aneurysm are to relieve symptoms if present, prevent rupture (thereby prolonging life), and restore arterial continuity. These goals are best accomplished when operations are performed electively under optimal conditions. This is obviously not always possible.

Emergent operation is indicated for almost all patients with known or suspected *rupture*, regardless of the size of the aneurysm or age of the patient. The coexistence of another fatal illness, such as metastatic cancer, may be sufficient reason for choosing a nonoperative approach. Emergent or urgent operation is also indicated for *symptomatic aneurysms* in the absence of signs of rupture. It is frequently impossible to determine whether an aneurysm has in fact ruptured or is just expanding. Although CT and MRI scans can be relied upon to detect the presence of periaortic blood in most cases, the absence of this finding should not lead to unnecessary delays in operating, since actual rupture can occur at any time. In addition, the location of these imaging units in many hospitals is in an area where close monitoring of the patient is difficult.

Elective aneurysm repair should be recommended for *asymptomatic patients* with aneurysms 5.0 cm or larger in diameter who are acceptable operative risks and who have an estimated life expectancy of 2 years or more. Elective operation should also be considered for smaller aneurysms, those less than 5.0 cm in maximum diameter, in good-risk patients, especially if they are hypertensive or live in a remote area where proper medical care would not be readily available should signs and symptoms of rupture develop. Aneurysms between 4.0 and 5.0 cm in diameter that have shown documented enlargement of more than 0.5 cm in less than 6 to 12 months by serial imaging studies should also be treated surgically.

High-risk patients (very old, nonreconstructible coronary disease, poor left ventricular function with congestive heart failure, severe obstructive lung disease) with small aneurysms should be observed until the aneurysm becomes symptomatic or large. High-risk patients with large aneurysms require thorough evaluation for the condition that puts them in the high-risk category.[68,88] Frequently, such evaluations will fail to substantiate the original degree of presumed risk, and it has been reported that fewer than 50 per cent of these patients die of the disease for which they were initially denied aneurysm repair.

Because of excessively high operative mortality in some very high-risk patients with large abdominal aneurysms, several surgeons proposed extraanatomic bypass in conjunction with induced thrombosis of the aneurysm.[110] Thrombosis of the aneurysm, it was argued, would eliminate the risk of rupture and the extraanatomic bypass would lower operative mortality by avoiding the risks of a major intraabdominal operation. Unfortunately, nonresective therapy has not been as successful as originally hoped. Rupture still occurs in about 20 per cent of patients so treated and operative mortality has been over 10 per cent, a figure far in excess of the mortality reported in similar but highly selected groups of patients subjected to conventional aneurysm operations.[88,111–113] Fortunately, this nonresective form of surgical therapy for abdominal aneurysms is being abandoned, even by some of its earlier proponents. The natural history (unoperated) of abdominal aortic aneurysms and the excellent results currently achievable for conventional surgical treatment justify a vigorous diagnostic and therapeutic approach.

OPERATIVE TECHNIQUE

Incision and Exposure

There are three options for the incision for abdominal aortic aneurysm operations. The *full-length midline incision* provides access to the entire abdominal cavity, including the supraceliac aorta and iliac arteries, is rapid to make and close, and provides the fewest limitations. For the treatment of supra- or pararenal aneurysms, medial-visceral rotation can be added and will usually provide adequate exposure of the entire suprarenal segment of the abdominal aorta. This maneuver involves mobilization, from lateral to medial, of the left colon, spleen, and pancreas in what is normally an avascular plane. Significant splenic injury requiring splenectomy occurs about 25 per cent of the time when this is done, and there is an increased risk of pancreatic injury.

A *wide transverse incision*, extending from flank to flank and curved either above or below the umbilicus, depending upon the aortic and iliac pathology, also provides excellent exposure for aortic aneurysm repair and is the preference of many surgeons. It is more time consuming to create and close than a midline incision and is said to be stronger, although proof of superiority in terms of wound dehiscence is lacking. Transverse incisions are less painful and therefore interfere less with respiratory function postoperatively because they cut across fewer intercostal nerves.

Both of these incisions offer wide access to the peritoneal cavity and the retroperitoneum and their contents. They permit a thorough abdominal exploration that should be performed as a preliminary step in all elective operations, since there is a significant incidence of coexisting pathology, including colon tumors and gallstones.

Retroperitoneal exposure of the aorta can also be achieved through an *oblique incision* extending from the left 11th intercostal space to the edge of the rectus abdominus muscle.[114–116] For this, the patient is placed in a semilateral position but with the hips allowed to rotate back to the supine position. This allows access to both femoral arteries. Through this retroperitoneal exposure the suprarenal aorta can be controlled if necessary, but access to the right iliac artery is often very limited, especially if the aortic aneurysm is large or if there is a large iliac aneurysm. Among the advantages claimed for the retroperitoneal approach are less postoperative respiratory compromise, lower intravenous fluid volume requirements, less intraoperative hypothermia, shorter period of postoperative ileus, and avoidance, in many cases, of the need for postoperative nasogastric intubation. Although it has been perceived that these patients generally "do better" than those operated upon through a midline incision, when the two incisions were compared in prospective studies, no significant important differences were found.[114-116] One major disadvantage of the retroperitoneal approach is that the contents of the peritoneal cavity are not available for inspection. Nevertheless, many surgeons prefer this approach for elective aneurysm operations and even use it for ruptured aneurysms that are contained because of the ability to achieve rapid control of the upper abdominal aorta in this way.[117]

The choice of incision is a matter of personal preference. Factors to consider in making this choice include the extent of the aneurysm, the status of the iliac arteries, the degree of obesity and pulmonary disease, previous abdominal operations, the necessity to inspect intraperitoneal structures, especially in patients with atypical symptoms, and the speed with which aortic control must be attained. Surgeons should be familiar with all three approaches in order to take advantage of each when appropriate.

Extensive perioperative monitoring is indicated for patients undergoing abdominal aortic aneurysm repair.[68,118] This has contributed significantly to the improved results reported in large series of elective aneurysm repair. Monitoring usually includes continuous recording of ECG, intraarterial pressure, body temperature, urine output, and central venous or pulmonary artery pressures. In high-risk patients, especially if the aorta will be cross-clamped above the renal arteries, transesophageal two-dimensional echocardiographic monitoring of left ventricular function may be superior to measurements of pulmonary artery pressure for evaluation of intravascular volume status.[119] Various blood components should be monitored as well, including arterial oxygen and carbon dioxide content and pH, plasma glucose, electrolytes, and coagulation parameters and factors. Monitoring the clotting system is especially important in ruptured aneurysms and in other cases when there has been a need to infuse large volumes of blood and blood products. The use of autotransfusion should be routine in order to minimize the amount of homologous blood transfusion. For elective operations, patients should be encouraged to donate their own blood for autologous transfusion in the perioperative period.

When midline or transverse incisions are used, the aorta is exposed by a retroperitoneal incision slightly to the right of the midline. The duodenum must be carefully reflected laterally along with the rest of the small bowel. The left renal vein usually marks the cephalad extent of the dissection unless the aneurysm extends to (juxtarenal) or involves the renal arteries (pararenal aneurysm). In this situation, aortic clamping will have to be suprarenal and the left renal

vein must be thoroughly mobilized so that it can be retracted cephalad or caudad to facilitate adequate exposure of the aorta.[120] It is sometimes necessary to divide the left renal vein. This is usually well tolerated if the left adrenal and gonadal veins are not ligated. Reanastomosis of the transected renal vein is optional.

Distally the dissection should avoid the fibroareolar tissue overlying the left common iliac artery because it contains branch vessels of the inferior mesenteric artery and the autonomic nerves that control sexual function in men. If the common iliac arteries are relatively normal (i.e., not aneurysmal, stenotic, or heavily calcified) they can be clamped and a straight tube graft used. Significant disease of the common iliac arteries makes a bifurcated graft preferable. Control of the iliac arteries in these situations is best achieved by mobilizing the external and internal iliac arteries and clamping them individually. Particular care must be paid in this location to avoid injury to accompanying venous structures, as well as the ureters, which cross anterior to the common iliac bifurcation. Every effort should be made to ensure antegrade perfusion in at least one hypogastric artery in order to minimize the risk of postoperative ischemia of the left colon. This sometimes requires construction of end-to-side anastomoses between the graft limbs and the external iliac artery when anastomosis to the common iliac is not possible.

Aneurysm Repair

Regardless of the extent of the aortic aneurysm, the proximal graft anastomosis should be made as close as possible to the renal arteries in order to prevent recurrent aortic pathology. The degree of disease in the iliac arteries determines the distal extent of the graft. In some recent series, up to 80 per cent of patients were successfully treated with a straight tube graft, although in the experience of others only about one third of patients have suitable anatomy for this approach. There does not appear to be a significant incidence of subsequent iliac aneurysm formation when tube grafts are used.

The choice of graft material, Dacron or polytetrafluoroethylene (PTFE), and its construction, knitted or woven, are controversial but relatively unimportant issues. There is no proven superiority of one graft type when used for aortic replacement. Most surgeons find knitted grafts easier to handle, but preclotting is a necessary and sometimes time-consuming step. Preclotted grafts often leak a substantial amount of blood, which increases the need for transfusion. Knitted Dacron grafts sealed with collagen or gelatin do not require preclotting and are gaining in popularity. For ruptured aneurysms, nonporous grafts are clearly preferable because of savings in time and interstitial blood loss. Many surgeons routinely use woven Dacron or extruded PTFE grafts for elective aneurysm repair for the same reason.

Systemic heparin is nearly universally administered during the occlusive phase of aneurysm operations, since most surgeons believe its use provides an added margin of safety from distal thrombosis. The distal clamps should be applied before the proximal aortic clamp to prevent distal embolization. The aorta is opened longitudinally and either partially or completely transected at the site of the proximal anastomosis. If there is a very short neck (juxtarenal aneurysm), temporary proximal aortic clamping above the renal arteries will be required for infrarenal repair (Fig. 23–3). The proximal anastomosis can be done with a continuous or interrupted suture technique; the former is quicker. If the aorta is especially weak or friable, the sutures can be supported with Teflon-felt pledgets.

The distal anastomoses can be end-to-end or end-to-side depending on their location and the status of the common and internal iliac arteries. All mural thrombus and atheroma should be débrided from the aneurysm wall. Several studies have shown a surprisingly high incidence of positive bacterial cultures of this material, varying from 10 to 15 per cent to 40 per cent of patients. The significance of these positive cultures is unknown, but most of them have been due to coagulase-negative *Staphylococcus* species, an organism commonly found in aortic graft infections.[121] Back-bleeding lumbar vessels can be the source of significant blood loss and should be suture-ligated from within the aortic sac. If the inferior mesenteric artery is patent and actively back-bleeding, it can also be ligated within the aneurysm sac, but if back-bleeding is meager, the vessel should be preserved and reassessed after distal flow is reestablished, especially if internal iliac flow is compromised. Reimplantation of the inferior mesenteric artery is relatively easy to perform when necessary using the Carrel patch technique.

All anastomoses should be constructed with permanent, synthetic sutures. Braided Dacron and monofilament polypropylene are the most commonly used. Theoretical fears about late fracture of polypropylene sutures have not been substantiated in clinical practice. If suprarenal clamping is necessary, the clamp should be moved onto the graft below the renal arteries to minimize renal ischemia after ensuring that the proximal anastomosis is secure. The distal anastomoses are then constructed as indicated by the iliac artery disease. It is sometimes easier to control iliac artery back-bleeding by the use of intraluminal balloon catheters and to oversew the common iliac arteries from within the opened aortic and/or iliac aneurysm. In unusual circumstances, external iliac disease will necessitate making the distal anastomosis to the common femoral artery.

Declamping hypotension is now an unusual event in elective aortic aneurysm surgery. It is essential to maintain excellent communication with the anesthesiology team so that depth of anesthesia and blood and fluid replacement can be adjusted in anticipation of lower extremity reperfusion. Even though the graft and native vessels are flushed and back-bled prior to reestablishing distal flow, it is preferable to reestablish flow first into one hypogastric artery to minimize the chances of distal embolization to the leg. Prior to abdominal closure, adequacy of lower extremity and left colon perfusion should be ensured by direct inspection or noninvasive instrumentation. The graft should be insulated from the overlying bowel by careful closure of the aneurysm sac over the graft. This is sometimes impossible when the aneurysm is small, and in these situations rotation of a flap of the aneurysm wall or use of a vascularized omental pedicle can be employed to separate the graft from the duodenum.

It is beyond the scope of this chapter to discuss all of the technical details that might be encountered in the course of the surgical treatment of an aortic aneurysm. The principles outlined above are generally applicable for most cases. If additional vascular procedures are required, such as renal or visceral artery reconstruction, appropriate modifications in technique will be required.[122]

Repair of Ruptured Aneurysm

For ruptured aneurysms, the first priority is to control the hemorrhage by gaining proximal control of the aorta. Usually it is better to have the patient prepped and draped, with the surgical team ready to make a rapid entry into the abdomen, prior to induction of anesthesia. The induction of anesthesia in these circumstances is often associated with sudden and severe hypotension when the tamponade effects are relieved by relaxation of the abdominal wall. If the rupture is contained, proximal aortic control is best achieved at the level of the supraceliac aorta through the lesser omentum. The hematoma can then be entered and the clamp repositioned distally after the aortic neck is identified. The hematoma usually makes this portion of the dissection relatively easy, but caution must be exercised to avoid injury to major venous structures, since this is one of the commonest causes of excessive hemorrhage and subsequent death. If there is a free intraperitoneal rupture, the aorta can be quickly compressed at the diaphragm with an assistant's hand or a commercial compression device without formally dissecting this area. An infrarenal clamp or an intraluminal occluding balloon catheter can be substituted as soon as possible. After bleeding is controlled, adequate blood and volume replenishment should be achieved before attempting to restore flow to the lower extremities. Heparin is best avoided in ruptured aneurysm patients, since bleeding and coagulopathy are frequently associated with the shock, hypothermia, and massive blood loss and replacement that occur. The proper use of blood and blood products, including platelets and fresh-frozen plasma, is essential for survival of these patients.

COMPLICATIONS OF AORTIC ANEURYSM REPAIR

Survival following aortic aneurysm surgery has been discussed earlier in this chapter. Mortality ranges from 0 to 3 per cent for patients with uncomplicated aneurysms operated upon electively to over 80 per cent for patients with rupture, hypotension, and oliguria. The most frequent cause of death is myocardial dysfunction, usually ischemic in origin. Nonfatal myocardial infarction is also fairly common following even elective aortic aneurysm repair, occurring in from 3.1 to 16 per cent (average 6.9 per cent) of patients in reported cases.[8] The varying incidence is due to varying criteria used to define myocardial infarction.

Several other major complications can occur during or following aortic aneurysm operations. *Hemorrhage* is a constant threat, most often from injury to iliac or lumbar veins. It can be severe and extremely difficult to control, especially if it involves the left common iliac vein where it passes beneath the right common iliac artery. Extreme care must be taken when mobilizing the iliac arteries, especially if they are aneurysmal, in which case they are especially likely to be adherent to the underlying veins. Injury to the left renal vein or one of its tributaries is also associated with brisk bleeding. This is particularly likely when there are venous anomalies such as a retroaortic left renal vein or a circumaortic venous collar. These anomalies should be suspected when, during cephalad dissection of the aortic neck, either a small or no left renal is encountered. Postoperative hemorrhage can occur in any patient, and hemodynamic instability and evidence of continued blood loss should lead to early reexploration of the abdomen.

Declamping hypotension is not as frequent or severe a problem as it once was. Better understanding of its physiology, more aggressive management of intravascular volume, and better monitoring and anesthetic techniques have all contributed to the reduction in the incidence and seriousness of this problem. The surgeon can contribute to minimization of this condition by giving the anesthesiologist advance notification of plans to restore distal perfusion and then doing it gradually. In spite of these precautions, declamping hypotension can still be a serious problem, especially in the setting of a ruptured aneurysm in a cold, hypovolemic patient with poor cardiac performance.

Renal failure is another serious but now infrequent complication. At one time, 3 to 12 per cent of operative deaths following elective abdominal aortic aneurysm operations and an even higher percentage after emergency operations for rupture were attributable to acute renal failure.[123] Renal failure or less severe degrees of renal functional impairment can occur even when there is no hypotension and the proximal aortic clamp has been infrarenal in location. The etiology of renal dysfunction in these situations is poorly understood but is thought to involve reflex renal vasoconstriction and intrarenal redistribution of blood flow. Atheromatous embolization from clamping or manipulation of the perirenal aorta is also a potential contributing factor, as is temporary suprarenal clamping. Sometimes the large contrast load of an aortogram performed a day or two preoperatively can cause renal dysfunction that only becomes apparent postoperatively. Mannitol is commonly administered prior to aortic cross-clamping to increase urine output and prevent renal failure. Although this seems reasonable, studies have shown that intraoperative urine volume does not predict postoperative renal function.[124] Renal failure due to acute tubular necrosis is much more common following ruptured aortic aneurysms, occurring in 21 per cent of survivors of operation in one series. Unfortunately, the mortality associated with this complication still varies from 50 to 70 per cent in spite of the use of acute hemodialysis and adequate nutritional support.

Technical injury to the bowel or ureters can cause catastrophic infectious complications involving the newly implanted prosthetic graft. This is most likely to occur when there are adhesions from previous operations or the structures are in an unusual position (i.e., the ureters displaced anteriorly and laterally by the aneurysm). Such injuries should be meticulously repaired and the area irrigated with antibiotic solution. Ureteral injuries should be stented. In some situations, nephrectomy will be the safest course in order to avoid possible graft contamination.

Gastrointestinal complications of a functional nature regularly occur after aortic aneurysm surgery. Ileus is the rule for at least 3 to 4 days after transperitoneal surgery. Typically, gastric and colonic ileus persists longer than small bowel ileus. Occasionally, duodenal obstruction will persist for longer periods of time. Hematoma and edema in the vicinity of the proximal anastomosis is thought to contribute to this problem. Postoperative pancreatitis is relatively common, as determined by elevation of serum amylase, although clinically apparent pancreatitis is unusual. The pancreas can be injured by retractors, however, and a few patients will have serious consequences of these seemingly minor injuries.

The most serious gastrointestinal complication is ischemia of the left colon and rectum. The incidence of ischemic colitis following aortic reconstruction is about 2 per cent (range 0.2 to 10 per cent).[125] It is three to four times more common following operations for aortic aneurysm than operations for occlusive disease, and the incidence is several times higher in patients studied prospectively with colonoscopy after sustaining a ruptured aneurysm. Ligation of the inferior mesenteric artery is thought to be an important pathophysiological mechanism, but the inferior mesenteric artery is already occluded in the majority of patients with abdominal aneurysms. Improper ligation of the inferior mesenteric artery too far away from the wall of the aneurysm can contribute to this complication by interfering with collateral blood supply to the rectosigmoid.[126] This also emphasizes the importance of maintaining antegrade perfusion in at least one internal iliac artery following arterial reconstruction for aortic aneurysm. Even though most patients with occlusion of both internal iliac arteries and the inferior mesenteric artery will have adequate colonic perfusion, postoperative hypotension, bowel distention, and mesenteric vessel compression by hematoma can all contribute to postoperative colonic ischemia.

Postoperative colon ischemia can involve the mucosa only, which usually causes a transient, mild form of ischemic colitis, or it can involve mucosa and muscularis, which may result in fibrous healing and stricture formation. The most severe and dreaded form is transmural ischemia, which occurs in over 60 per cent of the reported cases.[127] The clinical manifestations of bowel ischemia depend on the severity of ischemia. Diarrhea, especially if it is bloody, is one of the earliest manifestations and usually begins within 48 hours of operation. It is an indication for colonoscopy to assess the status of the colonic mucosa. Other findings indicative of bowel gangrene and peritonitis may be present and demand prompt reoperation, resection of all compromised bowel, and creation of appropriate stomas. During bowel resection, efforts should be made to isolate the underlying aortic prosthesis from the surgical field, although this is usually impossible, setting the stage for subsequent prosthetic infection. If the graft becomes grossly contaminated, it should be removed and lower extremity perfusion restored by axillofemoral bypass. Less severe degrees of colonic ischemia can be managed nonoperatively, although subsequent correction of a colonic stricture may be required. A high index of suspicion of this complication must be maintained in order to detect and treat it in a timely fashion.

The mortality for postoperative colon ischemia following aortic aneurysm surgery is about 50 per cent overall, but increases to 90 per cent when full-thickness colonic gangrene and peritonitis occur. Preoperative evaluation of the blood supply to the colon and intraoperative assessment of colonic perfusion by Doppler or inferior mesenteric artery back-pressure measurements might help identify patients at highest risk for this disastrous complication so that preventive measures can be taken.

Paraplegia due to *spinal cord ischemia*, a well-recognized complication of thoracoabdominal aneurysm repair, is a rare event after operations confined to the infrarenal aorta, with only slightly more than 50 cases reported. Szilagyi et al. noted an incidence of 0.2 per cent in over 3000 aortic operations and it occurred 10 times more frequently in patients with ruptured aneurysms.[128] This suggests that hypotension is a contributing factor in most cases even though injury to an unusually located arteria magna radicularis (artery of Adamkiewicz) to the spinal cord may be the primary event. Unfortunately, this complication is not preventable, predictable, or treatable. Although the severity of the clinical manifestations

varies and approximately 50 per cent of affected survivors recover some neurologic function, there is a 50 per cent mortality associated with this complication.

Ischemia of the lower extremities can also occur following aortic aneurysm surgery. This may be due to embolization of dislodged mural thrombus from the aneurysm itself, thrombosis of a vessel due to distal stasis, creation of an intimal flap, or crushed atherosclerotic plaque. The use of heparin during the occlusive phase of aneurysm repair will not prevent the embolic events from occurring but may limit the propagation of thrombus, and should prevent formation of stasis thrombi in the distal vascular beds. Before closing the abdomen, the surgeon must be satisfied with the perfusion status of the lower extremities.

Microembolization can also occur, resulting in small patchy areas of ischemia, usually on the plantar aspect of the feet. Pedal pulses are usually still palpable in this situation. Euphemistically, this is known as "trash foot," and if recognized intraoperatively, the passage of small balloon catheters can sometimes retrieve at least some of the atheromatous debris. Lumbar symphathectomy may also be beneficial in limiting or preventing full-thickness tissue loss.

Infection involving the prosthetic graft used to restore aortic continuity occurs in from less than 1 to about 6 per cent of patients. It is more common after treating ruptured aneurysms. It may be associated with graft-enteric fistula, which is more common following surgery for aortic aneurysm than aortic occlusive disease. These infections usually become manifest months to years following graft implantation and are discussed in detail in Chapter 38.

UNUSUAL PROBLEMS ASSOCIATED WITH ABDOMINAL AORTIC ANEURYSMS

Several anatomical and pathological conditions can complicate the management of abdominal aortic aneurysms and adversely affect the outcome.

Venous Anomalies

There are several anomalies of the inferior vena cava and left renal vein that are important in aortic surgery. The inferior vena cava may be entirely on the left side (without situs inversus), or may be duplicated, with one on each side of the aorta. Double vena cava is estimated to occur in up to 3 per cent of patients, and the isolated left-sided vena cava occurs in only 0.2 to 0.5 per cent.[129,130] An isolated left-sided vena cava crosses obliquely in front of the aorta and may be joined by a short, immobile right renal vein. It can also cross from left to right behind the aorta. These anomalies can be especially troublesome if the aorta is approached retroperitoneally from the patient's left side. Near the neck of an aortic aneurysm, these anomalously positioned veins are prone to injury. Sometimes a crossing left inferior vena cava will have to be divided to enable satisfactory handling of the proximal aortic anastomosis. With a duplicated inferior vena cava, the left-sided one can be ligated if necessary, but care must be exercised to ensure that adequate venous drainage of the adrenal gland and left kidney are provided.

A retroaortic left renal vein, either alone or in association with an anterior vein in the usual location, is another rare anomaly that can lead to exsanguinating hemorrhage if it is injured during dissection or clamping of the aortic neck.[131] The incidence of this anomaly is 1.8 to 2.4 per cent. As mentioned earlier, when the surgeon cannot find the left renal vein in its usual preaortic location, he or she should assume that it is retroaortic and limit dissection in that area. Great care must be taken when applying the aortic cross-clamp to avoid tearing these posterior veins. If such a vein is injured, transection of the aorta is usually required to expose it well enough to control the bleeding.

Circumaortic venous collar is more common, occurring in up to 8.7 per cent of cases.[132] This anomaly is even more prone to injury, since the anterior component can be normal in size, leading the surgeon to disregard the possibility of a second, posterior renal vein.

Inflammatory Aneurysm

Nearly 5 per cent of abdominal aortic aneurysms are associated with a dense inflammatory, fibrotic reaction in the retroperitoneum that incorporates adjacent structures.[133,134] This appears to be a distinct clinicopathological entity of unknown etiology but characterized histologically by marked thickening of the adventitia and media (in contrast to other aortic aneurysms, which have a thinned, attenuated medial layer). Both layers are infiltrated with a prominent acute and chronic inflammatory reaction that include giant cells. The majority of the inflammatory cells are activated T-lymphocytes. The desmoplastic inflammatory reaction involves the duodenum in 90 per cent of cases, the inferior vena cava and left renal vein in over 50 per cent, and the ureters in about 25 per cent.[135] These aneurysms tend to be large and most patients are symptomatic (pain) in the absence of rupture. A majority of the patients have an elevated erythrocyte sedimentation rate of uncertain significance and many have lost weight. The diagnosis can be suspected on the CT scan where the periaortic fibrous tissue can be easily seen obliterating tissue planes and a typical halo effect of this tissue appears after intravenous contrast administration. MRI also shows a characteristic appearance of inflammatory aneurysm consisting of several concentric rings surrounding the aortic lumen. Either of these imaging techniques can establish the presence of an inflammatory aneurysm in a high percentage of cases. Recently published reports have pointed out several

advantages of the left-sided retroperitoneal approach for these lesions, and establishing this diagnosis preoperatively makes possible the selection of this technique. In cases of ureteric involvement, the ureters are pulled medially and may be obstructed (again in contrast to other large aneurysms, which tend to push the ureters laterally). At laparotomy, the diagnosis can be immediately established by recognition of the dense, shiny, white, highly vascular reaction in the retroperitoneum, centered over the aortic aneurysm. Once recognized, the usual maneuvers of aneurysmorrhaphy should be modified in order to avoid injury to adherent structures, especially the duodenum. The aorta should be exposed cephalad to the renal vein or at the diaphragm and opened without dissecting the duodenum off the wall. Concomitant ureterolysis is seldom necessary, since the inflammatory reaction usually resolves postoperatively. Ureteral catheterization is a useful adjunct, however, and helps to avoid intraoperative ureteral injury. Although the transfusion requirements and operative mortality are slightly higher than for noninflammatory aneurysms, the long-term outlook for these patients is comparable to that for patients with ordinary abdominal aortic aneurysms, and the usual criteria for recommending elective operation should be applied, since these aneurysms can rupture in spite of their very thick anterior wall.[136]

Horseshoe Kidney

Horseshoe kidney occurs in from 1:400 to 1:1000 of the general population. Its association with abdominal aortic aneurysm is rare, but it complicates graft replacement because the kidney mass is usually fused anterior to the aorta, the collecting system and ureters are medially displaced, and there are frequently multiple renal arteries arising from the aorta, including the aneurysmal part, and/or the iliac arteries.[137,138] It has been estimated that in 60 per cent of cases the anomalous renal blood supply will require some form of surgical correction.[139] Preoperative arteriography is essential for the proper evaluation of these renal arteries but, unless it is performed as a matter of routine, it will not usually be considered unless the diagnosis is suspected from an intravenous pyelogram or CT or ultrasound scan. The isthmus of a horseshoe kidney seldom needs to be or should be divided, since the aortic graft can be passed behind it. If renal arteries arise from the aneurysm, they can be reimplanted into the graft as a Carrel patch. If recognized preoperatively, a left retroperitoneal approach allows easier management of the multiple and accessory renal arteries.

Associated Intraabdominal Pathology and Concomitant Surgical Procedures

Occasionally, there will be stenotic atherosclerotic lesions in aortic branches that require surgical correction at the time of aortic aneurysm repair. This most often involves the renal arteries in patients with renovascular hypertension or impaired renal function.[140,141] Rarely, chronic visceral ischemia will necessitate concomitant visceral artery repair and aneurysmorrhaphy. In most series, the morbidity and mortality of combined procedures exceeds that of elective aneurysm alone, so caution is urged in the performance of purely prophylactic procedures in this setting.

Malignant tumors are unexpectedly found in 4 to 5 per cent of patients undergoing operation for abdominal aneurysm. Most of these are colonic. Since operating on the colon converts a clean into a contaminated procedure with its potential for prosthetic graft infection, the decision is not always easy regarding how to treat each lesion (aneurysm, colon mass). It is sometimes difficult to distinguish cancer from inflammatory lesions intraoperatively. In addition, most vascular surgeons do not employ a formal bowel prep for patients undergoing elective aortic aneurysm surgery. For these reasons, unless there are compelling reasons for treating the colonic lesion (perforation, obstruction, hemorrhage), the aneurysm procedure should be completed and the colon left alone. The colonic lesion can then be properly evaluated and treated postoperatively. Generally, it is possible to perform an elective colon operation sooner after an aortic aneurysm repair than the opposite, especially if there has been a septic complication (common following colon surgery but rare after aortic surgery).

Asymptomatic gallstones is a far more common condition found unexpectedly in from 5 to 20 per cent of patients undergoing aortic surgery. Several series have been published attesting to the safety of concomitant cholecystectomy and aortic repair.[142,143] A major impetus for this philosophy is the postulated high incidence of postoperative cholecystitis in such patients who have only their aortic pathology treated. In the series reported by String there was only one documented late graft infection in 34 patients who underwent combined procedures.[142] However, the follow-up was rather short, especially when one considers the usual long intervals between aortic grafting and the first manifestations of graft infection. In addition, the incidence of positive cultures from bile of patients with cholelithiasis is as high as 33 per cent. As with colonic lesions, performance of elective cholecystectomy, which could possibly lead to contamination of a newly implanted aortic prosthesis, should not be performed in conjunction with vascular grafting operations.[144] The consequences of infection of the aortic graft are so grave that the risk of doing so is unjustified for an elective operation.

Aortocaval Fistula

Abdominal aortic aneurysms can rupture into the inferior vena cava or iliac veins. This is the most frequent cause of aortocaval fistula and occurs in from 0.2 to 1.3 per cent of patients with atherosclerotic (degenerative) abdominal aortic aneurysms.[145–148] The incidence is at least twice as high in cases of ruptured aneurysms. The most frequent site of fistulization is the distal aorta at or just above the confluence of the iliac veins. Almost all aortocaval fistulas are symptomatic, and impaired renal function is common. Abdominal and/or back pain is present in over 80 per cent of patients and most have a palpable mass; 75 per cent have an audible bruit, but only about 25 per cent have a palpable thrill. Venous hypertension can affect the gastrointestinal tract as well as the lower extremities, and lower gastrointestinal tract bleeding as well as hematuria are common.

In spite of these protean manifestations, the diagnosis of aortocaval fistula is usually not made clinically. Aortography is the best diagnostic modality, although the fistulas can sometimes be documented by CT, MRI, or ultrasound scans. The natural history of aortocaval fistula is progressive cardiac decompensation and death. Surgical correction offers the only hope for survival and should be undertaken promptly. A conventional infrarenal aortic aneurysm operation with oversewing of the fistula from within the opened aorta will cure the fistula. Hemodynamic improvement is immediate and renal function usually recovers rapidly. Nevertheless, reported mortality rates have been between 22 and 51 per cent, largely as a result of blood loss, cardiac decompensation, and pulmonary embolism.[148]

MYCOTIC AORTIC ANEURYSMS

Mycotic aneurysm refers to an aneurysm of infectious although not necessarily fungal etiology. The term mycotic is derived from the mushroom-shaped false aneurysm of the arterial wall that is typically found. They usually occur as a consequence of bacterial or septic emboli loading at a point on the intimal surface of an artery in sufficient number to produce a locally invasive infection that then spreads to become a transmural arteritis. Although this can occur in normal arteries, it more commonly affects large, major atherosclerotic vessels and their branches. A septic embolus may also lodge in vasa vasorum and initiate a necrotic process in the arterial wall. A third mechanism is arterial invasion from a septic focus adjacent to a major artery. In recent years, traumatic contamination of an artery has replaced endocarditis as the most common etiology, often as a result of drug abuse.

In the largest collective review of mycotic aneurysms, the abdominal aorta was the second most frequent site of involvement (31 per cent), exceeded only by the femoral artery (38 per cent).[149] Chan et al. have recently reported a series of 22 mycotic aortic aneurysms out of a series of 2585 patients, an incidence of 0.85 per cent).[150] Coincident with the change in etiology, there has been a change in the bacteriology of mycotic aneurysms, with *Salmonella* species declining while *Staphylococcus* species are increasing, but, together, these are still the most frequently cultured organisms from aortic mycotic aneurysms.[151] The predilection for the infrarenal abdominal aorta probably relates to the frequent occurrence of atherosclerotic plaques in this location.

Most patients present with a nonspecific febrile illness of variable duration and many do not have a palpable aneurysm. Only about one third have abdominal pain. The triad of abdominal pain, fever, and a pulsatile abdominal mass should suggest the diagnosis of mycotic aneurysm. Leukocytosis is a common finding. Mycotic aneurysms are often detected by CT scans performed for evaluation of undiagnosed fever. They appear as a mass located on one side of the aorta rather than a circumferential enlargement.[149,151] They enhance with intravenously administered contrast, but the significance of this can be difficult to appreciate. Angiography will demonstrate the characteristic lobulated saccular aneurysm, which may be multiple and contiguous. These are false aneurysms, contained by compressed periaortic tissue. The aneurysm wall tends to be thin and friable and associated with contiguous lymphadenopathy and obvious inflammation. Blood clot of varying age is present both within and outside the aneurysmal sac, because there is a high incidence of rupture, although it is usually contained. Periaortic abscess may also be present. The opening between the aorta and the aneurysm tends to be irregular or ragged.

Mycotic aneurysms are a fulminant infectious process and must be treated vigorously and promptly.[150,152,153] Control of clinical sepsis does not appear to be necessary for successful surgical treatment and delays in operative intervention are associated with aneurysmal rupture. Proper antibiotic therapy must be combined with resection of the infected arterial segments, débridement of all adjacent necrotic tissue, and arterial reconstruction. Control of infection by antibiotics does not prevent rupture of the aneurysm, and excision is mandatory and should be carried out promptly. Many of these aneurysms involve the upper abdominal aorta, where it is not always possible to avoid use of prosthetic arterial grafts. In situ prosthetic replacement is necessary when renal or visceral perfusion would be compromised by aortic excision. For the infrarenal aorta, if the intraoperative Gram's stains are negative and there is no periaortic purulence, in situ prosthetic grafting is also the procedure of choice. It should be followed with 6 to 8 weeks of specific antibiotic therapy, and, in the case of *Salmonella* infections, probably lifelong antibiotics. When there is frank periaortic pus and/ or positive Gram's stain of an infrarenal mycotic aneurysm, management can be either aortic débridement and ligation, extraanatomic bypass, and a shorter course of antibiotics, or alternatively by the in situ grafting technique described above. Recent data tend to favor the in situ method. Using these principles, Crawford's group has reported an operative survival rate of 86 per cent, with only one recurrent infection.[150]

ILIAC ARTERY ANEURYSMS

Common iliac artery aneurysms occur frequently in continuity or in association with abdominal aortic aneurysms. As isolated lesions they are uncommon, accounting for less than 1 per cent of all aneurysms involving the aortoiliac segment.[154-158] They are most often atherosclerotic (degenerative) in nature, and therefore most occur in the atherosclerosis age group, but some have developed during pregnancy in the absence of atherosclerosis. Mycotic iliac aneurysms have been reported, as have traumatic ones, usually following lumbar disk or hip surgery. Iliac aneurysms usually involve the common or internal iliac arteries. They are multiple in over 33 per cent of patients. Isolated external iliac aneurysms are rare. Since these lesions are in the pelvis, they are difficult to detect by abdominal examination so they tend to be quite large or symptomatic when they are eventually discovered. This also accounts for the unusually high incidence of rupture, which averages 33 per cent in collected series, but was 51 per cent in the largest review.[143] Symptoms are most often due to rupture (77 per cent) and/or pressure on adjacent pelvic structures (urinary tract, lower gastrointestinal tract, lumbosacral nerves, pelvic veins, etc.).[159] Lower abdominal, flank, and groin pain are common. Most of the symptoms are not those usually attributed to the arterial system, which contributes to delay in diagnosis.

Even though iliac aneurysms are difficult to detect by routine abdominal examination, large ones can be palpated on abdominal, rectal, or pelvic examination. Common iliac aneurysms are generally more readily palpable abdominally and internal iliac aneurysms more easily palpable rectally. Other tests useful in the diagnosis of iliac aneurysms are proctoscopy, barium enema, cystoscopy, and plain abdominal x-ray. CT, ultrasound, and MRI can be expected to establish the correct diagnosis in the majority of patients. Arteriography documents the presence of most iliac aneurysms but, as with aneurysms elsewhere, often underestimates the size because of laminated thrombus.

Iliac aneurysms tend to be large when diagnosed. In Shuler and Flanigan's collected review, the average size at operation or autopsy was 8.5 cm, and the incidence of rupture of the entire series of 83 iliac aneurysms was 51 per cent.[154]

The natural history of iliac aneurysms appears to be unfavorable.[160] Probably because of their large size when diagnosed, there is a high rate of rupture within a few months of diagnosis. Operative mortality in patients with ruptured aneurysms is high (59 per cent in Schuler and Flanigan's review), compared to only 11 per cent for elective operations. Thus, isolated iliac aneurysms should be treated surgically when they are discovered in order to avoid the high mortality associated with rupture. For the common iliac artery, a diameter of 3.0 cm appears to be the size for which surgical treatment is prudent.

The treatment of choice for internal iliac aneurysms is proximal ligation and endoaneurysmorrhaphy. For aneurysmal involvement of the common iliac artery, graft replacement is recommended, and since the external iliac artery is almost never aneurysmal, these grafts can be confined to the abdomen. If both common iliac arteries are aneurysmal or the aneurysm extends to the aortic bifurcation, an aortoiliac bifurcation graft should be inserted.

REFERENCES

1. Bickerstaff LK, Hollier LH, Van Peenen HJ, et al: Abdominal aortic aneurysm: The changing natural history. J Vasc Surg 1:6–12, 1984.
2. Castelden W, Mercer J: Abdominal aortic aneurysms in western Australia: Descriptive epidemiology and patterns of rupture. Br J Surg 72:109–112, 1985.
3. Melton L, Bickerstaff L, Hollier LH, et al: Changing incidence of abdominal aortic aneurysms: A population based study. Am J Epidemiol 120:379–386, 1984.
4. Norman PE, Castleden WM, Hockey RL: Prevalance of abdominal aortic aneurysm in Western Australia. Br J Surg 78:1118–1121, 1991.
5. Darling RC, Messina CR, Brewster DC, Ottinger LW: Autopsy study of unoperated aortic aneurysms. Circulation 56(suppl 2):161–164, 1977.
6. Cabellon S, Moncreif CL, Pierre DR, Cavanaugh DG: Incidence of abdominal aortic aneurysms in patients with atheromatous arterial disease. Am J Surg 146:575–576, 1983.
7. Thurmond AS, Semler JH: Abdominal aortic aneurysm. Incidence in a population at risk. J Cardiovasc Surg 27:457–460, 1986.
8. Taylor LM, Porter JM: Basic data related to clinical decision-making in abdominal aortic aneurysms. Ann Vasc Surg 1:502–504, 1980.
9. Graham LM, Zelenock GB, Whitehouse WM, et al: Clinical significance of atherosclerotic femoral artery aneurysms. Arch Surg 155:502–507, 1980.
10. Vermilion BD, Kimmins SA, Pace WG, Evans WE: A review of 147 popliteal aneurysms with long-term follow-up. Surgery 90:1009–1014, 1981.
11. Bengtsson H, Bergqvist D, Ekberg O, Janzon L: A population based screening of abdominal aortic aneurysms (AAA). Eur J Vasc Surg 5:53–57, 1991.
12. Scott RAP, Ashton HA, Kay DN: Abdominal aortic aneurysm in 4237 screened patients: Prevalence, development and management over 6 years. Br J Surg 78:1122–1125, 1991.
13. Johnston KW, Rutherford RB, Tilson MD, et al: Suggested standards for reporting on arterial aneurysms. J Vasc Surg 13:452–458, 1991.
14. Steinberg CR, Morton A, Steinberg I: Measurement of the abdominal aorta after intravenous aortography in health and arteriosclerotic peripheral vascular disease. AJR 95:703–708, 1965.
15. Hollier LH, Stanson AW, Glovicski P, et al: Arteriomegaly: Classifications and morbid implications of diffuse aneurysmal disease. Surgery 93:700, 1983.
16. Bengtsson H, Ekberg O, Aspelin P, et al: Abdominal aortic dilatation in patients operated on for carotid artery stenosis. Acta Chir Scand 154:441–445, 1988.
17. Mukherjee D, Mayberry JC, Inahara T, Greig JD: The relationship of the abdominal aortic aneurysm to the tortuous internal carotid artery. Is there one? Arch Surg 124:955–956, 1989.
18. Cohen J: Pathogenesis of aortic aneurysms. Perspect Vasc Surg 3:103–111, 1990.
19. Tilson DM, Stansel HC: Differences in results for aneurysm vs. occlusive disease after bifurcation grafts. Results of 100 elective grafts. Arch Surg 107:1173–1175, 1980.
20. Dobrin PB: Pathophysiology and pathogenesis of aortic aneurysms. Current concept. Surg Clin North Am 69:687–703, 1989.
21. Zarins CK, Glagov S: Aneurysms and obstructive plaques: Differing local responses to atherosclerosis. In Bergan JJ, Yao JST (eds): Aneurysms: Diagnosis and Treatment. New York, Grune & Stratton, 1982, pp 61–82.
22. Busuttil RW, Abou-Zamzam AM, Machleder HI: Collagenase activity of the human aorta: Comparisons of patients with and without abdominal aortic aneurysms. Arch Surg 115:1373–1378, 1980.
23. Busuttil RW, Heinrich R, Flesher A: Elastase activity: The role of elastase in aortic aneurysm formation. J Surg Res 32:214–217, 1982.
24. Dobrin PB, Baker WH, Gley WC: Elastolytic and collagenolytic studies of arteries: Implications for the mechanical properties of aneurysms. Arch Surg 119:405–409, 1984.
25. Dobrin PB, Baker WH, Schwarcz TH: Mechanisms of arterial and aneurysmal tortuosity. Surgery 104:568–571, 1988.
26. Cohen J, Mandell C, Chang JB, Wise L: Elastin metabolism of the infrarenal aorta. J Vasc Surg 7:210–214, 1988.
27. Cronenwett JL, Murphy TF, Zelenock GB, et al: Actuarial analysis of variables associated with rupture of small aortic aneurysms. Surgery 98:472–483, 1985.
28. Majumder PP, St. Jean PL, Ferrell RE, et al: On the inheritance of abdominal aortic aneurysm. Am J Hum Genet 48:164–170, 1991.
29. Tilson MD, Seashore MR: Human genetics of the abdominal aortic aneurysm. Surg Gynecol Obstet 158:129–132, 1984.
30. Tilson MD: Decreased hepatic copper levels: A possible chemical marker for the pathogenesis of aortic aneurysms in man. Arch Surg 117:1212–1213, 1982.
31. Tilson MD: Generalized arteriomegaly: A possible predisposition to the formation of abdominal aortic aneurysms. Arch Surg 116:1030–1032, 1981.
32. Collin J, Walton J: Is abdominal aortic aneurysm familial? Br Med J 299:493, 1989.
33. Johansen K, Koepsell T: Familial tendency for abdominal aortic aneurysms. JAMA 256:1934–1936, 1986.
34. Clifton MA: Familial abdominal aortic aneurysms. Br J Surg 64:765–766, 1977.
35. Szilagyi DE: Clinical diagnosis of intact and ruptured abdominal aortic aneurysms. In Bergan JJ, Yao JST (eds): Aneurysms: Diagnosis and Treatment. New York, Grune & Stratton, 1982, pp 205–215.
36. Sterpetti AV, Feldhaus RJ, Schultz RD, Blair EA: Identification of abdominal aortic aneurysm patients with different clinical features and clinical outcomes. Am J Surg 156:466–473, 1988.
37. Lawrie GM, Crawford ES, Morris GC Jr, Howell JF: Progress in the treatment of ruptured abdominal aortic aneurysm. World J Surg 4:653–660, 1980.
38. Rutherford RB, McCroskey BL: Ruptured abdominal aortic

aneurysms. Special considerations. Surg Clin North Am 69(4):859–868, 1989.

39. Bower TC, Cherry KJ Jr, Pairolero PC: Unusual manifestations of abdominal aneurysms. Surg Clin North Am 69:745–753, 1989.

40. Moran KT, Persson AV, Jewell ER: Chronic rupture of abdominal aortic aneurysms. Am Surg 55:485–487, 1989.

41. Rich NM, Clagett GP, Salander JM, et al: Role of arteriography in the evaluation of aortic aneurysms. *In* Bergan JJ, Yao JST (eds): Aneurysms: Diagnosis and Treatment. New York, Grune & Stratton, 1982, pp 233–241.

42. Friedman SG, Kerner BA, Krishnasastry KV, Doscher W, Deckoff SL, Friedman MS: Abdominal aortic aneurysmectomy without preoperative angiography: A prospective study. NY State J Med 90(1):176–178, 1990.

43. Gaspar MR: Role of arteriography in the evaluation of aortic aneurysms. The case against. *In* Bergan JY, Yao JST (eds): Aneurysms: Diagnosis and Treatment. New York, Grune & Stratton, 1982, pp 243–254.

44. Goldstone J: Vascular imaging techniques. *In* Rutherford RB (ed): Vascular Surgery, 3rd ed. Philadelphia, WB Saunders Company, 1989, pp 119–128.

45. Quill DS, Colgan MP, Summer DS: Ultrasonic screening for the detection of abdominal aortic aneurysms. Surg Clin North Am 69(4):713–720, 1989.

46. Bluth EI: Ultrasound of the abdominal aorta. Arch Intern Med 144:377, 1984.

47. Gomes MN, Choyke PL: Pre-operative evaluation of abdominal aortic aneurysms: Ultrasound or computed tomography? J Cardiovasc Surg 28:159–165, 1987.

48. Greatorex RA, Dixon AK, Flower CDR, Pulvertaft RW: Limitations of computed tomography in leaking abdominal aortic systems. Br Med J 297:284–285, 1988.

49. Amparo EG, Hoddick WK, Hricak H, et al: Comparison of magnetic resonance imaging and ultrasonography in the evaluation of abdominal aortic aneurysms. Radiology 154:451, 1985.

50. Clayton MJ, Walsh JW, Brewer WH: Contained rupture of abdominal aortic aneurysms: Sonographic and CT diagnosis. AJR 138:154, 1982.

51. Weinbaum FI, Dubner S, Turner JW, et al: The accuracy of computed tomography in the diagnosis of retroperitoneal blood in the presence of abdominal aortic aneurysm. J Vasc Surg 6:11, 1987.

52. Lee JKT, Ling D, Heiken JP, et al: Magnetic resonance imaging of abdominal aneurysms. AJR 143:1197, 1984.

53. Estes JE Jr: Abdominal aortic aneurysm: A study of 102 cases. Circulation 2:258–264, 1950.

54. Wright IS, Urdenata E, Wright B: Re-opening the case of the abdominal aortic aneurysm. Circulation 13:754–768, 1956.

55. Szilagyi DE, Smith RF, De Russo FJ, et al: Contribution of abdominal aortic aneurysmectomy to prolongation of life. Ann Surg 164:678–689, 1966.

56. Bernstein EF, Chan EL: Abdominal aortic aneurysm in high risk patients: Outcome of selective management based on size and expansion rate. Ann Surg 200:255–263, 1984.

57. Szilagyi DE, Elliott JP, Smith RF: Clinical fate of the patient with asymptomatic abdominal aortic aneurysm and unfit surgical treatment. Arch Surg 104:600–606, 1972.

58. Foster JH, Bolasny BL, Gobbel WG, Scott HW: Comparative study of elective resection and expectant treatment of abdominal aortic aneurysm. Surg Gynecol Obstet 129:1–9, 1969.

59. Nevitt MP, Ballard DJ, Hallett JW Jr: Prognosis of abdominal aortic aneurysms. N Engl J Med 321:1009–1014, 1989.

60. Glimåker H, Holmberg L, Elvin A, Nybacka O, Almgren B, Björck CG, Eriksson I: Natural history of patients with abdominal aortic aneurysm. Eur J Vasc Surg 5:125–130, 1991.

61. Johansson G, Nydahl S, Olofsson P, Swedenborg J: Survival in patients with abdominal aortic aneurysms. Comparison between operative and nonoperative management. Eur J Vasc Surg 4:497–502, 1990.

62. Walsh AKM, Briffa N, Nash JR, Callum KG: The natural history of small abdominal aortic aneurysms: An ultrasound study. Eur J Vasc Surg 4:459–461, 1990.

63. Cronenwett JL, Sargent SK, Wall MH, et al: Variables that affect the expansion rate and outcome of small abdominal aortic aneurysms. J Vasc Surg 11:260–269, 1990.

64. Collin J, Heather B, Walton J: Growth rates of subclinical abdominal aortic aneurysms—implications for review and rescreening programmes. Eur J Vasc Surg 5:141–144, 1991.

65. Thompson JE, Hollier LH, Putment RD, Person AV: Surgical management of abdominal aortic aneurysms. Ann Surg 181:654–660, 1975.

66. Baird RJ, Gurry JF, Kellam JF, Wilson DR: Abdominal aortic aneurysms: Recent experience with 210 patients. Can Med Assoc J 118:1229–1235, 1978.

67. Crawford ES, Saleh SA, Babb JW III, et al: Infrarenal abdominal aortic aneurysm. Factors influencing survival after operation performed over a 25 year period. Ann Surg 193:699–709, 1981.

68. Whittemore AD, Clowes AW, Hechtman HB, Mannik JA: Aortic aneurysm repair reduced operative mortality associated with maintenance of optimal cardiac performance. Ann Surg 120:414–421, 1980.

69. Ramos TK, Goldstone J: Should small abdominal aortic aneurysms be operated on? *In* Veith F (ed): Current Critical Problems in Vascular Surgery, vol 4. St. Louis, Quality Medical Publishing, 1992, pp 197–206.

70. Pairolero PC: Repair of abdominal aortic aneurysms in high-risk patients. Surg Clin North Am 69:755–763, 1989.

71. Pilcher DB, Davis JH, Ashileoga T, et al: Treatment of abdominal aortic aneurysm in an entire state over 7½ years. Ann J Surg 139:487–494, 1980.

72. Hertzer NR, Avellone JC, Farrel CJ, et al: The risk of vascular surgery in a metropolitan community. J Vasc Surg 1:13–21, 1984.

73. DeBakey ME, Crawford ES, Cooley DA, et al: Aneurysm of abdominal aorta. Analysis of results of graft replacement therapy one to eleven years after operation. Ann Surg 169:622, 1964.

74. Robson AK, Currie IC, Poskitt KR, Scott DJA, Baird RN, Horrocks M: Abdominal aortic aneurysm repair in the over eighties. Br J Surg 76:1018–1020, 1989.

75. Vasko JS, Spencer FC, Bahnson HT: Aneurysm of the aorta treated by excision: Review of 237 cases followed up to seven years. Am J Surg 105:793, 1963.

76. Cannon JA, Van De Water J, Barker WF: Experience with the surgical management of 100 consecutive cases of abdominal aortic aneurysm. Am J Surg 106:128, 1963.

77. Voorhees AB, McAllister FF: Long term results following resection of arteriosclerotic abdominal aortic aneurysms. Surg Gynecol Obstet 117:355, 1963.

78. Levy JF, Kouchoukos NT, Walker WB, Butcher HR: Abdominal aortic aneurysmectomy: A study of 100 cases. Arch Surg 92:498, 1966.

79. May AG, DeWeese JA, Frank I, Mahoney EB, Rob CG: Surgical treatment of abdominal aortic aneurysms. Surgery 63:711, 1968.

80. Baker AG, Roberts B: Long-term survival following abdominal aortic aneurysmectomy. JAMA 212:445, 1970.

81. Stokes J, Butcher HR: Abdominal aortic aneurysms: Factors influencing operative mortality and criteria of operability. Arch Surg 107:297, 1973.

82. Hicks GL, Eastland MW, DeWeese JA, May AG, Rob CG: Survival improvement following aortic aneurysm resection. Ann Surg 181:863, 1975.

83. O'Donnell TF, Darling RC, Linton RR: Is 80 years too old for aneurysmectomy? Arch Surg 111:1250–1257, 1976.

84. Crawford ES, Saleh SA, Babb JW III, Glaeser DH, Vaccaro PS, Silvers A: Infrarenal abdominal aortic aneurysm: Factors influencing survival after operations performed over a 25-year period. Ann Surg 193:699, 1981.

85. Reigel MM, Hollier LH, Kazmier FJ, O'Brien PC, Pairolero PC, Cherry KJ, Hallett JW: Late survival in abdominal aortic aneurysm patients: The role of selective myocardial

revascularization on the basis of clinical systems. J Vasc Surg 5:222, 1987.

86. Bernstein EF, Dilley RB, Randolph HF III: The improving long term outlook for patients 70 years of age with abdominal aortic aneurysms. Ann Surg 207:318, 1988.

87. Hollier LH, Taylor LM, Ochsner J: Recommended indications for operative treatment of abdominal aortic aneurysms. Report of a subcommittee of the Joint Council of the Society for Vascular Surgery and the North American Chapter of the International Society for Cardiovascular Surgery. J Vasc Surg 15:1046–1056, 1992.

88. Hollier LH, Reigel MM, Kozmier FJ, et al: Conventional repair of abdominal aortic aneurysm in the high-risk patient: A plea for abandonment of nonresective treatment. J Vasc Surg 3:712–717, 1986.

89. Hiatt JCG, Barker WF, Machleder HI, Baker JD, Busuttil RW, Moore WS: Determinants of failure in the treatment of ruptured abdominal aortic aneurysms. Arch Surg 119:1264–1268, 1984.

90. Fielding JWL, Black J, Ashton F, Slaney G: Ruptured aortic aneurysms: Postoperative complications and their aetiology. Br J Surg 72:487–491, 1984.

91. Donaldson MC, Rosenberg JM, Bucknam CA: Factors affecting survival after ruptured abdominal aortic aneurysm. J Vasc Surg 2:564–570, 1985.

92. Hoffman M, Avellone JC, Plecha FR, et al: Operation for ruptured abdominal aortic aneurysm: A community-wide experience. Surgery 91:597–602, 1982.

93. Burnham SJ, Johnson G Jr, Curri JA: Mortality risks for survivors of vascular reconstructive procedures. Surgery 92:107, 1982.

94. Johnson G Jr, Gurri JA, Burnham SJ: Life expectancy after abdominal aortic aneurysm repair. *In* Bergan JJ, Yao JST (eds): Aneurysms: Diagnosis and Treatment. New York, Grune & Stratton, 1982, pp 279–285.

95. Hollier LH, Plate G, O'Brien PC, et al: Late survival after abdominal aortic aneurysm repair. Influence of coronary artery disease. J Vasc Surg 1:290–299, 1984.

96. Hertzer NR: Fatal myocardial infarction following abdominal aortic aneurysm resection: 343 patients followed 6–11 years post-operative. Ann Surg 190:667–673, 1980.

97. Hertzer NR: Clinical experience with pre-operative coronary angiography. J Vasc Surg 2:510–512, 1985.

98. Hertzer NR, Young JR, Bevan EG, et al: Late results of coronary bypass in patients with infra-renal aortic aneurysms. The Cleveland Clinic Study. Ann Surg 205:360–367, 1987.

99. Crawford ES, Morris GC Jr, Howell JF, et al: Operative risk in patients with previous coronary artery bypass. Ann Thorac Surg 26:215–221, 1978.

100. Ruby ST, Whittemore AD, Couch NP, et al: Coronary artery disease in patients requiring abdominal aortic aneurysm repair. Selective use of a combined operation. Arch Surg 201:758–764, 1985.

101. Reul G Jr, Cooley DA, Duncan MJ, et al: The effect of coronary bypass on the outcome of peripheral vascular operation in 1093 patients. J Vasc Surg 3:788–798, 1986.

102. Bevan EG: Routine coronary angiography in patients undergoing surgery for abdominal aortic aneurysm and lower extremity occlusive disease. J Vasc Surg 3:682–684, 1986.

103. Yeager RA, Moneta GL: Assessing cardiac risk in vascular surgical patients: Current status. Perspect Vasc Surg 2:18–39, 1989.

104. Blomberg PA, Ferguson IA, Rosengarten DS, et al: The role of coronary artery disease in complications of abdominal aortic aneurysm repair. Surgery 101:150–155, 1987.

105. Goldman L: Cardiac risks and complications of non-cardiac surgery. Ann Surg 198:780–791, 1983.

106. Golden MA, Whittemore AD, Donaldson MC, Mannick JA: Selective evaluation and management of coronary artery disease in patients undergoing repair of abdominal aortic aneurysms: A 16-year experience. Ann Surg 212:415–423, 1990.

107. McPhail NV, Ruddy TD, Calvin JE, Davies RA, Barber GG: A complication of dipyridamole-thallium imaging and exercise testing in the prediction of post-operative cardiac complications in patients requiring arterial reconstruction. J Vasc Surg 10:51–56, 1989.

108. Boucher CA, Brewster DC, Darling RC, et al: Determination of cardiac risk by dipyridamole-thallium imaging before peripheral vascular surgery. N Engl J Med 312:389–394, 1985.

109. Cheitlin MD: Finding the high-risk patient with coronary artery disease. JAMA 259:2271–2277, 1988.

110. Karmody AM, Leather RP, Goldman M, et al: The current position of non-resective treatment for abdominal aortic aneurysm. Surgery 94:591–597, 1983.

111. Schwartz RA, Nichols WK, Silver D: Is thrombosis of the infrarenal abdominal aortic aneurysm an acceptable alternative? J Vasc Surg 3:448–455, 1986.

112. Cho SI, Johnson WC, Buch HL Jr, et al: Lethal complications associated with nonresective treatment of abdominal aortic aneurysms. Arch Surg 117:1214–1217, 1982.

113. Inahara T, Beary GL, Mukherjee D, Egan JM: The contrary position to the nonresective treatment for abdominal aortic aneurysm. J Vasc Surg 2:42–48, 1985.

114. Sicard GA, Allen BJ, Munn JS, Anderson CB: Retroperitoneal vs. transperitoneal approach for repair of abdominal aortic aneurysms. Surg Clin North Am 69:795–806, 1989.

115. Cambria RP, Brewster DC, Abbott WM, et al: Transperitoneal versus retroperitoneal approach for aortic reconstruction. A randomized, prospective study. J Vasc Surg 11:314–325, 1990.

116. Cambria RP, Brewster DC: Advantages of the retroperitoneal approach for aortic surgery: Fact or fancy? Perspect Vasc Surg 3:52–69, 1990.

117. Chang BB, Shan DJ, Paty PS, Kaufman JL, Leather RP: Can the retroperitoneal approach be used for ruptured abdominal aortic aneurysms? J Vasc Surg 11:326–330, 1990.

118. Goldstone J: Intraoperative monitoring in aortic surgery. *In* Bergan JJ, Yao JST (eds): Arterial Surgery. New Diagnostic and Operative Techniques. Orlando, FL, Grune & Stratton, 1988, pp 257–271.

119. Roizen MF, Beaupre PN, Albert RA, et al: Monitoring with two-dimensional transesophageal echocardiography. J Vasc Surg 1:300–305, 1984.

120. Budden J, Hollier LH: Management of aneurysms that involve the juxtarenal or suprarenal aorta. Surg Clin North Am 69:837–844, 1989.

121. Macbeth GA, Rubin JR, McIntyre KE, et al: The relevance of arterial wall microbiology to the treatment of prosthetic graft infections. Graft infection vs. arterial infection. J Vasc Surg 1:754–756, 1984.

122. Schwarcz TH, Flanigan DP: Repair of abdominal aortic aneurysms in patients with renal, iliac, or distal arterial occlusive disease. Surg Clin North Am 69:845–857, 1989.

123. Castronuovo JJ Jr, Flanigan DP: Renal failure complicating vascular surgery. *In* Bernhard VM, Towne JB (eds): Complications in Vascular Surgery, 2nd ed. Orlando, FL, Grune & Stratton, 1985, pp 259–273.

124. Alpert RA, Roizen MF, Hamilton WK, et al: Intraoperative urinary output does not predict postoperative renal function in patients undergoing abdominal aortic revascularization. Surgery 95:707–711, 1984.

125. Ernst CB, Hagihara PF, Daughorty ME, et al: Ischemic colitis incidence following abdominal aortic reconstruction: A prospective study. Surgery 80:417, 1976.

126. Ernst CB: Prevention of intestinal ischemia following abdominal aortic reconstruction. Surgery 93:102, 1983.

127. Schroeder T, Christofferson JK, Anderson J, et al: Ischemic colitis complicating reconstruction of the abdominal aorta. Surg Gynecol Obstet 160:299, 1985.

128. Szilagyi DE, Hagemen JH, Smith RF, et al: Spinal cord damage in surgery of the abdominal aorta. Surgery 83:38, 1978.

129. Bartle EJ, Pearce WH, Sun JH, et al: Infrarenal venous anomalies and aortic surgery. J Vasc Surg 6:590–593, 1987.

130. Giordano JM, Trout HH: Anomalies of the inferior vena cava. J Vasc Surg 3:924–928, 1986.
131. Brener BJ, Darling C, Frederick PL, et al: Major venous anomalies complicating abdominal aortic surgery. Arch Surg 108:160–165, 1974.
132. Kunkel JM, Weinstein ES: Preoperative detection of potential hazards in aortic surgery. Perspect Vasc Surg 2:1–17, 1989.
133. Goldstone J, Malone JM, Moore WS: Inflammatory aneurysms of the abdominal aorta. Surgery 83:425–430, 1978.
134. Goldstone J: Inflammatory aneurysms of the abdominal aorta. Semin Vasc Surg 1:165–173, 1988.
135. Crawford JL, Stowe CL, Safitt J, et al: Inflammatory aneurysms of the aorta. J Vasc Surg 2:113–124, 1985.
136. Pennell RC, Hollier LH, Lie JT, et al: Inflammatory abdominal aortic aneurysms: A thirty year review. J Vasc Surg 2:859–869, 1985.
137. Conelly TL, McKinnon W, Smith RB III, et al: Abdominal aortic surgery and horseshoe kidney. Arch Surg 115:1459–1463, 1980.
138. Starr DS, Foster WJ, Morris GC Jr: Resection of abdominal aortic aneurysm in the presence of horseshoe kidney. Surgery 89:387–389, 1981.
139. Hollis HW, Rutherford RB: Abdominal aortic aneurysms associated with horseshoe or ectopic kidneys. Techniques of renal preservation. Semin Vasc Surg 1:148–159, 1988.
140. Tarazi RY, Hertzer NR, Bevan EG, et al: Simultaneous aortic reconstruction and renal revascularization: Risk factors and late results in 89 patients. J Vasc Surg 5:707–714, 1987.
141. Stewart MT, Smith RB III, Fulenwider JT, Perdue GD, Wells JO: Concomitant renal revascularization in patients undergoing aortic surgery. J Vasc Surg 2:400–405, 1985.
142. String ST: Cholelithiasis and aortic reconstruction. J Vasc Surg 1:664–669, 1984.
143. Ouriel K, Ricotta JJ, Adams JT, DeWeese JA: Management of cholelithiasis in patients with abdominal aortic aneurysms. Ann Surg 198:717–719, 1983.
144. Goldstone J, Effeny DJ: Prevention of arterial graft infection. In Bernhard VM, Towne JB (eds): Complications in Vascular Surgery, 2nd ed. Orlando, FL, Grune & Stratton, 1985, pp 487–498.
145. Alexander JJ, Imbebo AL: Aorta-vena cava fistula. Surgery 105:1–12, 1989.
146. Salo JA, Verkkala K, Perhoniemi V, Harjola PT: Diagnosis and treatment of spontaneous aortocaval fistula. J Cardiovasc Surg 28:180–183, 1987.
147. Baker WH, Sharzer LA, Ehrenhaft JL: Aortocaval fistula as a complication of aortic aneurysms. Surgery 72:933–938, 1972.
148. Harrington EB, Schwartz M, Haimov M, et al: Aorto-caval fistula: A clinical spectrum. J Cardiovasc Surg 30:579–583, 1989.
149. Brown SL, Busuttil RW, Baker JD, et al: Bacteriologic and surgical determinants of survival in patients with mycotic aneurysms. J Vasc Surg 1:541–547, 1984.
150. Chan FY, Crawford ES, Coselli JS, et al: In situ prosthetic graft replacement for mycotic aneurysms of the aorta. Ann Thorac Surg 47:193–203, 1989.
151. Parson R, Gregory J, Palmer DL: Salmonella infections of the abdominal aorta. Rev Infect Dis 5:227–231, 1983.
152. Reddy DJ, Lee RE, Oh HK: Suprarenal mycotic aortic aneurysm: Surgical management and follow-up. J Vasc Surg 3:917–920, 1986.
153. Scher LA, Brenner BJ, Goldenkranz RJ, et al: Infected aneurysms of the abdominal aorta. Arch Surg 115:975–978, 1980.
154. Schuler JJ, Flanigan DP: Iliac artery aneurysms. In Bergan JJ, Yao JST (eds): Aneurysms: Diagnosis and Treatment. New York, Grune & Stratton, 1982, pp 469–485.
155. Lowry SF, Kraft RO: Isolated aneurysms of the iliac artery. Arch Surg 113:1289–1293, 1978.
156. Eisenman JI, Doering RB, Finck EJ: The isolated iliac artery aneurysm. Vasc Surg 1:202–204, 1967.
157. McCready RA, Pairolero PC, Gilmore JC, et al: Isolated iliac artery aneurysms. Surgery 93:688–693, 1983.
158. Nachbur BH, Inderbitzi RGC, Bär W: Isolated iliac aneurysms. Eur J Vasc Surg 5:375–381, 1991.
159. Marino R, Mooppan UMM, Zein TA, et al: Urologic manifestations of isolated iliac artery aneurysms. J Urol 137:232–234, 1987.
160. Richardson JW, Greenfield LJ: Natural history and management of iliac aneurysms. J Vasc Surg 8:165–171, 1988.

REVIEW QUESTIONS

1. Factors considered to be involved in the pathogenesis of abdominal aortic aneurysms include all of the following except:

   (a) heredity
   (b) atherosclerosis
   (c) enzyme deficiencies
   (d) enzyme excess
   (e) hormones

2. The incidence of abdominal aortic aneurysm is highest among patients with the following:

   (a) femoral aneurysm
   (b) aortoiliac occlusive disease
   (c) thoracic aortic aneurysm
   (d) bilateral popliteal aneurysm
   (e) isolated iliac artery aneurysm

3. The risk of rupture of infrarenal abdominal aortic aneurysms

   (a) increases with increasing size of the aneurysm
   (b) increases with increasing age of the patient
   (c) is negligible for aneurysms less than 5 cm in diameter

   (d) is not affected by blood pressure
   (e) is related to plasma lipoprotein levels

4. The most common cause of late death following surgical treatment of abdominal aortic aneurysm is:

   (a) renal failure
   (b) respiratory failure
   (c) myocardial ischemia
   (d) graft infection
   (e) malignancy

5. The true mortality for ruptured abdominal aortic aneurysms, including prehospital deaths, is approximately

   (a) 15 per cent
   (b) 30 per cent
   (c) 50 per cent
   (d) 75 per cent
   (e) 90 per cent

6. Which of the following is true when the surgeon fails to see the left renal vein during exposure of an abdominal aortic aneurysm?

(a) the dissection should be extended above the superior mesenteric artery
(b) the neck of the aneurysm should be thoroughly mobilized
(c) the interior mesenteric vein should be carefully preserved
(d) the surgeon can relax because the left renal vein is probably congenitally absent
(e) extra care must be paid to the application of the aortic cross-clamp

7. Aorto caval fistulae:
(a) are usually infectious in origin
(b) are usually symptomatic
(c) usually occur just below the left renal vein
(d) all of the above
(e) none of the above

8. Which of the following statements is/are true about complications of aortic aneurysm repair?
(a) colon ischemia is associated with a mortality rate of about 50 per cent
(b) renal failure does not occur if the aortic cross-clamp is totally infrarenal
(c) paraplegia occurs only with suprarenal clamping

(d) myocardial dysfunction is now an uncommon cause of postoperative death
(e) the use of autotransfusion devices has greatly reduced the degree of postoperative hemorrhage

9. All of the following statements are true about inflammatory aneurysms except:
(a) thick fibrous walls
(b) frequently associated with abdominal tenderness in the area of the aneurysm
(c) requires CT scanning for definitive preoperative diagnosis
(d) frequently ruptures
(e) frequently associated with ureteral obstruction

10. All of the following statements about iliac artery aneurysms are true except:
(a) arteriosclerosis is the most common etiology
(b) most are associated with or an extension of infrarenal abdominal aortic aneurysms
(c) most isolated iliac aneurysms present with symptoms prior to rupture
(d) may be diagnosed by digital examination of the vagina and rectum
(e) most can be palpated by abdominal examination

ANSWERS

1. e	2. d	3. a	4. c	5. e	6. e	7. b
8. a	9. d	10. c				

24

ANEURYSMS OF THE PERIPHERAL ARTERIES

D. PRESTON FLANIGAN

Peripheral arterial aneurysms are distinctly less common than aortic aneurysms but, nevertheless, can cause significant morbidity. Although occasionally these lesions may lead to death, the most common serious complication is usually that of end-organ loss or dysfunction. For the purposes of this chapter, peripheral aneurysms include the upper extremity arteries distal to and including the subclavian artery, the lower extremity arteries distal to and including the femoral artery, and the extracranial carotid arteries. Mycotic aneurysms affecting these vessels are also included.

NONMYCOTIC PERIPHERAL ANEURYSMS

Incidence and Etiology

Overall, the most common cause of nonmycotic peripheral aneurysms is atherosclerosis. However, when based on location, this is not true for all peripheral aneurysms. In general, all peripheral aneurysms can be considered rare. In descending order, the relative frequency of these aneurysms is probably popliteal, femoral, subclavian/axillary, and carotid. More reports on distal aneurysms involving the brachial, radial, ulnar, profunda femoris, and tibial/peroneal arteries are limited to small series or case reports. Although true aneurysms have been reported in these areas,[1,2] for the most part, forearm and hand aneurysms are secondary to trauma or are mycotic in origin.[3]

Age and sex distribution is dependent on etiology. Atherosclerotic aneurysms tend to occur primarily in men over 50 years of age. Aneurysms due to trauma are also more common in men but occur at a younger age. Aneurysms secondary to thoracic outlet syndrome are most commonly seen in middle-aged females (75 per cent).

Extracranial Carotid Artery Aneurysms

The rarity of extracranial carotid aneurysms is demonstrated by numerous publications reporting insti-

tutional experiences with aneurysm patients. In 2300 aneurysms reported from Baylor University there were only seven extracranial carotid aneurysms.[5] In a 30-year experience at Johns Hopkins only 12 such aneurysms were seen.[5] Only eight carotid aneurysms were demonstrated by Houser and Baker in performing 5000 cerebral arteriograms.[6] The largest single series of patients with extracranial carotid aneurysms was reported by McCollum.[7] In this latter series 37 aneurysms were seen over a 21-year period.

Currently, the common carotid artery is the most often affected. This is followed by the internal carotid artery; the external carotid artery rarely being involved.[8]

The most common cause of extracranial carotid aneurysms is atherosclerosis. These aneurysms tend to be fusiform in nature and are almost always associated with arterial hypertension. Most of the patients also have evidence of generalized atherosclerosis.[8] Another cause of carotid aneurysm is trauma, both blunt and penetrating.[9] False aneurysms of the carotid artery have been reported following carotid endarterectomy.[10] More rare etiologies include cystic medial necrosis, Marfan's syndrome, fibromuscular dysplasia, medial arteriopathy, granulomatous disease, radiation, and congenital defects.[9]

Subclavian/Axillary Aneurysms

Aneurysms of the subclavian and axillary arteries are also rare. Hobson et al. recently reviewed the world literature on the subject and found only 195 aneurysms in these locations.[11] This accounts for only 1 per cent of all peripheral aneurysms. Of the 195 cases, 88 per cent involved the subclavian artery. Subclavian/axillary aneurysms are rarely due to atherosclerosis, with this etiology accounting for only 15 per cent of the aneurysms. Thoracic outlet syndrome is primarily responsible for the majority of subclavian artery aneurysms (74 per cent), while crutch trauma accounts for most of the cases of axillary aneurysms (54 per cent). Other more rare etiologies have also been reported (Table 24–1).

**TABLE 24–1. ETIOLOGY OF SUBCLAVIAN/
AXILLARY ANEURYSMS**

Etiology	Subclavian	Axillary	Total
Thoracic outlet syndrome	127	1	128
Crutch trauma		13	13
Atherosclerosis	24	5	29
Pseudoaneurysm	5	2	7
Blunt trauma	2		2
Fibromuscular dysplasia		2	2
Dissection		1	1
Other	13		13
Total	171	24	195

Forearm/Hand Aneurysms

True aneurysms in the forearm and hand are quite rare. During a 10-year period, only 10 such patients were treated at the University of Chicago.[2] Half of true aneurysms in these areas are associated with occupational or recreational trauma. Most forearm and hand aneurysms are false aneurysms secondary to penetrating trauma.[3]

Femoral/Popliteal Artery Aneurysms

Femoral and popliteal artery aneurysms are grouped together because of their similar etiology, their similar clinical behavior, and their frequent association.

Aside from trauma and rare degenerative and congenital disorders, femoral and popliteal aneurysms are almost exclusively atherosclerotic in origin.[12,13] Together, these two types of aneurysms account for over 90 per cent of peripheral aneurysms.[14] Femoral aneurysms may involve the common femoral artery in the groin, but occasionally these aneurysms may be limited to the superficial femoral artery in the midthigh. These latter lesions are not unusual and are often seen in patients with arteriomegaly and/or "aneurysmosis."

Dent has shown an association between popliteal and femoral aneurysms and other aneurysms of atherosclerotic origin.[15] Most commonly, these associated aneurysms are located in the aortoiliac vessels, but more rarely they involve the renal, splanchnic, and brachiocephalic vessels. In patients with at least one peripheral aneurysm, 83 per cent had multiple aneurysms. Of patients with a common femoral aneurysm 95 per cent had a second aneurysm, 92 per cent had an aortoiliac aneurysm, and 59 per cent had bilateral femoral aneurysms. Of patients with a popliteal aneurysm, 78 per cent had a second aneurysm, 64 per cent had an aortoiliac aneurysm, and 47 per cent had bilateral popliteal artery aneurysms.

Natural History

As with aortic aneurysms, peripheral aneurysms can be asymptomatic or may lead to significant complications. Unlike aortic aneurysms, which tend to rupture, peripheral aneurysms most commonly thrombose or give rise to arterial emboli.

Extracranial Carotid Artery Aneurysms

Central neurologic events are very common in these patients. Rhodes reported that 13 of the 19 carotid aneurysms reported in the University of Michigan series had amaurosis fugax, transient ischemic attacks, stroke, or vague neurologic symptoms such as dizziness.[8] Most of these symptoms are thought to be secondary to embolization. Cranial nerve compression leads to local neurologic dysfunction and can include facial pain (Vth nerve), oculomotor palsies (VIth), auricular pain (IXth), and hoarseness (Xth). Horner's syndrome can also be seen from compression of the sympathetic chain. As cervical carotid aneurysms enlarge they can cause dysphagia, cranial nerve compression, and pain. Hemorrhage has also been seen as a complication of these aneurysms; however, rupture is uncommon.

Subclavian/Axillary Artery Aneurysms

Only 10 per cent of patients with known subclavian/axillary aneurysms are found to be asymptomatic.[11] Good natural history studies are not available, probably due to the small number of patients seen with this problem. It is inferred that, since 90 per cent of patients are symptomatic at the time of presentation, the likelihood of complications subsequently occurring in asymptomatic aneurysms is great. The primary complication seen with subclavian/axillary aneurysms is embolization (68 per cent).[11] Thrombosis and rupture are rare but have been reported.[11,16]

Forearm/Hand Aneurysms

The most common presenting signs and symptoms of aneurysms in these areas are mass and pain. Distal embolization occurs in roughly one third of these patients.[2]

Femoral/Popliteal Artery Aneurysms

The natural history of unoperated femoral and popliteal aneurysms demonstrates a high incidence of thromboembolic events. Tolstedt reported a 43 per cent rate of thrombosis in conservatively followed femoral aneurysms, and in Cutler and Darling's series 47 per cent presented with major complications.[17,18] In Szilagyi et al.'s series of popliteal aneurysms, only 32 per cent of those followed conservatively remained without complication at 5 years.[12] Vermillion et al. followed 26 popliteal aneurysms an average of 3 years and demonstrated that 31 per cent suffered limb-threatening complications, with two patients requiring major amputation and two patients left with rest pain.[13] Rupture of femoral or popliteal aneurysms has only rarely been reported. Profunda femoris aneurysms are particularly prone to rupture, with rates of 50 per cent being reported.[1] Popliteal aneurysms have been shown to rupture, on occasion, into the popliteal vein.[19] Less catastrophic complications include pain secondary to tibial nerve compression and popliteal vein thrombosis secondary to popliteal vein compression.

Diagnosis

Most peripheral aneurysms can be diagnosed by simple palpation of the artery in question. More sophisticated studies such as ultrasound, computed tomography (CT) scans, and arteriography augment the diagnosis and allow for better preoperative planning.

Extracranial Carotid Artery Aneurysms

The most common presentation for carotid aneurysms is a palpable pulsatile, submandibular, lateral neck mass or a mass presenting in the tonsillar fossa. The former presentation is most often seen with common carotid aneurysms, whereas presentation in the tonsillar fossa is more often seen with internal carotid artery aneurysms. Because of the variability in the location of the carotid bifurcation the presentation can be only a rough guide to the artery involved. The differential diagnosis includes kinked or redundant carotid arteries, enlarged lymph nodes, salivary gland tumors, branchial cleft cysts, cystic hygromas, and carotid body tumors. When the diagnosis is not clear, CT scanning with contrast injection is usually diagnostic. Arteriography further aids in elucidating the diagnosis and is required for proper preoperative planning. Carotid duplex ultrasound scanning may also be helpful.

Subclavian/Axillary Artery Aneurysms

The most common presenting signs and symptoms are secondary to distal embolization (68 per cent). Other signs and symptoms include tissue loss, claudication, pain, and evidence of brachial plexus compression (Table 24–2).

When the aneurysm is secondary to thoracic outlet syndrome, it often cannot be palpated. Aneurysms secondary to atherosclerosis tend to be larger and are palpable in two thirds of patients at the time of presentation.[16] A bruit may be present in the subclavian fossa or in the axilla. Small punctate cyanotic lesions affecting the fingers and palm that are painful in nature and occur suddenly are often present as a result of distal embolization. Rarely, embolization will cause large axial artery occlusion. This event usually requires immediate embolectomy but may lead to claudication if the initial ischemia does not precipitate the need for immediate medical attention. With chronic small embolization, the distal radial and ulnar pulses may not be palpable due to buildup of embolic material. Repeated embolization may be associated with

distal digital ulceration or tissue loss and severe pain. Many patients present with vague shoulder pain. Rupture produces severe shoulder pain radiating into the upper arm and lower neck.

When all types of subclavian/axillary aneurysms are considered, only 16 per cent can be palpated.[11] Occasionally ultrasound can be applied in the diagnosis of subclavian artery aneurysms, but the bony cage of the thoracic outlet may preclude adequate exposure in some patients. CT scanning is also able to demonstrate subclavian/axillary aneurysms. However, since in most cases the diagnosis should be suspected on the basis of history and physical examination, arteriography is the most useful test, since it is also needed preoperatively for proper planning of the operative procedure.

Forearm/Hand Aneurysms

Forearm, and especially hand, aneurysms are most often diagnosed by palpation of a pulsatile mass. These aneurysms can also be diagnosed by ultrasound or CT scanning, but nonpalpable aneurysms generally are found on arteriography in patients being studied for embolization.

Femoral/Popliteal Artery Aneurysms

The diagnosis of femoral and popliteal aneurysms is usually made by palpation. This is particularly easy in the case of femoral aneurysms because of their superficial nature. Popliteal aneurysms are suspected in any patient in whom the popliteal pulse is widened and very easily felt. Femoral and popliteal aneurysms should be considered in any patient with an acute arterial occlusion in the leg or with embolic disease affecting the foot and lower leg. Many popliteal aneurysms are calcified and can be detected by plain roentgenograms of the popliteal fossa. Both femoral and popliteal aneurysms are easily diagnosed by ultrasound. CT scanning is particularly accurate in making the diagnosis (Fig. 24–1). Despite the presence of mural thrombus, arteriography usually will confirm the diagnosis and is necessary for proper operative planning. The status of the runoff vessels visualized arteriographically is particularly important in patients with popliteal aneurysms.

Indications for Operation

Unlike aortic aneurysms, for which size is the main determinant of the need for surgery, the presence of a peripheral aneurysm is often all that is required to suggest the need for operative correction. As with patients with aortic aneurysms, the decision to operate on a patient with a peripheral aneurysm must be tempered by the overall medical condition of the patient so that the risk of operation is considerably less than the risk of the natural history of the disease.

TABLE 24–2. CLINICAL FINDINGS IN SUBCLAVIAN/AXILLARY ARTERY ANEURYSMS

Finding	Number	Percent
Asymptomatic	20	10
Claudication	9	5
Pain	36	18
Brachial plexus palsy	24	12
Tissue loss	20	10
Embolization	136	68

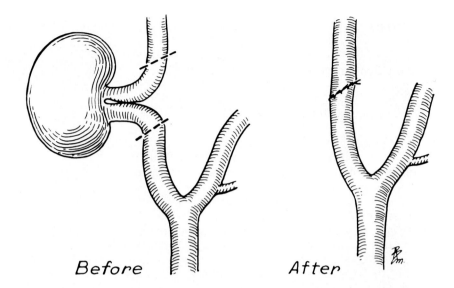

FIGURE 24–1. Method of end-to-end repair of a redundant internal carotid artery after aneurysm resection. (From Trippel OH, et al: Extracranial carotid aneurysms. *In* Bergan JJ, Yao JST (eds): Aneurysms. New York, Grune & Stratton, 1982, pp 493–503.)

Before   After

Extracranial Carotid Artery Aneurysms

The indication for operation in a patient with a cervical carotid artery aneurysm is usually the presence of the aneurysm. Since patients with this condition are rarely seen when asymptomatic, most patients are operated upon for the relief of symptoms. The high incidence of cranial nerve compression and central nervous system events in untreated patients, however, justifies surgery on asymptomatic carotid aneurysms as well (68 per cent in Rhodes et al.'s series[8]). This finding is common in nearly all reported studies, and the point is not a controversial one.

Subclavian/Axillary Artery Aneurysms

Generally speaking, the presence of a subclavian/axillary aneurysm is an indication for surgery. The anticipated natural history would indicate that these lesions are both life and limb threatening.[16] As is the case with carotid aneurysms, most patients are symptomatic at the time of presentation, however, and have clear indications for surgical intervention. Some controversy exists regarding the small fusiform post-stenotic subclavian dilatation often seen with thoracic outlet compression of the subclavian artery. The natural history of this lesion if not resected at the time of thoracic outlet decompression is not well established. In the four patients with subclavian artery aneurysms in Pairolero et al.'s series who had only thoracic outlet decompression, no subsequent thromboembolic events were seen in follow-up.[16]

Femoral/Popliteal Artery Aneurysms

It is generally thought that the presence of a femoral or popliteal aneurysm is an indication for surgery. This recommendation is based upon the high incidence of thromboembolic complications associated with these lesions as detailed above. Size is generally not used in assessing risk from these aneurysms, since even small aneurysms in these locations give rise to serious complications.

Treatment

There are only two primary objectives in the surgical management of peripheral aneurysms: exclusion of the aneurysm and restoration of arterial continuity. In most cases both objectives can be achieved. In some inaccessible aneurysms, however, exclusion alone must be accepted, since restoration of arterial continuity may not be possible.

Extracranial Carotid Artery Aneurysms

The techiques applied to the management of extracranial carotid aneurysms are ligation (or angiographic occlusion), endoaneurysmorrhaphy, resection with primary anastomosis, or resection with graft replacement.

The preferred treatment is resection with primary anastomosis or graft replacement. Redundancy of the carotid artery is not uncommon when aneurysm is present. In such cases resection of the aneurysm with mobilization of the carotid artery and primary anastomosis is sometimes quite easily accomplished (Fig. 24–2). This technique is most applicable to internal carotid artery aneurysms. An alternate technique for flow restoration following resection of an internal carotid artery aneurysm is to divide the distal external carotid artery and perform an end-to-end anastomosis between the proximal external carotid and the distal internal carotid arteries. Aneurysm of the external carotid artery is rare and can be resected without the need to restore arterial continuity. Aneurysms of the carotid bifurcation usually require resection with graft replacement between the common and internal carotid arteries. When the internal carotid is redundant, it can be mobilized and anastomosed end to end to the common carotid artery. In both these latter cases the external carotid is usually ligated. Aneurysms involving the common carotid artery are usually able to be treated by resection and primary anastomosis or graft replacement. All

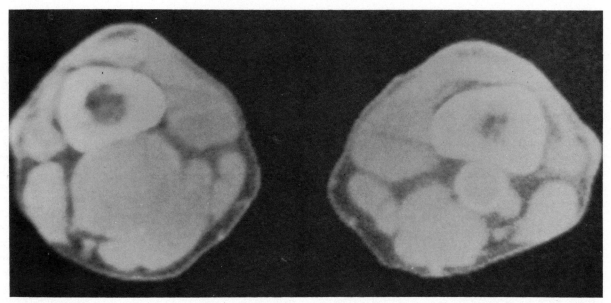

FIGURE 24–2. CT scan showing obvious right popliteal artery aneurysm and smaller left popliteal artery aneurysm.

of the above procedures can usually be performed through a standard neck incision such as is used for carotid endarterectomy.

The need for an indwelling carotid artery shunt is no better understood for aneurysm patients than it is for patients undergoing carotid endarterectomy. If the use of a shunt is desired, shunting can be accomplished in most patients. In patients undergoing resection with primary anastomosis, a shunt can be inserted into the open ends of the arteries to be anastomosed after opening of the aneurysm. If a graft is to be used, the shunt is placed through the graft prior to performing any anastomosis and inserted into the arterial ends after opening the aneurysm.

Aneurysms that involve the distal cervical internal carotid artery are often inaccessible using standard techniques. In some patients, mandibular subluxation or transection will allow the application of the above-mentioned methods of repair.[20] Alternative approaches are often required for high internal carotid lesions, however. In some patients, high fusiform aneurysms can be treated by aneurysmorrhaphy using an indwelling shunt for flow continuity and as a method of distal arterial control. In many cases distal lesions must be treated by ligation or balloon occlusion using angiographic techniques. Unfortunately, acute occlusion of the internal carotid artery in these patients is associated with high neurological morbidity. Stroke rates from 30 to 60 per cent have been reported following this procedure, with half of those patients sustaining a stroke dying as a result.[9] This morbidity and mortality clearly approaches the morbidity and mortality secondary to the natural history of the disease.

A way to select patients who may safely undergo carotid ligation is to measure carotid stump pressure. This can be done at surgery, but the preoperative knowledge of this pressure allows for better operative planning. The carotid stump pressure can also be measured by temporary balloon occlusion at the time of arteriography using an end-hole balloon catheter, or it can be assessed using carotid compression maneuvers during the measurement of ocular pressures using the Gee oculopneumoplethysmograph.[21] Stump pressures in excess of 70 mm Hg appear to be safe for patients undergoing carotid ligation. Since many strokes occurring after carotid ligation are not present immediately following the procedure but, rather, occur hours to days later, it has been recommended that these patients be maintained on heparin anticoagulation for 7 to 10 days postoperatively.

When stump pressure measurements indicate that carotid ligation is not safe, the performance of an extracranial-to-intracranial bypass using ipsilateral superficial temporal artery has been suggested.[20] Since this procedure is usually only necessary for high internal carotid lesions, the ipsilateral external carotid artery is usually preserved, thus allowing for adequate inflow into the superficial temporal artery.

Subclavian/Axillary Artery Aneurysms

The approach to the surgical treatment of subclavian/axillary aneurysms is dependent upon the etiology, size, and location of the aneurysm and the status of the distal circulation. Except in cases of small, asymptomatic subclavian artery aneurysms secondary to thoracic outlet syndrome, for which thoracic outlet decompression alone may be adequate, the aneurysm should be excluded and arterial continuity restored if possible. Proximal and distal ligation of these aneurysms has been reported. Although tissue loss does not usually occur following this procedure, claudication is not uncommon.[16]

When a symptomatic or large asymptomatic subclavian aneurysm is present as a result of thoracic outlet syndrome, repair of the aneurysm should be accompanied by thoracic outlet decompression. Although this combined approach has been reported through an axillary approach, the author prefers the supraclavicular approach. This latter approach allows for safe control of the artery, although the thoracic outlet decompression is more involved through this approach. Hobson et al. have recommended performing the aneurysm repair through the supraclavicular approach combined with a transaxillary approach to the first rib.[11]

Atherosclerotic and traumatic distal subclavian artery aneurysms or pseudoaneurysms can be approached through a supraclavicular approach. When the aneurysm is proximal enough that proximal control cannot be safely obtained through this approach a median sternotomy (right side) or a left-sided thoracotomy (left side) is needed, usually in combination with the supraclavicular approach. Midsubclavian lesions can often be managed through a supraclavicular approach with medial clavicular resection.

Primary anastomosis is usually not possible and graft replacement is required. This is most commonly performed as an interposition graft using either saphenous vein or prosthetics. Prosthetics are more commonly used because of the size of the subclavian artery. The vertebral artery should be preserved when possible. In patients with a dominant contralateral vertebral artery, this may not be necessary.

High-risk patients with proximal aneurysms who are thought too frail to undergo a major procedure can be treated with distal ligation and axilloaxillary bypass.

Management of axillary artery aneurysms often may be accomplished through the axillary approach. In many patients, proximal control must be obtained through an infraclavicular approach. With more proximal lesions or lesions involving both the subclavian and axillary arteries, a combined supraclavicular and infraclavicular approach must be used. Aneurysms involving the axillary artery are often intimately involved with the cords of the brachial plexus and resection may be hazardous. When there are symptoms of brachial plexus compression, resection and interposition grafting may be indicated. For smaller lesions, however, proximal and distal ligation combined with bypass can be performed, thus avoiding dissection around the brachial plexus.

When subclavian/axillary aneurysms are complicated by embolization and ischemia, revascularization of the arm may be required in combination with aneurysm repair. This is usually accomplished by autogenous vein bypass from proximal to the aneurysm to the most appropriate distal artery. In this situation, the aneurysm can either be ligated, if appropriate, or resected.

Forearm/Hand Aneurysms

Aneurysms of the forearm arteries may be treated by ligation if the remaining vessels provide adequate collateral circulation to the hand. More often, however, vein interposition grafting is performed, since it is simple to accomplish. Aneurysms of vessels in the hand tend to be less well collateralized and vein graft repair is usually necessary.[1]

Femoral/Popliteal Artery Aneurysms

The treatment of femoral artery aneurysms is usually resection and graft interposition. Because of the size of the common femoral artery, a prosthetic graft is preferred. When the profunda femoris artery is involved, the graft may be sewn end to end to the superficial femoral artery, and the origin of the profunda implanted into the side of the graft. When femoral aneurysms are being treated concomitantly with an inflow or outflow procedure, it is still best, in most cases, to replace the common femoral artery with an interposition graft. Inflow or outflow grafts are then anastomosed to the interposition graft in an end-to-side fashion (Fig. 24–3). Repair of profunda femoris aneurysms is dictated by the patency of the superficial femoral artery and how distal the aneurysm is located in the profunda femoris artery. Approximately 50 per cent of profunda femoris aneurysms can be safely ligated, while 50 per cent require reestablishing arterial continuity.[1]

Superficial femoral and popliteal aneurysms are preferably bypassed rather than resected. In most cases this means an above-knee–to–below-knee bypass using autogenous vein through a medial approach. In some patients, the popliteal aneurysm may extend proximal into the superficial femoral artery. In these patients the proximal anastomosis can be made to the common femoral artery or, more commonly, to the mid–superficial femoral artery proximal to the adductor canal.

When there has been extensive embolization leading to obliteration of the outflow tract of the popliteal artery, popliteal-to-tibial or popliteal-to-peroneal bypass is required. This should be performed using autogenous vein.

When popliteal aneurysms are sufficiently large to cause symptomatic compression of the surrounding nerve and vein, consideration should be given to resection of the aneurysm with interposition grafting. The risk of damage to these structures is greater, but, if this is not done, many patients will remain symptomatic postoperatively. This procedure is best performed through a posterior approach as long as both anastomoses are within the limitations of the operative field.

Results of Therapy

Since most patients with peripheral aneurysms do not have occlusive disease, the results of reconstructive vascular procedures are usually excellent. In some cases, however, embolization from the aneurysm can lead to obliteration of some or all of the outflow tract, leading to poor results.

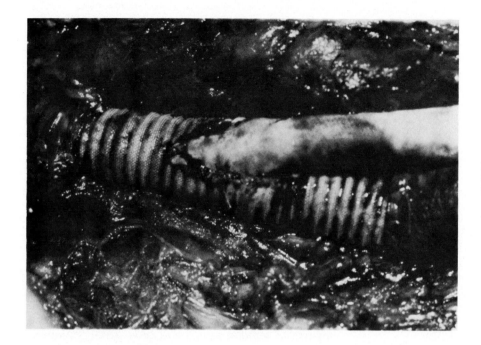

FIGURE 24–3. Concomitant repair of femoral aneurysm followed by prosthetic femoropopliteal bypass.

Extracranial Carotid Artery Aneurysms

The small number of patients in reports assessing the results of surgical therapy for carotid aneurysm makes the calculation of morbidity and mortality statistics somewhat unreliable. Most reports, however, have indicated that these procedures can be performed with safety. In Rhodes et al.'s series from Michigan, 1 of 19 aneurysm operations resulted in a stroke, which was thought to be due to intraoperative embolization. There was no operative death.[8] Excision of large and distal aneurysms is associated with an increased incidence of cranial nerve injury. Long-term results are sparsely reported but, when reported, have been excellent. All investigators agree that the results of surgery are vastly superior to the natural history of the disease.

Subclavian/Axillary Artery Aneurysms

The results of surgery for subclavian/axillary aneurysms are similar to those for upper extremity reconstruction for occlusive disease.[16,22] Pairolero et al. showed that 18 of 18 patients undergoing aneurysm resection with restoration of arterial continuity remained with patent reconstructions during an average 9.2-year follow-up.[16] This is most likely due to the lack of distal occlusive disease. Patients with obliteration of their radial and ulnar arteries, however, have a high failure rate following arm revascularization.[22] This latter point further emphasizes the need for early surgical intervention in these patients.

Forearm/Hand Aneurysms

Both ligation in the presence of adequate collateral circulation and vein graft repair are quite successful in the treatment of forearm and hand aneurysms. Clark reported 100 per cent patency at 7 years for vein graft repairs in the forearm and hand.[2]

Femoral/Popliteal Artery Aneurysms

When femoral and popliteal aneurysms are treated before complications arise, the results are excellent. The 18 asymptomatic patients with femoral aneurysms in Cutler and Darling's series all had excellent early and late results (no graft occlusions). However, of the 45 symptomatic patients with femoral aneurysms, four had amputations and 17 remained symptomatic despite therapy.[18] In Lilly et al.'s series of 48 popliteal aneurysms, the 5-year patency rate for reconstructions for asymptomatic lesions was 91 per cent compared to 54 per cent for symptomatic lesions.[23] These differing results were directly related to the status of the tibial runoff vessels. In a series of 51 popliteal aneurysms reported by Shortell et al., results were dependent upon the clinical presentation and the status of the runoff vessels.[24] Patients presenting with limb-threatening ischemia had a graft patency rate of 69 per cent at 1 year, while all electively performed grafts were patent at 1 year. After 3 years, runoff dictated patency, as grafts with good runoff had a patency rate of 89 per cent while poor runoff was associated with a 3-year patency rate of only 30 per cent.

Dawson et al. compared operative and nonoperative approaches to 71 popliteal aneurysms.[25] Thromboembolic complications developed in 57 per cent of asymptomatic popliteal aneurysms over a mean follow-up period of 5 years. In aneurysms followed a full 5 years, the complication rate was 74 per cent. In comparison, operated patients had graft patency and limb salvage of 64 per cent and 95 per cent, respectively, at 10-year follow-up.

Dawson et al. also showed a high risk for subsequently developing aneurysms in these patients. At 5-year follow-up, 32 per cent of patients developed additional aneurysms, and at 10 years, 49 per cent had new aneurysms.

The above reports strongly support the early surgical treatment of asymptomatic popliteal aneurysms and underscore the need for careful follow-up of these patients for the development of new aneurysms.

MYCOTIC ANEURYSMS

Mycotic aneurysms are considered separately because they generally have a different etiology, affect arteries in a different distribution, require different treatment, and have poorer outcomes than bland aneurysms. Despite the term, mycotic aneurysms are considered to be any true or false aneurysm that is infected.

Etiology

Numerous classifications for mycotic aneurysms have been proposed and are nicely described by Moore and Malone[26] and Wilson et al.[27] Pastel and Johnston have indicated that the source of infection must be either endogenous or exogenous. Endogenous sources include embolism, septicemia, or direct extension; exogenous sources include trauma and iatrogenic injury. They have further suggested that classifications be based upon the preexisting status of the artery: normal, atherosclerotic, aneurysmal, or prosthetic. Any classification must consider these factors.[28]

Normal axial arteries are seldom infected primarily, but clumps of bacteria or fungi may lodge in smaller vessels and cause transmural necrosis and aneurysm formation. Normal, larger arteries can be infected, however, by organisms lodging in the vaso vasorum. Arteries that are diseased with atherosclerosis or aneurysm, and prosthetic grafts, are subject to local invasion by circulating organisms. The process is similar to that described above in that infection leads to arterial wall weakening and subsequent aneurysm formation. Infection may spread to arterial walls from outside the vessel through direct contact with abscesses, wound infections, salivary glands, and the like. Exogenous sources of arterial infections include diagnostic and therapeutic catheterizations, penetrating trauma, and drug abuse. Graft infections may also lead to infected pseudoaneurysm formation, usually as a result of disruption of an anastomosis.

Mycotic aneurysms have been reported in essentially all arteries. The location of mycotic aneurysms is primarily a result of the etiology. Mycotic aneurysms secondary to bacterial endocarditis favor the superior mesenteric artery followed by the aorta and femoral arteries. Those mycotic aneurysms that follow trauma most commonly involve the extremities. Mycotic aneurysms occurring as a result of infection of already present atherosclerotic aneurysms will commonly affect the aorta, femoral, and popliteal arteries. Those secondary to atherosclerosis alone will involve the aorta and superficial femoral arteries as well as other common atherosclerotic sites. Those secondary to catheters and drug abuse involve the brachial, radial, and, most commonly, the femoral arteries. For unknown reasons, *Salmonella* species favor the infrarenal aorta.

The organisms most commonly involved in mycotic aneurysms vary depending upon the source of the organism. When bacterial endocarditis is the source, *Streptococcus* and *Staphylococcus* prevail. *Salmonella*, *Staphylococcus*, and *Escherichia coli* are the most common organisms causing mycotic aneurysms secondary to bacteremia. Mycotic aneurysms secondary to direct extension of infections are predominantly caused by *Salmonella*, *Staphylococcus*, *Mycobacterium*, and fungi.[26] *Staphylococcus aureus* and *E. coli* are the most common organisms seen in mycotic aneurysms secondary to trauma (all types).[29]

In the preantibiotic era, most mycotic aneurysms were secondary to bacterial endocarditis and syphilis. Today, most mycotic aneurysms are probably secondary to trauma (including drug abuse, surgery, and arterial catheterization). This change is most likely due to the use of antibiotic therapy for endocarditis, the significant decrease in the prevalence of syphilis, the increasing use of diagnostic catheterization, the increase in violent trauma, and widespread drug abuse. In the author's experience, these forces have now made common femoral artery mycotic aneurysms the most common type currently encountered.

Natural History

Once established, the natural course of a mycotic aneurysm is to enlarge and eventually rupture in most known cases. Occasionally, spontaneous thrombosis may occur with resolution of the septic process; however, the thrombosed aneurysm may serve as a continuing septic focus. Septic emboli arising from the aneurysm are not uncommon and can lead to miliary abscesses and septic arthritis.

Diagnosis

Patients with mycotic aneurysms may present with catastrophic illness or with insidious disease. Most patients have some combination of fever, malaise, weight loss, chills, night sweats, pain, leukocytosis, positive downstream blood cultures, and elevated sedimentation rate. There is usually a history of trauma, or a recent infectious disease. When the aneurysm is superficial, as most peripheral aneurysms are, it can be palpated in 90 per cent of cases.[30] The aneurysm may appear bland but, more commonly, will show signs of erythema, warmth, and tenderness. Particularly large aneurysms may also present with skin necrosis with imminent rupture (Fig. 24–4). Petechial lesions in the skin may be seen distal

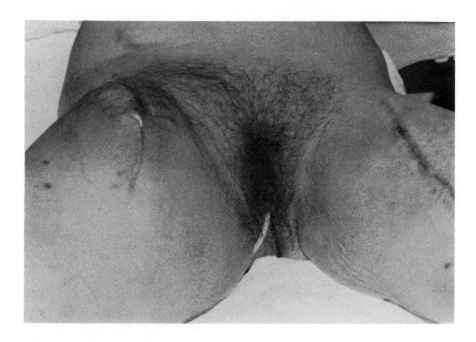

FIGURE 24–4. Mycotic aneurysm in right groin with overlying skin necrosis and imminent rupture.

to the aneurysm when embolization has occurred. Many patients present with rupture.

The diagnosis of mycotic aneurysm is often deduced by combining the findings of history and physical examination with test findings. In some patients, the history and physical examination may be sufficient, such as in the patient shown in Figure 24–4 who had a retained Dacron chimney left attached to her right femoral artery following removal of an intraaortic balloon catheter. In other patients, the diagnosis is made by the finding of sepsis and an aneurysm in a patient in whom no other septic focus can be found.

Ultrasound and CT scans may be used to visualize mycotic aneurysms. CT scans have the advantage of being able to more clearly demonstrate surrounding fluid or gas, a finding consistent with infection. Gallium scans and radioactively tagged white cell scans are usually positive with mycotic aneurysms. Arteriography is usually required in preoperative planning, except in emergency situations, and usually demonstrates a saccular aneurysm or pseudoaneurysm (Fig. 24–5).

Treatment

The indication for treatment of a mycotic aneurysm is its presence. Antibiotic therapy, guided by culture results when available, should be employed in all patients. Antibiotics alone are not sufficient, and surgical removal of the mycotic aneurysm is required in nearly all cases. Basic surgical principles dictate that all infected tissue must be removed and adequate circulation must remain or be provided when possible.

Extracranial Carotid Artery Mycotic Aneurysms

As noted above, cervical carotid aneurysms are rare. It follows, then, that cervical carotid mycotic aneurysms are extremely rare. Jones and Frusha recently reviewed the English literature and found only 23 bacteriologically proven cases.[31] More recently, Jebara et al. added an additional four cases.[32]

Treatment of these lesions requires complete excision of the artery, under antibiotic coverage, and débridement of all infected tissue. Vascular reconstruction should be avoided if possible, since reconstruction in an infected field yields less than optimal results.[33] Patients should be selected for arterial ligation based upon carotid stump pressure as described above. Heparin should be continued for 7 to 10 days postoperatively when ligation is employed. If ligation is not safe, then reconstruction using autogenous vein is the treatment of choice. In Jones and Frusha's review, the overall mortality rate was 23 per cent. The death rate was 27 per cent in the ligation group compared to 11 per cent in the grafted group. Extracranial-intracranial bypass has not been reported in these patients.

Subclavian/Axillary Artery Mycotic Aneurysms

Mycotic aneurysms in this area are also quite rare and usually are the result of trauma and drug abuse. The approach to the subclavian artery depends on the side and distal and proximal extent of the aneurysm as mentioned above for bland aneurysms in this location. In this location, complete excision of the aneurysm may be too risky in view of the proximity of the brachial plexus and subclavian vein. Successful treatment with arterial ligation and incision and drainage of the aneurysm has been reported.[34] Proximal subclavian artery ligation usually does not lead to the need for revascularization.

Axillary mycotic aneurysms are usually palpable. The principles of management of subclavian mycotic aneurysms probably apply for axillary lesions. Axillary artery ligation may be associated with ischemia

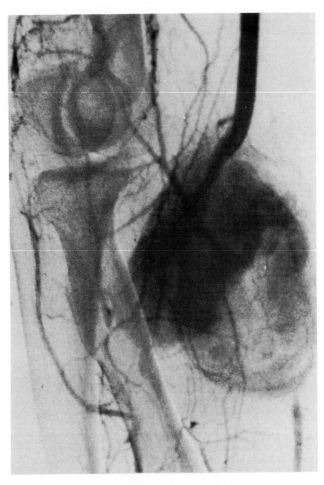

FIGURE 24-5. Arteriogram of a mycotic popliteal artery aneurysm.

more often, however, and extraanatomic bypass may be required in some patients. This can usually be performed in clean tissue planes about the shoulder using autogenous vein.

Forearm/Hand Artery Mycotic Aneurysms

Treatment of mycotic aneurysms in these areas follows the general guidelines for other mycotic aneurysms. Arterial ligation with aneurysm excision is generally all that is required. In the rare situation where distal ischemia might occur, autogenous revascularization in clean planes is required.

Femoral/Popliteal Artery Mycotic Aneurysms

The treatment of infected groin aneurysms has evolved through several stages. Although most of

these lesions seen today are secondary to trauma and drug abuse, the principles applied to the management of groin mycotic aneurysms secondary to other causes should probably be the same in most cases.

Several options are available, including remote bypass followed by aneurysm resection, aneurysm resection followed by remote bypass if needed, aneurysm resection alone, or aneurysm resection with in situ autogenous reconstruction.

Initial obturator bypass followed by aneurysm resection usually requires the use of prosthetic material, since most of these patients are drug addicts whose saphenous veins have been destroyed. Reddy et al. showed this approach to be associated with a 100 per cent graft infection rate in drug addicts.[29] In other patients, vein is often available and this approach is preferred. Buerger and Feldman have reported that revascularization is not effective in reducing the amputation rate after aneurysm resection in drug addicts (17 per cent in their series) and may occasionally be a fatal approach. In Buerger and Feldman's series, the same amputation rate was achieved without any death when aneurysm excision and ligation alone was used.[35] Reddy et al. obtained a similar amputation rate (19 per cent) with excision and ligation.[29] They reported that excision and ligation of only one of the three femoral arteries in the groin can be performed without limb loss, but that when the common femoral bifurcation is involved, thus necessitating the ligation of all three vessels, the amputation rate is very high. They suggested that, as an alternative in these latter patients, immediate autogenous vein reconstruction with sartorius muscle flap coverage may be used when adequate débridement can be performed to control sepsis. Using this approach they reported a 9 per cent amputation rate without mortality. Reddy et al. have found that, even in drug addicts, there is usually satisfactory saphenous vein in the thigh for femoral artery reconstruction. Ligation and excision with postoperative observation to assess the need for subsequent revascularization did not yield satisfactory results in Reddy et al.'s series.[29]

Mycotic aneurysms involving the popliteal artery are uncommon and few guidelines are provided in the vascular surgical literature. In the author's experience aneurysm excision with in situ autogenous interposition grafting has worked well. Most of these patients have normal tibial artery runoff, facilitating long-term patency, and the readily available soft tissue coverage afforded by the muscles in the popliteal space facilitates healing of the surgical wound without complication.

REFERENCES

1. Tait WF, Vohra RK, Carr HMH, Thomson GJL, Waker MG: True profunda femoris aneurysms: Are they more dangerous than other atherosclerotic aneurysms of the femoropopliteal segment? Ann Vasc Surg 5:92–95, 1991.

2. Clark ET, Mass DP, Bassiouny HS, Zarins CK, Gewertz BL: True aneurysmal disease in the hand and upper extremity. Ann Vasc Surg 5:276–281, 1991.

3. Flinn WR, Yao JST, Bergan JJ: Aneurysms of secondary and

tertiary branches of major arteries. *In* Bergan JJ, Yao JST (eds): Aneurysms. New York, Grune & Stratton, 1982, pp 449–467.

4. Beall AC, Crawford ES, Cooley DA, et al: Extracranial aneurysms of the carotid artery. Report of seven cases. Postgrad Med 32:93, 1962.

5. Reid MR: Aneurysms in the Johns Hopkins Hospital. Arch Surg 12:1, 1926.

6. Houser OW, Baker HL Jr: Fibromuscular dysplasia and other uncommon diseases of the cervical carotid artery: Angiographic aspects. Am J Roentgenol Radium Ther Nucl Med 104:201, 1968.

7. McCollum CH, Wheeler WG, Noon GP, et al: Aneurysms of the extracranial carotid artery: Twenty-one year's experience. Am J Surg 137:196, 1979.

8. Rhodes EL, Stanley JC, Hoffman GL, et al: Aneurysms of extracranial carotid arteries. Arch Surg 111:339, 1976.

9. Goldstone J: Aneurysms of the extracranial carotid artery. *In* Rutherford RB (ed): Vascular Surgery. Philadelphia, WB Saunders Company, 1984, pp 1279–1287.

10. Ehrenfeld WK, Hays RJ: False aneurysm after carotid endarterectomy. Arch Surg 104:288, 1972.

11. Hobson RW II, Isreal MR, Lynch TG: Axillosubclavian arterial aneurysms. *In* Bergan JJ, Yao JST (eds): Aneurysms. New York, Grune & Stratton, 1982, pp 435–447.

12. Szilagyi DE, Schwartz RL, Reddy DJ: Popliteal arterial aneurysms. Their natural history and management. Arch Surg 116:724, 1981.

13. Vermilion BD, Kimmins SA, Pace WG, et al: A review of one hundred forty seven popliteal aneurysms with long-term follow-up. Surgery 90:1009, 1981.

14. Evans WE, Vermilion BD: Popliteal and femoral aneurysms. *In* Rutherford RB (ed): Vascular Surgery. Philadelphia, WB Saunders Company, 1984, pp 814–827.

15. Dent TL, Lindenaur SM, Ernst CB, et al: Multiple arteriosclerotic arterial aneurysms. Arch Surg 105:338, 1972.

16. Pairolero PC, Walls JT, Payne WS, et al: Subclavian-axillary artery aneurysms. Surgery 90:757, 1981.

17. Tolstedt GE, Radke HM, Bell JW: Late sequelae of arteriosclerotic femoral aneurysms. Angiology 12:601, 1961.

18. Cutler BS, Darling RC: Surgical management of arteriosclerotic femoral aneurysms. Surgery 74:764, 1973.

19. Reed MK, Smith BM: Popliteal aneurysm with spontaneous arteriovenous fistula. J Cardiovasc Surg 32:482–484, 1991.

20. Stoney RJ, Qvarfordt PG: Accessible and inaccessible aneurysms of the extracranial carotid artery. *In* Moore WS (ed): Surgery for Cerebrovascular Disease. New York, Churchill Livingstone, 1987, pp 567–577.

21. Gee W, Mehigan JT, Wylie EJ: Measurement of collateral cerebral hemispheric blood pressure by ocular pneumoplethysmography. Am J Surg 130:121, 1975.

22. Gross WS, Flanigan DP, Kraft RO, et al: Chronic upper extremity: Etiology, manifestations, and treatment. Arch Surg 84:417, 1978.

23. Lilly MP, Flinn WR, McCarthy WJ, et al: The effect of distal arterial anatomy on the success of popliteal aneurysm repair. J Vasc Surg 7:653, 1988.

24. Shortell CK, DeWeese JA, Ouriel K, Green RM: Popliteal artery aneurysms: A 25 year experience. J Vasc Surg 14:771–779, 1991.

25. Dawson I, van Bockel H, Brand R, Terpstra JL: Popliteal artery aneurysms: Long-term follow-up of aneurysmal disease and results of surgical treatment. J Vasc Surg 13:398–407, 1991.

26. Moore WS, Malone JM: Mycotic aneurysms. *In* Bergan JJ, Yao JST (eds): Aneurysms. New York, Grune & Stratton, 1982, pp 581–595.

27. Wilson SE, Wagenen PV, Passaro E Jr: Arterial infection. Curr Probl Surg 15:9, 1978.

28. Patel S, Johnston KW: Classification and management of mycotic aneurysms. Surg Gynecol Obstet 144:691, 1977.

29. Reddy DJ, Smith RF, Elliot JP, et al: Infected femoral artery false aneurysms in drug addicts: Evolution of selective vascular reconstruction. J Vasc Surg 3:718, 1986.

30. Anderson CB: Mycotic aneurysms. *In* Rutherford RB (ed): Vascular Surgery. Philadelphia, WB Saunders Company, 1984, pp 835–847.

31. Jones TR, Frusha JD: Mycotic cervical carotid artery aneurysms: A case report and review of the literature. Ann Vasc Surg 2:373, 1988.

32. Jebara VA, Acar C, Dervanian P, et al: Mycotic aneurysms of the carotid arteries: Case report and review of the literature. J Vasc Surg 14:215–219, 1991.

33. Howell HS, Baburano T, Graziano J: Mycotic cervical carotid aneurysm. Surgery 81:357, 1977.

34. Miller CM, Sangiuolo P, Schanzer H: Infected false aneurysms of the subclavian artery: A complication in drug addicts. J Vasc Surg 1:684, 1984.

35. Buerger R, Feldman AJ: Infected groin aneurysms from heroin addiction. *In* Bergan JJ, Yao JST (eds): Aneurysms. New York, Grune & Stratton, 1982, pp 643–655.

25

SPLANCHNIC AND RENAL ARTERY ANEURYSMS

JAMES C. STANLEY, LOUIS M. MESSINA,
and GERALD B. ZELENOCK

Aneurysms of the major visceral branches of the abdominal aorta have been recognized with increasing frequency. More than 3000 splanchnic and renal aneurysms have been described in the English literature, of which over half have been reported during the past two decades. The cumulative experience with these unusual lesions documents splanchnic aneurysms to be approximately twice as common as renal aneurysms. Splanchnic and renal artery aneurysms are best addressed individually because of the marked variability in their biologic character and clinical relevance.

SPLANCHNIC ARTERY ANEURYSMS

Splanchnic artery aneurysms are an uncommon but serious vascular disease (Table 25–1A and B). Nearly 22 per cent of these aneurysms present as surgical emergencies, including 8.5 per cent that result in death.[1] The major splanchnic vessels involved with these macroaneurysms, in decreasing order of frequency, include: the splenic, hepatic, superior mesenteric, celiac, gastric-gastroepiploic, jejunal-ileal-colic, pancreaticoduodenal-pancreatic, and gastroduodenal arteries (Tables 25–1A and B). The natural history of splanchnic artery aneurysms has become better defined with their more frequent clinical recognition.[2–8]

Splenic Artery Aneurysms

Splenic artery aneurysms account for 60 per cent of all splanchnic artery aneurysms.[6–9] The frequency of these lesions in the general population probably approaches the 0.78 per cent incidence noted in nearly 3600 consecutive abdominal arteriographic studies performed for reasons other than suspected aneurysmal disease.[6] Women are four times more likely than men to develop these aneurysms because of hormone-related events associated with these lesions.

Three distinct, preexisting conditions may contribute to the development of splenic artery aneurysms. The first is medial fibrodysplasia, usually manifest by hypertension secondary to renal artery involvement. The coexistence of renal artery medial fibrodysplasia and splenic artery aneurysms has only been identified in women. Approximately 2 per cent of patients with the former renal artery disease have splenic artery aneurysms. Second are the deleterious effects of increased splenic blood flow and the altered levels of reproductive hormones on elastic vascular tissue that accompany repeated pregnancies. Approximately 40 per cent of women harboring these lesions have been reported to be grand multiparous.[6] Third, portal hypertension with splenomegaly has been associated with splenic artery macroaneurysms in nearly 10 per cent of patients.[6,10] This may reflect both increased splenic blood flow,[11] as well as increased estrogen activity associated with cirrhosis. A female sex predilection does not exist in this subgroup of patients with splenic artery aneurysms. Recently, there has been an increased recognition of these aneurysms in patients following orthotopic liver transplantation.[12,13]

Although certain splenic artery aneurysms exhibit arteriosclerotic disease, the typical calcific arteriosclerotic changes in many of these aneurysms is more likely a secondary event, rather than a primary etiologic process.[6] Inflammatory disease, such as chronic pancreatitis, and penetrating trauma are less common causes of these aneurysms. Microaneurysms within the spleen are usually associated with generalized vasculitis, such as polyarteritis nodosa, and are of less clinical importance than extraparenchymal aneurysms.

Most splenic artery aneurysms associated with arterial fibrodysplasia, multiple pregnancies, or portal hypertension are saccular and occur at vessel branchings[6]

TABLE 25–1A. SPLANCHNIC ARTERY MACROANEURYSMS

Aneurysm Location	Frequency Within Splanchnic Circulation	Male:Female Ratio	Contributing Factors
Splenic artery	60%	1:4	Medial degeneration; arterial fibrodysplasia; multiple pregnancies; portal hypertension; chronic pancreatitis with arterial erosion by pseudocysts
Hepatic artery	20%	2:1	Medial degeneration; blunt and penetrating liver trauma; infection related to intravenous substance abuse
Superior mesenteric artery	5.5%	1:1	Infection related to bacterial endocarditis, often associated with nonhemolytic streptococci and more recently with intravenous substance abuse; medial degeneration
Celiac artery	4%	1:1	Medial degeneration
Gastric and gastroepiploic arteries	4%	3:1	Periarterial inflammation; medial degeneration
Jejunal, ileal, and colic arteries	3%	1:1	Medial degeneration; connective tissue diseases
Pancreaticoduodenal and pancreatic arteries and gastroduodenal arteries	2% 1.5%	4:1	Pancreatitis-related arterial necrosis and arterial erosion by pseudocysts (60% of gastroduodenal, 30% of pancreaticoduodenal artery aneurysms); medial degeneration

(Fig. 25–1). It is at such sites that discontinuities exist in the internal elastic lamina of normal vessels, and certainly subsequent degenerative effects involving elastic tissue, such as occur with pregnancy, are apt to produce aneurysmal changes in these locations. These aneurysms are multiple 20 per cent of the time. Splenic artery aneurysms associated with pancreatitis usually involve the main splenic artery (Fig. 25–2).

Vascular calcifications evident on plain abdominal radiographs are often the first clinical evidence of a splenic artery aneurysm's presence. The most characteristic of these calcifications have a signet-ring appearance. Diagnosis in contemporary times usually results from arteriographic demonstration of the aneurysm during studies being undertaken for some other disease state. Ultrasonography, computed tomography (CT) scanning, and magnetic resonance imaging (MRI) are occasionally useful for establishing the presence of these lesions and are often helpful in identifying bleeding aneurysms.[8,14] In select circumstances, these noninvasive studies are valuable for following size changes in asymptomatic (bland) aneurysms.

Symptoms of left upper quadrant or epigastric pain occur in a minority of individuals with splenic artery aneurysms, although abdominal discomfort has been described in as many as 20 per cent of these patients.[6] Bleeding from a ruptured splenic artery aneurysm is usually initially contained within the lesser sac. Right lower quadrant pain in such cases may reflect the presence of blood exiting through the foramen of Winslow and collecting along the right paracolic gutter. Eventually, free hemorrhage into the peritoneal cavity occurs and causes vascular collapse. This represents the so-called double-rupture phenomenon.

Pancreatitis-related aneurysms are often a source of intestinal hemorrhage following their erosion into the stomach or pancreatic ductal system.[15–19] Arteriovenous fistula formation from rupture of a splenic artery aneurysm into the adjacent splenic vein is a rare but recognized cause of gastrointestinal hemorrhage from esophageal varices due to left-sided portal hypertension.[20]

The risk of splenic artery aneurysm rupture must take into account the etiology of these lesions. Rupture of bland aneurysms occurs in less than 2 per cent of cases.[6] Contrary to certain earlier misconceptions regarding these lesions, rupture has been just as likely to occur when the aneurysm is calcified, occurs in a normotensive patient, or affects the very elderly. Bland aneurysms in liver transplant recipients may be at greater risk for rupture than those in other patients.[13] Nearly 95 per cent of aneurysms first recognized during pregnancy have ruptured.[6,21–24] Maternal mortality in these cases approaches 70 per cent, and fetal mortality exceeds 75 per cent. However, these data are somewhat misleading in that most women develop their aneurysms during repeated pregnancies, and although the rupture rate during pregnancy as reported in the literature is very high, most splenic artery aneurysms in pregnant women do not rupture. Nevertheless, splenic artery aneurysms recognized during pregnancy, even though asymptomatic, are a serious threat to the health of the mother and fetus.

The surgical mortality from rupture of a splenic artery aneurysm is 25 per cent.[7] Most nonpregnant patients experiencing aneurysmal rupture undergo operation. Thus, it would seem ill-advised to undertake elective operative intervention for the usual small

TABLE 25–1B.   SPLANCHNIC ARTERY MACROANEURYSMS

Aneurysm Location	Frequency of Reported Rupture	Site of Rupture	Mortality with Rupture	Usual Treatment Options
Splenic artery	2% (bland aneurysms)	Intraperitoneal within lesser sac; Intragastric with pancreatitis-related inflammatory aneurysms	25% bland and unassociated with pregnancy; during pregnancy 70% maternal and 75% fetal	Splenectomy; aneurysm exclusion or excision without splenectomy
Hepatic artery	20%	Intraperitoneal and biliary tract with equal frequency	35%	Aneurysmectomy with and without hepatic artery reconstruction; hepatic territory resection; transcatheter aneurysm obliteration
Superior mesenteric artery	Uncommon (thrombosis more common)	Intraperitoneal and retroperitoneal	50%	Aneurysmectomy with superior mesenteric artery reconstruction; ligation if collateral circulation is adequate
Celiac artery	13%	Intraperitoneal	50%	Aneurysmectomy with celiac artery reconstruction; ligation if circulation is adequate
Gastric and gastroepiploic arteries	90%	Intraperitoneal (30%); Intestinal tract (70%)	70%	Aneurysm excision with involved gastric tissue; ligation if extramural
Jejunal, ileal, and colic arteries	30%	Intestinal tract common; Intraperitoneal uncommon	20%	Aneurysm excision with involved intestine; ligation if extramural
Pancreaticoduodenal, pancreatic, and gastroduodenal arteries	75% inflammatory 50% noninflammatory	Intestinal tract (85%); Intraperitoneal (15%)	50%	Aneurysm ligation within false aneurysms (pseudocyst-related); pancreatic resection; ligation if extrapancreatic

asymptomatic splenic artery aneurysm when the risk of operative death might predictably be greater than 0.5 per cent (this figure representing the product of the 25 per cent mortality and 2 per cent rupture rate of bland aneurysms). When intervention is otherwise deemed necessary in higher risk patients, percutaneous transcatheter embolization of splenic artery aneurysms may represent a reasonable alternative.[25–27]

Splenectomy for splenic artery aneurysms has been the most common form of surgical therapy in the past. With contemporary recognition of the immunologic importance of splenic preservation even in the aged, simple ligature obliteration or excision of these aneurysms appears preferable to splenectomy.[28] This would clearly be appropriate in the management of most proximal and many distal splenic artery aneurysms. Occasional splenic artery aneurysms embedded in the pancreas are best treated by distal pancreatectomy. Other aneurysms, especially false

aneurysms associated with pseudocyst erosion into the adjacent artery, are most easily treated by incising the aneurysmal sac and ligation of entering and exiting vessels from within.[19] Undertaking pancreatic resection or cyst drainage in the latter cases must be individualized, and often depends on the degree of associated pancreatic inflammation and general condition of the patient.

Hepatic Artery Aneurysms

Hepatic artery aneurysms account for 20 per cent of all splanchnic artery aneurysms.[4,8,29] Men are twice as likely to be affected as women. Nontraumatic and nonmycotic aneurysms are most often discovered during the sixth decade of life. The cause of many hepatic artery aneurysms is poorly defined. In the past these lesions have been attributed to arterio-

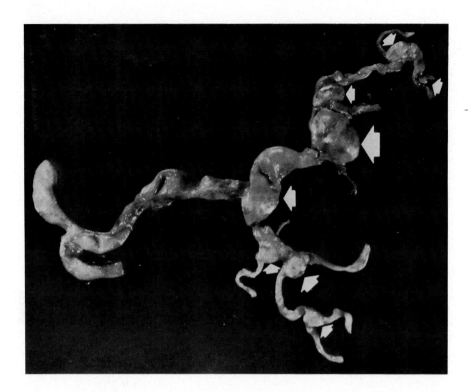

FIGURE 25–1. Multiple splenic artery aneurysms (arrows) occurring at each bifurcation of the distal artery in a grand multiparous female patient. (From Stanley JC, Thompson NW, Fry WI: Splanchnic artery aneurysms. Arch Surg *101*:689–697, 1970.)

sclerosis (32 per cent), medial degeneration (24 per cent), trauma (22 per cent), and infection, especially associated with intravenous drug abuse–related sepsis endocarditis (10 per cent). Two facts regarding the etiology of these aneurysms are noteworthy. First, arteriosclerosis, in all likelihood, represents a secondary event rather than an actual cause of these aneurysms. Second, with increasing societal violence and substance abuse there has been a marked increase in the number of reported traumatic and infection-related aneurysms. Iatrogenic false aneurysms secondary to biliary tract operative trauma remain very uncommon.[30] Connective tissue arteriopathies, such as periarteritis nodosa, have also been incriminated as a cause of occasional macroaneurysms involving the hepatic vessels.[31] Hepatic artery aneurysms are usually solitary, being extrahepatic in nearly 80 per cent of cases and intrahepatic in 20 per cent. In general, these aneurysms are fusiform when less than 2 cm in diameter and saccular when larger (Fig. 25–3).

In the past most hepatic artery aneurysms were initially suspected because of displacement and indentations on intestinal structures noted during barium contrast studies. In more contemporary times they have been recognized as incidental findings during arteriography, CT scans, or ultrasonography for other illnesses.[32,33] Very few hepatic artery aneurysms are symptomatic, but when such is the case, they characteristically present with right upper quadrant and epigastric pain. Acute expansion of hepatic artery aneurysms can cause severe upper abdominal discomfort similar to that of pancreatitis. Large aneurysms have been reported to cause obstructive

jaundice.[34] However, most hepatic artery aneurysms are too small to compress the biliary ducts. Similarly, these lesions rarely present as pulsatile abdominal masses.

The reported incidence of rupture of hepatic artery aneurysms in contemporary times is close to 20 per cent, but the true incidence may be considerably less. This is in contrast to a rupture rate of 44 per cent described in cases encountered from 1960 to 1970.[7] Mortality rates attending aneurysm rupture have not changed and continue to be approximately 35 per cent. Bleeding from ruptured hepatic artery aneurysms occurs equally into the biliary tract and into the peritoneal cavity. In the case of the former, hemobilia, manifest by biliary colic, hematemesis, and jaundice, is often evident.[35,36] Chronic gastrointestinal hemorrhage is an uncommon sequela of aneurysm rupture into the biliary tract. Intraperitoneal bleeding is most often associated with false aneurysms caused by periarterial inflammatory processes eroding into the hepatic vessels.

Common hepatic artery aneurysms have been most often treated by aneurysmectomy or aneurysm exclusion, without arterial reconstruction.[4] The extensive collateral circulation to the liver and the ability of portal venous flow to increase in most cases, usually ensures adequate blood flow to the liver despite interruption of the proximal hepatic artery. Hepatic ischemia is most likely to accompany treatment of aneurysms involving the more distal hepatic artery. However, in the absence of coexisting liver disease, complex arterial reconstructions should be avoided and simple ligation undertaken if temporary operative occlusion of the aneurysmal artery does not cause

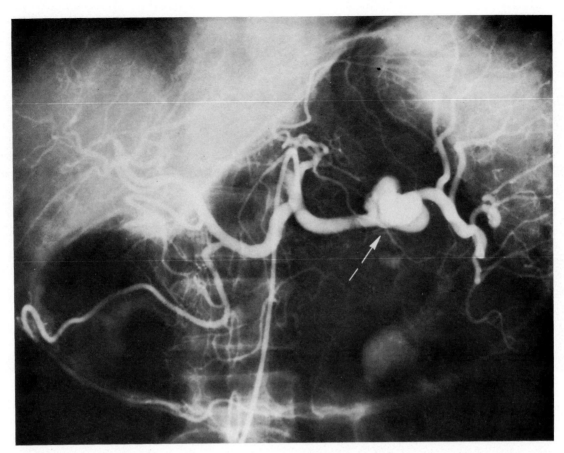

FIGURE 25–2. Solitary splenic artery aneurysm affecting the midportion of the vessel, caused by arterial erosion from a pancreatic pseudocyst in an alcoholic patient. (From Stanley JC, Frey CF, Miller TA, Lindenauer SM, Child CG: Major arterial hemorrhage. A complication of pancreatic pseudocysts and chronic pancreatitis. Arch Surg *111*:435–440, 1976.)

obvious major hepatic ischemia. If compromised liver blood flow becomes apparent with such a maneuver, then direct vascular reconstruction must be undertaken with either prosthetic or autologous grafts. Casual ligation of extrahepatic branches to control bleeding from intrahepatic aneurysms may cause liver necrosis.[4] Because of this potential complication, hepatic territory resection for intrahepatic aneurysms may prove to be the most appropriate therapy in select patients. In high-risk cases, percutaneous transcatheter obliteration of the aneurysm with balloons, coils, or thrombogenic particulate matter may be a reasonable alternative to surgical intervention.[25,37–40]

Superior Mesenteric Artery Aneurysms

Aneurysms of the proximal superior mesenteric artery are the third most common splanchnic artery aneurysm, accounting for 5.5 per cent of these lesions.[8] Men and women are affected equally. Mycotic aneurysms secondary to bacterial endocarditis continue to be a common lesion affecting this vessel.[41] Nonhemolytic streptococci and a variety of pathogens associated with parenteral substance abuse account for these latter lesions. Superior mesenteric artery aneurysms have also been related to medial degeneration, periarterial inflammation, and trauma. Arteriosclerosis, when present, has been considered a secondary event rather than an etiologic process. Superior mesenteric artery aneurysms are initially recognized most often during CT scans and arteriographic studies for nonvascular disease. A majority of reported superior mesenteric artery aneurysms have been symptomatic. In these patients, abdominal discomfort varies from mild to severe pain, and is often suggestive of intestinal angina.

Rupture of superior mesenteric aneurysms is very unusual,[42] and aneurysmal dissection is uncommon.[43] Gastrointestinal hemorrhage associated with these aneurysms usually reflects their acute occlusion and bleeding from areas of intestinal infarction.[7] The unique location of these aneurysms near the origins of the inferior pancreaticoduodenal and middle colic arteries effectively isolates the distal mesenteric circulation should aneurysmal dissection or occlusion occur. It is in this setting that intestinal ischemia occurs, because the usual collateral network from the adjacent celiac and inferior mesenteric arterial circulations is ineffective.

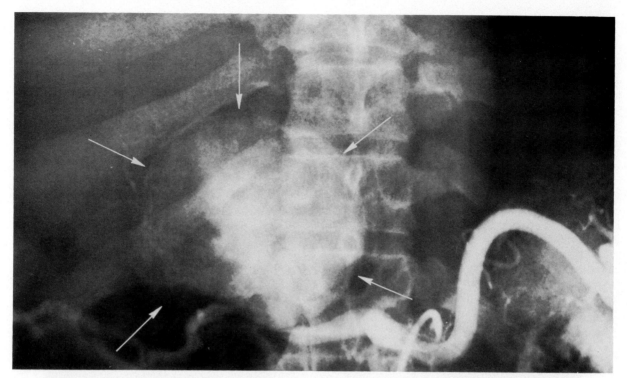

FIGURE 25–3.　Large hepatic artery aneurysm affecting the proximal artery in a patient with an underlying connective tissue disorder. (From Stanley JC, Whitehouse WM Jr: Aneurysms of splanchnic and renal arteries. *In* Bergan JJ, Yao JST (eds): Surgery of the Aorta and Its Body Branches. New York, Grune & Stratton, 1979, pp 497–519.)

Operative management of superior mesenteric artery aneurysms carries the potential complication of profound intestinal ischemia. Aneurysmectomy or simple ligation of vessels entering and exiting an aneurysm without arterial reconstruction may prove catastrophic. Intestinal revascularization by means of an aortomesenteric graft or some other bypass is often necessary, but has been accomplished infrequently. Because of the potential for graft infection if bowel ischemia is present, autologous vein or artery is favored over prosthetic conduits for these reconstructions.

Ligation of superior mesenteric artery aneurysms without arterial reconstruction may prove possible in certain cases, especially those associated with prior arterial obstruction in patients who have developed an adequate collateral circulation to their midgut structures.[8] Surprisingly, ligation and aneurysmorrhaphy have been the most commonly reported means of managing these superior mesenteric artery lesions.[44–46] Temporary occlusion of the superior mesenteric artery and Doppler assessment of blood flow along the intestine's antimesenteric border will assist in defining the adequacy of collateral vessels in these circumstances.

Celiac Artery Aneurysms

Celiac artery aneurysms account for 4 per cent of all splanchnic artery aneurysms.[8] In recent times men and women appear equally affected with these lesions.[47] Half of the celiac artery aneurysms encountered prior to 1950 had an infectious cause. More recently most aneurysms have been associated with medial defects. Arteriosclerosis is a frequent finding but, as in the case of other splanchnic artery aneurysms, is considered a secondary process. Celiac artery aneurysms are usually saccular, affecting the distal trunk of this vessel (Fig. 25–4).

Most contemporary celiac artery aneurysms have been asymptomatic or have been associated with vague abdominal discomfort. Antemortem diagnoses most often are the result of these aneurysms being recognized as incidental findings during ultrasonography, angiography, or other imaging studies for nonvascular diseases. In more recent times, rupture has been reported to affect 13 per cent of these aneurysms and carries a mortality of 50 per cent.[47] In contrast to this contemporary experience are previously published rupture rates greater than 80 per cent.[48] Celiac artery aneurysm rupture usually causes exsanguinating hemorrhage, first into the lesser space and then into the general peritoneal cavity. Although rare, gastrointestinal bleeding may follow aneurysm rupture into the stomach or pancreatic ducts.

Operative treatment is advocated in the management of all celiac artery aneurysms, unless prohibitive surgical risks exist.[47] In the presence of acute

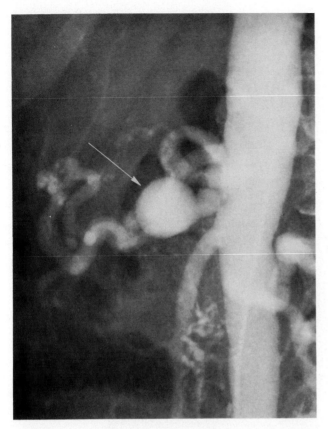

FIGURE 25–4. Celiac artery aneurysm affecting the distal trunk of the vessel. (From Whitehouse WM Jr, Graham LM, Stanley JC: Aneurysms of the celiac, hepatic, and splenic arteries. *In* Bergan JJ, Yao JST (eds): Aneurysms. Diagnosis and Treatment. New York, Grune & Stratton, 1981, pp 405–415.)

expansion or rupture, these lesions are best approached through a thoracoabdominal incision extending from the left midaxillary line within the seventh intercostal space, across the costal margin inferiorly in a midline or a right subcostal route. Most nonruptured aneurysms may be treated using only an abdominal approach, usually through a supraumbilical transverse incision extending from the midaxillary line on one side to a similar point on the opposite side, followed by medial visceral rotation to the right and exposure of the celiac artery at its aortic origin.

Aneurysmectomy with arterial reconstruction of the celiac trunk is the preferred treatment for most celiac artery aneurysms, although successful exclusion of an aneurysm with ligation of the branches entering and exiting the aneurysm has been performed in select patients.[47,49] If simple ligature is undertaken, the foregut collateral blood flow to the liver must first be documented to be sufficient to prevent hepatic necrosis. If such is not the case, hepatic revascularization is mandatory. An aortoceliac artery bypass under those circumstances is usually undertaken with autologous vein or prosthetic grafts. Successful outcomes of surgical therapy in contemporary times have

been reported in greater than 90 per cent of celiac artery aneurysms treated operatively.[47]

Gastric and Gastroepiploic Artery Aneurysms

Gastric and gastroepiploic artery aneurysms account for 4 per cent of splanchnic artery aneurysms.[8] Gastric artery aneurysms are ten times more common than gastroepiploic artery aneurysms. Men are three times more likely than women to have these aneurysms. The majority of these perigastric lesions affect patients over 50 years of age. Most of these aneurysms are solitary and are acquired, either as a result of periarterial inflammation or medial degeneration. Arteriosclerosis, when present, is a secondary accompaniment of these lesions.

Surprisingly few gastric or gastroepiploic artery aneurysms have been asymptomatic when initially recognized. In fact, these perigastric aneurysms usually present as emergencies without preceding symptoms. Rupture has occurred in greater than 90 per cent of reported cases. Gastrointestinal bleeding has occurred slightly more than twice as often as intraperitoneal hemorrhage. That rupture of these aneurysms is catastrophic is emphasized by the reported 70 per cent mortality of such an event.[7]

Surgical treatment of gastric and gastroepiploic artery aneurysms does not involve vascular reconstructive surgery. Intramural gastric aneurysms require excision with the involved portion of the stomach. Extramural aneurysms should be treated by arterial ligation alone, with or without aneurysm excision. Many of these perigastric aneurysms are very small, and a search for them is often tedious if preoperative localization has not been established by arteriographic studies.[7,19]

Jejunal, Ileal, and Colic Artery Aneurysms

Aneurysms of the jejunal, ileal, and colic arteries account for 3 per cent of splanchnic artery aneurysms.[8] They are usually recognized in patients older than 60 years of age. Men and women are affected equally. Multiple aneurysms have been reported in 10 per cent of cases. Acquired medial defects are responsible for most lesions. Arteriosclerosis, present in 20 per cent of these aneurysms, is considered a secondary event rather than a causative process. These aneurysms occasionally evolve as sequelae of infected emboli associated with subacute bacterial endocarditis.[50] Periarteritis nodosa and other connective tissue diseases are additional causes of multiple aneurysms affecting these intestinal branch arteries.[51]

Many of these aneurysms are undoubtedly asymptomatic and are recognized as incidental findings during arteriography for gastrointestinal bleeding (Fig. 25–5).[52] Although most reported intestinal branch aneurysms have ruptured, actual rupture rates are

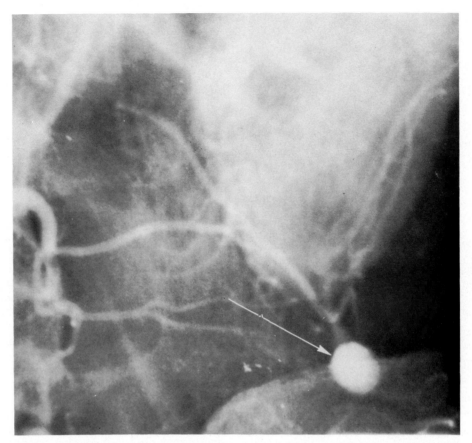

FIGURE 25–5. Ileal artery branch aneurysm. (From Stanley JC, Whitehouse WM Jr: Aneurysms of splanchnic and renal arteries. *In* Bergan JJ, Yao JST (eds): Surgery of the Aorta and Its Body Branches. New York, Grune & Stratton, 1979, pp 497–519.)

probably close to 30 per cent. Aneurysms of ileal branches are probably more apt to rupture, with jejunal branch aneurysm rupture being relatively rare.[53] This complication is associated with a mortality of approximately 20 per cent.[8] Ruptured aneurysms are usually associated with gastrointestinal hemorrhage. Rupture into the mesentery or the free peritoneal cavity is very uncommon. Nevertheless, small mesenteric branch aneurysms are more apt to rupture and cause abdominal apoplexy than any other splanchnic artery aneurysm.

Operation for intestinal branch aneurysms requires careful localization by preoperative arteriographic studies. Arterial ligation, with or without aneurysmectomy, is usually adequate therapy for extraintestinal lesions. Intramural aneurysms or those associated with bowel infarction will necessitate resection of the involved segment of intestine. Aneurysms of the inferior mesenteric artery are quite rare and definition of their clinical importance is anecdotal at best.[54]

Pancreaticoduodenal, Pancreatic, and Gastroduodenal Artery Aneurysms

Pancreatic and pancreaticoduodenal artery aneurysms account for 2 per cent, and gastroduodenal artery aneurysms represent an additional 1.5 per cent of all splanchnic artery aneurysms.[8] Men are four times more likely than women to exhibit these lesions. Most patients with these lesions are older than 50 years of age. These peripancreatic aneurysms, in general, are the most difficult to treat of all splanchnic artery aneurysms.[19,55–60] The most common cause of these aneurysms is pancreatitis-related vascular necrosis or vessel erosion by an adjacent pancreatic pseudocyst (Fig. 25–6). Medial degenerative and traumatic lesions are less common, and arteriosclerosis is invariably a secondary, not a causative process. Occasional aneurysms may evolve as a consequence of increased collateral flow within affected vessels of patients having celiac artery stenoses.[61]

The vast majority of patients with these aneurysms experience epigastric pain and discomfort. This may be due to underlying pancreatic disease, in that approximately 60 per cent of gastroduodenal and 30 per cent of pancreaticoduodenal artery aneurysms are pancreatitis related. Asymptomatic aneurysms of these arteries are unusual.

Gastroduodenal and pancreaticoduodenal aneurysm rupture has been described in nearly half the reported cases.[8] Bleeding in these circumstances has been reported in 75 per cent of inflammatory and 50

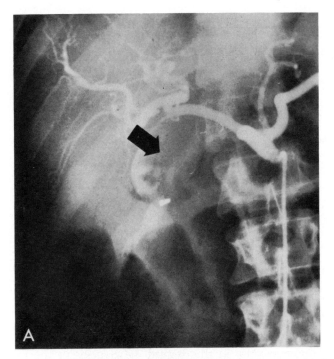 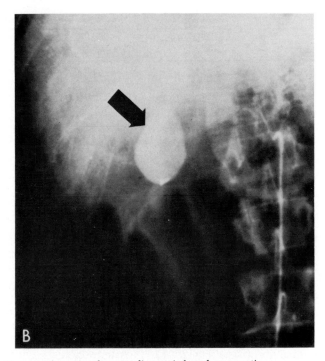

FIGURE 25–6. Gastroduodenal aneurysm associated with arterial erosion by an adjacent infected pancreatic pseudocyst. *A,* Early phase selective celiac arteriogram. *B,* Late phase with contrast collection in the false aneurysm.

per cent of noninflammatory lesions. The site of hemorrhage may be the stomach, the biliary tract, or the pancreatic ductal system in these patients. Hemorrhage into the peritoneal cavity is less common, being a complication accompanying approximately 15 per cent of these aneurysms. Arteriography is necessary to confirm the existence of these lesions. CT scanning and MRI are of increasing importance in recognizing these aneurysms, and are helpful in detecting the presence of rupture or associated pancreatic pathology. Mortality rates with rupture, despite aggressive surgical therapy, approach 50 per cent.

Operative intervention is mandatory in all but the poorest risk patients with gastroduodenal, pancreaticoduodenal, or pancreatic arterial aneurysms.[19,55,56,62] Surgical treatment of pancreatitis-related false aneurysms is often best accomplished by arterial ligation from within the aneurysmal sac rather than extra-aneurysmal arterial ligation. Extensive dissection of the pancreas involved in dense inflammatory adhesions is hazardous. If a pancreatic pseudocyst or abscess has eroded into an artery and caused a false aneurysm, then some form of drainage procedure should accompany ligature control of the affected vessel. Pancreatic resections, including distal pancreatectomy or pancreaticoduodenectomy, are the safest therapy for select patients.[19,63] Transcatheter embolization and electrocoagulation have been employed in very high risk patients to ablate certain aneurysms.[64,67] Unfortunately, rebleeding and late aneurysmal rupture with such therapy can occur and restrict its universal use.[68]

RENAL ARTERY MACROANEURYSMS

Renal artery aneurysms represent an uncommon vascular disease (Table 25–2). Although our understanding of these aneurysms has been better defined in recent years, considerable controversy persists concerning their clinical importance.[69–77] Any discussion of these lesions must take into consideration the differences between true and dissecting aneurysms of the renal artery.

Renal Artery Aneurysms

The incidence of true renal artery aneurysms probably approaches 0.1 per cent, a figure derived from the incidence of these aneurysms in approximately 8500 patients subjected to arteriographic studies for nonrenal disease.[77] Women are more likely than men to have renal artery aneurysms. However, when aneurysms in patients having renal arterial dysplasia are excluded, there is no sex predilection. The fact that the right renal artery is more likely to develop aneurysms than the left may reflect the greater incidence of dysplastic disease known to affect the right renal artery.[77]

Most renal artery aneurysms are saccular (Fig. 25–7). Seventy-five per cent are located at primary or secondary renal artery bifurcations. Most aneurysms have diameters less than 1.5 cm. Fusiform aneurysms do not usually involve bifurcations. Intraparenchymal lesions occur in less than 10 per cent of cases.

Renal artery aneurysms usually appear to be caused

TABLE 25–2. RENAL ARTERY MACROANEURYSMS

Lesion	Male:Female Ratio	Contributing Factors	Frequency of Reported Rupture	Mortality with Rupture	Usual Treatment Options
Renal artery aneurysm	1:1.2	Medial degeneration arterial fibrodysplasia; hypertension	3% (bland aneurysms)	10% (bland aneurysms); during pregnancy 55% maternal, 85% fetal	Aneurysmectomy with renal artery reconstruction; nephrectomy for ruptured aneurysms
Renal artery dissection	10:1	Blunt abdominal trauma; intraarterial catheterization; medial degeneration	Uncommon (thrombosis more common)	Undefined	Renal artery reconstruction

by a medial degenerative process.[77] Internal elastic lamina fragmentation is invariably present. Excessive accumulations of collagen and ground substances, with a paucity of medial smooth muscle, are characteristic of these aneurysms. Systemic arterial hypertension may contribute to certain of these aneurysms. In many instances these aneurysms appear to be part of the dysplastic process associated with medial fibroplasia (Fig. 25–8).[71,77] Arteriosclerosis, with hemorrhage, calcium deposition, collections of cholesterol, and necrotic cellular debris within a matrix of fibrous tissue, affects a third of these aneurysms.

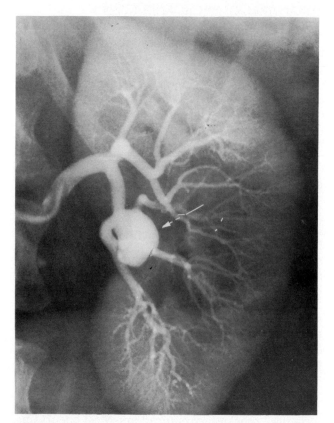

FIGURE 25–7. Saccular renal aneurysm occurring at a segmental branching. (From Stanley JC, Whitehouse WM Jr: Renal artery macroaneurysms. *In* Bergan JJ, Yao JST (eds): Aneurysms. Diagnosis and Treatment. New York, Grune & Stratton, 1981, pp 417–431.)

However, similar changes of the adjacent renal artery are very uncommon and the former findings are thought to represent a secondary event, rather than a primary process. Importantly, arteriosclerosis in some but not all aneurysms in the same patients suggests a nonarteriosclerotic cause of these lesions.[77] Evidence exists that both congenital and acquired factors contribute to the evolution of most renal artery macroaneurysms. In this regard deficiencies in the internal elastic lamina of muscular arteries appear to be congenital, but the reported increase in aneurysm appearance with increasing age indicates the presence of acquired factors. Microaneurysms secondary to necrotizing arteritides, such as polyarteritis nodosa, may become relatively large.[79]

The majority of renal artery aneurysms are asymptomatic.[77] Some have suggested that few of these aneurysms ever evolve serious clinical complications.[71,78,80] Nevertheless, aneurysmal expansion or renal infarction from dislodged thrombus may occasionally account for symptoms attributed to these lesions. Hematuria and abdominal bruits, when present in these cases, are unlikely to be related to aneurysmal disease. Similarly, because of their small size, very few aneurysms present as pulsatile masses on physical examination.

Rupture represents the most serious complication attending renal artery aneurysms. Such an event is likely to affect fewer than 3 per cent of cases. Aneurysm rupture has been reported by some to be 20 to 40 per cent with intrarenal lesions,[81] but such a common frequency is not in keeping with most clinical experiences. Importantly, exsanguinating hemorrhage and death following rupture occurs less often than reported earlier.[70,72,76,81,82] Mortality in such circumstances is approximately 10 per cent. However, loss of a kidney is an almost inevitable outcome of aneurysm rupture.[77,83,84] Renal artery aneurysm rupture during pregnancy is an exception regarding the life-threatening nature of these lesions.[85–88] Rupture of these aneurysms during pregnancy has not appeared related to patient age, presence of hypertension, or parity.[89] Aneurysm rupture in pregnancy has caused nearly an 85 per cent fetal mortality and resulted in approximately a 45 per cent maternal mortality.[87] The affected kidney has been salvaged in

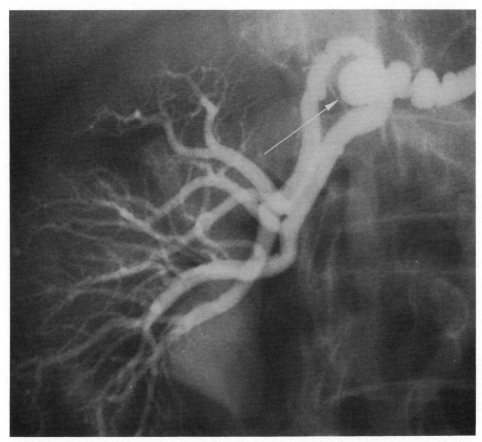

FIGURE 25–8. Renal artery macroaneurysm affecting the primary bifurcation of a vessel exhibiting medial fibrodysplasia. (From Stanley JC, Whitehouse WM Jr: Renal artery macroaneurysms. *In* Bergan JJ, Yao JST (eds): Aneurysms. Diagnosis and Treatment. New York, Grune & Stratton, 1981, pp 417–431.)

nearly 20 per cent of surviving women. It has been suggested that aneurysms greater than 1.5 cm in diameter, noncalcified aneurysms, and those occurring in hypertensive patients are more likely to rupture. This has not proven to be the case.

The cause-effect association of renal artery aneurysms to elevated arterial blood pressure is controversial.[74,84,90–92] It is possible that aneurysmal thrombus may embolize or propagate and occlude a distal artery, thereby producing renal ischemia and renovascular hypertension.[73,77] Extensive atheromatous disease within large aneurysmal sacs may predispose to thrombotic events, yet small nonarteriosclerotic aneurysms also have been recognized as the source of distal cortical embolization. Aneurysmal compression of adjacent arteries has been proposed as an additional cause of renovascular hypertension, but such is very uncommon. However, intrinsic stenotic disease adjacent to an aneurysm, which is not always evident on preoperative arteriograms, may be the cause of secondary hypertension in many of these cases. Determination of renal-systemic renin indexes in patients with hypertension and isolated renal artery aneurysms may better define the presence or absence of reninmediated renovascular hypertension.[94]

Indications for operative treatment of renal artery macroaneurysms have become better defined. Certainly, all symptomatic patients with suspected aneurysmal expansion should be subjected to operation. Similarly, aneurysms coexisting with functionally important renal artery stenoses are best treated operatively. Surgical therapy is also warranted for aneurysms that contain thrombus, if distal embolization is evident. Lastly, because of the potential for catastrophic rupture during pregnancy, operative therapy is recommended for aneurysms in all women of childbearing age who might possibly conceive in the future.

Surgical therapy is directed at elimination of the aneurysm without loss of the kidney or compromise of normal renal blood flow.[73,77,95] An exception exists in the management of ruptured aneurysms, where nephrectomy may be the only logical therapy. Large aneurysms of the main renal artery may often be excised with simple primary repair of the artery. Excision of smaller aneurysms usually necessitates an angioplastic vein patch arterial closure, or implantation of the involved artery into an adjacent uninvolved artery. In situ renal artery reconstructions with autogenous saphenous vein, or internal iliac artery grafts for bifurcation aneurysms, or lesions associated with functionally important stenoses are perhaps the most common means of treating patients with these lesions.[77,96] In select instances, ex vivo repairs are appropriate.[96-98] Partial nephrectomy may be necessary for intraparenchymal aneurysms. These latter lesions may occasionally be treated by transcatheter embolization.[73] Patients not subjected to operation must be followed carefully with serial CT scans or arteriography. Particular attention should be directed to controlling hypertension in patients not subjected to surgical therapy.

Renal Artery Dissections

Isolated dissections of the renal arteries are usually classified as (1) those due to blunt abdominal trauma or intraluminal catheter–induced injury, and (2) those occurring spontaneously.[99,100] All forms of dissections may be associated with false aneurysm formation (Fig. 25–9). Interestingly, the renal artery exhibits spontaneous dissections more than any other peripheral artery.[101] Men are ten times more likely than women to exhibit dissections of the renal artery.[102] The right renal artery is much more often affected than the left. This may reflect increased physical stresses on this artery due to greater ptosis of the right kidney compared to the left. Approximately one third of renal artery dissections are bilateral.

Two primary mechanisms contribute to renal artery dissections due to blunt abdominal trauma. The first is displacement of the kidney during deceleration, with marked stretching of the vascular pedicle.[103,104] Fracture of the intima, which is the least elastic arterial wall component, in these circumstances leads to subintimal dissections. The second relates to direct trauma of the renal artery over the unyielding posteriorly located vertebral bodies.[105] Medial hemorrhage and false aneurysm formation may occur in this setting. Renal artery injury during arteriography appears to be a very uncommon but important cause of dissections. In the University of Michigan experience, only four renal artery catheter–related dissections were encountered among more than 11,000 abdominal arteriographic examinations, including more than 2200 selective renal arteriograms.[99]

The second major subcategory of renal artery dissections are those associated with spontaneous vessel wall disruption. Surprisingly, spontaneous dissections affect the renal arteries more than any other peripheral artery. They usually appear related to coexistent renovascular disease.[93,106] Spontaneous dissections have been reported in 0.5 per cent of patients having renal artery dysplasia in the University of Michigan experience.[99] Differences in defining dissections may account for such disparate observations.

Spontaneous dissections are most apt to extend

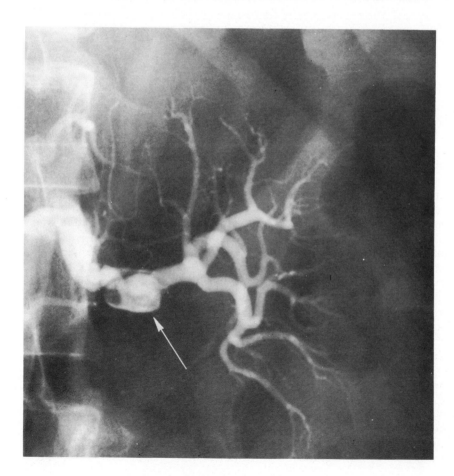

FIGURE 25–9. Renal artery dissection with associated false aneurysm. (From Gewertz BL, Stanley JC, Fry WI: Renal artery dissections. Arch Surg *112:*409–414, 1977.)

within the outer media.[104,107,108] This is in contrast to subintimal and inner medial location of most traumatic dissections. In certain instances, these spontaneous dissections have been attributed to rupture of abnormal vasa vasorum. Under such circumstances the dissecting mural hematoma may increase vessel wall ischemia and further compromise its integrity. Spontaneous renal artery dissections most often originate in the proximal vessels and terminate proximal to first-order branchings.

Pain, hematuria, and elevated blood pressure are frequent manifestations of acute renal artery dissections, regardless of their cause.[99] Chronic manifestations of these dissections are often associated with compromised renal function and renovascular hypertension. Delayed rupture is uncommon. An incorrect initial clinical diagnosis is common, occurring in nearly 60 per cent of patients with renal artery dissections.[99] Rapid infusion urography, often with tomography, may be useful in establishing the presence of renal ischemia in these cases, but the accuracy of this study is limited.[109,110] Certainly, delays in obtaining urograms lessens their usefulness. Because prompt diagnosis may improve results of surgical therapy, intravenous urography should be deferred in favor of prompt arteriography.[99,111] Criteria for arteriographic diagnosis of renal artery dissections include: (1) luminal irregularities with aneurysmal dilatation or saccular dissections associated with segmental stenoses; (2) predilection of dissections to extend distally to the first renal artery bifurcation; (3) cuffing at branchings causing a "rolled-down sock" appearance; and (4) variable degrees of reversibility documented by serial studies.[93]

Kidney preservation is of prime importance in patients exhibiting renal artery dissections.[99,100] This is particularly relevant in that renal artery disease involves the contralateral kidney in half the patients exhibiting spontaneous dissections.[99] Arterial reconstructions utilizing autogenous saphenous vein or hypogastric artery may be complex, and ex vivo repairs are appropriate in select cases. Dissections secondary to severe blunt trauma usually necessitate emergent arterial reconstructions. Delayed repair becomes necessary when hypertension persists or renal function deteriorates in instances of seemingly minor injury. Some physicians have taken a cautious nonsurgical approach in managing traumatic dissections in that operation in the acute setting often results in nephrectomy. Treatment using an endovascular stent has appeal, but as of yet, remains an unproven therapy.[112] In contrast, spontaneous dissecting aneurysms should all be subjected to surgical therapy once hemodynamically significant stenoses or occlusions are recognized as causing renovascular hypertension or deterioration in renal function.[99,102]

REFERENCES

1. Stanley JC: Abdominal visceral aneurysms. *In* Haimovici H (ed): Vascular Emergencies. New York, Appleton-Century-Crofts, 1981, pp 387–397.
2. Busuttil RW, Brin BJ: The diagnosis and management of visceral artery aneurysms. Surgery *88*:619–630, 1980.
3. Graham JM, McCollum CH, DeBakey ME: Aneurysms of the splanchnic arteries. Am J Surg *140*:797–801, 1980.
4. Iseki J, Tada Y, Wada T, Nobori M: Hepatic artery aneurysm. Report of a case and review of the literature. Gastroenterol Jpn *18*:84–92, 1983.
5. Jorgensen BA: Visceral artery aneurysms. A review. Dan Med Bull *32*:237–242, 1985.
6. Stanley JC, Fry WJ: Pathogenesis and clinical significance of splenic artery aneurysms. Surgery *76*:889–909, 1974.
7. Stanley JC, Thompson NW, Fry WJ: Splanchnic artery aneurysms. Arch Surg *101*:689–697, 1970.
8. Stanley JC, Zelenock GB: Splanchnic artery aneurysms. *In* Rutherford RB (ed): Vascular Surgery, 3rd ed. Philadelphia, WB Saunders Company, 1989, pp 969–983.
9. Trastek VF, Pairolero PC, Joyce JW, Hollier LH, Bernatz PE: Splenic artery aneurysms. Surgery *91*:694–699, 1982.
10. Puttini M, Aseni P, Brambilla G, Belli L: Splenic artery aneurysms in portal hypertension. J Cardiovasc Surg *23*:490–493, 1982.
11. Nishida O, Moriyasu F, Nakamura T, Ban N, Miura K, Sakai M, Uchino H, Miyake T: Hemodynamics of splenic artery aneurysm. Gastroenterology *90*:1042–1046, 1986.
12. Ayalon A, Wiesner RH, Perkins JD, Tominaga S, Hayes DH, Krom RA: Splenic artery aneurysms in liver transplant patients. Transplantation *45*:386–389, 1988.
13. Bronsther O, Merhav H, Van Thiel D, Starzl TE: Splenic artery aneurysms occurring in liver transplant recipients. Transplantation *52*:723–756, 1991.
14. Martin KW, Morian JP Jr, Lee JK, Scharp DW: Demonstration of a splenic artery pseudoaneurysm by MR imaging. J Comput Assist Tomogr *9*:190–192, 1985.
15. Clay RP, Farnell MB, Lancester JR, Weiland LH, Gostout CJ: Hemosuccus pancreaticus. An unusual cause of upper gastrointestinal bleeding. Ann Surg *202*:75–79, 1985.
16. deVries JE, Schattenkerk ME, Malt RA: Complications of splenic artery aneurysm other than intraperitoneal rupture. Surgery *91*:200–204, 1982.
17. Harper PC, Gamelli RL, Kaye MD: Recurrent hemorrhage into the pancreatic duct from a splenic artery aneurysm. Gastroenterology *87*:417–420, 1984.
18. Stabile BE, Wilson SE, Debas HT: Reduced mortality from bleeding pseudocysts and pseudoaneurysms caused by pancreatitis. Arch Surg *118*:45–51, 1983.
19. Stanley JC, Frey CF, Miller TA, Lindenauer SM, Child CG III: Major arterial hemorrhage. A complication of pancreatic pseudocysts and chronic pancreatitis. Arch Surg *111*:435–440, 1976.
20. Williams DB, Payne SP, Foulk WT, Johnson CM: Case report. Splenic arteriovenous fistula. Mayo Clin Proc *55*:383–386, 1980.
21. Lowry SM, O'Dea TP, Gallagher DI, Mozenter R: Splenic artery aneurysm rupture: The seventh instance of maternal and fetal survival. Obstet Gynecol *67*:291–292, 1986.
22. MacFarlane JR, Thorbjarnason B: Rupture of splenic artery aneurysm during pregnancy. Am J Obstet Gynecol *95*:1025–1037, 1966.
23. O'Grady JP, Day EJ, Toole AL, Paust JC: Splenic artery aneurysm rupture in pregnancy. A review and case report. Obstet Gynecol *50*:627–630, 1977.
24. Vassalotti SB, Schaller JA: Spontaneous rupture of splenic artery aneurysm in pregnancy. Report of first known antepartum rupture with maternal fetal survival. Obstet Gynecol *30*:264–268, 1967.

25. Baker KS, Tisnado J, Cho SR, Beachley MC: Splanchnic artery aneurysms and pseudoaneurysms: Transcatheter embolization. Radiology 163:135–159, 1987.

26. Probst P, Castaneda-Zuniga WR, Gomes AS, Yonehiro EG, Delaney JP, Amplatz K: Nonsurgical treatment of splenic-artery aneurysms. Radiology 128:619–623, 1978.

27. Waltman AC, Luers PR, Athanasoulis CA, Warshaw AL: Massive arterial hemorrhage in patients with pancreatitis. Complementary roles of surgery and transcatheter occlusive techniques. Arch Surg 121:439–443, 1986.

28. Taylor JL, Woodward DA: Splenic conservation and the management of splenic artery aneurysm. Ann R Coll Surg Engl 69:179–180, 1987.

29. Guida PM, Moore SW: Aneurysm of the hepatic artery. Report of five cases with a brief review of the previously reported cases. Surgery 60:299–310, 1966.

30. Jeans PL: Hepatic artery aneurysms and biliary surgery. Two cases and a literature review. Aust N Z J Surg 58:889–894, 1988.

31. Parangi S, Oz MC, Blume RS, Bixon R, Laffey KF, Perzin KH, Buda JA, Markowitz AM, Nowygrod R: Hepatobiliary complications of polyarteritis nodosa. Arch Surg 126:909–912, 1991.

32. Athey PA, Sax SL, Lamki N, Cadavid G: Sonography in the diagnosis of hepatic artery aneurysms. Am J Roentgenol 147:725–727, 1986.

33. Kibbler CC, Cohen DL, Cruicshank JK, Kushwaha SS, Morgan MY, Dick RD: Use of CAT scanning in the diagnosis and management of hepatic artery aneurysm. Gut 26:752–756, 1985.

34. Lal RB, Strohl JA, Piazza S, Aslam M, Ball D, Patel K: Hepatic artery aneurysm. J Cardiovasc Surg 30:509–513, 1989.

35. Harlaftis NN, Akin JT: Hemobilia from ruptured hepatic artery aneurysm: Report of a case and review of the literature. Am J Surg 133:229–232, 1977.

36. Stauffer JT, Weinman MD, Bynum TE: Hemobilia in a patient with multiple hepatic artery aneurysms: A case report and review of the literature. Am J Gastroenterol 84:59–62, 1989.

37. Goldblatt M, Goldin AR, Shaff MI: Percutaneous embolization for the management of hepatic artery aneurysms. Gastroenterology 73:1142–1144, 1977.

38. Jonsson K, Bjernstad A, Eriksson B: Treatment of a hepatic artery aneurysm by coil occlusion of the hepatic artery. Am J Roentgenol 134:1245–1247, 1980.

39. Kadir S, Athansoulis CA, Ring EJ, Greenfield A: Transcatheter embolization of intrahepatic arterial aneurysms. Radiology 134:335–339, 1980.

40. Okazaki M, Higashihara H, Ono H, Koganemaru F, Hoashi T, Inada S, Kuroda Y: Percutaneous embolization of ruptured splanchnic artery pseudoaneurysms. Acta Radiologica 32:349–354, 1991.

41. Friedman SG, Pogo GJ, Moccio CG: Mycotic aneurysm of the superior mesenteric artery. J Vasc Surg 6:87–90, 1987.

42. Blumenberg RM, David D, Skovak J: Abdominal apoplexy due to rupture of a superior mesenteric artery aneurysm: Clip aneurysmorrhaphy with survival. Arch Surg 108:223–226, 1974.

43. Cormier F, Ferry J, Artru B, Wechsler B, Cormier JM: Dissecting aneurysms of the main trunk of the superior mesenteric artery. J Vasc Surg 15:424–430, 1992.

44. DeBakey ME, Cooley DA: Successful resection of mycotic aneurysm of superior mesenteric artery: Case report and review of the literature. Am Surg 19:202–212, 1953.

45. Geelkerken RH, van Bockel JH, de Roos WK, Hermans J: Surgical treatment of intestinal artery aneurysms. Eur J Vasc Surg 4:563–567, 1990.

46. Olcott C, Ehrenfeld WK: Endoaneurysmorrhaphy for visceral artery aneurysms. Am J Surg 133:636–639, 1977.

47. Graham LM, Stanley JC, Whitehouse WM Jr, Zelenock GB, Cronenwett JL, Lindenauer SM: Celiac artery aneurysms: Historical (1745–1949) versus contemporary (1950–1984)

differences in etiology and clinical importance. J Vasc Surg 2:757–764, 1985.

48. Shumacker HB Jr, Siderys H: Excisional treatment of aneurysm of celiac artery. Ann Surg 148:885–889, 1958.

49. Hertzer NR, Mullally PH: Celiac artery aneurysmectomy with hepatic artery ligation. Arch Surg 104:337–339, 1972.

50. Trevisani MF, Ricci MA, Michaels RM, Meyer KK: Multiple mesenteric aneurysms complicating subacute bacterial endocarditis. Arch Surg 122:823–824, 1987.

51. Selke FW, Williams GB, Donovan DL, Clarke RE: Management of intra-abdominal aneurysms associated with periarteritis nodosa. J Vasc Surg 4:294–298, 1986.

52. Bleichrodt RP, Smulders TAE, Schreuder F, Tinbergen W, Muller WFH: Aneurysms of the jejunal artery. J Cardiovasc Surg 25:376–377, 1984.

53. Diettrich NA, Cacioppo JC, Ying DPW: Massive gastrointestinal hemorrhage caused by rupture of a jejunal branch artery aneurysm. J Vasc Surg 8:187–189, 1988.

54. Graham LM, Hay MR, Cho KJ, Stanley JC: Interior mesenteric artery aneurysms. Surgery 97:158–163, 1985.

55. Eckhauser FE, Stanley JC, Zelenock GB, Freier DT, Lindenauer SM: Gastroduodenal and pancreaticoduodenal artery aneurysms: A complication of pancreatitis causing spontaneous gastrointestinal hemorrhage. Surgery 88:335–355, 1980.

56. Gadacz TR, Trunkey D, Kieffer RF: Visceral vessel erosion associated with pancreatitis. Case reports and a review of the literature. Arch Surg 113:1438–1440, 1978.

57. Gangahar DM, Carveth SW, Reese HE, Buchman RJ, Breiner MA: True aneurysm of the pancreaticoduodenal artery: A case report and review of the literature. J Vasc Surg 2:741–742, 1985.

58. Spanos PK, Kloppedal EA, Murray CA: Aneurysms of the gastroduodenal and pancreaticoduodenal arteries. Am J Surg 127:345–348, 1974.

59. Taheri SA, Mueller G: Surgical approach and review of literature on gastroduodenal aneurysm: A case report. Angiology 36:895–898, 1985.

60. Verta MJ Jr, Dean RH, Yao JST, Conn J Jr, Mehn WH, Bergan JJ: Pancreaticoduodenal artery aneurysms. Ann Surg 186:111–114, 1977.

61. Quandalle P, Chambon JP, Marache P, Saudemont A, Maes B: Pancreaticoduodenal artery aneurysms associated with celiac axis stenosis: Report of two cases and review of the literature. Ann Vasc Surg 4:540–545, 1990.

62. Granke K, Hollier LH, Bowen JC: Pancreaticoduodenal artery aneurysms: Changing patterns. South Med J 83:918–921, 1990.

63. Pitkaranta P, Haapianinen R, Kivisaari L, Schroder T: Diagnostic evaluation and aggressive surgical approach in bleeding pseudoaneurysms associated with pancreatic pseudocysts. Scand J Gastroenterol 26:58–64, 1991.

64. Mandel SR, Jaques PF, Mauro MA, Sanofsky S: Nonoperative management of peripancreatic arterial aneurysms. A 10-year experience. Ann Surg 205:126–128, 1987.

65. Prasad JK, Chatterjee KS, Jonston DWB: Unusual case of massive gastrointestinal bleeding-pseudoaneurysm of the head of the pancreas. Can J Surg 18:490–492, 1975.

66. Thakker RB, Gajjar B, Wilkins RA, Levi AJ: Embolization of gastroduodenal artery aneurysm caused by chronic pancreatitis. Gut 24:1094–1098, 1983.

67. Vujic I, Anderson MC, Meredith HC, Cullon JW: Successful embolization of the dorsal pancreatic artery to control massive upper gastrointestinal hemorrhage. Ann Surg 46:184–186, 1980.

68. Lina JR, Jaques P, Mandell V: Aneurysm rupture secondary to transcatheter embolization. Am J Roentgenol 132:553–556, 1979.

69. DeBakey ME, Lefrak EA, Garcia-Rinaldi R, Noon GP: Aneurysm of the renal artery: A vascular reconstructive approach. Arch Surg 106:438–443, 1973.

70. Hageman JH, Smith RF, Szilagyi DE, Elliott JP: Aneurysms

of the renal artery: Problems of prognosis and surgical management. Surgery 84:563–572, 1978.

71. Henriksson C, Lukes P, Nilson AE, Pettersson S: Angiographically discovered, nonoperated renal artery aneurysms. Scand J Urol Neprhol 18:59–62, 1984.
72. Hubert JP Jr, Pairolero PC, Kazmier FJ: Solitary renal artery aneurysm. Surgery 88:557–565, 1980.
73. Hupp T, Allenberg JR, Post K, Roeren T, Meier M, Clorius JH: Renal artery aneurysm: Surgical indications and results. Eur J Vasc Surg 6:477–486, 1992.
74. Martin RS III, Meacham PW, Ditesheim JA, Mulherin JL Jr, Edwards WH: Renal artery aneurysm: Selective treatment for hypertension and prevention of rupture. J Vasc Surg 9:26–34, 1989.
75. Smith JN, Hinman F Jr: Intrarenal aneurysms. J Urol 97:990–996, 1968.
76. Poutasse EF: Renal artery aneurysms. J Urol 113:443–449, 1974.
77. Stanley JC, Rhodes EL, Gewertz BL, Chang CY, Walter JF, Fry WJ: Renal artery aneurysms: Significance of macroaneurysms exclusive of dissections and fibrodysplastic mural dilations. Arch Surg 110:1327–1333, 1975.
78. Tham G, Ekelund L, Herrlin K, Lindstedt EL, Olin T, Bergentz SE: Renal artery aneurysms. Natural history and prognosis. Ann Surg 197:348–352, 1983.
79. Smith DL, Wernick R: Spontaneous rupture of a renal artery aneurysm in polyarteritis nodosa: Critical review of the literature and report of a case. Am J Med 87:464–467, 1989.
80. Henriksson C, Bjorkerud S, Nilson AE, Pettersson S: Natural history of renal artery aneurysm elucidated by repeated angiography and pathoanatomical studies. Eur Urol 11:244–248, 1985.
81. Mohamed A, Yalla SV, Ivker M, Burros HM: Intrapelvic rupture of an infrarenal arterial aneurysm. J Urol 110:277–279, 1973.
82. Hogbin BM, Scorer CG: Spontaneous rupture of an aneurysm of the renal artery with survival. Br J Urol 41:218–221, 1969.
83. Poutasse EF: Renal artery aneurysms: Their natural history and surgery. J Urol 95:297–306, 1966.
84. Vaughan TJ, Barry WF, Jeffords DL, Johnsrude IS: Renal artery aneurysms and hypertension. Radiology 99:287–293, 1971.
85. Burt RL, Johnson FF, Silverthorne RG, Lock FR, Dickerson A: Ruptured renal artery aneurysm in pregnancy: Report of a case with survival. Obstet Gynecol 7:229–233, 1956.
86. Cohen SG, Cashdan A, Burger R: Spontaneous rupture of a renal artery aneurysm during pregnancy. Obstet Gynecol 39:897–902, 1972.
87. Dayton B, Helgerson RB, Sollinger HW, Acher CW: Ruptured renal artery aneurysm in a pregnant uninephric patient: Successful ex vivo repair and autotransplantation. Surgery 107(6):708–711, 1990.
88. Schoon IM, Seeman T, Niemand D, Lindell D, Andersch B, Bjorkerud S: Rupture of renal arterial aneurysm in pregnancy. Acta Chir Scand 154:593–597, 1988.
89. Cohen JR, Shamash FS: Ruptured renal artery aneurysms during pregnancy. J Vasc Surg 6:51–59, 1987.
90. Cummings KB, Lecky JW, Kaufman JJ: Renal artery aneurysms and hypertension. J Urol 109:144–148, 1973.
91. Ruberti U, Miani S, Scorza R, Mingazzini P, Biasi GM: Aneurysms of the renal artery. Int Angiol 6:407–414, 1987.
92. Soussou ID, Starr DS, Lawrie GM, Morris GM Jr: Renal artery aneurysm: Long-term relief of renovascular hypertension by in situ operative correction. Arch Surg 114:1410–1415, 1979.
93. Hare WSC, Kincaid-Smith P: Dissecting aneurysm of the renal artery. Radiology 97:255–263, 1970.
94. Stanley JC, Fry WJ: Surgical treatment of renovascular hypertension. Arch Surg 112:1291–1297, 1977.
95. Mercier C, Piquet P, Piligian F, Ferdani M: Aneurysms of the renal artery and its branches. Ann Vasc Surg 1:321–327, 1986.
96. Ortenberg J, Novick AC, Straffon RA, Stewart BH: Surgical treatment of renal artery aneurysms. Br J Urol 55:341–346, 1983.
97. Bugge-Asperheim B, Sdal G, Flatmark A: Renal artery aneurysm. Ex vivo repair and autotransplantation. Scand J Urol Nephrol 18:63–66, 1984.
98. Dubernard JM, Martin X, Gelet A, Mongin D: Aneurysms of the renal artery: Surgical management with special reference to extracorporeal surgery and autotransplantation. Eur Urol 11:26–30, 1985.
99. Gewertz BL, Stanley JC, Fry WJ: Renal artery dissections. Arch Surg 112:409–414, 1977.
100. Reilly LM, Cunningham CG, Maggisano R, Ehrenfeld WK, Stoney RJ: The role of arterial reconstruction in spontaneous renal artery dissection. J Vasc Surg 14(4):468–479, 1991.
101. Foord AG, Lewis RD: Primary dissecting aneurysms of peripheral and pulmonary arteries. Dissecting hemorrhage of media. Arch Pathol 68:553–557, 1959.
102. Edwards BS, Stanson AW, Holley KE, Sheps SG: Isolated renal artery dissection: Presentation evaluation management and pathology. Mayo Clin Proc 57:564–571, 1982.
103. Caponegro PJ, Leadbetter GW: Traumatic subintimal hemorrhage of the renal artery. J Urol 105:330–334, 1971.
104. Henry L, Burke WD: Isolated dissecting aneurysms of the renal artery. Angiology 14:269–276, 1963.
105. Stables DP, Fouche RF, DeVilliers Van Neiker JP, Cremin BJ, Holt SA, Peterson NE: Traumatic renal artery occlusion: Twenty-one cases. J Urol 115:229–233, 1976.
106. Stanley JC, Gewertz BL, Bove EL, Sottiurai VS, Fry WJ: Arterial fibrodysplasia: Histopathologic character and current etiologic concepts. Arch Surg 110:561–566, 1975.
107. Rosenblum WI: Isolated dissecting aneurysm of the renal artery. J Urol 95:135–138, 1966.
108. Watson AJ: Dissecting aneurysms of arteries other than the aorta. J Pathol Bacteriol 72:439–449, 1956.
109. Scott R Jr, Carlton CE Jr, Goldman M: Penetrating injuries of the kidney: An analysis of 181 patients. J Urol 101:247–253, 1969.
110. Wein AJ, Arger PH, Murphy JJ: Controversial aspects of blunt renal trauma. J Trauma 17:662–666, 1977.
111. Stables DP: Unilateral absence of excretion at urography after abdominal trauma. Radiology 121:609–615, 1976.
112. Mali WP, Geyskes GG, Thalman R: Dissecting renal artery aneurysm: Treatment with an endovascular stent. Am J Roentgenol 153:623–614, 1989.

REVIEW QUESTIONS

1. Which of the following represents the proper order of splanchnic artery aneurysm in order of decreasing frequency?
   (a) splenic, hepatic, SMA, celiac
   (b) hepatic, splenic, celiac, SMA
   (c) intestinal, celiac, hepatic, splenic
   (d) splenic, hepatic, celiac, SMA

2. Splenic artery aneurysms:
   (a) are more common in women than men
   (b) tend to be saccular and occur at vessel branching
   (c) may exhibit a "double-rupture" phenomenon

(d) all of the above

3. Hepatic artery aneurysms:
   (a) account for 20 per cent of splanchnic artery aneurysms
   (b) often present with obstructive jaundice
   (c) have ruptured in 20 per cent of reported cases with approximately a 50 per cent mortality accompanying rupture
   (d) are twice as likely to rupture into the biliary tract as the peritoneal cavity

4. Aneurysms of the superior mesenteric artery:
   (a) are the third most common splanchnic aneurysm, accounting for 4 per cent of all such aneurysms
   (b) are commonly mycotic in origin
   (c) affect men twice as often as women
   (d) have ruptured in 12 per cent of reported cases

5. Celiac artery aneurysms:
   (a) are best treated by simple ligation with or without aneurysmectomy
   (b) are rarely diagnosed prior to rupture in contemporary times
   (c) are associated with a 50 per cent mortality when they do rupture
   (d) are more likely to affect women than men

6. Jejunal, ileal, and colic aneurysms:
   (a) are most commonly due to atherosclerosis
   (b) occur most commonly in women
   (c) when multiple tend to be associated with subacute bacterial endocarditis or periarteritis nodosa

(d) carry a risk of rupture of 30 per cent

7. Renal artery aneurysms:
   (a) are demonstrated in 0.1 per cent of patients undergoing angiography for nonrenal indications
   (b) tend to be fusiform and occur at branchings of the main renal artery
   (c) are usually caused by atherosclerosis
   (d) cause hypertension in approximately 15 per cent of cases

8. Ruptured renal artery aneurysms:
   (a) usually present with hematuria
   (b) have a mortality approaching 10 per cent
   (c) are most commonly treated by arterial reconstruction
   (d) are more likely to occur with noncalcified than calcified lesions

9. Renal artery aneurysms may be associated with hypertension due to:
   (a) depulsatile blood flow beyond the aneurysm
   (b) common compression of adjacent arteries
   (c) intrinsic stenotic disease adjacent to the aneurysm
   (d) contralateral release of renal renin

10. Spontaneous dissections of the renal artery:
    (a) are a rare form of arterial dissection
    (b) occur most often in women
    (c) are bilateral in a third of cases
    (d) rarely require surgical therapy

ANSWERS _____

1. d	2. d	3. a	4. b	5. c	6. c	7. a
8. b	9. c	10. c				

26

AORTOILIAC OCCLUSIVE DISEASE

ANTHONY D. WHITTEMORE, MAGRUDER C. DONALDSON, and
JOHN A. MANNICK

Arteriosclerotic occlusive disease of the abdominal aorta and iliac arteries is a common cause of ischemic symptoms in the lower extremities of middle-aged and elderly patients in the western world. While not as common as occlusive disease of the femoropopliteal arterial system, with which it may be combined, aortoiliac occlusive disease may be more disabling because of the greater number of muscle groups subjected to diminished perfusion. The initial manifestation of occlusive disease of the distal aorta and/or iliac arteries is intermittent claudication with symptoms involving muscles of the thigh, hip, and buttock as well as the calf. Since the calf muscles are usually the only muscle groups affected by intermittent claudication caused by superficial femoral artery occlusion, the involvement of more proximal muscles in the symptom complex may help to distinguish aortoiliac occlusive disease from femoropopliteal occlusive disease. Unfortunately, there is a sizeable minority of patients with aortoiliac disease who complain only of calf claudication. In addition to claudication, male patients with aortoiliac occlusive disease may complain of difficulty in achieving and maintaining an erection because of inadequate perfusion of the internal pudendal arteries. The Leriche syndrome consists of the manifestations of aortoiliac occlusive disease in the male and includes claudication of the muscles of the thigh, hip, and buttocks; atrophy of the leg muscles; impotence; and diminished femoral pulses.[1]

Aortoiliac occlusive disease per se is rarely the cause of ischemia at rest or ischemic tissue loss, except by embolization. The collateral circulation that develops around the occlusive process in the aorta and iliac arteries is usually rich and sufficient to supply the lower extremities with adequate quantities of arterial blood to ensure good resting tissue perfusion. However, arteriosclerotic plaques in the aorta and iliac arteries may cause the so-called blue toe syndrome (i.e., microembolization of arteriosclerotic debris to the terminal vessels in the foot).[2–5] Such symptoms may appear in a patient who otherwise appears to have adequate distal arterial supply, including, in

some instances, palpable pedal pulses. Under these circumstances, a search must be made by angiography for a proximal source of microembolization.

When aortoiliac occlusive disease is combined with femoropopliteal occlusive disease, a finding more common in elderly patients, resting ischemia may result.[6] As in any arterial system, tandem lesions in the arteries supplying the extremities are more significant than single lesions.

The risk factors for aortoiliac occlusive disease are those for atherosclerosis in general and include cigarette smoking, hypertension, elevated serum cholesterol, and diabetes.[7–18] In our experience, patients reporting symptoms of claudication caused by aortoiliac occlusive disease are on the average nearly a decade younger than those complaining of claudication on the basis of superficial femoral artery occlusion. However, patients with ischemia at rest from the combination of aortoiliac and femoropopliteal occlusive disease are in general in the seventh decade of life and are not notably younger than those who develop ischemic rest pain from femoropopliteal disease.

The initial lesions of aortoiliac occlusive disease in most patients appear to begin at the terminal aorta and the proximal portions of the common iliac arteries and/or at the bifurcations of the common iliacs (Fig. 26–1). The lesions then progress proximally and distally. Approximately one third of the patients we have operated on for symptomatic aortoiliac disease have had disease at the origin of the profunda femoris arteries in the groin and more than 40 per cent have had superficial femoral artery occlusions. The natural history of aortoiliac occlusive disease is one of slow progression.[19,20] The ultimate anatomic result of progressive aortoiliac atherosclerosis is occlusion of the distal abdominal aorta with progression of the thrombus up to the level of the renal arteries (Fig. 26–2B). While occlusion of the terminal aorta, once it occurs, may remain stable for years, it does not always have a benign course, as indicated in the report by Strarrett and Stoney, who observed that more than one third of a series of patients with aortic

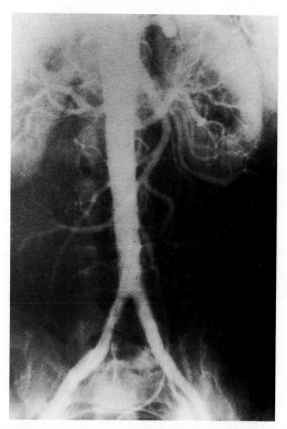

FIGURE 26–1. The earliest manifestations of aortoiliac occlusive disease are evident in the terminal aorta and proximal common iliac vessels.

occlusion went on to thrombose the renal arteries over a period of 5 to 10 years[21] (see Fig. 26–3).

There are variants in the pattern of aortoiliac occlusive disease, including relatively circumscribed occlusive lesion of the midabdominal aorta described in early middle-aged females who are heavy cigarette smokers (Fig. 26–4). While the upper abdominal aorta is ordinarily spared in patients with aortoiliac occlusive disease, a minority of such patients have marked involvement of this aortic segment with occlusive disease of the origins of the major visceral vessels and renal arteries (Fig. 26–5).

DIAGNOSIS

The diagnosis of aortoiliac occlusive disease is ordinarily easily made on the basis of the patient's symptoms. Complaints of high claudication, with or without accompanying sexual dysfunction in the male, certainly suggest this disease process. Claudication symptoms, however, must be distinguished from symptoms of nerve root irritation caused by spinal stenosis or intervertebral disk herniation, which may be associated with activity and relieved by sitting or lying down in some individuals.[22] These patients can ordinarily be distinguished quite easily from patients with true claudication by the fact that their symptoms

are produced as much by standing still as by walking, and by the typical sciatic distribution of their pain.

The patient with intermittent claudication on the basis of aortoiliac disease will ordinarily have lower extremities that appear healthy and well perfused at rest, although the muscles may be somewhat atrophic from disuse. Diminished or even absent femoral pulses are often a principal clue as to the level of the occlusive process. Bruits heard in the groins can also call attention to proximal occlusive lesions. However, stenotic lesions at the origins of the superficial femoral or profunda femoris arteries can also cause femoral bruits. Easily palpable pedal pulses at rest may be found in patients with severe claudication from aortoiliac occlusive disease even when the femoral pulses are barely discernible. This reflects the rich collateral circulation that is ordinarily present in such patients. Segmental Doppler pressures at all levels in the lower extremity are ordinarily lower than the brachial pressure. If there is no accompanying superficial femoral occlusive disease, there will not be an impressive gradient between the high thigh pressure and the ankle pressures; however, disabling symptoms may occur in patients with aortoiliac disease who have resting ankle pressures in the near-normal range and a normal ankle-brachial pressure index. Thus, in evaluating these patients, it is often wise to repeat the pressure measurements after a period of graded exercise.[23] A marked fall in ankle pressure immediately after exercise will be found if the patient's symptoms are on the basis of significant aortoiliac occlusive disease. More sophisticated Doppler waveform analysis and/or the use of a pulse volume recorder may reveal patterns suggestive of proximal occlusive lesions.[24–26] We have, however, found resting and postexercise Doppler pressure measurements satisfactory for the evaluation of the vast majority of patients.

The indications for surgery in symptomatic aortoiliac occlusive disease are disabling claudication and ischemia at rest manifested by rest pain in the foot, ischemic ulceration, or pregangrenous skin changes. Patients with aortoiliac disease and ischemia at rest ordinarily have accompanying femoropopliteal disease unless the ischemic lesions are the result of microemboli, as noted earlier.

PREOPERATIVE EVALUATION

Preoperative evaluation of the patient with aortoiliac occlusive disease includes a careful evaluation of any accompanying cardiac and pulmonary disease. In our experience, approximately 40 per cent of patients presenting with symptomatic aortoiliac occlusive disease will have clear-cut clinical and electrocardiographic evidence of coronary artery disease. Symptomatic unstable coronary artery disease in such individuals clearly demands investigation, including cardiac catheterization and coronary angiography in many cases. If coronary artery reconstruction is in-

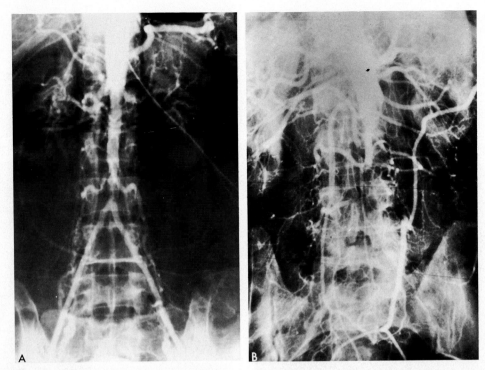

FIGURE 26–2. Aortoiliac occlusive disease results in a variable degree of collateralization shown as a discreet channel from a lumbar to the deep iliac circumflex artery (*A*) and as a multiplicity of small vessels that supply the hemorrhoidal and gluteal arteries that reconstitute the femoral vessels via iliac and femoral circumflex arteries (*B*).

dicated, this procedure should clearly be done first and the aortoiliac occlusive disease repaired as a second procedure. Patients with mild or stable coronary artery disease can ordinarily undergo aortoiliac reconstruction without great risk. Elderly patients with severe cardiopulmonary disease, who are not good candidates for coronary artery reconstruction, are probably best managed by extraanatomic bypass procedures of lesser magnitude than formal aortoiliac or aortofemoral reconstruction. Patients with severe restrictive pulmonary disease may require a period of preoperative preparation, which includes abstinence from cigarette smoking, bronchodilators, and broad-spectrum antibiotics.

Angiography, which is an essential part of the preoperative evaluation in the patient with symptomatic aortoiliac disease, can, in a surprising number of instances, be performed by the retrograde Seldinger technique using the femoral approach.[27] When this is not possible, studies by the translumbar or transaxillary route are performed.[28,29] The goal of the x-ray examination is to provide views of the entire abdominal aorta in two planes in order to demonstrate unexpected lesions of the celiac axis or superior mesenteric artery origins, to provide anteroposterior and oblique views of the pelvis to define any iliac artery lesions in more than one plane, and to demonstrate possible lesions at the origins of the profunda femoris arteries. Views should also be obtained of the vessels in the thighs, at the knees, and in the calves in order to demonstrate associated femoro-

popliteal occlusive disease and the quality of the run-off. At the time of angiography, it is very useful to obtain pull-back pressures across iliac artery lesions of doubtful significance, since this technique can demonstrate directly whether or not such lesions are likely to interfere with flow. Measurements should be taken at rest and after papaverine injection or during a period of reactive hyperemia following tourniquet ischemia to mimic the hemodynamic situation that occurs during exercise.[30] Intravenous digital subtraction angiography may be used for initial evaluation of patients with aortoiliac occlusive disease. The intravenous digital method does suffer from the problems of limited size of the x-ray field and a requirement for large volumes of contrast medium along with occasionally inadequate resolution of abdominal and pelvic vessels, particularly in obese individuals. However, intraarterial digital subtraction angiography has become quite useful for evaluation of the aortoiliac arterial segment. This technique has the advantage of the use of very small amounts of contrast medium and good resolution of the vessels studied.

AORTOFEMORAL BYPASS GRAFT

History

During the past decade, the aortofemoral bypass graft has become the preferred method of treatment

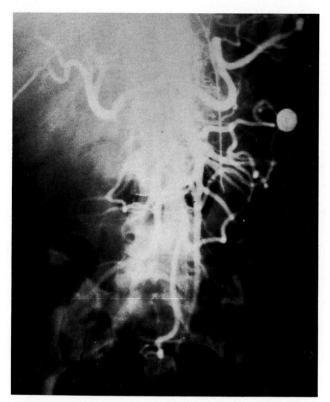

FIGURE 26–3. The end result of aortoiliac occlusive disease consists of total aortic thrombosis, which may include the origins of the renal arteries.

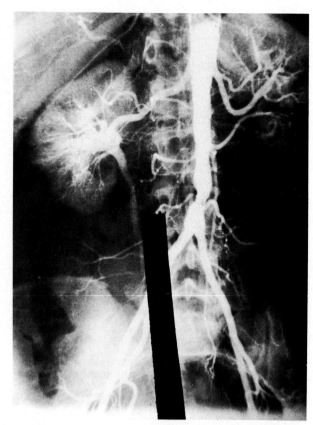

FIGURE 26–4. Aortoiliac occlusive disease may consist of a short segment circumferential lesion, especially common in younger females. Such a lesion might be amenable to localized endarterectomy.

of symptomatic aortoiliac occlusive disease and has, to a considerable degree, supplanted a more limited aortoiliac bypass in the hands of most surgeons. The 5 to 8 per cent, 30-day operative mortality rate for this procedure prevalent in the early 1970s has been reduced in our own experience to under 2 per cent over the past decade, a level consistent with reports from other surgeons and similar to that observed in patients undergoing elective abdominal aortic aneurysm repair.[31–37] It is well recognized that arterial insufficiency of the lower extremities is a manifestation of a systemic process that results in clinically evident coronary artery disease in approximately 50 per cent of these patients.[38–40] It might be anticipated then that the reduced operative mortality observed in recent years has been associated with a concomitant reduction in the number of early cardiac deaths. This indeed appears to be the case. The improved perioperative management of the patient with a diseased heart has resulted from a number of factors, which include selective employment of preliminary cardiac surgery in certain individuals, sophisticated pharmacologic management of the damaged myocardium, and more precise perioperative fluid management tailored to the individual patient's myocardial reserve.[37]

Initial aortobifemoral graft limb patency rates now approach 100 per cent, and the 5-year patency is greater than 80 per cent in a number of recent re-

ports.[31,32,34,41,42] Long-term patency has also improved to an anticipated 75 per cent at 10 years.[31] A number of refinements of operative technique may be responsible for the low incidence of graft limb thrombosis seen in recent years. The more prevalent use of the aortobifemoral graft as opposed to an aortoiliac bypass or extended aortoiliofemoral endarterectomy has negated the effect of unsuspected or progressive atherosclerosis in the external iliac vessels. Meticulous avoidance of graft limb redundancy and an awareness of the desirability of compatibility of the diameter of the graft limb and the vessel into which it is implanted have also probably helped to maintain long-term patency.

Surgical Procedures

The knitted Dacron prosthesis is the standard graft material employed by most surgeons with experience in aortoiliac reconstruction. This material, with or without a velour construction, may provide a more stable pseudointima than woven prostheses.[43,44] An important factor contributing to improved results has undoubtedly been the recognition of the critical role played by the deep femoral artery in providing sustained patency of the aortofemoral graft limb.[31,34,45,46] The current practice of extending the distal anasto-

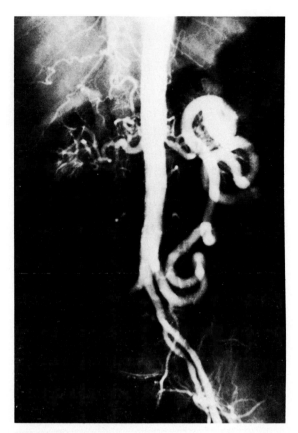

FIGURE 26–5. A large meandering mesenteric artery associated with total superior mesenteric artery celiac occlusion, renal artery stenosis, complete occlusion of the right common iliac, and distal left external iliac stenoses with a single patent hypogastric. End-to-side proximal anastomosis might best preserve both mesenteric and pelvic circulation.

geons probably favor the end-to-end technique of proximal anastomosis with transection of the aorta between clamps about 1 to 2 inches below the renal arteries and oversewing or stapling the distal end (Fig. 26–6). This permits an endarterectomy or thrombectomy of the proximal aortic stump under direct vision prior to constructing the anastomosis. It also has the advantage of not requiring flow to be reestablished in the more distal aorta where arteriosclerotic plaque and mural thrombus may have been loosened by application of the distal clamp. This may have advantages in avoiding intraoperative emboli to the lower extremities. The end-to-end technique has also been claimed by some authors to reduce the incidence of aortoduodenal fistulas because the end-to-end anastomosis does not project anteriorly as does an end-to-side aortofemoral reconstruction. Unfortunately, such controlled studies as are available do not indicate that the end-to-end technique gives results significantly superior to the end-to-side techniques. Therefore, we have taken the position that the end-to-end technique is probably most appropriate for those patients who will not suffer any hemodynamic disadvantage from interruption of forward flow in the abdominal aorta. This technique also appears desirable for those patients who have already suffered complete aortic occlusion. The end-to-side technique (illustrated in Fig. 26–7) is reserved for those individuals who would lose perfusion of an important hypogastric or inferior mesenteric artery if forward flow in the aorta were sacrificed at the time of surgery.[52] Arteriographic studies in patients with indication for an end-to-side anastomosis are shown in Figures 26–5 and 26–8.

While aortofemoral reconstruction has the potential of restoring potency to males with sexual dysfunction on the basis of inadequate hypogastric artery perfusion,[52] surgical dissection in the area of the terminal aorta and proximal left common iliac artery can also cause difficulty with both erection and ejaculation by interfering with the autonomic nervous plexus, which sweeps over these vessels. In performing aortofemoral bypass grafting, therefore, we have chosen to confine the dissection of the aorta to the area between the renal arteries and the inferior mesenteric artery. The aorta is exposed anteriorly and laterally without distorting the vessel to avoid embolization of arteriosclerotic debris. After systemic heparinization the distal clamp is placed proximal to the inferior mesenteric artery and then the aorta is cross-clamped below the renal arteries where the aortic wall is likely to be considerably less diseased. The aorta is divided transversely and the distal end bevelled and oversewn. In the case of an end-to-side anastomosis, the longitudinal aortotomy is placed high up near the renals in the more normal aorta and great care is taken to remove all loose debris and mural thrombus from the lumen in the excluded aortic segment. At completion of an end-to-side anastomosis great care is also given to adequate back-flushing of all loosened debris and clot from the distal aorta before forward

mosis down over the origin of the profunda femoris to ensure an adequate outflow tract has been widely accepted and is undoubtedly important in patients with tandem superficial femoral occlusions and in patients with stenosis of the profunda origin. We have found, however, that if extensive profundaplasty or profunda endarterectomy is necessary, it is better to close this vessel with an autogenous tissue patch of saphenous vein or endarterectomized superficial femoral artery than to attempt to make a long profunda femoris patch with the distal end of an aortofemoral prosthesis.[45] The incidence of graft infection has been minimized with preoperative and intraoperative antibiotics.[31,47–49] It is also recognized that aortoenteric fistulas can be prevented by closure of retroperitoneal tissue and the posterior parietal peritoneum over the graft and proximal suture line to prevent erosion of the graft into the duodenum.[31,50,51] The abandonment of the use of silk sutures in favor of permanent prosthetic suture material has undoubtedly helped reduce the incidence of false aneurysm formation.

There remains a good deal of controversy as to the proper method of performing the proximal anastomosis of an aortobifemoral graft.[31,50–52] Most sur-

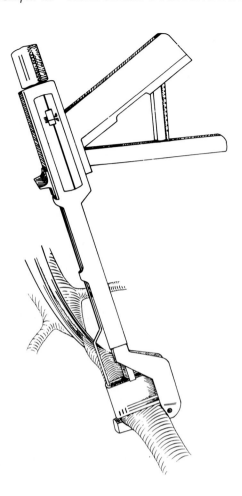

a

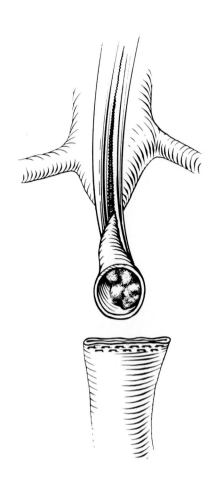

b

FIGURE 26–6. End-to-end proximal anastomosis for aortofemoral reconstruction may be initiated with the infrarenal aortic
cross clamp placed in anterior/posterior direction with minimal
dissection as close to the origin of the renal arteries as possible.
The aorta is then stapled or occluded with a second clamp just
proximal to the origin of the inferior mesenteric artery as illustrated
(*a*). Following transection of the infrarenal aorta and complete
thromboendarterectomy of the proximal infrarenal aortic cuff (*b*),
end-to-end anastomosis is completed with continuous 3-0 polypropylene suture (*c*).

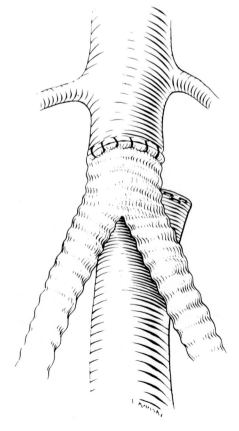

c

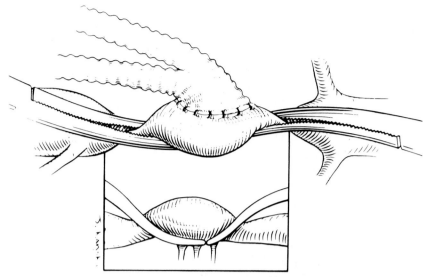

FIGURE 26–7. End-to-side proximal anastomosis for aortofemoral reconstruction is required to preserve antigrade pelvic perfusion in situations where retrograde perfusion from distal femoral anastomoses is doubtful. The infrarenal aorta is occluded proximal to the origin of the inferior mesenteric artery and just distal to the origin of the renal arteries. Following longitudinal arteriotomy and thorough thromboendarterectomy if required, the anastomosis is constructed using continuous polypropylene suture.

flow is reestablished. In performing either type of proximal anastomosis a short stem of a graft is sutured to the aorta with a running suture of 3-0 polypropylene. Knitted Dacron prostheses are invariably used and the size is selected so that the limb diameter

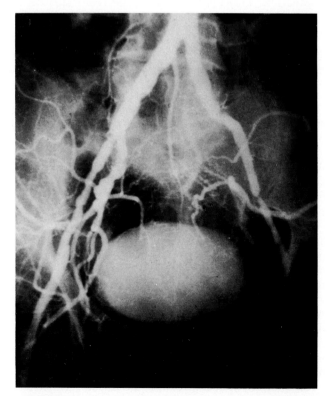

FIGURE 26–8. Diffuse aortoiliac disease with left hypogastric occlusion and minimal left pelvic collateralization might warrant end-to-side proximal anastomosis to preserve right hypogastric system.

will correspond to the diameter of the patient's common femoral arteries. The average prosthesis size used for males is 14 × 7 mm or, in larger individuals, 16 × 8 mm. For females, the most commonly used sizes are 12 × 6 mm and 13 × 6.5 mm. After completion of the proximal anastomosis, the limbs are tunneled retroperitoneally into the groins. On the left the tunnel ordinarily passes beneath the sigmoid mesentery and into the groin in a rather lateral channel that avoids trauma to the nerve plexuses at the terminal aorta. On the right, the tunnel is made along the course of the right common iliac artery beneath the ureter. In the groins, end-to-side anastomoses are fashioned in the distal common femoral with 5-0 polypropylene. The anastomoses are carried down into the profunda femoris arteries for a short distance if there is any evidence of incipient stenosis of the origins of these vessels or if the superficial femorals are occluded. The end of the graft thus acts as a patch, widening the orifice of the profunda femoris.

Results

While excellent results have been achieved with aortoiliac endarterectomy for occlusive disease, this operation, even in the hands of enthusiasts, is now confined to those individuals whose disease ends distally near the bifurcation of the common iliac arteries[31] (see Figs. 26–4 and 26–9). Endarterectomy of the external iliac has proven to be tedious and unrewarding for most surgeons. There is at present little evidence to suggest that endarterectomy is superior to a properly performed aortofemoral bypass graft in terms of the early or late results. In our practice, aortoiliac endarterectomy is confined to a

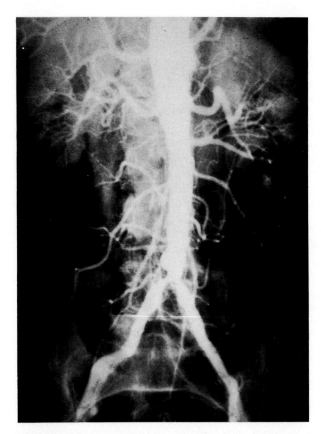

FIGURE 26–9. Aortoiliac occlusive disease with significant lesion confined to the origin of the right common iliac artery, amenable to either local endarterectomy or percutaneous transluminal angioplasty.

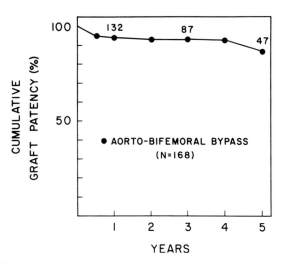

FIGURE 26–10. For 168 aortobifemoral graft limbs inserted in 84 consecutive patients, the 5-year cumulative patency was 86 per cent.

minority of individuals who appear to have principally aortic disease with little involvement of the iliac arteries. This group of patients is characteristically early middle-aged females with occlusive disease of the midabdominal aorta, which ends at the aortic bifurcation or in the proximal portions of the common iliac arteries. We have avoided aortoiliac endarterectomy in males because of concern over interference with the autonomic nerves at the terminal aorta and proximal left common iliac artery.

The authors' results with aortofemoral bypass grafting are illustrated in Figure 26–10. The 5-year cumulative patency of 86 per cent is comparable to that reported in a number of other recent studies.[31,32,34,41] Thirty-day operative mortality was slightly less than 1 per cent. This low mortality rate undoubtedly reflects careful patient selection as well as improved operative management and anesthetic technique. However, since aortoiliac occlusive disease is rarely life threatening, although it may be limb threatening, we have preferred to treat high-risk patients with procedures of lesser magnitude.

Although the excellent graft patency rates for aortofemoral bypass grafts do not necessarily reflect functional results, approximately 95 per cent of patients are initially rendered asymptomatic or improved, and after 5 years about 80 per cent remain

in this category.[34,41] A study from Britain indicates that of patients fully employed prior to aortobifemoral bypass, 85 per cent return to full employment an average of 4 months following surgery and more than 50 per cent of those not previously employed were returned to work following bypass.[53] The 5-year cumulative survival rate for patients undergoing aortofemoral bypass grafting remains some 14 per cent lower than that anticipated for a normal age-corrected population. However, nearly 80 per cent survive 5 years while less than 50 per cent survive 10 years.[39]

Concomitant Distal Reconstructions

When patients have threatened limb loss from a combination of aortoiliac and femoropopliteal occlusive disease, it is clear that the repair of the proximal or inflow lesions is necessary in order to permit salvage of the extremity. However, it is not always clear whether or not concomitant distal reconstructions, such as a femoropopliteal bypass, should be performed at the time of the initial operation. Results reported in the literature and our own experience suggest that in the majority of patients with ischemia at rest, on the basis of combined aortoiliac and femoropopliteal disease, repair of the aortoiliac occlusive disease, and restoration of normal perfusion to the profunda femoris arteries will achieve limb salvage in the vast majority, probably 80 per cent of patients.[46,54] However, in those patients, particularly diabetics, with extensive tissue necrosis of the skin of the forefoot or heel, restoration of pulsatile flow in the foot may be necessary in order to achieve healing. Under these circumstances we believe that a combination of both proximal and distal reconstructive procedures may be necessary at the initial operation. The combined procedure has the disadvantage of increasing the operating time and surgical trauma in a group of patients who are likely to be elderly with a high incidence of coronary artery disease; however, with modern anesthetic management and a two-team operative approach, this combined reconstruction can be performed safely and within a reasonable period of time.

ALTERNATIVES FOR THE HIGH-RISK PATIENT

Although transabdominal arterial reconstruction for aortoiliac occlusive disease can be performed successfully with low morbidity and mortality in many patients, less extensive procedures may be preferable in patients who are at high risk for major surgery under general anesthesia. In such patients, distal aortic and proximal iliac arterial occlusions may be treated by axillofemoral bypass grafts, which will be discussed subsequently.[55–59] If the occlusive disease is limited to one common or external iliac artery, alternatives to axillofemoral bypass are warranted in poor-risk individuals because use of the patent iliac system as an origin for a bypass will permit a shorter graft segment and will afford better long-term patency. The femorofemoral bypass is an example of such a procedure.[60] However, an anatomically similar procedure, the iliofemoral graft, has received little attention in the literature.

Ilioiliac and Iliofemoral Bypass Grafts

We have recently reviewed our experience over the past decade with 94 patients undergoing ilioiliac or iliofemoral bypass grafting. Poor-risk patients, particularly those with severe cardiopulmonary impairment, who had no important occlusive disease in the aorta or in the proximal segment of at least one common iliac artery, were considered for reconstruction using a patent common or external iliac artery for the proximal anastomosis (Fig. 26–5). The iliac site for anastomosis has several technical advantages, which include exposure through an oblique suprainguinal, "renal transplant" incision, which is quite simple technically even in obese patients. The graft is more deeply placed and therefore more cushioned than in the femorofemoral position. Ilioilial grafts are shorter than femorofemoral grafts, and there is no disturbance of inguinal lymph nodes or lymphatics. The femoral artery on the donor side is left undisturbed for later use as the origin for a distal bypass if indicated.

The mean age of the 94 patients undergoing ilioiliac or iliofemoral bypass was 60 years, and 26 per cent had diabetes mellitus. Forty-one per cent had clearcut clinical and electrocardiographic evidence of coronary artery disease, and 43 per cent had significant hypertension. Fifty-eight per cent of the patients were operated on for claudication and 42 per cent for limb salvage. Twenty-three patients had ilioilial grafts and 71 patients had iliofemoral grafts. Fifty-seven ilio-

unifemoral grafts and 14 iliobifemoral grafts were performed.

In patients subjected to iliac arterial reconstruction, the patent iliac arterial segment was exposed extraperitoneally through a curvilinear incision parallel to and above the inguinal ligament, identical to the approach for renal transplantation. Limited iliac endarterectomy was necessary in a few instances. Separate vertical groin incisions were made to expose the common femoral arteries. For ilioiliac bypass, symmetrical incisions were made to expose the iliac vessels and the graft was positioned in the retroperitoneum (Fig. 26–11A). The grafts to the femoral arteries were placed under the inguinal ligament (Fig. 26–11B and C). For patients undergoing bilateral iliofemoral reconstruction, the crossover limb was placed from the iliofemoral graft retroperitoneally in the iliac fossa or, in a few cases, subcutaneously to the contralateral femoral artery (Fig. 26–11C).

The 30-day operative mortality for these procedures was zero. The 4-year cumulative patency for the ilioiliac grafts (23 limbs) was 96 per cent; that for the iliofemoral grafts (91 limbs) was 72 per cent. The 4-year patency for iliobifemoral grafts (28 limbs) was 72 per cent, and for iliounifemoral grafts (63 limbs), 71 per cent (Fig. 26–12). When both the superficial and deep femoral arteries were patent, the cumulative patency rate for iliofemoral grafts was higher (85 per cent) at 4 years than when only the deep femoral artery was patent (62 per cent). It was not possible to demonstrate a statistically significant difference in late patency between aortofemoral grafts and iliofemoral grafts, although the aortofemoral grafts had numerically superior 4- and 5-year patencies. We thus believe that the iliofemoral bypass is an adequate substitute for aortofemoral bypass in certain elderly and poor-risk individuals who have their proximal occlusive disease confined largely to the external iliac arteries or to one iliac system.

Femorofemoral Bypass Graft

In patients whose occlusive disease is confined to one iliac artery, and whose aorta and contralateral iliac system is free of hemodynamically significant lesions, the femorofemoral bypass is often employed. Brief, Plecha, Vetto, and our own group have demonstrated that these operations yield quite satisfactory long-term results (60 per cent to more than 80 per cent 5-year patency).[58,60–62] Failure of these grafts because of progressive worsening of proximal atherosclerosis has been uncommon. It has been suggested that such worsening may be retarded by increased flow through the donor iliac system, which is required to supply both the lower extremities with blood. Berguer, Faulkner, and Rittgers have reported experimental support for this hypothesis by demonstrating in animals that intimal hyperplasia correlates inversely with blood flow and sheer stress.[63]

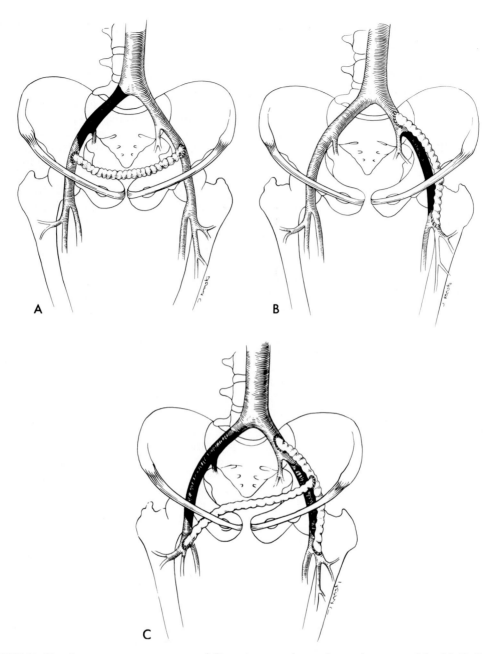

FIGURE 26–11. A patent common or external iliac artery may be used as a donor vessel for (*A*) ilioiliac, (*B*) iliofemoral, or (*C*) iliobifemoral bypasses in appropriate patients who would otherwise require axillofemoral reconstruction.

However, experimental results yielding the opposite conclusion have also been reported.[64]

The femorofemoral graft is particularly applicable to high-risk patients, since it can be performed easily under epidural or spinal anesthesia. The two common femoral arteries are exposed through short vertical groin incisions. The groin incisions are connected by a subcutaneous suprapubic tunnel created by blunt dissection on the deep fascia. We prefer to have the graft form a "C" configuration, with the anastomoses placed in the distal common femoral arteries and the graft traveling proximally up through the suprapubic tunnel and down to the opposite common femoral (Fig. 26–13). Over the past decade we have had experience with femorofemoral grafts in 53 patients. Sixty per cent of these were operated on for limb salvage and 40 per cent for disabling claudication. The average age of these patients was 61 years. Forty-one per cent had clinical evidence of coronary artery disease, 33 per cent were diabetic, and 44 per cent had significant hypertension. There was one postoperative mortality in this group of patients, from a pulmonary embolus. The 5-year cumulative graft patency was 80 per cent (Fig. 26–14).

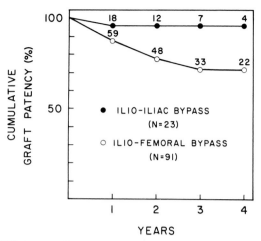

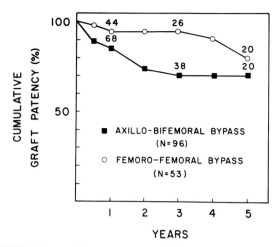

FIGURE 26–12. Using a patent iliac vessel as the donor artery, the 4-year cumulative graft patency for 23 ilioiliac grafts was 96 per cent, while the patency for 91 iliofemoral graft limbs was 72 per cent.

FIGURE 26–14. The 4-year cumulative graft patency for 53 femorofemoral grafts was 80 per cent, and the patency for 48 axillobifemoral grafts (96 limbs) was 70 per cent.

The late patency rate is not statistically significantly different from that achieved with aortofemoral bypass in our hands, but it is slightly numerically inferior.

The reasonably good long-term results, the ease of performance, and the low morbidity associated with the femorofemoral bypass suggest that it might logically be employed in good-risk as well as poor-risk patients who have their proximal occlusive disease confined to one iliac arterial segment. While it is difficult to argue against this point of view, the fact that the groins have been operated on and the common femoral arteries dissected during the course of performing a femorofemoral graft makes an aortobifemoral reconstruction in such individuals techni-

cally more difficult if progression of proximal disease causes return of symptoms or late failure of the femorofemoral bypass. Therefore, in good-risk patients with evidence of arteriosclerotic disease in the aorta or in the patent iliac system, we recommend aortobifemoral bypass at the outset in an attempt to avoid the need for possible future reoperation.

Axillofemoral Bypass Graft

In very elderly and high-risk patients, who are in danger of limb loss from a combination of aortoiliac and femoropopliteal occlusive diseases and whose proximal occlusive lesions involve the aorta and proximal iliac arteries, the axillofemoral bypass graft is the logical alternative to aortoiliac reconstruction or primary amputation. Extraanatomic reconstruction may also prove useful for patients with multiple prior abdominal procedures, multiple adhesions, or previous pelvic irradiation. Intraabdominal sepsis, not infrequently resulting from an infected aortic graft, is another common indication. If an axillofemoral graft is chosen for such individuals, the axillobifemoral graft is preferred to the axillounifemoral graft because several reports, beginning with that of LoGerfo et al., have shown that the axillobifemoral graft has a decidedly better 5-year cumulative patency.[57,59] The probable reason for this finding is that the axillobifemoral graft has approximately double the flow rate in its axillary limb as has the axillounifemoral graft.

In constructing an axillobifemoral graft, the first portion of the axillary artery is exposed by an incision placed beneath the clavicle on the side selected for the proximal anastomosis (Fig. 26–15). We ordinarily split the pectoralis major and divide the pectoralis minor muscle to provide better operative exposure and more space for the graft as it emerges from the axilla into the subcutaneous plane. The common fem-

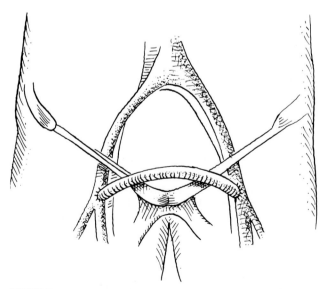

FIGURE 26–13. The femorofemoral bypass graft is illustrated with the preferred "C" configuration of the subcutaneous tunnel constructed well above the pubis.

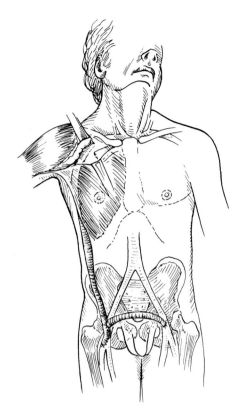

FIGURE 26–15. Subcutaneous axillobifemoral bypass graft completed with proximal anastomosis to the right axillary artery, right distal anastomosis to the common and deep femoral arteries, and extension of the prosthesis with side limb to left common femoral artery.

oral arteries are exposed through bilateral short groin incisions.

A DeBakey tunneling instrument can then be passed from the infraclavicular incision laterally to a subcutaneous plane in the midaxillary line. The curve in the tunneler can then be used to direct the tunnel anteriorly above the iliac crest and then in front of the inguinal ligament into the ipsilateral groin incision. A Dacron or polytetrafluoroethylene (PTFE) prosthesis, usually 8 mm in diameter, is attached to the tunneling instrument and drawn back through the tunnel into the axillary incision for anastomosis with the first portion of the axillary artery. A side limb is attached to the graft in the ipsilateral groin incision just proximal to the anastomosis with the common femoral artery. The side limb is then passed through a subcutaneous suprapubic tunnel into the opposite groin in a manner similar to that employed for a femorofemoral graft.

Since neither the thoracic nor the abdominal cavity is "entered" in performing an axillofemoral graft, this procedure usually does not interfere with the patient's ability to breathe, cough, or take oral feedings. On the first postoperative day, most patients are ambulatory and on a regular diet. During the past decade we have performed axillobifemoral grafts electively in 48 poor-risk patients for symptomatic aortoiliac occlusive disease. All but two of these individuals

were operated on for limb salvage from a combination of far-advanced aortoiliac and femoropopliteal disease. The 5-year cumulative graft patency in this group of patients was 70 per cent (Fig. 26–14). While this figure is not completely discouraging, it is statistically significantly inferior to the results achieved with aortofemoral bypass grafting during the same time period. We therefore believe that axillofemoral grafts should be offered only to poor-risk individuals in danger of limb loss and should not be utilized for the treatment of symptoms of claudication alone.

When axillofemoral grafts do fail, they can frequently be reopened by thrombectomy under local anesthesia if the patient presents himself promptly after graft thrombosis has occurred. About 25 per cent of grafts thrombectomized in this fashion will go on to long-term patency.[57] Thus, the functional good results achieved with axillobifemoral grafting may be somewhat higher than the 70 per cent graft patency figure would indicate.

Patency rates associated with axillofemoral reconstruction range from a low of 30 per cent to a high of 85 per cent in the recent literature.[65,66] The reasons for this extraordinary variability are in large part explained by patient selection, indication, and status of the outflow vessels. Extraanatomic reconstruction for nonocclusive disease, as is the case for patients with intraabdominal sepsis or an infected aneurysm repair, will achieve better patency rates than patients operated on primarily for occlusive disease. Claudicants will fare better than those requiring limb salvage due to inherent outflow restriction in the latter group. In similar fashion, patients who undergo simultaneous distal femoropopliteal reconstruction will achieve better results than those whose infrainguinal disease is not addressed. Finally, in some series, axillobifemoral grafts sustain a significantly better 5-year patency than unilateral reconstructions. It has been shown that flow through the descending axillary limb in bilateral reconstructions is twice that of axillounilateral grafts, perhaps explaining the improvement in some series. Other investigators have found no significant difference whatsoever between bilateral and unilateral reconstructions, again in all probability reflecting patient selection and status of outflow. Thus, the most favorable results achieved thus far, as reported by Harris et al. in 1990, demonstrate an 85 per cent patency rate after 4 years in a group of 76 patients, 26 per cent of which were operated on for nonocclusive disease, and 20 per cent of whom underwent simultaneous outflow reconstruction and all of whom had axillobifemoral grafts.[65] This series was also carried out in a single institution using a technique that has been standardized for many years. In contrast, a less favorable patency rate (29 per cent) was reported by Donaldson et al. in 72 patients carried out in several institutions by a group of 30 surgeons operating on patients with predominately occlusive disease.[66] Finally, many authors have reported secondary patency rates, either exclusively or in addition to primary rates, which further confuse the statistics. It is clear from all of these series that the secondary patency rate is significantly better than the primary, attesting to the fact that as many as 25 per cent of axillobifemoral grafts will require subsequent thrombectomy in order to maintain patency.

PERCUTANEOUS TRANSLUMINAL ANGIOPLASTY

Percutaneous catheter dilation of atheromatous vascular stenoses was introduced by Dotter in 1963.[67] However, this technique did not become widely applied until Gruntzig designed and developed the double-lumen balloon catheter for percutaneous transluminal angioplasty in the early 1970s. In the Gruntzig technique, the balloon catheter is inserted into a stenotic arterial region with the Seldinger technique and is expanded to a fixed diameter. In one of Gruntzig's original reports in 1977, percutaneous dilation was attempted in 41 patients with isolated iliac artery stenosis and proved to be initially successful in 91 per cent.[68]

Early success is not necessarily sustained, as evidenced by the lower 50 to 60 per cent 5-year success rate reported by Johnston among 684 iliac angioplasties carried out in Toronto between 1978 and 1986.[69] If initial technical failures are excluded, however, success rates improve by 10 to 15 per cent as confirmed in a randomized prospective multicenter trial reported by Wilson.[70] This study demonstrated that successful results were sustained for 3 years in 73 per cent of dilated iliac lesions, not significantly different from the 82 per cent success rate observed with conventional surgery. Success rates for percutaneous transluminal angioplasty are maximal when indicated for claudication resulting from common iliac stenosis with excellent runoff (75 per cent) and minimal when carried out for critical ischemia caused by external iliac occlusion with poor runoff (19 per cent). Our own experience with this technique in selected patients has been encouraging. We have not found the technique useful in patients with complete iliac artery occlusion or with stenotic arterial segments longer than 5 cm. However, this technique has been very useful in the initial management of patients with symptomatic short segmental iliac stenoses (Fig. 26–9). High-risk patients with appropriate lesions can be palliated effectively without undergoing anesthesia and major surgery. Even in good-risk patients percutaneous transluminal angioplasty has an advantage, as initial therapy for symptomatic lesions, in that it does not in any way jeopardize future surgical approach to the aorta or iliac arteries if the angioplasty ultimately fails. The cost effectiveness of a successful procedure is unquestionable, since patients may be discharged from the hospital the day following dilation. It should be emphasized that effective use of transluminal angioplasty can be achieved only through a cooperative effort on the part of both angiographers and vascular surgeons. Such cooperation is important with regard to proper patient selection, the appropriate combination or staging of procedures, and the prompt treatment of complications.

REFERENCES

1. Lerich R, Morel A: The syndrome of thrombotic obliteration of the aortic bifurcation. Ann Surg 127:193, 1948.
2. Crane C: Atherothrombotic embolism to lower extremities in arteriosclerosis. Arch Surg 94:96, 1967.
3. Karmody AM, Powers SR, Monaco VJ, et al: "Blue toe" syndrome. Arch Surg 111:1263, 1976.
4. Moldveen-Geronimus M, Merriam JC Jr: Cholesterol embolization: From pathological curiosity to clinical entity. Circulation 35:946, 1967.
5. Williams GM, Harrington D, Burdick J, White RI: Mural thrombus of the aorta. Am Surg 194:737, 1981.
6. Brewster DC, Perier BA, Robison JG, et al: Aortofemoral graft for multilevel occlusive disease: Predictors of success and need for distal bypass. Arch Surg 117:1593, 1982.
7. Ballantyne D, Lawrie TDV: Hyperlipoproteinemia and peripheral vascular disease. Clin Chim Acta 47:269, 1973.
8. Cox FC, Rifking B, Robinson J, et al: Primary hyperlipoproteinaemias in myocardial infarction. In Peeters H (ed): Protides of the Biological Fluids, vol 19. New York, American Elsevier, 1972, p 279.
9. Doyle JT, Dawber TR, Kannel WB, et al: The relationship of cigarette smoking to coronary heart disease: The second report of the combined experience of the Albany, N.Y., and Framingham, Mass., studies. JAMA 190:886, 1964.
10. Greenhalgh RM, Rosengarten DS, Mervant I, et al: Serum lipids and lipoproteins in peripheral vascular disease. Lancet 2:947, 1971.
11. Kannel WB, Castelli WP, Gordon T, et al: Serum cholesterol lipoproteins and the risk of coronary heart disease. Ann Intern Med 74:1, 1971.
12. Kannel WB, Dawber TR, Friedman GD, et al: Risk factors in coronary artery disease. Ann Intern Med 61:888, 1964.
13. Oberman A, Harlan WR, Smith M, et al: The cardiovascular risk: Associated with different levels and types of elevated blood pressure. Minn Med 52:1283, 1969.
14. Paterson D, Slack J: Lipid abnormalities in male and female survivors of myocardial infarction and their first degree relatives. Lancet 1:393, 1972.
15. Paul O: Physical inactivity: The associated cardiovascular risk. Minn Med 52:1327, 1969.
16. Sirtori CR, Biasi G, Vercellio G, et al: Diets, lipids and lipoproteins in patients with peripheral vascular disease. Am J Med Sci 268:325, 1974.
17. Strong JP, Eggen DA: Risk factors and atherosclerotic lesions. In Jones RJ (ed): Atherosclerosis: Proceedings of the Second International Symposium. New York, Springer-Verlag, 1970, pp 355–364.
18. Vogelberg KH, Berchtold P, Berger H, et al: Primary hyperlipoproteinemias as risk factors in peripheral artery disease documented by arteriography. Atherosclerosis 22:271, 1975.
19. Boyd AM: The natural course of arteriosclerosis of the lower extremities. Proc R Soc Med 55:591, 1962.
20. Imparato AM, Kim G, Davidson T, et al: In intermittent claudication: Its natural course. Surgery 78:795, 1975.
21. Starrett RW, Stoney RJ: Juxta-renal aortic occlusion. Surgery 76:890, 1974.

22. Karayannacos PE, Yashon D, Vasko JS: Narrow lumbar spinal canal with "vascular" syndromes. Arch Surg 111:803, 1976.

23. Raines JK, Darling RC, Both J, et al: Vascular laboratory criteria for the management of peripheral vascular disease of the lower extremities. Surgery 79:21, 1976.

24. Darling RC, Raines JK, Brener BJ, et al: Quantitative segmental pulse volume recorder: A clinical tool. Surgery 72:873, 1972.

25. Winsor T, Sibley AE, Fisher EK, et al: Peripheral pulse contours in arterial occlusive disease. Vasc Dis 5:61, 1968.

26. Yao JST: Haemodynamic studies in peripheral arterial disease. Br J Surg 57:761, 1970.

27. Seldinger SE: Catheter replacement of needle in percutaneous arteriography: New technique. Acta Radiol 39:368, 1953.

28. Beschoor Plug MH, Westra D: Complications in catheterization of the axillary artery. Radiol Clin Biol 42:510, 1973.

29. McAfee JG, Wilson JKV: A review of the complications of translumbar aortography. Am J Roentgenol 75:956, 1956.

30. Udoff EJ, Barth KH, Harrington DP, et al: Hemodynamic significance of iliac artery stenosis: Pressure measurements during angiography. Radiology 132:289, 1979.

31. Brewster DC, Darling RC: Optimal methods of aortoiliac reconstruction. Surgery 84:739, 1978.

32. Crawford ES, Bomberger RA, Glaeser DH, et al: Aortoiliac occlusive disease: Factors influencing survival and function following reconstructive operation over a twenty-five-year period. Surgery 90:1055, 1981.

33. DeBakey ME, Crawford ES, Cooley DA, et al: Surgical considerations of occlusive disease of the abdominal aorta and iliac and femoral arteries: Analysis of 803 cases. Am Surg 148:306, 1958.

34. Malone JM, Moore WS, Goldstone J: The natural history of bilateral aortofemoral bypass grafts for ischemia of the lower extremities. Arch Surg 110:1300, 1975.

35. Moore WS, Caferata HT, Hall AD, et al: In defense of grafts across the inguinal ligament: An evaluation of early and late results of aortofemoral bypass grafts. Ann Surg 168:207, 1968.

36. Perdue GD, Long WT, Smith RB III: Perspective concerning aortofemoral arterial reconstruction. Ann Surg 173:940, 1971.

37. Whittemore AD, Clowes AW, Hechtman HB, et al: Aortic aneurysm repair: Reduced operative mortality associated with maintenance of optimal cardiac performance. Ann Surg 192:414, 1980.

38. Kannel WB, Skinner JJ Jr, Schwartz MJ, et al: Intermittent claudication: Incidence in the Framingham study. Circulation 41:857, 1970.

39. Malone JM, Moore WJ, Goldstone J: Life expectancy following aorto-femoral arterial grafting. Surgery 81:551, 1977.

40. McAllister FF: The fate of patients with intermittent claudication managed non-operatively. Am J Surg 132:593, 1976.

41. Mozersky DJ, Summer DS, Strandness DE: Long-term results of reconstructive aortoiliac surgery. Am J Surg 123:503, 1972.

42. Whittemore AD, Mannick JA: The ischemic leg. *In* McLean LD (ed): Advances in Surgery. Chicago, Year Book Medical Publishers, 1981, p 293.

43. Cooley DA, Wukasch DC, Bennett JG, et al: Double velour knitted Dacron grafts for aortoiliac vascular replacements. Paper presented at Vascular Graft Symposium, National Institutes of Health, Bethesda, MD, November 5, 1976.

44. Yates SG, Barros D'Sa AA, Berger K, et al: The preclotting of porous arterial prosthesis. Ann Surg 188:611, 1978.

45. Malone JM, Goldstone J, Moore WS: Autogenous profundaplasty: The key to long-term patency in secondary repair of aortofemoral graft occlusion. Ann Surg 188:817, 1978.

46. Morris GC Jr, Edwards W, Cooley DA, et al: Surgical importance of profunda femoris artery. Arch Surg 82:32, 1961.

47. Kaiser AB, Clayson KR, Mulherin JL, et al: Antibiotic prophylaxis in vascular surgery. Ann Surg 188:283, 1978.

48. Lindenauer SM, Fry WJ, Schaub G, et al: The use of antibiotics in the prevention of vascular graft infections. Surgery 62:487, 1967.

49. Szilagyi DE, Smith RF, Elliott JP, et al: Infection in arterial reconstruction with synthetic grafts. Ann Surg 176:321, 1972.

50. Knox GW: Peripheral vascular anastomotic aneurysms. Ann Surg 183:120, 1976.

51. Stoney RJ, Albo EJ, Wylie EJ: False aneurysms occurring after arterial grafting operations. Am J Surg 110:153, 1965.

52. Pierce GE, Turrentine M, Stringfield S, et al: Evaluation of end-to-side v end-to-end proximal anastomosis in aorto-bifemoral bypass. Arch Surg 117:1580, 1982.

53. Waters KJ, Proud G: Return to work after aortofemoral bypass surgery. Br Med J 2:556, 1977.

54. Royster TS, Lynn R, Mulcare RJ: Combined aortoiliac and femoropopliteal occlusive disease. Surg Gynecol Obstet 143:949, 1976.

55. Blaisdell FW, Hall AD, Lim RC Jr, et al: Aortoiliac substitution utilizing subcutaneus grafts. Ann Surg 172:775, 1970.

56. Eugene J, Goldstone J, Moore WS: Fifteen year experience with subcutaneous bypass grafts for lower extremity ischemia. Ann Surg 186:177, 1977.

57. LoGerfo FW, Johnson WC, Carson JD, et al: A comparison of the late patency rates of axillobilateral femoral and axillounilateral femoral grafts. Surgery 81:33, 1977.

58. Maini BS, Mannick JA: Effect of arterial reconstruction on limb salvage. Arch Surg 113:1297, 1978.

59. Mannick JA, Williams LE, Nabseth DC: The late results of axillofemoral grafts. Surgery 68:1038, 1970.

60. Vetto RM: The treatment of unilateral iliac artery obstruction with a transabdominal, subcutaneous, femorofemoral graft. Surgery 52:342, 1962.

61. Brief DK, Brener FJ, Alpert J, Parsonnet V: Cross-over femoro-femoral grafts followed up five years or more. Arch Surg 110:1294, 1975.

62. Plecha FR, Pories WJ: Extra-anatomic bypasses for aortoiliac disease in high risk patients. Surgery 80:480, 1976.

63. Berguer R, Higgins RF, Reddy DJ: Intimal hyperplasia. An experimental study. Arch Surg 115:332, 1980.

64. Towne JB, Quinn K, Salles-Cunha S, et al: Effect of increased arterial blood flow on localization and progression of atherosclerosis. Arch Surg 117:1469, 1982.

65. Donaldson MC, Louras JC, Bucknam CA: Axillofemoral bypass: A tool with a limited role. J Vasc Surg 3:757–763, 1986.

66. Harris EJ, Taylor LM, McConnell DB, et al: Clinical results of axillobifemoral bypass using externally supported polytetrafluoroethylene. J Vasc Surg 12:416–421, 1990.

67. Dotter CT, Judkins MD: Transluminal treatment of arteriosclerotic obstruction. Description of a technique and a preliminary report of its application. Circulation 30:654, 1964.

68. Gruntzig A: Die Perkutane Transluminale Rekanalisation Chronischer Arterienversch Lusse mit einer Neven Dilatationstechnik. Baden-Baden, G. Witzstrock Verlag, 1977.

69. Johnston KW, Rae M, Hogg-Johnston SA, et al: Five year results of a prospective study of percutaneous transluminal angioplasty. Ann Surg 206:403–413, 1987.

70. Wilson SE, Wolf GL, Cross AP, et al: Percutaneous transluminal angioplasty versus operation for peripheral arteriosclerosis. J Vasc Surg 9:1–8, 1989.

27

FEMORAL-POPLITEAL-TIBIAL OCCLUSIVE DISEASE

FRANK J. VEITH

Arteriosclerosis may involve the common femoral popliteal artery, any of the infrapopliteal arteries including their terminal branches, or any combination of these arteries. This involvement generally begins early in adult life and progresses slowly to the point where a flow-reducing stenosis or occlusion occurs in one or more of the arteries below the inguinal ligament. As the average age of our population increases, the number of individuals with this hemodynamically significant infrainguinal arteriosclerosis also increases. This chapter deals with the present status of treatment for arteriosclerotic occlusive disease of the femoral, popliteal, and tibial arterial systems.

Obviously, this disease is associated in varying degrees with arteriosclerotic involvement elsewhere in the body, and this fact must constantly be considered when making therapeutic decisions in afflicted patients. It is this consideration that guides the surgeon correctly to a lesser intervention or operation that maintains function rather than one that will restore a normal circulation. The generalized and slowly progressive nature of the disease process and the imperfect results of all interventional treatments should also deter any who might be unwisely tempted to treat asymptomatic or minimally disabling arteriosclerotic occlusive lesions. In the management of the increasingly common entity of infrainguinal arteriosclerosis, diagnostic and therapeutic restraint and the desire to minimize risks and avoid doing harm must be paramount principles if the disease is not producing major functional impairment or tissue necrosis. On the other hand, despite the advanced age and poor generalized condition of the afflicted population, aggressive intervention for both diagnosis and treatment is justified if limb loss is truly threatened by the disease process.

CLINICAL PRESENTATION

The reserve of the human arterial system is enormous. Hemodynamically significant stenoses or major artery occlusions can exist in the infrainguinal arterial tree with no or only minimal symptoms. This is particularly true if collateral pathways are normal or the patient's activity level is limited by coronary arteriosclerosis or other disease processes. Accordingly, the most common manifestation of a short segmental occlusion of the superficial femoral artery, the most common site of major arteriosclerotic involvement below the inguinal ligament, will be mild intermittent claudication. Similarly, this lesion will often be totally asymptomatic, and this is usually the case if only one or two tibial arteries are occluded without other significant lesions. Thus the usual patient who presents with severe disabling intermittent claudication or tissue necrosis has multiple sequential occlusions or so-called combined segment disease with hemodynamically significant lesions at the aortoiliac level and the superficial femoral/popliteal level, or either or both of these combined with severe infrapopliteal disease as well.[1]

Staging

Patients with hemodynamically significant infrainguinal arteriosclerosis may be classified into one of five stages depending on their clinical presentation as indicated in Table 27–1. Patients in stages III and IV are those whose limbs may be considered imminently threatened, although some patients with mild ischemic rest pain may remain stable for many years and an occasional patient with a small patch of gangrene or an ischemic ulcer will heal his lesion with conservative in-hospital treatment. With the exception of these few patients, invasive diagnostic procedures such as angiography are easily justified for those with stages III and IV disease, which is usually associated with disease at several levels.

Rest pain as an isolated symptom in patients with infrainguinal arteriosclerosis can be difficult to evaluate unless it is accompanied by other findings. Many patients with significant arterial lesions have pain at

TABLE 27–1. STAGING OF INFRAINGUINAL ARTERIOSCLEROSIS WITH HEMODYNAMICALLY SIGNIFICANT STENOSIS OR OCCLUSIONS

	Stage Presentation	Invasive Diagnostic and Therapeutic Intervention
0	No signs or symptoms	Never justified
I	Intermittent claudication (> 1 block) No physical changes	Usually unjustified
II	Severe claudication (< 1/2 block) Dependent rubor Decreased temperature	Sometimes justified Not always necesary May remain stable
III	Rest pain Atrophy, cyanosis Dependent rubor	Usually indicated but may do well for long periods without revascularization
IV	Nonhealing ischemic ulcer or gangrene	Usually indicated

rest from causes other than their arteriosclerosis, such as arthritis or neuritis. Such pain will not be relieved by even a successful revascularization. Significant ischemic rest pain must be associated not only with decreased pulses but also with other objective manifestations of ischemia, such as atrophy, decreased skin temperature when compared to the other extremity, and marked rubor and relief of pain with dependency. In some patients with a complex etiology to their rest pain, it may be necessary to perform a noninvasive laboratory and angiographic evaluation before the predominant cause of the symptom can be determined and appropriate treatment instituted. Every patient with pain at rest and decreased pulses is not a candidate for angiography and an arterial bypass. Some of these patients will be relieved by appropriate treatment for gout or osteoarthritis. Others can be well managed with simple analgesics and reassurance that their limb is not in jeopardy. Such reassurance generally suffices for patients with stage I disease and those with stage II disease who are elderly (over 80 years) or at high risk because of intercurrent disease or atherosclerotic involvement of other organs such as the heart, the kidneys, or the brain.

This conservative approach to patients with stage I involvement from infrainguinal arteriosclerosis is becoming increasingly widespread, albeit not universally so.[2] Conservatism appears to be clearly justified by the numerous reports of the benignancy and slow progression of stage I disease to more advanced stages.[3–5] Without treatment, 10 to 15 per cent of patients in stage I will improve over 5 years, and 60 to 70 per cent will not progress over the same period. The 10 to 15 per cent who do worsen are, in our opinion, best treated with a primary operation or other therapeutic intervention *after* their disease progresses. We further believe that this conservative approach to stage I disease is justified by the greater surgical difficulty encountered when a procedure for claudication fails in the early or remote postoperative

period and the patient then has a threatened limb, a situation that we have observed all too frequently.

The fact that some patients in stage II and a few in stage III or IV may remain stable and easily managed without operation for protracted periods of 1 or more years justifies a cautiously conservative nonoperative approach to selected patients in these stages. This often requires hospitalization so that the patient and the progress of his ischemia can be assessed. Moreover, this conservative nonoperative approach is particularly indicated if the patient is elderly and a poor surgical risk from a systemic and a local point of view. An example of this would be an octogenarian with intractable congestive failure in whom a difficult distal small vessel bypass would be required to alleviate stage III signs and symptoms. Close observation can and often should be the preferred management for such a patient for several months or even years; however, we would not hesitate to revascularize such a patient when his rest pain became intolerable or he developed a small progressive patch of gangrene.[1,6]

Impact of Newer Interventional Treatments on Threshold for Therapy

The relative simplicity of percutaneous balloon angioplasty alone or in combination with other newer endovascular treatments using laser ablation or atherectomy devices (see Chapter 16) to remove arteriosclerotic plaque has prompted some physicians or surgeons to recommend lowering of the therapeutic thresholds for infrainguinal atherosclerosis. Some surgeons, radiologists, and particularly cardiologists new to the peripheral vascular field and armed with these new techniques and devices have used them routinely to treat stage I and even stage 0 disease detected incidentally during physical examination or coronary arteriography. This practice is to be condemned at this time for many reasons. Most importantly, the mid- and long-term results of these newer treatments remain totally unknown. Even if they are successful immediately, they can initiate a healing process in the artery that causes late failure or, worse, an acceleration of the occlusive process and ultimately net harm to the patient. Therefore, they subject patients to risks they may not fully appreciate. In fact, one has to question the motives of practitioners who treat these relatively early, minimally symptomatic lesions before more is known about these newer high-tech treatments. Although they are all exciting and interesting to patients and doctors alike and although they may prove to be safe and effective, this has not yet been shown. Accordingly, there is no justification as yet to lower the threshold for intervening in patients with infrainguinal arteriosclerosis. This fact should be communicated freely to patients to offset the unjustified marketing efforts of uninformed practitioners.

Differential Diagnosis

Intermittent claudication, or pain brought on by exertion and relieved by rest, is a fairly distinct symptom and usually a manifestation of arteriosclerotic occlusive disease, although mild calf claudication can be produced by a significant stenotic lesion in the superficial femoral or popliteal artery. An occasional patient will describe his claudication as a sense of heaviness, weakness, or fatigue in the limb without pain, and such patients may be mistakenly diagnosed as having neuromuscular disorders. Sometimes claudication-like symptoms can be produced by lesions compressing the lower spinal cord or cauda equina.[7,8] Such *pseudoclaudication* is most often produced by spinal stenosis and can easily be suspected when peripheral pulses are normal. Occasionally, neurologic problems will coexist with arterial occlusive disease, making an exact determination of the cause of the patient's symptoms a difficult challenge for the neurologist and the vascular surgeon. In such circumstances, angiography, CT scan of the lumbar spine, and myelography may be necessary.

Some of the difficulties that can be encountered in differentiating pain at rest from true *ischemic rest pain* have already been discussed. Again, these difficulties are greatest when arterial occlusive disease coexists with other pathology. Similar difficulties can be encountered in determining the primary cause of ulcerating lesions in the ankle region and on the foot. The typical *venous ulcer* poses no problem in deferential diagnosis. It occurs in a setting of chronic venous disease, is associated with stasis changes and normal arterial pulses, is usually relatively painless, and heals with elevation and compressive measures. The typical *arterial* or *ischemic ulcer* is far more painful and is associated with other manifestations of ischemia. It usually has a more necrotic base and is located at an area of chronic pressure or trauma, such as over the malleoli or the bunion area. Both conditions may be improved by hospitalization, bed rest, and local care. Differential diagnosis is usually only difficult when chronic venous and arterial disease coexist. Venography and arteriography may be required. In some patients the primary cause of the ulcer can only be determined when arterial reconstruction produces healing after a period of intense conservative management has failed to do so.

When a patient presents with a gangrenous (black) or pregangrenous (blue) toe, several etiologies other than progression of chronic arteriosclerotic occlusive disease must be considered. *Local infection* can be the sole or a contributing cause of the toe lesion. This is particularly common in diabetics. If foot pulses or noninvasive tests of arterial function are normal, the gangrenous condition can be presumed to result from local arterial or arteriolar thrombosis secondary to infection. Radical local *excision* and drainage of all involved tissue will usually result in a healed foot. Diagnosis is more difficult when infection coexists with arterial occlusive disease. Noninvasive studies and arteriography are usually required before it can be determined whether treatment should consist of excision and drainage alone or in combination with an arterial reconstruction. Decision making under these conditions can be among the most difficult in vascular surgery.

Patients with black or blue toes may also have them as the result of embolic processes. Such emboli may originate from the heart, a proximal aneurysm, or any proximal atherosclerotic lesion. In the latter circumstance, small cholesterol, platelet, or fibrin emboli may lodge in interosseous or digital arteries. Peripheral pedal pulses may be normal, and spontaneous improvement of the resulting blue toe often occurs. This sequence of events has been termed the "blue toe syndrome," and its pathogenesis is thought to be analogous to that of transient ischemic attacks from atherosclerotic disease at the carotid bifurcation.[9] If a single dominant arterial lesion can be identified by angiography, it should be treated by endarterectomy or more commonly by an appropriate bypass. However, in our experience, it has been difficult to identify a single lesion in the arterial tree of these patients, and we have usually operated on them only after they have had multiple embolic episodes.

In any patient whose ischemia developed suddenly, the possibility of a major embolus from the heart or a proximal aneurysm must be considered. In such circumstances, angiography is indicated even if limb viability is not in question, since major emboli should be removed as soon as they are identified. In the last several decades with progress in cardiac surgery for rheumatic heart disease, almost all patients that we have seen with major arterial emboli and acute arterial occlusions have had them superimposed on extensive arteriosclerosis. Even with angiography, *which we employ routinely in such cases*, the diagnosis and treatment of embolic disease is difficult and the results imperfect.[10] The only certain diagnostic feature of embolus is multiplicity. Furthermore, the location of the embolus may be atypical, and the vascular surgeon treating a presumed embolus in the presence of extensive arteriosclerosis must be prepared to perform an extensive arterial reconstruction or bypass even if the operation is undertaken soon after the acute event.[10] Because of these facts and because acute thrombosis sometimes cannot be differentiated in any way from embolus, complete preoperative angiography should be mandatory in any suspected embolic occlusion of the lower extremity in a patient who could have arteriosclerosis. Exploration of the distal popliteal artery is usually the best surgical approach in patients with severe ischemia due to an acute occlusion of the popliteal or the distal superficial femoral arteries,[11] although use of intraarterially administered lytic agents, particularly urokinase, may have significant therapeutic advantages in the management of acute thromboembolic occlusions of native lower extremity arteries, especially those with some underlying atherosclerosis. Moreover, the care and surgical treatment of such cases should only be undertaken by an experienced vascular surgeon. A more complete discussion of the management of acute thromboembolic arterial occlusions appears in Chapter 36.

PATIENT EVALUATION

Local Factors and Extremity Physical Examination

As already indicated, the findings on physical examination of the involved extremity contribute to the staging of the atherosclerotic process and provide a rough guide to whether diagnostic or therapeutic intervention is justified and needed. Physical examination by revealing discoloration and swelling should also provide evidence of the presence and extent of infection in the involved foot. As a general rule, the extent of infection and necrosis deep to the skin is greater than one might expect from an examination of the skin. Reexamination after a short period of soaking to soften the epidermis and dried exudate may also be helpful in revealing purulent collections and subcutaneous necrosis. Exploration of suspicious areas can sometimes be carried out without anesthesia if the patient has diminished sensation from diabetic neuropathy. If not, such exploration and necessary débridement should be performed in the operating room with anesthesia.

In the initial examination of a patient with suspected infrainguinal arterial disease, careful inspection for previous operative scars is essential, since patients may be unaware of a prior sympathectomy or the nature and extent of previous arterial surgery. The site of scars can provide clues as to whether the arteries below the knee were violated, whether ipsilateral saphenous vein was utilized, and if so, how much is left. Physical examination can also provide evidence of associated chronic disease. In evaluating an ischemic limb, particular attention must be given to careful inspection of the heel and between the toes where unsuspected ischemic ulcers or infection may be present. A flashlight is extremely helpful in this regard. The uninvolved extremity must also be examined carefully. Because of the symmetry of atherosclerosis, the opposite extremity may harbor unsuspected ischemic lesions. Moreover, such findings as coolness and bluish discoloration are far more meaningful if they are asymmetrical, since cool dusky extremities may sometimes be present without major arterial disease.

Pulse examination in the lower extremities of a patient with suspected ischemia is extremely important. It requires considerable experience and must be performed with care. The strength of a pulse as assessed by an experienced examiner is a valuable semiquantitative assessment of the arterial circulation at that level. Pulses are graded from 0 to 4+, and a pulse cannot be described as "plus or minus" or "questionable." The latter indicates an incomplete exam.

A 0 pulse cannot be felt. A 1+ pulse is definitely present but definitely diminished. Both 2+ and 3+ are normal intensities, and 4+ is an abnormally strong pulse, as with an aneurysm or aortic insufficiency. If a pulse is 2+ on one side and 3+ on the opposite side, the 2+ is a decreased pulse, and arterial pressure at that site is probably decreased (unless the 3+ pulse is due to an aneurysm).

In examining a patient with diminished pulses it is extremely helpful to count the pulse to an assistant who is palpating the patient's radial pulse to be sure the examiner is not feeling his own pulse or spurious muscular activity. Before one describes a pulse as being absent, considerable time and effort must be expended and ectopic localization of pulses, such as the lateral tarsal artery pulse, must be examined. In this era of too frequently performed noninvasive arterial tests, the value of a carefully performed and recorded pulse exam cannot be overemphasized. It provides a basis for comparison if subsequent disease progression occurs, and it is a simple way of accurately assessing the arterial circulation in the lower extremities at a given point in time. It also provides an indicator of what type of approach will be required to save a threatened foot.

Many examples of this value can be cited. If a patient with a gangrenous toe lesion has a pedal pulse, local treatment without reconstructive arterial surgery will almost always be the correct approach to achieve a healed foot. If a patient with an ischemic foot lesion has a normal popliteal pulse but no pedal pulses, some form of infrapopliteal or small vessel bypass will almost always be the correct approach to obtain a healed foot. If a patient with an ischemic foot lesion has a normal ipsilateral femoral pulse without distal pulses, some form of infrainguinal arterial reconstruction, hopefully a femoropopliteal bypass, will be the correct approach to achieve a healed foot. If such a patient has a diminished femoral pulse, often with an associated bruit, some form of proximal arterial reconstruction or angioplasty above the inguinal ligament will almost certainly be required.

Systemic Factors

Systemic factors that are important in the patient who is a candidate for interventional treatment for infrainguinal arteriosclerosis include all those in the history, physical examination, and routine laboratory tests that might indicate major organ failure. Most important are evidence of heart disease, diabetes, kidney disease, hypertension, chronic pulmonary disease, and atherosclerotic involvement of arteries to the brain. All these intercurrent diseases, if present, require appropriate medical management before, during, and after diagnostic and therapeutic interventions so that risks will be minimized. A detailed discussion of this management is beyond the scope of this chapter. However, since all patients with infrainguinal arteriosclerosis also have some degree of coronary involvement and since myocardial infarction is the principal cause of operative as well as late mortality in this group of patients, some details of cardiac evaluation and management should be mentioned. Evidence of myocardial ischemia and congestive failure should be sought. Thallium-persantin stress tests may be a useful screening evaluation. If marked abnormalities or severe angina pectoris are present, some patients should be subjected to coronary arteriography and aortocoronary bypass prior to treating their limb ischemia. Patients with recent myocardial infarctions and those in congestive heart failure should have a Swan-Ganz catheter inserted and have their fluid and volume replacement optimized before, during, and after operation on the basis of appropriate cardiac output and pressure measurements.[12] It is also especially important to monitor renal function repetitively after any angiographic procedure, since transient renal failure is common. If detected and appropriately treated, this is almost always reversible and rarely a serious problem.

Noninvasive Vascular Laboratory Tests

Although the nature and value of these tests are discussed in depth in Chapter 13, there are several relevant points that should be made here regarding their role in patients with infrainguinal arteriosclerosis. In the early stages, in which interventional measures are not required, segmental arterial pressures and pulse volume recordings provide an objective and semiquantitative assessment of the circulation and help to confirm the diagnosis made by the history and physical examination, including a careful pulse exam. These tests also provide a baseline against which future changes can be measured. They also provide a rough index of the localization of occlusive lesions and the degree of ischemia in the foot. However, the correlation is not absolute, and flat ankle and forefoot wave tracings with ankle pressures less than 35 mm Hg can be unassociated with foot lesions or serious symptomatology. In addition, decreased thigh waveforms and pressures may be associated entirely with disease below the inguinal ligament as well as aortoiliac disease. The differentiation between these two types of lesions can only be made by femoral pulse examination and direct pressure measurements, and exact localization and definition of lesions can only be made when angiography, sometimes in two planes, is added to these two determinations.

Noninvasive testing can be extremely helpful in predicting when a toe amputation or local procedure on the foot has virtually no chance of healing. A flatline forefoot tracing with an ankle pressure below 50 mm Hg indicates that a toe amputation or other foot operation for an ischemic lesion will not heal without prior revascularization. Because these tests do not evaluate the severity or extent of infection, the opposite is not always true. Good forefoot pulse waves and ankle pressures do not guarantee healing of foot operations, although they suggest it will occur if infection can be eliminated. Furthermore, there is a gray zone in intermediate values in which the noninvasive tests are of little value and a therapeutic trial of a local foot procedure is justified and appropriate.

Angiographic Evaluation

As in other areas of vascular surgery, proper high-quality *arteriography* is essential to make the most accurate diagnosis of infrainguinal arteriosclerosis, to determine whether therapeutic intervention is possible and justified by its risk, and to allow planning of the optimal form that this intervention should take.[5] Adequate arteriography also defines the localization and extent of arteriosclerotic involvement in the infrarenal aorta and iliac arteries, although for optimal accuracy it may have to be supplemented by direct pressure measurements taken at the time of arteriography or operation.

To provide adequate information, the arterial tree from the groin to the forefoot should be well visualized in continuity, preferably by the transfemoral route. This is generally possible only if a long film changer, multiple exposures, large boluses of contrast, and other technical modifications described elsewhere[13] are employed. Oblique views may be required to visualize completely the origin and proximal portion of the deep femoral artery. Good preoperative distal artery visualization is, in our opinion, the key to performing optimal bypass surgery to arteries in the foot and lower leg. Reactive hyperemia, digitally augmented views, and delayed films may be necessary to achieve the needed visualization. Although others have advocated intraoperative arteriography to achieve this end,[14] we have found it less effective and rarely necessary. Recently, magnetic resonance imaging (MRI) of flowing blood (MR angiography) has provided preoperative evaluation of patent distal leg and foot arteries without the need for dye injection. However, these techniques are not yet generally available.

Saphenous venography and *duplex ultrasonography* have also been helpful in planning long bypasses.[15,16] They may also show a vein defect preoperatively and thereby spare the patient and the surgeon the needless effort of harvesting a saphenous vein that cannot be used. These techniques are particularly indicated in patients who have undergone prior prosthetic bypasses, since many of these patients have had their vein erroneously injured at their first operation. However, neither method is totally accurate, and surgical exploration is the only way to assess vein quality with certainty.

TREATMENT: PRINCIPLES, PROCEDURES, AND JUDGMENTAL ISSUES

In general our approach, which is detailed below, represents the most aggressive effort to salvage limbs that are threatened because of infrainguinal arteriosclerosis. Patients who have ischemic foot lesions or pain but who can be treated successfully by aortofemoral, femorofemoral, or axillofemoral bypass alone should be treated. These patients are excluded from the following discussion even though many of them have infrainguinal arteriosclerosis in addition to their more proximal disease.

General Considerations

According to our aggressive approach to patients whose limbs are threatened because of infrainguinal arteriosclerosis, limb salvage should be considered and attempted if feasible, unless gangrene extends into the deeper tissues of the tarsal region of the foot or unless the patient has severe organic mental syndrome with inability to ambulate, communicate, or provide self-care.[1,6] Patients in the latter categories should undergo primary below- or above-knee amputation. Primary above-knee amputation should also be employed if a patient with foot gangrene is unable to stand or walk because of long-standing severe flexion contractures.

Medical Considerations

As expected, there is in these patients a high incidence of other arteriosclerotic manifestations, and more than 60 per cent may have diabetes mellitus.[6] The mean age is over 70 years, and many patients are in their eighties. Many have suffered documented myocardial infarction, some are in uncompensated congestive heart or renal failure, some have had myocardial infarctions within 3 weeks of presentation,[6,17] and some have concurrent carcinomas.[2]

The general plan of medical management is to achieve maximal improvement of cardiac, renal, and diabetic status before proceeding with arteriographic examination and operation. In some instances, the urgency of the ischemic situation, coupled with progressive infection in the foot, make it necessary to perform angiographic examination and operation before ideal medical control can be achieved. In these patients decisions to proceed are made jointly by the surgeon and internist. Almost without exception, age, medical status, incurable malignancy, and/or a contralateral amputation are not considered reasons to withhold arterial reconstruction.[1,6]

Surgical Considerations and Criteria for Reconstructability

Femoropopliteal Bypass

Patients whose limbs are clearly threatened and who have undergone arteriographic examination should undergo femoropopliteal bypass when the superficial femoral or popliteal artery is occluded and the patent popliteal artery segment distal to the occlusion has luminal continuity, on arteriographic examination, with any of its three terminal branches. This is true even if one or more of these branches ends in an occlusion anywhere in the leg. Even if the popliteal artery segment into which the graft is to be inserted is occluded distally, femoropopliteal bypass to this *isolated segment*[18] is the procedure of choice. If the isolated popliteal segment is less than 7 cm in length or there is extensive gangrene of infection in the foot, a femoral-to-popliteal-to-distal artery bypass or *sequential bypass* is sometimes performed, in one or two stages.[19,20] All femoropopliteal bypasses can be classified on the basis of their relationship to the knee joint and runoff from the popliteal artery, as determined radiographically by previously described criteria.[20] However, it should be noted that all angiographic evaluations of popliteal runoff are imperfect and correlated in only a limited way with outflow resistance and bypass patency.[21]

Infrapopliteal Bypass

Bypasses to arteries beyond the popliteal (small vessel bypasses) are performed only when femoropopliteal bypass is not deemed possible, according to the foregoing criteria. These small vessel bypasses are performed to the posterior tibial, the anterior tibial, or the peroneal arteries, in the order of preference. A tibial artery is generally used only if its lumen runs without obstruction into the foot, although short vein bypasses to isolated tibial artery segments and other disadvantaged outflow tracts have been performed and remained patent over 4 years.[22,23] A peroneal artery is usually used only if it is continuous with one or two of its terminal branches, which then run into the foot. Absence of a plantar arch and vascular calcification *are not* considered contraindications to a reconstruction.[6,22] Some patients require a bypass to an artery or arterial branch in the foot.[1,6,22,23] Very few patients fail to have in their leg or foot an artery that meets these requirements, so that less than 1 per cent of our patients are now considered unreconstructible on the basis of angiographic findings.[1]

With both femoropopliteal and small vessel bypasses, stenosis of less than 50 per cent of the diameter of the vessel is acceptable at or distal to the site chosen for the distal anastomosis. Although an effort is made to find the most disease-free segment of artery to use for the distal anastomosis, this may be tempered by the advisability of using the most proximal patent segment possible, to shorten the length of the bypass. For example, we believe that a mildly diseased proximal popliteal artery should be used for a distal anastomosis in preference to a nondiseased distal popliteal artery.

The common femoral artery has been generally used as the site of origin for all bypasses to the popliteal and more distal arteries. However, over the last

18 years, we have also used as inflow sites the superficial femoral, popliteal, or tibial arteries when these vessels were relatively undiseased or vein length was limited.[22,24] The superficial femoral and popliteal arteries are now used preferentially if possible; that is, if there is no proximal luminal stenosis in excess of 40 per cent of the cross-sectional diameter.

Axillopopliteal Bypass

This operation is employed only when amputation is imminent and a more standard arterial reconstruction is not feasible because of groin infection, previous operative scarring, or extensive bilateral arteriosclerotic involvement of the iliac and femoral artery systems.[25,26]

Profundaplasty

Endarterectomy of the origin and proximal portion of the deep femoral artery is chiefly of value in salvaging threatened limbs when it is combined with some form of inflow operation, such as an aortofemoral or axillofemoral bypass.[27] As an isolated procedure in patients whose limbs are threatened because of infrainguinal arteriosclerosis, we have found profundaplasty to be of little value. Perhaps it is occasionally justified as the sole procedure if the patient has rest pain without necrosis *and* a tight stenosis or occlusion of the deep femoral artery with a demonstrable pressure gradient across the lesion at operation. In practice we have employed a short vein bypass to the distal deep femoral artery more frequently than an isolated profundaplasty.

Graft Material

Until 1976, reversed autologous saphenous vein (ASV) grafts were clearly the graft material of choice, with a variety of Dacron grafts serving as the alternate material if the vein was unavailable. Tubular expanded polytetrafluoroethylene (PTFE) grafts became available in 1976 and were first used only when ipsilateral saphenous vein was unavailable or unusable. Promising early and intermediate results with this material in femoropopliteal bypasses[28-30] prompted liberalization of the indications for its use in this operation to include patients whose probable life expectancy is less than 3 years, and some surgeons, after adequately analyzing their results, still advocate the preferential use of PTFE grafts for femoropopliteal bypass.[31]

In 1986 we completed, with Drs. Bergan, Bernhard, Yao, Flinn, Towne, and others, a cooperative, randomized, prospective study comparing ASV to PTFE grafts in all infrainguinal bypass operations.[32,33] ASV and PTFE grafts were compared in 845 infrainguinal bypass operations, 485 to the popliteal artery and 360 to infrapopliteal arteries. Life-table primary patency rates for randomized PTFE grafts to the popliteal artery parallel those for randomized ASV grafts to the same level for 2 years and then became significantly different [4-year patency of 68 ± 8 per cent ($\pm$S.E.) for ASV versus 47 ± 9 per cent for PTFE, $p <$

.025]. Four-year patency differences for randomized above-knee grafts were not statistically significant (61 ± 12 per cent for ASV versus 38 ± 13 per cent for PTFE, $p > .25$), but were for randomized below-knee grafts (76 ± 9 per cent for ASV versus 45 ± 11 per cent for PTFE, $p < .05$). Four-year limb salvage rates after bypasses to the popliteal artery for critical ischemia did not differ for the two types of randomized grafts (75 ± 10 per cent for ASV versus 7 ± 10 per cent for PTFE, $p > .25$). Although primary patency rates for randomized PTFE grafts and obligatory PTFE grafts to the popliteal artery were significantly different ($p < .025$), 4-year limb salvage rates were not (70 ± 10 per cent versus 68 ± 20 per cent, $p < .25$). Primary patency rates at 4 years for infrapopliteal bypasses with randomized ASV were significantly better than those with randomized PTFE (49 ± 10 per cent versus 12 ± 7 per cent, $p < .001$). Three and one-half–year limb salvage rates for infrapopliteal bypasses with both randomized grafts (57 ± 10 per cent for ASV and 61 ± 10 per cent for PTFE) were better than those for obligatory infrapopliteal PTFE grafts (38 ± 11 per cent, $p < .01$). These results fail to support the routine preferential use of PTFE grafts for either femoropopliteal or more distal bypasses. However, this graft may be used preferentially in selected poor-risk patients for femoropopliteal bypasses, particularly those that do not cross the knee. Although every effort should be made to use autologous vein for infrapopliteal bypasses, a PTFE distal bypass is a better option than a primary major amputation. This study provides much more data and justifies many additional important conclusions, some of which may depend on an individual surgeon's interpretation of the study and its data. The reader is therefore well advised to evaluate the original reports of this study[33,33] before drawing his or her own final conclusions.

Although we believe that PTFE grafts are the best currently available alternative arterial prosthetic if the ipsilateral ASV is not available for femoropopliteal bypass or if no vein is available for infrapopliteal bypasses, other grafts have also been used with some success. The tanned umbilical vein graft has received the greatest attention, and patency rates similar to those of PTFE grafts have been reported in both the femoropopliteal and infrapopliteal positions.[34] A number of randomized comparisons of the two grafts have been completed. However, many of these studies were flawed or yielded inconclusive differences. In addition, reports of a high incidence of aneurysmal degeneration occurring in umbilical vein grafts after even a few years are worrisome and suggest that this graft be employed with caution even though the manufacturers have recently strengthened the external Dacron mesh.[35]

Another alternative prosthetic that may have some usefulness in infrainguinal bypasses is the externally supported Dacron fabric graft.[36] It is thought that the external ring support provides kink resistance as the graft is flexed at joints such as the knee. However, more long-term comparative data will have to be obtained before the relative merits of these supported grafts are known with certainty. At present it is clearly wrong to use any new prosthetic grafts *in preference* to ipsilateral ASV until appropriate randomized prospective studies comparing the prosthetic to vein have been completed. Many surgeons often find it too easy to succumb to the temptation of finding a rationale to use a prosthetic graft preferentially. We believe this temptation must be resisted and encourage randomized study of all promising new prosthetics before they are used preferentially. Sixty to 80 per cent of patients will have a usable vein if a real effort is made to find it.[16,37] On the other hand, many patients do not have an adequate autologous vein, and use of a prosthetic graft is far better than an unwise attempt to use a small (less than 3.0 mm in distended diameter), fibrotic, or otherwise inadequate autologous vein.[37,38] These considerations should be kept in mind when evaluating the "all-autologous policy" espoused by some capable vascular surgeons.[39] As more and more secondary operations become necessary to save limbs, the proportion of patients who do not have an adequate autologous vein conduit will increase. In such patients a prosthetic (PTFE) graft will yield better results than ill advised use of a poor or intrinsically diseased vein.

In Situ Versus Reversed Saphenous Vein Grafts

The in situ saphenous vein graft was described as an infrainguinal arterial prosthetic by Hall in 1962.[40] It has several theoretical advantages over the more commonly used reversed saphenous vein graft, although the technique is demanding and requires elimination of all venous valves and occlusion of branches. In the last several years, Leather and Karmody have devised new methods for rendering the venous valves incompetent, and the Albany group and Gruss of West Germany have popularized the use of in situ vein grafts for infrainguinal arterial reconstructions.[41–43] Recently a number of claims have been made regarding the superiority of in situ vein grafts to reversed vein grafts, particularly for tibial and peroneal bypasses. While better endothelial preservation may be possible with in situ veins and while they may offer advantages when long bypasses with small veins are required, superior patency rates in comparable situations have never been proven. Comparisons using historical controls are not valid. In an ongoing multicenter prospective randomized comparison of in situ and reversed vein grafts that we are carrying out with Gregor Jhanik of Dublin and Peter Harris of Liverpool, no significant patency differences have yet emerged. Moreover, we have shown that many of the striking results that can be accomplished with in situ vein grafts can also be successfully accomplished with reversed vein grafts.[22] This includes the use of small-caliber veins to disadvantaged outflow tracts (Figs. 27–1, 27–2, and 27–

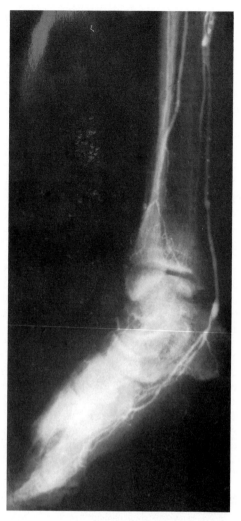

FIGURE 27–1. Arteriogram performed on patient 3 years after posterior tibial-to-posterior tibial bypass. The plantar arch is incomplete. (From Veith FJ, Ascer E, Gupta SK, et al: Tibiotibial vein bypass grafts: A new operation for limb salvage. J Vasc Surg 2:552–557, 1985.)

3). In addition, many patients who have autologous vein suitable for an *ectopic* reversed vein graft do not have a vein suitable for an in situ graft. Patients without any remaining major superficial vein in the ipsilateral lower extremity but with a good vein in the opposite leg or an arm are one example. Thus, until the superiority of in situ grafts is clearly documented by adequately controlled studies, we will adhere to the belief that the technical perfection of the operation and the commitment of the surgeon and his colleagues to the limb salvage goal are far more important in achieving good results than whether the vein graft is of the reversed or in situ type.

In the last few years, Taylor and his colleagues have published their recent results with infrainguinal reversed vein bypasses and claim that reversed vein grafts are better than in situ grafts.[44] However, more than 20 per cent of the patients whom these authors include in their cases were operated on for indications other than limb salvage. Thus their claims of

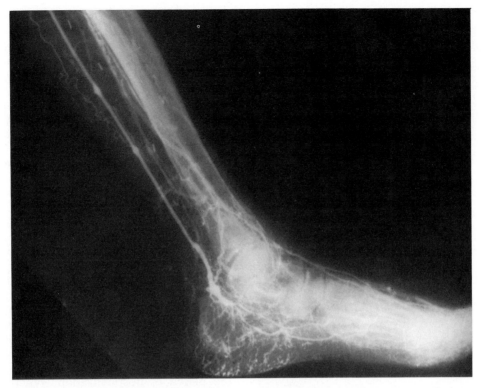

FIGURE 27–2. Intraoperative arteriogram after bypass from tibioperoneal trunk to posterior tibial artery at its bifurcation in the foot. Note small size of vein graft and intact plantar arch. (From Veith FJ, Ascer E, Gupta SK, et al: Tibiotibial vein bypass grafts: A new operation for limb salvage. J Vasc Surg 2:552–557, 1985.)

superiority for reversed vein grafts are based on data without comparable, concurrent controls, the same defect that they noted in the reports of others who claimed that the in situ technique gave superior results. Thus, the question of which type of vein graft is best remains an unanswered one that will require further study. On this basis, we continue to randomize the type of vein graft used in our long distal bypasses to infrapopliteal arteries. However, we have recently noted extremely poor late patency rates for long reversed vein grafts less than 3.5 mm in diameter and short vein grafts less than 3.0 mm in diameter.[45] Since similar poor patency has not been reported in small-diameter in situ grafts,[46] the in situ technique may be superior in patients whose vein is less than 3.0 mm in distended diameter.

Upper Extremity Veins

The cephalic and basilic veins from the upper extremities have been advocated for use as a graft when lower extremity autologous vein is unavailable. Although the work of Schulman and Dabley and many others suggest that arm veins are inferior to the saphenous vein in infrainguinal bypasses,[47] other observations indicate that the cephalic vein can be used with good success in lower extremity arterial reconstructions.[48] However, arm veins are more thin walled and more difficult to work with than is the saphenous

vein. Moreover, in our experience arm veins can have frequent fibrotic, recanalized segments from previous trauma and venipunctures. When several healthy segments are joined to form a composite graft, poorer patency results. On this basis and because of the high degree of symmetry in infrainguinal arteriosclerosis, we believe it is presently justified to use a prosthetic graft in the femoropopliteal position if the ipsilateral saphenous vein is unsuitable or unavailable. However, for infrapopliteal bypasses, every effort should be made to find usable autogenous vein. In this regard, lesser saphenous veins, accessory saphenous veins, and veins from the opposite thigh and upper extremities may all be useful, and we use them in that order of preference.

Operative Technique

All operations are performed with the patient under light general or epidural anesthesia. Care is taken to protect the opposite heel by placing a small pillow under the Achilles tendon. The arterial blood pressure is monitored by a radial artery catheter. Surgical techniques are detailed elsewhere,[26,30,49] and illustrated in Figures 27–4 and 27–5. Vessels are occluded with a minimum of force and distortion. Recently, we have found tourniquet occlusion, as recommended by Bernhard and Towne, to also be useful during the distal anastomosis. Anastomoses are meticulously constructed with continuous 6-0 polypropylene sutures, with particular care to take small,

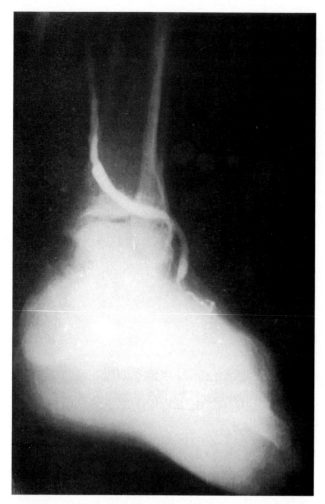

FIGURE 27–3. Postoperative arteriogram after bypass to the lateral tarsal artery, which appears to end in a total occlusion. There is also no patent plantar arch. (From Veith FJ, Ascer E, Gupta SK, et al: Tibiotibial vein bypass grafts: A new operation for limb salvage. J Vasc Surg 2:552–557, 1985.)

evenly spaced bites of all layers of the vessel wall, and to exclude all adventitia from the anastomotic lumen. Intraoperative angiographic examination is performed after most small vessel bypasses, but only if special problems are encountered after a femoropopliteal bypass. Although many vascular surgeons think of completion angiography as a panacea, it is not. Defects can be overlooked or not visualized because the proximal portion of the reconstruction is not included on the film. Moreover, "pseudo-defects" may be visualized and may prompt time-consuming, needless, and harmful further manipulation.

Bypasses to Ankle or Foot Arteries

For many years, our group has advocated the effectiveness of performing bypasses to arteries near the ankle or in the foot in patients who have no usable patent artery for distal bypass insertion at a more proximal level.[6,22] With adequate preoperative arteriography, these very distal arteries can usually be visualized if they are patent. Indeed, visualization

of such arteries and using them for bypass insertion has been a major factor in reducing the proportion of patients whose arterial disease was so distal that they were "unsuitable for an attempt at limb salvage" or inoperable. Although our advocacy of these very distal perimalleolar and inframalleolar bypasses was at first greeted with skepticism, these procedures are now being performed and advocated more widely, and the midterm effectiveness of bypasses to pedal arteries and their main branches (Fig. 27–6) has been documented[22,23] (Figs. 27–1, 27–2, and 27–3).

Perioperative and Postoperative Drug Treatment

All patients receive prophylactic antibiotic treatment with 1 gm of cefazolin 12 hours preoperatively, during operation, and 12 and 24 hours after operation. All receive heparin, 100 to 150 units/kg, during periods of vascular occlusion.

Based on the experimental observations of Oblath et al.,[50] all patients are given 325 mg of aspirin and 125 mg of dipyridamole three times daily, beginning 48 hours before operation and continued throughout the period of hospitalization. When the patient is discharged from the hospital, the aspirin and dipyridamole dosages are reduced to 325 mg and 50 mg, respectively, once daily; one of these drugs, usually aspirin, is continued indefinitely if possible.

Management of Foot Lesions

Approximately 75 per cent of our patients have gangrenous or necrotic foot or toe lesions.[1,6] Small (less than 2 sq cm), uninfected gangrenous lesions on the toe or foot are not treated. Larger gangrenous lesions and any area of infection associated with necrosis are usually extensively débrided at the end of any arterial reconstruction. These débridements often require excision of one or more toes, and frequently consist of a partial (medial or lateral) transmetatarsal amputation. An attempt is made to excise enough bone so there is overhanging skin and soft tissue. These wounds are usually left open, and drying of the soft tissues is prevented by placing the involved portion of the foot in a normal saline wet dressing within a plastic bag or plastic seal. Subsequent débridement of foot lesions is often required on the ward or in the operating room. This is performed to remove all infected or necrotic tissue and exposed cartilage without regard for anatomic landmarks. It is sometimes necessary, particularly in diabetics, to perform multiple secondary operative procedures (up to seven) to achieve a healed foot. Skin grafts are used to cover large cutaneous defects but are placed only when the wound is rendered entirely clean and granulating by débridement and frequent dressing changes. In some patients, particularly those with extensive foot gangrene or infection and a femoropop-

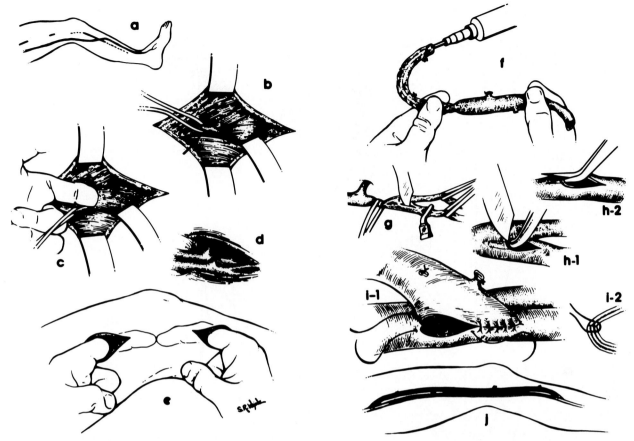

FIGURE 27–4. Small vessel bypass in the upper and middle third of the leg. This may be performed to the tibioperoneal trunk, the posterior tibial artery, or the peroneal artery using a medial approach below the knee joint to gain access to these vessels. The anterior tibial artery requires an additional anterior incision (shown in Fig. 27–5). *A,* In heavy lines, the position of the incisions required to perform bypasses from the femoral artery to the tibioperoneal trunk or the peroneal or posterior tibial arteries in the upper third of the leg. The upper incision provides access to the common or superficial femoral artery. The above-knee incision allows tunneling under the sartorius muscle and along the course of the popliteal vessels behind the knee. The dashed extension to the lower incision provides access to the posterior tibial and peroneal arteries in the middle third of the leg. If the saphenous vein is to be used, all incisions should be placed over the vein as shown by the double line, and access to deeper structures obtained when needed by raising thick flaps.

B, The below-knee incision opened through the skin, subcutaneous fat, and deep fascia of the popliteal space. The gastrocnemius muscle is retracted posteriorly. The more superficial popliteal vein is encircled with a Silastic loop to facilitate dissection of the underlying popliteal artery (arrow), which can be seen disappearing deep to the fibers of the soleus muscle. *C,* A finger or right-angle clamp being placed deep to the soleus muscle prior to cutting it at its origin from the fibrous band that attaches to the back of the tibia. This exposes the origin of the anterior tibial artery and its accompanying vein or veins. *D,* Division of these veins allows further retraction of overlying veins and exposure of the tibioperoneal trunk and its terminal branches. *E,* Tunnels are fashioned by finger dissection.

F, Details of vein preparation using a long (6-inch) cannula to permit the vein to be distended in segments so that leaks can be controlled and recanalized segments detected. *G,* Elevation of the arteries by Silastic vessel loops and the beginning of the scalpel incision in the artery. In this view only the taut Silastic loops are required to control bleeding, except for the posterior tibial artery, which also has a microvascular clip applied to it. *H,* Placement of a mosquito clamp to facilitate extension of the initial opening in the artery (1). Alternatively, a microvascular scissors may be used to extend the arteriotomy if the vessel is thin walled and normal (2). *I,* Details of the anastomotic suturing, which is begun at the distal end and continued to the midportion of each side of the anastomosis of the artery and the saphenous vein graft. Equal bites of all layers of each vessel are included in each stitch, which is always placed under direct vision. *J,* Completed graft in place. If more distal exposure of the posterior tibial or peroneal arteries is required, further separation of the soleus muscle from the posterior surface of the tibia and its overlying muscles provides access to the neurovascular bundles. Careful dissection of the veins with ligation of crossing branches provides access to the more deeply placed arteries. These can be dissected free, taking great care to preserve all branches, so that an appropriate segment of artery can be elevated and controlled to perform the distal anastomosis. (From Veith FJ, Gupta SK: Femoral-distal artery bypasses. *In* Bergan JJ, Yao JST (eds): Operative Techniques in Vascular Surgery. New York, Grune & Stratton, 1980, pp 141–150.)

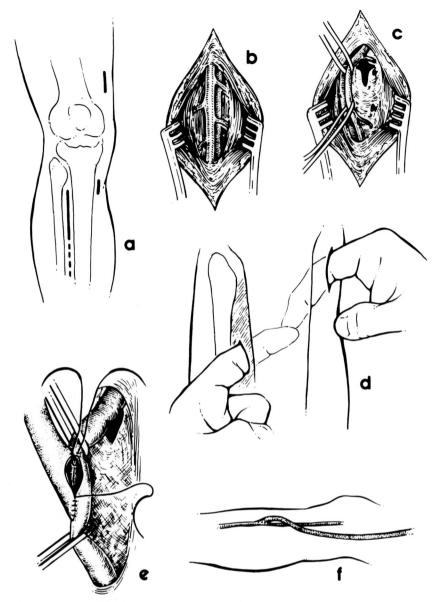

FIGURE 27–5. Bypass to the anterior tibial artery in the upper and middle thirds of the leg. *A*, This requires an anterolateral incision in the leg midway between the tibia and fibula over the appropriate segment of patent artery. Additional small medial incisions are also required for tunneling. *B*, The anterior incision is carried through the deep fascia, and the fibers of the anterior tibial muscle and the long extensors of the toes are separated to reveal the neurovascular bundle. Mobilization of accompanying veins with division of branches allows visualization of the anterior tibial artery, which can then be carefully mobilized. *C*, After the artery is freed, it is elevated and retracted along with the accompanying veins by Silastic loops. This permits further posterior dissection, which allows the interosseous membrane to be visualized and incised in a cruciate fashion. *D*, Careful blunt finger dissection from this anterior approach and from the popliteal fossa via the medial incision facilitates creation of a tunnel without injuring the numerous veins in the area. Alternatively, the tunnel for the bypass may be placed lateral to the knee in a subcutaneous plane. *E*, By elevating the anterior tibial artery, a meticulous distal anastomosis can be constructed as already described. *F*, The resulting graft in place. The anterior tibial artery can also be approached by a lateral incision with fibulectomy, but we believe this approach to be bloodier and more time consuming than the one we have described. (From Veith FJ, Gupta SK: Femoral-distal artery bypasses. *In* Bergan JJ, Yao JST (eds): Operative Techniques in Vascular Surgery. New York, Grune & Stratton, 1980, pp 141–150.)

liteal bypass that is inserted into an isolated popliteal artery segment, it is impossible to achieve healing at the metatarsal or even tarsal level, and below-knee amputation is required even though the bypass is patent. In some similar instances, it has been possible to obtain foot healing by performing a secondary bypass to an artery distal to the popliteal segment.[20] However, in the occasional patient with extensive infection and necrosis a healed foot cannot be obtained even with straight-line arterial flow into pedal arteries. This is particularly common in patients with end stage kidney disease and diabetes.

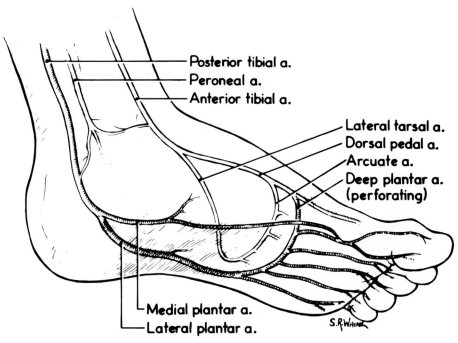

FIGURE 27-6. Diagram of named arteries in the ankle region and foot. Any of the main arteries or their branches, if patent, may be approached surgically and used as the distal outflow for a limb salvage bypass. (From Ascer E, Veith FJ, Gupta SK: Bypasses to plantar arteries and other tibial branches: An extended approach to limb salvage. J Vasc Surg 8:434–441, 1988.)

Reoperation

All patients whose bypasses thrombose in the first month after operation undergo reoperation. The techniques employed have been described elsewhere.[51] Intraoperative angiographic examination is used routinely after graft thrombectomy. Vein grafts that failed immediately after operation usually require interposition of a segment of PTFE or total replacement with this material, although in our experience an occasional thrombectomized vein graft will remain patent if no etiologic lesion is present.

Patients whose bypasses thrombose after the first postoperative month are considered for aggressive reoperation and femoral angiography is usually performed; however, the patients are subjected to reoperation only if the bypass failure is associated with a renewed threat to limb viability. If the patient has originally undergone operation elsewhere and details of the first operation are not known or the distal anastomosis is at or below the knee joint, a totally new bypass is performed. This is best accomplished using a variety of unusual approaches that permit access to infrainguinal arteries via unscarred, uninfected tissue planes.[51,52] These unusual approaches include a direct approach to the distal two thirds of the deep femoral artery (Figs. 27–7 and 27–8),[53] lateral approaches to the popliteal artery above and below the knee,[54] and medial or lateral approaches to all three of the infrapopliteal arteries. In addition to permitting dissection in virginal tissue planes, these unusual access routes facilitate use of shorter grafts,

which enable the surgeon to use the patient's remaining segments of good vein when his ipsilateral greater saphenous vein has been used or injured by the primary operation.

If the surgeon elects to salvage an old PTFE graft, which may be appropriate if the original distal anastomosis was above the knee and the patient's veins are poor as determined by venography or duplex ultrasonography, appropriate surgical techniques are critical to obtaining a favorable outcome.[51,52] The prior distal incision is opened and the distal end of the graft, the distal anastomosis, and the proximal and distal artery are dissected free. The graft is opened with a longitudinal incision to within a few millimeters of its distal tip (Fig. 27–9). The graft is then thrombectomized by passage of balloon catheters. Thrombus is gently removed from the distal anastomosis under direct vision, and balloon catheters are passed proximally and distally in the artery using extreme gentleness and care. If no disease or defect is seen within the anastomotic lumen, the opening in the graft is closed and an arteriogram is obtained. If no lesion is found, the operation is terminated. If intimal hyperplasia or other disease is noted at or just distal to the anastomosis, the opening in the graft is extended across its toe and down the artery to a point beyond the disease. A patch graft is placed to close this opening, and an intraoperative arteriogram is performed. If graft thrombosis has resulted from progression of arteriosclerosis proximal or distal to an anastomosis, and appropriate graft extension is constructed after removing all clot. Failed below-knee

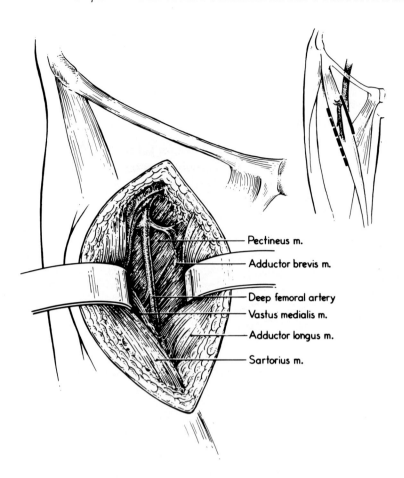

— Pectineus m.

— Adductor brevis m.

— Deep femoral artery

— Vastus medialis m.

— Adductor longus m.

— Sartorius m.

FIGURE 27–7. Incisions and anatomy for direct approaches to the distal two thirds of the deep femoral artery. (From Nunez A, Veith FJ, Collier P, et al: Direct approach to the distal portions of the deep femoral artery for limb salvage bypasses. J Vasc Surg 8:576–581, 1988.)

PTFE femoropopliteal and small vessel bypasses can be similarly managed but are probably best treated by performance of an entirely new bypass, preferably with vein and using previously undissected arteries if possible.

Failing Graft Concept

Intimal hyperplasia, progression of proximal or distal disease, or lesions within the graft itself can produce signs and symptoms of hemodynamic deterioration in patients with a prior arterial reconstruction without producing concomitant thrombosis of the bypass graft.[55–57] We have referred to this condition as a "failing graft" because, if the lesion is not corrected, graft thrombosis will almost certainly occur.[56] The importance of this failing graft concept lies in the fact that many difficult lower extremity revascularizations can be salvaged for protracted periods by relatively simple interventions if the lesion responsible for the circulatory determination and diminished graft blood flow can be detected before graft thrombosis occurs.

We have now been able to detect more than 200 failing grafts and to correct the lesions before graft thrombosis has occurred. The majority of these grafts were vein grafts, but approximately one third were PTFE or Dacron grafts. Invariably the corrective pro-

cedure is simpler than the secondary operation that would be required if the bypass went on to thrombose. Some lesions responsible for the failing state could be remedied by percutaneous transluminal angioplasty (PTA), although many required a vein patch angioplasty, a short bypass of a graft lesion, or a proximal or distal graft extension. Some of the transluminal angioplasties of these lesions have failed and required a second reintervention; others have remained effective in correcting the responsible lesion, as documented by arteriography more than 2 to 5 years later. If the failing graft is a vein bypass, detection of the failing state permits accurate localization and definition of the responsible lesion by arteriography and salvage of any undiseased vein. In contrast, if the graft is permitted to thrombose, the responsible lesion may be difficult to identify; the vein may be difficult or impossible to thrombectomize; and the patient's best graft, the ipsilateral greater saphenous vein, may have to be sacrificed, rendering the secondary operation even more difficult and more likely to fail with associated limb loss. Most importantly, the results of reinterventions for failing grafts, in terms of both continued cumulative patency and limb salvage rates, have been far superior to the results of reinterventions for grafts that have thrombosed and failed.[56–58]

This difference in results together with the ease of

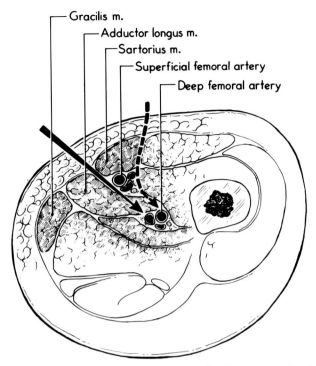

FIGURE 27–8. Cross-sectional anatomy for direct approaches to the distal two thirds of the deep femoral artery. (From Nunez A, Veith FJ, Collier P, et al: Direct approach to the distal portions of the deep femoral artery for limb salvage bypass. J Vasc Surg 8:576–581, 1988.)

reintervention for failing grafts mandate that surgeons performing infrainguinal bypass operations follow their patients closely in the postoperative period and indefinitely thereafter. Ideally noninvasive laboratory tests, including duplex studies, should be performed with similar frequency.[58] If the patient has any recurrence of symptoms or the surgeon detects *any* change in peripheral pulse examination or other manifestations of ischemia, the circulatory deterioration must be confirmed by noninvasive parameters and *urgent arteriography*. If a lesion is detected as a cause of the failing state, it is corrected urgently by PTA or operation. Recently we have tended to reoperate for vein graft lesions except for those less than 1.5 cm in length. PTA may be effective for some of these lesions. However, it can be ineffective and lead to graft thrombosis in other angiographically similar appearing lesions.

Role of Angioplasty

Opinions regarding the usefulness of this modality vary considerably, and its exact role in the treatment of infrainguinal arteriosclerosis is still somewhat controversial. Our own[1,59] and others' experience[60,61] suggests that with appropriate patient selection and in skilled hands, the complication rate is low. Moreover when complications or failure of PTA do occur, they can generally be well treated by relatively simple

surgical procedures with little if any increased patient morbidity or mortality.[59]

On this basis we presently will attempt a PTA on any patient with sufficiently severe disease and ischemia (usually stage III or IV) to warrant intervention and in whom the procedure is deemed suitable. Patients with stage III or IV ischemia who have a hemodynamically significant segmental iliac stenosis and infrainguinal arteriosclerosis generally have a PTA of the iliac lesion as their first therapeutic intervention. If the PTA is unsuccessful, a bypass to the femoral level is performed. If the PTA is successful, further arterial intervention, usually some form of femorodistal bypass, is performed only if the ischemia is unrelieved and a healed foot cannot be obtained. We do not hesitate to perform a bypass distal to an iliac artery treated by PTA, and subsequent experience has borne out the effectiveness of the approach.[1,6,62,63]

PTA is also used as the primary therapeutic intervention in patients without hemodynamically significant iliac artery disease who have a short (5 cm) segmental stenosis of the superficial femoral or popliteal artery, if this lesion is judged hemodynamically significant on the basis of pulse examination or noninvasive testing. In slightly less than half of our cases treated by angioplasty, some form of direct arterial surgery has also been required, usually for bypass of a second lesion distal to the one successfully treated by angioplasty.[1,6]

PTA has also been effective in the treatment of stenotic lesions in tibial arteries and stenoses developing in or proximal or distal to a still-functioning vein or PTFE graft.[1,56,61]

RESULTS OF TREATMENT

Arteriosclerotic involvement is generally less, both in regard to extent and multiplicity of lesions, in patients with intermittent claudication than in those whose limb is threatened. It is therefore not surprising that the short-term and long-term patency results of infrainguinal arterial bypasses performed for intermittent claudication are generally better than those done for limb salvage, and this difference has been documented by virtually every author who evaluated his results on the basis of operative indications.[37,64] Since we believe that femoropopliteal bypass should rarely be performed for intermittent claudication and that the other infrainguinal bypasses should never be performed for this indication alone, we will restrict our discussion of results to operations performed because of severe ischemic rest pain, a nonhealing ulcer, or gangrene. However, it is true that many respected vascular surgeons still believe that femoropopliteal bypasses for truly disabling claudication are justified by their good results and low risk rate,[2] and we do not disagree with this opinion, provided the patient is informed of the risks of intervention. In our ex-

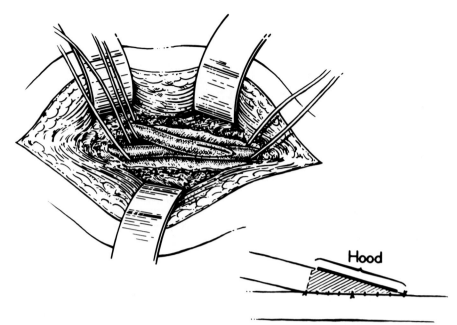

FIGURE 27–9. Technique for a reoperation in which graft salvage will be attempted. Control of the artery proximal and distal to the anastomosis must be obtained. The opening in the graft is placed so that the interior of the anastomosis can be visualized.

perience, when patients are so informed, they usually opt for noninterventional treatment.

Results of infrainguinal bypasses clearly vary with the training, technical skill, and commitment of the surgeon. These operations are demanding and should be performed only by surgeons doing them regularly and, more importantly, by surgeons with the skill and commitment to reoperate successfully should a bypass fail in the early or late postoperative period. In deciding whether these operations and an aggressive approach to limb salvage are in fact justified in a given setting, every vascular surgeon should continually examine his or her own results to see if they are good enough to justify continued application of these sometimes difficult operations in these often brittle patients.

Operative Mortality

The 30-day mortality for all patients undergoing infrainguinal arterial reconstructions for threatened limbs ranges from 2 to 6 per cent.[1,6,65] Operative mortality is slightly greater for infrapopliteal and axillopopliteal bypasses than for femoropopliteal bypasses, probably because the former operations are required in patients with more advanced generalized as well as lower extremity disease. The principal cause of death from these operations is myocardial infarction.

These low operative mortalities contrast with the high late-death rates reflected in Figure 27–10, which shows that only 48 per cent of all patients that had arterial reconstructions were alive 5 years later. Almost all late deaths were unrelated to the original operation, most being due to intercurrent arteriosclerotic events, chiefly myocardial infarction. These findings again reflect the advanced stage of generalized arteriosclerosis present in these patients.

Limb Salvage

When the aggressive approach already outlined for the management of patients whose limbs are threatened by infrainguinal arteriosclerosis was used and when only those patients who had organic mental syndrome and extensive local gangrene were excluded, 96 per cent of patients underwent arteriographic examination.[6] Ninety-four per cent of patients who underwent arteriography were suitable candidates for some form of arterial revascularization procedure. With recent technical advances only 1 to 2 per cent of patients undergoing arteriography do not have some patent distal artery suitable for use in an attempt at revascularization, and most of these are patients who have previous failed operations.[1]

Immediate Limb Salvage

Defined as relief of ischemia and healing of ischemic lesions for 1 month after the first revascularization procedure, immediate limb salvage was achieved in 86 per cent of patients in whom revascularization was possible.[6] This immediate limb salvage rate was calculated by subtracting from the number of patients who could undergo revascularization procedures those patients who died or whose arterial reconstructive operation and/or angioplasty failed irretrievably within 1 month of the primary

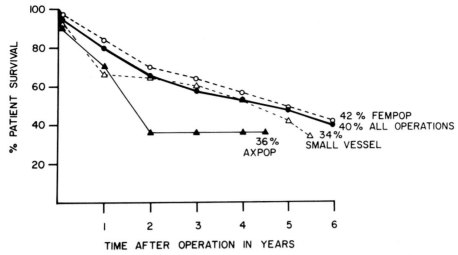

FIGURE 27–10. Cumulative life-table patient survival rates after 318 femoropopliteal (*FEMPOP*), 204 small vessel (infrapopliteal), and 29 axillopopliteal (*AXPOP*) bypasses. Fifty-two per cent of all patients undergoing all reconstructive arterial operations for limb-threatening infrainguinal arteriosclerosis were dead within 5 years. (From Veith FJ, Gupta SK, Samson RH, et al: Progress in limb salvage by reconstructive arterial surgery combined with new or improved adjunctive procedures. Ann Surg *194*:386–400, 1981.)

procedure, and those patients who required major amputations despite a successful revascularization procedure. Multiple (four to seven) local operations and 2 to 4 months of hospitalization were required to achieve foot healing in 7 per cent of our patients. Heel and forefoot gangrene did not preclude ultimate limb salvage, although they could, if extensive, contribute to the need for prolonged periods of hospitalization. Even when the initial procedure attempted to achieve limb salvage failed immediately, the involved extremity could often be saved by promptly performing some secondary procedure.[1,6,57] This was particularly common if a PTA was technically unsuccessful or failed to improve the arterial supply to the foot.[1,6,59]

Late Limb Salvage

The cumulative limb salvage rates for all patients having arterial reconstructive operations are shown in Figure 27–11. Sixty-six per cent of the patients who survived 5 years after a reconstructive arterial operation below the inguinal ligament for limb salvage had an intact limb up to that time. The limb salvage rates were better after femoropopliteal bypass than after a small vessel bypass or an axillopopliteal bypass (*p* < .25) (Fig. 27–12). Even though all operations were performed because the limb was threatened, limb salvage rates (Fig. 27–12) could not be equated by bypass patency rates (Fig. 27–13). In some patients, gangrene and infection had been healed by the original operation and the limb remained intact when the bypass thrombosed; moreover, in many instances when the limb was rethreatened, bypass patency could be restored by appropriate reoperation. This was particularly common if the original procedure had been a femoropopliteal bypass.[51] On the other hand, limb salvage rates could be rendered lower than bypass

patency rates if a major amputation was required despite a patent arterial reconstruction.

Patency of Arterial Reconstructive Operations

Older cumulative life-table patency rates for reconstructive arterial operations are shown in Figure 27–13. More recent patency rates have improved somewhat and continue to be significantly better for femoropopliteal bypasses than for small vessel or axillopopliteal bypasses (*p* < .01). Our small vessel bypass patency rate was not affected by age, sex, hypertensive or diabetic status, or previous ipsilateral bypass. In contrast to reports from other groups, an incomplete plantar arch, a heavily calcified bypass insertion site, an unusable saphenous vein, and a very low ankle pressure did not preclude long-term success, although these factors were associated with a somewhat higher early failure rate.[1,6]

Recent Results

Several recent reports have documented better late limb salvage and bypass patency results than those presented. While some of these apparently improved results may reflect more refined surgical and management techniques, these more optimistic recent reports have generally only included patients operated on by a particular surgical technique, such as reversed vein bypass or in situ vein bypass. Since these techniques, although ideal, are not applicable to all patients with a threatened lower extremity, it is probable that the older statistics that are presented above are still representative of the overall results that can be achieved

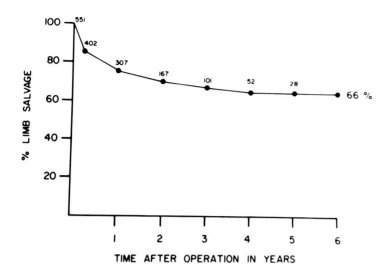

FIGURE 27–11. Cumulative life-table limb salvage rates of all patients undergoing reconstructive arterial operations for limb-threatening infrainguinal arteriosclerosis. The number with each point indicates the number of cases observed with intact limbs for that length of time. (From Veith FJ, Gupta SK, Samson RH, et al: Progress in limb salvage by reconstructive arterial surgery combined with new or improved adjunctive procedures. Ann Surg *194*:386–400, 1981.)

in an entire group of patients undergoing lower limb arterial reconstruction to save an extremity. Moreover, some of the more recent articles with favorable late bypass patency results are actually reporting secondary patency figures that are achievable with a more aggressive policy of detecting and reintervening on failing bypasses; and some recent reports include results on substantial numbers of patients undergoing operation for intermittent claudication. Thus, while some recent improvements in results may be real, much of it is due to patient selection and differences in the methods of reporting or analyzing results.

Angioplasty Durability

Eleven per cent of our iliac angioplasties and 8 per cent of our femoropopliteal angioplasties were initially unsuccessful. If one considers the durability of those angioplasties that were initially successful, cumulative life-table patency at 4 years was 78 per cent for the iliac angioplasties and 50 per cent for the femoropopliteal angioplasties. Repeat angioplasty after late failure had a poor durable success record, and we no longer consider secondary angioplasty with enthusiasm. However, appropriate surgery when an angioplasty failed and a limb was rethreatened resulted in protracted limb salvage in more than 70 per cent of cases. Generally, the operative procedure was the same one that would have been performed had the angioplasty not been selected as the initial interventional treatment. These facts, coupled with our angioplasty mortality of 1 per cent in this elderly, sick group of patients, indicate that the risk of angioplasty failure is not excessive. We therefore continue

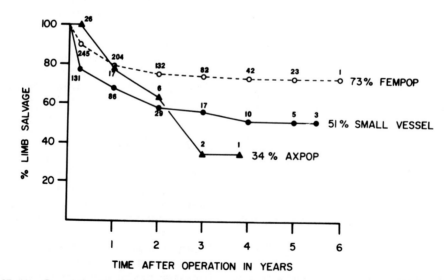

FIGURE 27–12. Cumulative life-table limb salvage rates of 318 femoropopliteal (*FEMPOP*), 204 small vessel, and 29 axillopopliteal (*AXPOP*) bypasses performed for limb-threatening infrainguinal arteriosclerosis. The number with each point indicates the number of cases observed with intact limbs for that length of time. (From Veith FJ, Gupta SK, Samson RH, et al: Progress in limb salvage by reconstructive arterial surgery combined with new or improved adjunctive procedures. Ann Surg *194*:386–400, 1981.)

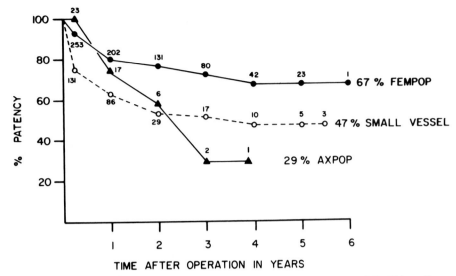

FIGURE 27–13.   Cumulative life-table patency rates of 318 femoropopliteal (*FEMPOP*), 204 small vessel, and 29 axillopopliteal (*AXPOP*) bypasses performed for limb-threatening infrainguinal arteriosclerosis. The number with each point indicates the number of cases observed to be patent for that length of time. (From Veith FJ, Gupta SK, Samson RH, et al: Progress in limb salvage by reconstructive arterial surgery combined with new or improved adjunctive procedures. Ann Surg *194*:386–400, 1981.)

to regard PTA, when performed by a committed radiology-surgery team, as an important part of an aggressive approach to salvaging limbs.[1] However, 81 per cent of patients with threatened limbs will require operative treatment at some point in their course; only 19 per cent can be treated by PTA alone.[1]

Reoperations

Our policy of performing a graft thrombectomy on all thrombosed small vessel and axillopopliteal bypasses, if and when the thrombosis was associated with a threat to the limb, has not resulted in any operative deaths, but has generally been unrewarding. The majority of such reoperated grafts rethrombosed within a few days, weeks, or months. In occasional instances, comprising approximately 10 per cent of such reoperated cases, patency was restored and persisted more than 3 years.

Thus, our present policy for the treatment of failed small vessel bypass if the limb is rethreatened is to perform an entirely new bypass to another unoperated segment of an infrapopliteal artery. Our results with such secondary small vessel bypasses have not differed greatly from those of primary procedures, although others have not had a similar experience.

The results of aggressive reoperation for failed vein and nonvein *femoropopliteal bypasses* have been surprisingly good.[1,6,51,57,66,67] In our series of 318 femoropopliteal bypasses, 13 failed *during the first month after operation* and all were treated by reoperation. There was one postoperative death and two late deaths among the patients with patent bypasses, 3 and 14 months after operation. Eight of the 10 other bypasses have been patent for 2 to 44 months (mean:

25 months). The ninth patient has a viable limb 26 months after the original operation, although the graft rethrombosed 1 year ago, and the tenth patient also has a viable limb 4 months after the original operation, although her graft reoccluded 2 months after her reoperation.

Thirty-nine of our femoropopliteal bypasses failed *more than 1 month after operation* and were considered for aggressive reoperation. A conservative approach to a failed bypass that did not place the limb in jeopardy has been justified by the continued viability for 2 to 72 months of all eight limbs in this category. Reoperation was performed in the remaining 31 patients with threatened limbs. In 28 patients, bypass patency was reestablished for at least 2 months. In 20 patients, graft patency has persisted until death or the present. The range of patency after reoperation in this group of 20 patients is 2 to 48 months, with a mean of over 17 months, although seven patients have required a secondary reoperation to maintain bypass patency and limb viability. Sixteen grafts have remained open more than 1 year after reoperation. Only 8 of the 39 patients in whom late graft occlusion occurred ultimately required a major amputation, and in all but two instances this could be successfully performed below the knee. One of the 31 patients died within 1 month of the reoperation.

The sustained effectiveness of appropriate reoperations when limb salvage femoropopliteal bypasses fail in the early or late postoperative period is illustrated by Figure 27–14, which shows that reoperation increased overall patency rates by 15 per cent at 5 years. When the same calculations were applied to 440 cases with longer periods of follow-up, this difference between primary and secondary patency rates at 5 years fell to 8 per cent. Limb salvage rates are,

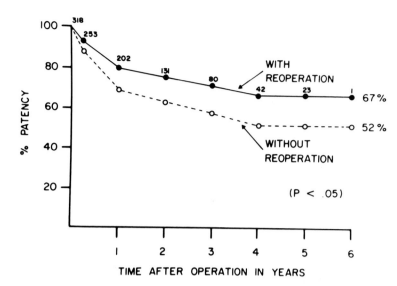

FIGURE 27–14. Cumulative life-table patency rates of 318 femoropopliteal bypasses performed for limb salvage. The upper curve was calculated without regard to whether or not a reoperation was required to maintain patency. The lower curve was calculated on the basis of time to first bypass occlusion even if reoperation restored patency. The number with each point indicates the number of cases observed to be patent for that length of time. (From Veith FJ, Gupta SK, Samson RH, et al: Progress in limb salvage by reconstructive arterial surgery combined with new or improved adjunctive procedures. Ann Surg 194:386–400, 1981.)

of course, similarly increased by effective reoperations. The efficacy of such reoperations in maintaining durable patency is further shown by the cumulative life-table 4- to 6-year patency rate of 56 per cent for our 44 femoropopliteal bypasses requiring reoperation for thrombosis. Limb salvage rates were even higher. Similar patency rates and limb salvage rates have also been achieved by Whittemore and his colleagues, who employed reoperations in the management of a group of patients with failed vein femoropopliteal bypasses and threatened limbs.[57] Both Whittemore's group, we, and many other groups have found that detection of *failing* reconstructions *before* graft thrombosis has occurred permits simpler corrective measures to be used and results in much better long-term graft patency and limb salvage.[55–57]

Although Craver and his colleagues showed many years ago that reoperation for early postoperative thrombosis of femoropopliteal vein grafts was associated with poor long-term patency rates,[68] we have found this not to be the case with PTFE bypasses above the knee,[51] and Whittemore and his associates have reported similar protracted successes after reoperation for failure of saphenous vein femoropopliteal grafts.[57] Appropriate use of intraoperative angiography and other technical details of these reoperations are important in achieving the reported good results. In both series, surgical clot removal from thrombosed vein and PTFE grafts sometimes allows these conduits to be used effectively for protracted periods if all other lesions encroaching substantially on the lumen are corrected or bypassed.[51,57]

Lytic Agents

Recently a number of reports have appeared advocating the use of intraarterially administered streptokinase and particularly urokinase to restore patency to thrombosed infrainguinal grafts. While these agents may ultimately prove to be useful to treat failed grafts

and to detect the cause of failure, PTA or surgical graft revision is almost always required to correct the lesion causing thrombosis. Moreover, the long-term efficacy of such combined procedures remains to be demonstrated, and in most patients we still believe that a totally new bypass is the best treatment for a thrombosed graft that is associated with limb-threatening ischemia.

Arteriographic Outflow Characteristics of the Popliteal Artery and Patency

With significant numbers of patients now followed for 5 years or more, patency rates of femoropopliteal bypasses inserted into popliteal artery segments that appeared on arteriograms to be occluded at both ends were not significantly different from those of bypasses inserted into popliteal arteries that appeared to be continuous with one or more of their main terminal branches. These results support the use of femoropopliteal bypass to isolated segments of popliteal artery in preference to small vessel bypass in most circumstances.[20,69] This appears to be true even when the absence of a usable saphenous vein makes it necessary to use a PTFE graft. A major disadvantage of such use of isolated popliteal segments is the high incidence of continued threat to the limb despite a patent bypass. This is particularly common if there is extensive gangrene or infection in the foot.[20] In such circumstances, a femoral-to-popliteal-to-small vessel bypass or sequential bypass is indicated and it is best to perform the distal-most portion of this complex bypass with autologous vein if it is available in any of the patient's extremities.[19,20,70,71]

Relationship of Position of Anastomosis to Patency

In our hands, femoropopliteal bypass patency was not significantly influenced solely by the position of the distal anastomosis relative to the knee joint. This was true with both PTFE and vein grafts. Other patient-related factors are probably more important in determining patency than is the location of the popliteal anastomosis. These factors are not controlled in any study comparing above-knee and below-knee results, thereby rendering the comparisons meaningless in terms of selecting the best level of popliteal artery to use if it is patent above and below the knee in a given patient.

Amputation Level

When major amputation was required after a revascularization procedure had been performed, every effort was made to perform it at the below-knee level. This was possible in all 18 patients who required amputation despite a patent bypass, in 90 per cent of patients who required a major amputation when a femoropopliteal bypass occluded, in 69 per cent of patients who required a major amputation after a failed small vessel bypass, and in 30 per cent of major amputations required after thrombosis of an axillopopliteal bypass.[6] Operative mortality rate for these secondary amputations was 4 per cent.

ANALYSIS OF COST-BENEFIT RATIO OF AGGRESSIVE EFFORTS AT LIMB SALVAGE

Our results indicate that more than 98 per cent of patients whose limbs are threatened because of infrainguinal arteriosclerosis have a distribution of occlusive and stenotic arterial lesions that is suitable for reconstructive arterial surgery, which can relieve the ischemia at least partially and salvage the limb. The results also show that it is possible to obtain immediate limb salvage in more than 85 per cent of the patients in whom revascularization is possible, with an operative mortality rate of less than 4 per cent and a low morbidity rate despite the existence in many patients of local and systemic factors that might, in the past, have precluded attempts at revascularization and limb salvage. These factors include advanced age, recent congestive heart failure or myocardial infarction, concurrent malignancy, expensive forefoot or heel gangrene, a contralateral amputation, an isolated popliteal artery segment, absence of usable saphenous vein, and the presence of a popliteal pulse with three-vessel occlusive disease in the upper, middle, and lower thirds of the leg.

The fact that limbs can now be saved in such circumstances is of interest. Alone it does not mean that limb salvage attempts, which may require multiple operations and prolonged periods of hospitalization to obtain a healed foot, are justified in this group of patients, whose life expectancy is known to be poor. Is the cost-benefit ratio such that attempts at limb salvage are worthwhile in these patients?

This is a difficult question to answer with certainty since, in part, the answer depends on one's philosophy and perspective and on subjective factors such as quality of life and the ability to live and function independently. However, certain objective parameters are relevant. Among these are the durability of limb salvage in surviving patients and the longevity of the patients. Figure 27–10 is an index of patient longevity. Figure 27–11 is a measure of the durability of limb salvage in surviving patients. Of the 48 per cent of patients who survived 5 years after operation, two thirds retained their limb at least that long. It is also relevant to know that of every 100 patients who underwent operation, 68 lived at least 1 year after operation with an intact limb, and 54 lived at least 2 years with a viable, usable extremity. Moreover, of the 52 per cent of the patients who died within 5 years, 88 per cent (81 to 95 per cent) retained the salvaged limb until they died (Fig. 27–15). Both we and almost all of our patients believe that these benefits outweigh the risks and costs of an aggressive attempt at limb salvage, even if this attempt entails a lengthy period of hospitalization with several operative procedures to achieve a healed foot. Similar conclusions have been reached by Reichle and Tyson, Maini and Marnick, and Perdue, Bartlett, and Auer and their colleagues in their analyses of patients with limb-threatening ischemia.[65,66,72–74]

A case can also be made for performing a primary below-knee amputation in some or all of these patients, and relatively rapid rehabilitation may be achieved with such a procedure.[75,76] However, our experience has shown that the older, poor-risk patients do not ambulate easily or quickly with a below-knee prosthesis. Such patients may never walk and, if they do, they may require 2 or 3 months of institutional training to learn. For some patients, limb salvage offers the only opportunity for them to care for themselves, maintain their independence, and avoid permanent admission to an institution. Furthermore, in many patients the opposite limb soon becomes threatened because of the symmetry of the disease process, and salvage of at least one limb is critical for the patient to maintain independence. Finally, the point has been made that unsuccessful attempts at limb salvage result in a high incidence of loss of the knee.[37,76,77] Our data fail to confirm this except after failed axillopopliteal bypass, a procedure performed in patients with the most advanced disease. Thus, we believe that limb salvage should be attempted if suitable vessels for revascularization are present, unless the patient has severe organic mental syndrome or gangrene and infection proximal to the midfoot.

Economic Impact of Limb Salvage

The dollar cost of an aggressive approach to salvage limbs is high, with a mean cost of $19,000 for femoropopliteal bypass and $29,000 for small vessel bypass. These figures include all physician, hospital,

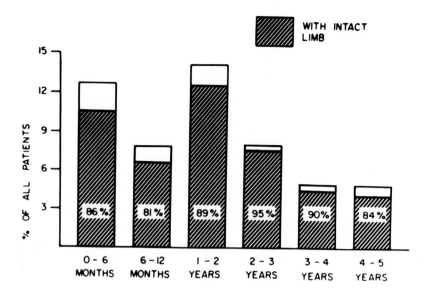

FIGURE 27–15. Percentage of all patients who underwent limb salvage attempts and who died in the various intervals after operation. The cross-hatched areas indicate the proportion of these patients who died without losing their previously threatened limb. (From Veith FJ, Gupta SK, Samson RH, et al: Progress in limb salvage by reconstructive arterial surgery combined with new or improved adjunctive procedures. Ann Surg 194:386–400, 1981.)

and rehabilitation costs, including those of reoperations. On the other hand, the mean total cost of below-knee amputation, which in 26 per cent of our patients resulted in failed rehabilitation with a need for chronic institutional care or professional assistance at home, was $27,000. Thus, limb salvage surgery is expensive but no more so than the less attractive alternative of amputation.[78]

NEW DEVELOPMENTS

Clearly all the principles and practices outlined thus far describe our present attitudes toward the treatment of a complex disease process. As we have tried to point out, many of these attitudes are controversial. More importantly, they are all in a state of constant evolution. As more data and newer methodology become available, our attitudes and those of others interested in the problems of femoral-popliteal-tibial arteriosclerosis should and will change. In this section we will describe briefly some of the new developments that have the greatest likelihood of leading to future therapeutic improvements.

Digital (Computer-Assisted) Venous Angiography and Arteriography

This method of visualizing the arterial tree using computer-augmented imaging after a central venous injection of contrast medium holds great promise, since it avoids some of the risks associated with an arterial puncture. However, it has not achieved great utility as a guide to the treatment of infrainguinal arteriosclerosis because the field of visualization is small and the resolution less than that of the standard arteriography already described. Digital studies have been and may become increasingly useful in assessing graft patency and following patterns of disease

progression at and just proximal and distal to anastomotic sites. Moreover, digital image augmentation can improve the visualization of distal small arteries following an intraarterial contrast injection, although we have seldom found it necessary for these purposes except to help visualize patent arterial segments near the ankle or in the foot in an occasional patient.

Improvements in Arterial Prosthetics

Endothelial seeding of prosthetic grafts is probably the most interesting recent development in vascular prosthetics. Methods have been developed to seed fabric prostheses and expanded PTFE grafts with autologous endothelial cells.[79] These cells migrate preferentially to and cover the luminal surface of the graft and may decrease the tendency for thrombosis and intimal hyperplasia. This technique offers hope of leading to a substantial improvement in vascular prosthetics. However, this promise must be validated in clinical trials, and such validation has yet to be reported.

Outflow Resistance Measurements

In an effort to predict which infrainguinal bypasses will fail with greater accuracy than has heretofore been possible, our group and others have measured outflow resistance during femoropopliteal and infrapopliteal bypasses.[21] This work, which is based on a simple intraoperative method of measurement, has shown that this parameter is an accurate predictor of early success and failure. Outflow resistance has correlated poorly with angiographic evaluation of so-called runoff characteristics.[21] This probably explains why angiographically determined factors have been such a poor predictor of graft patency. Although of little value in femoropopliteal bypasses, outflow resistance measurements have been helpful in small vessel bypasses in which they can serve as a guide to which patients should have sequential bypasses and which patients should *not* be subjected to reoperation for early graft failure.[21] However, the method is still time consuming and cumbersome. It has, therefore, not gained widespread acceptance.

Other New Developments in Tibial Bypass

Over the last 12 years, because of some of the promising results already discussed, we have been evaluating other procedures to simplify or extend the limits of operability for limb salvage. Some of these procedures show sufficient promise to deserve mention.

Tibiotibial bypasses are an extension of our concept of using more distal arteries as bypass origins than were previously thought optimal.[24] All these distal origin procedures allow shorter segments of saphenous vein to be used, shorten operative time, avoid dissection in obese or infected groins, and may have superior patency. We have now performed more than 70 distal vein bypasses to the lower third of the leg or foot using the infrapopliteal (tibial arteries) as inflow sites.[22] Many of these grafts remained patent more than 4 years despite their insertion into isolated tibial artery segments and the fact that they were performed with saphenous veins 2.5 to 3.0 mm in smallest diameter (Figs. 27–1, 27–2, 27–3).

Small vessel bypasses to blind tibial artery segments have been performed in some patients facing imminent amputation. These operations have been done in patients in whom no other procedures were possible because of the arterial anatomy or local infection in the foot. Again, vein grafts were used. Several of these bypasses have remained patent over 2 years and many otherwise unsalvageable limbs have been saved.[22]

Use of heavily calcified tibial arteries for distal bypass insertion sites has been possible with a variety of techniques that include crushing of the involved artery to permit occlusion, incision, and suture placement. Acceptable early and midterm patency has resulted.[6]

Intraoperative Transluminal Angioplasty

Intraoperative transluminal angioplasty is now possible with a variety of different techniques.[80] This procedure should be useful in patients with combined segment disease. The intraoperative dilation of stenoses proximal or distal to an occlusive lesion should make shorter bypasses possible. Although such procedures have considerable theoretical appeal, their value remains to be demonstrated by comparison with standard operative procedures and with standard, separate PTA combined with standard operations.

REFERENCES

1. Veith FJ, Gupta SK, Wengerter KR, et al: Changing arteriosclerotic disease patterns and management strategies in lower limb-threatening ischemia. Ann Surg 212:402–414, 1990.
2. Donaldson MC, Mannick JA: Femoropopliteal bypass grafting for intermittent claudication. Is pessimism warranted? Arch Surg 115:724–727, 1980.
3. Boyd AM: The natural course of arteriosclerosis of the lower extremities. Proc R Soc Med 55:591–593, 1962.
4. Coran AG, Warren R: Arteriographic changes in femoropopliteal arteriosclerosis obliterans: A five year follow-up study. N Engl J Med 274:643–645, 1966.
5. Imparato AM, Kim GE, Davidson T, Crowley JG: Intermittent claudication: Its natural course. Surgery 78:795–797, 1975.
6. Veith FJ, Gupta SK, Samson RH, et al: Progress in limb salvage by reconstructive arterial surgery combined with new or improved adjunctive procedures. Ann Surg 194:386–401, 1981.
7. Goodreau JJ, Greasy JK, Flanigan DP, et al: Rational approach to the differentiation of vascular and neurogenic claudication. Surgery 84:749–757, 1978.
8. Kavanaugh GJ, Svien HJ, Holman CB, Johnson RM: "Pseudoclaudication" syndrome produced by compression of the cauda equina. JAMA 206:2477–2481, 1968.
9. Karmody AM, Powers SR, Monaco VJ, Leather RP: Blue toe syndrome: An indication for limb salvage surgery. Arch Surg 111:1263–1268, 1976.
10. Haimovici HC, Moss CM, Veith FJ: Arterial embolectomy revisited. Surgery 78:409–411, 1975.
11. Gupta SK, Samson RH, Veith FJ: Embolectomy of the distal part of the popliteal artery. Surg Gynecol Obstet 153:254–258, 1981.
12. Whittemore AD, Clowes AW, Hechtman HB, Mannick JA: Aortic aneurysm repair: Reduced operative mortality associated with maintenance of optimal cardiac performance. Ann Surg 192:414–420, 1980.
13. Sprayregen S: Principles of angiography. In Haimovici H (ed): Vascular Surgery, Principles and Techniques. New York, McGraw-Hill, 1976, pp 39–66.
14. Flanigan DP, Williams LR, Keifer T, et al: Prebypass operative arteriography. Surgery 92:627–633, 1982.
15. Sapala JA, Szilagyi DE: A simple aid in greater saphenous phlebography. Surg Gynecol Obstet 140:265–266, 1975.
16. Veith FJ, Moss CM, Sprayregen S, Montefusco CM: Preoperative saphenous venography in arterial reconstructive surgery of the lower extremity. Surgery 85:253–255, 1979.
17. Rivers SP, Scher LA, Gupta SK, Veith FJ: Safety of peripheral vascular surgery after recent myocardial infarction. J Vasc Surg 11:70–76, 1990.
18. Mannick JA, Jackson BT, Coffman JD: Success of bypass vein grafts in patients with isolated popliteal artery segments. Surgery 61:17–35, 1967.
19. Flinn WR, Flanigan DP, Verta MJ, et al: Sequential femoral-tibial bypass for severe limb ischemia. Surgery 88:357–365, 1980.
20. Veith FJ, Gupta SK, Daly V: Femoropopliteal bypass to the isolated popliteal segment: Is polytetrafluoroethylene graft acceptable? Surgery 89:296–303, 1981.
21. Ascer E, Veith FJ, Morin B, et al: Components of outflow resistance and their correlation with graft patency in lower extremity arterial reconstructions. J Vasc Surg 1:817–825, 1984.

22. Veith FJ, Ascer E, Gupta SK, et al: Tibiotibial vein bypass grafts: A new operation for limb salvage. J Vasc Surg 2:552–557, 1985.

23. Ascer E, Veith FJ, Gupta SK: Bypasses to plantar arteries and other tibial branches: An extended approach to limb salvage. J Vasc Surg 8:434–441, 1988.

24. Veith FJ, Gupta SK, Samson RH, et al: Superficial femoral and popliteal arteries as inflow site for distal bypasses. Surgery 90:980–990, 1981.

25. Gupta SK, Veith FJ, Ascer E, et al: Five year experience with axillopopliteal bypass for limb salvage. J Cardiovasc Surg 26:321–324, 1985.

26. Veith FJ, Moss CM, Daly V, et al: New approaches in limb salvage by extended extraanatomic bypasses and prosthetic reconstructions to foot arteries. Surgery 84:764–774, 1978.

27. Towne JB, Bernhard VM, Rollins DL, Baum PL: Profundaplasty in perspective: Limitations in the long-term management of limb ischemia. Surgery 90:1037–1046, 1981.

28. Campbell CD, Brook DH, Webster MW, et al: Expanded microporous polytetrafluoroethylene as a vascular substitute: A two-year follow-up. Surgery 85:177–183, 1979.

29. Gupta SK, Veith FJ: Three year experience with expanded polytetrafluoroethylene arterial grafts for limb salvage. Am J Surg 140:214–217, 1980.

30. Veith FJ, Moss CM, Fell SC, et al: Comparison of expanded polytetrafluoroethylene and autologous saphenous vein grafts in high risk arterial reconstructions for limb salvage. Surg Gynecol Obstet 147:749–752, 1978.

31. Quiñones-Baldrich WJ, Busuttil RW, Baker JD, et al: Is the preferential use of polytetrafluoroethylene grafts for femoropopliteal bypass justified? J Vasc Surg 8:219–228, 1988.

32. Bergan JJ, Veith FJ, Bernhard VM, et al: Randomization of autogenous vein and polytetrafluoroethylene grafts in femoral-distal reconstruction. Surgery 92:921–930, 1982.

33. Veith FJ, Gupta SK, Ascer E, et al: Six year prospective multicenter randomized comparison of autologous saphenous vein and expanded polytetrafluoroethylene grafts in infrainguinal arterial reconstructions. J Vasc Surg 3:104–114, 1986.

34. Dardik H, Baier RE, Meenaghan M, et al: Morphologic and biophysical assessment of long term human umbilical cord vein implants used as vascular conduits. Surg Gynecol Obstet 154:17–26, 1982.

35. Cranley JJ, Karkow WS, Hafner CD, Flanagan LD: Aneurysmal dilatation in umbilical vein grafts. In Bergan JJ, Yao JST (eds): Reoperative Arterial Surgery. Orlando, FL, Grune & Stratton, 1986, pp 343–358.

36. Kenney AD, Sauvage LR, Wood SJ, et al: Comparison of noncrimped, externally supported (EXS) and crimped, nonsupported Dacron prosthesis for axillofemoral and above knee femoropopliteal bypasses. Surgery 92:931–946, 1982.

37. Szilagyi DE, Hageman JH, Smith RF, et al: Autogenous vein grafting in femoropopliteal atherosclerosis. The limits of its effectiveness. Surgery 86:836–851, 1979.

38. Szilagyi DE, Smith RF, Elliot JP, Hageman JH: The biologic fate of autogenous vein implants as arterial substitutes: Clinical, angiographic and histopathologic observations in femoropopliteal operations for atherosclerosis. Ann Surg 178:232–244, 1973.

39. Kent KC, Whittemore AD, Mannick JA: Short-term and midterm results of an all autologous tissue policy for infrainguinal reconstruction. J Vasc Surg 9:107–114, 1989.

40. Hall KV: The great saphenous vein used "in-situ" as an arterial shunt after extirpation of the vein valves. Surgery 51:492–495, 1962.

41. Leather RP, Shah DM, Karmody AM: Infrapopliteal bypass for limb salvage: Increased patency and utilization of the saphenous vein used "in situ." Surgery 90:1000–1008, 1981.

42. Leather RP, Shah DM, Chang BB, et al: Resurrection of the in situ vein bypass: 1000 cases later. Ann Surg 205:435–442, 1988.

43. Gruss JD, Bartels D, Vargas H, et al: Arterial reconstruction for distal disease of the lower extremities by the in situ vein graft technique. J Cardiovasc Surg 23:231–234, 1982.

44. Taylor LM, Edward JM, Porter JM: Present status of reversed vein bypass: Five year results of a modern series. J Vasc Surg 11:207–215, 1990.

45. Wengerter KR, Gupta SK, Veith FJ, et al: Critical vein diameter for infrainguinal arterial reconstructions. J Cardiovasc Surg 28:109, 1987.

46. Towne JB, Schmidt DD, Seabrook GR, Bandyk DF: The effect of vein diameter on early patency and durability of in situ bypass grafts. J Cardiovasc Surg 30:64, 1989.

47. Schulman ML, Bradley MR: Late results and angiographic evaluation of arm veins as long bypass grafts. Surgery 92:1032–1041, 1982.

48. Harris RW, Andros G, Dulana LB, et al: Successful long-term limb salvage using cephalic vein bypass grafts. Ann Surg 200:785–794, 1984.

49. Veith FJ, Gupta SK: Femoral-distal artery bypasses. In Bergan JJ, Yao JST (eds): Operative Techniques in Vascular Surgery. New York, Grune & Stratton, 1980, pp 141–150.

50. Oblath RW, Buckley FO, Green RM, et al: Prevention of platelet aggregation and adherence to prosthetic vascular grafts by aspirin and dypyridamole. Surgery 84:37–44, 1978.

51. Veith FJ, Gupta SK, Ascer E, Rivers SP, Wengerter KR: Improved strategies for secondary operations on infrainguinal arteries. Ann Vasc Surg 4:85–93, 1990.

52. Veith FJ, Ascer E, Nunez A, et al: Unusual approaches to infrainguinal arteries. J Cardiovasc Surg 28:58, 1987.

53. Nunez A, Veith FJ, Collier P, et al: Direct approach to the distal portions of the deep femoral artery for limb salvage bypasses. J Vasc Surg 8:576–581, 1988.

54. Veith FJ, Ascer E, Gupta SK, Wengerter KR: Lateral approach to the popliteal artery. J Vasc Surg 6:119–123, 1987.

55. O'Mara CS, Flinn WR, Johnson ND, et al: Recognition and surgical management of patent but hemodynamically failed arterial grafts. Ann Surg 193:467–476, 1981.

56. Veith FJ, Weiser RK, Gupta SK, et al: Diagnosis and management of failing lower extremity arterial reconstructions. J Cardiovasc Surg 25:381–384, 1984.

57. Whittemore AD, Clowes AW, Couch NP, Mannick JA: Secondary femoropopliteal reconstruction. Ann Surg 193:35–42, 1981.

58. Bandyk DF, Cata RF, Towne JB: A low flow velocity predicts failure of femoro-popliteal and femoro-tibial bypass grafts. Surgery 98:799–809, 1985.

59. Samson RH, Sprayregen S, Veith FJ, et al: Management of angioplasty complication, unsuccessful procedures and early and late failures. Ann Surg 199:234–240, 1984.

60. Gruntzig A, Kumpe DA: Technique of percutaneous transluminal angioplasty with the Gruntzig balloon catheter. Am J Roentgenol 132:547–552, 1979.

61. Ring EJ, Alpert JR, Frieman DB, et al: Early experience with percutaneous transluminal angioplasty using a vinyl balloon catheter. An Surg 191:438–442, 1980.

62. Alpert JR, Ring EJ, Freiman DB, et al: Balloon dilatation of iliac stenosis with distal arterial surgery. Arch Surg 115:715–717, 1980.

63. Kadir S, Smith GW, White RI Jr, et al: Percutaneous transluminal angioplasty as an adjunct to the surgical management of peripheral vascular disease. Ann Surg 195:786–795, 1982.

64. DeWeese JA, Robb CG: Autogenous venous grafts ten years later. Surgery 82:775–784, 1977.

65. Reichle FA, Tyson R: Comparison of long-term results of 364 femoropopliteal or femorotibial bypasses for revascularization of severely ischemic lower extremities. Ann Surg 182:449–455, 1975.

66. Bartlett ST, Olinde AJ, Flinn WR, et al: The reoperative potential of infrainguinal bypass: Long-term limb and patient survival. J Vasc Surg 5:170–179, 1987.

67. Boontje AH: Occlusion of femoropopliteal bypasses (Biograft). J Cardiovasc Surg 25:385–390, 1984.
68. Craver JM, Ottinger LW, Darling RC, et al: Hemorrhage and thrombosis as early complications of femoropopliteal bypass grafts: Causes, treatment and prognostic implications. Surgery 74:839–845, 1973.
69. Davis RC, Davies WT, Mannick JA: Bypass vein grafts in patients with distal popliteal artery occlusion. Am J Surg 129:421–425, 1975.
70. DeLaurentis DA, Friedman P: Arterial reconstruction above and below the knee. Another look. Am J Surg 121:392–397, 1971.
71. Edwards WS, Gerety E, Larkin J, Hoyt TW: Multiple sequential femoral tibial grafting for severe ischemia. Surgery 80:722–728, 1976.
72. Auer AI, Hurley JJ, Binnington HB, et al: Distal tibial vein grafts for limb salvage. Arch Surg 118:597–602, 1983.
73. Maini BS, Mannick JA: Effect of arterial reconstruction on limb salvage: A ten-year appraisal. Arch Surg 113:1297–1304, 1978.
74. Perdue GD, Smith RB, Veazey CR, Anslery JD: Revascularization for severe limb ischemia. Arch Surg 115:168–171, 1980.
75. Hobson RW, Lynch TG, Jamil Z, et al: Results of revascularization and amputation in severe lower extremity ischemia: A five-year clinical experience. J Vasc Surg 2:205–213, 1985.
76. Stoney RJ: Ultimate salvage for the patients with limb-threatening ischemia: Realistic goals. Am J Surg 136:228–232, 1978.
77. Ramsburgh SR, Lindenauer SM, Weber IR, et al: Femoropopliteal bypass for limb salvage surgery. Surgery 81:453–458, 1977.
78. Gupta SK, Veith FJ, Samson RH, et al: Cost analysis of operations for infrainguinal arteriosclerosis. Circulation 66(suppl II): II–9, 1982.
79. Stanley JC, Burkel WE, Ford JW, et al: Enhanced patency of small diameter, externally supported Dacron iliofemoral grafts seeded with endothelial cells. Surgery 92:994–1005, 1982.
80. Fogarty TJ, Chin A, Shoor PM, et al: Adjunctive intraoperative arterial dilatation: Simplified instrumentation technique. Arch Surg 116:1391–1398, 1981.

REVIEW QUESTIONS

1. Which of the following statements concerning arterial emboli is generally *not* true?
   (a) the only certain way to diagnose an embolic occlusion is the demonstration that the occlusive process is multifocal
   (b) emboli are often associated with moderate or severe atherosclerosis
   (c) the treatment of emboli is generally simple and results are almost uniformly good
   (d) angiography is usually indicated for lower extremity emboli
   (e) emboli can be effectively removed even after several days

2. Bypasses to arteries below the popliteal should be performed for limb salvage with PTFE grafts:
   (a) when there is no acceptable autologous vein in the involved lower extremity
   (b) only when there is no autologous vein available in any of the patient's four extremities
   (c) in no circumstances
   (d) only to the posterior tibial artery
   (e) none of the above

3. Heavily calcified incompressible tibial arteries are a contraindication to their use in limb salvage arterial bypasses. True or false?

4. It has been clearly shown that in situ vein bypasses are uniformly superior to reversed vein bypasses. True or false?

5. The standard arteriogram for femoropopliteal occlusive disease should visualize all arteries from the renals to the forefoot. True or false?

6. Preferential use of PTFE grafts for above-knee femoropopliteal bypass is justified in patients whose life expectancy is less than:
   (a) 1 year
   (b) 2 years
   (c) 3 years
   (d) 4 years
   (e) none of the above

7. Bypass to a tibial artery at the ankle level or in the foot is indicated for disabling intermittent claudication:
   (a) occasionally
   (b) almost never
   (c) rarely
   (d) infrequently
   (e) very infrequently

8. Toe amputation or foot débridement should never be combined with an arterial revascularization. True or false?

9. The presence of pedal pulses is evidence of sufficiently good circulation in the foot that a toe amputation for infection is likely to heal. True or false?

10. Patients who have had an infrainguinal bypass that fails and who again have a threatened limb have a poor chance of having the foot saved by a secondary revascularization. True or false?

ANSWERS

1. c 2. b 3. False 4. False 5. True 6. b 7. b
8. False 9. True 10. False

28

INFLUENCE OF DIABETES MELLITUS ON THE PATTERNS AND COMPLICATIONS OF VASCULAR OCCLUSIVE DISEASE

EDWARD A. STEMMER

The signs and symptoms of diabetes mellitus and even some of its complications have been known since ancient times. The Ebers papyrus (1500 B.C.) prescribes a treatment for polyuria, and writers in the Vedic literature (1500 to 200 B.C.) were aware that diabetic urine was sweet. Aretaeus, the Cappadocian, who lived in Alexandria in the first and second centuries A.D., is usually credited with the first systematic description of diabetes. He described the excessive thirst, constant need to urinate, dry mouth, parched skin, and loss of weight associated with the disease and coined the word "diabetes," which means "to run through a siphon." Japanese and Chinese physicians of the second and third centuries A.D. referred to diabetes as "the malady of thirst" and were aware that diabetics often developed furunculosis. Avicenna, a Persian physician at the turn of the 10th century, observed that diabetics were vulnerable to gangrene of the extremities.[1,2] The fact that diabetic urine is sweet was rediscovered in 1674 by an English physician, Thomas Willis. The possibility that diabetes might be a consequence of disease or injury of the pancreas was suggested in 1788 by another English physician, Thomas Cawley. At the same time, William Cullen added the qualifying adjective "mellitus" (from the Latin or Greek; "honey") to the term "diabetes," since glycosuria was a constant feature of the disease. Experimental confirmation of Cawley's hypothesis was accomplished by Von Mering in 1886 when he produced phloridzin diabetes. A Baltimore pathologist, George MacCallum, pointed out the relationship between the islets of Langerhans and glycosuria in 1909.[3] The isolation of insulin in 1921 by Banting, an orthopedic surgeon, and Best, then a medical student, was to have a profound effect not only on the lifespan of

the diabetic but on the incidence and mortality of vascular disease associated with diabetes mellitus.[4]

Prior to the isolation of insulin by Banting and Best in 1921, the average length of life of a diabetic after diagnosis was 4.9 years. Death was usually due to infection or diabetic coma. As diabetics lived longer, their greater vulnerability to vascular disease became apparent. At present, 84 per cent of diabetics who live longer than 20 years after diagnosis will have some form of vascular disease. Seventy-five per cent of diabetics now die of vascular disease or its complications, primarily myocardial infarction and stroke.[2,5]

DIABETES MELLITUS AND VASCULAR DISEASE

Although deficiency or impairment of the action of insulin is the essence of diabetes mellitus, it is clear that the disease is not a single entity but a group of diseases that have in common an inability of the body to utilize carbohydrate normally. It is also clear that diabetes mellitus involves more than a mere deficiency in the production of insulin by the body.[6] Diabetes mellitus can be produced by excessive activity of glucocorticoids, growth hormone, or catecholamines (and perhaps glucagon) as well as by pancreatitis and pancreatectomy. Most cases of diabetes mellitus, however, arise spontaneously for reasons that are not clearly known. Currently, the disease is characterized as either insulin-dependent diabetes mellitus (IDDM) or non–insulin-dependent diabetes mellitus (NIDDM). The first of these terms includes the older classification of type I or juvenile diabetes, whereas the second includes the older classifications of type II, adult- or maturity-onset diabetes. Genetic factors are clearly important in the etiology of both types of diabetes mellitus. For example, relatives of diabetics develop the disease 4 to 10 times more frequently than do relatives of nondiabetics.[1,7] Also, a family history of diabetes can be obtained in at least 25 per cent of diabetic patients. The incidence of diabetes in both of monozygotic twins is 70 per cent, in contrast to 10 per cent in dizygotic twins.[1,5] There are also racial differences in the incidence of diabetes. The disease is almost nonexistent in Eskimos, but affects 40 per cent of Pima Indians.[1]

For a time it was generally accepted that diabetes mellitus was inherited via a mendelian recessive gene. The heterozygous individual was prone to develop NIDDM, while the homozygous individual developed IDDM. Differences in outcome were attributed to differences in gene penetration.[8] At the present time, diabetes mellitus is thought to be multigenic in origin, with genetic heterogeneity characterizing both NIDDM and IDDM. Other factors also appear to be important to the clinical expression of diabetes in patients who are genetically vulnerable to the disease. Viral infections are associated with the development of juvenile diabetes, while obesity clearly plays a role in the development of adult-onset disease. In addition, it has been shown that there is a clear and consistent association of juvenile, insulindependent diabetes with specific human leukocyte antigen (HLA) loci.[8,9] The mixture of familial, genetic, metabolic, and immunologic factors involved in the development of diabetes mellitus has led to its description as a geneticist's nightmare.[10]

The reason for the increased incidence of vascular disease in the diabetic remains unknown. Although some believe that the association of vascular disease and diabetes mellitus is a chance occurrence, there seems to be little doubt now that vascular disease in the diabetic occurs earlier in life, is more extensive, is different in distribution, and is more likely to result in amputation and premature death than in the nondiabetic.[1,5,11–13] Three hypotheses have been proposed. The first hypothesis proposes that the vascular disease is secondary to the derangement of carbohydrate, protein, and fat metabolism. This hypothesis is based primarily on observations that the frequency of vascular lesions increases with the duration of diabetes and that the retinal and renal vascular disease characteristic of diabetes can occur in patients with nongenetic diabetes who have chronically elevated blood sugars. The second hypothesis proposes that the vascular disease seen in diabetics is due to genetic traits separate and independent from those responsible for the metabolic abnormality but inherited with some form of linkage. This hypothesis is based on the observations that some patients can have severe renal or retinal disease with only borderline, subclinical carbohydrate disorders and that two diabetic parents can produce offspring that have normal glucose tolerances but still have significant thickening of the capillary basement membranes, a lesion that is characteristic of the small vessel disease seen in clinical diabetics. Support for this second hypothesis was gained from a study of Mandrup-Poulson, who reported in 1984 that a genetic marker linked to the incidence of atherosclerosis was present proximal to the human insulin gene.[14] The third hypothesis proposes an immunologic cause of diabetic vascular disease because of the resemblance of small vessel disease in diabetics to that observed in patients with various immune disorders.[15]

Whatever the specific etiology of vascular disease in diabetics might be, the diabetic with vascular disease shares the risk factors that are commonly found in nondiabetics with vascular disease. These include abnormalities of lipid metabolism, obesity, hypertension, and a diet that is often high in fat content. Elevated triglyceride levels are commonly found in diabetics. In fact, triglyceride abnormalities are more commonly found in diabetics with arterial disease than is hypercholesterolemia. Conversely, the relatively few diabetics without vascular disease have triglyceride and cholesterol levels indistinguishable from nondiabetic patients without vascular disease. Obesity is a common finding in diabetics, particularly those with adult-onset diabetes. Joslin et al. reported that 77 per cent of 1000 diabetics were overweight at the time of diagnosis, while only 8 per cent were below normal weight.[16] Both systolic and diastolic hypertension are more common in diabetics than in nondiabetics, particularly in the 20- to 39-year age group. The restricted carbohydrate diet often prescribed for diabetics is necessarily higher in fat content if total calories are to remain unchanged. It is of interest to note that Japanese diabetics who consume a diet higher in carbohydrate but lower in fat than diabetics in western countries have very little coronary or peripheral atherosclerosis.[17] The Framingham Study, evaluating these factors in both diabetics and nondiabetics, concluded that while hypertension, obesity, and lipid abnormalities were present in the diabetic population with vascular disease, they could not completely explain the high incidence of vascular disease in these patients.[11,17,18]

There is little doubt that a unique linkage exists between vascular disease and diabetes mellitus. White, in the 1940s, noted that 50 per cent of children with diabetes for more than 15 years were found to have calcification of the leg vessels.[16] In contrast to experience in nondiabetics with vascular disease, the prevalence of atherosclerosis in diabetic women is the same as that in diabetic men at all ages. Moreover, diabetics of both sexes have a higher incidence of vascular disease than nondiabetics of the same age.[12,13] Wahlberg and Thomasson reported that 61 per cent of oral glucose tolerance tests and 55 per cent of intravenous glucose tolerance tests were abnormal in patients with atherosclerosis in the absence of overt or previously diagnosed diabetes mellitus.[19] The prognosis of the diabetic patient with vascular disease is much poorer than that of the nondiabetic with vascular disease. Silbert and Zazeela[20] reported that, in a series of 1198 patients with vascular disease, 10 per cent of nondiabetic patients were dead 10 years after diagnosis and 33 per cent were dead 15 years after the diagnosis of vascular disease was made. The corresponding figures for diabetics with vascular disease were 38 and 69 per cent, respectively.[20]

Vascular disease in the diabetic presents in two distinct forms. Macroangiopathy affects the large- and medium-sized arteries. It occurs most commonly in patients with maturity-onset diabetes (over 25 years of age), rarely produces clinical disease in the child or adolescent, and is morphologically indistinguishable from atherosclerosis occurring in nondiabetics. It typically produces disease of the coronary and cerebral arteries and the vessels supplying the lower limbs.[11,21,22] Microangiopathy is a pathologic process occurring almost exclusively in diabetics and most often affects the insulin-dependent or juvenile diabetic. The process takes place in the vessel wall of the capillary, precapillary arteriole, and postcapillary venule. It is characterized microscopically by thickening of the basement membranes of the involved vessels. On a clinical level, microangiopathy produces progressive disease primarily in three organ systems—the kidney, the eye, and the nervous system—although the process may contribute to diseases of the skin, peripheral circulation, and microcirculation of the heart (a small vessel disease). Microangiopathy is the process responsible for the formation of retinal microaneurysms and the development of nodular glomerulosclerosis (Kimmelstiel-Wilson syndrome).[11,22] Retinopathy and nephropathy due to microangiopathy become major problems in the younger patient and progress with increasing duration of diabetes.

While the duration of diabetes is strongly related to the incidence of macroangiopathy, the severity of diabetes and its degree of control have little or no relationship to the development of atherosclerosis. The development, incidence, and severity of microangiopathy does seem to be related to the degree and duration of hyperglycemia. Both forms of vascular disease often exist in the same patient, particularly as the diabetic ages.[1,15]

INSULIN IN DIABETIC VASCULAR DISEASE

The primary targets of insulin are the metabolic activities of the liver, muscle, and adipose tissue. Other tissues, such as the vascular intima and nerves, respond more slowly to changes in the blood level of insulin. Greatly simplified, the action of insulin in a normal individual can be described as follows: in response to an elevated blood sugar, elevated levels of insulin act on the liver, muscle, and fat depots to remove metabolic fuels from the circulation by consumption or storage; as the levels of insulin fall, the storage areas release their respective fuels into the circulation. Balodimos and Cahill describe this se-

quence of events as the feeding-fasting types of metabolism.[15]

In addition to its effects on blood sugar, insulin also plays an important role in protein and fat metabolism. It is essential for the uptake of dietarily derived triglyceride into the fat stores. In a normal individual, glucose is converted into fat by insulin acting in the fat storage areas. A lesser amount of glucose is converted into fat by the liver and then transported by the bloodstream. In an insulin-deficient or -resistant individual the liver takes over a larger share of fat synthesis, with the result that blood levels of triglycerides rise. At the same time the antilipolytic effects of insulin decrease or cease, also resulting in a rise of blood lipid levels. The implications of these two metabolic abnormalities in atherogenesis are obvious and may account in part for the earlier and more extensive atherosclerosis seen in diabetics.[1,15] The relatively greater hypertriglyceridemia seen in diabetics has already been described.

DIABETES MELLITUS AND SEPSIS

It is well known that diabetics are much more vulnerable to infection, particularly spreading infection, than are nondiabetics. Moreover, infection with the same organism may be more severe in the diabetic. For example, infection with *Escherichia coli* may present the picture of gas gangrene. Saprophytic fungi, which rarely cause disease in normal humans, can produce a spreading and even fatal infection in diabetics. Infection is the most common factor in the initiation of diabetic ketoacidosis. The combination of infection and ischemia can make treatment of vascular disease in the diabetic many times more difficult than in the nondiabetic and can adversely affect the outcome of surgery.

Increased tissue levels of glucose may be a factor in the increased incidence of spreading or progressive infection in the diabetic, but it seems more probable that the increased vulnerability of diabetics to infection is due to increased exposure to infectious agents or decreased ability to mobilize effective defenses.[1] Polymorphonuclear cell function, as measured by leukocyte chemotaxis, adherence to vascular endothelium, phagocytosis, or intracellular killing activity, is depressed in some diabetics, particularly those in ketosis. Serum opsonic activity and cell-mediated immunity are also depressed. Small vessel disease not only impairs the natural responses to infection but also makes chemotherapy of the infection less effective.[1,23]

Since the discovery of insulin, deaths from sepsis in the diabetic population have decreased markedly. Nevertheless, there is still disagreement as to whether strict control of the blood sugar offers better protection against sepsis than less strict but adequate control of the blood sugar. Studies by Rayfield indicate that tight control of the blood sugar in diabetics (less than 230 mg/dl) will help prevent certain infections and ensure normal host defense mechanisms.[23]

Management of insulin requirements in diabetics undergoing surgery, particularly those with infection, is of critical importance. Not infrequently, diabetics undergoing surgery for gangrene of an extremity or even those undergoing vascular reconstruction have major degrees of infection as well. Preoperatively, these patients may be toxic, with high insulin requirements. Following correction of the vascular problem and drainage or elimination of the associated infection, the insulin requirement may fall abruptly. Since many adult diabetics have associated coronary arterial and cerebrovascular disease, the goal of insulin management during the perioperative period in these patients should be prevention of ketoacidosis and avoidance of hypoglycemia, with its attendant hypotension. The safety zone for the blood sugar level during the perioperative period lies between 150 and 250 mg/dl.[24]

DIABETIC NEUROPATHY

The frequency with which the nervous system is affected in diabetics was responsible for the earlier view that diabetes was caused by disease of the nervous system. The converse was established by Calvi in 1864.[25]

The etiology of diabetic neuropathy has been variously ascribed to accumulation of sorbitol metabolites in the nerve tissues, decreased levels of myoinositol, defective myelin synthesis, malnourishment in poorly controlled diabetics, and/or microvascular disease of the nervous system.[1,25,26] The evidence best indicates that it is due to a combination of ischemia secondary to microvascular disease and the metabolic abnormalities that occur in poorly controlled diabetics. The disease can affect single or multiple motor and sensory nerves, cranial nerves, the spinal cord, and the autonomic nervous system in various patterns. Both demyelination and axonal disease occur in diabetic neuropathy as well as degeneration in the posterior columns of the spinal cord secondary to loss of dorsal root ganglion cells. Degeneration of sympathetic ganglion cells also occurs.[25] The disease is seen as a complication of early-onset insulin-dependent diabetes, maturity-onset diabetes, nonalcoholic pancreatic diabetes, and hemochromatosis.

The incidence of diabetic neuropathy varies from 5 to almost 100 per cent depending on the closeness of examination and the symptoms that are accepted as evidence of neuropathy. Five to 10 per cent of diabetics have weakness or sensory loss. Forty-five per cent of diabetics have pain and paresthesias. Thirteen to 21 per cent show abnormal signs such as loss of tendon reflexes in the legs, loss of vibration sense, loss of position sense, or loss of sensation. Radiographs may demonstrate rarefaction of bone and destruction of joints. The small joints of the feet are those most often affected, but the ankle and knee can also be involved. Charcot's joints may result from loss of sensation in the limb. Deep and usually painless trophic ulcers of the plantar surface of the foot are a common complication of diabetic neuropathy. If very sensitive methods of measurement are used, neuropathy may be detected in almost all diabetics. Nerve involvement is common by the 5th to 10th year of diabetes, although it is a rare finding in patients younger than 15 years of age.[1,15]

Clinical findings of neuropathy may be the first evidence of diabetes. The earliest and most common manifestation of neuropathy is a diffuse sensory disturbance usually involving both legs in a stockinglike distribution. Men and women are affected equally. Eighty-five per cent of clinical cases occur in patients over the age of 40 years. There seems to be a good correlation between the occurrence of neuropathy and the degree of control of diabetes, but the incidence of neuropathy does not correlate with the degree of atherosclerosis of large- or medium-sized vessels. Symptoms in the upper extremities are less common than those in the legs, but upper extremity involvement may be severe enough to prevent the diabetic from learning braille. Autosympathectomy of the lower extremities can result from involvement of the autonomic nervous system. Most of the morbidity related to diabetic neuropathy is a result of undetected injuries due to sensory loss.[27]

Treatment of diabetic neuropathy is, for the most part, unsatisfactory. Some motor lesions recover spontaneously and in many instances stricter control of the blood sugar will help diabetic amyotrophy. Quinine, 0.3 gm at bedtime, may relieve the nocturnal cramps associated with diabetic neuropathy. There are no satisfactory methods for relieving the hyperesthesias, paresthesias, and neuropathic pain. Vitamins are of no benefit in the treatment of diabetic neuropathy.

PATTERNS OF VASCULAR DISEASE

The life expectancy of diabetics at any age and in either sex is lower than that of the general population. However, the later in life that diabetes makes its clinical appearance, the less its effect on survival. For example, the median survival of female diabetics in whom the diagnosis is established before age 30 years is 25 years less than that of the general female population. For female diabetics in whom the diagnosis is established between the ages of 30 and 49 years, median survival is 12 years less than the general population. Female diabetics with onset of the disease between the ages of 50 and 69 years have a median survival 5 years less than the general population. After age 70 at diagnosis, survival in female diabetics is only 2 years less than the general population. Male diabetics follow the same pattern, although the differences in survival are not as great prior to age 70 and disappear after age 70.[28] The major cause of death in diabetics is arteriosclerosis. Fifty-four per cent of deaths are due to cardiac disease; 11 per cent to stroke; 7 per cent to renal disease, and 12 per cent to cancer. Less than 1 per cent of deaths are directly the result of gangrene. In the general population, the corresponding percentages are cardiac, 38 per cent; stroke, 11 per cent; renal, 0.5 per cent; and cancer, 17 per cent.[29] A unique characteristic of vascular disease in the diabetic is that the male-female ratio approaches 1 in all sites.[30] Clinically proven diabetics, who constitute 1 to 2 per cent of the general population, make up 30 to 50 per cent of all patients who are operated upon for peripheral vascular disease and 65 to 75 per cent of patients undergoing vascular reconstruction in the lower leg and malleolar areas.[31,32] Peripheral vascular disease is the most common indication for surgery in the diabetic.

Cerebrovascular Disease

Until recently, there was not general agreement that cerebrovascular accidents were more common in diabetics than in nondiabetics. Warren et al.[33] found no difference in the two groups, whereas Palumbo[34] stated that the incidence of both strokes and transient ischemic attacks was increased in diabetics. Balodimos, quoting Alex and Entmaker, reported that while there was no difference in the incidence of cerebral hemorrhage in diabetics and nondiabetics, cerebral infarction was found more commonly in diabetics.[15,35] Kannell, reporting the results of the Framingham Study, noted that in a population 45 to 74 years old the incidence of stroke was 2.7 times higher in diabetic males than in nondiabetic males. In females the ratio was 3.8:1. The increased rate of stroke for diabetics persisted even after correction for associated risk factors such as hypertension.[30] Aronow, reporting the results of a 36-month prospective study of 708 patients ranging in age from 62 to 103 years, noted that atherothrombotic brain infarction occurred 3 times more commonly in diabetic men and 2.3 times more commonly in diabetic women than in their nondiabetic counterparts.[36]

Diabetic Retinopathy

Diabetic retinopathy is one of the common sequelae of microangiopathy in the diabetic. Overall it affects approximately 25 per cent of diabetics and has become the third most common cause of blindness in the United States. Although fluorescein angiography can often demonstrate microaneurysms early in the course of diabetes, ophthalmoscopic evidence of retinopathy is unusual in the first 5 to 10 years of the disease. The frequency of retinopathy approaches 50 per cent in those who have had diabetes for more than 10 years. The incidence of retinopathy rises to 65 per cent after 15 years of disease and to 80 per

cent after 30 years of diabetes regardless of the age of onset. Proliferative retinopathy is less common than nonproliferative retinopathy, but its prognosis for useful vision is much graver. Photocoagulation and vitrectomy in selected patients can preserve or improve vision in a significant number of patients. If all causes of legal blindness are included, diabetes is the most common disease associated with new-onset blindness in patients aged 20 to 74 years. Patients with diabetes have a sixfold increased risk of blindness compared to nondiabetics.[37]

Coronary Arterial Disease

Clinical evidence of coronary arterial disease is present in approximately 40 per cent of all diabetics. Conversely, an abnormal glucose tolerance test is found in from 45 to 65 per cent of patients with coronary arterial disease. Sixteen to 20 per cent of patients operated upon for angina pectoris are clinical diabetics. The incidence of coronary arterial disease in the male diabetic is 1.7 times that in the nondiabetic male, while in the female diabetic the ratio is 2.7:1. Correction for factors other than diabetes does not change these ratios.[37] Not only is coronary arterial disease more frequent in diabetics than in nondiabetics, it is more severe and more diffuse. Hertzer et al., in 1984, reviewed a series of 1000 coronary angiograms performed in patients under consideration for peripheral vascular surgery. He noted that inoperable coronary arterial disease was discovered in 12 per cent of diabetics but only 4.5 per cent of nondiabetics.[38] At autopsy, myocardial infarction is found two to five times more frequently in diabetics than nondiabetics. Coronary arterial disease is the cause of death in over 50 per cent of diabetic patients above the age of 40 years.[15,39]

The risk of death following acute myocardial infarction is also significantly greater in the diabetic than in the nondiabetic. Even in modern coronary care units diabetics suffer a higher in-hospital mortality than do nondiabetics. In a combined series, Kereiakes reported a 31 per cent mortality in the diabetic compared to a 19 per cent mortality in the nondiabetic.[40] Moreover, there was an increased incidence of congestive heart failure and shock in the diabetic patients. Mortality for those patients receiving insulin or oral hypoglycemic therapy was greater than for those diabetics controlled by diet alone. Female diabetics had a 40 per cent greater mortality during acute infarction than male diabetics.[40] The reported 5-year survival for diabetics postinfarction is 25 to 38 per cent compared to 50 to 75 per cent for nondiabetics.[39–41] The causes of death in the diabetic with coronary arterial disease are primarily recurrent infarction, heart failure, and dysrhythmia. The microangiopathy that is characteristic of diabetes mellitus can also affect the heart, producing diabetic cardiomyopathy and congestive heart failure even in the absence of significant coronary arterial stenosis.[34,39]

Peripheral Vascular Disease

General Considerations

Intermittent claudication is the symptom that most frequently leads to a diagnosis of peripheral vascular disease.[20,42] Using claudication as an index, the prevalence of peripheral vascular disease in the diabetic population between the ages of 45 and 74 years is four to six times greater than that in the nondiabetic population even when corrections are made for risk factors other than diabetes. Herman et al. reported that peripheral vascular disease affected 10 per cent of the diabetic population in Rochester, Minnesota but only 2.6 per cent of the nondiabetic population.[37] Other studies have indicated that arteriosclerosis is 11 times more frequent in diabetics than in controls and develops about 10 years earlier in diabetic patients than in nondiabetic patients.[43] Moreover, diabetic vascular disease does not spare the female. Juergens et al. noted that in a series of nondiabetic patients with onset of symptoms of vascular disease before age 60 years, only 8 per cent of the patients were women.[44] By contrast, the ratio of males to females in diabetics with vascular disease approaches 1.[30,45]

Long-term survival is poorer in diabetics with vascular disease at all ages with or without vascular reconstruction. Silbert noted that the 10-year mortality for diabetics was 38 per cent compared to 11 per cent for nondiabetics.[20] The same authors found that survival of nondiabetics with peripheral vascular disease approximated that of the normal population without diabetes or peripheral vascular disease. Bartlett et al., reviewing the results of aortic reconstruction in 100 patients, noted a 36 per cent 9-year survival in diabetics compared to a 73 per cent survival in nondiabetics.[46] Imparato et al., reviewing 60 patients followed for 6 years after femorotibial bypass, noted a cumulative survival of 66 per cent in diabetics in contrast to 79 per cent in nondiabetics.[47] The major cause of death in both diabetic and nondiabetic patients was myocardial infarction.

Most authors who have studied vascular disease have noted that the disease is more diffuse in diabetics and is more distal in the arterial tree. For example, approximately 12 to 17 per cent of patients undergoing aortoiliac reconstruction are diabetic, while 65 to 75 per cent of patients undergoing femorotibial bypasses are diabetic.[31,32,48,49] Diabetics with vascular disease also present with different types of symptoms than do nondiabetics. Steer et al. found that, in a group of 332 patients, the incidence of ulceration or gangrene with or without rest pain among the diabetic group was 1.86 times greater than among the nondiabetic group.[50]

Intermittent Claudication

Intermittent claudication is generally believed to be a relatively benign symptom of peripheral vascular disease, since only infrequently does it lead to gangrene or amputation of the extremity. The classic study cited to support this opinion was performed in Manchester, England by Boyd in 1962. In that study, Boyd reported a 10-year follow-up of 1476 patients who presented with intermittent claudication but without gangrene or pregangrenous changes.[51] He found that the amputation rate for males averaged 1.4 per cent per year, with a 5-year amputation rate of 7 per cent and a 10-year amputation rate of 12 per cent. The survival rate of patients with intermittent claudication approximated that of a general population 10 years older. No mention is made of the number of diabetics in the study population.[51] The Framingham Study[52] (1970) and that of Imparato et al.[53] (1975) also support the conclusion that intermittent claudication, of itself, does not lead to limb loss very often.

The studies of Juergens et al. (1961) and Jonason and Ringqvist (1985), however, indicate that intermittent claudication may not be as benign a disease in diabetics as it is in nondiabetics. In Juergens et al.'s study the amputation rate in diabetics over a 9-year period was 27.1 per cent versus a 3.8 per cent incidence in uncomplicated nondiabetics (i.e., those without hypertension or angina).[54] In Jonason and Ringqvist's study 12.8 per cent of diabetics underwent amputation over a 6-year period of follow-up compared to only 0.5 per cent of nondiabetics.[55] This difference led Jonason and Ringqvist to state that a more aggressive surgical approach to intermittent claudication in the diabetic might prevent future amputations. They based their opinion, in part, on the observation that only 23 per cent of the diabetic patients with peripheral vascular complications had below-knee stenosis compared with 56 per cent of diabetics without complications. Patients with rest pain or gangrene at presentation were excluded from follow-up in the study by Jonason and Ringqvist. In both studies the survival of diabetics was markedly worse than the survival of nondiabetics (54.4 versus 75.7 per cent and 50 versus 74 per cent at 5 and 6 years in the respective studies).

Additional evidence for the more serious prognosis of intermittent claudication in the diabetic is provided by McAllister's study of 100 consecutive patients followed from 1 to 18 years for claudication.[56] Thirteen of the patients were diabetic. Symptoms of peripheral vascular disease worsened in 16 of the 87 nondiabetics (18 per cent) and 6 of the 13 diabetics (46 per cent) with an average follow-up of 6 years. Only one of the nondiabetics came to amputation (1 per cent) but six of the diabetics (46 per cent) required amputation during the study period.[56]

Aortoiliac Disease

In 1985, approximately 30,000 aortoiliofemoral bypass procedures were performed in the United States.[57] The relative incidence of aortoiliac disease in diabetics is about half that in nondiabetic patients, reflecting the greater incidence of distal disease in the diabetic.[58] Gensler et al. reported that 13.4 per cent of atherosclerotic lesions occurred in the aortoiliac region in diabetics, while 25 per cent of atherosclerotic lesions occurred in the aortoiliac region in nondiabetics.[59] While there is some variation between series, from 11 to 17 per cent of patients undergoing aortoiliofemoral surgery are diabetics.[48,60,61] Long-term graft patency and limb salvage rates are somewhat less in diabetics than in nondiabetics, but long-term survival is markedly reduced in diabetic patients (36 versus 73 per cent at 9 years).[46,61] Other authors have found that diabetics with iliac artery occlusion have a higher incidence of amputation than do nondiabetics with iliac arterial disease (46 versus 16 per cent).[20]

Profunda Femoris Disease

It is generally believed that the profunda femoris artery is spared in patients with atherosclerotic disease. Mavor, in a series of 104 patients, found the profunda femoris artery spared in all instances.[62] However, others have found arteriosclerotic changes in one third of those profunda femoris arteries examined in diabetics, in contrast to one tenth of those vessels in nondiabetic patients. In addition, 75 per cent of diabetic patients with disease at the orifice of the profunda femoris artery were found to have disease in the distal segments of that vessel.[63] There is a marked decrease in graft patency, limb salvage, and survival in diabetics when compared to nondiabetics undergoing profundaplasty.[64,65] Malone et al. reported that at 36 months 85 per cent of nondiabetics had patent profundaplasties, whereas the patency rate in diabetics was zero.[65] The poorer results in diabetics were clearly related to the more advanced stage of disease and greater distal involvement present in the diabetic group at the time of operation.

Femoropopliteal Disease

The relative incidence of femoropopliteal disease is essentially the same in diabetics and nondiabetics. However, the diabetic patient with arteriosclerosis has a much higher incidence of disease distal to the popliteal artery than does the nondiabetic. Conversely, the diabetic with tibioperoneal disease almost always has proximal arterial disease, with the femoropopliteal segment being the most frequent site.[66,67] Disease at the trifurcation is also more common in the diabetic compared with the nondiabetic (81 versus 71 per cent).[68] In instances of acute femoral artery occlusion, the overall amputation rate has been reported to be 18 per cent. As in the case of iliac occlusion, however, the diabetic is more likely to suffer an amputation following acute occlusion of the femoral artery (32 versus 12 per cent).[20] Long-term patency of femoropopliteal grafts and limb salvage are approximately the same in diabetics and nondiabetics, but the long-term survival of diabetics postoperatively is markedly decreased. Deweese and Rob reported that within 10 years, 92 per cent of diabetics were dead, in contrast to 65 per cent of nondiabetics.[69]

Tibioperoneal Disease

Occlusion of the leg arteries alone occurs in about 25 per cent of patients with atherosclerosis without diabetes. In the diabetic population, however, less than 5 per cent present with atherosclerotic disease restricted to the leg vessels. Moreover, the diabetic typically has more diffuse disease in the leg vessels than the nondiabetic. Involvement of a single leg vessel occurs in 65 per cent of nondiabetic patients but in only 31 per cent of diabetic patients. Conversely, occlusion of two or all three leg vessels occurs in 69 per cent of diabetic patients in contrast to 35 per cent of nondiabetic patients. The peroneal artery is the vessel most frequently spared.[66]

Sixty-five to 75 per cent of patients undergoing tibioperoneal reconstruction are clinical diabetics. Eighty-four per cent of the diabetic patients present with gangrene or nonhealing ulcers as the indication for surgery, in contrast to 66 per cent of the nondiabetics.[31] Rosenblatt et al., comparing distal lower extremity grafts placed in 89 diabetics and 82 nondiabetics, noted no statistically significant difference in graft patency at 4 years. Indications for surgery in the diabetics were more often rest pain, ulceration, or gangrene (93 per cent) than in the nondiabetics (71 per cent). Diabetics underwent a greater number of minor amputations than did the nondiabetics, but had fewer major amputations. Late deaths were more frequent in the diabetic group (18 versus 12 per cent).[70]

In evaluating either diabetic or nondiabetic patients for reconstructive arterial surgery, it is essential that patency and inflow to the pedal vascular arches be demonstrated angiographically. If the anterior or posterior tibial vessels can be shown to communicate with the pedal arch, an initial success rate of 90 to 95 per cent can be expected following reconstruction.[71] Most authors recommend tibioperoneal reconstruction only for limb salvage rather than for treatment of claudication.

THE DIABETIC FOOT

There are three major disease processes that produce what is commonly called the diabetic foot: ischemia, infection, and neuropathy. While each of the three processes may exist independently, they usually occur together in varying degrees, particularly in the older diabetic as the duration of diabetes increases. Approximately 20 per cent of all hospitalizations of the diabetic are for foot problems.

Preventive foot care is of extreme importance in the diabetic, since even seemingly trivial lesions, injuries, or minor infections can lead to loss of an extremity. These preventive measures include:

1. Daily inspection of the feet to detect small ulcerations or injury.
2. Daily washing of the feet and careful drying.
3. Cutting of toenails straight across to avoid ingrown toenails.

4. Avoidance of poorly fitting shoes.
5. Never walking barefoot.
6. Avoiding hot bath water or external application of heat.
7. Avoiding dry, cracking skin by using a skin lubricant (but never applied between the toes).
8. Treatment of epidermophytosis with appropriate antifungal ointment at night and powder during the day.
9. Prompt medical treatment for even the most minor lesions.

Adherence to these precautions can easily mean the difference between correction of an ingrown toenail or callus and a major amputation of an extremity.[1,15,72] The importance of patient education in the prevention of complications of diabetic foot problems is illustrated by Malone et al.'s study, in which a single educational session resulted in a threefold decrease in the number of amputations over the short term.[73]

Ischemic disease of the foot typically presents with cramps and rest pain, although in advanced cases the pain may be severe and unrelenting. Ischemia may be due to proximal arterial lesions, but is due more often to disease of the tibioperoneal vessels or the smaller vessels of the foot. Approximately 40 per cent of diabetics presenting with gangrene of the foot or lower leg will have a palpable popliteal pulse, while 25 to 30 per cent of such patients will have palpable posterior tibial or dorsalis pedis pulses.[74,75] Sixty per cent of diabetics undergoing amputation will have significant occlusive disease in the metatarsal arteries in contrast to 21 per cent of nondiabetics.[76] Ischemic ulcers are extremely painful and classically present over the toes. When they occur as a result of ill-fitting shoes, the ischemic ulcers occur over the medial aspect of the first metatarsal or the lateral aspect of the fifth metatarsal. Ulceration can occur in the pretibial area as a result of trauma or over the heels as a result of prolonged bed rest. Initially, the ischemic ulcers are superficial, but, untreated, they may progress to involve deeper structures. There is usually a prior history of progressive intermittent claudication.[77]

When the diabetic presents with impending or frank gangrene of the foot, the patient should not be treated on an ambulatory basis but should be hospitalized. Radiographs of the foot should be performed to demonstrate osteomyelitis or destruction of bone or joints due to neuropathic lesions.[15] If nonoperative treatment is unsuccessful, either vascular reconstruction for limb salvage or amputation will be necessary. Angiographic studies must include visualization of the leg vessels and pedal arches as described in the preceding section. Amputation should be performed at the lowest level possible as determined by physical exam, angiography, and noninvasive techniques for evaluating the circulation. In general, vascular reconstruction of the leg has a good short-term prognosis if inflow to the pedal vascular arches is present.[71]

Sepsis in the diabetic foot usually begins as a my-

cotic infection (epidermophytosis) leading to maceration between the toes and the development of interdigital fissures or ulcerations that become secondarily infected. Commonly, cultures show a mixture of two or three organisms, particularly *Staphylococcus aureus* and *albus*, hemolytic and nonhemolytic streptococci, and colonic organisms, often *E. coli*. Clostridial infection is rare, but nonclostridial organisms often produce gas in the tissues.[72] Because of the impaired circulation, relatively minor infections can progress to lymphangitis, cellulitis, deep tissue abscesses, osteomyelitis, and ultimately, gangrene. The main indication for surgery in the diabetic with foot infection is suppuration extending beyond the subcutaneous tissue into the subfascial planes and/or the adjacent joints.[78]

Diabetic neuropathy involving the foot presents with sensory disturbances, autonomic nerve involvement, trophic skin lesions, plantar ulceration, and degenerative arthropathy (Charcot's joints). Typically, neuropathic ulcers are deep and painless. Generally they are situated on the ball of the foot over the metatarsal heads or the plantar aspect of the great toe. Loss of pain sensation and repeated, undetected trauma are the most important factors in their development, but ischemia is a contributing factor.[25] When pedal pulses are present, there is no need for amputation unless infection has penetrated to the bone and produced osteomyelitis. Local surgery to provide drainage and avoidance of weight bearing will usually result in healing of the ulcers, although they tend to recur.[72]

GANGRENE AND AMPUTATION

At least 115,000 lower extremity amputations (50 per 100,000 general population) were performed in 1985. These included 31,000 above-knee, 29,000 below-knee, 12,000 foot, and 43,000 toe amputations.[57] Clinical diabetics, who make up approximately 2 per cent of the population, constitute 50 to 66 per cent of the population undergoing amputation.[74,79,80]

Approximately 40 per cent of diabetics who present with gangrene will have the process limited to the toes. In another 40 per cent, gangrene is limited to the foot. In the remaining 20 per cent, gangrene extends to the ankle or higher.[75] Light et al.,[81] reviewing a series of 90 patients who presented with gangrene of one or more toes, reported that 62 per cent of nondiabetic men required only toe amputation for limb salvage. The corresponding figure for diabetic men was 15 per cent. None of the women (diabetic or nondiabetic) achieved limb salvage by amputation alone. If inflow vascular procedures were performed in addition to toe amputation, diabetic men fared as well as nondiabetic men. Diabetic women did not fare as well as nondiabetic women even with the addition of an inflow procedure (73 versus 100 per cent limb salvage). Toe amputation alone did not succeed in any patient with an ankle-brachial index of less than 0.35.[81]

Silbert and Zazeela, following 1198 patients with peripheral vascular disease, observed that 34 per cent of diabetics underwent amputation as contrasted to only 8 per cent of nondiabetics.[20] The amputation rate in female patients was higher than in their male counterparts (male diabetics 29 per cent, male nondiabetics 7 per cent; female diabetics 44 per cent, female nondiabetics 11 per cent). The remaining limb is also in greater jeopardy in the diabetic. In Silbert and Zazeela's study, 30 per cent of diabetics undergoing amputation lost the second leg within 3 years and 51 per cent within 5 years.[20]

SYMPATHECTOMY

The effectiveness of lumbar sympathectomy as a primary or adjunctive treatment of ischemic limbs is controversial, with some studies showing good relief of symptoms and a high degree of limb salvage, while others have shown little or no beneficial effect on symptoms, amputation rate, or amputation level.[82,83] There is general agreement that while sympathectomy may increase blood flow to the skin, it does not improve blood flow to muscle. Even when cutaneous blood flow is increased, it may not be effective at the cellular level.[84] The problem is compounded in diabetics because of their high incidence of neuropathy. DeValle et al. noted a 5-year cumulative success rate of 19 per cent in diabetics as compared with a 51 per cent success rate in a general arteriosclerotic population following sympathectomy for similar indications.[85] Silbert and Zazeela found an 18 per cent amputation rate in nondiabetic patients and a 47 per cent amputation rate in diabetics following lumbar sympathectomy.[20]

Most authors state that lumbar sympathectomy can be considered in diabetic patients, provided arterial reconstruction is not feasible and diagnostic tests show that some degree of sympathetic activity still exists in the affected limb.[42,84,86]

DIABETES AND HEMODIALYSIS

Mortality from renal failure in diabetics is 17 times that of the general population. It is the major cause of death in almost one half of patients who develop diabetes before the age of 15 years.[87] By contrast, only about 6 per cent of maturity-onset diabetics die of nephropathy.[88] The earliest manifestations of nephropathy are found 10 to 15 years after the onset of diabetes. However, death occurs within 10 to 12 years after the onset of proteinuria.[15] Virtually all patients with diabetic nephropathy have diabetic neuropathy as well.

There is no question that maintaining an arteriovenous fistula or shunt in a diabetic patient is more difficult than in the nondiabetic. Peripheral flow, even in the upper extremities, of diabetics is poorer than in nondiabetics, and they tend to have heavy calcification of vessels at the wrist.[89] Infection of the fistula or shunt is three times more common in diabetics. Myocardial infarction and dialysis-related deaths due to fluid overload are eight times more common in diabetics than in nondiabetics.[90] The need to resite a shunt is also more common in diabetics.[91] Anticoagulation is a particular hazard in diabetics because of the increased risk of cerebral hemorrhage and the likelihood that the diabetic's retinopathy will progress if heparinization is employed.[88,91]

Because of these problems, some authors recommend that arteriovenous fistulas be used in diabetics in preference to shunts and that the fistulas be sited more proximally in the arm to obtain better flow.[89,91]

DISCUSSION AND SUMMARY

Diabetic patients of either sex have a higher mortality at any age with or without vascular reconstructive surgery. The differences in median survival are dependent on both the age at which diabetes is diagnosed and the duration of the disease, with diabetes having a lesser effect on survival in the older patient. The number of diabetics dying of vascular disease is increasing both because the incidence of diabetes mellitus is increasing and because diabetics are living longer. While the incidence of vascular disease rises with increasing duration of diabetes, severity of the diabetes or the strictness of its treatment has little or no effect on the development of macroangiopathy. Most surgical series underestimate the percentage of diabetics in the patient population because of the way the disease is recorded in these groups.

It is clear that peripheral vascular disease is more common in the diabetic, occurs earlier in life, is more likely to be diffuse, is more likely to involve the distal circulation, and is more likely to result in amputation, reamputation, and loss of the second limb than is vascular disease in the nondiabetic. Coronary arterial disease and cerebrovascular disease are more common in the diabetic patient and are more likely to have a fatal outcome. The usual male-female ratio of vascular disease is not seen in the diabetic. Not only does peripheral vascular disease differ in distribution in the diabetic and nondiabetic, but the diabetic is more likely to present with rest pain, ulceration, and gangrene. Even when the diabetic presents with claudication as the primary symptom, it is not the benign process so often observed in the nondiabetic. Whether vascular reconstruction in the diabetic has a poorer outcome than in the nondiabetic is not entirely clear. In almost every surgical series, long-term survival of the diabetic patient is clearly worse than that of the nondiabetic patient. In some series, graft patency rates and limb salvage rates are poorer in the diabetic than in the nondiabetic; but even when the differences reach statistical significance, it would appear that they are due to the more advanced disease present in the diabetic preoperatively. Since patients are usually selected for vascular reconstruction on the basis of preoperative or intraoperative arteriography, it is not surprising that graft patency and limb salvage would be comparable in diabetics and nondiabetics. The great majority of postoperative deaths in both diabetics and nondiabetics are the result of cardiac or cerebrovascular disease. From a practical point of view there is consensus among surgeons that diabetics should be selected for reconstructive vascular surgery using the same indications that are employed in nondiabetics.

REFERENCES

1. Felig P: Disorders of carbohydrate metabolism. *In* Bondy PK, Rosenberg LE (eds): Metabolic Control and Disease. Philadelphia, WB Saunders Company, 1980, pp 276–392.
2. Wellman KF, Volk BW: Historical review. *In* Volk BW, Wellman KF (eds): The Diabetic Pancreas. New York, Plenum Press, 1977, pp 1–14.
3. Schmidt JE: Medical Discoveries. Springfield, IL, Charles C. Thomas, 1959, pp 126–128.
4. Lowes E: Insulin, a case history in private research. Private Pract 4(8):31–33, 1972.
5. Loeb RF: Diabetes mellitus. *In* Cecil RL, Loeb RF (eds): Cecil's Textbook of Medicine. Philadelphia, WB Saunders Company, 1951, pp 615–638.
6. Anderson GE: Collier's Encyclopedia, vol 6. New York, PF Collier & Son, 1955, p 436.
7. Rimoin DL: Inheritance in diabetes mellitus. Med Clin North Am 55(4):807–819, 1971.
8. Iris FJM, Scott RS, Mann JI: Genetic factors in diabetes mellitus. *In* Davidson JK (ed): Clinical Diabetes Mellitus, A Problem Oriented Approach, 2nd ed. New York, Thieme Medical Publishing Inc, 1991, pp 58–67.
9. Rotter JI, Anderson CE, Rimoin DL: Genetics of diabetes mellitus. *In* Ellenberg M, Rifkin H (eds): Diabetes Mellitus, Theory and Practice. New York, Medical Examination Publishing Company Inc, 1983, pp 481–503.
10. Thompson JS, Thompson MW: Overview. *In* Thompson JS, Thompson MW (eds): Genetics in Medicine, 3rd ed. Philadelphia, WB Saunders Company, 1980, pp 331–347.
11. Stout RW, Bierman EL, Brunzell JD: Atherosclerosis and disorders of lipid metabolism in diabetes. *In* Vallance-Owen J (ed): Diabetes: Its Physiological and Biochemical Basis. Baltimore, University Park Press, 1975, pp 127–138.
12. Ostrander LD, Francis F, Hayner NS, et al: The relationship of cardiovascular disease to hyperglycemia. Ann Intern Med 62:1188–1198, 1965.
13. Wood P: Diseases of the Heart and Circulation. London, Eyre and Spottiswood, 1968.
14. Mandrup-Poulson T, Mortensen SA, Meinertz H, et al: DNA sequences flanking the insulin gene on chromosome 11 confer risk of atherosclerosis. Lancet 1:250–252, 1984.
15. Balodimos MC, Cahill GF Jr: Diabetes and vascular disease. *In* Conn HL Jr, Horwitz O (eds): Cardiac and Vascular Diseases. Philadelphia, Lea & Febiger, 1971, pp 1284–1294.
16. Joslin EP, Root HF, White P, et al: The Treatment of Diabetes Mellitus, 7th ed. Philadelphia, Lea & Febiger, 1940, p 783.
17. Keen H, Jarett RJ: Macroangiopathy, its prevalence in asymptomatic diabetes. Adv Metab Disord 14(suppl 2):3–9, 1973.
18. Garcia MJ, McNamara PM, Gordon T, et al: Morbidity and mortality in diabetics in the Framingham population. Sixteen year follow-up study. Diabetes 23:105–111, 1974.
19. Wahlberg F, Thomasson B: Glucose tolerance in ischemic cardiovascular disease. *In* Dickens F, Ravelle PJ, Whelan WJ (eds): Carbohydrate Metabolism and Its Disorders. London, Academic Press, 1968.
20. Silbert S, Zazeela H: Prognosis in arteriosclerotic peripheral vascular disease. JAMA 166:1816–1821, 1958.
21. Drash AL, Becker D: Diabetes mellitus in the child: Course, special problems and related disorders. *In* Katzen HM, Mahler RJ (eds): Diabetes, Obesity and Vascular Disease. Washington, DC, Hemisphere Publishing Corp, 1978, pp 615–643.
22. McMillan DE: Deterioration of the microcirculation in diabetes. Diabetes 24:944–957, 1975.
23. Rayfield EJ: Can strict glucose control prevent infections in diabetics? Drug Ther 8(2):33–42, 1983.
24. Levine R: Preparing the diabetic for surgery. Contemp Surg 19(2):41–43, 1981.
25. Thomas PK, Eliasson SG: Diabetic neuropathy. *In* Dyck PJ, Thomas PK, Lambert EH (eds): Peripheral Neuropathy. Philadelphia, WB Saunders Company, 1975, pp 956–981.
26. Greene DA, DeJesus PV, Winegrad AL: Effects of insulin and dietary myoinositol on impaired peripheral motor nerve conduction velocity in acute streptozotocin diabetes. J Clin Invest 55:1326–1336, 1975.
27. Boulton WJM, Knight G, Drury J, et al: The prevalence of symptomatic diabetic neuropathy in an insulin treated population. Diabetes Care 8(2):125–128, 1985.
28. Krowlewski AS, Warram JH, Christlieb AR: Onset, course, complications and prognosis of diabetes mellitus. *In* Marble A, Krall LP, Bradley RF, Christlieb AR, Soeldner JS (eds): Joslin's Diabetes Mellitus. Philadelphia, Lea & Febiger, 1985, pp 251–277.
29. Entmacher PS, Krall LP, Kranczer SN: Diabetes mortality from vital statistics. *In* Marble A, Krall LP, Bradley RF, Christlieb AR, Soeldner JS (eds): Joslin's Diabetes Mellitus. Philadelphia, Lea & Febiger, 1985, pp 278–297.
30. Kannel WB, McGee DL: Diabetes and vascular disease. The Framingham study. JAMA 241:2035–2038, 1979.
31. Andros G, Harris RW, Salles-Cunha SX, et al: Bypass grafts to the ankle and foot. J Vasc Surg 7:785–794, 1988.
32. Rosenbloom MS, Walsh JJ, Schuler JJ, et al: Long-term results of infragenicular bypasses with autogenous vein originating from the distal superficial femoral and popliteal arteries. J Vasc Surg 7:691–696, 1988.
33. Warren S, LeCompte PM, Legg MA: The Pathology of Diabetes Mellitus, 4th ed. Philadelphia, Lea & Febiger, 1966.
34. Palumbo PJ: How to treat maturity onset diabetes mellitus. Geriatrics 32(12):57–63, 1977.
35. Root HF: Prognosis in diabetes. Med Clin North Am 49(4):1147–1161, 1965.
36. Aronow WS, Gutstein H, Lee NH, Edwards M: Three-year follow-up of risk factors correlated with new atherothrombotic brain infarction in 708 elderly patients. Angiology 39:563–566, 1988.
37. Herman WH, Teutsch SM, Geiss LS: Closing the gap: The problem of diabetes mellitus in the United States. Diabetes Care 8:391–406, 1985.
38. Hertzer NR, Beven EG, Young JR, et al: Coronary artery disease in peripheral vascular patients. A classification of 1000 coronary angiograms and results of surgical management. Ann Surg 199:223–233, 1984.
39. Bradley RF, Partamian JO: Coronary heart disease in the diabetic patient. Med Clin North Am 49:1093–1103, 1965.
40. Kereiakes DJ: Myocardial infarction in the diabetic patient. Clin Cardiol 8:446–450, 1985.
41. Bradley RF, Bryfogle JW: Survival of diabetic patients after myocardial infarction. Am J Med 20:207–216, 1956.
42. Barker WF: Peripheral vascular disease in diabetes. Diagnosis and management. Med Clin North Am 55(4):1045–1055, 1971.
43. Dry TJ, Hines EA Jr: The role of diabetes in the development of degenerative vascular disease: With special reference to

the incidence of retinitis and peripheral neuritis. Ann Intern Med 14:1893–1902, 1941.

44. Juergens JL, Barker NW, Hines EA Jr: Arteriosclerosis obliterans: Review of 520 cases with special reference to pathogenic and prognostic factors. Circulation 21:188–195, 1960.

45. Ganda OP: Pathogenesis of macrovascular disease including the influence of lipids. In Marble A, Krall LP, Bradley RF, Christlieb AR, Soeldner JS (eds): Joslin's Diabetes Mellitus. Philadelphia, Lea & Febiger, 1985, pp 217–250.

46. Bartlett FF, Gibbons GW, Wheelcock FC Jr: Aortic reconstruction for occlusive disease. Arch Surg 121:1150–1153, 1986.

47. Imparato AM, Kim GE, Madayag M, Haveson S: Angiographic criteria for successful tibial arterial reconstruction. Surgery 74:830–838, 1973.

48. Crawford ES, Bomberger RA, Glaeser DH, et al: Aortoiliac occlusive disease: Factors influencing survival and function following reconstructive operation over a twenty-five year period. Surgery 90:1055–1067, 1981.

49. Szilagyi DE, Elliott JP Jr, Smith RF, et al: A thirty year survey of the reconstructive surgical treatment of aortoiliac occlusive disease. J Vasc Surg 3:421–436, 1986.

50. Steer HW, Cuckle HS, Franklin PM, Morris PJ: The influence of diabetes mellitus upon peripheral vascular disease. Surg Gynecol Obstet 157:64–72, 1983.

51. Boyd AM: The natural course of arteriosclerosis of the lower extremities. Proc Soc Med 55:591–593, 1962.

52. Kannel WB, Skinner JJ, Schwartz MJ, Shurtleff D: Intermittent claudication. Incidence in the Framingham study. Circulation 41:875–883, 1970.

53. Imparato AM, Kim G, Davidson T, Crowley JG: Intermittent claudication: Its natural course. Surgery 78:795–799, 1975.

54. Schadt DC, Hines EA Jr, Juergens JL, Barker NW: Chronic atherosclerotic occlusion of the femoral artery. JAMA 175:937–940, 1961.

55. Jonason T, Ringqvist I: Diabetes mellitus and intermittent claudication. Acta Med Scand 218:217–221, 1985.

56. McAllister FF: The fate of patients with intermittent claudication managed nonoperatively. Am J Surg 132:593–595, 1976.

57. Ernst CB, Rutkow IM, Cleveland RJ, et al: Vascular surgery in the United States. Report of the Joint Society for Vascular Surgery—International Society for Cardiovascular Surgery Committee on Vascular Surgical Manpower. J Vasc Surg 6:611–621, 1987.

58. Strandness DE, Priest RE, Gibbons GE: Combined clinical and pathologic study of diabetic and nondiabetic peripheral arterial disease. Diabetes 13:366–372, 1964.

59. Gensler SW, Haimovici H, Hoffert P, et al: Study of vascular lesions in diabetic, nondiabetic patients. Arch Surg 91:617–622, 1965.

60. Brewster DC, Darling RC: Optimal methods of aortoiliac reconstruction. Surgery 84:739–748, 1978.

61. Malone JM, Moore WS, Goldstone J: The natural history of bilateral aortofemoral bypass grafts for ischemia of the lower extremities. Arch Surg 110:1300–1306, 1975.

62. Mavor GE: Pattern of occlusion in atheroma of lower limb arteries. Br J Surg 43:352, 1956.

63. Haimovici H: Reconstruction of the profunda femoris artery. In Haimovici H (ed): Vascular Surgery Principles and Techniques. New York, McGraw-Hill, 1976, pp 480–492.

64. Cotton LT, Roberts VC: Extended deep femoral angioplasty: An alternative to femoropopliteal bypass. Br J Surg 62:340–343, 1975.

65. Malone JM, Goldstone J, Moore WS: Autogenous profundaplasty: The key to long-term patency in secondary repair of aortofemoral graft occlusion. Ann Surg 188:817–823, 1978.

66. Haimovici H: Arteriographic patterns of atherosclerotic occlusive disease of the lower extremity. In Haimovici H (ed): Vascular Surgery Principles and Techniques. New York, McGraw-Hill, 1976, pp 240–263.

67. Strandness DE Jr: Preoperative evaluation of vascular diseases. In Haimovici H (ed): Vascular Surgery Principles and Techniques. New York, McGraw-Hill, 1976, pp 17–38.

68. Kallero KS, Bergqvist D, Cederholm C, et al: Arteriosclerosis in popliteal artery trifurcation as a predictor for myocardial infarction after arterial reconstructive operation. Surg Gynecol Obstet 159:133–138, 1984.

69. DeWeese JA, Rob CG: Autogenous venous grafts ten years later. Surgery 82:775–784, 1977.

70. Rosenblatt MS, Quist WC, Sidawy AN, Paniszyn CC, LoGerfo FW: Results of vein graft reconstruction of the lower extremity in diabetic and nondiabetic patients. Surg Gynecol Obstet 171:331–335, 1990.

71. Dardik H: Tibial peroneal arterial reconstruction. Contemp Surg 14:83–117, 1979.

72. Pratt TC: Gangrene and infection in the diabetic. Med Clin North Am 49:987–1004, 1965.

73. Malone JM, Snyder M, Anderson G, Bernhard VM, Holloway GA Jr, Bunt TJ: Prevention of amputation by diabetic education. Am J Surg 158:520–524, 1989.

74. Gibbons GW: Management of the diabetic foot. Surg Rounds 9(1):55–59, 1986.

75. Gutman M, Kaplan O, Skornick Y, et al: Gangrene of the lower limbs in diabetic patients: A malignant complication. Am J Surg 154:305–308, 1987.

76. Ferrier TM: Comparative study of arterial disease in amputated lower limbs from diabetics and nondiabetics. Med J Aust 1:5, 1967.

77. Thiele BL: Evaluation of ulceration of the lower extremities. Vasc Diagn Ther 1(1):33–39, 1980.

78. Haimovici H: Amputation of lower extremity. In Haimovici H (ed): Vascular Surgery Principles and Techniques. New York, McGraw-Hill, 1976, pp 893–925.

79. Keagy BA, Schwartz JA, Kotb M, et al: Lower extremity amputation: The control series. J Vasc Surg 4:321–326, 1986.

80. Russels AS: Amputation, immediate postoperative fitting and early ambulation. In Haimovici H (ed): Vascular Surgery Principles and Techniques. New York, McGraw-Hill, 1976, pp 926–943.

81. Light JT Jr, Rice JC, Kerstein MD: Sequelae of limited amputation. Surgery 103:294–299, 1988.

82. Fulton RL, Blakely WR: Lumbar sympathectomy: A procedure of questionable value in the treatment of arteriosclerosis obliterans of the legs. Am J Surg 116:735–744, 1968.

83. Persson AV, Anderson L, Rodberg FT Jr: Selection of patients for lumbar sympathectomy. Surg Clin North Am 65:393–403, 1985.

84. MacCarty CS, Piepgras DG, Nauss LA: Sympathetic denervation of the extremities for peripheral vascular disease. In Juergens JL, Spittel JA Jr (eds): Textbook of Peripheral Vascular Disease. Philadelphia, WB Saunders Company, 1980, pp 903–919.

85. DeValle MJ, Baumann FG, Mintzer R, et al: Limited success of lumbar sympathectomy in the prevention of ischemic limb loss in diabetic patients. Surg Gynecol Obstet 152:784, 1981.

86. Towne JB: Management of foot lesions in the diabetic patient. In Rutherford RB (ed): Vascular Surgery, 2nd ed. Philadelphia, WB Saunders Company, 1984, pp 661–669.

87. Marble A (quoted in Churg J, Dolger H): Diabetic renal disease. In Strauss MB, Welt LG (eds): Diseases of the Kidney. Boston, Little, Brown & Company, 1963, p 882.

88. Lundgren G, Groth C, Gunnarson R, et al: Dialysis and renal transplantation in end stage diabetic nephropathy. Acta Med Scand [Suppl] 639:59–63, 1980.

89. Haimov M, Burrows L, Casey JD, et al: Problems of vascular access for hemodialysis—experience with 214 patients. Proc Eur Dial Transplant Assoc 9:173–177, 1972.

90. Kjellstrand CM, Simmons RL, Goetz FC, et al: Mortality and morbidity in diabetic patients accepted for renal transplantation. Proc Eur Dial Transplant Assoc 9:345–358, 1972.

91. White N, Snowden SA, Parsons V, et al: The management of terminal renal failure in diabetic patients by regular dialysis therapy. Nephron 11:261–275, 1973.

REVIEW QUESTIONS

1. Which of the following statements most accurately reflects the course of the diabetic patient following the discovery of insulin?
   (a) the diabetic lives longer
   (b) mortality from coma and sepsis has decreased
   (c) mortality from vascular disease has increased
   (d) adequate therapy of the carbohydrate defect does not prevent the development of vascular complications
   (e) all of the above

2. Abnormal glucose tolerances are found more frequently in:
   (a) relatives of the diabetics
   (b) monozygotic twins than dizygotic twins
   (c) some races than others
   (d) patients with vascular disease
   (e) all of the above

3. Which statement is most true?
   (a) long-term hemodialysis should not be performed in diabetics because of poor long-term results and complications of blood access procedures
   (b) neuropathic foot ulcers are typically shallow and painful when first seen
   (c) small vessel disease is not a common occurrence in diabetics
   (d) long-term results of peripheral vascular surgery are poorer in diabetics than in nondiabetics because of the higher incidence of disease in the more distal vessels and concomitant illnesses

4. Which statement about myocardial infarction in the diabetic is the least true?
   (a) it is the most common cause of death in the maturity-onset diabetic
   (b) the incidence and mortality of perioperative infarction is higher in diabetics
   (c) long-term survival is poorer in the diabetic
   (d) myocardial infarction is often due to disease in the microcirculation
   (e) the incidence of infarction is unaffected by physiologic control of the blood sugar

5. Which statement is most true in patients with diabetes mellitus?
   (a) atherosclerosis of large and medium-sized arteries does not differ in morphology or distribution in the diabetic and nondiabetic patient
   (b) duration of diabetes is unrelated to the incidence of vascular disease
   (c) severity of diabetes is unrelated to the incidence of vascular disease in the diabetic
   (d) disease in the microcirculation rarely requires surgical intervention

6. Strict control of the blood sugar in the diabetic will most probably:
   (a) decrease the incidence and severity of vascular disease
   (b) decrease the incidence and severity of sepsis
   (c) decrease the incidence of perioperative complications
   (d) not affect the occurrence of neuropathy

7. Which statement is most true of diabetic neuropathy?
   (a) diabetic neuropathy can result in bone rarefaction and Charcot's joints
   (b) the degree of control of diabetes does not affect the incidence of neuropathy
   (c) diabetic neuropathy will usually improve with improved management of the diabetic
   (d) diabetic neuropathy is uncommon in the feet of patients with palpable pedal pulses

8. The distribution of vascular disease in the diabetic:
   (a) is relatively more frequent in the aortoiliac area
   (b) is relatively more frequent in the tibioperoneal circulation
   (c) produces symptoms in the upper extremities as frequently as in the lower extremities
   (d) spares the profunda femoris vessels
   (e) does not result in a greater mortality from stroke

9. Which statement or statements is/are true of gangrene and amputation in the diabetic?
   (a) reamputation is more common in the diabetic
   (b) they are more frequent in the diabetic
   (c) they more frequently affect the opposite leg than in the nondiabetic
   (d) amputation occurs or is necessary in 20 to 30 per cent of diabetics
   (e) all of the above

10. Which of the following statements is most true of the indications for vascular reconstruction in the diabetic?
    (a) should be performed primarily for limb salvage rather than for claudication
    (b) should be avoided in patients with vascular disease and severe neuropathy in the lower extremity
    (c) should be performed less frequently in the diabetic because of poorer long-term results
    (d) should be performed more often with concomitant sympathectomy because of the higher incidence of small vessel disease in the diabetic
    (e) should be performed for the same indications in diabetics and nondiabetics

ANSWERS

1. e   2. e   3. d   4. d   5. c   6. b   7. a
8. b   9. e   10. e

29

RENOVASCULAR HYPERTENSION

RICHARD H. DEAN

Although hypertension has been recognized for centuries, the importance of its identification and treatment has been appreciated only during the past 150 years. Most commonly, hypertension is a silent process and is manifested only by sequelae of acceleration in the rate of atherogenesis and frequency of cardiovascular morbid and mortal events. Uncommonly, the hypertension may be so severe that the elevated pressure itself produces vessel wall injury and the clinical picture of malignant hypertension. Although most physicians appreciate the potentially lethal nature of this malignant variety and the importance of its control, physician apathy towards the merits of aggressive diagnostic evaluation and management of asymptomatic patients with less severe hypertension continues to limit the impact of current knowledge on population-wide success of treatment of this disorder.

Richard Bright of Guy's Hospital, London[1] called attention to the association of hypertension and renal disease in 1836. He observed the apparent association between hardness of the pulse, "dropsy," albuminuria, and granular shrunken kidneys. This is especially remarkable, since the modern sphygmomanometer was not described until 1896. Although Bright's observation stimulated much interest in the kidney, 70 years passed before Tigerstedt and Bergman,[2] in 1987, discovered a renal pressor substance in the rabbit. They called this crude extract "renin." Confirmation of a renovascular source of hypertension, however, awaited Goldblatt's classic experiment.[3] In 1934, he and his coworkers showed that constriction of the renal artery produced atrophy of the kidney and hypertension in the dog. Following this documentation of a renovascular origin for hypertension, many patients were treated by nephrectomy on the basis of hypertension and a small kidney or intravenous pyelography. Curiously, there was rarely any interest in documenting a renal artery occlusive lesion in any of these patients. Dissatisfaction with the results of this form of treatment prompted Smith,[4] in 1956, to review 575 cases treated in this manner. He found only a 26 per cent cure of hypertension by nephrectomy using these criteria. This led him to suggest that nephrectomy should be limited to strict urologic indications. Two years previously, however, Freeman and his associates[5] performed an aortic and bilateral renal artery thromboendarterectomy on a hypertensive patient with resultant resolution of hypertension. This was the first cure of hypertension by renal revascularization.

DeCamp and Birchall,[6] Morris et al.,[7] and others[8,9] soon followed with additional descriptions of relief of hypertension by renal revascularization. Concomitant with these reports, aortography began to be widely used. During the late 1950s many centers were demonstrating renal artery stenosis in hypertensive patients by aortography and then performing either aortorenal bypass or thromboendarterectomy. Nevertheless, by 1960 it became apparent that revascularization in hypertensive individuals with renal artery stenosis was associated with reduction of blood pressure in less than 50 per cent. General pessimism followed regarding the merits of operative treatment of hypertension.

As this experience pointed out, the coexistence of renal artery stenosis and hypertension does not establish a causal relationship. Many normotensive patients, especially those past the age of 50, have renal artery stenosis. Obviously, special studies are required to establish the functional significance of renal artery lesions. The most recent era in the history of operative treatment of renovascular hypertension began with the introduction of meaningful tests of split renal function by Howard and Conner[10] and by Stamey et al.[11] Furthermore, the work of Page and Helmes[12] and others[13-15] in the identification of the renin-angiotension system of blood pressure control added a new dimension to our understanding of renovascular hypertension. With the later addition of accurate methods of measuring plasma renin activity, the physician now can accurately predict which renal artery lesion is producing renovascular hypertension. Our experience has shown that if the split renal function studies or renal vein renin assays are positive, one can expect a good response in blood pressure following successful operation in over 95 per cent of the cases.[16]

The incidence of renovascular hypertension (RVH), the necessity of its identification, and the value of interventional management, however, remain poorly defined. In this chapter, diagnostic studies and methods of management of the respective causes of renovascular disease and RVH will be reviewed, with emphasis to be placed on the current status of their value and results of their use.

PATHOLOGY

Occlusive lesions of the renal artery can be divided into two groups: atherosclerotic and fibromuscular dysplasia. There is nothing peculiar to atherosclerosis of the renal artery. The pathogenesis parallels atherosclerotic lesions elsewhere, with cholesterol-rich lipid deposition and intimal thickening. Later, this "atheroma" may undergo central degeneration and even calcification. They typically occur at or near the renal artery ostium (Fig. 29–1), are most commonly found on the left, and account for about 70 per cent of patients with renovascular hypertension. Often, there is arteriographic evidence of asymptomatic simultaneous involvement of the abdominal aorta and its bifurcation. Occasionally, the renal artery stenosis is only one manifestation of severe end-stage generalized atherosclerosis.

Fibromuscular dysplasia of the renal artery encompasses a variety of hyperplastic and fibrosing lesions of the intima, media, and/or adventitia. They are most frequently seen in young women. This is of no predictive value, however, because fibrodysplastic lesions can be found at any age and in either sex. The right renal artery is more commonly affected than the left, but bilateral involvement is present in the vast majority of patients. The basic cause of fibromuscular dysplasia remains unknown, but its frequent occurrence in multiple arteries suggests a common etiologic agent. Embryologic variations, hormonal influences, autoimmune mechanisms, and even recurrent trauma during youth have been suggested as possible etiologic factors. None of these explanations are adequate, however, and the evidence in their support remains mostly conjectural.

Based on the angiographic appearance of fibromuscular disease, several methods of categorization have been suggested. To establish a uniform terminology, Harrison and McCormack[17] combined their experience and developed a classification of these lesions correlating the morphologic and angiographic appearance. Depending on the layer predominantly involved, lesions may either be intimal, medial, or adventitial. Clinically, however, it may be difficult to segregate individual lesions into one of their respective categories. The most common variety of fibromuscular dysplasia is medial fibroplasia with mural aneurysms (Fig. 29–2). This variety accounts for about 70 per cent of all renal artery dysplasias. It often involves long segments of the renal artery and its branches, producing a characteristic "string-of-beads" appearance angiographically. Less commonly, the dysplastic lesions may be a single mural stenosis (Fig. 29–3), which may be an intimal or subadventitial variety.

PATHOPHYSIOLOGY

The kidney, by its influence on circulating plasma volume as well as on modulation of vasomotor tone, is a dominant site of blood pressure regulation. To examine the pathophysiology of RVH, it is appropriate to review the normal homeostatic activities of the kidney in regulation of blood pressure.

Renin-Angiotensin-Aldosterone System

The renin-angiotensin-aldosterone system is a complex feedback mechanism normally acting to maintain a stable blood pressure and blood volume under varying conditions. Richly innervated modified smooth muscle cells located along the afferent arterioles in juxtaposition to the renal glomerulus (juxtaglomerular apparatus) are sensitive monitors of perfusion pressure. Diminished perfusion pressure stimulates these cells to release renin, a proteolytic enzyme. Renin, in turn, interacts with an α-globulin (angiotensinogen) manufactured in the liver to pro-

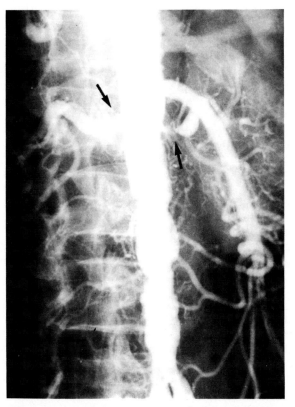

FIGURE 29–1. Arteriogram showing typical appearance of atherosclerotic renal artery stenosis located at the origin of the vessel.

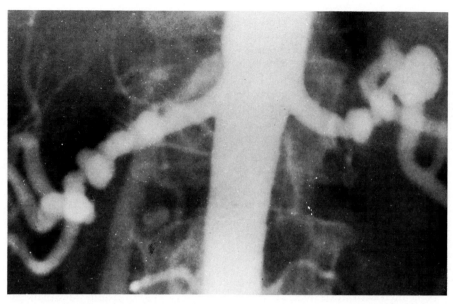

FIGURE 29–2. Arteriogram demonstrating typical "string-of-beads" appearance of medial fibromuscular dysplasia with microaneurysm.

duce angiotensin I. Angiotensin I, an inactive and labile decapeptide, is converted to the potent vasoconstrictor angiotensin II by converting enzyme found primarily in the lungs. In addition to its potent vasoconstrictor properties, angiotensin II also increases blood pressure through its stimulation of aldosterone release from the zona glomerulosa of the adrenal cortex. This, in turn, increases plasma volume by increasing sodium and water resorption in the renal tubules. Through these actions of angiotensin II, blood

pressure, plasma volume, and plasma sodium content are increased. In addition, the adjacent cells of the distal convoluted tubule (macula densa) may play a role by acting as sensors of sodium concentration in the distal tubules and exerting a positive feedback mechanism on renin release. As these mechanisms increase perfusion pressure to the juxtaglomerular cells, further renin production and release is suppressed, and blood pressure is modulated within a narrow range. This scheme is a simplistic representation of a very complex mechanism.

Many intermediate steps remain unknown. The role of the prostaglandins in the regulation of renin release remains unsettled. Their action in blood pressure control, and specifically the part they play in RVH, is the focus of intensive investigation. The medullary interstitial cells are normally rich in prostaglandin content. A reduction in their prostaglandin content is seen in experimental RVH. This may suggest a loss of some intrarenal inhibitory feedback mechanism of renin production or release as a result of the reduction in prostaglandin content. This is highly speculative, and much more investigation is required before the interactions between the intrarenal content of prostaglandin and renin release can be identified.

Cause of Hypertension (Two Forms)

Potentially, two forms of hypertension may be produced by the development of renovascular disease: (1) renin-dependent hypertension and (2) volume-dependent hypertension. Through the mechanisms just described, decreased perfusion activates the renin-angiotensin-aldosterone axis of vasoconstriction and volume expansion. Current information regarding the

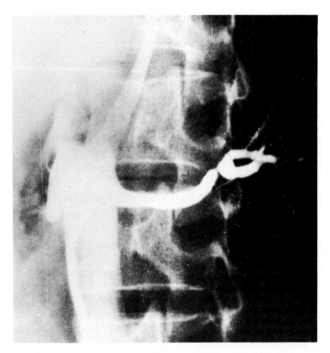

FIGURE 29–3. Appearance of single mural fibromuscular dysplastic lesion on arteriogram.

nature of RVH suggests that a functionally significant unilateral renal artery stenosis activates both the angiotensin II–mediated increase in peripheral resistance and blood pressure as well as aldosterone-mediated volume expansion. When the contralateral renal artery and kidney are normal, the feedback mechanisms in the normal kidney produce an effect natriuresis and compensatory reduction in circulating plasma volume. In this scheme, an angiotensin II–vasoconstrictive source of hypertension is created.

In contrast, when the contralateral renal artery or kidney is also diseased, this compensatory diuresis is lost and volume expansion occurs, producing an angiotensin-aldosterone–mediated, volume-dependent hypertension. Modification of renal perfusion by renal revascularization can effectively diminish or abolish the underlying mechanism producing either of these varieties of renovascular hypertension.

INCIDENCE OF RENOVASCULAR HYPERTENSION

Renovascular hypertension is generally thought to account for 5 to 10 per cent of the hypertensive population. Recently, Tucker and Labarthe[18] have suggested an even lower prevalence. Likewise, Shapiro et al.[19] have suggested that the identification and successful operative treatment of RVH in patients over the age of 50 years is so unlikely that diagnostic investigation for a correctable cause in that group should be undertaken only when hypertension is severe and uncontrollable. Estimates of the prevalence of hypertension in the United States from all causes vary from 45 to 60 million people; and it may be present in 10 to 15 per cent of the adult population. Indeed, the incidence of RVH is undoubtedly low in this general hypertensive population if all patients with even mild hypertension are included. Since RVH tends to produce relatively severe hypertension, its prevalence in the large subpopulation of mildly hypertensive patients (diastolic blood pressure 105 mm Hg) is probably negligible. In contrast, however, it is a frequent cause of hypertension in the smaller group of severely hypertensive people. Hollifield (unpublished data) investigated 137 patients with previously unrecognized hypertension who were identified in a shopping center screening program (Table 29–1). Diagnostic study in these patients included arteriography and, when appropriate, renal vein renin assays and split renal function studies. This study revealed that 9 of the 22 (41 per cent) white patients with severe diastolic hypertension (118 mm Hg or greater) had RVH. Similarly, Davis et al. have shown a 31 per cent incidence of RVH in 85 patients initially evaluated in our center for malignant hypertension.[20]

In our experience, the presence of severe hypertension at the two extremes of life carries the highest probability of being RVH. Our review of the causes of hypertension in 74 children admitted for diagnostic

TABLE 29–1. RESULTS OF SCREENING 137 NEW HYPERTENSIVE PATIENTS[a]

Diastolic Blood Pressure	No. of Patients	No. with RVH	Percentage
90–115 mm Hg	102	0	
>117 mm Hg	35	9	26
Black	13	0	
White	22	9	41

[a]From J. W. Hollifield (unpublished data).

evaluation over a 5-year period showed that 78 per cent of the children less than 5 years old had a correctable renovascular origin (Table 29–2).[21] Interestingly, after childhood, the age group that has the next highest probability of having RVH is the elderly. In our center, 33 per cent of patients over 60 years old admitted for evaluation have had RVH. Certainly, the elderly age group admitted for evaluation is skewed toward the more severe end of the spectrum of hypertension, because less severe levels likely would not have led to referral of such patients to our center.

From these data it is inappropriate to view hypertensive patients as a homogeneous group with respect to the prevalence of RVH. Rather, the probability of finding RVH correlates with the severity of hypertension. Accordingly, the search for RVH should be directed to the subset of patients who have the more severe degree of hypertension. It must be remembered, however, that severity of hypertension is based on its level without medication interference and does not refer to the difficulty of control by drug therapy.

CHARACTERISTICS OF RENOVASCULAR HYPERTENSION

Because of the relative infrequency of RVH in the entire hypertensive population, many reports have focused on the value of demographic factors, physical findings, and screening tests as discriminates between essential hypertension (EH) and RVH on which to base the decision for further diagnostic study. Most frequently quoted as discriminate factors suggesting the presence of RVH and a need for further study are recent onset of hypertension, young age, lack of family history of hypertension, and the presence of an abdominal bruit. The most complete study com-

TABLE 29–2. CLASSIFICATION OF HYPERTENSION IN 74 CHILDREN[a]

	0–5 Yr	6–10 Yr	11–15 Yr	16–20 Yr
Total no. of children	9	9	29	27
Essential	1	5	24	24
Correctable	8 (78%)	4 (44%)	5 (17%)	6 (22%)

[a]From Lawson JD, Boerth RK, Foster JH, et al: Diagnosis and management of renovascular hypertension in children. Arch Surg 112:1307, 1977.

paring the clinical characteristics of patients with RVH to those with EH was the Cooperative Study of Renovascular Hypertension.[22] In that study, the prevalence of certain clinical characteristics in 339 patients with EH was compared to their prevalence in 175 patients with RVH secondary to atherosclerotic lesions (91 patients) and fibromuscular dysplasia (84 patients). Although the prevalence of several characteristics is significantly different when RVH is compared to EH, none of the characteristics has sufficient discriminate value to be used to exclude patients from further diagnostic investigation for RVH. Certainly the finding of an epigastric bruit in a young white female with malignant hypertension is strongly suggestive of a renovascular origin of the hypertension. The absence of such criteria, however, does not exclude the presence of RVH, and such criteria should not be used to eliminate patients from further diagnostic study.

In a review of the first 122 patients with RVH treated in our center, 52 per cent had family histories of hypertension, 46 per cent had no audible abdominal bruit, and ages ranged from 4 months to 69 years (mean: 46 years).[23] Since RVH can be secondary to any of several processes affecting the renal artery and since each of these diseases has its own clinical characteristics, it is not surprising that the use of demographic or physical findings such as age, abdominal bruit, and duration of hypertension as discriminates to exclude patients from study have a high risk of inappropriately excluding patients with RVH from further study. Therefore, one should base the decision for diagnostic study on the severity of hypertension. Mild hypertension has a minimal chance of being renovascular in origin. In contrast, the more severe the hypertension, the higher the probability that it is from a correctable cause. With this in mind, we submit all patients with diastolic blood pressures greater than 105 mm Hg who would be acceptable operative candidates to evaluation for a correctable origin of hypertension.

DIAGNOSTIC EVALUATION

The selection and appropriate sequence of diagnostic studies in the evaluation of hypertensive patients remain ill defined. Continued modifications of attitudes toward the merits of evaluation and introduction of new techniques prevent a definitive statement on which studies to employ in all patients. The general evaluation of all hypertensive patients should include a careful medical history, physical examination, serum electrolytes and creatinine, and an electrocardiogram. Electrocardiography is important to gauge the extent of secondary myocardial hypertrophy or associated ischemic heart disease. Serum electrolytes and serial serum potassium determinations can effectively exclude patients with primary aldosteronism if potassium levels are greater than 3.0 mg/dl. One must remember, however, that hypokalemia

is often due to salt-depleting diets and previous diuretic therapy. Finally, estimation of renal function is mandatory. Preexisting renal disease may reduce renal function and cause hypertension. Further, hypertension from any cause may produce intrarenal arteriolar nephrosclerosis and subsequent depression of renal function.

Screening Studies

Identification of a noninvasive screening test that will accurately identify all patients with renovascular disease that might require interventional management remains an elusive goal. Prior methods such as peripheral plasma renin activity, rapid sequence intravenous pyelography, and saralasin infusion are examples of such tests that have been abandoned. Isotope renography continues to be proposed as a valuable screening test, yet the methods employed are continuously modified with the hope of improving the sensitivity and specificity. The newest versions of isotope renography consist of renal scans performed before and after exercise or captopril infusion. In these methods, a test is interpreted as positive when there is augmentation of derangements in renal perfusion following exercise or captopril infusion. Although these methods have improved specificity of isotope renography, their reliance on activation of the renin-angiotensin system leads to an unacceptable incidence of false-negative results.

Our bias is that screening tests that image the vascular anatomy and assess hemodynamics of renal flow are the most promising methods for widespread screening for renovascular disease. In this regard vascular images using magnetic resonance imaging (MRI) or positron emission tomography (PET) may hold great promise. Current expense, lack of widespread availability, and limitations of patient selection criteria prevent its application as a screening tool except in the most unusual circumstances.

Renal duplex sonography (RDS) has been proposed by several investigators as a useful screening test with which candidates for arteriography can be identified. We have reported our experience with duplex sonography and evaluated its sensitivity and specificity for identification of renovascular occlusive disease.[24] The study population for RDS validity analysis consisted of 74 consecutive patients who had 77 comparative RDS and standard angiographic studies of the arterial anatomy to 148 kidneys. Renal duplex sonography results from six kidneys (4 per cent) were considered inadequate for interpretation. This study population contained 26 patients (35 per cent) with severe renal insufficiency (mean serum creatinine: 3.6 mg/dl) and 67 individuals with hypertension (91 per cent). Fourteen patients (19 per cent) had 20 kidneys with multiple renal arteries. Renal duplex sonography correctly identified the presence of renovascular disease in 41 of 44 patients with angiographically proven lesions, and renovascular disease was not identified in any patient free of disease. When single renal arteries were present (122 kidneys), RDS proved to have a 93 per cent sensitivity, 98 per cent specificity, 98 per cent positive predictive value, 94 per cent negative predictive value, and an overall accuracy of 96 per cent. These results were adversely affected when kidneys with multiple (polar) renal arteries were examined. Although the end-diastolic ratio was inversely correlated with serum creatinine ($r = .30773$, $p = .009$), low end-diastolic ratio in 35 patients submitted to renovascular reconstruction did not preclude beneficial blood pressure or renal function response. We concluded from this analysis that RDS can be a valuable screening test in the search for correctable renovascular disease causing global renal ischemia and secondary renal insufficiency (ischemic nephropathy). Renal duplex sonography does not, however, exclude polar vessel renovascular disease causing hypertension alone, nor does it predict hypertension or renal function response after correction of renovascular disease.

With these results in mind, we now use RDS as the screening tool of choice. Nevertheless, since it does not accurately identify accessory vessels or branch vessel disease we will proceed to arteriography when hypertension is severe, difficult to control, or is occurring in pediatric-age patients. Finally, when unilateral disease is identified by angiography, we believe confirmation of the physiologic importance of the lesion by performance of renal vein renin assays is appropriate. As a standard rule, we will not recommend revascularization of unilateral disease unless renin values lateralize to the involved side.

Renal Arteriography

There continues to be controversy over the use of aortography and renal arteriography in the routine screening of hypertensive individuals. Some believe it should be reserved for select groups of patients. We do not share this conservative view and proceed with arteriography in circumstances summarized in the previous section.

Both aortography and selective renal arteriography using multiple projections may be necessary to adequately examine the entire renal artery. As is shown in Figure 29–4, the proximal third of the left renal artery usually courses anteriorly, the middle third transversely, and the distal third posteriorly, whereas the right renal artery pursues a more consistent posterior course. Lesions in the renal artery that are coursing anteriorly or posteriorly are frequently not seen or may appear insignificant in an anteroposterior (AP) aortogram. Oblique aortography or oblique selective renal arteriography will project these portions of the vessels in profile and identify the stenosis. Figure 29–5 shows how the delicate septal lesions of fibromuscular dysplasia may be unrecognizable or appear insignificant in the AP projection, whereas in the oblique projection the true severity is demonstrated.

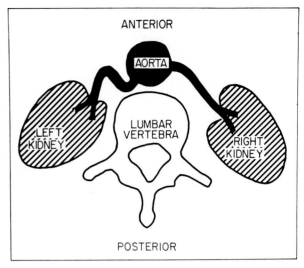

FIGURE 29–4. The usual course of the renal arteries on sagittal section.

A common cause of false-positive angiography is the creation of renal artery spasm at the tip of the arteriogram catheter during selective renal angiography (Fig. 29–6). In most cases this phenomenon is easily recognized when the area in question is studied on the flush AP or oblique aortogram. Occasionally, however, instillation of a vasodilator and repeat study after repositioning the catheter may be necessary to distinguish it from a true renal artery stenosis.

The introduction of digital subtraction angiography (DSA) has broadened enthusiasm for the use of angiography in screening for renovascular disease. Although the intravenous route of contrast injection for DSA was initially thought to be useful for this eval-

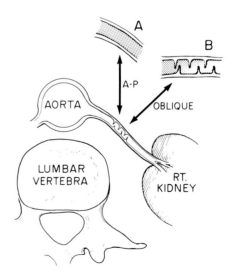

FIGURE 29–5. Graphic illustration of how the septa of fibromuscular dysplasia can be missed. *A*, When the vessel is viewed with an AP arteriogram, the septa are masked by the overlying dye column. *B*, They are demonstrated by oblique projection placing the direction of the vessel in a perpendicular direction and the septa parallel to the direction of the x-ray.

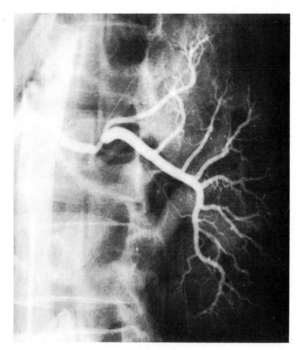

FIGURE 29–6. Arteriogram demonstrating spasm of the renal artery induced by the catheter tip.

uation, this method provides such poor delineation that many fibromuscular lesions are missed and one cannot examine branch vessels with any accuracy. In addition, the amount of contrast material used for intravenous DSA is contraindicated in patients with reduced renal function. In contrast, intraarterial DSA can be performed as an outpatient procedure and is useful in some patients. Depending on resolution, however, even this technique can miss some lesions and inadequately define branch disease. For these reasons, we continue to primarily rely on standard "cut film" arteriography for most evaluations.

Functional Studies

Two tests, renal vein renin assays and split renal function studies, have proven valuable in confirming the functional significance of renal artery stenosis. Neither have great value, however, when severe bilateral disease or disease in the renal artery supplying a single kidney is present. In these circumstances, the decision for operation is based on the severity of hypertension and the degree of renal insufficiency.

Renal Vein Renin Assays

When an obstructive lesion is found by renal arteriography, its functional significance should be evaluated. Most centers now rely solely on renal vein renin assays (RVRAs) to establish the diagnosis of RVH. The unfortunate consequence of this trend is that one must presume that all patients with RVH will have lateralizing RVRAs. Results of evaluation of this study in our center underscore the fallacy of

this presumption. There are many factors that affect the results of RVRA that, if not properly managed, will lead to erroneous results.

The effect of antihypertensive medications and unrestricted sodium intake on renin release, and thereby RVRA, is widely recognized. Many antihypertensive medications, especially those that function through β-adrenergic blockade, suppress renin output and can lead to false nonlateralization of RVRA. Most common of these β-blockers in use today are α-methyldopa and propranolol. Before one can consider that there is no drug interference in the release of renin, all such medications must have been withheld for at least 5 days or, preferably, 2 weeks prior to the measurement of RVRA. Similar effects on renin levels are seen when sodium intake is not restricted. For this reason, the patient must be on no more than a 2-gm sodium diet for at least 2 weeks prior to the study. The preparation of patients for RVRA in our center is summarized in Table 29–3.

The technical aspects of performing RVRA cannot be overemphasized as a potential source of error. Since the left renal vein contains not only renal venous effluent but also adrenal, gonadal, and lumbar venous effluent, misplacement of the venous catheter into the origin of one of the nonrenal branches or sampling in the proximal renal vein where a mixture from these other sources is present may dilute the renin activity coming from the kidney. This will lead to erroneously low measurements of renin activity and produce a false interpretation of RVRA.

The time of sampling the two renal veins for renin activity is also a potential source of error in RVRA. In studies performed with a single catheter, several minutes may elapse between sampling the two renal veins as the catheter is switched from one side to the other. Furthermore, catheter manipulation and patient discomfort may affect renin release. It is not surprising, therefore, that when the single catheter is employed, both false-positive and false-negative renal vein renin ratios are frequent.

Several methods of stimulating renin release have been suggested over the past 15 years. These include tilting the patient to the upright posture during the study, stimulation with intravenous apresoline, and, more recently, nitroprusside stimulation. Although all of these methods increase renin release, they also increase false-positive determinations and reduce reliability of RVRA to unacceptable levels.

Vaughn et al. stressed the importance of express-

TABLE 29–3. PATIENT PREPARATION FOR RENAL VEIN RENIN ASSAYS

1. Chronic salt restriction (2-gm sodium diet)
2. Discontinue all antihypertensive drugs except diuretics for at least 5 days prior to study
3. Oral furosemide (40 mg) diuresis night before the study
4. Nothing by mouth for 8 hours prior to study
5. Strictly flat bed rest for 4 hours before and during study
6. Prestudy sedation with intramuscular Valium (5 mg)

ing RVRA in relation to the systemic renin activity rather than simply evaluating the ratio of renin activity between the two renal veins.[25] In patients with RVH secondary to unilateral renal artery stenosis, one should find hypersecretion of renin from the ischemic kidney and suppression of renin secretion from the normal kidney. Through application of this hypothesis, Stanley and Fry have shown a statistically significant difference in the renal-systemic renin indices in patients who were cured of RVH by operation when compared to those who were only improved.[26] Although this method has appeal as a predictor of the extent of benefit, its value in patients with bilateral renal artery lesions is limited. Since both lesions may be producing RVH, both this method and renal vein renin ratios have reduced validity as predictors of response to operation. Furthermore, the risk of hypertension is more directly related to its severity rather than its absolute presence or absence. If one bases the decision for operative management solely on whether or not absolute cure is to be expected, then many patients who would receive the benefit of reduction in severity of hypertension to a mild, easily controlled level would be dropped from consideration as operative candidates. Therefore, this method of RVRA interpretation should be considered only as an additional predictive tool and not an alternative to the evaluation of renal vein renin ratios.

Renal vein renin assays also may be spuriously unrevealing in patients with accessory or segmental renal artery stenosis if renal venous sampling is limited to the main renal vein. Since recognition of renin hypersecretion depends on sampling the ischemic areas of the kidneys, selective segmental venous sampling must be done in these patients. When segmental sampling is required, the renin activity from the segment sampled is compared to the simultaneously collected contralateral main renal vein sample to calculate the renal vein renin ratio.

Split Renal Function Studies

With the advent of RVRAs, most centers have stopped using split renal function studies because of the associated discomfort, possible complications, and confusing results. Valuable information can be obtained from split renal function studies that is not obtained from RVRAs. Information regarding the likelihood of viability of a severely ischemic kidney and data suggesting the most severely affected side in bilaterally stenotic kidneys are among the benefits of split renal function studies. Classically, a positive test shows a 40 per cent reduction in urine volume, a 50 per cent increase in creatinine concentration, and a 100 per cent increase in *para*-aminohippuric acid concentration on the involved side. Nevertheless, we consider this test positive if there is consistent lateralization in each of three samples with a decrease in urine volume and an increase in *para*-aminohippuric acid and creatinine concentration. When either the RVRA or the split renal function

study is positive, the diagnosis of renovascular hypertension is established.

THERAPEUTIC OPTIONS

Identification of the optimal method of treating patients with RVH remains an elusive goal. Advocates of drug therapy, operative management, and more recently, percutaneous transluminal angioplasty (PTA) separately defend their viewpoints with selective data from the literature to strengthen the validity of their argument. A majority of the medical community still only evaluate patients for RVH when medications are not tolerated and hypertension remains severe and uncontrolled. Although we are currently conducting a randomized, prospective study comparing drug therapy to surgery, it is not completed; and no similar randomized comparative trial is available in the literature. The study by Hunt and Strong[27] is the most informative study currently available to assess the comparative value of drug therapy and operation. In their study, they compared the results of operative treatment in 100 patients with the results of drug therapy in 114 similar patients. After 7 to 14 years of follow-up, 84 per cent of the operated group were alive as compared to 66 per cent in the drug therapy group. Furthermore, of the 84 patients alive in the operated group, 93 were cured or significantly improved, whereas 16 (21 per cent) of the patients alive in the drug therapy group had required operation for uncontrollable hypertension. Another seven patients remained uncontrolled without operation. Death during follow-up was twice as common in the medically treated group. These differences were statistically significant ($p < .01$) in both patients with atherosclerotic lesions and those with fibromuscular lesions of the renal artery.

Additional information influencing the decision for operative management of RVH in the atherosclerotic patient is the anatomic and renal function changes that occur during drug therapy. We have reported the results of serial renal function studies, which were performed on 41 patients with RVH secondary to atherosclerotic renal artery disease who had been randomly selected for nonoperative management (Table 29–4).[28] In 19 patients, serum creatinine levels increased between 25 and 50 per cent. The glomerular filtration rates dropped between 25 and 50 per cent in 12 patients. Fourteen patients (37 per cent) lost more than 10 per cent of renal length. In four patients (12 per cent), a significant stenosis progressed to total occlusion. Seventeen patients (41 per cent) had deterioration of renal function or loss of renal size that led to operation. One patient required removal of a previously reconstructable kidney. Of the 17 patients with deterioration, 15 had acceptable blood pressure control during the period of nonoperative observation. Therefore, we believe that progressive deterioration of renal function in nonoperatively treated patients with atherosclerotic renal artery stenosis and

TABLE 29–4. FREQUENCY OF SEVERE DETERIORATION IN PARAMETERS OF RENAL FUNCTION DURING DRUG THERAPY (41 PATIENTS)[a]

Parameter	Patients Followed	Mean Follow-up	Failure Event	Number Affected	Percentage Affected
Renal length	38	33 mo	≥ 10% decrease	14	37
Serum creatinine	41	25 mo	≥100% increase	2	5
Glomerular filtration rate or creatinine clearance	30	19 mo	≥ 50% decrease	1	3
Totals	41			17	41

[a]From Dean RH, Kieffer RW, Smith BM, et al: Renovascular hypertension. Arch Surg *116*:1408, 1981.

RVH is indicated, even in the presence of blood pressure control with drugs.

The detrimental changes that occur during drug therapy and the current excellent results of operative management[16] argue for an aggressive attitude toward the merits of renal revascularization in the treatment of RVH. Our indications for operative management of RVH have been outlined in detail elsewhere.[29] Nevertheless, in brief, all patients with severe, difficult-to-control hypertension should be considered for operation. This includes patients with complicating factors such as branch lesions or extrarenal vascular disease and patients with associated cardiovascular disease that would be improved by blood pressure reduction.

Young patients with moderate hypertension and no complicating diseases who have an easily correctable atherosclerotic or fibromuscular main renal artery stenosis also are candidates for operation. The chance for cure of moderate hypertension is quite good in such patients who have no complicating factors. It remains to be proven that drug control is ever as good as the complete cure of hypertension. In fact, one might argue that reduction in the driving pressure of blood flow across the stenosis by successful drug therapy might accelerate deterioration in renal function by further reducing renal perfusion.

Finally, there is no clear evidence that age (at least under 60 years), type of lesion (whether atherosclerotic or fibromuscular), duration of hypertension, or the presence of bilateral lesions by themselves have proven value as determinants of operative risk or likelihood of successful operative management. Therefore, they should not be used as deterrents to such management.

Preoperative Preparation

Antihypertensive medications are reduced during the preoperative period to the minimum necessary for blood pressure control. Frequently, patients requiring large doses of multiple medications for control will have significantly reduced requirements while hospitalized. If continued therapy is required, then α-methyldopa or vasodilators (e.g., Procardia) are the drugs of choice. There is little effect on hemodynamics when these agents are combined with anesthesia. We have also commonly continued low-dose

propranolol therapy as well without any adverse effects. If the patient's diastolic blood pressure is 120 to 140 mm Hg, it is essential that the pressure be brought under control and that operative treatment be postponed until this is accomplished. Recently, if blood pressure has been difficult to control, we have transferred the patient to the intensive care unit, where intravenous nitroprusside therapy with continuous intraarterial monitoring of blood pressure is instituted for the 24 hours prior to operation. Similarly, if the patient has a significant history of heart disease, pulmonary artery wedge pressure and cardiac output are monitored to maintain optimal cardiac hemodynamics and recognize and correct adverse changes before they become clinically significant.

Operative Techniques

A variety of operative techniques have been used to correct renal artery stenoses. From a practical standpoint, two basic operations have been most frequently utilized: aortorenal bypass and thromboendarterectomy. We favor aortorenal bypass, preferably with saphenous vein, and limit endarterectomy to orificial lesions of accessory renal arteries or in an occasional case with severe bilateral orificial stenoses. Uncommonly, the renal artery will be redundant after it has been circumferentially mobilized. In such patients with orificial lesions, renal artery reimplantation also has been used with gratifying results (Fig. 29–7).

Certain measures and maneuvers are applicable in almost all renal arterial operations. Mannitol, 12.5 gm, is administered intravenously early in the operation. Just prior to renal artery cross-clamping, heparin, 75 mg or 7500 units, is given intravenously. Protamine is occasionally required for reversal of the heparin at the end of the reconstruction.

Mobilization and Dissection

Through a midline xiphoid-to-pubis incision, the posterior peritoneum overlying the aorta is incised longitudinally and the duodenum is reflected to the patient's right to expose the left renal artery. By extending the posterior peritoneal incision to the left along the inferior border of the pancreas, an avascular plane behind the pancreas can be entered (Fig. 29–8) to expose the entire renal hilum on the left.

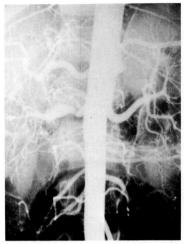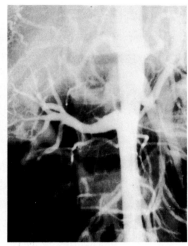

FIGURE 29–7. Preoperative and postoperative arteriograms in a 5-year-old child who underwent right renal artery reimplantation.

This exposure is of special significance when there are also distal lesions to be managed. The left renal artery lies behind the left renal vein. In some cases, the vein can be retracted cephalad to expose the artery; in other cases, caudal retraction of the vein provides better access. Usually, the gonadal and adrenal veins, which enter the left renal vein, must be ligated and divided to facilitate exposure of the artery. Frequently a lumbar vein enters the posterior wall of the left renal vein, and it can be avulsed easily unless special care is taken while mobilizing the renal vein. The proximal portion of the right renal artery can be exposed through the base of the mesentery by ligating two or more pairs of lumbar veins and retracting the left renal vein cephalad and the vena cava to the patient's right. However, the distal portion of the right renal artery is best exposed by mobilizing the duodenum and right colon medially (Fig. 29–9). Then the right renal vein is mobilized and usually retracted cephalad in order to expose the artery.

When bilateral renal artery lesions are to be cor-
rected and when correction of a right renal artery lesion or bilateral lesions is combined with aortic reconstruction, we modify these exposure techniques. First, we extend the base of the mesentery exposure to allow complete evisceration of the entire small bowel, right colon, and transverse colon; in this exposure, the posterior peritoneal incision begins with division of the ligament of Treitz and proceeds along the base of the mesentery to the cecum and then up the lateral gutter to the foramen of Winslow (Fig. 29–10). Second, we extend the incision to the left along the inferior border of the pancreas to enter a retropancreatic plane, thereby exposing the aorta to a point above the superior mesenteric artery. Through

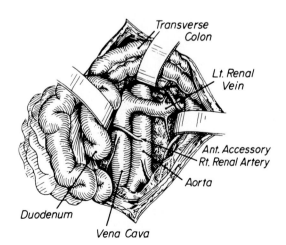

FIGURE 29–8. Exposure of the retroperitoneum through the base of the mesentery.

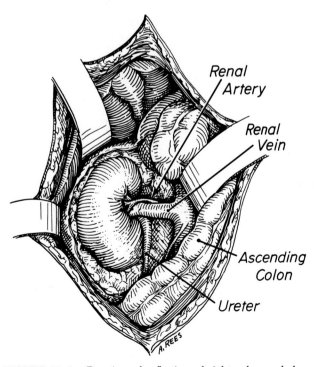

FIGURE 29–9. Drawing of reflection of right colon and duodenum to the left to expose the distal right renal artery.

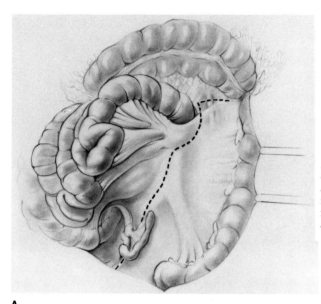

A

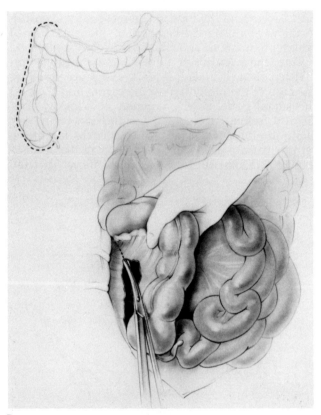

B

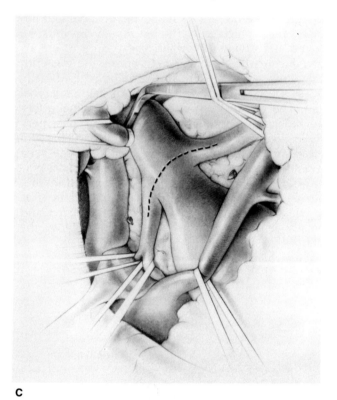

C

FIGURE 29–10.   Drawing of evisceration for bilateral renal artery exposure. Incision begins at base of mesentery (*A*), and continues around the cecum and up the right lateral mesocolon peritoneal reflection (*B*). Through this technique the entire small bowel and right colon is eviscerated for exposure of entire juxtarenal aorta and both renal arteries (*C*).

this modified exposure, simultaneous bilateral renal endarterectomies, aortorenal grafting, or renal artery attachment to the aortic graft can be performed with wide visualization of the entire area.

One other technique that we sometimes use is partially dividing both diaphragmatic crura as they pass behind the renal arteries to their paravertebral attachment. By this partial division of the crura, the aorta above the superior mesenteric artery is easily

visualized and can be mobilized for suprarenal cross-clamping.

Aortorenal Bypass

Three types of graft are usually available for aortorenal bypass: autologous saphenous vein, autologous hypogastric artery, and synthetic prosthesis. The decision as to which graft should be used depends on a number of factors. We use the saphenous vein preferentially. However, if it is small (less than 4 mm in diameter), the hypogastric artery or a synthetic prosthesis may be preferable. A 6-mm polytetrafluoroethylene graft is quite satisfactory when the distal renal artery is of large caliber.

When an end-to-side renal artery bypass is used, the anastomosis between the renal artery and the graft is done first. Silastic slings can be used to occlude the renal artery distally. This method of vessel occlusion is especially applicable to this procedure. In contrast to vascular clamps, these slings are essentially atraumatic to the delicate renal artery. The absence of clamps in the operative field is also advantageous. Furthermore, when tension is applied to the slings, they lift the vessel out of the retroperitoneal soft tissue for more accurate visualization.

The length of the arteriotomy should be at least three times the diameter of the renal artery to guard against late suture-line stenosis. A 6-0 or 7-0 monofilament polypropylene (Prolene; Ethicon) suture material is employed with loop magnification.

After the renal artery anastomosis is completed, the occluding clamps and slings are removed from the artery and a small bulldog clamp is placed across the vein graft adjacent to the anastomosis. The aortic anastomosis is then done. First, an ellipse of the anterolateral aortic wall is removed, and then the anastomosis is performed. If the graft is too long, kinking of the vein and subsequent thrombosis may result. If there is any element of kinking or twisting of the graft after both anastomoses are completed, the aortic anastomosis should be taken down and redone after appropriate shortening or reorientation of the graft. In certain instances, an end-to-end anastomosis between the graft and the renal artery provides a better reconstruction. Fry et al.[30] prefer the end-to-end anastomosis. We routinely employ end-to-end renal artery anastomosis when combining aortic replacement with renal revascularization. In this circumstance, the saphenous vein is attached to the Dacron aortic graft prior to its insertion. After the aortic graft is attached and flow is restored to the distal extremities, the renal artery can be transected and attached to the end of the saphenous vein graft without interrupting aortic flow.

Thromboendarterectomy

Thromboendarterectomy is only for atherosclerotic renal artery stenosis. It is not applicable in fibromuscular disease. Transaortic endarterectomy of bilateral main renal artery lesions has been strongly advocated by Wylie et al.[31] In this procedure, the proximal aortic clamp must usually be placed above the superior mesenteric artery. If it is placed below this artery, it will seriously compromise the exposure of the orifices of the renal arteries. Visualization of the distal end of the renal artery endarterectomy, however, is often difficult or impossible with this procedure. Because of this, we currently prefer a transverse aortotomy, carrying the incision across the stenoses and into each renal artery. By this method,

the entire endarterectomy can be performed under direct vision (Fig. 29–11).

Ex Vivo Reconstruction

Ex vivo management is necessary in patients with fibromuscular dysplasia and aneurysms or stenoses involving renal artery branches; patients with fibromuscular dysplasia and renal artery dissection and branch occlusion; patients with congenital arteriovenous fistulas of renal artery branches requiring partial resection; and patients with degeneration of previously placed grafts to the distal renal artery. Several methods of ex vivo hypothermic perfusion and reconstruction are available. A midline xiphoid-to-pubic incision is used for most renovascular procedures and is preferred when autotransplantation of the reconstructed kidney or combined aortic reconstructions are to be performed. An extended flank incision made parallel to the lower rib margin and carried to the posterior axillary line is used for complex branch renal artery repairs, and is our preferred approach for ex vivo reconstructions without autotransplantation. The ureter is always mobilized, but left intact, and an elastic sling or noncrushing clamp is placed around it to prevent collateral perfusion, inadvertent rewarming, or continued blood loss through the ureter.

After the kidney is mobilized and the vessels divided, the kidney is placed on the abdominal wall and perfused with a renal preservation solution. Continuous perfusion during the period of total renal ischemia is possible with complex perfusion pump systems, and may be superior for prolonged renal preservation during storage periods. However, simple intermittent flushing with a chilled preservation solution provides equal protection during the shorter periods (2 to 3 hours) required for ex vivo dissection and complex renal artery reconstructions. For intermittent flushing, we refrigerate the preservative overnight, add the additional components (Table 29–5)

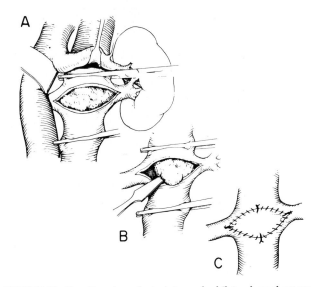

FIGURE 29–11. Drawing of arteriotomy for bilateral renal artery thromboendarterectomies.

TABLE 29–5.   ELECTROLYTE SOLUTION[a] FOR INTERMITTENT FLUSHING

Composition (gm/l)		Ionic Concentration (mEq/l)		Additives at Time of Use to 930 ml of Solution
Component	Amount	Electrolyte	Concentration	
K_2HPO_4	7.4	Potassium	115	50% dextrose: 70 ml
KH_2PO_4	2.04	Sodium	10	Sodium heparin: 2000 units
KCl	1.12	Phosphate (HPO_4-)	85	
$NaHCO_3$	0.84	Phosphate (H_2PO_4-)	15	
		Chloride	15	
		Bicarbonate	10	

[a]Electrolyte solution for kidney preservation supplied by Travenol Labs, Inc, Deerfield, IL.

immediately before use to make up a liter of solution, and hang the chilled (5° to 10°C) solution on an intravenous stand to provide gravitational perfusion pressure of at least 2 m. Five hundred milliliters of solution are flushed through the kidney immediately after its removal from the renal fossa. As each anastomosis is completed, an additional 150 to 200 ml of solution are flushed through the kidney, a procedure that also shows any leaks at the suture line.

Surface hypothermia is used to maintain constant hypothermia during ex vivo renal artery reconstruction. Our method of surface hypothermia consists of the following steps. We place 2-liter bottles of normal saline solution in ice slush overnight. When we remove the kidney, we place it in a watertight plastic sheet from which excess saline solution can be suctioned away, and place laparotomy pads over the kidney, keeping it cool and moist by a constant drip of the chilled saline solution. With this technique, we can maintain renal core temperatures of 10° to 15°C throughout the period of ischemia. We do not believe that autotransplantation to the iliac fossa is necessary for most ex vivo reconstructions, even though it is the accepted method for reattachment of the ex vivo reconstructed renal artery. Autotransplantation of the reconstructed kidney to the iliac fossa was borrowed from the renal transplant surgeon without thought being given to significant difference between the two patient populations. Reduction in the magnitude of the operative exposure, manual palpation of the transplanted kidney, potential use of irradiation for episodes of rejection, and ease of removal when treatment of rejection has failed are all historic and practical reasons for placing the transplanted kidney into the recipient's iliac fossa, but none of these advantages apply to the patient requiring ex vivo reconstruction. Rather, the factors most important in this patient are related to improving the predictability of permanent patency after revascularization. Because many ex vivo procedures are performed in relatively young patients, the durability of operation should be measured in terms of decades. For this reason, attachment of the kidney to the iliac arterial system within or below sites that are highly susceptible to significant atherosclerotic occlusive disease subjects the repaired vessels to disease that may, in time, threaten their patency. Furthermore, subsequent management of peripheral vascular dis-

ease may be complicated by the presence of the autotransplanted kidney. Finally, if the kidney is replaced in the renal fossa and the renal artery graft is properly attached to the aorta at a proximal infrarenal site, the result should mimic that of the standard aortorenal bypass and thus carry a high probability of technical success and long-term durability.

For replacement of the kidney in its original site, Gerota's capsule must be removed from the kidney during mobilization. Before transection of the renal vein begins, a large vascular clamp is placed to partially occlude the vena cava where it is entered by the renal vein. An ellipse of vena cava containing the entrance site of the renal vein is then excised, and the kidney is removed for ex vivo perfusion and reconstruction (Fig. 29–12). When the renal artery–graft anastomoses are completed and the kidney is replaced in its bed, the ellipse of vena cava is reattached (Fig. 29–13). This technique protects against stenosis of the renal vein anastomosis as a result of

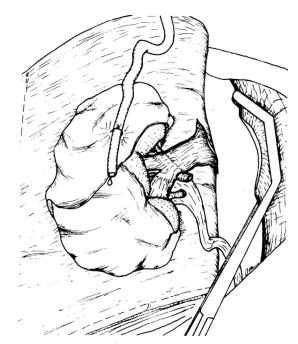

FIGURE 29–12.   Drawing of mobilized kidney and divided renal artery and vein for ex vivo repair. Note that a partial occlusion clamp is used on the lateral vena cava to excise an ellipse that includes the origin of the renal vein.

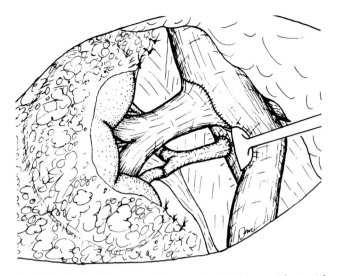

FIGURE 29–13. Drawing of the reimplanted kidney with arterial and venous attachments completed. The envelope of Gerota's fascia is reattached to secure the kidney in its original position.

technical error. The renal artery graft is then attached to the aorta in the standard manner.

Nephrectomy

Nephrectomy is a procedure that should be limited to a subgroup of patients with RVH in whom the kidney responsible for the hypertension has nonreconstructable vessels and negligible or no residual excretory function. In these circumstances of unretrievable renal function, nephrectomy can provide benefit in control of hypertension while not diminishing overall excretory function. In all other circumstances in which there is significant residual excretory renal function, the price of nephrectomy (loss of functioning renal mass) is greater than the potential benefit. Exception to this rule occurs only when hypertension is uncontrollable on maximal drug therapy and residual pressures consistently are severely elevated (greater than 120 mm Hg). This extreme conservatism for the role of nephrectomy is based on the knowledge that greater than 35 per cent of patients with atherosclerotic lesions will develop contralateral severe lesions during follow-up. Such lesions will place such a patient at risk for clinically severe renal failure and recurrent hypertension. This is of even greater importance in children, in whom 50 per cent of those who initially present with a unilateral lesion subsequently will develop contralateral disease.

EFFECT OF OPERATION ON HYPERTENSION

Most of the controversy surrounding the role of operative treatment of RVH relates to the risk of operation, unacceptable frequency of technical failures, and a low rate of favorable blood pressure response to operation. Certainly the literature ade-

quately documents the fact that poorly performed operations in poorly selected patients will result in an infrequent favorable blood pressure response. Current results of operative intervention in centers experienced with management of RVH, however, underscore the predictability of success. Although our experience spans over 25 years and includes the operative management of over 700 patients, review of the results on a recent series of 200 consecutive patients exemplifies current experience. The evolution of the patient population presenting for management is shown by comparing this group to the first 122 patients reported by the author over 20 years ago (Table 29–6).

In the most recent experience, during a 54-month period, atherosclerotic renovascular disease (RVD) was the predominant pathologic condition, accounting for 78 per cent of patients, 83 per cent of renal artery lesions repaired, and 100 per cent of the operative (3.1 per cent) and follow-up patient mortality rates (17.1 per cent). Despite the frequent need for extensive vascular repair (69 per cent) superimposed on diffuse or extreme atherosclerotic disease (85 per cent) and organ-specific damage (94 per cent), beneficial hypertension response was observed in 90 per cent of patients with atherosclerotic RVD patients. Note that the contemporary group is considerably older and more diffusely atherosclerotic than the patients treated in the earlier era.

Among patients with nonatherosclerotic RVD, 92

TABLE 29–6. COMPARISON OF EARLIER SURGICAL EXPERIENCE WITH CURRENT SERIES

	1961–1972[a]	1987–1991[b]
No. of patients	122	200
Mean age (yr)[e]		
NAs-RVD	33	38
As-RVD	50	62
Duration hypertension (yr)		
NAs-RVD	4.6	11.2
As-RVD	5.1	15.0
Renal artery disease (%)		
NAs-RVD	35%	21%
As-RVD	65%	79%
Renal artery repair (%)		
Unilateral	80%	60%
Bilateral	20%	40%
Combined[c]	13%	32%
Renal insufficiency (%)		
Not dependent on dialysis	8%	65%
Dependent on dialysis	0%	6%
Graft failure (%)	16%	3%
Hypertension response (%)		
NAs-RVD		
Cured	72%[d]	43%
Improved	24%[d]	49%
AS-RVD		
Cured	53%[d]	15%
Improved	36%[d]	75%

[a]Data derived from Foster et al. (1973).
[b]Current series.
[c]Combined aortic repair for occlusive or aneurysmal disease.
[d]Hypertension response excluding technical failures.
[e]NAs, nonatherosclerotic.

per cent demonstrated a beneficial hypertension response; however, only 43 per cent were considered cured, a figure below cure rates reported from earlier surgical series.[23,25] This difference may be explained by the number of older patients, the number of patients with uncorrected contralateral lesions, and the duration of hypertension in many of these patients with nonatherosclerotic RVD. In contrast to the blood pressure results obtained in the entire group, patients less than 55 years of age who had all anatomic renal artery lesions corrected and who had been hypertensive for less than 5 years had a cure rate of 68 per cent and an improvement rate of 32 per cent. This response rate is comparable to results from earlier reports. We speculate that previous surgical series included patients with nonatherosclerotic RVD who had surgical repair earlier in their course than did the contemporary population admitted for operative management.

Although operation was accomplished in the non-atherosclerotic RVD group without death and with minimal morbidity (8.5 per cent), the operative (3.1 per cent) and later mortality (17.1 per cent) among 157 patients with atherosclerotic RVD was high. Twenty-six of 32 operative and late deaths occurred in patients considered to have extreme atherosclerotic disease. The presence of near end-stage renal insufficiency (mean EGFR: 13.7 ml/min) accounted for this significant association with follow-up death. Furthermore, follow-up death was significantly influenced by renal function response to operation and progression to dependence on dialysis. Patients with extreme disease but improved EGFR after operation demonstrated improved survival and decreased risk of eventual dependence on dialysis compared with patients with no change in EGFR. Nevertheless, the low actuarial survival among patients with extreme atherosclerotic RVD (49 per cent at 48 months) raises the question of whether death within this group was actually accelerated by operation. Since no parallel patient group with extreme atherosclerotic RVD was medically managed, data to provide an answer to this question are lacking.

EFFECT OF RENAL REVASCULARIZATION ON ISCHEMIC NEPHROPATHY

Traditionally, study of the sequelae of renovascular occlusive disease has centered on the pathophysiology and management of the resultant renovascular hypertension. Recently, however, the potential for simultaneous retrieval of excretory function in some patients with combined hypertension and renal insufficiency has been recognized. These observations have renewed awareness of this functional consequence of renal ischemia and have led to the coinage of the term "ischemic nephropathy." By definition, ischemic nephropathy reflects the presence of anatomically severe occlusive disease of the extrapar-

enchymal renal artery in a patient with excretory renal insufficiency.

Little information is available in the literature that accurately describes the incidence, prevalence, spectrum of clinical presentations, or the natural history of ischemic nephropathy. Nevertheless, circumstantial evidence suggests that it may be a more common cause of progressive renal failure in the atherosclerotic age group than previously recognized. In a 1986 survey, 73 per cent of end-stage renal disease (ESRD) patients were in the atherosclerotic age.[32] In a report by Mailloux et al.,[33] a presumed renal vascular cause of ESRD increased in frequency from 6.7 per cent for the period 1978 to 1981 to a frequency of 16.5 per cent for the period 1982 to 1985. The median age at onset of ESRD for that group was the oldest of all groups, falling in the seventh decade of life.

To improve our understanding of ischemic nephropathy we recently undertook a retrospective review of data collected during a recent 42-month period from 58 consecutive patients with ischemic nephropathy submitted to operative management in our center[34] to examine the rate of decline in their renal function during the period before intervention and to examine the impact of operation on their outcome. The ages ranged from 22 years to 79 years (mean: 69 years). Based on serum creatinine values, immediate preoperative EGFR ranged from 0 to 46 ml/min (mean: 23.85 ± 9.76 ml/min). Eight patients were dialysis dependent or anuric at the time of operation. Patients with at least three sequential measurements for calculations of EGFR changes during the 6 months before operation ($n = 50$) and the first 12 months after operation ($n = 32$) were used to describe the preoperative rate of decline in EGFR and the impact of operation on this decrease in the operative survivors. In addition, comparative analyses of data from patients with unilateral versus bilateral lesions and patients classified as having improvement in EGFR versus no improvement after operation were performed. Comparison of the immediate preoperative EGFR with the immediate postoperative EGFR for the entire group showed significant improvement in response to operation (Fig. 29–14). Likewise, the rate of deterioration in EGFR for the total group was improved after operation (Fig. 29–15). A similar improvement in the rate of deterioration in EGFR was seen in the subgroup of patients who received an immediate improvement in EGFR in response to operation (Fig. 29–16). The results of revascularization in dialysis-dependent patients is shown in Table 29–7. Note that all patients with unilateral lesions were removed from dialysis.

From this review we found that bilaterality of occlusions, normality of distal vessels, and rapidity of deterioration in renal function were valuable positive predictors of benefit in renal function by operation. Conversely, unilateral disease, absence of severe hypertension, and diffuse branch vessel occlusive disease were negative predictors of such benefit.

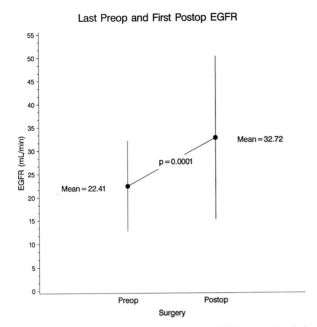

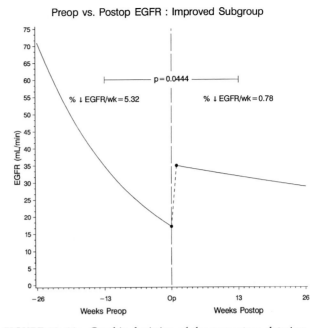

FIGURE 29–14. Comparison of the mean EGFR immediately before and at least 1 week after operation. The *p* value for the differences is determined using *t* test for unpaired data.

FIGURE 29–16. Graphic depiction of the percentage deterioration of EGFR per week during the 6 months before (*n* = 23) and after (*n* = 25) operation in the group of patients who received at least a 20 per cent improvement in EGFR following operation. The immediate effect of operation on EGFR in this group is also depicted. The *p* values for differences are determined using *t* test for unpaired data. Note the improvement in the slope of decline in EGFR after operation in this group.

Further, the data presented in this retrospective review argue that ischemic nephropathy is a rapidly progressive form of renal insufficiency. The effect of renal revascularization on renal function, however, was heterogeneous. Nevertheless, the frequency of both retrieval of renal function and slowing of the

rate of its deterioration during follow-up was gratifying and encourages enthusiasm for the continued study of the role of operation in properly selected patients. Most importantly, the results argue that a carefully controlled prospective randomized trial comparing operation with medical therapy is necessary to confirm the value of operation in patients with controlled hypertension. Only through this method could one accurately clarify the role of operation in the prolongation of the period of dialysis independence and long-term survival in patients with ischemic nephropathy.

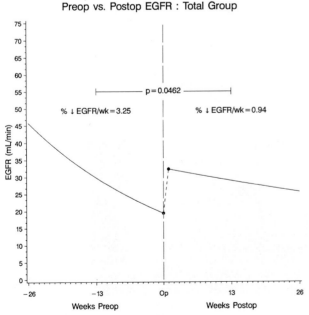

FIGURE 29–15. Graphic depiction of the percentage deterioration of EGFR per week for the entire group during the 6 months before (*n* = 50) and after (*n* = 32) operation. The immediate effect of operation on EGFR is also depicted. The *p* values for differences are determined using *t* test for unpaired data. Note the improvement in the slope of decline in EGFR after operation.

TABLE 29–7.   RESULTS IN DIALYSIS-DEPENDENT GROUP

Age (Yrs)	Sex	Dialysis Duration	Immediate Postoperative EGFR	Site of Operation
51	F	11 days	32.7	Bilateral
63	M	32 days	34.6	Bilateral
65	M	6 days	44.5	Bilateral
59	M	30 days	49.0	Bilateral
76	M	10 days	30.7	Bilateral
61	F	0[a]	13.5	Bilateral
66	M	6 days	CD[b]	Unilateral
75	M	54 days	CD[b]	Unilateral

[a]Patient had developed anuria; operation undertaken without dialysis.
[b]CD, continued on dialysis.

TABLE 29–8. SEQUENTIAL 1- TO 23-YEAR FOLLOW-UP ARTERIOGRAPHY (198 RECONSTRUCTIONS)

Status	No. of Grafts	Percentage
No adverse change	174	88
Aneurysmal dilation	7	3.5
Stenosis	10	5.0
Occlusion	4	2.0
False aneurysm	3	1.5

LATE FOLLOW-UP RECONSTRUCTIONS

From our experience with the operative management of RVH, 1- to 23-year follow-up sequential angiography of 198 reconstructions is available for evaluation (Table 29–8). Five saphenous vein grafts and two hypogastric autografts have undergone aneurysmal dilatation. Only one of these, a hypogastric autograft, has required replacement (Fig. 29–17). The remaining six have stabilized, and the patients have remained cured of hypertension. Aneurysmal dilatation of autogenous grafts (vein or artery) has occurred only in the young children in our experience. This suggests that the immature saphenous vein is particularly susceptible to this phenomenon. For this reason, we prefer the normal hypogastric artery as the conduit of choice in this group. In the two instances of autogenous arterial graft aneurysmal degeneration, fibromuscular dysplasia of the donor hypogastric artery was identified in retrospective microscopic evaluation.

Ten grafts have developed suture-line or midgraft stenoses requiring revision from 1 to 8 years after the initial operation (Fig. 29–18). Four patients have had graft occlusions during follow-up and probably represent missed graft stenoses, which progressed to occlusion. Three grafts required correction of aortic anastomotic false aneurysms of Dacron grafts in two patients 8 and 20 years postoperatively. The remaining grafts (88 per cent) have had no untoward changes and continued patency of the reconstruction during follow-up (Fig. 29–19).

Follow-up angiography also has shown progression of mild to moderate contralateral renovascular disease in 38 per cent of the patients. This is most important in children, in whom 7 of 15 with fibromuscular dysplasia had bilateral involvement.[21] Only three of these seven children had the contralateral disease demonstrated at the time of the initial evaluation and operation. The remaining four children had documentation of the development and progression of contralateral disease subsequently. This occurrence of subsequent contralateral stenosis has led us to perform nephrectomy in children only if blood pressure is uncontrollable and revascularization is impossible. Since the longest follow-up group is only 10 years, the true incidence of subsequent contralateral disease requires additional longitudinal follow-up.

EFFECT OF BLOOD PRESSURE RESPONSE ON LONG-TERM SURVIVAL

Since the logic for management of hypertension of any cause is to improve long-term cardiovascular morbidity and event-free survival, we recently reviewed the outcome of 71 patients who underwent operative management of RVH from 15 to 23 years previously.[35] Complete follow-up was available in 66 of the 68 patients who survived operation. Comparison of the initial blood pressure response to operation (1 to 6 months postoperatively) to the blood pressure status at the time of death or current date (up to 23 years later) shows that the effect of operative treatment is maintained over long-term follow-up (Fig. 29–20). In those patients who required repeat renovascular operation for recurrent RVH during follow-up, the majority of the operations were performed for the management of contralateral lesions that had progressed to functional significance (i.e., produced RVH).

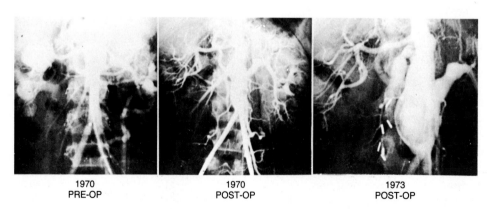

| 1970 PRE-OP | 1970 POST-OP | 1973 POST-OP |

FIGURE 29–17. Sequential follow-up arteriogram of a 10-year-old child who underwent a hypogastric autograft to the left renal artery and an iliac vein autograft to the superior mesenteric artery. Ultimately, both grafts required replacements.

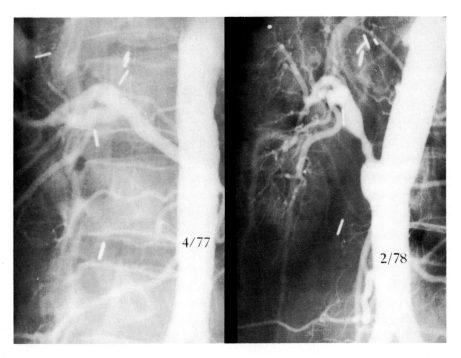

FIGURE 29–18.   Postoperative arteriograms showing fibrous narrowing of the saphenous vein graft secondary to subendothelial fibroblastic proliferation.

Assessment of the effect of blood pressure response on late survival produced results that are not surprising. Although the subgroup of nonresponders is small, they experienced a significantly more rapid death rate during follow-up than did those patients who had a blood pressure response to operation (Fig. 29–21). This confirms the validity of the premise that inadequate management of RVH leaves the patient at higher risk of early death from cardiovascular events. The presence of angiographically diffuse atheroscle-

rosis at the time of evaluation and operation was predictive of a more rapid rate of death during follow-up (Fig. 29–22).

This difference in subsequent death rate was present, even though comparison between patients with diffuse atherosclerotic disease (ASD) and focal atherosclerotic disease (ASF) was undertaken only in patients experiencing a significant blood pressure response. In view of the suggestion by some physicians that the presence of diffuse disease precludes a high

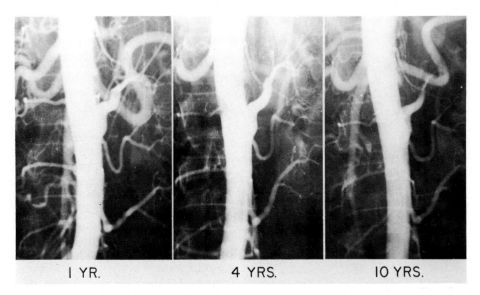

FIGURE 29–19.   Sequential follow-up arteriograms after autogenous vein aortorenal bypass showing its long-term durability.

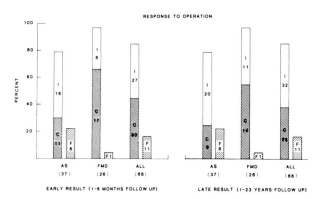

FIGURE 29–20. Bar graphs comparing initial benefit with late blood pressure response in the respective types of lesions. *AS,* arteriosclerotic lesion; *FMD,* fibromuscular dysplasia.

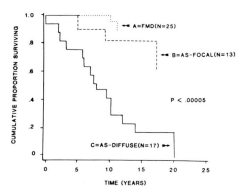

FIGURE 29–22. Kaplan-Meier life-table analysis of survival of patients benefited from operation by type and stage of disease, with 55 patients cured or improved (deaths from cardiovascular causes). *FMD,* fibromuscular dysplasia; *AS-Focal,* focal atherosclerosis; *AS-Diffuse,* diffuse atherosclerosis.

rate of blood pressure response to operation, it is worthwhile to stress that there was no significant difference in frequency of response between the ASF (80 per cent) and ASD (77 per cent) groups in this study. In addition, although the presence of ASD was associated with a more rapid death rate, it does not preclude the probability of a longer survival in this subgroup when compared with a similar group of patients who either did not undergo operation or received no blood pressure benefit from such intervention. Furthermore, if one considers that ASD is only a later stage of ASF, it is not surprising that the end point of clinically significant disease, namely death from cardiovascular events, arrives sooner when one begins follow-up or removes a risk factor, which causes its acceleration later in its natural history.

Finally, our evaluation of other preoperative markers potentially predictive of a more rapid occurrence of cardiovascular morbid and mortal events requires comment. Clinically meaningful results from our statistical assessment of such parameters as smoking, hyperlipidemia, prior history or evidence of cardiac disease, or obesity were minimized by the limited patient population and dominant influence of the type of disease (fibromuscular dysplasia versus ath-

erosclerosis) and stage of disease (ASF versus ASD) in this analysis. Through inclusion of more recently managed patients in our analysis, we are hopeful that a more accurate prediction of symptom-free survival or, alternatively, of early death regardless of blood pressure response will be obtained. Indeed, some of these risk factors have also been reviewed among a group of patients in our more recent operative experience. These 114 patients, who had operation during the 5-year period from 1975 to 1980, were evaluated for preoperative markers predictive of reduced survival and event-free survival. Those risk factors found to be statistically significant determinants of earlier death included electrocardiographic evidence of left ventricular hypertrophy (with and without strain) or previous myocardial infarction and history of angina. Such information, in conjunction with the results of prospective randomized comparisons of the respective therapeutic regimens currently available for management of RVH, will resolve the continuing controversy regarding the preferred method of treatment.

PERCUTANEOUS TRANSLUMINAL ANGIOPLASTY

The introduction of the alternative interventional modality percutaneous transluminal angioplasty by Grüntzig in 1978[36] has led to a new era in the management of hypertensive patients with renal artery stenosis. This technique employs the principle of coaxial dilatation of the vessel by inflation of a balloon-tipped catheter that has been introduced across the stenotic renal artery lesion. The stenotic lesion is disrupted, and, by stretching the vessel wall itself, portions of the media are disrupted as well, leaving the vessel at a greater diameter than its dimension prior to dilatation. The increased luminal diameter is primarily created by disruption of the intima, the atherosclerotic or fibrodysplastic lesion, and portions of the media. Early reports of the results of this tech-

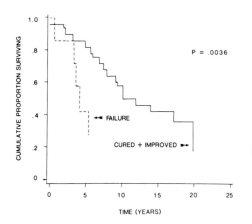

FIGURE 29–21. Kaplan-Meier life-table analysis: Survival by response to operation in 37 arteriosclerotic patients (deaths from cardiovascular causes).

nique showed that stenotic renal arteries frequently could be dilated successfully with immediate improvement in levels of hypertension in patients with RVH.

By reviewing the reported experience with PTA and the observations from the operative management of unsuccessful PTA, one can formulate indications for the preferential use of each procedure in the treatment of RVH. Reported experience with PTA of fibrodysplastic lesions has results similar to those of open surgical repairs. Beneficial blood pressure responses have been reported to be as high as 100 per cent following PTA in properly selected cases, and although vessel perforation, hemorrhage, and branch occlusions have been reported, their incidence has been less than 5 per cent.[37] One would anticipate that such complications would be most likely in patients with diffuse fibromuscular dysplasia affecting both the distal main renal artery and its branches. The cure rate after PTA of fibromuscular dysplasia, even when the procedure is performed by experienced surgeons, varies from 37 to 51 per cent.[38] In contrast, 77 per cent of patients with fibrodysplastic lesions on whom we have operated have been cured of hypertension. Having routinely found that angiography underestimates the distal extent of fibromuscular dysplasia, we believe this difference in cure rates represents residual, inadequately managed disease in the PTA group. For this reason, we believe that fibromuscular dysplasia extending to the branch level is best managed primarily by an open operative approach and that PTA should be reserved for the subgroup of medial dysplastic lesions that are clearly limited to the main renal artery.

Stenotic lesions occurring in children are usually discrete narrowings and therefore would appear ideal for PTA. However, the stenotic area is commonly a congenital narrowing of the entire vessel wall and is predominantly composed of elastic tissue. When such a vessel is submitted to PTA, the original diameter returns after dilatation or, if the vessel has been overdistended, rupture of the entire vessel wall is likely. Therefore, we believe that PTA is an inappropriate method of intervention in children with renal artery stenosis and that success is best achieved by operative correction.

Finally, a review of series reporting results with PTA for atherosclerotic lesions dramatizes the frequency of failure with this lesion as well. Miller et al.[39] reported that only 45 per cent of ostial and mixed lesions were improved after 6 months; Sos et al.[38] reported only a 14 per cent benefit rate when bilateral ostial lesions were treated. These results show that PTA has little value in the treatment of this variety of lesion, for one must accept the risks of cholesterol embolization, vessel thrombosis, and loss of renal function, while expecting only a minimal chance for prolonged benefit.

To summarize, experience with the liberal use of PTA has helped to clarify its role as one of the therapeutic options in the treatment of renovascular hypertension, but the data now accumulated argue for its selective application. In this regard, PTA of nonorificial atherosclerotic lesions and medial fibrodysplastic lesions limited to the main renal artery yields results comparable to those of operation if carried out by surgeons experienced in the technique. In contrast, the use of PTA for the treatment of congenital stenotic lesions, fibrodysplastic lesions involving renal artery branches, and ostial atherosclerotic lesions is associated with inferior results and with increased risk of complications. For this reason, we believe that operation remains the initial treatment of choice for patients in these groups, and that the type of interventional therapy for RVH must always be individualized.

REFERENCES

1. Bright R: Cases and observations illustrative of renal disease accompanied with the secretion of albuminous urine. Guy's Hospital Rep 1:388, 1836.
2. Tigerstedt R, Bergman PG: Niere und Kreislauf. Scand Arch Physiol 8:223, 1898.
3. Goldblatt H: Studies on experimental hypertension. J Exp Med 59:347, 1934.
4. Smith HW: Unilateral nephrectomy in hypertensive disease. J Urol 76:685, 1956.
5. Freeman N: Thromboendarterectomy for hypertension due to renal artery occlusion. JAMA 157:1077, 1973.
6. DeCamp PT, Birchall R: Recognition and treatment of renal arterial stenosis associated with hypertension. Surgery 43:134, 1958.
7. Morris GC Jr, Cooley DA, Crawford ES, et al: Renal revascularization for hypertension. Clinical and physiologic studies in 32 cases. Surgery 48:95, 1960.
8. Hurwitt ES, Seidenburg B, Hainovoco H, et al: Splenorenal arterial anastomosis. Circulation 14:537, 1956.
9. Luke JC, Levitan BA: Revascularization of the kidney in hypertension due to renal artery stenosis. Arch Surg 79:269, 1959.
10. Howard JE, Conner TB: Use of differential renal function studies in the diagnosis of renovascular hypertension. Am J Surg 107:58, 1964.
11. Stamey TA, Nudelman IJ, Good PH, et al: Functional characteristics of renovascular hypertension. Medicine 40:347, 1961.
12. Page IH, Helmes OM: A crystalline pressor substance (angiotensin) resulting from the reaction between renin and renin activator. J Exp Med 71:29, 1940.
13. Braun-Menendez E, Fasciolo JC, Lelois LF, et al: La substancia hypertensora de la sangre del rinon, isquemiado. Rev Soc Argent Biol 15:420, 1939.
14. Lentz KE, Skeggs LT Jr, Woods KR, et al: The amino acid composition of hypertensin II and its biochemical relationship to hypertension. Int J Exp Med 104:183, 1956.
15. Tobian L: Relationship of juxtaglomerular apparatus to renin and angiotensin. Circulation 25:189, 1962.
16. Dean RH: Operative management of renovascular hypertension. *In* Bergan JJ, Yao JST (eds): Surgery of the Aorta and its Body Branches. New York, Grune & Stratton, 1979, p 377.
17. Harrison EG Jr, McCormack LJ: Pathologic classification of

renal arterial disease in renovascular hypertension. Mayo Clin Proc 46:161, 1971.

18. Tucker RM, Labarthe DR: Frequency of surgical treatment for hypertension in adults at the Mayo Clinic from 1973 through 1975. Mayo Clin Proc 52:549, 1977.

19. Shapiro AP, Perez-Stable E, Scheib ET, et al: Renal artery stenosis and hypertension. Am J Med 47:175, 1969.

20. Davis BA, Crook JE, Vestal RE, Oates JA: Prevalence of renovascular hypertension in patients with Grade III or IV hypertensive retinopathy. N Engl J Med 301:1273, 1979.

21. Lawson JD, Boerth RK, Foster JH, et al: Diagnosis and management of renovascular hypertension in children. Arch Surg 112:1307, 1977.

22. Simon N, Franklin SS, Bleifer KH, Maxwell MH: Clinical characteristics of renovascular hypertension. JAMA 220:1209, 1972.

23. Foster JH, Dean RH, Pinkerton JA, et al: Ten years experience with the surgical management of renovascular hypertension. Ann Surg 177:755, 1973.

24. Vaughn ED, Buhler FR, Larach JH, et al: Renovascular hypertension: Renin measurements to indicate hypersecretion and contralateral suppression, estimate renal plasma flow, and score for surgical curability. Am J Med 55:402, 1973.

25. Stanley JC, Fry WJ: Surgical treatment of renovascular hypertension. Arch Surg 112:1291, 1977.

26. Davidson J, Lowe B, Dean RH, Rhamy RK: Variability of split renal function studies in essential and renovascular hypertension. Surg Forum 30:574, 1979.

27. Hunt JC, Strong CG: Renovascular hypertension. Mechanisms, natural history and treatment. Am J Cardiol 32:562, 1973.

28. Dean RH, Kieffer RW, Smith BM, et al: Renovascular hypertension. Arch Surg 116:1408, 1981.

29. Dean RH: Indications for operative management of renovascular hypertension. J So Carolina Med Assoc Dec:523, 1977.

30. Fry WJ, Brink BE, Thompson NW: New techniques in the treatment of extensive fibromuscular disease involving the renal arteries. Surgery 68:959, 1970.

31. Wylie EJ, Perloff DL, Stoney RJ: Autogenous tissue revascularization techniques in surgery for renovascular hypertension. Ann Surg 170:416, 1969.

32. Eggers PW: Effect of transplantation on the medicare end-stage renal disease program. Transplant Medicare ESRD Prog 318:223, 1988.

33. Mailloux LU, Bellucci AG, Mossey RT, et al: Predictors of survival in patients undergoing dialysis. Am J Med 84:855–862, 1988.

34. Dean RH, Tribble RW, Hansen KJ, et al: Evolution of renal insufficiency in ischemic nephropathy. Ann Surg 213:446–456, 1991.

35. Dean RH, Krueger TC, Whiteneck JM, et al: Operative management of renovascular hypertension: Results after 15–23 years follow-up. J Vasc Surg 1:234, 1984.

36. Grüntzig A, Vetter W, Meier B, et al: Treatment of renovascular hypertension with transluminal dilatation of a renal artery stenosis. Lancet 1:801, 1978.

37. Tegtmeyer CJ, Kellum D, Ayers C: Percutaneous transluminal angioplasty of the renal artery. Results and long-term follow-up. Radiology 153:77–84, 1984.

38. Sos TA, Pickering TG, Sniderman K, Saddekni S, Case DB, Silane MF, Vaughan ED Jr, Laragh JH: Percutaneous transluminal renal angioplasty in renovascular hypertension due to atheroma of fibromuscular dysplasia. N Engl J Med 309:274–279, 1983.

39. Miller GA, Ford KK, Braun SD, Newman GE, Moore AV Jr, Malone R, Dunnick NR: Percutaneous transluminal angioplasty vs. surgery for renovascular hypertension. AJR 144:447–450, 1985.

30

VISCERAL ISCHEMIC SYNDROMES

JOHN J. BERGAN

. . . for 71 years, your mesenteric artery will have performed perfectly . . . until today [when] a brown, stony mass of blood will obstruct the circulation to your intestine.

Carlos Fuentes
"The Death of Artemio Cruz"

Thus does a poetic author describe the end of the life of an adventurous revolutionary, romantic, poetic rancher whose life and love was intermingled with the Mexican Revolution and Pancho Villa. He describes the hopelessness of the situation when the abdomen is ". . . swollen, hard, full of blood. They find the area of gangrene bathed in fetid liquid. Mesenteric infarct. They look at . . . dilated intestine, deep scarlet, almost black." In this vivid description is the experience of every surgeon who has seen this condition. Hopelessness is implied, frustration evident.

Mesenteric ischemia bridges the gap between general surgery and vascular surgery. The discipline of general surgery is inseparably bound to vascular surgery in syndromes of the intestinal circulation. Patients with weight loss, the hallmark of visceral ischemia, present to physicians and general surgeons for diagnosis. Patients suffering acute abdominal catastrophes of sudden mesenteric artery occlusion present to general surgeons for emergent diagnosis and therapy. However, repair of the blood vessels of the viscera is taxing, meticulous, and fraught with problems that lead to reocclusion of the newly restored blood supply. In short, revascularization of viscera requires expert vascular reconstructive skills.

Knowledge of the syndromes of visceral ischemia can be organized in systematic fashion; however, no single laboratory test makes an absolute diagnosis.[1-4] In situations of chronic and acute intestinal ischemia, knowledge and interpretative skills spiced with a dash of intuition are necessary. A little experience with visceral ischemia, both good and bad, is a great help. In this chapter, syndromes of visceral ischemia will encompass chronic visceral ischemia; acute intestinal ischemia due to embolic, thrombotic, and nonorganic cause; and mesenteric venous thrombosis.

ANATOMIC PATTERNS

Anatomically and embryologically, the three main sources of arterial blood supply to the viscera derive from the main artery of the foregut (the celiac axis), the midgut (the superior mesenteric artery), and the hindgut (the inferior mesenteric artery). The arborizations and interconnections of these arteries vary so greatly that it is hard to define what is normal with regard to anatomic distribution. Nevertheless, there is no doubt that the superior mesenteric artery is the most important of the vessels to the alimentary tract. At its origin in the upper portion of the abdominal cavity, it is surrounded by pancreas and sympathetic nerve fibers adjacent to the portal vein and duodenum. It is in one of the most inaccessible areas of the human body. To expose the aorta and the origin of the superior mesenteric artery is difficult. However, as the artery emerges from behind the duodenum, it is easily accessible in the root of the small bowel mesentery, where the first branch beyond the inferior pancreaticoduodenal artery is the middle colic artery. Beyond these are the intestinal arteries, which vary from 3 to 20 in number and which, in turn, supply the intestinal arcades. Because of its angle of emergence from the aorta, the superior mesenteric artery easily receives emboli originating from the heart.

In contrast to the angulation of the superior mesenteric artery, the celiac axis pokes straight forward from the aorta, where its origin is also obscured. It is crossed by dense fibers of the arcuate ligament of the diaphragm and by a network of sympathetic nerves. Entrapment of the vessel by the arcuate ligament may markedly narrow its origin and even allow poststenotic dilatation to appear. The axis divides immediately into its three branches, the left gastric artery, the hepatic artery, and the splenic artery. However, in nearly 20 per cent of patients, the right hepatic artery originates from the superior mesenteric artery.

The inferior mesenteric artery origin from the aorta is also obscured, but in this instance by the aortic wall itself. As much as 2 cm of the artery may be intramural. In visceral ischemic syndromes, the most important branch of the inferior mesenteric artery is the left colic, which gives rise to three to four vasa recta before continuing as the ascending branch of the left colic artery. This is the important collateral to the superior mesenteric artery that elongates and widens in response to increased blood flow (Fig. 30–1). Thus, it becomes the meandering mesenteric artery. Anatomically, the ascending branch of the left colic artery bifurcates to join in formation of the marginal artery (of Drummond). The other branch forms an arcade with the middle colic artery, called the arc of Riolan.

The descending branch of the left colic artery bifurcates into the two superior hemorrhoidal arteries. Their inverted "Y" appearance is characteristically found on many aortograms.

CHRONIC VISCERAL ISCHEMIA

Clinical Picture

Clinical manifestations of chronic intestinal ischemia include pain with or without diarrhea or constipation, cachexia, a systolic bruit in the abdomen, and coincidental coronary and/or cerebrovascular insufficiency and claudication.[5] Diarrhea may be explained by the increased motility stimulated by ischemia. The resulting decrease in intact food may lead the patient into a pattern of constipation.

The pain is abdominal in location, with occasional radiation to the back. It may vary from a nauseating cramp to an acute colic. At first it is of short duration. but gradually, as the ischemia worsens, it persists for a longer period of time until the patient may be pain free only briefly between meals. Consciously or by reflex, the patient decreases food intake, which immediately leads to weight loss and appearance of malignant cachexia. Because the pain has many similarities to the pain of infiltrating pancreatic carcinoma, carcinoma of the stomach, or peptic ulcer disease, focus on diagnosis of these conditions becomes dominant. The combination of weight loss, absence of such carcinoma, and the presence of symptomatic arteriosclerotic occlusive disease should suggest chronic visceral ischemia. These findings are important because such patients are demonstrating failure of collateral circulation. When further ischemia supervenes, an abdominal catastrophe is inevitable.

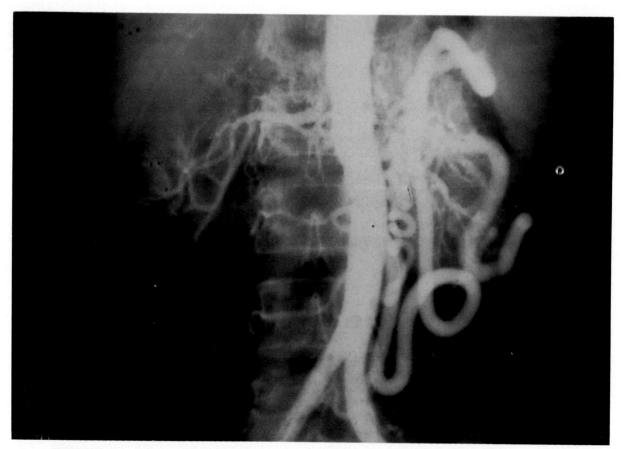

FIGURE 30–1. Aortogram showing the meandering mesenteric artery ascending as a branch of the left colic artery and then joining in formation of the marginal artery. As this joins the arborization of the superior mesenteric artery, the connection is called the arc of Riolan. Thus, the inferior mesenteric artery becomes a part of the collateral circulation to the superior mesenteric arterial bed.

Investigations

Although the history of chronic intestinal ischemia becomes clear in retrospect, there is not any one symptom that triggers an early diagnosis. The problem is compounded by the fact that the symptoms are not unique. They mimic other more common gastrointestinal disorders. Physical examination is not helpful. Therefore, diagnosis depends upon intuition, suspecting the condition, and ordering appropriate investigations. Noninvasively, duplex ultrasound scans[6-8] are easily performed and are reliable. Should these studies prove diagnostic, aortography will reveal the anatomic pattern of the lesions and provide a guideline for therapy.

Surgical Approaches

The fact that many differing surgical techniques have evolved to correct visceral artery obstructive disease means that no single technique has emerged as definitive. Direct arterial reconstruction includes open endarterectomy, reimplantation of visceral vessels, bypass operations from infrarenal aorta to visceral arteries, suprarenal aorta-to-visceral artery bypasses, iliac artery-to-visceral artery bypasses, single and multiple intestinal artery reconstructions, and combined aortic reconstruction with intestinal artery reconstruction.[9,10]

At this time, in the evolution of arterial reconstructive surgery, three general techniques are favored. These include transaortic endarterectomy, infrarenal aortic-to-visceral bypass, and more recently, suprarenal-to-visceral artery bypass. Thromboendarterectomy demands a thoracoabdominal approach in which the aorta is cross-clamped above and below the major visceral arteries. A "U"-shaped aortotomy is created surrounding the orifices of the celiac axis and superior mesenteric artery. The atheroma is removed using an extraction eversion endarterectomy. This may be combined with renal thromboendarterectomy.[11]

Because high-risk patients are excluded from such surgery, aortovisceral bypass grafting is favored by many. Autogenous vein or prosthetic graft can be used alternatively. A transabdominal approach is used for bypass grafting, and a choice is made between supraceliac or infrarenal origin of the grafts. What is absolutely necessary is an undiseased aortic segment. This fact tips the scales toward supraceliac origin of grafts (Figs. 30–2 through 30–4). This also allows a better orientation of the graft and avoidance of kinking. If this approach is chosen, a vertical midline or transverse, subcostal, bilateral incision can be used to give wide exposure of the upper abdomen. The attachments of the left lobe of the liver are cut and the left lobe is retracted to the right. The stomach is retracted to the left and inferiorly and the lesser omental bursa is entered, carefully protecting the vagus nerves. The crural tissue enveloping the aorta is split, thus exposing the supraceliac aorta. Here the

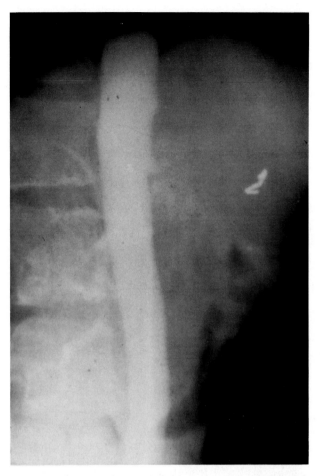

FIGURE 30–2. Lateral aortogram showing no true origins of the celiac axis, superior mesenteric artery, or inferior mesenteric artery. On the other hand, surgical clips are seen in the upper abdomen. Thus, a syndrome is suggested. This is a young woman who is taking contraceptive pills and smoking cigarettes; she has had obstruction of the main arteries to the intestinal vascular beds and acalculus cholecystitis, which led to cholecystectomy and placement of the surgical clips. Her chronic indigestion (postprandial pain) and weight loss led to the investigation shown here.

aorta is circumferentially freed of investing tissues so as to allow proximal distal clamping for the graft origin anastomosis. The common hepatic and splenic arteries are dissected free from the investing sympathetic nerve fibers and elevated from their position at the upper border of the pancreas. Further dissection caudally exposes the origin of the superior mesenteric artery, and this is freed for an appropriate distance. If saphenous vein is chosen it is harvested and either reversed or nonreversed vein used. A longitudinal aortotomy will allow the grafts to be sewn in an end of graft-to-side of aorta manner, and two saphenous veins can be anastomosed to one another. The anastomosis to the visceral vessels can be end to end or end to side.

Surgical Risk

Although patients requiring visceral revascularization are at increased risk compared to general sur-

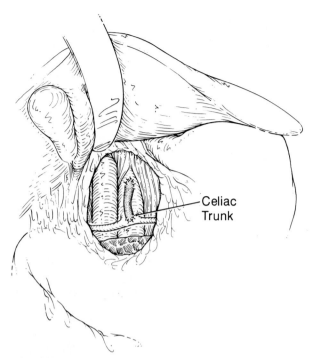

FIGURE 30–3. After the crus of the diaphragm is incised, the supraceliac aorta is encircled and skeletonized so that the aorta-to-celiac axis graft shown here can be placed. The graft may be prosthetic (polytetrafluoroethylene) or autogenous vein.

gical patients, in fact the operation can be performed with minimal morbidity. Because of the preoperative weight loss, which makes the operation easier, nutritional repletion should be considered prior to operation. If supraceliac aortic clamping is contemplated, myocardial protection should be considered and cardiac afterload reduction provided.

If the infrarenal bypass technique is chosen, the saphenous veins may be attached to the infrarenal, easily accessible aorta, and tunneled in the retropan-

creatic anatomic plane to the celiac axis in the lesser omental sac, or directly to the superior mesenteric artery.[12] Care must be taken in placing the aorto-mesenteric graft. If it is too short occlusion will occur, and if it is too long redundancy will allow twisting and kinking.

Some surgeons have favored a "C"-shaped configuration, directing the graft superiorly and toward the left shoulder before curving it medially and then to the superior mesenteric artery in an antegrade direction.[13]

Although antegrade revascularization is currently favored, a disturbing report of postoperative vasospasm after such surgery has been recorded. In patients observed, episodes of abdominal pain occurred 5 to 20 days after revascularization, and immediate angiography revealed patent grafts with diffuse mesenteric vasospasm. Treatment with nifedipine and reduction in oral intake was effective. The cause of this syndrome appeared to be a heightened myogenetic response of a formerly protected vascular bed when suddenly exposed to high perfusion pressures.[14]

Mesenteric Angioplasty

As percutaneous transluminal angioplasty has evolved, it was inevitable that mesenteric artery stenoses would be treated. Diagnosis in such patients is dependent upon angiography, and the chronicity of the condition allows contemplation of this less invasive technique in treatment.[15–17] Success of this procedure can be predicted, as can frequent recurrent stenoses. What is less obvious is the fact that these patients being treated are demonstrating lack of collateral circulation. Acute occlusion of the dilated artery may produce a fatal abdominal catastrophe. Emergent revascularization in circumstances that are

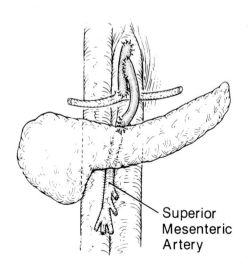

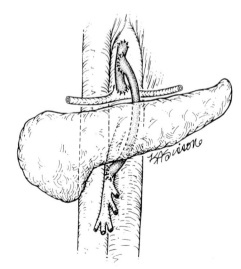

FIGURE 30–4. Either the supraceliac aorta itself or the primary aortoceliac graft can be used as an origin for further grafting to the superior mesenteric artery above the pancreas (*A*) or below the pancreas (*B*).

less than favorable would be required in such a situation.

In an experience with 10 patients, 19 arteries were treated with an immediate technical failure rate of 20 per cent, and symptoms recurred in five patients within 6 to 22 months. This high rate of recurrence of symptoms within such a short time is manifestly unsatisfactory.[17]

Confirmation of restenosis of mesenteric vessels subject to angioplasty has now been reported.[18] Simultaneously, angioplasty has been extended to relief of total mesenteric artery occlusion. Long-term follow-up of patients so treated will be necessary to judge the place of percutaneous transluminal angioplasty in treatment of visceral arterial occlusions.[19]

ACUTE VISCERAL ARTERY OCCLUSION

The fact that acute intestinal infarction produced a treatment mortality of 70 to 100 per cent in the 1930s and a mortality of 70 to 100 per cent in the late 1980s indicates both the severity of this condition and the lack of progress in treating it.[20,21] When it is considered that aggressive diagnostic and therapeutic approaches have been attempted recently and a great many surgeons trained in vascular techniques have been involved in the care of these patients, persistence of such a high mortality is difficult to rationalize.[22,23] Improved survival and decreased mortality in treating this condition in the future will depend on a clear understanding of diagnosis as well as extremely aggressive management of the postoperative situation. This is the subject of this portion of the chapter.

Clinical Manifestations

There are certain similarities between embolic occlusion of the mesenteric arteries, thrombotic occlusion of the visceral vessels, and nonorganic occlusion.[24,25] These similarities are: severe abdominal pain commonly out of proportion to physical findings; profound leukocytosis generally in excess of 14,000 except in aged patients unable to mount a leukocytosis; and gut emptying characterized by vomiting and defecation.[1,17,26] Further clinical manifestations common to these conditions include a change from normal stool to melena and late, usually fatal, peritonitis.

Embolic Occlusion

Gradually, it has become recognized that mesenteric embolization is among the commonest causes of mesenteric infarction.[3,5,27] This is important. The dramatic onset of mesenteric embolization allows prompt intervention with salvage of bowel and patients. Typical, is Vollmar's report from Ulm in which

38 patients were seen with mesenteric infarction, 26 due to arterial emboli and only six to arterial thrombosis. The other six were divided between venous thrombosis (four) and nonocclusive disease (two). This report can be taken to be indicative of the most modern diagnostic approaches.[27]

The triad of acute intestinal ischemia credited to Klass consists of sudden abdominal pain, bowel emptying, and a cardiac source for the embolization. This can be expanded to include history of prior embolic events and profound leukocytosis. All of these are characteristic of acute occlusion of the mesenteric artery by embolus. Onset of the ischemia can be ascribed to the beginning of symptoms.

Because no specific noninvasive diagnostic tests are reliable,[4] the diagnosis must be based upon angiography or laparotomy. This is of crucial importance, since it is within the first 6 to 12 hours that the ischemic bowel may retain viability. The seromuscular layers are particularly resistant to ischemia, although the mucosa may slough following as little as 4 to 6 hours of ischemia. Immediate aortography will reveal the classical mercury meniscus sign within the mesenteric artery distal to its origin. Collateral circulation may reconstitute the distal intestinal arteries and arcades. Segmental occlusions of these vessels may be seen if the embolus has shattered in its progress through the mesenteric artery. Survival following surgery is directly related to early diagnosis which, in turn, is dependent upon emergency mesenteric arteriography.[8]

At laparotomy, inspection of the compromised intestine will give a clue to diagnosis. Very early after acute arterial occlusion of mesenteric vessels, the bowel may appear sufficiently normal for mesenteric artery occlusion to be missed. However, close inspection of the bowel will show it to be grayer than usual and lacking in normal sheen. The vasa recta of the terminal ileum may be pulseless; those proximal to the jejunum remain pulsatile. Later on, there is hemorrhage into the mesentery. When this occurs, the entire intestine becomes deeply cyanotic. Later, frankly necrotic intestine is identified.

Careful inspection of the bowel and its mesentery will define the diagnosis. Since embolus lodges peripherally at the level of the mid-colic artery or distally, the first jejunal branches and their arcades are patent and pulsatile. This allows the first portion of the jejunum, distal to the ligament of Treitz, to be normal. Visible pulsations in the first three or four arcade vessels must be searched for. This is a finding of great importance. In contrast, if the main body of the embolus has shattered, segmental necrosis of the bowel is seen with skip areas of normal bowel interspersed. These findings are in contrast to the appearance of thrombotic occlusion of the mesenteric vessels as described later in this chapter.[29]

Embolectomy

The mesenteric artery should be identified in the mesenteric root by palpation. The pulse stops abruptly at the site of the embolus near the origin of the mid-colic artery. There the artery is skeletonized, overlying veins divided, jejunal branches controlled with atraumatic slings, and an arteriotomy made. Alternatively, the mesenteric artery can be approached by dividing the gastrocolic mesentery and the mesenteric artery identified at the inferior border of the pancreas. In either approach, a transverse arteriotomy allows closure of the vessel without narrowing. A no. 3 Fogarty catheter may be used for removal of distal propagated thrombus.[12] Thorough irrigation with heparinized saline solution may liberate other clot fragments. Revascularization must precede resection. Then, after closure of the arteriotomy, attention can be given to the extent of proposed intestinal resection.

It is unclear at the cellular level whether severe damage occurs during ischemia or during reperfusion. It is known that as blood flow falls below a critical level, adenosine triphosphate is depleted and elevated concentrations of adenosine monophosphate are found. This is catabolized to adenosine, inosine, and hypoxanthine. At this time xanthine dehydrogenase is converted to xanthine oxidase. With reperfusion, the superoxide radical is produced and this may be a mediator of further tissue damage. Experimentally, both the ischemic period and the extent of revascularization/reperfusion tissue damage may be modified by administration of superoxide dismutase, allopurinol, or dimethylsulfoxide. Allopurinol acts to block xanthine oxidase, whereas dimethylsulfoxide scavenges oxygen free radicals.[30-35] Clinical relevance of these observations has yet to become established.[36,37]

Assessment of Intestinal Viability

Clinically, an experienced surgeon judges intestinal viability with great regularity and accuracy. Surgical observation is subjective but accurate. It is dependent upon the surgeon's ability to assess color, motility, and presence of pulses. Bowel with peristalsis is viable. Bowel with relatively little peristalsis may be viable. Pulses in the mesentery are relatively unreliable but reassuring.

However, assessment of intestinal viability has entered an objective quantitative phase. Perhaps this will allow more accurate assessment of viability. Among the methods advocated are continuous-wave Doppler, fluorescein infusion, surface oximetry, and photoplethysmography.[31,38-41] The Doppler technique is attractive because of its simplicity. The sterilized probe can be placed on the antimesenteric border of the bowel and pulses detected. If they are detected, the bowel is very likely viable and can be left in place despite its appearance.

Second-Look Procedure

Although the role of the second-look procedure is not clarified, it is clear that postoperative management provides the best opportunity to salvage patients with acute mesenteric infarction. Preoperative delay in diagnosis is so often dependent upon factors occurring before the patient reaches the hospital; factors which remain outside of the sphere of influence of the surgeon. However, aggressive care following the primary operation may improve surgical results by decreasing mortality. In the Swedish experience addressing this point, 80 patients were operated upon for mesenteric vascular occlusion.[20] Only five had mesenteric revascularization; 50 required some intestinal resection, and anastomotic insufficiency or gangrene necessitated additional resection. Dehiscence of intestinal anastomosis was seen in patients without intestinal revascularization.[17]

The decision to perform a second-look operation must be made at the time of the primary operation. This should be an irrevocable decision because the postoperative condition of the patient, and his subsequent clinical course, will be of no help in deciding for or against a second-look procedure.

Further Aggressive Therapy

Gradually, surgeons interested in bettering results of treatment of mesenteric infarction have realized that patients surviving primary operation and second-look procedures occasionally abruptly worsen later. In the University Hospital Basel experience, an interesting observation can be gleaned by careful analysis of the data presented.[23] Eighty-one patients were operated upon for mesenteric infarction. Forty-four were treated with curative intent at the first operation. Fourteen of these (32 per cent) died of early recurrence of mesenteric infarction. Within this group were five patients initially treated only by embolectomy. This experience, added to clinical experience in this country, suggests that a highly aggressive postoperative posture should be adopted in the future. Relaparotomy and/or repeat angiography may clarify sudden worsening of patient status.

The following case is illustrative of several major considerations in treatment of mesenteric infarction as described in the text in this section.

An 84-year-old man was operated upon for an acute abdominal catastrophe. A suspected diagnosis was mesenteric infarction due to embolus from intermittent arrhythmia. At the first operation, a segment of intestinal necrosis was resected, the bowel carefully inspected and ascertained to be entirely viable, and anastomosis performed. Leukocytosis persisted and abdominal pain was severe. A mesenteric arteriogram was performed showing embolic occlusion of the mesenteric artery distal to the midcolic. Relaparotomy revealed dehiscence of the intestinal anastomosis and cyanosis of the adjacent bowel. Embolectomy was performed.

MESENTERIC THROMBOSIS

Clinical manifestations of thrombotic occlusion of the mesenteric artery are exactly the same as those described above with the exception that the onset of the condition is not sudden nor dramatic. In fact, it is insidious. Furthermore, the patient may be aged, infirm, and carrying the stigmata of advanced peripheral atherosclerosis or its treatment. In the worst cases, the patients have been institutionalized for severe incapacity, senility, or both. Many of these are patients thought to have inoperable lesions, late diagnosis, and predicted failure to survive the diagnostic and therapeutic manipulations required. In short, fate has determined that mesenteric infarction will be the mode of exodus of these patients from life. They cannot be saved.

However, thrombotic occlusion of the mesenteric artery occurs in patients who may be salvageable. Diagnosis by noninvasive means is not yet possible, nor is there a serum analysis that will provide a clue to diagnosis. Only laparotomy or angiography are helpful. Angiography will show mesenteric artery occlusions near the aortic origin of the celiac axis and superior mesenteric artery with or without inferior mesenteric artery occlusion. It is these patients who will have a history of intestinal angina if it is searched for. This is in sharp contrast to patients with embolic occlusion of the mesenteric artery, who will have no such history of intestinal angina or weight loss.

Laparotomy may show findings different from embolic occlusion. Usually, the area of compromised bowel is confluent and not segmental. Furthermore, the first portion of jejunum may be ischemic, in contrast to the viable jejunal first portion found with embolic occlusion. Precise diagnosis is important because Fogarty catheter thromboembolectomy is unsuccessful in thrombotic occlusion of the mesenteric vessels.

Revascularization

Methods of revascularization described earlier apply to thrombotic occlusion of the mesenteric arteries. Bypass techniques must be employed because thromboendarterectomy is too traumatic and embolectomy is not acceptable.

Revascularization must precede bowel resection for the reasons indicated earlier. A second-look procedure must be contemplated at the time of the primary operation and relaparotomy or angiography pursued vigorously in the postoperative course.

NONOCCLUSIVE MESENTERIC ISCHEMIA

Nonocclusive mesenteric ischemia is simply a low-flow state. Fortunately, it is disappearing as a clinical entity, as more efficient cardiac resuscitation is carried out in medical intensive care units. Many clinical conditions produce the low-flow state. These include cardiac failure, cardiac arrhythmia, myocardial infarction, shock, hypovolemia, extensive body burns, trauma, aortic valvular insufficiency, and inotropic drugs. Fixed vasoconstriction in such states is a compensatory mech-

anism designed to improve perfusion to vital structures such as the brain and kidneys. The vasoconstriction will remain fixed unless treated by intraarterial vasodilating drugs such as papaverine or glucagon.

Angiographic findings include spasm of segmental branches of the superior mesenteric artery, either diffuse, focal, or concentric. Spastic areas are uniformly smooth, and contrast media reflux into the aorta with the mesenteric injection is often seen.

Clinical manifestations of nonocclusive bowel ischemia are exactly the same as those mentioned earlier because the response of the intestine to ischemia is uniform regardless of the etiologic mechanism.

If papaverine is chosen as the vasodilating agent, a test dose of 30 mg is rapidly infused into the mesenteric artery catheter and a repeat arteriogram done. If benefit is demonstrated, the infusion is continued at a rate of 30 to 60 mg/hr. The drug is diluted to a concentration of 1 mg/ml and the infusion continues for 24 hours. A repeat arteriogram is performed and a decision is made for continuation or cessation of the infusion. The patient must be monitored for hypotension and tachycardia, although these are seldom seen with intraarterial infusion of the drug because 90 per cent of it is inactivated with each pass through the liver. Laparotomy may be necessary if the patient develops signs of peritonitis.

MESENTERIC VENOUS THROMBOSIS

Until recently, mesenteric venous thrombosis was thought to be a condition of insidious onset, with long duration of symptoms consisting of vague abdominal pain, distention, change in bowel habits, nausea, and mild fever. Often, this would follow a viral or flulike illness. Mild abdominal tenderness was seen, as well as hypoactive bowel sounds and leukocytosis, with features of an acute abdomen prompting laparotomy. In such a condition, diagnosis by angiography included findings of reflux of contrast into the aorta, spasm of the superior mesenteric artery, prolongation of the arterial phase, and often intense opacification of the thickened bowel wall. Characteristic of the thinking about venous thrombosis in the past is the statement by Marston: "Mesenteric venous thrombosis is a surgical emergency and the need for early operation must be stressed."[42] Now, computed tomography scanning with contrast infusion and duplex visualization of the portal vein allow diagnosis before peritonitis has occurred.[43] Because such a condition is often a coagulopathy, a history of previous thrombophlebitis and family history of venous thrombosis must be vigorously sought for. Treatment can be by heparin anticoagulation without laparotomy unless signs of peritonitis occur.[44,45]

Thus, new findings in portal and mesenteric vein imaging have clarified a spectrum of atypical gastrointestinal symptomatology suggesting a triad of miscellaneous digestive complaints, history of recurrent thrombophlebitis, and splanchnic venous thrombosis that should be treated by prompt, long-term anticoagulation. Laparotomy with bowel resection can be employed infrequently.[43]

CONCLUSION

Visceral ischemic syndromes can be clarified and rendered less confusing. Chronic ischemia is rare and may masquerade as malignancy, perforated diverticulitis, or other conditions. Acute ischemia is catastrophic but early intervention may save gut. Patient survival is dependent upon aggressive, intensive care and relaparotomy. Mesenteric venous thrombosis, in contrast, may prove largely benign if early imaging is done and heparin anticoagulation instituted.

REFERENCES

1. Bergan JJ: Recognition and treatment of intestinal ischemia. Surg Clin North Am 47:109, 1967.
2. Bergan JJ: Recognition and treatment of superior mesenteric artery embolization. Geriatrics 24:118, 1969.
3. Bergan JJ, Dry L, Conn J Jr, Trippel OH: Intestinal ischemic syndromes. Ann Surg 169:120, 1969.
4. Bounous G, McArdle AH: Release of intestinal enzymes in acute mesenteric ischemia. J Surg Res 9:339, 1969.
5. Marston A: Chronic intestinal ischemia. Acta Chir Scand [Suppl] 555:237–243, 1990.
6. Lilly MP, Harward TRS, Flinn WR, et al: Duplex ultrasound measurement of changes in mesenteric blood flow. J Vasc Surg 9:18–25, 1989.
7. Eidt JF, Harward T, Cook JM, Kahn MB, Troillett R: Current status of duplex Doppler ultrasound in the examination of the abdominal vasculature. Am J Surg 160:604–609, 1990.
8. LaBombard FE, Musson A, Browersox JC, Zwolak RM: Hepatic artery duplex as an adjunct in the evaluation of chronic mesenteric ischemia. J Vasc Technol 16(1):7–11, 1992.
9. Cormier JM, Fichelle JM, Vennin J, Laurian C, Gigou F: Atherosclerotic occlusive disease of the superior mesenteric artery: Late results of reconstructive surgery. Ann Vasc Surg 5:510–518, 1991.
10. Kieny R, Batellier J, Kretz JG: Aortic reimplantation of the superior mesenteric artery for atherosclerotic lesions of visceral arteries: Sixty cases. Ann Vasc Surg 4:122–125, 1990.
11. Stoney RJ, Schneider PA: Technical aspects of visceral artery revascularization. In Bergan JJ, Yao JST (eds): Techniques in Arterial Surgery. Philadelphia, WB Saunders Company, 1990.
12. Bergan JJ: Operative procedures in acute mesenteric infarction. In Bergan JJ, Yao JST (eds): Operative Techniques in Vascular Surgery. Orlando, FL, Grune & Stratton, 1980.
13. Yao JST, Bergan JJ: Operative procedures in visceral ischemia. In Bergan JJ, Yao JST (eds): Techniques in Arterial Surgery. Philadelphia, WB Saunders Company, 1990.
14. Gewertz BL, Zarins CK: Postoperative vasospasm after antegrade mesenteric revascularization: A report of three cases. J Vasc Surg 14:382–385, 1991.
15. Levy PJ, Haskell L, Gordon RL: Percutaneous transluminal angioplasty of splanchnic arteries. Eur J Radiol 7:239–242, 1987.
16. Mani J, Courtheoux P, Mercier V, Alachkar F, Maiza D, Theron J: Endoluminal angioplasty of atheromatous stenoses of gastrointestinal arteries. Ann Radiol 29:589–592, 1986.
17. Odurny A, Sniderman KW, Colapinto RF: Intestinal angina: Percutaneous transluminal angioplasty of celiac and superior mesenteric arteries. Radiology 167:59–62, 1988.
18. McShane MD, Proctor A, Spencer P, Cumberland DC, Welsh CL: Mesenteric angioplasty for chronic intestinal ischaemia. Eur J Vasc Surg 6:333–336, 1992.
19. Warnock NG, Gaines PA, Beard JD, Cumberland DC: Treatment of intestinal angina by percutaneous transluminal angioplasty of a superior mesenteric artery occlusion. Clin Radiol 45:18–19, 1992.
20. Lindblad B, Hakansson H: Rationale for second-look operation in mesenteric vessel occlusion. Acta Chir Scand 153:531–533, 1987.
21. Wilson C, Gupta R, Gilmour DG, Imrie CW: Acute superior mesenteric ischemia. Br J Surg 74:279–281, 1987.
22. Boley SJ, Sprayregen S, Siegelman SS, Veith FJ: Initial results from an aggressive roentgenological and surgical approach to acute mesenteric ischemia. Surgery 82:848, 1977.
23. Clavian PA, Muller C, Harder F: Treatment of mesenteric infarction. Br J Surg 74:500–503, 1987.
24. Bergan JJ, Flinn WR, McCarthy WJ III, Yao JST: Acute mesenteric ischemia. In Bergan JJ, Yao JST (eds): Vascular Surgical Emergencies. Orlando, FL, Grune & Stratton, 1987, pp 401–413.
25. Bergan JJ, McCarthy W, Flinn WR, Yao JST: Nontraumatic mesenteric vascular emergencies. J Vasc Surg 5:903, 1987.
26. Bergan JJ, Haid SP, Conn J Jr: Systemic effects of intestinal revascularization. Am J Surg 117:235, 1969.
27. Paes E, Vollmar JF, Hutschenreiter S, et al: Der Mesenterial Ianfarkt. Chirurg 59:828–835, 1988.
28. Batellier J, Kieny R: Superior mesenteric artery embolism: Eighty-two cases. Ann Vasc Surg 4:112–116, 1990.
29. Bergann JJ: Unexpected vascular problems at laparotomy. Probl Gen Surg 1:190–199, 1984.
30. Boley SJ, Feinstein FR, Sammartano R, et al: New concepts in the management of emboli of the superior mesenteric artery. Surg Gynecol Obstet 153:561, 1981.
31. Bulkley GB, Zuidema GD, O'Mara CS, et al: Intraoperative determination of viability following ischemic injury: A prospective, controlled trial of adjuvant methods (Doppler and fluorescein) compared to standard clinical judgment. Ann Surg 193:628, 1981.
32. Bulkley GB, Kveitz PR, Granger DN: Relation between intestinal blood flow and oxygen uptake. Am J Physiol 224:6605, 1983.
33. McCord JM: Oxygen-derived free radicals in post-ischemic tissue injury. N Engl J Med 312:159, 1985.
34. Parks DA, Bulkley GB, Granger DN: Role of oxygen derived free radicals in digestive tract diseases. Surgery 94:415, 1983.
35. Parks DA, Bulkley GB, Granger DN, et al: Ischemic injury in the cat small intestine: Role of superoxide radicals. Gastroenterology 82:9, 1982.
36. Garcia-Garcia J, Martin-Rollan C, de la Cruz L, Garcia-Criado J, Gomez-Alonso A: The protective effect of superoxide dismutase (SOD) in intestinal ischemia. Res Surg 3:184–187, 1991.
37. Dyess DL, Bruner BW, Donnell CA, Ferrara JJ, Powell RW: Intraoperative evaluation of intestinal ischemia: A comparison of methods. South Med J 84:966–974, 1991.
38. Cooperman M, Martin EW Jr, Carey LC: Evaluation of ischemic intestine by Doppler ultrasound. Am J Surg 139:73, 1980.
39. Locke R, Hauser CJ, Shoemaker WC: The use of surface oximetry to assess bowel viability. Arch Surg 119:1252, 1984.
40. Whitehill TA, Pearce WH, Rosales C, et al: Detection thresholds of nonocclusive intestinal hypoperfusion by Doppler ultrasound, photoplethysmography, and fluorescein. J Vasc Surg 8:28, 1988.
41. Wright CB, Hobson RW: Prediction of intestinal viability using Doppler ultrasound technique. Am J Surg 129:642, 1975.

42. Marston A: Vascular Disease of the Gastrointestinal Tract. Baltimore, Williams & Wilkins, 1986.
43. Harward TRS, Green D, Bergan JJ, et al: Mesenteric venous thrombosis. J Vasc Surg 9:328–333, 1989.
44. Green D, Ganger DR, Blei AT: Protein-C deficiency in splanchnic venous thrombosis. Am J Med 82:1171–1174, 1987.
45. Maung R, Kelly JK, Schneider MP, et al: Mesenteric venous thrombosis due to antithrombin III deficiency. Arch Pathol Lab Med 112:37–39, 1988.
46. Grieshop RJ, Dalsing MC, Cikrit DF, Lalka SG, Sawchuk AP: Acute mesenteric venous thrombosis. Revisted in a time of diagnostic clarity. Am Surg 57:573–578, 1991.

REVIEW QUESTIONS

1. Chronic visceral ischemia is diagnosed by:
   - (a) aortography
   - (b) absorption studies
   - (c) large and small bowel contrast studies
   - (d) none of the above

2. Mesenteric venous thrombosis usually:
   - (a) leads to bowel necrosis
   - (b) always requires intestinal resection
   - (c) may be effectively treated by anticoagulation
   - (d) has an identifiable etiology

3. Acute mesenteric ischemia has the lowest mortality when caused by:
   - (a) mesenteric embolus
   - (b) mesenteric thrombosis
   - (c) mesenteric vasculitis
   - (d) nonorganic occlusion

4. Chronic visceral ischemia:
   - (a) clinically appears as undiagnosed malignancy
   - (b) appears with weight loss
   - (c) is best treated by multiple bypasses
   - (d) all of the above

5. In the patient with acute mesenteric ischemia:
   - (a) plain film of the abdomen is diagnostic
   - (b) clinical diagnosis is made early
   - (c) arteriography should not be done because the patient is too sick
   - (d) arteriography identifies nonorganic ischemia

6. Acute mesenteric infarction sparing the jejunum is usually caused by:
   - (a) mesenteric thrombosis
   - (b) mesenteric embolus
   - (c) nonorganic occlusion
   - (d) mesenteric venous thrombosis

7. Chronic visceral ischemia leading to mesenteric infarction is caused by:
   - (a) mesenteric embolus
   - (b) mesenteric venous thrombosis
   - (c) superior mesenteric artery thrombosis
   - (d) celiac axis and superior mesenteric artery thrombosis

8. Nonorganic mesenteric ischemia is associated with:
   - (a) angiographically demonstrated concentric stenoses
   - (b) digitalis dose manipulation
   - (c) severe aortic valvular insufficiency
   - (d) all of the above

9. Abdominal pain, defecation, vomiting, and leukocytosis are characteristic of:
   - (a) mesenteric embolus
   - (b) nonorganic mesenteric ischemia
   - (c) mesenteric artery thrombosis
   - (d) all of the above

10. Chronic visceral ischemia demonstrates:
    - (a) characteristic mucosal changes on biopsy
    - (b) peristaltic motility abnormalities
    - (c) malabsorption
    - (d) all of the above
    - (e) none of the above

ANSWERS

1. d	2. c	3. a	4. d	5. d	6. b	7. d
8. d	9. d	10. e				

31

EXTRACRANIAL CEREBROVASCULAR DISEASE—The Carotid Artery

WESLEY S. MOORE

HISTORICAL REVIEW

The development of surgery on the extracranial cerebrovascular circulation was dependent upon three principal factors: (1) recognition of the pathologic relationship between extracranial cerebrovascular disease and subsequent cerebral infarction, (2) the introduction of cerebral angiography to identify lesions prior to the patient's death, and (3) the development of vascular surgical techniques that could be applied to the extracranial vessels once the anatomic patterns of disease were understood and described.

The earliest report linking cervical carotid artery disease with stroke is credited to Savory, who, in 1856, described a young woman with left monocular symptoms in combination with a right hemiplegia and dysesthesia.[1] Postmortem examination demonstrated an occlusion of the cervical portion of the left internal carotid artery together with bilateral subclavian artery occlusions. Gowers, in 1875, reported a similar case,[2] and subsequent reports of individual cases were made by Chiari in 1905,[3] Guthrie and Mayou in 1908,[4] and Cadwater in 1912.[5] By 1914, Ramsey Hunt, in an important publication, emphasized the relationship between extracranial carotid artery disease and stroke.[6] He also described the phenomenon of intermittent cerebral symptoms associated with partial occlusion and used the term "cerebral intermittent claudication" as a characterizing analogy. Hunt also pointed out that the clinicopathologic observations in patients with stroke were hampered by the fact that routine autopsies did not include examination of the cervical carotid arteries (as is often the case today because of the desire to maintain access to the external carotid artery for the mortician). He emphasized that no examination of cerebral infarction can be considered complete without examination of the neck vessels.[6]

The next major step in the evolution of the management of extracranial cerebral vascular disease came with the development of carotid angiography by Moniz

in 1927.[7] By 1937, Moniz and colleagues described four cases of internal carotid occlusion diagnosed by angiography.[8] In 1938, Chao and colleagues[9] added two additional cases, and by 1951, Johnson and Walker had collected a total of 101 cases of occlusion of the cervical carotid artery diagnosed by angiography from the world literature.[10] In spite of these early observations, the medical world was still slow to appreciate the relationship between extracranial cerebral vascular disease and cerebral symptoms, as emphasized by the fact that when cerebral angiography came into common use for neurologic diagnosis in the 1950s and 1960s, only the intracranial vessels were included on films. The area of the carotid bifurcation was seldom looked at. By the late 1950s, it was still common to have patients admitted with a hemiplegia and to be diagnosed as having a "middle cerebral artery thrombosis" without considering the carotid bifurcation as a source of the problem.

The next major steps in the evolution of understanding came from reports by Miller Fisher in 1951 and 1954.[11,12] Fisher reemphasized the relationship between extracranial arterial occlusive disease and cerebral symptoms. He also pointed out that the lesions could either be total occlusion or stenosis. His most important observation, however, was that the disease was often quite localized to a short segment of the carotid artery, and Fisher predicted that surgical correction might be possible if patients could be identified in the early stages of the clinical syndrome. Fisher stated that "It is even conceivable that some day vascular surgery will find a way to bypass the occluded portion of the artery during the period of ominous fleeting symptoms. Anastomosis of the external carotid artery or one of its branches with the internal carotid artery above the area of narrowing should be feasible."

The surgical phase of understanding and management of extracranial cerebral vascular disease probably began in 1951, but was actually not reported in the literature until 1955. This early report by Carrea,

Molins, and Murphy[13] from Buenos Aires described their experience with the management of a patient with carotid artery stenosis. They resected the diseased internal carotid artery and performed an anastomosis between the external carotid artery and the distal internal carotid as predicted earlier by Miller Fisher. In 1953, Strully, Hurwitt, and Blakenberg[14] attempted a thromboendarterectomy of a totally thrombosed internal carotid artery. This was unsuccessful, but the authors suggested that thromboendarterectomy should be technically feasible prior to thrombosis as long as the internal carotid artery was patent distally. The first carotid endarterectomy was probably performed by DeBakey and colleagues in an operation done on August 7, 1953, but was not actually written up until 1959,[15] and then subsequently reviewed again in 1975.[16] The report that was most important in calling the world's attention to the feasibility of carotid artery reconstruction came from Eastcott, Pickering, and Rob, who published their experience in *The Lancet* in November, 1954.[17] Their operation was performed on May 19, 1954 on a patient who was having hemispheric transient ischemic attacks (TIAs), with demonstrable disease at the carotid bifurcation, using direct, end-to-end anastomosis between the common carotid artery and the internal carotid artery distal to the atherosclerotic lesion.

While operations on the carotid artery were in the early phase of development, surgical attack was also considered feasible on occlusive lesions of the major arch vessels. In 1956, Davis, Grove, and Julian reported their experience with endarterectomy of the innominate artery done on a patient of March 20, 1954.[8] In 1957, Warren and Triedman reported the second case.

By this time, the stage was set for explosive development in the aggressive surgical approach for managing extracranial cerebral vascular disease as a means of preventing or treating cerebral infarction.

NATURAL HISTORY OF EXTRACRANIAL ARTERIAL OCCLUSIVE DISEASE

Therapy aimed at prevention of cerebral infarction must be compared to the natural history of the disease process. The prognosis of a patient with extracranial arterial occlusive disease will differ depending on the presence or absence of symptoms. When a permanent neurologic deficit is present the outlook worsens, thus underscoring the importance of prevention. A thorough understanding of the natural history of the disease is essential in formulating a rational and effective therapeutic program. The physician needs to be familiar with the expected results of each available option. This implies that no one alternative is applicable to all situations and that individualization is the key to effective prevention.

There are approximately 500,000 new stroke victims in the United States each year. In 200,000 of these cases death follows, but at any one time there are around 1,000,000 stroke victims alive and disabled. In 1976, it was estimated that the annual direct and indirect cost of stroke was $7,363,784,000.[20] Thirteen years later, with inflation and the accelerating cost of medical care, this cost has probably quadrupled. The incalculable morbidity of the affected individual adds further to the magnitude of this problem. Prevention remains the most plausible alternative.

The initial mortality of an ischemic stroke ranges between 15 and 33 per cent.[21-23] Survivors remain at an inordinately high risk of subsequent stroke, estimated between 4.8 and 20 per cent year year.[24,25] This implies that half of the patients will experience a second event within 5 years.[22,26,27] The average reported in the literature is between 6 and 12 per cent each year. It is well known that the most common cause of death in patients with extracranial arterial occlusive disease is myocardial infarction. In an analysis of 535 stroke victims, however, the leading cause of death was recurrent stroke, as opposed to the expected myocardial mortality.[25]

Since 1973, public health statistics have documented an accelerating decline in stroke mortality.[28] This has led to the erroneous assumption that there has also been a decline in stroke incidence, which may or may not be the case.

In 1989, Wolf and colleagues reported the epidemiologic data from the Framingham Study to the 14th International Joint Conference on Stroke and Cerebral Circulation. They reviewed the experience from three successive decades, beginning in 1953. A decline in stroke fatality in both men and women was observed. However, the 10-year prevalence of stroke actually rose, and the incidence of stroke rose in men from 5.7 to 7.6 per cent, to 7.9 per cent, without any apparent change in women. The authors postulated that falling case fatality rates may result from changes in diagnostic criteria, a lessening in stroke severity, or improved care of stroke patients.[29]

Harmsen and colleagues reviewed the experience of stroke incidence and fatality in Göteborg, Sweden, between 1971 and 1987. They noted that the stroke incidence remained the same during that interval but that the stroke fatality rate declined in both sexes. This was more marked for intracerebral hemorrhage and subarachnoid hemorrhage rather than infarction. They concluded that the decline in stroke fatality rates may be related to decreases in smoking habits or better management of blood pressure. They had no explanation as to why there was not a corresponding decline in stroke incidence.[30] Finally, Modan and Wagener examined the epidemiologic aspects of stroke based upon death certificate information available from the National Center for Health Statistics compressed mortality file for all 50 states and the District of Columbia for the period 1968 to 1988. They noted that there was a decline in stroke mortality that continued through the 1970s and 1980s, whereas the morbidity remained constant and possibly even increased. They noted similar morbidity and mortality rates in both sexes. They concluded that the observed decrease in stroke mortality rates resulted from an improved survival rather than a decline in incidence.[31]

A variety of reasons for decline in stroke mortality have been postulated, including the more aggressive treatment of hypertension. It is of interest that no one has suggested that the decline of stroke mortality may be related to the increasing use of carotid endarterectomy. Figure 31–1 compares the declining incidence in stroke mortality with the accelerating incidence of carotid endarterectomy. While this is not proof of a relationship, neither should a possible relationship be discounted.

Two clinical syndromes deserve special emphasis because of their dismal natural history. *Stroke-in-evolution*, also known as progressing stroke or incomplete stroke, represents an acute neurologic deficit of modest degree that within hours or days progresses to a major cerebral infarct. This can happen in a sequential series of acute exacerbations or in a pattern of waxing and waning in signs and symptoms over hours or days, with incomplete recovery eventually leading to a major fixed neurologic deficit. *Crescendo TIAs* is that pattern that allows complete recovery between ischemic events, suggesting repeated frequent embolization from a point arterial source in the affected territory. In a review of the literature, Mentzer et al. identified 263 reported cases of stroke-in-evolution managed conservatively.[32] Twenty-three per cent had complete resolution or mild neurologic deficit on follow-up. Sixty-two per cent had a moderate to severe deficit in the early recovery phase, and the overall mortality was 14.5 per cent. In their own series, there were 26 patients with stroke-in-evolution treated conservatively. Mortality was 15 per cent, but, more importantly, 66 per cent suffered moderate

to severe permanent neurologic deficit, with only 5 patients recovering completely or experiencing a mild neurologic dysfunction. This compared with a series of 17 patients operated on emergently for stroke-in-evolution. None had worsening of the preoperative neurologic deficit, four (24 per cent) remain unchanged, and 12 (70 per cent) had complete recovery.[32] In 1972, Millikan reviewed the natural history of patients with progressing stroke.[33] Of 204 patients, 12 per cent were normal at 14 days, 7 per cent had developed moderate to severe neurologic deficits, and 14 per cent had died. Thus, stroke-in-evolution treated conservatively carries a poor prognosis. More than half of the patients will develop a severe permanent neurologic deficit within a few days of the onset and around 15 per cent will die as a result. Only 10 to 20 per cent will recover full or partial neurologic function.[33]

Patients who experienced TIAs are also at a higher risk of developing a stroke. In the Mayo Clinic population study,[34] 118 patients with TIAs were followed as a control group without therapy. The stroke rates at 1, 3, and 5 years were 23, 37, and 45 per cent, respectively. Most permanent deficits occurred during the first year. This represents a 16-fold increased risk of stroke when compared to an age- and sex-adjusted population. The Oxfordshire project reported an actuarial risk of stroke during the first year following the onset of TIAs to be 11 to 16 per cent. For each subsequent year, the rate was 5 to 9 per cent per year.[35] Some series[36,37] have reported lower figures, but the average reported in the literature is on the order of 30 to 35 per cent at 5 years, or 10 per cent the first year and 6 per cent each year thereafter. Finally, Toole, in his Willis Lecture, reminded us that there is a surprising frequency of cerebral

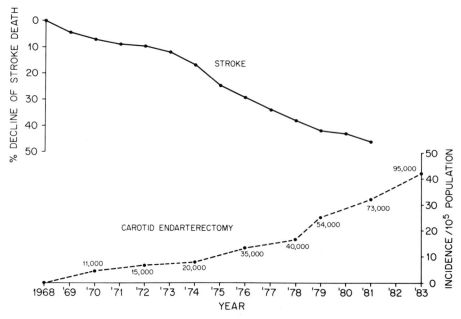

FIGURE 31–1. The declining incidence of stroke-related death from 1968 to 1981 is compared to the accelerating frequency with which carotid endarterectomy was performed during the same time interval.

infarction in TIA patients that goes unrecognized by either patient or physician. These lesions are now identified by better neuroimaging techniques and raises the question of whether or not TIAs are actually small strokes.[38] If a TIA is actually a small stroke, the implied benignity of TIA will have to be reexamined. Thus it may be equally important to prevent TIA, as it may be a small stroke. This consideration is further strengthened by the observations of Grogg and colleagues, who correlated cerebral infarction and atrophy as a function of TIAs as percentage stenosis. They graded carotid stenosis in symptomatic patients from A (no stenosis) to E (occlusion). In patients with amaurosis fugax, the incidence of cerebral infarction rose from 2 per cent in patients with stenoses grades A, B, and C; to 40 per cent in grade D; and 58 per cent in grade E. The incidence of atrophy increased in parallel from 10 per cent in grade A to 30 per cent in grade E.[39]

The natural history of asymptomatic patients with significant extracranial or arterial occlusive disease is most difficult to accurately predict. Most studies that have addressed this problem have used the presence of a cervical bruit as the sole criterion for inclusion. This will inevitably include patients without significant occlusive disease and omit others without cervical bruit but with high-risk lesions in their extracranial circulation.

As noninvasive studies have developed, it is possible to detect hemodynamically significant lesions in the carotid system. Kartchner and McRae[40] followed 1130 patients who either were asymptomatic or had nonhemispheric symptoms for a mean of 24 months. Of 303 patients with hemodynamically significant lesions, 11.9 per cent had strokes at 2 years. The group with negative noninvasive studies had a much lower stroke rate, on the order of 3 per cent over the same follow-up period. Busuttil et al.[41] noted an unfavorable trend toward higher stroke rates in asymptomatic patients with hemodynamically significant lesions in the carotid bifurcation.

In a report by Roederer et al., 167 asymptomatic patients with cervical bruits were followed with serial duplex scanning regardless of the degree of the stenosis at the time of presentation.[42] During follow-up, 10 patients became symptomatic. The development of symptoms was accompanied by disease progression in 80 per cent of patients. By life-table analysis, the annual rate of symptom occurrence was 4 per cent; however, the presence of progression graded at 80 per cent stenosis was highly correlated with either the development of total occlusion of the internal carotid artery or new symptoms. Thus 89 per cent of the symptoms were preceded by progression of the lesion to a greater than 80 per cent stenosis. Progression of a lesion to more than 80 per cent stenosis was an important warning observation, since it carried a 35 per cent risk of ischemic symptoms or internal carotid occlusion within 6 months and 46 per cent risk at 12 months. Conversely, only 1.5 per cent of the lesions that remained in a less

than 80 per cent stenosis category developed such a complication. These data suggest that careful follow-up with repeated noninvasive evaluation is of great assistance in determining the appropriate management of the asymptomatic carotid lesion.[42]

In an analysis of 294 asymptomatic and nonhemispheric patients submitted to cerebrovascular testing, Moore et al. found a 15 per cent stroke incidence during the first 2 years in patients with greater than 50 per cent stenosis.[43] This compared to a 3 per cent incidence at 2 years in patients with 1 to 49 per cent stenosis. This was found to be statistically significant ($p < .05$). The 5-year cumulative stroke incidence was 21 per cent with greater than 50 per cent stenosis, 14 per cent with 1 to 49 per cent stenosis, and 9 per cent in patients without noninvasive evidence of carotid artery disease.[43]

Chambers and Norris have been following a group of 500 asymptomatic clinical patients with noninvasive studies and clinical evaluation. They have identified two high-risk groups: those with stenosis greater than 75 per cent and those who show disease progression between studies. For patients with a greater than 75 per cent stenosis, the 1-year neurologic event rate (TIA and stroke) was 22 per cent. The 1-year stroke rate alone was 5 per cent.[44] In a more recent publication, the authors continue to note that neurologic events correlate with increasing percentage stenosis as well as disease progression between test intervals. In the study viewed over 5 years, the annual average neurologic event rate was 10 to 15 per cent, with the highest event rate occurring within the first year of diagnosis.[45] Finally, the incidence of silent cerebral infarction as documented on computed tomographic (CT) scan was studied in the same patient population. The authors noted a 10 per cent incidence of cerebral infarction among patients with mild (35 to 50 per cent) stenosis; 17 per cent in moderate (50 to 75 per cent) stenosis; and 30 per cent in patients with severe (greater than 75 per cent) stenosis. The authors concluded that silent cerebral infarction may be an indication for carotid endarterectomy in asymptomatic patients.[46]

Although the natural history of the asymptomatic carotid stenosis remains controversial, recent studies using serial noninvasive cerebrovascular testing have concluded that there is an increased risk of stroke ipsilateral to a 50 per cent or greater carotid artery stenosis. These lesions appear to carry a risk of subsequent stroke on the order of 4 per cent per year. In addition, progression of the disease carries an even higher risk of stroke, with lesions greater than 80 per cent stenosis carrying a 35 per cent risk of subsequent symptoms or carotid occlusion at 2 years. Other studies have suggested that the composition of the plaque influences the stroke risk of carotid artery lesions. In one analysis, 297 carotid patients with stenosis greater than 75 per cent at the time of initial study were at higher risk than peers without significant narrowing or developing symptoms ipsilateral to the lesion.[47] Even those patients with less than 75 per cent stenosis were at a greater risk if the associated plaque was less organized (i.e., soft). This was determined by B mode ultrasound, by which plaques were classified as dense, calcified, or soft. A definite trend toward higher risk was seen in plaques of lower density. Only 10 per cent of those patients with calcified plaque in significantly stenotic vessels developed symptoms, whereas 92 per cent of patients with soft plaques and tight stenosis developed symptoms within the first 3 years of follow-up.[47] The morphology of the atherosclerotic plaque, as documented by B mode ultrasound, is emerging as one of the more important factors associated with embolic potential and stroke risk. Two recent studies conclude that a heterogeneous plaque carries an increased risk of stroke and is an independent variable from carotid stenosis alone.[48,49]

The embolic potential of ulcerated carotid lesions has been well documented.[50–52] Patients who experience symptoms from these probably have the same prognosis as patients with occlusive lesions. Whether the former patient group responds more favorably to platelet antiaggregants remains to be determined. Moore and coworkers first pointed out the fact that asymptomatic patients with significant ulceration in a carotid plaque in the absence of stenosis appeared to be at a higher risk of stroke.[53] In a subsequent report, they expanded their series to 153 patients with asymptomatic nonstenotic ulcerative lesions in the carotid bifurcation. Patients with deep or complex ulcerations were followed and found to have a stroke rate of 4.5 and 7.5 per cent each year, respectively.[54] Other reports have suggested a similar stroke risk for complete ulcerations in the carotid bulb. However, a much lower stroke risk was reported for deep ulcerations with no significant added risk of stroke observed in these patients. Controversy still exists about the deep ulceration without complex morphology. However, there is agreement that complex ulcerations in the carotid bulb do increase the risk of stroke for asymptomatic patients.[55]

The presence of an asymptomatic hemodynamically significant stenosis may increase the risk of stroke during major surgery. Kartchner and McRae reported their experience with 234 patients, 41 of whom had evidence of significant carotid artery stenosis by oculoplethysmography.[56] Seven postoperative strokes developed in the group with positive criteria (17 per cent), whereas postoperative cerebral infarction developed in 2 (1 per cent) of 192 patients with negative noninvasive studies. The mechanisms of stroke and the territory involved were not specifically reported. This high incidence of permanent neurologic deficits led the authors to conclude that prophylactic carotid endarterectomy should be considered in patients with hemodynamically significant carotid stenosis undergoing a major cardiovascular procedure.[56] Other series have reported results to the contrary.[57–60] Using noninvasive vascular evaluation and in one series angiography, patients with 50 per cent or greater stenosis in the carotid bifurcation were compared to patients with lesser degrees of stenosis undergoing cardiovascular surgery. No increased incidence of perioperative strokes was found in patients with positive criteria. Most of these investigators, however, have excluded the preocclusive stenosis in their considerations. Lesions of 90 per cent or greater stenosis were excluded from these series and subjected to prophylactic endarterectomy prior to their cardiovascular operation. This perhaps suggests the appropriate management of the patient with combined carotid and coronary artery disease.

Review of the available literature reveals a dichotomy of outcome in patients with asymptomatic carotid stenosis who undergo a noncardiac operation. Those patients who undergo a cardiac operation do not have an increase in stroke risk, whereas those who undergo a noncardiac operation in the presence of an uncorrected carotid lesion do have an increased stroke risk. One possible explanation for this difference is the fact that the cardiac patient is protected from emboli of carotid origin by anticoagulation and hemodilution with the pump-run and postoperative hypocoagulability.

Cardiac surgeons have long been concerned about the presence of carotid stenosis in a patient who will be going on bypass with decrease in pump perfusion pressure, believing that there will be a corresponding and unacceptable drop in cerebral blood flow. In fact, the opposite is the case. Von Reutern and colleagues used transcranial Doppler to study middle cerebral artery blood flow before and during cardiopulmonary bypass in patients with and without carotid artery disease.[61] Surprisingly, middle cerebral artery blood flow actually increases during cardiopulmonary bypass. While the increase is not as great in patients with carotid artery disease, it is clearly an increase over baseline. This observation should dispel the concern about a potential drop in cerebral flood flow in patients with carotid stenosis while on the pump.[61]

The natural history of extracranial arterial occlusive disease cannot be complete without including the natural history of frequently associated conditions such as coronary artery disease, hypertension, and diabetes. Myocardial infarction remains the most frequent cause of death in these patients. It is therefore important to include these variables in the equation when one is formulating a treatment plan for a particular patient. The goal of therapy should be the prevention of a permanent neurologic deficit. The most effective way to achieve this must consider the life expectancy of the patient and the inherent risk of each particular form of therapy.

PATHOLOGY OF EXTRACRANIAL ARTERIAL OCCLUSIVE DISEASE

The pathology of cerebral vascular disease of extracranial origin can be divided into flow-restrictive lesions and lesions with embolic potential. Each of these can be further subdivided into occlusive or aneurysmal lesions. All entities that have been described as etiologic in extracranial disease will fall within these categories.

Atherosclerosis

By far the most common lesion found in patients with extracranial cerebral vascular disease is an atherosclerotic plaque in the carotid bifurcation. This can produce symptoms by reducing blood flow to the hemisphere supplied or, more commonly, by releasing embolic material. This can be either clot, platelet aggregates, or cholesterol crystals.

The carotid bifurcation appears to be susceptible to the development of atherosclerotic plaques.[62] Frequently, severe changes at the carotid bifurcation occur with minimal or no changes present in the common or internal carotid artery.[63] Several investigators have proposed conflicting theories based on hemodynamic observations in various models. High shear stress and fluctuations in shear stress,[64] disordered or turbulent flow, flow separation, and high and low flow velocity have all been implicated.[65-68] Which of these mechanisms is responsible for plaque formation is not known. Zarins et al.[69] used a model of the human carotid bifurcation under steady flow and compared its hemodynamics with those of cadaver specimens. They concluded that carotid lesions localize in regions of low flow velocity and flow separation rather than in regions of high velocity and increased shear stress. They used their model to explain the propensity of the outer wall of the carotid sinus opposite the divider to develop atherosclerotic plaques (Fig. 31–2). This may have further clinical implications in that an enlarged carotid bulb after endarterectomy may create a region of reduced flow

velocity with increased separation that may favor recurrent plaque deposition.

Once the initial intimal injury is produced by these forces, platelet deposition, smooth-muscle cell proliferation, and the slow accumulation of lipoproteins will be involved in the reparative process (Fig. 31–3). These will eventually lead to plaque formation, which will further alter the hemodynamics of the system and favor further injury.

The contribution of platelets to atheroma formation may take several forms.[70] Platelets may adhere to one another, to the diseased vessel, or both. This can lead to thrombus formation. This process may narrow the vessel lumen, or it may dislodge, resulting in distal embolization. Vasoactive substances stored in granules within the platelet may be released, causing vasospasm and further contributing to compromise of the arterial lumen. The platelets' interaction with collagen, exposed in an injured intima, may include elaboration of a smooth muscle growth factor that can lead to intimal thickening. The activation of enzymes in platelets, by their contact with collagen, will initiate the production of highly active prostaglandins. It appears that the production of thromboxane A_2 represents the final common pathway of platelet response to diverse stimuli.[71] This substance is a potent stimulant of platelet aggregation and a powerful vasoconstrictor, and it is believed to be important in the pathophysiology of plaque formation and/or symptoms from already established atheroma.

Hemorrhage into a plaque may also play a significant role in the development of symptoms from an atherosclerotic lesion. Imbalances in wall tension secondary to asymmetric deposition of plaques can lead to the sudden development of plaque fracture and intraplaque hemorrhage.[72] These can lead to sudden expansion of the atheroma with acute restriction of flow or breakdown of the intimal surface and concomitant embolization. An alternative mechanism for sudden intraplaque hemorrhage may be related to an increase in neovascularity within the plaque substance. Hypertension may be responsible for precipitating rupture of neovascular vessels, leading to intraplaque hemorrhage and expansion.[73] This process may be responsible for a large number of symptomatic lesions. In a prospective evaluation[74] of 79 atheromatous plaques removed from 69 patients undergoing carotid endarterectomy, 49 of 53 (92.5 per cent) symptomatic patients had evidence of intramural hemorrhage. In contrast, only 7 of 26 (27 per cent) asymptomatic patients demonstrated recent or acute intraplaque hemorrhage. Rupture of an atherosclerotic plaque with intraluminal release of atheromatous debris has also been correlated with acute stroke and internal carotid occlusion in an autopsy study.[75]

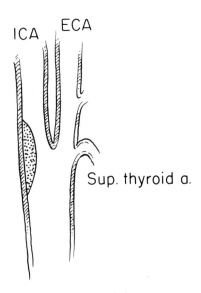

FIGURE 31–2. Artist's concept of the common carotid artery bifurcation; the most common site for atherosclerotic plaque deposition is located on the wall opposite the divider. *ECA*, external carotid artery; *ICA*, internal carotid artery.

Fibromuscular Dysplasia

Fibromuscular dysplasia is a nonatherosclerotic process that affects medium-sized arteries. It was first

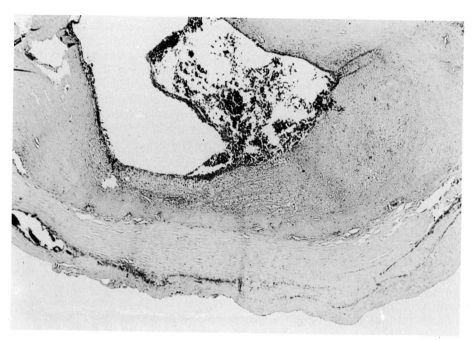

FIGURE 31–3. Microscopic section of an atherosclerotic plaque removed from the carotid bifurcation. Notice the fibrointimal proliferation with cholesterol cleft formation. Thrombotic material is adherent to the luminal surface of the plaque.

described in the carotid artery in 1964,[76] and since then it has been recognized as a cause of cerebrovascular symptoms.[77] It may also affect the intracranial arteries, and around 30 per cent of patients with cervical involvement have associated intracranial aneurysms.[78] Up to 65 per cent of patients will have bilateral disease[78] and 25 per cent will have associated atherosclerotic changes.[79]

Four histologic types of fibromuscular dysplasia have been described[80]:

1. *Intimal fibroplasia* accounts for about 5 per cent of cases and affects both sexes equally. It usually presents as long tubular stenoses in young patients and as focal stenoses in older patients. It results from an accumulation of irregularly arranged subendothelial mesenchymal cells with a loose matrix of connective tissue. Medial and adventitial structures are always normal.

2. *Medial hyperplasia* is a rare form of the disease that produces focal stenoses. The intima and adventitia remain normal, while the media shows excess smooth muscle.

3. *Medial fibroplasia* is the most common pattern of fibromuscular dysplasia, accounting for most if not all internal carotid involvement. It may present as a focal stenosis or multiple lesions with intervening aneurysmal outpouchings. Histologically, the disease is limited to the media, with replacement of smooth muscle with compact fibrous connective tissue. The inner media may show accumulation of collagen and ground substance separating disorganized smooth muscle cells. Gradation of these changes correlates with the severity of the lesion. Mural dilations and microaneurysms are common.

4. *Perimedial dysplasia* is characterized by accumulation of elastic tissue between the media and the adventitia. It affects renal arteries and is associated with macroaneurysms.

Fibromuscular dysplasia preferentially affects long arteries with few primary branches. Hormonal effects on medial tissue, mechanical stresses on the vessel wall, and unusual distribution of the vasa vasorum in these arteries seem to play an etiologic role.[80] The fact that women are most commonly affected (92 per cent of cases),[79] and some experimental evidence,[81] support a possible role of hormones in this process. The normal paucity of vasa vasorum in long nonbranching arterial segments, such as the extracranial carotid artery and the renal artery, in the appropriate hormonal environment may predispose to mural ischemia and the initiation of the fibroplastic process. Experimental evidence supports this concept.[82]

The exact cause of symptoms is controversial. Thromboembolism from clot and/or platelets, decreased flow due to a critical stenosis or a series of noncritical narrowings, intracranial involvement with or without aneurysm formation, and hypertension have been implicated.[79]

Coils and Kinks of the Extracranial Arteries

Coils and kinks of the extracranial system on occasion have been associated with fibromuscular dysplasia.[79] More commonly, these are due to embryologic events and changes that occur in the aging process. Neurologic manifestations from these have been reported in children[83] and in adults.[84-86] Embryologically, the internal carotid artery is derived from the third aortic arch and the dorsal aortic root. In its early stages, a normally occurring kink is straightened as the heart and great vessels descend in the mediastinum. Failure of this process may account for the occurrence of coils and loops in children and for its bilaterality in about 50 per cent of cases.[86]

In adults, kinking of the extracranial vessels is almost always associated with atherosclerosis. In the aging process, there is loss of elasticity of the vessel wall, which, in combination with lateral stresses, causes elongation between fixed points, the skull and the thoracic inlet. This will produce bowing with eventual formation of coils and kinks. Between 5 and 16 per cent of patients submitted for angiographic evaluation will have coiling or kinking of one of the extracranial vessels.[84,86] The kinking of the artery is more likely to produce symptoms due either to flow reduction or to concomitant plaque formation with distal embolization. Kinking is considered as an angle of less than 90 degrees between arterial segments (Fig. 31–4). It is unlikely that flow restriction exists in the absence of this configuration. This acute angulation is more likely to occur when the head is turned to the ipsilateral side.[83] In other cases, contralateral rotation, neck flexion, and extension may exaggerate the abnormality to markedly reduce flow. A history of TIAs associated with head motion should lead the clinician to suspect the presence of kink. Abnormal pulsations in the neck, sometimes suggesting an aneurysmal dilatation, may be present on physical examination. Secondary arteriosclerotic changes may occur because of abnormal flow patterns that predispose to plaque formation and ulceration, accounting for the development of neurologic symptoms. Rarely will the vertebral circulation be affected by a kink.[84]

Aneurysms

Aneurysms of the carotid artery can cause neurologic symptoms by several mechanisms. Thrombosis and rupture are rare, but embolization is a frequent event.[87] Pressure of cranial nerves can be seen when expansion is rapid, but more frequently this is associated with acute dissection.

Most extracranial aneurysms are secondary to atherosclerosis. Internal elastic lamina disruption and medial thinning are frequent histologic findings.[88] Two types are recognized: fusiform and saccular. Fusiform aneurysms are the most common. These are frequently bilateral and associated with other arterial aneurysms. Saccular aneurysms are often unilateral and tend to involve the common or internal arteries more often. They may also have a congenital, degenerative, or traumatic etiology.[89] Atherosclerotic aneurysms of the extracranial circulation are almost always associated with hypertension.[88]

Trauma is a frequent cause of carotid aneurysms. These are usually saccular and most commonly result from blunt rather than penetrating injury. Hyperextension and rotation of the neck cause compression of the internal carotid artery on the transverse process of the atlas.[90] An intimal injury is produced that frequently leads to thrombosis but that may also produce aneurysmal dilation.[88]

Mycotic aneurysms are rare. Syphilis and peritonsillar abscess were once common causes of these aneurysms.[91] *Staphylococcus aureus* is the responsible organism at present.

False aneurysms of the carotid artery may form after penetrating injury, but the most frequent cause at present is previous carotid surgery. They are more common after patch closure of the artery than primary closure.[87] Disruption of the suture line by infection, suture failure, and technical error are believed to be responsible for their formation. False aneurysms can expand, thrombose, rupture, or lead to distal embolization. The diagnosis is an indication for surgical repair.

Acute dissection of the carotid artery with or without aneurysm formation is another cause of neurologic events resulting from pathology in the extracranial circulation. It can occur secondary to atherosclerosis, fibromuscular dysplasia, or cystic medial necrosis.[92] A history of trauma may or may not be present. On gross inspection, a sharply demarcated transition between the normal color and size of the carotid artery and the dark blue and cylindrical dilation in the dissected segment are noted.[93] More commonly, the internal carotid artery is affected, and frequently the end of the dissection is not surgically accessible. A double lumen is usually present, with the dissection occurring in the outer layers of the media. Smooth muscle cells are widely separated, and there is degeneration and fragmentation of the internal elastic membrane.[93] The most frequent presentation is a sudden onset of temporal headache or cervical pain associated with a neurologic or visual deficit and/or Horner's syndrome. The acute expansion may cause compression of cranial nerves IX, X, XI, or XII, with concomitant dysfunction.[92] Horner's syndrome is thought to be secondary to disruption of periadventitial sympathetic fibers. The carotid artery is far more frequently affected than the vertebral. Only a few cases of the latter have been reported, with involvement of the segment between C1 and C2 noted consistently.[92]

Takayasu's Arteritis

In 1908, Takayasu[94] described ocular changes in a 21-year-old woman with nonspecific arteritis. These consisted of a peculiar capillary flush with rustlike arteriovenous anastomoses around the papilla and blindness due to cataracts. Similar cases were later

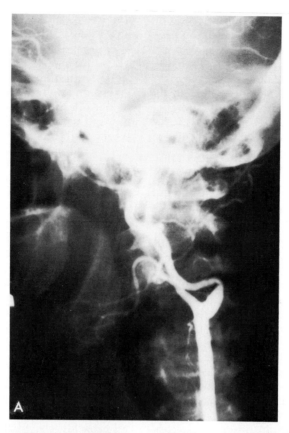

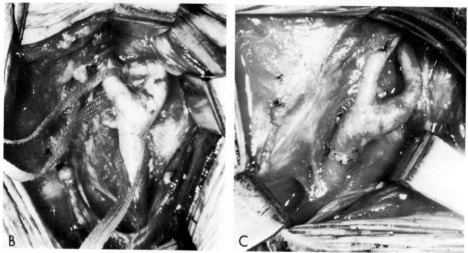

FIGURE 31–4.   *A,* Selective left carotid arteriogram demonstrating kink of the internal carotid artery. Note the angulation of less than 90 degrees and the paucity of contrast material beyond the kink. *B,* Operative appearance of the internal carotid artery kink. *C,* Operative appearance of the internal carotid artery following connection of the kink by mobilization and segmental resection of the common carotid artery. The carotid bifurcation is pulled down and an end-to-end anastomosis is constructed.

described with the absence of pulses in the arm. Since then, Takayasu's arteritis has been recognized as a cause of neurologic symptoms secondary to a nonspecific inflammatory process of unknown etiology affecting segmentally the aorta and its main branches. The end result of this process is a constriction or occlusion and occasional aneurysm formation of the affected vessels secondary to marked fibrosis and thickening of the arterial wall.[95] Originally thought to be rare in this hemisphere, it is now well recognized that many cases of atypical coarctations of the aorta and other unusual lesions of its main branches are indeed Takayasu's arteritis. This explains the many eponyms given to this syndrome.[96]

Four varieties of the disease are recognized.[97] In type 1, the involvement is localized to the aortic arch and its branches. Type 2 does not have arch involvement; the lesions are confined to the descending and abdominal aorta. Type 3 has features of both, and type 4 describes any of the above with involvement of the pulmonary artery.

In a retrospective study of 107 patients,[97] 84 per cent were female, and 80 per cent were ages 11 to 30. Two phases of the disease are recognized. In the acute or prepulseless stage, systemic symptoms of a nonspecific nature are present. Skin rashes, fever, myalgia, arthralgias, pleuritis, generalized weakness, and other nonspecific symptoms develop, making the diagnosis difficult. This may resolve and go unrecognized by the patient or physician until months or years later, when the second or occlusive stage evolves. It is then that symptoms of obstruction of the main aortic branches develop. These lesions are not easily managed by endarterectomy. This makes bypass surgery the treatment of choice.

Other forms of arteritis, specifically giant cell arteritis, can cause neurologic symptoms because of extra- or intracranial involvement. Patients are older then those with Takayasu's arteritis, and both sexes appear to be equally affected.[96] Systemic symptoms are usually present. Tenderness over the carotid or other affected areas may occur.[98] The histologic picture is characteristic, with changes confined to the media, where a large number of giant cells interspersed with lymphocytes are seen. Early diagnosis is important, because corticosteroid therapy may abort the latter stages of the process.[98]

Radiation Therapy Injury

External cervical radiation therapy is now recognized as a cause of accelerated atherosclerotic changes in the extracranial circulation. Experimentally,[99] atherosclerotic lesions similar to the naturally occurring one can be produced in the abdominal aorta in dogs by x-ray and electron beam radiation. Injury to the endothelial cell, ground substance, elastic lamina, and smooth muscle appears to alter the vessel wall, increasing its permeability to circulating lipids and impairing its ability to repair elastic tissue, leading to formation of a plaque characterized by fibrosis, fatty infiltration, and intimal destruction.[100] These changes may occur months to years after completion of therapy. Lesions occur in locations unusual for atherosclerosis (Fig. 31–5). Blowout of the affected carotid may occur, but it is more frequent when surgery is combined with radiation in treating cervical malignancies. Hyperlipidemia and hypercholesterolemia appear to predispose patients receiving radiation therapy to the development of these accelerated changes.[101] Endarterectomy of the affected segments is somewhat more difficult but can be carried out safely.[100,102] Moritz et al. reported their experience with 53 patients who underwent radiation therapy to the neck an average of 28 months previously and compared them with 38 patients who did not have radiation and served as a control group. Thirty per cent of the radiated group had moderate to severe lesions of the carotid bifurcation as detected by duplex scanning in contrast to only 6 per cent of the control group. Five patients in the radiated group were symptomatic. The authors conclude that patients who receive carotid radiation should undergo follow-up periodic duplex scanning of the carotid arteries.[103]

Recurrent Carotid Stenosis

Recurrent carotid stenosis has been reported to occur in a range from 1 to 21 per cent,[104–109] and may yield an incidence of hemodynamically significant stenosis as high as 32 per cent after 7 years.[104] This can lead to neurologic symptoms by producing emboli or restricting flow. The most common lesion developing within the first 2 years after surgery is myointimal fibroplasia. Histologically, there is a concentric lesion with no calcium or lipid deposits. Dense accumulation of collagen and mucopolysaccharides surrounds cellular elements. These substances are produced by the myointimal cell in the normal healing process. An accelerated production seems responsible for the development of the fibroplastic lesion leading to stenosis of the lumen. An endarterectomy plane is almost impossible to develop.

The morphologic characteristics of the early (less than 2 years) restenosis suggest a lower risk of stroke when compared to arteriosclerotic lesion of similar degree.[110] In addition, regression of stenosis documented by noninvasive tests has been reported. Thus, controversy exists as to the management of the early recurrent stenosis following carotid endarterectomy.[111] In the asymptomatic stage, a restenosis documented by successive noninvasive testing should lead the surgeon to consider surgical intervention if there is progression of persistent stenosis greater than 80 per cent of the diameter. Recurrent symptoms are certainly an indication for reoperation unless a different etiology is suspected. Interestingly, Bernstein et al. showed an inverse correlation between a greater than 50 per cent recurrent stenosis, late stroke, and death. Their data suggested that patients with early recurrent stenosis had a better long-term prognosis than those who did not develop recurrent stenosis.[112]

When a stenotic lesion develops more than 2 years after carotid endarterectomy, atherosclerosis is usually the etiologic process. Injury to the vessel by vascular clamps may play a role. Elevated serum cholesterol has been shown to have a statistically significant association with recurrent carotid stenosis.[105]

These lesions probably carry the same stroke risk as primary arteriosclerotic lesions in the carotid bifurcation. Recommendation for reoperation thus is based on the known risk factors of similar primary arteriosclerotic lesions.

Some investigators have suggested that patch closure at the time of the initial carotid endarterectomy may prevent recurrent stenosis. This remains controversial.

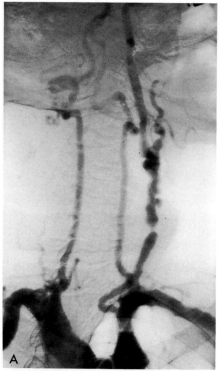

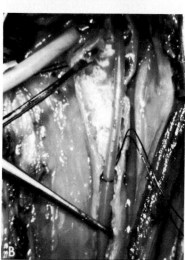

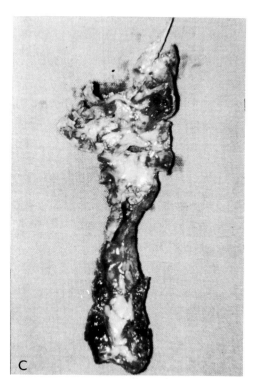

FIGURE 31–5. *A*, Arch angiogram demonstrating carotid artery disease secondary to external cervical radiation. Note complete occlusion of the right common carotid artery. There are multiple stenoses of the left common carotid artery, an unusual site for primary atherosclerosis. *B*, Operative appearance of the lesion secondary to external radiation. *C*, Intimectomy specimen of the lesion produced by external cervical radiation.

Several prospective randomized studies, either completed or in progress, suggest a lower incidence of restenosis with the use of patch angioplasty.[106,113–116] However, a significant benefit of patch angioplasty appears to be a reduction in technical end point problems. Therefore, patching may be more important in preventing occurrence rather than recurrence. The same objective can be achieved by preventing or correcting technical error at the time of operation when identified with completion angiography. Data obtained from experimental hemodynamic studies suggest that an enlarged bulb that would follow after patch closure of an endarterectomy site may predispose to areas of low shear stress and therefore recurrent disease. Factors associated with early recurrence include incomplete in-

timectomy (occurrence), the use of distal tacking sutures, female gender, continued cigarette smoking, and primary closure of an anatomically small internal carotid artery.[117,118]

PATHOGENETIC MECHANISMS OF TRANSIENT ISCHEMIC ATTACKS AND CEREBRAL INFARCTION

In reviewing the mechanisms for TIA and cerebral infarction, emphasis will be placed on those events related to disease in the extracranial vessels. Hemorrhagic stroke will be excluded. Cerebral ischemic events related to hypertension and cardiac emboli will be briefly reviewed because of their importance in differential diagnosis and workup of the symptomatic patient. Finally, from a pathogenetic standpoint, the difference between TIA and fixed deficit is a matter of degree, duration, and presence of actual infarction. The mechanisms of occurrence are essentially the same. Therefore, for purposes of discussion, we will use the general inclusive term "ischemic event."

Arterial Thrombosis

When an atherosclerotic plaque expands to produce a critical reduction in blood flow, the vessel will ultimately undergo thrombosis. In the case of the internal carotid artery, if this column of thrombus stops at the ophthalmic artery and remains stable, and if there is sufficient collateral circulation via the circle of Willis, the thrombotic event may be entirely asymptomatic (Fig. 31–6). If the thrombus propagates beyond the ophthalmic artery to occlude the middle cerebral artery (Fig. 31–7), however, or if small thrombi rather than a thrombotic column form and are subsequently carried to the intracranial vessels by continuous blood flow (Fig. 31–8), then the patient will experience cerebral symptoms that can vary from transient ocular or hemispheric events to a profound hemiplegia, depending upon the extent of propagated thrombus or embolus. In addition, if

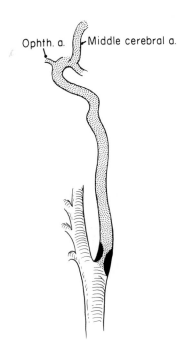

FIGURE 31–7. In this instance, the thrombus that develops secondary to an occlusive atherosclerotic lesion of the internal carotid artery progresses beyond the ophthalmic artery to involve the middle cerebral artery.

the collateral circulation to the circle of Willis is poor, the sudden loss of flow through a diseased internal carotid artery may incite a precipitous drop in flow to the hemisphere, resulting in ischemic infarction as a consequence of inadequate proximal blood flow.

Flow-Related Ischemic Events

While this mechanism used to be considered the most common cause for transient ischemic events, it is actually a rather rare occurrence. Transient drops in hemispheric blood flow or the development of a chronic low-flow state can be responsible for nonspecific symptoms of lightheadedness, presyncopy, or intellectual deterioration.[1,119] It must also be recognized, however, that there are other causes for these symptoms that are nonvascular and probably more frequent.

The collateral blood flow to the brain, via the circle of Willis, is an extremely efficient system. There have been multiple observations of patients with bilateral internal carotid artery occlusion, perhaps combined with occlusion of the vertebral artery, who were totally asymptomatic from a central neurologic point of view. Experience obtained performing carotid endarterectomy under local anesthesia has shown that only about 10 per cent of patients will experience neurologic symptoms when the carotid artery is clamped.[52] It is this 10 per cent who can have symptoms on the basis of compromised blood flow when the stenosis progresses or goes on to complete occlusion. Another circumstance that can produce

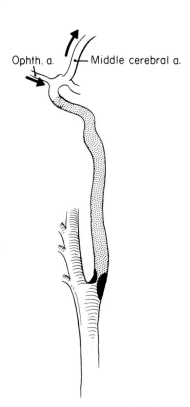

FIGURE 31–6. Artist's concept of a thrombus occurring distal to an occlusive lesion of the internal carotid artery. Notice the column thrombus stops short of the ophthalmic artery, with maintenance of patency of the middle cerebral artery.

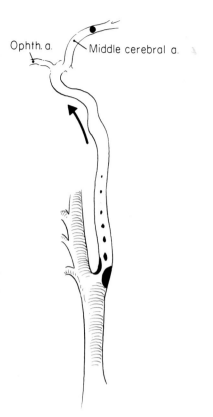

FIGURE 31–8. Emboli released from a plaque strategically placed at the origin of the internal carotid artery can pass into the middle cerebral artery and lodge in the terminal branch. This will result in either a temporary or a permanent neurologic deficit in the distribution appropriate to the arterial occlusion.

symptoms of global ischemia would be simultaneous stenosis or occlusion in more than one extracranial vessel; for example, a carotid occlusion on one side combined with a high-grade stenosis in the contralateral carotid artery. Under these circumstances, transient drops in blood pressure, perhaps posturally related, can produce either global or focal ischemic symptoms. Rarely, patients with unilateral carotid occlusion may have a downstream vascular bed that is marginally perfused. Postural changes under these circumstances can also produce focal ischemia and result in a flow-related TIA. Under these conditions, a patient would be a good candidate for extracranial-to-intracranial bypass grafting.

Flow-restricting lesions in the vertebral arteries or in major vessels proximal to the vertebral origin, such as the innominate or subclavian arteries, can produce symptoms related to hypoperfusion in the posterior circulation. One of the most dramatic anatomic observations is the so-called subclavian steal syndrome. If there is a stenosis or occlusion of the subclavian artery proximal to the vertebral artery takeoff, the pressure drop distal to the obstruction will cause its branches to serve as sources of collateral blood flow by reversing the normal flow direction. The branches now contribute to the flow of the main trunk rather than receiving flow from the proximally affected ar-

tery. The vessels that contribute to collateral blood flow of the distal subclavian artery by reversing flow include the vertebral artery. Under these circumstances, the vertebral artery not only is deprived of the usual antegrade flow, but actually siphons off blood flow from the basilar artery circulation because of flow reversal. This siphoning off of blood may be entirely without symptoms if there are abundant sources of inflow from the other vertebral artery or from the anterior circulation. On the other hand, if the opposite vertebral artery is small or occluded, there may be a deficiency in basilar artery flow that results in symptoms of basilar artery insufficiency. These symptoms may first appear or become exaggerated if the demand for flow in the affected subclavian artery increases, such as results from doing active exercise of the arm (Fig. 31–9).

Cerebral Emboli

The most common causes of cerebral ischemic events are embolic phenomena, primarily arterial in origin and secondarily from cardiac sources. The emboli of arterial origin occur as a consequence of morphologic change present on the luminal surface of a critical artery.[51,52,120,121] These changes most often are associated with atheromatous plaques but can also occur

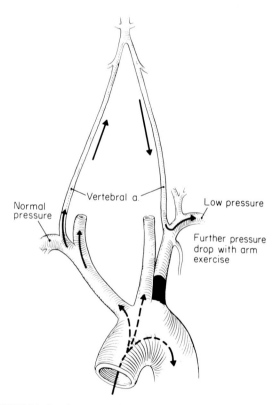

FIGURE 31–9. Artist's concept of the mechanism of the subclavian steal syndrome. Note the occlusion in the origin of the left subclavian artery. This produces a pressure gradient with reversal of blood flow in the left vertebral artery, producing a siphoning or steal from the basilar artery.

with other lesions, such as fibromuscular dysplasia. When there is an irregular surface producing turbulence, there is a stimulus for platelet aggregation. If the platelet aggregates become large enough and embolize to an important vessel in the brain, symptoms will occur. If the platelet aggregates break up quickly from mechanical forces or from the effect of arterial prostacyclin, the symptoms will be transient. If the embolic fragment persists, however, it can lead to focal infarction (Fig. 31–10).

An atherosclerotic plaque may undergo central degeneration or softening. When this occurs, there may be bleeding into the plaque substance, leading to sudden plaque expansion[48,73,108,122] with intraluminal rupture, or the plaque may spontaneously rupture into the lumen, discharging its contents into the arterial stream. The plaque contents consists of degenerative atheromatous debris, including various mixtures of cholesterol crystals, calcific material, or thrombotic remnants. If the atherosclerotic plaque is located at a critical point, such as the origin of the internal carotid artery, there is considerable likelihood that embolic atheromatous fragments will be carried to important vascular beds of the brain, producing either transient or permanent neurologic events (Fig. 31–11). These events are to be considered primary embolic events of atherosclerotic plaque origin.

After the plaque has ruptured, a defect is left behind, which is called an ulcer (Fig. 31–12). Further primary emboli can continue to escape from the raw

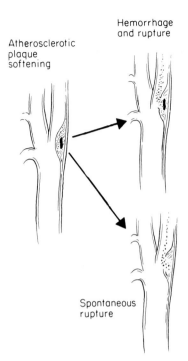

FIGURE 31–11. Artist's concept of an atherosclerotic plaque undergoing central softening. There may be spontaneous hemorrhage into the center of the plaque, producing rupture and discharge of embolic fragments, or the plaque may spontaneously rupture as a result of hydrostatic forces, releasing necrotic, embolic debris.

ulcerated surface, or the ulcer itself may serve as a focal point for thrombus or platelet aggregate material to form. These platelet or thrombotic aggregates may secondarily dislodge, owing to blood flow turbulence, and embolize to the brain (Fig. 31–13). Thus it must be remembered that the embolic material from an atherosclerotic plaque can consist of atheromatous debris, platelet aggregates, or blood clot. The emboli of arterial origin can be primary, occurring with plaque rupture or occurring on thrombogenic arterial plaque surfaces,[121,123] or secondary, having developed within ulcerative lesions from previous plaque rupture.[124]

Embolic events may produce the more dramatic focal neurologic events that will be immediately appreciated by the patient, or the embolic fragments may travel to more silent areas of the brain, in which

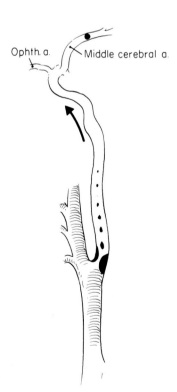

FIGURE 31–10. An embolic fragment in the middle cerebral artery. If this persists, it will lead to focal infarction. If the fragment breaks up and distributes itself through the microcirculation, the ischemic event will be transient.

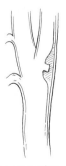

FIGURE 31–12. Following evacuation of an atherosclerotic plaque, a defect or ulcer is left behind.

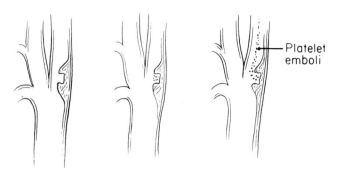

FIGURE 31–13. The ulcerated lesion within an atheromatous plaque can serve as a nidus for platelet aggregate or thrombotic material. These aggregates can secondarily embolize from the ulcer crypt.

case the results will be more subtle and appreciated on a chronic basis, such as cerebral atrophy or multiinfarct dementia.[125,126] The use of transcranial Doppler has provided more objective evidence of emboli from carotid plaques by discerning discrete noise as an embolic particle passes a point of Doppler insonation.[127] Finally, the occurrence of TIAs in a hemisphere distal to a carotid occlusion raises the question of the relationship of decreased flow to arterial border zones. Recent experimental data, however, have demonstrated that emboli originating from a contralateral carotid artery can cross through the circle of Willis and produce focal infarcts in the hemisphere distal to a carotid occlusion.[128] Thus the contralateral patent carotid artery should always be considered a possible source of emboli when a patient with a carotid occlusion begins to experience symptoms in the hemisphere distal to the occlusion.

Emboli can also occur from cardiac sources, which include aortic valvular disease, mitral valve prolapse, cardiac arrhythmias, and mural thrombus following myocardial infarction.

Lacunar Infarction

Focal areas of cerebral necrosis occurring in the basal ganglia, internal capsule, or pons have been described as a consequence of end-vessel occlusive disease involving the lenticulostriate or thalamoperforant arteries. The underlying etiology is related to uncontrolled hypertension, and the resulting neurologic deficit is often clinically identified as a pure motor or pure sensory stroke.[129] While descriptions of this phenomenon date back to the early 1900s, its current understanding and popularity are due to the efforts and writings of C. Miller Fisher.[130]

The clinical picture may often be confused with arterial-arterial emboli in that there may be antecedent TIAs. The differential diagnosis is best made by the very focal neurologic deficit seen clinically and the typical anatomic location as seen on CT brain scan. More recent evidence, however, suggests that so-called lacunes may, in fact, be the consequence of

emboli of arterial origin.[131–134] Thus the presence of symptoms with imaging of a deep white matter infarct does not rule out the carotid bifurcation as a cause of the event.

CLINICAL SYNDROMES OF EXTRACRANIAL ARTERIAL OCCLUSIVE DISEASE

Extracranial arterial occlusive disease may present with varying symptoms or in other instances may be completely asymptomatic. It is of utmost importance to obtain a thorough history, because this alone may provide clues as to the specific nature of the event in question. Often one will discover that symptoms exist that the patient has ignored. A complete review of symptoms is mandatory, because this in itself may alter the therapeutic alternatives available. Risk factors for atherosclerosis should be specifically recorded.

Patients can be divided into three categories. Asymptomatic patients represent that group in which a hemodynamically significant lesion or a nonocclusive ulcerated arteriosclerotic plaque in the extracranial circulation has been discovered in the absence of transient or permanent neurologic symptoms. The presence or absence of a bruit in the cervical area should not be a criterion for inclusion in this category. It should be recorded as a general marker of a patient at high risk for atherosclerosis.[135]

In an analysis of 1287 patients with cervical bruits, less than one third of the bruits proved to be hemodynamically significant by noninvasive criteria.[40] The fact that significant lesions can occur in the absence of a bruit and vice versa is important. The available data on the natural history of asymptomatic bruits cannot be applied to patients with these lesions. This group of patients is usually discovered by angiography in studying other conditions or by noninvasive studies carried out because of the presence of a bruit or screening prior to major surgical procedures. Because of what is known of the natural history of these lesions, as discussed later, therapeutic intervention in the asymptomatic stage may be beneficial.

The other two categories of symptomatic patients with extracranial arterial occlusive disease will be discussed separately.

Transient Ischemic Attacks

General Considerations

Transient ischemic attacks are defined as temporary focal neurologic deficits lasting not more than 24 hours, with complete recovery. The event is caused by ischemia in the territory of the brain supplied by a particular artery or branch. Clinically, symptoms are of sudden onset, without aura, and resolution is often within minutes. When symptoms last longer than 6 hours, a permanent abnormality is more likely, although it may not be clinically detectable.[136] Because of its territorial nature, symptoms tend to be stereotyped. Disappearance of symptoms is swift, ordinarily taking only a few minutes.[137] The frequency of attacks is variable. The patient may experience only one episode or multiple attacks, with variable symptom-free intervals. The most common cause of these transient territorial deficits is extracranial arterial occlusive lesions. The pathology of this has been discussed. Other important causes in the differential diagnosis include heart disease, hematologic disorders such as systemic lupus erythematosus, hyperglobulinemia, polycythemia and sickle cell disease, disseminated intravascular coagulation, subacute bacterial endocarditis, paroxysmal embolism, and several rare connective tissue disorders, such as pseudoxanthoma elasticum and Ehlers-Danlos syndrome.[136] Migraine, especially when associated with transient neurologic deficit, can be confused with a TIA. A history of migraine in the family, the throbbing quality of the headache, and its occurrence upon recovery from the neurologic deficit can be helpful in this situation.

An important concept when evaluating patients with symptoms suggestive of TIA is that those secondary to emboli from a point source such as the extracranial circulation will have the same symptoms with every attack. In contrast, patients who are embolizing from the heart will tend to have variable symptoms.

Since only about 9 per cent of patients with TIAs are seen by a physician during an attack,[138] the history remains the main factor in establishing the diagnosis. In this regard, family members may be extremely helpful.

Two important syndromes deserve mention. Occasionally, a patient will experience frequent repeated attacks of a specific neurologic deficit without the interval allowing time for complete recovery. If the deficit is the same with each attack and no deterioration in function is seen, this is known as crescendo TIAs. If progressive deterioration is seen with each successive attack, a stroke-in-evolution may be present. In any case, evaluation must proceed on an emergency basis. If a surgically correctable lesion is present and the neurologic deficit is not dense (no loss of consciousness or dense hemiparesis), serious consideration should be given to proceeding with emergency operation.

Carotid Artery Transient Ischemic Attacks

Manifestations of a transient ischemic episode in the territory of the carotid artery include deficits in areas supplied by the anterior and middle cerebral arteries. It must be remembered that in older individuals both anterior cerebral arteries and posterior arteries may be supplied by one carotid artery.[136]

Ischemia in a cerebral hemisphere often produces contralateral symptoms. Motor dysfunction can include weakness, paralysis, or clumsiness of one or both limbs contralateral to the affected hemisphere. Sensory alterations will include numbness, loss of sensation, or paresthesia in the opposite side of the face or in one or both limbs. When examined during an attack, this sensory loss may not be objectively demonstrable.[138]

Ninety-five per cent of patients have a dominant left hemisphere. Both receptive and motor aphasia can occur. When the former is present, the patient or family may interpret it as confusion. Dysarthria may occur as a function of the nondominant hemisphere, but when it is present as the sole symptom, it is more common in vertebrobasilar TIAs. Other functions of the nondominant side include inattention to the patient's own person and environment on the contralateral side.[136] Loss of function of these areas may also be interpreted as confusion.

Transient visual loss (amaurosis fugax) or blurring of vision in the ipsilateral eye is one of the most reliable symptoms of carotid artery TIAs.[139] This may be described as a curtain coming down (altitudinal) or as quadrant field defects. Conjugate eye deviation, as occurs in seizures or completed strokes, is not seen. Homonymous hemianopsia in combination with any of the above-mentioned symptoms suggests carotid TIAs. This is the result of ischemia in the area of the optic radiation emanating from the optic chiasm. This will produce loss of vision in the ipsilateral temporal visual field and the contralateral nasal visual field. When they occur secondary to carotid artery disease, these visual field defects usually are limited to a quadrant corresponding to the distribution of the optic radiation. When hemianopsia is complete, it cannot be distinguished from a vertebrobasilar TIA.[136]

Ischemic optic neuropathy is a condition characterized by blindness and is associated with giant cell arteritis in about 10 per cent of cases. In the other 90 per cent of cases, it has been labeled idiopathic. Berguer found a significant correlation between extracranial occlusive disease and idiopathic optic neuropathy.[140] In fact, of 20 symptomatic eyes examined, significant extracranial arterial occlusive disease was found in 60 per cent. An embolic mechanism was suggested as the etiology of the optic nerve infarct. A more severe form is seen in patients with very severe extracranial disease, usually occlusion on one side and a high degree of stenosis on the other. These patients will develop an ischemic ophthalmopathy characterized by neovascularization of the iris. The term "rubeosis" has been used to characterize this entity. This suggests that patients with idiopathic optic neuropathy not found to be secondary to giant cell arteritis should undergo extracranial vascular evaluation.[140]

Convulsions can occur but are more suggestive of a completed or hemorrhagic stroke. When sensory or motor symptoms are present, they appear all at one time, without a march suggestive of focal seizure activity.[137] A combination of symptoms may carry more reliability than a single symptom alone. In right carotid artery TIA, the combination of ipsilateral visual loss and any contralateral arm symptoms has an increased relationship. In left carotid TIA, diagnostic reliability is increased when language disturbance is combined with right face and/or extremity weakness or sensory loss.[139]

Altered consciousness or syncope can occur, but as the only symptom it is extremely rare, and more often is associated with other illnesses such as cardiac arrhythmias.[136] Other symptoms that represent difficulty in the initial evaluation are dizziness, amnesia, or confusion and impaired vision with alteration in consciousness. These, without other more specific symptoms, are not to be considered as manifestations of TIAs, because they occur most often with other illnesses.

Vertebrobasilar System Transient Ischemic Attacks

Transient ischemia of the area in the brain supplied by the vertebrobasilar system can occur owing to flow restriction or emboli from lesions in the vertebral or basilar arteries. Emboli from other sources may also affect this system.

An occlusive lesion at the origin of the subclavian artery can cause vertebrobasilar symptoms as the affected arm is exercised and reversal of flow occurs in the vertebral circulation. This subclavian steal is often accompanied by exertional pain in the arm of the affected side.[136]

Alternating hemipareses or hemisensory symptoms in repetitive attacks and bilateral circumoral sensory symptoms associated with unilateral arm or leg weakness or ataxia are highly suggestive of vertebrobasilar TIAs. Symptoms may change from one side to the other with different attacks and may even involve all four limbs at one time. Drop attacks, or falling precipitously to the ground without premonitory symptoms, occur in less than 4 per cent of patients.[139] In this syndrome, loss of consciousness is absent or so brief that the patient remembers striking the ground, a feature not present in syncope or seizure.[136]

Equilibratory gait or postural disturbance not associated with vertigo can occur. Complete or partial loss of vision in both homonymous fields or homonymous hemianopsia alone is highly suggestive. Vertigo alone, when not associated with other of the above specific symptoms, should not be considered indicative of TIA. When it occurs in clear relationship to focal weakness of the face, arm, or leg or to ataxia, or to persistent diplopia, the existence of TIA is likely. Tinnitus is not a feature of vertigo of a vertebrobasilar TIA and is suggestive of labyrinthine vertigo. Single occurrences of bilateral visual blurring, dysarthria, hoarseness, diplopia, dysphasia, confusion, hiccups, vomiting, loss of consciousness, and vital sign alteration may be manifestations of vertebrobasilar TIAs. These symptoms have so many other causes, however, that the diagnosis will be uncertain unless they occur in combination or with additional signs of focal brainstem or posterior hemisphere dysfunction.

Cerebral Infarction

A completed cerebral infarction with or without a clinically apparent neurologic deficit can be another manifestation of extracranial arterial occlusive disease. The specific deficits that will be clinically detectable are the same as those discussed as manifestations of TIAs.

It is difficult to estimate accurately what percentage of all strokes are secondary to lesions in the extracranial circulation. Available studies differ in population, criteria for diagnosis, and therapeutic approach, and thus the estimates range from 15 to 52 per cent.[141,142] It is generally accepted that extracranial vascular lesions play a major role in the occurrence of cerebral infarction. Approximately 50 per cent of these events will be preceded by TIAs, thus providing a clue for the diagnosis.[143]

Lacunar infarcts, emboli from a cardiac source, intracerebral or intracranial bleeding, and some hematologic disorders as causes of stroke should be included in the differential diagnosis. Cerebrospinal fluid examination, electroencephalography, echocardiograms, Holter monitors, and brain CT are helpful adjuncts in reaching etiologic explanation. Angiography should be considered, because noninvasive studies will not exclude ulcerative lesions in the extracranial circulation that may be responsible for the embolic infarction.

It is important to recognize that identification of a cause for the stroke is essential, because these patients remain at a high risk of developing a subsequent cerebral infarction.

ROLE OF THE VASCULAR LABORATORY

The vascular laboratory from the standpoint of methodology, accuracy, and interpretation is covered in detail in Chapter 13. The role of the vascular laboratory in this evaluation of patients with suspect cerebral vascular disease has been disputed by some and perhaps misused by others. It is our opinion that the vascular laboratory has an important role in the evaluation of patients with cerebral vascular disease, and we will endeavor to review its current application.

Asymptomatic Patients

Patients without symptoms may come to our attention as possible candidates for extracranial cerebral vascular disease because of the presence of one or more associated risk factors (cigarette smoking, hypertension, diabetes mellitus, coronary artery disease, or peripheral vascular disease) or by the presence of a bruit heard over the carotid artery bifurcation. The occurrence of a preocclusive carotid stenosis in the past could be ascertained only by proceeding with carotid angiography, yet the incidence of finding a lesion of significance by angiographic screening was only 20 to 30 per cent. That means that 70 per cent of the suspect population were subject to the costly and needless hospitalization, plus the risk and discomfort of angiography. Currently, with the available vascular laboratory modalities, the presence or absence of a hemodynamically significant lesion can be ascertained in an inexpensive, noninvasive manner with an accuracy of greater than 95 per cent. Those patients with positive findings can then be referred for angiographic survey prior to prophylactic operation, and those patients with a negative screening examination can be reassured, for the time being, and marked for periodic follow-up.

Symptomatic Patients

Patients may present with territorial neurologic events typical of carotid artery or vertebrobasilar disease, or they may have symptoms that are entirely nonspecific or atypical. In the case of the patient with nonspecific symptoms, such as "dizzy spells," these symptoms may be related to global ischemic events as a consequence of decreased blood flow associated with multiple extracranial occlusive lesions, or they may be due to a myriad of disorders unrelated to cerebral vascular disease. The vascular laboratory serves as an effective screen for these patients and can result in avoiding many negative and hence useless angiograms.

For patients with focal or territorial neurologic events, angiography is mandatory regardless of the findings in the noninvasive laboratory. The reason for this statement is that the patients can have embolic events from low-profile, nonhemodynamically significant plaques that cannot be identified in the vascular laboratory, since most tests are oriented toward the diagnosis of hemodynamically significant stenoses. In spite of the fact that angiography is the primary diagnostic test for this group of patients, the vascular laboratory still has a role. For example, if the noninvasive examination is strongly positive, the surgeon may wish to make himself available during the conduct of angiography in case the degree of stenosis is severe enough to mandate urgent or emergent carotid endarterectomy. This information, available prior to angiography, will permit appropriate planning. In addition, the preoperative baseline data from the vascular laboratory are extremely helpful in following patients immediately after operation as well as in the late follow-up interval. A conversion from a positive to a negative test following operation is expected. If this does not occur, a technical problem is suggested that may require investigation and management. Also, an abnormal study 6 months or a year after surgery in a patient who had a normal study following operation will alert the surgeon to the possibility of recurrent stenosis, often before the onset of symptoms. Finally, the importance of obtaining baseline data on the opposite, asymptomatic carotid artery should not be overlooked. Late strokes that occur in patients having undergone successful carotid endarterectomy are most often related to the nonoperated side. Early identification of progression on the contralateral side will permit earlier intervention as a means of preventing contralateral stroke.

BRAIN SCANS AND ANGIOGRAPHY

The advent of CT and magnetic resonance imaging (MRI) for head scanning has been a benefit in the evaluation of patients with cerebral vascular disease and has virtually eliminated the use of radionuclide scanning. Intracranial space-occupying lesions such as neoplasms, vascular malformations, or subdural hematomas enter into the differential diagnosis of patients with even the most convincing symptoms of transient cerebral ischemia. CT and MRI scanning are quick, noninvasive means of ruling out alternative pathology during patient workup.

The patient who presents with TIAs may have actually suffered a small cerebral infarction. CT or MRI scanning will identify an unsuspected cerebral infarction as well as establish a baseline status prior to operation. The advance knowledge that a small infarction exists is helpful information with respect to intraoperative and postoperative management.

While head scanning may not currently be routine in preoperative workup, it should become a standard part of patient evaluation prior to proceeding with angiography. MRI is replacing CT in some centers. It does not require ionizing radiation or contrast. It can identify acute cerebral infarction sooner than CT and can image smaller infarcts than CT. Finally, newer acquisition programs have enabled magnetic resonance to be used to reconstruct cervical and intracranial arterial anatomy, so-called magnetic resonance angiography (MRA).

Those patients who present with a clinically overt cerebral infarction should have a CT or MRI scan to document infarct size and to differentiate between an ischemic and hemorrhagic infarction. A hemorrhagic infarction will be promptly visible on CT scan, whereas an ischemic infarction may take several days of evolution before its low-density character will be visualized. CT scan data are necessary in decisions concerning the proper timing of operation following acute stroke in patients who have experienced a good neurologic recovery. In fact, of 245 patients with persistent neurologic deficits seen by Dosick et al., 171 were found to have negative CT scans.[144] Appropriate carotid lesions were found in 110 (64 per cent) of this group. All 110 patients underwent carotid endarterectomy within 14 days of the initial onset of their neurologic deficits. The perioperative morbidity was 0.9 per cent. These investigators concluded that angiography and carotid endarterectomy may be safely performed when indicated in patients with negative CT scans within the first 2 weeks following a prolonged neurologic deficit.[144]

The electroencephalogram (EEG) has generally not been considered helpful in the workup of patients with cerebrovascular disease, with the exception of ruling out seizure disorder in the differential diagnosis. However, a new application of cerebral electrical activity, so-called computerized brain mapping, has been shown to be of value. This modality utilizes 32 electrodes (rather than 16 used with EEG) arranged over both hemispheres. The data are digitized and color coded. The information is computer analyzed, and hard copy integrated data are generated. In a recent report comparing CT, MRI, and brain mapping, brain mapping was found to be more sensitive in identifying small areas of cortical dysfunction.[145] Aortocranial angiography is the cornerstone for diagnosis in the workup of patients with suspected cerebral vascular disease. It cannot be emphasized enough that the angiogram is a preoperative study. An angiogram should not be ordered unless the patient and surgeon are prepared to proceed promptly with operation. There is no place for the use of angiography as a routine data base item unless the information obtained is going to be used for therapeutic decision making. Noninvasive studies are now sophisticated enough for diagnosis. The angiogram should be used to confirm the presence of a surgically accessible lesion and a satisfactory distal vascular bed.

The extent of angiographic visualization required for proper evaluation in patients with cerebral vascular disease is controversial. The options include: (1) visualization of the aortic arch and extracranial vessels in two oblique views; (2) selective injection of both common carotid arteries in anteroposterior and lateral projections to obtain both extracranial and intracranial carotid visualization; (3) combined arch and selective carotid angiograms; (4) the possible addition of subclavian-vertebral angiography for both extracranial and intracranial visualization; and (5) digital intravenous or intraarterial subtraction angiography. Good arguments exist for any of these approaches to the exclusion of the alternates. It is the author's practice to choose the angiographic alternative on an individual basis rather than having a set routine. The generous use of noninvasive screening combined with CT scanning makes individual angiographic programming feasible. Patients who present with TIAs in the carotid distribution, who have a noninvasive screen consistent with a hemodynamically significant lesion in the appropriate carotid artery and have a negative CT scan, can be studied with an arch aortogram with two good oblique projections. This will visualize the arch vessels as well as the extracranial extent of the carotid and vertebral arteries. It is unlikely that a hemodynamically significant lesion of the carotid bifurcation will be missed on one of the two oblique views of the arch injection. The arch studies should give good

documentation of the location and extent of all extracranial lesions. An alternative for those institutions with good intravenous digital subtraction equipment is to use this method of visualization. It should be kept in mind, however, that the reported correlation between digital intravenous subtraction angiography and conventional angiography ranges from 60 to 85 per cent, with a significant incidence of false-negative as well as false-positive data.

For those patients with carotid territory symptoms and a negative noninvasive study, selective carotid injections are indicated. The presumed pathology is an ulcerative lesion of the carotid bifurcation in the absence of a hemodynamically significant stenosis. This lesion may be seen only on one view of a selective angiogram, and the arteriographer may have to obtain several views of the bifurcation area before the ulceration is visualized. Likewise, the possibility exists that an intracranial lesion is responsible for the symptoms and the region must be visualized with selective injection to rule out that site for significant pathology.

When patients present with vertebrobasilar symptoms and/or physical findings consistent with subclavian occlusive disease, the optimum study is an arch injection followed by selective subclavian-vertebral views, including the intracranial distribution of those arteries.

Patients who have been assessed for asymptomatic carotid stenosis can be adequately studied by arch aortography or digital subtraction angiography. The intraarterial injection of contrast with digital subtraction technique provides excellent views of the extracranial vascular system. This technique is especially suitable for those patients with compromised renal status, in whom the total amount of contrast used is of concern. The resolution of the intraarterial digital method is limited, and thus not appropriate in the evaluation of patients suspected of having nonhemodynamically ulcerative lesions in the carotid system.

The routine preoperative use of angiography has been questioned in the recent literature. A highly selected group of patients with hemodynamically significant lesions as determined by noninvasive evaluation, who may or may not be symptomatic in the ipsilateral hemisphere, may be candidates for endarterectomy without preoperative angiography. This remains a controversial issue and at present should be limited to those patients in whom a relative contraindication to angiography (i.e., renal insufficiency) is present.[146]

Those patients who are identified as having carotid stenosis in excess of 90 per cent occlusion are at significant risk of undergoing thrombosis within the next 12 hours following study. It is the author's practice either to proceed with emergency operation or to start intravenous systemic heparin therapy with the scheduling of urgent operation the following morning. Patients who suffer an iatrogenic plaque dissection progressing to occlusion, with or without neurologic deficit, should be taken promptly to the operating room for surgical repair.

It would be optimal to have total visualization of all vessels both extracranially and intracranially; however, this extensive angiographic survey increases the risk of morbidity and mortality of the procedure. It is debatable whether arch injection carries a greater or lesser risk than selective carotid angiography. It should be kept in mind, however, that in the atherosclerotic age group, with the presence of friable plaques, the risk of stroke following angiography has been reported to vary from 0.1 to 1.5 per cent. For this reason, angiography should be employed only when clinically indicated, as a preoperative study, and with the carefully informed consent of the patient.

SURGICAL CONSIDERATIONS AND TECHNIQUE

Anesthesia and Hemodynamic Monitoring

Patients about to undergo cerebral vascular surgery are probably best managed under general anesthesia. Although some surgeons still prefer to do carotid endarterectomy under local or cervical block anesthesia,[147] general anesthesia has the advantage of reducing the cerebral metabolic demand of the brain while increasing cerebral blood flow. General anesthesia also provides for good airway control, reduced patient anxiety, and a quiet surgical field.

Intraoperative blood pressure control and oxygenation are particularly critical during periods of arterial clamping. These parameters are best monitored with an arterial line, usually placed in the radial artery. The judicious use of nitroprusside or vasopressors by the anesthesiologist to maintain blood pressure in the patient's optimum physiologic range is of paramount importance.

Two primary options are available to monitor cerebral perfusion as might be required, particularly during trial clamping of the carotid artery prior to a decision to use an internal shunt. These options are the measurement of internal carotid artery backpressure[148,149] and the intraoperative use of electroencephalography.[150] While controversy exists as to which is more effective, excellent results have been reported with both techniques. EEG/CT brain mapping has been shown to be a sensitive and accurate means of identifying patients that require shunting.[145,151] A new technique, that of somatosensory-evoked potentials, has been investigated and does not appear to be as sensitive as EEG.[152] Finally, there are proponents of no monitoring, some advocating the routine use of an intraluminal shunt,[153] and others advocating routine operation without a shunt but done in an expeditious manner.[154,155] The literature currently supports either selective shunting based on clinical and monitoring criteria or routine shunting.

The general consensus is that either of these techniques will provide for the safest operation with best outcome.[156,157]

The argument in favor of selective shunting is that since only 15 per cent of patients actually require an intraluminal shunt, as judged by observation of operations carried out under local anesthesia, why expose the other 85 per cent of patients to the risks of an internal shunt, which include (1) possible air or atheroma embolisms, (2) scuffing or dissection of distal intima, (3) difficulty with end point visualization, and (4) risk of leaving an intimal flap that may lead to thromboembolic complications? The arguments in favor of the routine use of an intraluminal shunt are that (1) with routine use, there is increased operator facility with the technique and less likelihood of incurring complications, and (2) the presence of the intraluminal shunt acts as a stent that can aid in the closure of the internal carotid portion of the arteriotomy.

The criteria for selective shunting based on back-pressure measurement, as originally described by Moore and colleagues,[148,149] include patients who have had a prior cerebral infarction on the side of operation (regardless of back-pressure value) or patients without a prior cerebral infarction but with a back-pressure measured to be 25 mm Hg or less in the otherwise neurologically intact patient. The EEG criteria for shunt use include a loss of amplitude or slowing of rhythm during trial clamping of the carotid artery.

Carotid Bifurcation Endarterectomy

Indications

The indications for carotid endarterectomy have undergone considerable review and analysis. Data based upon retrospective reviews, prospective randomized trials, and committee discussion based upon expert opinion have been brought together to define the current indications for carotid endarterectomy.[158–160] Based upon analysis of current data, the indications for carotid endarterectomy can be divided into three major categories: general agreement, relative agreement, and controversial.

I. General agreement
    A. Asymptomatic patients with greater than 70 per cent stenosis in the presence of a contralateral occlusion or high-grade stenosis
    B. Symptomatic patients
       1. Single focal (ipsilateral) TIA with greater than 70 per cent stenosis
       2. Multiple focal (ipsilateral) TIA
          a. Greater than 70 per cent stenosis
          b. Greater than 50 per cent stenosis with ulceration
          c. Greater than 50 per cent stenosis—symptoms continue while on aspirin

3. Prior stroke (ipsilateral—mild)
    a. Greater than 70 per cent stenosis
    b. Greater than 50 per cent with large ulcer
4. Prior stroke (ipsilateral—moderate)
    a. Greater than 70 per cent stenosis with contralateral occlusion
5. Stroke-in-evolution
    a. Greater than 70 per cent stenosis (ipsilateral) with or without clot

II. Relative agreement
    A. Symptomatic patients
        1. Multiple TIAs
            a. Acute ipsilateral occlusion
            b. 50 to 69 per cent stenosis (crescendo TIAs)
        2. Recurrent TIAs (aspirin failure)
            a. 50 to 69 per cent stenosis with or without ulcer
    B. Asymptomatic patients
        1. Greater than 80 per cent stenosis
        2. Large ulceration with greater than 50 per cent stenosis
III. Controversial
    A. Symptomatic patients
        1. Multiple TIAs
            a. 30 to 69 per cent stenosis with or without ulcer
        2. Prior stroke—mild
            a. 30 to 69 per cent stenosis with or without ulcer
        3. Global symptoms
            a. Greater than 70 per cent carotid stenosis with uncorrectable vertebral-basilar disease

Technique

Following the induction of satisfactory anesthesia and the placement of appropriate access and monitoring lines, the patient is positioned supine on the operating table with the head turned away from the side of operation. The neck is moderately extended on the shoulders. The head of the table is flexed about 10 degrees to reduce venous pressure, which will minimize bleeding. The author prefers a longitudinal incision placed along the anterior border of the sternocleidomastoid muscle and centered over the carotid bifurcation, as best judged from the arteriogram. This incision can be extended proximally to the sternal notch for more proximal exposure of the common carotid artery and distally to the mastoid process for extensile exposure of the internal carotid artery, when needed. The dissection plane is maintained along the anterior border of the sternocleidomastoid muscle, which will permit anterior mobilization of the tail of the parotid gland rather than the bloody division of its substance, with risk of salivary fistula. The sternocleidomastoid muscle is mobilized off the carotid sheath, and self-retaining retractors are placed. The jugular vein is visualized through the carotid sheath, and the sheath is open

along the anterior border of the vein. The vein is mobilized until the large tributary, the common facial vein, is identified. The common facial vein, when present, is a relatively constant landmark for the carotid bifurcation. The common facial vein is divided between ligatures. In the case of a high carotid bifurcation, particular care must be taken to make sure that the hypoglossal nerve is not lurking behind the common facial vein, because this may lead to its inadvertent injury. Once the common facial vein is divided, the jugular vein can be mobilized laterally off the carotid bifurcation, providing excellent exposure. The vagus nerve usually lies in the posterior portion of the carotid sheath, but on occasion may spiral anteriorly. Particular care must be taken to watch for this anomalous course in order to avoid nerve injury. Another anomaly is the occasional presence of a nonrecurrent laryngeal nerve that comes directly off the vagus on the way to innervate the vocal cord. This nerve can cross anterior to the carotid artery and may be mistaken for a part of the ansa hypoglossi, resulting in mistaken division and cord paralysis. This anomaly most often occurs on the left side of the neck, but has also been described on the right side.

The common carotid artery is mobilized for sufficient length to get proximal to the atheromatous lesion as well as to provide sufficient length in case an internal shunt is required. When the dissection approaches the area of the carotid bifurcation, it may be necessary to inject a local anesthetic in the area of the carotid bifurcation in order to block the nerve to the carotid body to prevent or reverse reflex bradycardia. The external and internal carotid arteries are then mobilized for sufficient length to get completely beyond the atheromatous plaque and to a point where the vessels are completely normal circumferentially. When mobilizing the internal carotid artery, particular care must be taken to avoid injury to the hypoglossal nerve (Fig. 31–14).

In the case of a high bifurcation or an extensive lesion, it may be necessary to mobilize the internal carotid artery for its maximum extracranial length. Several maneuvers are available to gain additional length. The first and most important maneuver is to extend the skin incision all the way up to the mastoid process, with complete mobilization of the sternocleidomastoid muscle toward its tendinous insertion on the mastoid process. Care must be taken to avoid injury to the spinal accessory (XIth cranial) nerve, which enters the substance of the sternocleidomastoid muscle at that level. The posterior belly of the digastric muscle will come into view. This muscle can be divided with impunity, giving additional exposure of the internal carotid artery. If further exposure is needed, the limiting structures are the styloid process and the ramus of the mandible. The styloid process, after suitable preparation, can be divided with bone rongeurs, and the mandible can be displaced anteriorly. Techniques have also been described for dividing the ramus of the mandible in

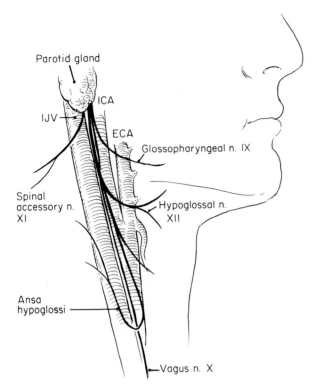

FIGURE 31–14. Artist's concept of the anatomic relationship between the carotid bifurcation and the cranial nerves in the neck. Note the intimate relationship between the hypoglossal nerve and the upper portion of the internal carotid artery (*ICA*). *ECA*, external carotid artery; *IJV*, internal jugular vein.

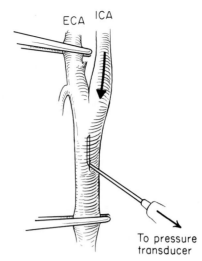

FIGURE 31–15. Techniques of measuring the internal carotid artery back-pressure. Note the needle placement and the needle angulation so as to maintain the tip of the needle in an axial plane with the common carotid artery. A disease-free portion of the common carotid artery is chosen for arterial puncture.

order to gain additional exposure, but we have not found this maneuver necessary.

Once the carotid artery has been sufficiently mobilized, 5000 to 10,000 units of heparin are administered systemically.

If the decision has been made to selectively shunt the patient based on back-pressure criteria, a 22-gauge needle is connected to rigid pressure tubing and hooked up to an arterial pressure transducer. The tubing is flushed with saline, and a zero-pressure level is obtained adjacent to the carotid bifurcation. The needle is carefully bent at a 45-degree angle and inserted into the common carotid artery so that the axis of the distal needle is parallel with the axis of the artery and lies freely within the lumen. The free carotid artery pressure is measured and compared with the radial artery pressure in order to ensure accurate reading. When the patient's blood pressure is stable and at the optimum level, the common carotid artery is clamped proximal to the needle, and the external carotid artery is also clamped, thus permitting the reading of the internal carotid artery back-pressure (Fig. 31–15). If the back-pressure is greater than 25 mm Hg, the internal carotid artery is clamped and the needle withdrawn. If the pressure is less than 25 mm Hg, the clamps on the common and external carotid arteries are temporarily removed, the needle withdrawn, and preparations made for the use of an internal shunt.

With the common, external, and internal carotid arteries clamped, an arteriotomy is made on the lateral portion of the common carotid artery with a no. 11 blade and is extended toward the plaque and up the internal carotid artery with Pott's scissors. The arteriotomy is extended as far as necessary up the internal carotid artery in order to get beyond the plaque and to expose relatively normal artery. An intimectomy plane is then established between the diseased intima and the internal elastic lamina, attempting to leave the circular medial fibers attached to the arterial adventitia. This will facilitate getting a clean distal end point. The proximal end point is obtained by sharply dividing the plaque. The intimectomy surface is copiously irrigated with heparinized saline solution so as to visualize all bits of debris and facilitate their removal.

The arteriotomy can be closed primarily or with patch angioplasty. There is evidence to suggest that female patients, patients with small internal carotid arteries, and patients who continue to smoke are at increased risk for recurrent carotid stenosis.[117,118] The use of patch angioplasty in these patients may reduce the risk of recurrent stenosis. Patch angioplasty should be routinely used when the indication for operation is recurrent stenosis.

Flow is established first to the external and then to the internal carotid artery. The author recommends the use of routine completion angiography, since there is a reported 5 to 8 per cent incidence of technical error identified by this technique and unsuspected until proved by angiography.[161,162] Completion angiography is used, primarily, to identify technical error involving the internal carotid artery. Intimal flaps in the external carotid artery occur more commonly but were considered to be of no consequence. Recently, we reported three cases of postoperative stroke secondary to intimal flaps in the external carotid artery. Clot formed, propagated retrograde, and then embolized up the internal carotid artery.[163] For this reason we advocate correction of intimal flaps of the external as well as the internal carotid artery. Following satisfactory arteriographic visualization, the wound is closed.

Internal Carotid Artery Dilation

Indications

This technique is uniquely applicable to fibromuscular dysplasia of the carotid artery. It represents a major technical advance in simplifying the surgical correction of this lesion.

Technique

The carotid bifurcation is exposed in the usual manner. The internal carotid artery is exposed for maximal length so that dilation can be carried out under visual and palpable control. Heparin is administered systemically, and the artery is clamped. A vertical arteriotomy, approximately 1 cm in length, is made in the carotid bulb, adjacent to the internal carotid artery. Coronary artery dilators are introduced and gently passed toward the base of the skull. The author usually starts with a 2-mm dilator and progresses at 0.5-mm increments to a 4-mm dilator. The surgeon will have a sensation of intraluminal septal "popping" as the dilator is passed to the base of the skull. Back-bleeding is allowed to occur after each passage (Fig. 31–16). Upon completion, the arteriotomy is closed, blood flow is restored, and a completion angiogram obtained to ensure adequate dilation. As an alternative, intraoperative balloon angioplasty of the affected segment of the internal carotid artery may be carried out. This technique is probably safer because traction injury of the intima is avoided. Assistance from a radiologist familiar with balloon angioplasty may be very helpful. The intraoperative use, through an open arteriotomy, avoids the possibility of forward embolization from the angioplasty site. After the balloon angioplasty is completed, vigorous back-bleeding of the vessel is allowed to retrieve any debris loosened by the dilation. As with progressive dilation of the vessel, completion angiography is highly recommended to assure an adequate technical result. The author does not favor percutaneous balloon dilatation of fibromuscular dysplastic segments of the extracranial vessels.

On occasion, the surgeon may not be sure that the dilator has been advanced fully to the base of the skull. It is helpful, under these circumstances, to obtain a plain x-ray film with the dilator in place and compare that film with the preoperative angiogram to ensure that the dilator has been passed sufficiently far distally.

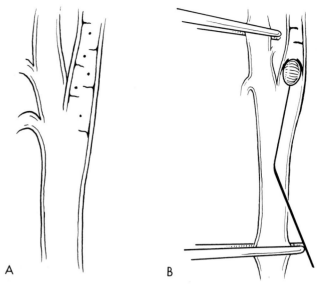

FIGURE 31–16. *A,* Artist's concept of the septated lesion of fibromuscular dysplasia. This kind of irregularity leads to symptoms from platelet aggregation and embolization. *B,* A coronary dilator is introduced through a small arteriotomy and advanced up the internal carotid artery. The olive tip of the dilator disrupts the small septae of the fibromuscular dysplastic segment. With an open arteriotomy, there is the opportunity for back-bleeding to occur, which will flush any residual intimal segments or platelet aggregates.

Correction of Kinking of the Internal Carotid Artery

Indications

This procedure is indicated by (1) symptomatic kinking of the internal carotid artery and (2) excessive redundancy of the internal carotid artery following mobilization of that vessel for endarterectomy.

Technique

Redundancy of the internal carotid artery can be corrected in a variety of ways, including (1) resection of the redundant internal carotid artery with end-to-end anastomosis, (2) division of the internal carotid artery with reimplantation onto the proximal common carotid artery, and (3) resection of a segment of the common carotid artery, thus permitting the redundant internal carotid artery to straighten when the carotid bifurcation is brought down for end-to-end anastomosis (Fig. 31–17).

In the author's experience, the easiest repair is resection of a segment of the common carotid artery, since the anastomosis is the easiest to perform. This will require mobilization of the external carotid artery in order to move the entire bifurcation proximally.

External Carotid Endarterectomy

Indications

This procedure is indicated (1) in the case of TIAs from embolization or flow reduction and (2) for cor-

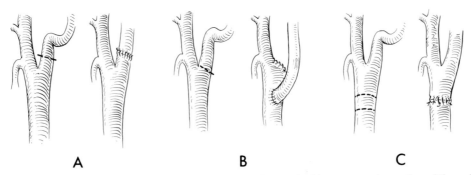

A **B** **C**

FIGURE 31–17. *A,* A kink of the internal carotid artery can be repaired by segmental resection of the redundant portion of the internal carotid artery and direct end-to-end anastomosis. *B,* The redundant internal carotid artery can be straightened by dividing it at its origin and moving it proximally to the common carotid artery for end-to-side anastomosis. *C,* The kinked internal carotid artery can be straightened by mobilization of the carotid bifurcation, resection of a segment of the common carotid artery, and direct end-to-end anastomosis, resulting in straightening of the kinked vessel.

rection of significant stenosis or ulceration prior to extracranial-to-intracranial bypass grafting.

Technique

The carotid bifurcation is dissected out in the usual manner. The internal carotid artery distal to the obstructed plaque is carefully examined because, on occasion, the vessel may still be patent, thus permitting a standard endarterectomy to be performed with restoration of blood flow to the internal carotid artery. If the internal carotid artery is confirmed to be occluded, it is divided flush with the carotid bifurcation. An arteriotomy is positioned on the posterior lateral aspect of the common carotid artery so that its distal extension will pass through the divided orifice of the internal carotid artery and onto the external carotid artery, beyond the atherosclerotic plaque in that vessel. An endarterectomy is then performed. The arteriotomy then may be closed primarily, leaving a smooth, tapered transition from the common carotid to the external carotid artery (Fig. 31–18). If the external carotid artery is particularly small, it may be necessary to use a patch. The patch

may be of prosthetic material, a vein, or a segment of the occluded internal carotid artery that has been resected and opened. This will serve nicely as autogenous arterial patch.

Postoperative Care

The first 12 hours are the most critical in the management of the patient following cerebral vascular reconstruction. In addition to the usual management of a patient recovering from a general anesthetic, the most important factors are observation of the patient's neurologic status, blood pressure control (either hypotension or hypertension must be appropriately treated), and close wound observation. An expanding hematoma should be identified early and the patient promptly returned to the operating room. These parameters are best observed in an intensive care unit setting. Usually by the morning after operation, under conditions of hemodynamic stability, the patient may be returned to routine care in a ward setting. It is the author's practice to resume antiplatelet drugs, and we recommend that, in the case of men, aspirin or, in the case of women, Persantine be continued to prevent platelet aggregation and embolization from the new intimectomy site as well as to serve as prophylaxis in the case of residual, unoperated atherosclerotic plaques in other critical cerebral vessels.

COMPLICATIONS FOLLOWING CAROTID ENDARTERECTOMY

Few vascular operations are as well tolerated as uncomplicated carotid endarterectomy. The operative trauma, blood loss, and recovery period are minimal following a successful reconstruction. On the other hand, the benefits of the procedure, especially in asymptomatic patients, can be negated by a high complication rate. The justification for surgical repair

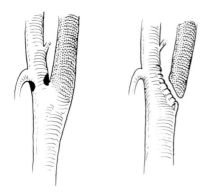

FIGURE 31–18. An external carotid endarterectomy can be performed by removing the occluded internal carotid artery and continuing the arteriotomy past the stenotic lesion. This permits endarterectomy under direct vision and primary closure, leaving a smooth taper between the common and the external carotid artery.

requires that the morbidity of the procedure be kept to a minimum. Possible intraoperative and postoperative complications, their prevention, and management will be discussed.

Intraoperative Complications

One of the most important steps in the prevention of intraoperative problems is adequate preoperative preparation of the patient. Hypertensive patients should have their blood pressure well controlled prior to the procedure. Patients must be well hydrated, especially if an angiographic procedure has been done within 24 to 48 hours, or if they have been on chronic diuretic therapy. Their myocardial status must be ascertained by careful history, electrocardiography, and other studies as indicated. The use of nitrates during the procedure should be considered in patients with coronary artery disease.

Intraoperative monitoring includes electrocardiographic and frequent or continuous blood pressure readings. The author routinely uses an intraarterial line to obtain continuous readouts and promptly recognize fluctuations in the patient's blood pressure. The use of Swan-Ganz catheters should be considered in selected patients.

Hypertension/Hypotension

Hypertension and hypotension are frequent during and immediately following carotid endarterectomy. Bove et al.[164] found significant hypertension in 19 per cent and hypotension in 28 per cent of 100 consecutive carotid endarterectomies and reported a 9 per cent incidence of neurologic deficits in this group, as opposed to no neurologic morbidity in normotensive patients. This fact plus their deleterious effects on myocardial function underscores the importance of early recognition and immediate treatment of extremes of blood pressure. Taking into account the minimal trauma and blood loss that occur during carotid endarterectomy, other factors must play a role in the development of this fluctuation. Some investigators[165] have found a significant increase in incidence of this problem in chronically hypertensive patients not well controlled preoperatively. The interference with the baroreceptor mechanisms at the carotid sinus may contribute to postoperative blood pressure fluctuations. The postendarterectomy bulb, which is now distensible, may also play a role.[166] Increased cerebral renin production during carotid cross-clamping has been implicated in the development of postendarterectomy hypertension.[167] In a retrospective study of 100 patients, we have found a correlation between the use of halogenated fluorocarbon general anesthesia and the development of postendarterectomy hypertension.[168] In a subsequent study we demonstrated that there was correlation between cranial norepinephrine levels in jugular venous blood, and not renin, in patients who developed postoperative hypertension.[169]

It is important to recognize that bradycardia during carotid manipulation will usually respond to the local injection of 0.5 per cent Xylocaine in the soft tissues comprising the carotid sinus. Failure of this maneuver to restore normal heart rate and blood pressure should be followed by immediate investigation and correction of other possible causes. Ranson et al.[170] have suggested that an uncorrected preoperative deficit in intravascular volume is a critical factor in the development of hypotension and bradycardia. Blocking the reflex arch by the administration of atropine sulfate while volume deficits are corrected will frequently return the blood pressure to within normal limits. If no response is seen after this, the use of vasoconstrictor agents should be considered, and they should be routinely available for immediate administration. It is important to recognize that the use of these drugs can be deleterious to myocardial function in the presence of hypovolemia.[136,171] The author's preference has been the use of dopamine hydrochloride titrated by an infusion pump.

Hypertension during or following endarterectomy should also be promptly treated. The author's preference is the use of sodium nitroprusside by infusion pump. It is usually started in normotensive patients when the systolic blood pressure is above 160 mm Hg, and in chronically hypertensive patients, above 180 mm Hg. It is titrated to keep the systolic levels between 140 and 160 mm Hg, respectively. In any case, diastolic pressure is kept below 100 mm Hg. The need for intravenous antihypertensive therapy is usually less than 24 hours. In patients with essential hypertension, their oral medications are restarted within that period.

Technical Complications

Technical problems during the procedure can be avoided by careful dissection and adherence to a proven established routine. The occurrence of intimal flaps at the distal end point of the endarterectomized segment usually results from incomplete removal of the plaque or too deep a plane of dissection in the media. Several steps must be taken to ensure that no distal intimal flap develops. Careful angiographic assessment and gentle palpation of the internal carotid will reveal the distal end of the plaque. The arteriotomy should be carried beyond this point. If a shunt is to be inserted, this becomes of critical importance.[172] Only in this manner can the lesion be completely removed under direct vision. As the endarterectomy is carried distally in the internal carotid artery, the most superficial plane in the media that will allow complete removal of the plaque should be chosen. In this manner, a tapered end is almost always encountered, and tacking sutures are virtually never required. The use of intraoperative completion angiograms is encouraged so that distal end point defects are recognized and corrected prior to completion of the procedure.

Emboli during or after carotid endarterectomy are probably the most frequent cause of a neurologic deficit seen following the procedure. Intraoperatively, these can occur during artery mobilization or shunt insertion, or after arteriotomy closure. Care should be taken in the distal insertion of the shunt so that it is done beyond the end of the lesion, as previously mentioned. Failure to do this will result in fragmentation of the plaque with embolization or elevation and wrinkling of the intima. Allowing the shunt to back-bleed freely will ensure adequate position and removal of all air. The author prefers proximal insertion with the shunt fully clamped so that slow careful release will allow immediate reclamping if any air or debris is seen flowing through the shunt.

After the endarterectomy is completed, the area should be free of any loose fragments. Careful irrigation with heparinized saline will ensure this. Prior to completion of the arteriotomy closure, the internal, external, and common carotid arteries should be allowed to bleed freely. When completed, flow should be established to the external circulation first so as to ensure that any debris that may be present will preferentially go to this system.

Emboli in the immediate postoperative period in the absence of an intimal flap or other technical error are likely to be from fibrin and platelet aggregates formed in the endarterectomized segment. Antiplatelet agents such as aspirin or dextran 40 may prevent such occurrences.

Occasionally, when the procedure is completed, one finds that a kink is now present in the endarterectomized portion of the internal carotid artery. If the angle between the segments is less than 90 degrees, flow restriction may occur, and disturbances that promote recurrent stenosis are likely. Many times this can be anticipated when an elongated or coiled artery is present prior to the endarterectomy. The author does not feel comfortable when this situation develops, and in severe cases prefers to correct the problem by some angioplastic procedure. The author's preference is resection of a segment of the common carotid with pull down and primary anastomosis (Fig. 31–17C). Ligation of the external carotid artery is rarely required, because dissection of the trunk and main branches will allow sufficient mobility to correct the kink. Ligation and division of the nerve of Herring and surrounding bifurcation tissues is always necessary.

A carotid–cavernous sinus fistula is a feared complication of embolectomy with balloon catheters of the internal carotid artery. On the rare occasions when this is necessary, several maneuvers should be attempted prior to the use of balloon catheters. The clot should be carefully separated from the intima and gently pulled down. The internal carotid backpressure is sometimes helpful in this process, and shunting the external circulation may make the difference necessary to extract the clot. If the use of balloon catheters becomes necessary, they should never be inserted beyond the proximal intracranial portion of the artery, and forcefulness is to be condemned. Although it is possible to perforate the carotid artery intracranially with the balloon catheter, the most common mechanism of injury that will create a carotid–cavernous sinus fistula is that of traction with the balloon catheter. This shearing force will create a transverse tear in that portion of the intracranial carotid that is intimately adherent to the cavernous sinus and fixed to the petrous portion of the skull. Therefore, traction on the inflated balloon catheter should be gentle. Fluoroscopic guidance may be helpful. Failure of these maneuvers makes abandonment of the procedure mandatory and requires consideration of an extracranial-to-intracranial bypass.

Cranial Nerve Injury

Peripheral cranial nerve injury is another source of morbidity following carotid endarterectomy. In a prospective analysis, Hertzer et al.[173] found a 16 per cent incidence of cranial nerve dysfunction following this procedure. Only 60 per cent of injuries were symptomatic. The rest would have gone unnoticed by the patient or physician had further detailed examination been omitted. A similar overall incidence was found by Evans et al.[174] on clinical grounds, but when speech pathologists were added as part of the evaluation, the incidence increased to 39 per cent, mostly related to superior laryngeal and recurrent laryngeal dysfunction. The great majority of these deficits were temporary, and when evaluation was repeated in 6 weeks, the incidence was between 1 and 4 per cent. These injuries can be avoided with careful dissection, the principle being to stay in the plane of the artery and to be familiar with the anatomy of the area, including well-recognized anomalies (Fig. 31–19).

The *hypoglossal nerve* is almost always visualized during carotid endarterectomy. It can be seen descending along the course of the internal carotid, then crossing the external carotid in a more superficial plan. Mobilization of this nerve is necessary only when a high bifurcation is present or when the lesion extends high in the internal carotid. This is accomplished by careful division of small veins that tent the nerve downward. A branch of the external carotid to the sternocleidomastoid muscle is frequently present and requires division. The ansa hypoglossi can frequently be retracted medially, but on occasion will require division as it comes off the hypoglossal. Traction or retractor injury to the hypoglossal nerve should be avoided. Clinically the deficit is manifested by deviation of the tongue to the ipsilateral side. Speech, deglutition, and mastication problems have been reported.[173]

The *spinal accessory nerve* is rarely seen during this dissection but on high dissections will be seen entering the sternocleidomastoid muscle superiorly. It can be left attached and retracted with the muscle, but care should be taken not to compress it with the retractor.

The *vagus nerve* is always seen, usually posterolateral to the carotid artery, between the latter and the jugular vein. On occasion it will lie anteromedial to the artery. Keeping the dissection close to the artery

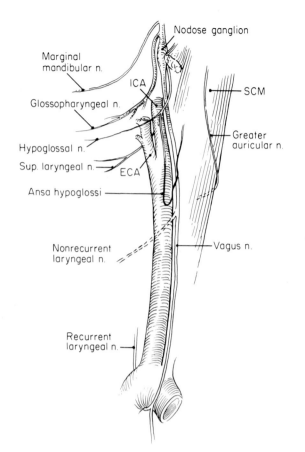

FIGURE 31–19. The surgical anatomy and relationship of structures encountered during exposure of the carotid bifurcation. *ECA,* external carotid artery; *ICA,* internal carotid artery; *SCM,* sternocleidomastoid muscle.

will avoid injury to this nerve. The recurrent laryngeal nerve usually lies within the trunk of the vagus at this level, but a nonrecurrent laryngeal nerve will on occasion traverse posterior to the common carotid artery. Injury to these structures can be asymptomatic or manifested with hoarseness. The importance of the asymptomatic injury gains significance when bilateral staged reconstructions are planned. On the other hand, hoarseness in the postoperative period will be due to vocal cord paresis in about half of the patients.[173] This underscores the importance of laryngoscopic examination in reaching a specific diagnosis. When staged bilateral carotid endarterectomy is planned, routine laryngoscopic visualization of the vocal cords is highly recommended. Detection of a paralyzed vocal cord mandates delaying of the procedure until recovery is complete. If vocal cord paralysis is permanent, appropriate precautions should be taken to avoid bilateral injury and perioperative airway management should be given special consideration.

The *superior laryngeal nerve* leaves the inferior ganglion of the vagus (nodose ganglion) and courses behind the internal carotid artery, bifurcating into an internal and an external branch. The internal branch is sensitive to the larynx, and the external innervates the inferior constrictor and cricothyroid muscles. The latter is responsible for the quality of voice, specifically the higher pitches. Injury to this nerve can be avoided by again keeping the dissection close to the arterial wall, specifically when controlling the superior thyroid artery.

The *glossopharyngeal nerve* is usually not seen in the dissection but can be injured when dissections are carried high, especially those requiring division of the digastric muscles.[175,176] This nerve courses posterior to the high portion of the internal carotid artery and can be injured with the application of a vascular clamp that includes other tissues than the artery itself. Again, dissection close to the arterial wall is the key in prevention. Clinically, the dysfunction is evident when tasks requiring oral pharyngeal muscle activity, mostly deglutition, are examined. Horner's syndrome may be produced by injury to the ascending sympathetic fibers in the area of the glossopharyngeal nerve.

The *cervical branch of the facial nerve* lies beneath the platysma inferior to the angle of the jaw. In some patients, this nerve sends branches to the mandibular branch, and its injury will produce sagging of the ipsilateral corner of the lower lip. The marginal mandibular branch can itself be injured when the incision is carried too close to the jaw. Both of these injuries can be avoided by curving the upper portion of the incision toward the mastoid process.[172] Self-retaining retractors should be carefully placed in this area.

The greater auricular nerve courses deep to the platysma over the sternocleidomastoid muscle at an angle toward the ear in the upper portion of the dissection. Its division should be avoided, but it is frequently necessary in high dissections. Numbness of the earlobe is the usual consequence, although, surprisingly, some patients have no complaints following its deliberate division.

The *parotid gland* lies in the superior portion of the incision anterior to the sternocleidomastoid muscle. Again, curving the incision toward the mastoid process will avoid injury in high dissections. Troublesome bleeding and the risk of a parotid fistula can be prevented by this maneuver.

Postoperative Complications

Upon completion of the operation, if done under general anesthesia, the patient is awakened in the operating room. A gross neurologic examination is performed. If no deficit is found, the patient is transferred to the recovery room, where a more detailed examination is performed.

Stroke is the most feared complication following carotid endarterectomy. In experienced hands, this will occur in between 1 and 3 per cent of cases, depending on the indication for the procedure.[177] Most of the low rates of stroke have been reported from specialized centers. Unfortunately, pooled data from community surveys have shown rates of combined stroke morbidity and mortality ranging from 6.5 to 21 per cent.[178–180] Since carotid endarterectomy is a prophylactic operation employed to prevent stroke, these higher complication rates erase most benefits and are clearly unacceptable. Recently, a committee of the Stroke Council of the American Heart Association reviewed this problem and set standards for upper acceptable limits of stroke and death as a function of indication for operation. Thus, for patients undergoing carotid endarterectomy for asymptomatic carotid stenosis, the combined operative stroke morbidity and mortality should not exceed 3 per cent; for TIA as an indication, 5 per cent; for prior stroke as an indication, 7 per cent; and for recurrent carotid stenosis, 10 per cent.[181] A mechanism for individual surgeon audit was described and recommended.

Transient ischemic attacks in the first postoperative week have been reported with a frequency as high as 8 per cent. When a neurologic deficit is found upon awakening the patient, the main question that needs to be resolved regards patency of the internal carotid artery. If a completion angiogram was obtained and no abnormalities seen, the event is likely to be embolic, and immediate reoperation would be of no benefit. If no angiographic data are available, patency of the vessel should be assessed by noninvasive means.[182] If occlusion is suggested, immediate reoperation may reverse the deficit.[183] If the vessel appears patent by noninvasive tests, the surgeon needs to determine whether the emboli occurred during the operation or whether a source is now present in the operated segment. This is also the case in a patient who is neurologically intact and who develops an event in the ipsilateral hemisphere hours or days after surgery. Once patency is evidenced by noninvasive means, immediate angiography is indicated. Reoperation is necessary if a significant defect or any clot is present. Otherwise conservative therapy with anticoagulation and/or antiplatelet agents is warranted. This excludes a patient experiencing repeated or progressive neurologic events, in whom immediate reoperation should be considered. Other factors will inevitably influence the decision to reoperate or observe the patient. The difficulty of the initial reconstruction, the patient's general status, and the availability and reliability of ancillary facilities will affect this difficult decision (see algorithm in Fig. 31–20).

The mortality following carotid endarterectomy has declined significantly as the incidence of postoperative stroke has diminished. Pulmonary problems, renal insufficiency, or sepsis are extremely unusual complications owing to the nature of this procedure. Myocardial infarction remains the most frequent cause of death in the early postoperative period, more so in patients with suspected coronary artery disease.[184] Because of this, preoperative assessment is of paramount importance. Postoperatively, electrocardiographic monitoring for the first 24 hours and a 12-lead electrocardiographic tracing should be obtained. Any suspicion of a myocardial event should be investigated and treated aggressively.

Wound infections following carotid endarterectomy are extremely rare. Routine use of prophylactic antibiotics should be limited to procedures in which the use of a prosthetic material is anticipated.

Taking into account that the procedure is done under full heparinization and that many patients have received platelet antiaggregates preoperatively, the incidence of wound bleeding is low. In Thompson's personal series, reoperation for this problem was required in 0.7 per cent of 1022 patients.[177]

Large cervical hematomas may form, and reoperation and drainage should be strongly considered in the otherwise stable patient. The routine use of a Silastic drain may reduce the incidence of this complication. Rarely will bleeding occur from the suture line. More often, a diffuse ooze will be present requiring reversal of anticoagulation. In any case, drainage of the hematoma and correction of its cause will prevent chronic draining wounds, infection, and the rare occurrence of pseudoaneurysm formation. The latter is more frequent when closure is performed with a patch.[177]

Headache following carotid endarterectomy is not unusual. It may be associated with a neurologic deficit, in which case a CT scan should be performed. In the majority of cases, however, it runs a self-limited course and is probably related to altered autoregulatory dysfunction of the cerebral circulation. The use of Inderal has been effective in treating troublesome headache.

Complications following carotid endarterectomy may be prevented by careful patient preparation, meticulous technique, and adherence to a rational well-established routine. An uneventful operation is the only way to effectively change the natural history of extracranial arterial occlusive disease.

RESULTS OF SURGICAL TREATMENT FOR EXTRACRANIAL ARTERIAL OCCLUSIVE DISEASE

The most frequently performed operation for extracranial arterial occlusive disease is endarterectomy of the carotid bifurcation. As experience is gained with this procedure, results have improved, and in experienced hands it can be done with morbidity and mortality rates well below the Stroke Council guidelines. In recommending this procedure, the results of the particular surgeon or institution are to be considered, because a higher morbidity and mortality may negate any beneficial effects of surgery.

The first multiinstitutional study that compared surgical and medical treatment in a prospectively randomized fashion comes from the joint Study on Extracranial Arterial Occlusion,[185] in which 1225 symptomatic patients with extracranial arterial occlusive disease were randomized to either medical or surgical therapy. Long-term survival of as long as 42 months was better in the surgically treated group with unilateral carotid stenosis who were experiencing TIAs

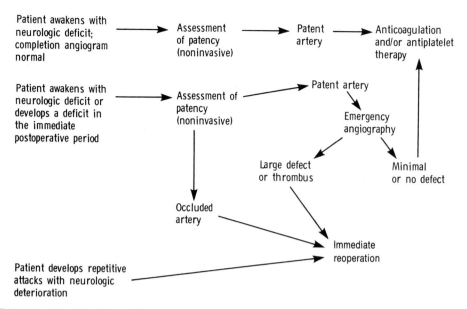

FIGURE 31–20.   Algorithm that can be applied to the management of the patient who awakens with postoperative neurologic deficit following carotid endarterectomy.

or cerebral infarction with minimal residual deficit. The neurologic morbidity in 316 patients who were identified as having hemispheric TIAs as an indication for inclusion in the study was evaluated. The incidence of cerebral infarction at 42 months was reduced in the surgical group. Recurrent TIAs or cerebral infarction usually affected the nonoperated side in the surgical patients, in contrast to the medically treated group, in whom neurologic events chiefly occurred in the distribution of the symptomatic artery at the time of randomization. The differences were statistically significant. It is important to emphasize that the combined postoperative morbidity and mortality in the surgically treated group was around 8 per cent, which is considered high by today's standards. This may have affected the results of this study in favor of medical therapy.

It has become evident that the preoperative neurologic status of the patient will affect the immediate postoperative results. Asymptomatic patients fare better than patients with TIAs, and the latter, in turn, have lower morbidity than patients with a completed stroke. In fact, late results may be similarly affected. Bernstein and colleagues[186] reported a series of 456 carotid endarterectomies followed for between 1 and 11 years, with an average follow-up of 45.3 months. Operated asymptomatic patients had a 1.6 per cent incidence of TIAs and 3.2 per cent incidence of stroke on late follow-up. Those operated on because of TIAs had a 19.5 and 5.2 per cent incidence of recurrent TIAs or stroke, respectively. Patients with a permanent neurologic deficit preoperatively had an incidence of TIAs of 7.9 per cent, and 11.0 per cent developed a stroke on late follow-up.

Similar results have been reported by Hertzer and Arison[187] in 329 patients followed a minimum of 10 years after carotid endarterectomy. The cumulative incidence of stroke by life-table method was 24 per cent at 10 years after operation. Only 10 per cent of patients sustained strokes that clearly involved the ipsilateral cerebral hemisphere. Hypertension, preoperative stroke as an indication, and patients with recognized contralateral carotid stenosis had a much higher incidence of stroke on long-term follow-up. Contralateral hemispheric strokes occurred in 36 per cent of patients with uncorrected contralateral lesions, compared with 8 per cent of those who had elective bilateral reconstruction. This was statistically significant. Elective myocardial revascularization produced a significant increase in long-term survival when compared to patients with uncorrected coronary artery disease. These results suggest that the annual incidence of late stroke, specifically involving the cerebral hemisphere ipsilateral to previous carotid repair, is 1.1 per cent, a figure within the expected range for the normal population. Stroke in the subset of patients with bilateral carotid arterial disease was five times more common in the contralateral than in the ipsilateral cerebral hemisphere. Therefore, staged contralateral endarterectomy should be seriously considered in patients with documented but otherwise asymptomatic advanced contralateral carotid stenosis.[187]

Analysis of the available surgical series with long-term follow-up reveals that a successfully performed carotid endarterectomy will place the patient at a significantly lower risk of stroke. The results of the various available surgical series are summarized in Table 31–1 according to the indications for operation. Asymptomatic patients will have a 1.2 per cent per year stroke risk, including perioperative morbidity and mortality. Patients whose indication for endarterectomy is TIAs will have an initial perioperative morbidity and mortality of about 3 per cent, with a

TABLE 31–1.   RESULTS OF CAROTID ENDARTERECTOMY ACCORDING TO THE INDICATION FOR OPERATION[a]

Indication	Reference	No. of Patients	Follow-Up	Operative		Recurrent TIAs Ipsilateral (%)	Stroke	
				Morbidity (%)	Mortality (%)		Ipsilateral (%)	Contralateral (%)
Asymptomatic	Thompson et al.[153]	132	55.1	1.2	0	0.75	4.7[b]	NS
	Sergeant et al.[188]	43	64.8 mo	2.3	2.3	0	0	0
	Moore et al.[189]	72	6–180 mo	0	0	2.7	5.6[c]	2.7
	Bernstein et al.[190]	87[d]	43 mo	NS[e]	0	NS	6.3[f]	NS
	Hertzer and Arison[187]	126	10–14 yr	NS	NS	NS	9[l]	7[l]
	Lord[191]	226	30–144 mo	2.6	1.1	NS	0.4	1.1
TIA	Bernstein et al.[190]	370[i]	12–132 mo	NS	0	19.5[i]	5.2	NS
	DeWeese et al.[192]	103	60-mo minimum	6.0	0.97	18.4[g]	7.7[h]	10.6
	Thompson et al.[193]	293	To 156 mo	2.7	1.4	16.3	4.7	0.6
	Takolander et al.[194]	142	5-yr actuarial	4.9	1.8	14.7	6.5	4.0
	Hertzer and Arison[187]	123	10–14 yr	NS	NS	NS	6[l]	9[l]
Stroke	Thompson et al.[193]	217	up to 156 mo	5.0	7.4		8.2	NS
	Eriksson et al.[195]	55	21-mo avg	3.7	3.7		3.8	NS
	Bardin et al.[196]	127	56-mo avg	3.9	3.1		20	NS
	Takolander et al.[194]	60	5-yr actuarial	4.9	5.9	11.6[f]	10	NS
	McCullough et al.[197]	50	41-mo avg	3.4	1.7		3.3	NS
	Hertzer and Arison[187]	80	40–14 yr	NS	NS	NS	6[l]	13

[a]NS, not specified.
[b]Side of stroke not specified; three strokes were fatal.
[c]Two patients suffered transient postoperative deficits with complete recovery.
[d]Number of procedures; exact number of patients not specified.
[e]Perioperative stroke rate of 3 per cent in the entire series of 370 patients.
[f]Side of neurologic event not specified; risk of stroke at 5 years by life-table analysis.
[g]Includes patients with nonterritorial symptoms.
[h]Includes operative morbidity.
[i]Total number of patients in series, including TIA patients.
[j]Territory affected not specified.
[k]Includes operations for acute strokes.
[l]Does not include perioperative strokes.

long-term risk of stroke of 2 per cent per year. Patients whose indication for operation is cerebral infarction have a higher perioperative morbidity, averaging about 5 per cent. Long-term results suggest that these patients have an annual stroke rate of approximately 4 per cent per year. The average recurrence of TIAs is on the order of 8 to 10 per cent at 5 years for all indications. These results compare favorably with the natural history of the disease but underscore the importance of maintaining the operative stroke rate at acceptable levels for the various indications. A higher figure will negate the early and late beneficial results of surgical therapy.

The results of carotid endarterectomy for nonhemispheric symptoms are less predictable. In a series of 107 patients subjected to carotid endarterectomy, the initial perioperative morbidity and mortality were similar to those in patients with specific indications for operation. Carotid endarterectomy was successful in ameliorating symptoms in patients with nonhemispheric symptoms who had greater than 60 per cent diameter reduction of the carotid artery and classic vertebrobasilar insufficiency.[198] The use of complete cerebral angiography can also be very helpful in selecting these patients. The presence of a posterior communicating artery suggests that the anterior circulation may be a major contributor to the vertebrobasilar system. Its presence would suggest that removal of a hemodynamically significant lesion in the carotid territory would be beneficial in alleviating posterior circulation systems.

In the absence of significant extracranial carotid artery disease, direct vertebral artery reconstruction is the procedure of choice for patients with vertebrobasilar systems secondary to extracranial occlusive disease. The results with direct vertebral artery reconstruction have been good, although the experience is not as extensive as that with carotid artery surgery. In a series of 109 vertebral artery operations, Imparato reported an operative mortality of 3 per cent.[199] Other complications included temporary hemidiaphragm paralysis and Horner's syndrome. Two thromboses of the reconstruction occurred. There were no perioperative strokes. Long-term follow-up revealed a stroke incidence of 1.5 per cent per year of follow-up. No controlled series on the natural history of these patients is available for comparison.[199]

The experience with external carotid revascularization has been limited and therefore long-term results are not available. In a series of 42 external carotid artery reconstructions, O'Hara et al. reported no early morbidity or mortality when the operation was limited to external carotid artery endarterectomy and patch angioplasty.[200] When the procedure was combined with bypass to the external carotid artery or with an extracranial-to-intracranial bypass, however, a 33 per cent incidence of stroke was observed. No neurologic symptoms have occurred in 60 per cent of the entire series on follow-up ranging from 1 to 72 months (mean: 27 months). These authors concluded that external carotid artery and endarterectomy can be performed with acceptable risks and long-term effectiveness. When the reconstruction involves bypass to the external carotid artery or extracranial-to-intracranial bypass, a higher operative risk can be expected.[200] A similar note of caution was expressed by Halstuk et al., reporting 49 external carotid revascularization procedures performed in 36 patients.[201] Indications included ipsilateral TIAs, amaurosis fugax, and procedure in anticipation of extracranial-to-intracranial bypass. Twenty patients had preoperative strokes. Twenty-nine patients underwent unilateral external carotid endarterectomy, with the remaining patients undergoing other procedures in addition to the external revascularization. There was a 13.8 per cent incidence of postoperative strokes within 8 days of external carotid revascularization. There was one operative death, for a mortality rate of 2.7 per cent. Long-term follow-up ranging from 1 to 75 months (mean: 29 months) revealed a 14.2 per cent incidence of late neurologic ischemic events. Three of these were TIAs, one was a reversible ischemic neurologic deficit, and one patient had a stroke 50 months after his initial operation. These results suggested caution in recommending external carotid artery surgery, especially when the revascularization is to involve more than just endarterectomy with patch closure.[201]

CURRENT STATUS OF THE PROSPECTIVE RANDOMIZED TRIALS

In spite of the fact that retrospective data analysis clearly demonstrates superiority of carotid endarterectomy over medical management with respect to stroke prevention, a number of well-meaning critics point out that retrospective data analysis can be misleading. Retrospective studies compare surgical results with available natural history data. The natural history of a particular disease process can change, often for the better, leaving the basis of comparison invalid. Likewise, retrospective reviews are often performed in centers of excellence, where surgical complication rates may be lower than the actual risk of operation as judged by analyzing community results. For this reason, several prospective randomized trials were initiated in North America and Europe. The objective of the trials was to scientifically evaluate the efficacy (or lack thereof) of carotid endarterectomy in preventing stroke for a variety of indications when compared with a true control group. The trials can be generally categorized into two major classifications: asymptomatic and symptomatic carotid artery disease.

There are three asymptomatic trials that are currently in progress or have recently completed their data acquisition and reported results. These are as follows: (1) the Veterans Administration Asympto-

matic Carotid Stenosis Study; (2) The Carotid Surgery versus Medical Therapy in Asymptomatic Carotid Stenosis (CASANOVA); and (3) the Asymptomatic Carotid Artery Stenosis Study (ACAS). There are three symptomatic trials in various stages of completion, and these are as follows: (1) the North American Symptomatic Carotid Endarterectomy Trial (NASCET); (2) the MRC European Carotid Surgery Trial (ECST); and (3) The Veterans Administration Symptomatic Trial.

Asymptomatic Trials

Veterans Administration Asymptomatic Carotid Stenosis Study

Ten Veterans Administration medical centers entered into a prospective randomized trial designed to test the hypothesis that carotid endarterectomy plus best medical management (aspirin and risk factor control) would result in fewer transient ischemic attacks, and fewer fatal and nonfatal strokes than patients treated with best medical management alone. The design of the study was published in 1986.[202] Angiography was performed in 713 patients, of whom three (0.4 per cent) sustained a neurologic deficit.[203]

Four hundred forty-four patients were randomized over a 54-month interval. Two hundred eleven carotid endarterectomies were performed in the surgical group and received aspirin therapy. Two hundred thirty-three patients were treated with aspirin alone. The study spanned a total of 8 years. The 30-day mortality rate was 1.9 per cent, and the incidence of stroke was 2.4 per cent. The combined stroke and mortality rate was 4.3 per cent.[204] The study has now been completed and the data analyzed. At the time of this writing, the manuscript has been accepted for publication in the *New England Journal of Medicine* for early 1993. The results were positive for the surgery group in the hypothesis being tested. The data analysis demonstrated that all neurologic events in any distribution including the study artery combined with deaths showed a total event number of 30 in the carotid endarterectomy group, which represented 14.2 per cent of the population. This included all deaths, strokes, TIAs, and amaurosis. For the patients treated medically, there were a total of 55 events, for an event rate of 23.6 per cent. This difference is statistically significant ($p < .006$). When the data were analyzed for deaths plus ipsilateral events only, there were a total of 21 events, for an incidence of 10 per cent in the carotid endarterectomy group, in contrast to 46 events, for an incidence of 19.7 per cent in the medically treated group. Once again, this difference was statistically significant ($p < .002$). While the study was not designed to look at stroke alone with respect to a difference in event rate, this was done retrospectively. There were a total of 10 strokes in the carotid endarterectomy group ipsilateral to the study artery, for an incidence of 4.7 per cent. There were a total of 20 strokes in the study artery distribution in the medically treated group, for an incidence of

8.6 per cent. Once again, this difference was statistically significant in spite of the small sample size. There was no difference in survival rate between the surgically treated and medically treated groups. This is not surprising, since the major cause of death in this patient group is myocardial infarction, and it is unlikely that the prevention of stroke is going to have a beneficial effect at reducing fatal myocardial infarction. The absence of difference of survival between the surgically treated and medically treated groups should not be considered a negative when interpreting data results inasmuch as the objective of operation is to maintain the patient stroke free during the patient's remaining lifetime.

The CASANOVA Study

This is a multiinstitutional European study designed to test the hypothesis that asymptomatic patients with stenoses greater than 50 per cent but less than 90 per cent would have fewer strokes and deaths when treated with surgery plus aspirin and dipyridamole than a comparable group of patients treated with aspirin and dipyridamole alone. The end points were stroke and death. Transient ischemic attack was not considered an end point. Four hundred ten patients were randomly allocated to two groups. Group A, 206 patients, was the surgical group. Group B, 204 patients, was the control group treated with medical management alone. Patients with high-grade stenoses, 90 per cent or greater, were excluded from the study and presumably operated upon preferentially. The surgery group underwent unilateral operation if a unilateral lesion was present or bilateral operations if bilateral lesions were present. Unfortunately, the medical group also had significant indication for operation as well. If a patient randomized to medical management was found to have bilateral stenoses, surgery was done on the most affected side. If during the course of follow-up there was a progression of the medically randomized lesion to 90 per cent or greater, surgery was performed. In the medically managed group, if the patient developed bilateral stenoses that exceeded 50 per cent, one artery was operated upon. Finally, if patients in the medically managed group developed the onset of transient ischemic attacks, the patient was allowed to cross over and received operation. Unfortunately, from the standpoint of data analysis, none of these events were considered end points. Furthermore, the design of the study was "intent to treat." That means that even though the patients were allowed to cross over to operation, the patients were still analyzed as if they were being treated medically alone. As a result, there were 216 carotid endarterectomies performed on 204 patients in the surgical group and 118 operations performed on 206 patients in the so-called medical group. Not surprisingly, when the study was completed, there was no apparent difference between group A and group B. Group A experienced 22 end points, for an incidence of 10.7 per cent, and group B experienced 23 end points, for an incidence

of 11.3 per cent. The authors concluded that surgery is not recommended for patients with asymptomatic carotid stenosis less than 90 per cent. Unfortunately, this conclusion is unjustified, because of serious flaws in study design and data analysis. First of all, high-risk patients (those with 90 per cent stenoses or greater) were excluded from the randomization process. Second, patients with bilateral stenosis in the medical group received operation on the tighter (presumably higher risk) lesion but were still considered medically managed for purposes of analysis. Patients in the medical group were allowed to cross over to surgery if they developed a 90 per cent stenosis of the study artery, bilateral stenoses 50 per cent or greater, or the onset of TIAs. When they crossed over to surgery, they were not considered end points or treatment failures but continued to be analyzed as if they were managed medically. The net result was that 118 high-risk lesions were removed from the medical group and treated surgically but continued to be analyzed as if they were treated medically. It would appear, then, that this study was invalidated by a flawed design and method of statistical analysis. If any information is to be gained from this study it might be that patients selectively treated with carotid endarterectomy did as well as those routinely treated with carotid endarterectomy. That is, patients with 90 per cent carotid stenoses, bilateral carotid stenoses, disease progression, or onset of TIAs were selected for operation in contrast to applying routine operation to all patients with carotid artery stenosis. Unfortunately, when this interpretation is applied, we are missing the important control group, which would be those patients who received no operation at all in order to determine whether or not selective or routine carotid endarterectomy is any better than no operation.[205]

The Asymptomatic Carotid Atherosclerosis Study (ACAS)

The ACAS is the largest of the trials of asymptomatic carotid stenosis. This is a prospective randomized trial consisting of 34 centers in North America and sponsored by the National Institutes of Health (NIH). The hypothesis that is being tested is that carotid endarterectomy plus aspirin and risk factor control will result in fewer TIAs, strokes, and deaths than aspirin and risk factor control alone. The design of the study calls for randomization of 1500 patients into either of two treatment regimens. The analysis will be carried out utilizing a two-tailed *t* test. The ACAS began in the spring of 1988, and as of August, 1992, over 1300 patients had been randomized. It is anticipated that the randomization process will be complete by the spring of 1993, at which time the follow-up of these patients will be continued.[206] It is anticipated that when this study is complete, there will be a sufficient number of patients in the two treatment groups that a definitive statement will be made as to the efficacy of carotid endarterectomy in the management of the patient with carotid stenosis. To date, there is apparently no clear or dramatic difference between the two study groups inasmuch as the Oversight Committee for the NIH has recommended that the randomization process continue.

Symptomatic Trials

The North American Symptomatic Carotid Endarterectomy Trial (NASCET)

The NASCET study is a large prospective trial carried out in North America designed to test the hypothesis that symptomatic patients (TIA or prior mild stroke) with ipsilateral carotid stenosis (30 to 99 per cent) will have fewer fatal and nonfatal strokes following carotid endarterectomy than patients treated with medical management alone, including aspirin. It was anticipated that approximately 3000 patients would be randomized to either medical or surgical management and followed for a minimum of 5 years. The NASCET study also was stratified to follow two subsets of patients as a function of their degree of carotid occlusive disease. The first patient subset included those with 70 to 99 per cent stenoses, and the second subset included patients with more moderate lesions ranging from 30 to 69 per cent.[207] Included in the design of the trial and required by the granting institution (NIH) is the establishment of an Oversight Committee. The responsibility of the Oversight Committee is to review the results of the data, from time to time, and to call a halt to the study if during the course of the conduct of the study a clear difference appears between the two groups. On February 25, 1991, a clinical alert was issued by the Oversight Committee, who reported that a clear difference had developed between the two groups that indicated that carotid endarterectomy was superior to medical management in the high-grade stenosis category (70 to 99 per cent). No clear difference had yet occurred in the moderate stenosis group (30 to 69 per cent), and the latter continue to enter patients for randomization. In the high-grade stenosis category, there were 295 patients randomized to medical management and 300 patients randomized to surgical management. It is of interest to note that 16 of the medically randomized patients (5.4 per cent) actually crossed over to surgery. Once again, because of the "intent to treat" analysis design, these patients continue to be analyzed as if they were managed medically in spite of the fact that they had operation. Crossovers become important if the group that they are leaving in fact is a disadvantaged group as is the case in this study. The 30-day operative morbidity and stroke mortality for patients managed surgically was 5.0 per cent. The analysis at the end of 18 months of follow-up, which was the basis of the Oversight Committee calling a halt to this arm of the study, is as follows: In the surgical group including the perioperative morbidity and mortality, at the end of 18 months, there was a 7.0 per cent incidence of fatal and nonfatal strokes. In the medical group, there was a 24 per cent incidence of fatal and nonfatal strokes.

The difference was highly statistically significant ($p < .001$). This represents an absolute reduction in risk of 17 per cent in favor of surgical management and a relative risk reduction of 71 per cent comparing surgical management with medical management by the end of 18 months. A surprising finding occurred when the mortality rates were analyzed. To date, no study has shown that carotid endarterectomy patients enjoy greater longevity than those treated medically. However, at the end of 18 months, the mortality rate among the medically treated group was 12 per cent in contrast to the 5 per cent rate for the surgically treated group. Once again these differences were statistically significant ($p < .01$). This indicates that there is a relative mortality risk reduction of 58 per cent in favor of carotid endarterectomy. Further analysis demonstrated that for every 10 per cent increase in percentage stenosis between 70 and 99 per cent, there was a progressive increase in morbidity and mortality in the control group. The converse is also true; therefore, the moderate stenosis group (30 to 69 per cent) continues to enter patients for randomization and follow-up. This group is of critical importance in that it is likely that there will be some lesser percentage stenosis category below which the risks of operation may outweigh the benefits. To date, that number has not been established.[208]

MRC European Carotid Surgery Trial (ECST)

This is a large, multicenter European trial of symptomatic patients with carotid artery disease that was carried out over a 10-year interval and reported at approximately the same time as the NASCET study and which confirmed the results reported to date of the NASCET study: 2518 patients were randomized over a 10-year interval, providing a mean follow-up of 3 years. This trial stratified their data into three groups, including mild stenoses (10 to 29 per cent), moderate stenoses (30 to 69 per cent), and severe stenoses (70 to 99 per cent). In the mild stenoses category, there was no apparent benefit for carotid endarterectomy compared to the risk of operation. However, in the severe stenosis category, there was a highly significant benefit in favor of operation. Carotid endarterectomy, in spite of an upfront 7.5 per cent risk of death and stroke in the perioperative interval, resulted in a sixfold reduction in subsequent strokes in a 3-year interval. This difference was highly statistically significant ($p < .0001$). To date, the moderate stenoses category has not reached an end point, and the ECST continues to randomize patients in this group, as does the NASCET study.[209]

Veterans Administration Symptomatic Trial

This is a prospective randomized trial designed to test the hypothesis that patients with greater than 50 per cent ipsilateral internal carotid stenosis who were experiencing symptoms, including transient cerebral ischemia and mild stroke, would have fewer neurologic events including cerebral infarction or crescendo TIAs in the vascular distribution of the study artery following carotid endarterectomy plus best medical management versus best medical management alone. This study was just getting underway when the results of the ECST and NASCET studies were reported and therefore was brought to a halt earlier than anticipated. Nonetheless, 189 patients with symptomatic carotid stenoses were randomized to either medical or surgical management. When the results were analyzed to date, with a mean follow-up of 11.9 months, 7.7 per cent of the patients randomized to surgical care had experienced stroke or crescendo TIA during the perioperative or follow-up interval. In contrast, those patients randomized to medical management alone experienced a 19.4 per cent incidence of stroke or crescendo TIA. This difference was statistically significant ($p = .01$). It is of interest that the benefit of operation became apparent within 2 months of randomization when compared to the medically managed control group.[210]

ALTERNATIVES TO SURGICAL THERAPY

The pathophysiology in the development of a stroke from an extracranial lesion has been discussed. The rationale for current medical therapy has evolved around an attempt to alter factors responsible for the development of symptoms secondary to extracranial arterial occlusion. At present, two forms of therapy are considered the mainstays in the medical management of this disease. Antiplatelet agents and anticoagulation are the principal therapeutic alternatives in the medical management of these patients.

It is important to emphasize that any form of therapy aimed at stroke prevention must include control of commonly associated conditions such as hypertension, diabetes, arrhythmias, and coronary artery disease. In addition, cigarette smoking has been shown to be a major independent risk factor for development of carotid bifurcation disease and stroke.[211–213] Any approach to medical control of stroke risk must begin with advice to the patient to stop smoking.

Anticoagulation, mainly with Coumadin, has been evaluated in several reports in an attempt to determine if its use significantly altered the natural history of extracranial arterial lesions. Baker and associates[214] reported a randomized prospective study in patients who had TIAs treated with Coumadin. On follow-up, those treated with anticoagulation had a significant reduction in the number of TIAs when compared to control patients. A favorable trend for fewer strokes was noted in the treated group, although the difference in the incidence of cerebral infarction between treated and control patients was not statistically significant.

A reduction in stroke rate was observed in a retrospective study in the community of Rochester regarding the use of anticoagulants in cerebral ischemia.[34] In this study, the net probability of having a stroke within 5 years was around 20 per cent for those patients treated with anticoagulants. While this compares favorably with the probability in untreated controls (40 per cent), it represents a significant risk when compared to other forms of available therapy.

Two reports from Sweden have also shown a reduction in the development of TIAs and stroke in patients treated with anticoagulants. The study by Link et al.[215] showed a higher incidence of stroke when anticoagulants were discontinued, and thus long-term therapy was recommended. In the second study, by Terent and Anderson,[216] patients treated with anticoagulants showed an increased mortality rate. Unacceptably serious bleeding complications were also seen in this group. Finally, a metaanalysis of 16 randomized studies of anticoagulation failed to show any benefit in patients suffering from TIA or ischemic stroke when compared with untreated control groups. However, there is evidence to suggest that patients with thrombosis in evolution might benefit from anticoagulation.[217]

From the available evidence, it seems reasonable to conclude that, although reduced, the incidence of stroke and recurrent TIAs in patients treated with anticoagulants remains high as compared to other forms of available therapy. The need for long-term administration with its concomitant increased risk of complications makes anticoagulant therapy less desirable.

Antiplatelet agents, mainly aspirin, have been advocated for use in patients with extracranial arterial occlusive disease. The rationale for this therapy is based on available evidence that platelets play a major role in the pathophysiology of this disease. At present there are seven double-blind, randomized, prospective studies that compare the use of platelet antiaggregants with placebo in treating patients who suffered cerebral ischemia secondary to extracranial atherosclerosis. In the Canadian Cooperative Study Group,[218] 585 patients who evidenced cerebral ischemia of extracranial origin were prospectively randomized into four treatment regimens. Each regimen was taken four times daily and consisted of a 200-mg capsule of sulfinpyrazone plus placebo, a placebo tablet plus 325 mg of aspirin, both active drugs, or both placebos. Follow-up from 12 to 57 months revealed no statistically significant reduction in TIAs, stroke, or death for patients on sulfinpyrazone. Aspirin reduced risk for continuing ischemic episodes, strokes, or death by 19 per cent. When analysis was restricted to stroke or death alone, the risk reduction increased to 31 per cent, and when male patients were analyzed, the reduction was even higher. No statistically significant differences in stroke or death rate was found among female patients taking any of the four regimens. Considering this observation literally, the probability of stroke in men taking aspirin was in excess of 5 per cent each year and in women higher than 8 per cent each year.[219] It appears that platelet antiaggregants will reduce the incidence of stroke in patients with extracranial lesions. The question still remains if this reduction will equal that achieved by other forms of available therapy.

In 1972, a double-blind, randomized, prospective trial of aspirin versus placebo was started in several U.S. centers and continued for 37 months.[220] Sixty per cent of these patients had operable lesions in the extracranial territory. The treatment group received 10 grains of aspirin twice daily. At 6 months of follow-up, a statistically significant difference in favor of aspirin was seen when death, cerebral or retinal infarction, and TIAs were grouped together. When each group was considered separately, the difference did not achieve statistical significance. Patients for whom a decision was made to proceed with endarterectomy were also assigned to a randomized, double-blind trial of aspirin during the postoperative period. The results of this trial constitute a separate report.[221] Life-table analyses of the above-mentioned end points at 24 months did not reveal a statistical difference in favor of aspirin. When non–stroke-related deaths were eliminated, a significant difference in favor of aspirin emerged. A favorable trend was also noted when the occurrence of TIAs within the first 6 months of follow-up was taken into consideration. In the placebo group, there were eight brain infarcts among eight patients reaching an end point in the first 24 months. There were also eight patients reaching an end point in the aspirin group; however, only two of these suffered a neurologic event.

These two studies show a favorable trend toward a reduction in the stroke rate among patients receiving aspirin as the treatment for symptomatic lesions in the extracranial circulation. In the first, aspirin was used as the principal form of therapy; whereas in the second, aspirin was an adjunct to surgical therapy. In the surgically treated group, the absolute level of cases having an unfavorable outcome was about half the percentage of unfavorable cases in those treated medically only (11.3 versus 19.2 per cent). This differential may reflect the independent favorable effect of surgery.

Two other studies have evaluated the use of aspirin in a randomized, controlled, prospective fashion. In a study from France, 604 patients with arteriothrombotic cerebral ischemic events referable to the carotid or vertebrobasilar circulation were entered in a double-blind, randomized clinical trial comparing aspirin 1 gm/day, aspirin 1 gm/day plus dipyridamole (225 mg/day), and placebo. The comparison of placebo and aspirin groups showed a significant reduction ($p < .05$) of cerebral infarction in the aspirin group. Overall, 66 patients of the entire group suffered a cerebral infarction during the trial. This corresponds to a cumulative stroke rate for the placebo group of 18 per cent and a rate 10.5 per cent for each of the aspirin groups. No significant difference between aspirin plus dipyridamole was found. Thus, the incidence of stroke per year was on the order of 6 per cent for placebo versus 3 per cent per year for the treatment groups. This represents, again, a 50 per cent reduction in the stroke risk.[222] In the recently concluded dipyridamole-aspirin trial in cerebral ischemia, the American-Canadian Cooperative Study Group concluded that there

was no difference between the stroke risk in patients receiving aspirin or aspirin plus dipyridamole in the prevention of stroke during long-term follow-up. Interestingly, the stroke rate reported in patients treated with either aspirin or aspirin and dipyridamole was on the order of 20 per cent at 5 years. This yields a 4 per cent per year stroke risk, which is not dissimilar to the lower rates reported in natural history studies.[223]

In 1983, a Danish cooperative study comparing the outcomes of patients with extracranial occlusive disease treated with aspirin or placebo was reported. No favorable influence of aspirin could be determined in the prevention of ischemic attacks.[224] Unfortunately, only 203 patients were followed, which is probably insufficient numbers to achieve any statistically valid data. This study has been criticized and probably suffers from type II statistical error.[225]

The objective of any treatment regimen for carotid artery disease should be the reduction of stroke risk. While each of the prospective randomized trials of antiplatelet agents showed a trend toward stroke risk reduction, none achieved statistical significance with regard to that parameter. Only when the end points of TIA, stroke, and nonfatal and fatal myocardial infarction were lumped together did a statistically significant benefit in favor of aspirin emerge. Individual studies always lacked sufficient numbers of patients to show a reduction of stroke risk in favor of aspirin. A statistical technique known as meta-analysis permits the combination of patients from the various series. In doing this, the best that could be shown is a 15 per cent stroke risk reduction in favor of aspirin, and this still failed to achieve statistical significance.[226]

A new antiplatelet drug, ticlopidine hydrochloride, was compared with aspirin in a multicenter prospective randomized trial in 3069 patients with recent transient or mild persistant focal cerebral or retinal ischemia. The 3-year event rate for nonfatal stroke or death for any cause was 17 per cent for ticlopidine and 19 per cent for aspirin. The rates of fatal and nonfatal stroke at 3 years were 10 per cent for ticlopidine and 13 per cent for aspirin. The authors concluded that ticlopidine was somewhat more effective than aspirin in preventing stroke in their study population, but that the risks of side effects were greater.[227]

Failures of antiplatelet therapy in the treatment of symptomatic carotid artery disease have been reported.[228] Caution should be used in patients who are placed on platelet antiaggregants as primary therapy for this disease. Partial disappearance of their symptoms should be considered as a failure and alternative forms of treatment considered. Patients who experience complete relief of symptoms should be followed carefully with annual noninvasive studies. Progression of the lesion may be obscured because of suppression of symptoms by the therapy. In a recent review of 27 aspirin failures requiring urgent operation,[228] 12 of the surgical specimens showed fresh hemorrhage in the atherosclerotic plaque. Whether this was induced or aggravated by aspirin cannot be concluded. This incidence of fresh hemorrhage in an endarterectomy specimen appears high when compared to the findings in elective cases.

In conclusion, the available forms of medical management produced a reduction in the stroke rate in patients with significant atherosclerotic lesions of the extracranial circulation. This reduction does not appear to be as significant as that achieved by successful carotid endarterectomy. Medical treatment for symptomatic extracranial arterial disease should thus be reserved for patients with limited life expectancy or unidentified or surgically inaccessible lesions or for those who are poor surgical candidates.

NEW AND CONTROVERSIAL TOPICS IN CEREBRAL VASCULAR DISEASE

Carotid Endarterectomy for Acute Stroke

Emergency operation following acute stroke was used early in the history of endarterectomy. Because of several reports indicating that there was risk of converting an ischemic cerebral infarction into a hemorrhagic cerebral infarction, this procedure was abandoned. In reviewing those reports, it is evident that several factors are common to the patients having undergone those complications. These include patients being operated on with massive cerebral infarction and in obtunded states, patients in whom an attempt was made to open an occluded internal carotid artery several days to weeks after thrombosis, and patients being operated on with severe hypertension in whom the hypertension was inadequately controlled.[229]

Recent evidence suggests improved results if carotid artery surgery is delayed for at least 5 weeks following the acute event. Of 49 carotid endarterectomies done for acute cerebral infarction, 27 were performed within 5 weeks and 22 were done between 5 and 20 weeks following the acute neurologic event. In the latter group there was no morbidity or mortality, whereas in the patients undergoing early operation an 18.5 per cent incidence of new postoperative neurologic deficits was observed. The authors concluded that an unstable situation during the early phase of stroke contraindicated endarterectomy. No details as to the preoperative degree of neurologic deficit or recovery in these patients were available.[230] Following these guidelines, Dosick et al. noted a 21 per cent incidence of recurrent stroke during the 4- to 60-week observation interval.[144] This led these authors to select their patients on the basis of CT scans, proceeding with surgery if the CT scans were negative. One hundred ten patients underwent early endarterectomy following a persistent neurologic deficit with negative CT scans. No patient suffered a neurologic deficit in the territory of the operated artery and there was no mortality.[144] A similar experience was reported in 28 patients with small fixed neurologic deficits undergoing endarterectomy an

average of 11 days from the onset of symptoms. Whittemore et al. reported one postoperative death in this small group of patients and no new perioperative neurologic deficits. They recommended proceeding with endarterectomy early in this select group of patients with small cerebral infarct.[231]

In general, surgical intervention during the acute phase of a stroke in contraindicated. If the patient has a dense neurologic deficit, loss of consciousness, or cardiovascular instability, clearly surgery is not indicated. However, if the patient has a mild to moderate deficit and is fully conscious and otherwise stable, carotid endarterectomy of the responsible lesion can be undertaken soon after the patient has reached a plateau in his recovery. This may represent days or weeks after the onset of the event. In the small group of patients where a clinically unstable lesion exists, manifested by crescendo TIAs or stroke-in-evolution, emergency endarterectomy should be strongly considered.

Crescendo TIAs and Stroke-in-Evolution

These conditions used to be considered contraindications to operation. The author initially reported his experience with a select group of patients in whom stroke-in-evolution or crescendo TIA patients were acutely studied with angiography. If an unstable condition such as a free-floating thrombus or a propagating thrombus in the presence of a distally patent internal carotid artery was identified, these patients were taken promptly to the operating room for operation. The net result in a series of approximately 25 patients was no deaths and essentially a return to a normal neurologic status, in contrast to the natural history of stroke-in-evolution, which has approximately an 80 per cent expected mortality.[232]

A similar experience was reported by Mentzer et al.[32] with 17 patients operated on emergently for stroke-in-evolution. None had worsening of the preoperative neurologic deficit, four (24 per cent) remained unchanged, and 12 (70 per cent) had complete recovery. There was one death, for a 6 per cent operative mortality. This compared favorably with a parallel nonrandomized group of 26 patients with stroke-in-evolution treated conservatively. In the medical group there was a 15 per cent mortality, but more importantly, 17 patients (66 per cent) suffered moderate to severe permanent neurologic deficit. In this report, the collated operative results reported in the literature in 90 cases were presented. Following successful endarterectomy, 55 per cent were improved, 25 per cent had no change, and 10 per cent were worse. A 10 per cent mortality for the collated experience was reported. Thus, surgical intervention in the presence of stroke-in-evolution carries a significantly increased risk of both perioperative stroke and death. However, the results of surgical therapy are considerably better than the natural history of the untreated condition. It is important that a specific goal for surgical intervention be identified by pre-operative angiography. Indications for emergency endarterectomy include the presence of an unstable condition such as a free-floating thrombus or propagating thrombus in the presence of a distally patent internal carotid artery. Exclusion by the use of CT scan of other associated conditions that could present as stroke-in-evolution is highly recommended.

Possible Deleterious Effect of Antiplatelet Drugs

In patients with asymptomatic carotid bifurcation plaques or with minimal plaques and TIAs whom the physician elects to treat with antiplatelet drugs, instances have been reported of a progression, more rapid than expected, of the atheromatous lesion to near-total occlusion. Operation at that time has indicated a high degree of intraplaque hemorrhage. There is a suggestion that the antiplatelet drugs may precipitate intraplaque hemorrhage, with a progression of the lesion more rapid than anticipated.[228] A subsequent report compared plaque histopathology with the preoperative use of antiplatelet drugs. Those patients taking antiplatelet drugs were found to have an 80.1 per cent incidence of multiple intraplaque hemorrhage in contrast to 19.7 per cent incidence of intraplaque hemorrhage in patients not receiving antiplatelet drugs.[233]

Balloon Angioplasty

Several centers in the country have experimental protocols in which balloon angioplasty is being applied to occlusive disease of the aortic arch branches, including lesions of the internal carotid artery. We find this a particularly frightening prospect, because there is no question that balloon angioplasty releases a great deal of atheromatous debris, setting the stage for embolization into critical arteries. Experimental catheters are currently being designed to permit temporary distal internal carotid artery occlusion while angioplasty is being carried out in the hope of permitting the embolization to take place in the external carotid artery. In view of the relatively low morbidity and mortality in the properly performed carotid endarterectomy, we find no rationale for use of this technique.

Asymptomatic Carotid Ulceration

It is not uncommon to discover, serendipitously, a large nonstenotic, ulcerative lesion in a contralateral carotid artery at the time that the ipsilateral symptomatic carotid artery is being studied by angiography. A decision of whether or not to operate on this ulcerative lesion has often been questioned. The author has carried out two retrospective reviews of pa-

tients with identified nonstenotic, ulcerative lesions that have been followed without treatment. He observed that the medium or large ulcerative lesions carried a significant stroke risk, usually not preceded by warning TIAs.[53] In the most recent study, the risk of stroke in patients being followed expectantly with large ulcerative lesions was approximately 7.5 per cent each year of follow-up after initial identification.[54] The author currently recommends that medium "B" and large "C" ulcers, when identified serendipitously, undergo prophylactic repair.

Tandem Lesions

It is not uncommon to discover a stenosis of the origin of the internal carotid artery in conjunction with a significant lesion of the carotid siphon. The question is often raised whether, if the siphon lesion is more than the lesion of the internal carotid artery, it is justified to operate on the carotid artery alone. Several reports now indicate that even though tandem lesions exist, the embolic potential of the atherosclerotic plaque at the carotid bifurcation greatly outweighs the thrombotic or embolic risk of the lesion in the carotid siphon.[234] It is the author's practice to operate on the carotid bifurcation lesion in symptomatic patients in spite of the presence of a siphon lesion.[235] Recently, a retrospective review was reported in which the perioperative morbidity, mortality, and late results were compared in patients undergoing carotid endarterectomy with and without angiographically documented intracranial arterial occlusive disease. There was no difference in results between the two groups. The perioperative stroke rate was 1.9 versus 1.8 per cent; mortality was 0.5 versus 0.7 per cent; and the 3-, 5-, and 10-year stroke rates were 93 versus 92 per cent, 87 versus 90 per cent, 79 versus 85 per cent, respectively.[236]

Combined Carotid and Coronary Occlusive Disease

This area is particularly controversial and it depends upon whether or not symptoms exist in either vascular bed. In patients with symptomatic coronary artery disease and in whom an asymptomatic carotid stenosis is found, it is difficult to know whether the carotid artery should be fixed first, followed by coronary artery bypass; whether both lesions should be fixed simultaneously; or whether the carotid artery lesion should be put off until after coronary artery bypass. At present, the literature is quite controversial on this subject, and we are continuing to individualize patients depending upon which lesion appears to be most critical. For example, if a patient has triple coronary artery disease with unstable angina and an asymptomatic carotid stenosis, we usually recommend that the coronary artery surgery be performed first and that the carotid lesion be evaluated following recovery. On the other hand, if the patient has relatively stable angina and has symptomatic carotid artery disease or a preocclusive (greater than 90 per cent) stenosis, it may well be wise to operate on the carotid artery first and then manage the coronary artery lesions a few days later. Finally, if the patient has both symptomatic carotid artery disease and unstable angina, a simultaneous, combined approach would appear to be justified.

Intellectual Testing and Improvement with Carotid Endarterectomy

It has been a common observation that, following carotid endarterectomy, patients and their families often report that they appear to be intellectually brighter and are able to carry out tasks that have been alien to them for quite some time. Numerous attempts have been made to quantitate this intellectual improvement, usually without success. We must be careful not to regard intellectually impaired patients as being routine candidates for carotid endarterectomy, since the majority of those patients will be suffering from organic brain disease rather than compromised blood flow.

Extracranial-to-Intracranial Bypass Grafting

The technical development of connecting an extracranial arterial branch such as the temporal artery to a cortical branch of the middle cerebral artery has been developed over the past 10 years. To determine whether extracranial-to-intracranial (EC/IC) bypass surgery would benefit patients with symptomatic atherosclerotic disease of the internal carotid artery, an international randomized trial was begun in 1977 and completed in 1982: 1377 patients with recent hemispheric strokes, retinal infarction, or TIAs who had arterial narrowing or occlusion of the ipsilateral carotid artery or middle cerebral artery were randomized. Of these, 714 were assigned to the best medical care and 663 were assigned to the surgical group. An EC/IC arterial bypass was performed, with a patency rate on long-term follow-up of 96 per cent. The 30-day surgical mortality was 6.6 per cent, with a stroke morbidity of 2.5 per cent. Nonfatal and fatal strokes on long-term follow-up occurred both more frequently and earlier in patients treated with EC/IC bypass. Survival analysis comparing the two groups for major strokes and all deaths for all strokes and all deaths for ipsilateral ischemic strokes demonstrated a similar lack of benefit from surgery. Reduction in the number of TIAs was noted in 77 per cent of the surgical patients. An equal number (80 per cent) of the medical patients also showed reduc-

tion or disappearance of TIAs. In all parameters studied, EC/IC bypass failed to improve the results of medical therapy. The large number of patients with long-term follow-up, the uniformity of disease process in the population studied, the randomization method (which produced a balanced treatment group), and the presence of complete and accurate records of all entry and event dates and the achievement of the effective anastomosis with acceptably low morbidity and mortality suggest that this conclusion is not only statistically powerful but clinically significant.[237]

Magnetic Resonance Angiography

In the continuing quest to find a substitute for invasive, contrast angiography, the use of MRI of the vascular system has been developed, so-called magnetic resonance angiography (MRA). Various computer programs for postprocessing of MR images to delineate the vascular system are under active development. To date, excellent imaging of the cervical and intracranial vessels has been achievable. However, several limitations of MRA have been identified to date. There were several instances where the MR image suggested total occlusion when contrast angiograms showed a patent vessel with a string sign. MRA also tends to overcall percentage stenosis, making minimal lesions look like hemodynamically significant lesions. Finally, MRA cannot delineate surface irregularity or ulceration.[238-240]

Carotid Endarterectomy Without Angiography

There is no question that angiography carries an important risk in the workup of patients with extracranial arterial occlusive disease. With improved techniques of imaging the carotid bifurcation, there has been a slow but increasing use of noninvasive imaging as the sole substitute for preoperative angiography in patients scheduled for carotid endarterectomy. This began initially with the use of improved quality duplex scanning. It is continuing with the use of magnetic resonance angiography (MRA). Finally, recognizing the limitations of both of these techniques, the most recent suggestion has been to combine duplex scanning and MRA for preoperative assessment. Where there is clear agreement between the two techniques, it would appear that this is a safe substitute for contrast angiography. On the other hand, where there is conflicting information, or an unsatisfactory study, or a clinical picture that is unexplained by noninvasive imaging, then this would be an indication for the selective use of contrast angiography.[241-252]

REFERENCES

1. Savory WS: Case of a young woman in whom the main arteries of both upper extremities and of the left side of the neck were throughout completely obliterated. Med Chir Trans Lond 39:205–219, 1856.

2. Gowers WR: On a case of simultaneous embolism of central retinal and middle cerebral arteries. Lancet 2:794, 1875.

3. Chiari M: Ueber das verhalten des tei lungs-winkels der carotis communis bei der endarteritis chronica deformans. Verh Dtsch Ges Pathol 9:326–330, 1905.

4. Guthrie LG, Mayou S: Right hemiplegia and atrophy of left optic nerve. Proc R Soc Med 1:180, 1908.

5. Cadwater WB: Unilateral optic atrophy and contralateral hemiplegia consequent on occlusion of the cerebral vessels. JAMA 59:2248, 1912.

6. Hunt JR: The role of the carotid arteries in the causation of vascular lesions of the brain, with remarks on certain special features of the symptomatology. Am J Med Sci 147:704–713, 1914.

7. Moniz E: L'encephalographie arterielle: son importance dans la localisation des tumeurs cerebrales. Rev Neurol (Paris) 2:72–90, 1927.

8. Moniz E, Lima A, de Lacerda R: Hemiplegies par thrombose de la carotide interne. Proc Med 45:977–980, 1937.

9. Chao WH, Kwan ST, Lyman RS, et al: Thrombosis of the left internal carotid artery. Arch Surg 37:100–111, 1938.

10. Johnson HC, Walker AE: The angiographic diagnosis of spontaneous thrombosis of the internal and common carotid arteries. J Neurosurg 8:631–659, 1951.

11. Fisher M: Occlusion of the internal carotid artery. Arch Neurol Psychiatry 65:346–377, 1951.

12. Fisher M: Occlusion of the carotid arteries. Arch Neurol Psychiatry 72:187–204, 1954.

13. Carrea R, Molins M, Murphy G: Surgical treatment of spontaneous thrombosis of the internal carotid artery in the neck. Carotid-carotideal anastomosis. Report of a case. Acta Neurol Latinoam 1:71–78, 1955.

14. Strully KJ, Hurwitt ES, Blankenberg HW: Thromboendarterectomy for thrombosis of the internal carotid artery in the neck. J Neurosurg 10:474–482, 1953.

15. DeBakey ME, Crawford ES, Cooley DA, et al: Surgical considerations of occlusive disease of innominate, carotid, subclavian, and vertebral arteries. Ann Surg 149:690–710, 1959.

16. DeBakey ME: Successful carotid endarterectomy for cerebrovascular insufficiency. Nineteen-year follow-up. JAMA 233:1083, 1975.

17. Eastcott HHG, Pickering GW, Rob C: Reconstruction of internal carotid artery in a patient with intermittent attacks of hemiplegia. Lancet 2:994–996, 1954.

18. Davis JB, Grove WJ, Julian OC: Thrombic occlusion of the branches of the aortic arch, Martorell's syndrome: Report of a case treated surgically. Ann Surg 144:124–126, 1956.

19. Warren R, Triedman LJ: Pulseless disease and carotid artery thrombosis. N Engl J Med 257:685–690, 1957.

20. Adelman SM: Economic impact. In McDowell FM (ed): Report on the National Survey of Stroke (American Heart Association monograph number 75). Stroke 12:1, 1981.

21. Mohr JP, Caplan LR, Meski JW, et al: The Harvard Cooperative Stroke Registry: A prospective registry. Neurology 28:754, 1978.

22. Sacco RL, Wolf PA, Kannel WB, McNamara PM: Survival and recurrence following stroke: The Framingham Study. Stroke 13:290, 1982.

23. Soltero I, Lin K, Cooper R, et al: Trends in mortality from cerebrovascular diseases in the United States, 1960 to 1975. Stroke 9:549, 1978.

24. Enger E, Boysen S: Longterm anticoagulant therapy in patients with cerebral infarction: A controlled clinical study. Acta Med Scand 178(suppl 438):1–61, 1965.

25. Robinson RE, et al: Natural history of cerebral thrombosis. 9–19 year follow-up. J Chronic Dis 21:221, 1968.

26. Schmidt EV, Smirnov VE, Ryabova VS: Results of the seven-year prospective study of stroke patients. Stroke 19:942–949, 1988.

27. Swedish Cooperative Study: High-dose acetylsalicylic acid after cerebral infarction. Stroke 18:325–334, 1987.

28. Klag MJ, Whelton PK, Seidler AJ: Decline in US stroke mortality demographic trends and antihypertensive treatment. Stroke 20:14–21, 1989.

29. Wolf PA, O'Neal A, D'Agostino RB, Kannel WB, Case CS, Belanger AJ: Declining mortality not declining incidence of stroke: The Framingham Study. Stroke 20:29, 1989.

30. Harmsen P, Tsipogianni A, Wilhelmsen L: Stroke incidence rates were unchanged, while fatality rates declined, during 1971–1987 in Göteborg, Sweden. Stroke 23:1410–1415, 1992.

31. Moden B, Wagner DK: Some epidemiologic aspects of stroke: Mortality/morbidity trends, age, sex, race, socioeconomic status. Stroke 23:1230–1236, 1992.

32. Mentzer RM, et al: Emergency carotid endarterectomy for fluctuating neurologic deficits. Surgery 89:60, 1981.

33. Milikan CH: Discussion. In McDowell FH, Brennan RW (eds): Cerebral Vascular Diseases (Transactions of the Eighth Princeton Conference on Cerebral Vascular Disease). New York, Grune & Stratton, 1973, p 209.

34. Whisnant JP, Matsumoto M, Elveback LR: The effects of anticoagulant therapy on the prognosis of patients with transient cerebral ischemic attacks in a community. Rochester, Minnesota 1965–1969. Mayo Clin Proc 48:844, 1973.

35. Dennis M, Bamford J, Sandercock P, Warlow C. Prognosis of transient ischemic attacks in the Oxfordshire Community Stroke Project Stroke 21:848–853, 1990.

36. Hass WK, Jonas S: Caution falling rock zone: An analysis of the medical and surgical management of threatened stroke. Proc Inst Med 33:80, 1980.

37. Loeb C, Priano A, Albana C: Clinical features and long-term follow-up of patients with reversible ischemic attacks. Acta Neurol Scand 57:471, 1978.

38. Toole JF: The Willis Lecture: Transient ischemic attacks, scientific method, and new realities. Stroke 22:99–104, 1991.

39. Grigg MJ, Papadakis K, Nicolaides AN, Al-Rutoubi A, Williams MA, Dealon DFS, Sonecha T, Eastcott KHG: The significance of cerebral infarction and atrophy in patients with amaurosis fugax and transient ischemic attacks in relation to internal carotid artery stenosis. A preliminary report. J Vasc Surg 7:215–222, 1988.

40. Kartchner MM, McRae LP: Noninvasive evaluation and management of the asymptomatic carotid bruit. Surgery 82:840, 1977.

41. Busuttil RW, et al: Carotid artery stenosis: Hemodynamic significance and clinical course. JAMA 245:1438, 1981.

42. Roederer GO, Langlois YE, Jager KA, et al: The natural history of carotid arterial disease in asymptomatic patients with cervical bruits. Stroke 15:605–613, 1984.

43. Moore DJ, et al: Non-invasive assessment of stroke risk in asymptomatic and non hemispheric patients with suspected carotid disease: Five year follow-up of 294 unoperated and 81 operated patients. Ann Surg 202:491–504, 1985.

44. Chambers BR, Norris JW: Outcome in patients with asymptomatic neck bruits. N Engl J Med 315:860–865, 1986.

45. Norris JW, Zhu CZ, Bornstein NM, Chambers BR: Vascular risks of asymptomatic carotid stenosis. Stroke 22:1485–1490, 1991.

46. Norris JW, Zhu CZ: Silent stroke and carotid stenosis. Stroke 23:483–485, 1992.

47. Johnson JM, et al: Natural history of asymptomatic carotid plaque. Arch Surg 120:1010–1012, 1985.

48. Langsfeld M, Gray-Weale AC, Lusby RJ: The role of plaque morphology and diameter reduction in the development of new symptoms in asymptomatic carotid arteries. J Vasc Surg 9:548–557, 1989.

49. Sterpetti AV, Schultz RD, Feldhaus RJ, et al: Ultrasono-

graphic features of carotid plaque and the risk of subsequent neurologic deficits. Surgery 104:652–660, 1988.

50. Madison SE, Moore WS: Ulcerated atheroma of the carotid artery: Arteriographic appearance. AJR 107:530, 1969.

51. Moore WS, Hall AD: Ulcerated atheroma of the carotid artery: A cause of transient cerebral ischemia. Am J Surg 116:237, 1968.

52. Moore WS, Hall AD: Importance of emboli from carotid bifurcation in pathogenesis in cerebral ischemia attacks. Arch Surg 101:708, 1970.

53. Moore WS, et al: Natural history of nonstenotic asymptomatic ulcerative lesions of the carotid artery. Arch Surg 113:1352, 1978.

54. Dixon S, et al: Natural history of nonstenotic, asymptomatic ulcerative lesions of the carotid artery: A further analysis. Arch Surg 117:1493, 1982.

55. Harward TRS, et al: Natural history of asymptomatic ulcerative plaques of the carotid bifurcation. Am J Surg 146:208, 1983.

56. Katchner MM, McRae LP: Guidelines for non-invasive evaluation of asymptomatic carotid bruits. Clin Neurosurg 28:418–428, 1981.

57. Barnes RW, et al: Natural history of asymptomatic carotid disease in patients undergoing cardiovascular surgery. Surgery 90:1075–1083, 1981.

58. Breslau PJ, et al: Carotid arterial disease in patients undergoing coronary artery bypass operations. J Thorac Cardiovasc Surg 82:765–767, 1981.

59. Furlan AJ, Craciun AR: Risk in stroke during coronary artery bypass graft surgery in patients with internal carotid artery disease documented by angiography. Stroke 16:797–799, 1985.

60. Turnipseed WD, Berkoff HA, Belzer FO: Post-operative stroke in cardiac and peripheral vascular disease. Ann Surg 192:365–368, 1980.

61. Von Reutern G-M, Hetzel A, Birnbaum D, Schlosser V: Transcranial Doppler ultrasonography during cardiopulmonary bypass in patients with severe carotid stenosis or occlusion. Stroke 19:674–680, 1988.

62. Schwartz CJ, Mitchell JRA: Observations on localization of arterial plaques. Circ Res 11:63, 1962.

63. Heath D, et al: The atherosclerotic human carotid sinus. J Pathol 110:49, 1973.

64. Caro CG, Fitzgerald JN, Schroter RC: Atheroma and arterial wall shear: Observation, correlation and proposal of a shear-dependent mass transfer mechanism for atherogenesis. Proc R Soc Lond (Biol) 117:109, 1971.

65. Balasubramanian K, Giddens DP, Maybon RS: Steady flow at the carotid bifurcation. *In* Schneck DJ (ed): Biofluid Mechanics, vol 6. New York, Plenum Press, 1980, p 475.

66. Ferguson GG, Roach MR: Flow conditions at bifurcations as determined in glass models with reference to the focal distribution of vascular lesions. *In* Bergel DH (ed): Cardiovascular Fluid Dynamics, vol 2. New York, Academic Press, 1972.

67. Fox JA, Hugh AE: Static zones in the internal carotid artery: Correlations with boundary layer separation and stasis in mobile flows. Br J Radiol 43:370, 1976.

68. Logerfo EW, et al: Flow studies in a model carotid bifurcation. Arteriosclerosis 1:235, 1981.

69. Zarins CK, Giddens DB, Glagov S: Artherosclerotic plaque distribution and flow velocity profiles in the carotid bifurcation. *In* Bergan JJ, Yao JDT (eds): Cerebrovascular Insufficiency. New York, Grune & Stratton, 1982, p 19.

70. Salzman EW: Platelet-vessel interactions in cerebrovascular disease: The role of prostaglandins in cerebrovascular insufficiency. *In* Bergan JJ, Yao JST (eds): Cerebrovascular Insufficiency. New York, Grune & Stratton, 1983, p 31.

71. Meyers KM, et al: The dominant role of thromboxane formation in secondary aggregation of platelets. Nature 282:331, 1980.

72. Born BGR: Arterial thrombosis and its prevention. *In* Hayase S, Murao S (eds): Proceedings of the VIIIth World Congress of Cardiology. Tokyo, Amsterdam, Excerpta Medica, 1978, p 81.

73. Fryer JA, Myers PC, Appleberg M: Carotid intraplaque hemorrhage: The significance of neovascularity. J Vasc Surg 63:341–349, 1987.

74. Lusby RJ, Ferrell LD, Wylie EJ: The significance of intraplaque hemorrhage in the pathogenesis of carotid arteriosclerosis. *In* Bergan JJ, Yao JST (eds): Cerebrovascular Insufficiency. New York, Grune & Stratton, 1983, p 41.

75. Ogata J, Masuda J, Yutani C, Yamguchi T: Rupture of atheromatous plaque as a cause of thrombotic occlusion of stenotic internal carotid artery. Stroke 21:1740–1745, 1990.

76. Palubinskas AJ, Ripley HR: Fibromuscular hyperplasia in extrarenal arteries. Radiology 82:451, 1964.

77. Patman RD, et al: Natural history of fibromuscular dysplasia of the carotid artery. Stroke 2:135, 1980.

78. Osborn AG, Anderson RE: Angiographic spectrum of cervical and intracranial fibromuscular dysplasia. Stroke 8:617, 1977.

79. Effeney DJ, Ehrenfeld WK, Stoney RJ, et al: Fibromuscular dysplasia of the internal carotid artery. World J Surg 3:179, 1979.

80. Stanley JC, et al: Arterial fibrodysplasia: Histopathologic character and current etiologic concepts. Arch Surg 110:561, 1975.

81. Ross R, Klebanoff SJ: Fine structural changes in uterine smooth muscle and fibroblasts in response to estrogen. J Cell Biol 32:155, 1967.

82. Nakata Y: An experimental study on the vascular lesions caused by obstruction of the vasa vasorum. Jpn Circ J 31:275, 1967.

83. Sarkari NBS, Palms JM, Bickerstaff ER: Neurological manifestations associated with internal carotid loops and kinks in children. J Neurol Neurosurg Psychiatry 33:194, 1973.

84. Metz H, et al: Kinking of the internal carotid artery in relation to cerebrovascular disease. Lancet 1:424, 1961.

85. Quattlebaum JK Jr, Upson ET, Neville RL: Strokes associated with elongation and kinking of the internal carotid artery. Ann Surg 150:824, 1959.

86. Vannix RS, Joergenson EJ, Carter R: Kinking of the internal carotid artery. Clinical significance and surgical management. Am J Surg 134:82, 1977.

87. Busuttil RW, et al: Selective management of extracranial carotid arterial aneurysms. Am J Surg 140:85, 1980.

88. Rhodes EL, et al: Aneurysms of extracranial carotid arteries. Arch Surg 111:339, 1976.

89. Kaupp HA, et al: Aneurysms of the extracranial carotid artery. Surgery 72:946, 1972.

90. Boldrey E, Maass L, Miller E: The role of atlantoid compression in the etiology of internal carotid thrombosis. J Neurosurg 13:127, 1956.

91. Smith RF, Szilagyi DE, Colville JM: Surgical treatment of mycotic aneurysms. Arch Surg 85:663, 1962.

92. Bradac GB, et al: Spontaneous dissecting aneurysm of cervical cerebral arteries: Report of six cases and review of the literature. Neuroradiology 21:149, 1981.

93. Ehrenfeld WK, Wiley EJ: Spontaneous dissection of the internal carotid artery. Arch Surg 111:1294, 1976.

94. Takayasu M: Case with unusual changes of the central vessels of the retina. Acta Soc Ophthalmol Jpn 12:554, 1908.

95. Nasu T: Pathology of pulseless disease: Systematic study and critical review of 21 autopsy cases reported in Japan. Angiology 14:225, 1962.

96. Lande A, Berkmen YM: Aortitis: Pathologic, clinical and arteriographic review. Radiol Clin North Am 14(2):219, 1976.

97. Lupi-Herrera E, et al: Takayasu's arteritis. Clinical study of 107 cases. Am Heart J 93:94, 1977.

98. Hamrin B, Jousson N, Landberg T: Involvement of large vessels in polymyalgia arteritica. Lancet 1:1193, 1965.

99. Lindsay S, et al: Aortic arteriosclerosis in the dog after localized aortic irradiation with electrons. Circ Res 10:61, 1962.

100. Silverberg GD, Britt RH, Goffinet DR: Radiation-induced carotid artery disease. Cancer 41:132, 1978.
101. McCready RA, et al: Radiation-induced arterial injuries. Surgery 93(2):306, 1983.
102. Levinson SA, et al: Carotid artery occlusive disease following external cervical irradiation. Arch Surg 107:395, 1973.
103. Moritz MW, Higgins RF, Jacobs JR: Duplex imaging and incidence of carotid radiation injury after high-dose radiotherapy for tumors of the head and neck. Arch Surg 125:1181–1183, 1990.
104. DeGrotte RD, Lynch JG, Jamil Z, Hobson RW II: Carotid restenosis: Long term non-invasive follow-up after carotid endarterectomy. Stroke 18:1031–1036, 1987.
105. Hertzer NR, et al: Recurrent stenosis after carotid endarterectomy. Surg Gynecol Obstet 149:360, 1979.
106. Hertzer NR, Beven EG, O'Hara PJ, Krajewski LP: A prospective study of vein patch angioplasty during carotid endarterectomy. Ann Surg 206:628–635, 1987.
107. Lees CD, Hertzer NR: Postoperative stroke and late neurologic complications after endarterectomy. Arch Surg 116:1561, 1981.
108. Stoney RJ, String ST: Recurrent carotid stenosis. Surgery 80:705–710, 1976.
109. Zierler RE, Bandyk DF, Thiele BL, Strandness DE Jr: Carotid artery stenosis following endarterectomy. Arch Surg 117:1408–1415, 1982.
110. O'Donnell TF, et al: Ultrasound characteristics of recurrent carotid disease: Hypothesis explaining the low incidence of symptomatic recurrence. J Vasc Surg 2:26–41, 1985.
111. Nicholls SC, et al: Carotid endarterectomy: Relationship of outcome to early restenosis. J Vasc Surg 2:375–381, 1985.
112. Bernstein EF, Torem S, Dolley RB: Does carotid restenosis predict an increased risk of late symptoms, stroke, or death? Ann Surg 212:629–636, 1990.
113. Awad IA, Little JR: Patch angioplasty in carotid endarterectomy—advantages, concerns, and controversies. Stroke 20:417–422, 1989.
114. Curley S, Edwards WS, Jacob TP: Recurrent carotid stenosis after autologous tissue patching. J Vasc Surg 6:350–354, 1987.
115. Eikelboom BC, Ackerstaff RGA, Hoeneveld H, et al: Benefits of carotid patching: A randomized study. J Vasc Surg 7:240–247, 1988.
116. Lord RSA, Raj TB, Stary DL, et al: Comparison of saphenous vein patch, polytetrafluoroethylene patch, and direct arteriotomy closure after carotid endarterectomy. Part I—perioperative results. J Vasc Surg 9:521–529, 1989.
117. Salvian A, Baker JD, Machleder HI, Busuttil RW, Barker WF, Moore WS: Cause and noninvasive detection of restenosis after carotid endarterectomy. Am J Surg 146:29–34, 1983.
118. Gelabert HA, El-Massry S, Moore WS: Carotid endarterectomy with primary closure does not adversely affect the rate of recurrent stenosis. Arch Surg 1993 (in submission).
119. Crawford ES, et al: Hemodynamic alteration in patients with cerebral arterial insufficiency before and after operation. Surgery 48:76, 1960.
120. Gunning AJ, et al: Mural thrombosis of the internal carotid artery and subsequent embolism. Q J Med 33:155–195, 1964.
121. Hertzer NR, et al: Ultramicroscopic ulcerations and thrombi of the carotid bifurcation. Arch Surg 112:1394–1042, 1977.
122. Imparato AM, et al: The carotid bifurcation plaque: Pathology findings associated with cerebral ischemia. Stroke 10:238–245, 1979.
123. Edwards JR, et al: Angiographically undetected ulceration of the carotid bifurcation as a cause of embolic stroke. J Neuroradiology 132:369–373, 1979.
124. Sterpetti AV, Hunter WJ, Schultz RD: Importance of ulceration of carotid plaque in determining symptoms of cerebral ischemia. J Cardiovasc Surg 32:154–158, 1991.
125. Loeb C, Gandolfo C, Bino G: Intellectual impairment and cerebral lesions in multiple cerebral infarcts. Stroke 19:560–565, 1988.

126. Zukowski AJ, Nicolaides AN, Lewis RJ, et al: The correlation between carotid plaque ulceration and cerebral infarction seen on CT scan. J Vasc Surg 1:782–786, 1984.
127. Siebler M, Sitzer M, Steinmetz H: Detection of intracranial emboli in patients with symptomatic extracranial stroke 23:1652–1654, 1992.
128. Tietjen GE, Futrell N, Garcia JH, Millikan C: Platelet emboli in rat brain cross when the contralateral carotid artery is occluded. Stroke 22:1053–1058, 1991.
129. Mohr JP: Lacunes. Stroke 13:3–11, 1982.
130. Fisher C-M: Pure motor hemiplegia of vascular origin. Arch Neurol 13:30–44, 1965.
131. Pullicino P, Nelson RF, Kendall BE, Marshall J: Small deep infarcts diagnosed on computed tomography. Neurology 30:1090–1096, 1980.
132. Bladin PF, Berkovic SF: Striatocapsular infarction: Large infarcts in the lenticulostriate arterial territory. Neurology 34:1423–1430, 1984.
133. Bamford JM, Warlow CP: Evolution and testing of the lacunar hypothesis. Stroke 19:1074–1082, 1988.
134. Horowitz DR, Tuhrim S, Weinberger JM, Rudolph SJ: Mechanisms in lacunar infarction. Stroke 23:325–327, 1992.
135. Heyman A, et al: Risk of stroke in asymptomatic persons with cervical arterial bruits: A population study in Evans County, Georgia. N Engl J Med 302:838, 1980.
136. Reinmuth OM: Transient ischemic attacks. Curr Neurol 1(7):166, 1978.
137. Heyman A, et al: XI. Transient focal cerebral ischemia: Epidemiological and clinical aspects. Stroke 5:277, 1974.
138. Price TR, et al: Cooperative study of hospital frequency and character of transient ischemic attacks, VI. Patients examined during an attack. JAMA 238:2512, 1977.
139. Futty DE, et al: Cooperative study of hospital frequency and character of transient ischemic attacks. V. Symptom analysis. JAMA 238:2386, 1977.
140. Berguer R: Idiopathic ischemic syndrome of the retina and optic nerve and their carotid origin. J Vasc Surg 2:649–653, 1985.
141. Mohr JP: Transient ischemic attacks and the prevention of stroke. N Engl J Med 299:93, 1978.
142. Pessin MS, et al: Clinical and angiographic features of carotid transient ischemic attacks. N Engl J Med 296:358, 1977.
143. Yatsu SM, Coull BM: Stroke. Curr Neurol 3:159, 1981.
144. Dosick SM, et al: Carotid endarterectomy in the stroke patient: Computerized axial tomography to determine timing. J Vasc Surg 2:214–219, 1985.
145. Ahn SS, Jordan SE, Nuwer MR, et al: Compared electroencephalographic topographic brain mapping—a new and accurate monitor of cerebral circulation and function for patients having carotid endarterectomy. J Vasc Surg 8:247–254, 1988.
146. Moore WS, Ziomek S, Quiñones-Baldrich WJ, et al: Can clinical evaluation and non-invasive testing substitute for arteriography in the evaluation of carotid artery disease? Am J Surg 208:91–94, 1988.
147. Connolly JE: Carotid endarterectomy in the aware patient. Am J Surg 150:159, 1985.
148. Moore WS, Hall AD: Carotid artery back pressure. Arch Surg 99:702, 1969.
149. Moore WS, Yee TM-I, Hall AD: Collateral cerebral blood pressure: An index of tolerance to temporary carotid occlusion. Arch Surg 106:520, 1973.
150. Baker TD, et al: An evaluation of electroencephalographic monitoring for carotid surgery. Surgery 78:787, 1975.
151. Elmore JR, Eldrup-Jorgensen J, Leschey WH, Herbert WE, Dillihunt RC, Ray FS: Computerized tomographic brain mapping during carotid endarterectomy. Arch Surg 125:734–738, 1990.
152. Kearse LA Jr, Brown EN, McPeck K: Somatosensory evoked potentials sensitivity relative to electroencephalography for cerebral ischemia during carotid endarterectomy. Stroke 23:498–505, 1992.
153. Thompson JE, Patman RD, Talkington CM: Asymptomatic

carotid bruit: Long term outcome of patients having endarterectomy compared with unoperated controls. Ann Surg *188*:308, 1978.

154. Baker WM, Dorner DB, Barnes RW: Carotid endarterectomy: Is an indwelling shunt necessary? Surgery *82*:321, 1977.

155. Whitney DG, et al: Carotid surgery without a temporary indwelling shunt. 1,917 consecutive procedures. Arch Surg *115*:1393, 1980.

156. Archie JP Jr: Technique and clinical results of carotid stump back-pressure to determine selective shunting during carotid endarterectomy. J Vasc Surg *13*:319–327, 1991.

157. Halsey JH Jr: Risks and benefits of shunting in carotid endarterectomy. Stroke *23*:1583–1587, 1992.

158. Matchar DB, Goldstein LB, McCory DC, et al: Carotid endarterectomy: A literature review and ratings of appropriateness and necessity. Rand GRA-05, 1992.

159. Moore WS, Mohr JP, Najafi H, Robertson JT, Stoney RJ, Toole JF: Carotid endarterectomy: Practice guidelines. Report of the ad hoc committee to the joint council of the Society for Vascular Surgery and the North American Chapter of the International Society for Cardiovascular Surgery. J Vasc Surg *15*:469–479, 1992.

160. Moore WS: Current status of carotid endarterectomy for stroke prevention. West J Med (in submission).

161. Blaisdell FM, Lim R Jr, Hall AD: Technical results of carotid endarterectomy: Arteriographic assessment. Am J Surg *114*:239, 1967.

162. Gaspar MR, Movins HJ, Rosenthal JJ: Routine intraoperative arteriography in carotid artery surgery. J Cardiovasc Surg, Special Issue, 447, 1974.

163. Moore WS, Martello JY, Quiñones-Baldrich WJ, Ahn SS: Etiologic importance of the intimal flap of the external carotid artery in the development of post-carotid endarterectomy stroke. Stroke *21*:1497–1502, 1990.

164. Bove EL, et al: Hypotension and hypertension as consequences of baroreceptor dysfunction following carotid endarterectomy. Surgery *85*:633, 1979.

165. Towne JB, Bernard VM: The relationship of postoperative hypertension to complications following carotid endarterectomy. Surgery *88*:375, 1980.

166. Angell-James JE, Lumley JSP: The effects of carotid endarterectomy on the mechanical properties of the carotid sinus and carotid sinus nerve activity in atherosclerotic patients. Br J Surg *61*:805, 1974.

167. Smith BL: Hypertension following carotid endarterectomy: The role of cerebral renin production. J Vasc Surg *1*:623–627, 1984.

168. Skydell JL, Machleder HI, Baker JD, Busuttil RW, Moore WS: Incidence and mechanism of post-carotid endarterectomy hypertension. Arch Surg *122*:1153–1155, 1987.

169. Ahn SS, Marcus DR, Moore WS: Post-carotid endarterectomy hypertension: Associated with elevated cranial norepinephrine. J Vasc Surg *9*:351–350, 1989.

170. Ranson JHC, et al: Factors in the mortality and morbidity associated with surgical treatment of cerebrovascular insufficiency. Circulation *39*(suppl I):I-269, 1969.

171. Riles TL, Koppleman I, Imparato AM: Myocardial infarction following carotid endarterectomy. A review of 683 operations. Surgery *85*:249, 1979.

172. Matsumoto GH, Cossman D, Callow AD: Hazards and safeguards during carotid endarterectomy: Technical consideration. Am J Surg *133*:485, 1977.

173. Hertzer NR, et al: A prospective study of the incidence of injury to the cranial nerve during carotid endarterectomy. Surg Gynecol Obstet *151*:781, 1980.

174. Evans WE, et al: Motor speech deficit following carotid endarterectomy. Am Surg *196*:461, 1982.

175. Bryant MF: Complications associated with carotid endarterectomy. Am Surg *42*:665, 1976.

176. Verta MJ Jr, et al: Cranial nerve injury during carotid endarterectomy. Ann Surg *185*:192, 1977.

177. Thompson JE: Complications of endarterectomy and their prevention. World J Surg *3*:155, 1979.

178. Brott T, Thalinger K: The practice of carotid endarterectomy in a large metropolitan area. Stroke *15*:950–955, 1984.

179. Brott TG, Labutta RJ, Kempczinski RF: Changing patterns in the practice of carotid endarterectomy in a large metropolitan area. JAMA *225*:2609–2612, 1986.

180. Easton JD, Sherman DG: Stroke and mortality rate in carotid endarterectomy: 228 consecutive operations. Stroke *8*:565–568, 1977.

181. Beebe HG, Clagett GP, DeWeese JA, Moore WS, et al: Assessing risk associated with carotid endarterectomy. Stroke *20*:314–315, 1989.

182. Sundt TM Jr, et al: Carotid endarterectomy. Results, complications, and monitoring techniques. Adv Neurol *16*:97, 1977.

183. Kwaan JHM, Connelly JE, Sharefkin JB: Successful management of early stroke after carotid endarterectomy. Ann Surg *190*:676, 1979.

184. Hertzer NR, Lees CD: Fatal myocardial infarction following carotid endarterectomy. 335 patients followed 6–11 postoperative years. Ann Surg *194*:212–218, 1981.

185. Bauer RB, et al: Joint study of extracranial arterial occlusion. III. Progress report of controlled study of long-term survival in patients with and without operation. JAMA *208*:509, 1969.

186. Bernstein EF, et al: Influence of preoperative factors on late neurologic events after carotid endarterectomy. International Vascular Symposium Programs and Abstracts. New York, Macmillan Publishers, Ltd, 1981, p 460.

187. Hertzer NR, Arison R: Cumulative stroke and survival ten years after carotid endarterectomy. J Vasc Surg *2*:661–668, 1985.

188. Sergeant PT, et al: Carotid endarterectomy for cerebrovascular insufficiency: Long-term follow-up of 141 patients followed for up to 16 years. Acta Chir Belg *79*:309, 1979.

189. Moore WS, Boren C, Malone JM, et al: Asymptomatic carotid stenosis: Immediate and long term results after prophylactic endarterectomy. Am J Surg *138*:228, 1979.

190. Bernstein EF, Humber PB, Collins GM, et al: Life expectancy and late stroke following carotid endarterectomy. Ann Surg *198*:80, 1983.

191. Lord RSA: Later survival after carotid endarterectomy for transient ischemic attacks. J Vasc Surg *1*:512, 1984.

192. DeWeese JA, et al: Results of carotid endarterectomy for transient ischemic attacks—five years later. Ann Surg *178*:258, 1973.

193. Thompson JE, Austin BJ, Patman RD: Carotid endarterectomy for cerebrovascular insufficiency: Long-term results in 592 patients followed up to 13 years. Ann Surg *172*:663, 1970.

194. Takolander RJ, Bergentz SE, Ericsson BF: Carotid artery surgery in patients with minor stroke. Br J Surg *70*:13, 1983.

195. Eriksson SE, Link H, Alm A, et al: Results from eight-eight consecutive prophylactic carotid endarterectomy in cerebral infarction and transitory ischemic attacks. Acta Neurol Scand *63*:209, 1981.

196. Bardin JA, Bernstein EF, Humber PB, et al: Is carotid endarterectomy beneficial in prevention of recurrent stroke? Arch Surg *117*:1401, 1982.

197. McCullough JL, Mentzer RM, Harman PK, et al: Carotid endarterectomy after a completed stroke: Reduction in long term neurologic deterioration. J Vasc Surg *2*:7, 1985.

198. Ouriel K, et al: Carotid endarterectomy for nonhemispheric symptoms: Predictors of success. J Vasc Surg *1*:331–345, 1984.

199. Imparato AM: Vertebral arterial reconstruction: A nineteen year experience. J Vasc Surg *2*:626–533, 1985.

200. O'Hara PJ, Hertzer NR, Beven EG: External carotid revascularization: Review of a ten year experience. J Vasc Surg *2*:709–714, 1985.

201. Halstuk KS, Baker WH, Littooy FN: External carotid endarterectomy. J Vasc Surg *1*:398–402, 1984.

202. Veterans Administration: A Veterans Administration Cooperative Study: Role of carotid endarterectomy in asymptomatic carotid stenosis. Stroke *17*:534–539, 1986.

203. Hobson RW, Song IS, George AM, Weiss DG: Results of arteriography for asymptomatic carotid stenosis. Stroke *20*:135, 1989.
204. Towne JB, Weiss DG, Hobson RW: First phase report of cooperative Veterans Administration asymptomatic carotid stenosis study—operative morbidity and mortality. J Vasc Surg *11*:252–259, 1990.
205. The CASANOVA Study Group: Carotid surgery vs medical therapy in asymptomatic carotid stenosis. Stroke *22*:1229–1235, 1991.
206. The Asymptomatic Carotid Artery Stenosis Group: Study design for randomized prospective trial of carotid endarterectomy for asymptomatic atherosclerosis. Stroke *20*:844–849, 1989.
207. North American Symptomatic Carotid Endarterectomy Trial (NASCET) Steering Committee: North American Symptomatic Carotid Endarterectomy Trial: Methods, patient characteristics, and progress. Stroke *22*:711–720, 1991.
208. North American Symptomatic Carotid Endarterectomy Trial Collaborators: Beneficial effect of carotid endarterectomy in symptomatic patients with high-grade carotid stenosis. N Engl J Med *325*:445–453, 1991.
209. European Carotid Surgery Trialists' Collaborative Group: MRC European Carotid Surgery Trial: Interim results for patients with severe (70–99%) or with mild (0–29%) carotid stenosis. Lancet *337*:1235–1243, 1991.
210. Maybert MR, Wilson SE, Yatsu F, Weiss DG, Messina L, Hershey LA, Colling C, Eskridge J, Deykin D, Winn HR: Carotid endarterectomy and prevention of cerebral ischemia in symptomatic carotid stenosis. JAMA *266*:3289, 1991.
211. Wolf PA, D'Agostino RB, Kannel WB, Bonita R, Belanger AJ: Cigarette smoking as a risk factor for stroke: The Framingham Study. JAMA *259*:1025–1029, 1988.
212. Whisnant JP, Homer D, Ingall TJ, Baker HL Jr, O'Fallon WM, Wiebers DO: Duration of cigarette smoking is the strongest predictor of severe extracranial carotid artery atherosclerosis. Stroke *21*:707–714, 1990.
213. Dempsey RJ, Moore RW: Amount of smoking independently predicts carotid artery atherosclerosis severity. Stroke *23*:693–696, 1992.
214. Baker RN, Schwartz WS, Rose AS: Transient ischemic strokes: A report of a study of anticoagulant therapy. Neurology *16*:841, 1964.
215. Link H, et al: Prognosis in patients with infarction and TIA in carotid territory during and after anticoagulant therapy. Stroke *10*:529, 1979.
216. Terent A, Anderson B: The outcome of patients with transient ischemic attacks and stroke treated with anticoagulants. Acta Med Scand *208*:359, 1980.
217. Jonas S: Anticoagulant therapy in cerebrovascular disease: Review and meta-analysis. Stroke *19*:1043–1048, 1988.
218. The Canadian Cooperative Study Group: A randomized trial of aspirin and sulfinpyrazone in threatened strokes. N Engl J Med *299*:53, 1978.
219. Whisnant JP: The Canadian trial of aspirin and sulfinpyrazone in threatened strokes. Am Heart J *99*:129, 1980.
220. Fields WS, et al: Controlled trial of aspirin in cerebral ischemia. Stroke *8*:301, 1977.
221. Fields WS, et al: Controlled trial of aspirin in cerebral ischemia. Part 2: Surgical group. Stroke *9*:309, 1978.
222. Bousser MD, et al: AICLA controlled trial of aspirin and dipyridamole in the secondary prevention of arteriothrombotic cerebral ischemia. Stroke *14*:5–14, 1983.
223. The American Canadian Cooperative Study Group: Persantine—aspirin trial in cerebral ischemia. Part 2: End point results. Stroke *16*:405, 1985.
224. Sorenson PS, et al: Acetylsalicylic acid in the prevention of stroke in patients with reversible cerebral ischemic attacks. A Danish cooperative study. Stroke *14*:15–22, 1983.
225. Dyken ML: Editorial. Stroke *14*:2–4, 1983.
226. Sze PC, Reitman D, Pincus MM, et al: Antiplatelet agents in the secondary prevention of stroke: Meta-analysis of the randomized control trials. Stroke *19*:436–442, 1988.

227. Hass WK, Easton D, Adams MP Jr, et al: A randomized trial comparing ticlopidine hydrochloride with aspirin for the prevention of stroke in high-risk patients. N Engl J Med *321*:501–507, 1989.
228. Carson SN, et al: Aspirin failure in symptomatic arteriosclerotic carotid artery disease. Surgery *90*:1084, 1981.
229. Wylie EJ, Hein MF, Adams JE: Intracranial hemorrhage following surgical revascularization for treatment of acute strokes. J Neurosurg *21*:212–215, 1964.
230. Giordano JM, et al: Timing carotid arterial endarterectomy after stroke. J Vasc Surg *2*:250, 1985.
231. Whittemore AD, Ruby ST, Couch NP, et al: Early carotid endarterectomy in patients with small fixed neurologic deficits. J Vasc Surg *1*:795, 1984.
232. Goldstone J, Moore WS: Emergency carotid artery surgery in neurologically unstable patients. Arch Surg *111*:1284, 1976.
233. Abu Rahma AF, Boland JP, Robinson P, Delanio R: Antiplatelet therapy and carotid plaque hemorrhage and its clinical implications. J Cardiovasc Surg *31*:66–70, 1990.
234. Schuler JJ, et al: The effect of carotid siphon stenosis on stroke rate, death, and relief of symptoms following elective carotid endarterectomy. Surgery *92*:1058–1067, 1982.
235. Moore WS: Does tandem lesion mean tandem risk in patients with carotid artery disease? J Vasc Surgery *7*:454–455, 1988.
236. Mackey WC, O'Donnell JF Jr, Callow AD: Carotid endarterectomy in patients with intracranial vascular disease: Short-term risk and long-term outcome. J Vasc Surg *10*:432–438, 1989.
237. The EC/IC Bypass Study Group: Failure of extracranial—intracranial arterial bypass to reduce the risk of ischemic stroke: Results of an international randomized trial. N Engl J Med *313*:1191–1200, 1985.
238. Wilkerson DK, Keller I, Mezich R, Schroeder WB, Sebok D, Gronlund-Jacobs J, Conway R, Zatina MA: The comparative evaluation of three dimensional magnetic resonance for carotid artery disease. J Vasc Surg *14*:803–811, 1991.
239. Mattle HP, Kent KC, Adelman RR, Atkinson DJ, Skillman JJ: Evaluation of the extracranial carotid arteries: Correlation of magnetic resonance angiography, duplex ultrasonography, and conventional angiography. J Vasc Surg *13*:838–845, 1991.
240. Wiles TS, Eidelman EM, Litt AW, Pinto RS, Oldford F, Schwartzenberg GWST: Comparison of magnetic resonance angiography, conventional angiography, and duplex scanning. Stroke *23*:341–346, 1992.
241. Blackshear WM, Connar RG: Carotid endarterectomy without angiography. J Cardiovasc Surg *23*:477, 1982.
242. Sandmann W, Hennerici M, Nullen H, Aulich A, Knab K, Kremer K: Carotid artery surgery without angiography: Risk or progress? *In* Greenhalgh RM, Rose FC (eds): Progress in Stroke Research II. London, Pitman, 1983, pp 447–461.
243. Ricotta JJ, Holen J, Schenk E, et al: Is routine angiography necessary prior to carotid endarterectomy? J Vasc Surg *1*:96–102, 1984.
244. Crew JR, Dean M, Johnson JM, et al: Carotid surgery without angiography. Am J Surg *148*:217–220, 1984.
245. Walsh J, Markowitz I, Kerstein MD: Carotid endarterectomy for amaurosis fugax without angiography. Am J Surg *152*:172–174, 1986.
246. Marshall WG, Kouchoukos NT, Murphy SF, Pelate C: Carotid endarterectomy based on duplex scanning without preoperative arteriography. Circulation *78*(suppl I):I-1–I-5, 1988.
247. Moore WS, Ziomek S, Quiñones-Baldrich WJ, Machleder HI, Busuttil RW, Baker JD: Can clinical evaluation and noninvasive testing substitute for arteriography in the evaluation of carotid artery disease? Ann Surg *208*:91–94, 1988.
248. Gelabert HA, Moore WS: Carotid endarterectomy without angiography. Surg Clin North Am *70*:213–223, 1990.
249. Ranaboldo C, Davies J, Chant A: Duplex scanning alone

before carotid endarterectomy: A five-year experience. Eur J Vasc Surg 5:415–419, 1991.
250. Wagner WH, Treiman RL, Cossman DV, Foran RF, Levein PM, Cohen JL: The diminishing role of diagnostic arteriography in carotid artery disease: Duplex scanning as definitive preoperative study. Ann Vasc Surg 5:105–110, 1991.
251. Gertler JP, Cambria RP, Kistler JP, Geller SC, MacDonald NR, Brewster DC, Abbott WM: Carotid surgery without arteriography: Non-invasive selection of patients. Ann Vasc Surg 5:253–256, 1991.
252. Chervu A, Moore WS: Carotid endarterectomy without angiography: Personal series and review of the literature. Presented SVS/ISCVS Breakfast Session, June 1992. J Vasc Surg (in submission).

REVIEW QUESTIONS

1. The most common etiology for perioperative neurologic deficits following carotid endarterectomy is:
   (a) thrombosis of the repair
   (b) lack of cerebral perfusion
   (c) tandem lesions in the carotid system
   (d) low cardiac output
   (e) none of the above

2. Carotid endarterectomy for asymptomatic disease:
   1. remains controversial
   2. carries the lowest perioperative morbidity and mortality
   3. should be considered when progression to 80 per cent stenosis is documented
   4. may prevent stroke, which is the most common initial manifestation of symptomatic carotid disease
   (a) 1,2,3
   (b) 1,3
   (c) 2,4
   (d) 4 only
   (e) all of the above

3. Tandem lesions in the intracranial carotid system:
   (a) carry a similar stroke risk when compared to a carotid bifurcation lesion
   (b) carry a lower stroke risk than a similar extracranial bulb lesion
   (c) carry a higher risk than a similar extracranial bulb lesion
   (d) should deter the surgeon from recommending bifurcation endarterectomy
   (e) are more frequently the source of symptoms when combined intra- and extracranial disease is present

4. The following is/are true about fibromuscular dysplasia:
   1. best described as an atherosclerotic process affecting medium-sized arteries
   2. 30 per cent of patients with cervical involvement may have intracranial aneurysms
   3. medial hyperplasia is the most common type affecting the carotid system
   4. most commonly affects women, suggesting a hormonal factor
   (a) 1,2,3
   (b) 1,3
   (c) 2,4
   (d) 4 only
   (e) none of the above

5. Kinks of the carotid artery:
   (a) are frequently the cause of cerebrovascular symptoms
   (b) may be congenital
   (c) never cause symptoms
   (d) repair frequently requires excision and grafting
   (e) are rarely associated with atherosclerosis

6. Transient ischemic attacks:
   1. carry a 40 per cent risk of stroke over 5 years when secondary to extracranial arterial occlusive disease
   2. are always secondary to platelet emboli
   3. may be a manifestation of lacunar infarction
   4. as a manifestation of cardiac emboli, are usually stereotyped, with similar symptoms with each occurrence
   (a) 1,2,3
   (b) 1,3
   (c) 2,4
   (d) 4 only
   (e) all of the above

7. The use of an internal shunt during carotid endarterectomy:
   (a) is necessary in approximately 50 per cent of patients
   (b) may be predicted based on angiographic findings
   (c) carries no added risk
   (d) all of the above
   (e) none of the above

8. External carotid endarterectomy:
   (a) carries significant risks when combined with EC/IC bypass
   (b) rarely requires patch closure
   (c) will frequently relieve amaurosis, but rarely hemispheric TIAs
   (d) all of the above
   (e) none of the above

9. Stroke-in-evolution:
   1. may be a manifestation of lacunar infarction
   2. suggests an unstable process in which urgent evaluation and therapy are indicated
   3. has a 10 per cent mortality with surgical therapy
   4. prompt medical therapy is preferable in view of the increased risk of surgery
   (a) 1,2,3
   (b) 1,3
   (c) 2,4
   (d) 4 only
   (e) none of the above

10. The following is/are true statements regarding carotid endarterectomy for acute stroke:
1. the risks of surgical intervention during the acute phase of a stroke are high; therefore, surgery is never indicated
2. if a CT scan done within 12 hours of the event is negative, endarterectomy can be safely performed
3. level of consciousness, hypertension, and/or severity of the deficit should not influence timing of surgical intervention
4. if the patient shows continuous recovery without deterioration, endarterectomy may be safely performed once a plateau has been reached

(a) 1,2,3
(b) 1,3
(c) 2,4
(d) 4 only
(e) none of the above

ANSWERS

1. e	2. a	3. b	4. c	5. b	6. b	7. e
8. a	9. a	10. a				

32

RECONSTRUCTION OF THE SUPRA-AORTIC TRUNKS AND VERTEBROBASILAR SYSTEM

RAMON BERGUER

The supra-aortic trunks (SATs) are that segment of the neck arteries crossing through the mediastinum that begins at the arch of the aorta and ends short of the carotid bifurcation and of the origin of the vertebral arteries. The trunks defined within these limits carry the entire blood supply to the head and upper extremities. The vertebrobasilar system is comprised of the two vertebral arteries and the basilar artery and its branches to the brainstem, cerebellum, and occipital lobes.

Occlusive disease of the SATs may result in symptoms of hemispheric (carotid) distribution or in manifestations of vertebrobasilar ischemia or both. The vertebrobasilar insufficiency may be secondary to poor inflow through both carotids and vertebral arteries, to a reversal of blood flow in the vertebral arteries caused by a proximal subclavian artery occlusion (subclavian steal), or to a reversal of both carotid and vertebral artery flow from an innominate artery occlusion.

Vertebral artery occlusive disease may, by restricting inflow into the basilar artery, result in vertebrobasilar insufficiency. The latter is more likely if compensatory flow from the carotid system is not available because of internal carotid occlusion or the absence of a well-developed posterior communicating artery.

The SATs are involved by atherosclerosis in the late years of life. This results in the development of plaques that may obstruct flow or embolize. Aneurysmal atherosclerotic disease of the SATs is rare. In other latitudes the SATs are a common site for arteritis of the Takayasu type, usually in younger individuals. Trauma and mycotic aneurysms of the SATs are uncommon but life-threatening conditions.

The incidence of atherosclerotic disease is lower in the trunks than in the more distal vessels (internal carotid and vertebral artery origins). However, the extensive study of extracranial arterial disease reported by Hass[1] showed that one third of the patients in the Joint Study undergoing arteriography had a severe lesion involving one or more of the SATs. The morphology of the atherosclerotic lesions of the SATs is also less well known than that of the plaques found in the internal carotid. This is partly due to the fact that for years the SATs were not routinely visualized during arteriography of the cerebral vessels. In addition, they are not accessible to ultrasonic examination, which has given us important morphologic information in other areas, notably in the carotid bifurcation. Since we have a limited knowledge of the natural history of these lesions, the facts upon which we draw our surgical indications are partly inferred. In addition, SAT lesions are often found in individuals who already have developed carotid and/ or vertebral artery disease, a situation that confuses the determination of the culprit lesion.

Stenosing lesions of the SATs are usually located at the origin of these vessels and often involve more than one artery. Since these plaques are located in the ostia, they are often continuous, with plaques of atheroma extending over the dome of the aortic arch. Outlining the lesions of the SATs by arteriography requires an arch injection, preferably in two projections (right and left posterior obliques). If the anatomic circumstances permit, the arteriographic study should also include selective injections of both carotid and subclavian arteries (four-vessel arteriogram). The very high incidence of concomitant carotid and/or vertebral artery lesions makes it mandatory to outline the entire extra- and intracranial circulation. The use of arteriographic intraarterial digital techniques has brought a substantial improvement in that lesser volumes of contrast material are now needed for these studies.

SYMPTOMS

Patients with occlusive disease of the SATs may present with symptoms of carotid basilar, and upper extremity arterial ischemia. It is traditionally believed that in SAT lesions the mechanism for the production of cerebral symptoms is restriction of blood flow rather than microembolization, but there is in fact no pathologic evidence to support this view. In stenosing lesions of the subclavian artery, both mechanisms—hypoperfusion and embolization—are observed. In patients with SAT disease the hemispheric symptoms are the same as those seen in internal carotid artery disease: hemisensory or motor deficits and amaurosis fugax. Likewise, the symptoms of vertebrobasilar insufficiency are the same as those caused by vertebrobasilar stenosis or occlusion, since the pathogenesis is the same (see later in this chapter).

Obliteration of the SATs is suggested by absent pulses in the neck (subclavian, carotid) or arm (axillary, brachial), in one or both sides, and the recording of an unequal or abnormally low pressure in the upper extremities. Waveforms recorded by Doppler tracings will be dampened in those vessels whose origins are stenosed or occluded. Bruits may or may not be present. In patients with subclavian steal, a pulse lag may be felt between both radial arteries or, more precisely, a pulse wave delay of 30 msec may be measured by recording simultaneously both brachial artery waveforms.[2] Claudication of the arm and/or digital artery embolization may be present in subclavian artery disease.

A computed tomography (CT) scan of the brain is an essential part of the workup of these patients. It will often reveal clinically unsuspected cerebral infarctions due to extra- or intracranial arterial disease.

In symptomatic vertebral (or basilar) artery occlusive disease the patient presents with any combination of the following symptoms: dizziness, vertigo, diplopia, perioral numbness, blurring of vision, tinnitus, ataxia, bilateral sensory deficits, and drop attacks. In the evaluation of these patients the mechanism that triggers the symptom must be sought. Patients with orthostatic hypotension usually develop symptoms when they stand abruptly after sitting or lying down. A recording of their blood pressure immediately after standing up will show a drop in systolic pressure greater than 20 mm Hg. This mechanism is particularly common in diabetics with sympathetic paralysis and loss of venomotor tone, who pool a substantial amount of blood volume in their legs upon standing.

The presence of vertebrobasilar ischemia related to turning of the neck may indicate osteophytic compression on the vertebral arteries or inner ear disease. In general, in patients with labyrinthine disorders symptoms appear with brief and very rapid head motion. Patients who develop symptoms by extrinsic compression of the vertebral arteries usually require a few seconds with the neck rotated in a particular direction to develop symptoms. In addition to orthostatism and osteophytic compression, there are other conditions capable of causing vertebrobasilar ischemia that must be ruled out. The most common are inappropriate antihypertensive medication, car-diac arrhythmias, anemia, brain tumors, and subclavian steal.

INDICATIONS

There is no data bank for the atherosclerotic lesions of the SATs comparable to that available for internal carotid artery disease. We know from arteriograms and postmortem studies that their incidence of disease is lower than that of the carotid bifurcation. On the other hand, we do not have the ability to use ultrasound to define the composition of these plaques. The specimens obtained at operation show degenerative features similar to those seen in carotid plaques: surface thrombus, ulceration, and intraplaque hemorrhage. It seems sensible to infer that the same pathologic mechanisms that operate in carotid artery plaques take place in these SAT lesions. Until more precise information is available it appears reasonable to use criteria similar to those that we follow in carotid disease to advance guidelines for surgical treatment. These criteria are to be tempered by the fact that the risk of surgical reconstruction of the SATs is generally higher than that of carotid endarterectomy.

Our indications for surgical repair of lesions of the SATs are: (1) lesions encroaching on more than 75 per cent of the cross-sectional area or plaques with ulceration or surface irregularities in patients with appropriate symptoms (ipsilateral carotid or vertebrobasilar); (2) the same lesions plus ipsilateral internal carotid disease for which an endarterectomy is indicated (the operation should correct both); (3) the same lesions plus a nonacute ipsilateral hemispheric infarction (overt or silent); and (4) preocclusive (greater than 90 per cent cross-sectional area loss) lesions in asymptomatic patients who are good surgical risks and have more than 5 years of life expectancy. This latter indication is arbitrary, albeit reasonable.

The primary indication for reconstructing a vertebral artery is to treat vertebrobasilar ischemia. Vertebral artery occlusive disease is a frequent anatomic finding in individuals who do not have vertebrobasilar ischemia. On the other hand, there are many systemic causes of vertebrobasilar ischemia that are not related to vertebral artery disease. Therefore, the indication for reconstructing a vertebral artery must be based on the strong anatomic and clinical presumption that the symptom (vertebrobasilar ischemia) is secondary to the anatomic lesion (occlusive disease of the vertebral arteries).

Vertebrobasilar ischemia may be due to stenosis or occlusion of the vertebral or basilar arteries, causing hypoperfusion of the territory. This is the so-called hemodynamic mechanism. These patients often have repetitive transient ischemic attacks (TIAs) triggered by positional or postural mechanisms. Although their risk for stroke is lower than in carotid disease, they may suffer serious traumatic injuries due to loss of balance. Ischemia of the vertebrobasilar territory may also be due to microembolization contrary to the previous group. These patients are at high risk for infarctions in the brainstem, cerebellum, and occipital lobes. The mechanism here is microembolization from a plaque in the proximal subclavian or vertebral arteries or from an inflammatory lesion in the wall of the vertebral artery secondary to repetitive trauma from an osteophyte.

In patients with hemodynamic symptoms of ischemia in the vertebrobasilar territory the surgical indication rests on the assumption that the basilar artery is not receiving adequate inflow from the vertebral arteries.

Because there are usually two vertebral arteries supplying one basilar artery, the presence of a normal vertebral artery contraindicates an operation on its opposite regardless of the anatomic condition of the latter. It is clinically well established that a vertebral artery of normal caliber emptying into a basilar artery is enough to supply appropriately the basilar territory. This means that for a lesion in the vertebral arteries to be considered significant, not only must it be severe (greater than 75 per cent stenosis) but the opposite vertebral artery must be equally diseased, hypoplastic, or absent.

Our approach to the patient with vertebrobasilar ischemia is first to determine whether any of the clinical conditions listed earlier as capable of producing these symptoms are present. If so, they should be corrected. If symptoms persist after treatment, an arteriogram is indicated. If the arteriogram shows a lesion that fulfills the anatomic criteria listed previously and the operation appears technically feasible a reconstruction of the vertebral arteries is indicated.

In patients with vertebrobasilar ischemia secondary to microembolization the indication for surgery rests on the demonstration of the embologenic lesion, regardless of the condition of the opposite vertebral artery.

TECHNIQUES FOR RECONSTRUCTION OF THE SUPRA-AORTIC TRUNKS

The main decision in reconstruction of the SATs is whether to do the repair through the chest or through the neck. Cervical repairs are traditionally done by means of a bypass between a good donor vessel and the diseased one. Most of these bypasses run transversely either between vessels on the same side of the neck (carotid and subclavian) or across the neck (remote bypasses). These operations are being partially superseded by translocation procedures that present the advantage of a single arterial anastomosis without the need for a saphenous vein or a prosthetic tube. Transthoracic or axial repairs require a midsternotomy for the direct approach to these vessels. The lesions are dealt with by endarterectomy or, more commonly, by a bypass from the ascending aorta.

The choice between transthoracic (axial) and cervical repairs (transverse) can be made under the following general guidelines. Axial repairs are preferred in younger patients who have innominate artery lesions or multiple lesions (usually innominate and left common carotid). They are also the natural choice in patients in whom a simultaneous coronary bypass operation is indicated. In patients with atherosclerotic disease of the SAT and coronary arteries it is advisable to repair concomitant severe lesions of the first segment of the left subclavian artery even though there may be no symptoms from the stenosis of this vessel. This repair will later permit a myocardial revascularization using the left internal mammary artery. Cervical repairs are preferred in older patients or those who are at high risk for thoracotomy, or who have had previous transsternal procedures, presenting with a single arterial lesion (other than the innominate artery).

Cervical Repairs

In the early 1970s techniques for revascularization of the SATs consisting of the insertion of a transverse bypass between a donor and a recipient (diseased) vessel became popular. The insertion of a bypass between the carotid and subclavian arteries, although described in 1957,[3] became popular in the 1970s. These bypasses were tended between the midportion of the carotid artery and the second (retroscalene) or third portions of the subclavian artery. In some cases the carotid artery acted as the donor vessel and the bypass corrected a blockage of the first portion of the subclavian artery. In others, the subclavian artery was the donor vessel to bypass a common carotid artery lesion. The original concern that when the carotid artery was the donor vessel these bypasses might divert too much flow into the subclavian and reduce distal carotid flow did not materialize. In subclaviocarotid bypasses, in which the anastomosis to the carotid artery is of the end-to-side type, there is the possibility of proximal embolization (from the diseased proximal common carotid) or of extension of the proximal thrombus across the end-to-side anastomosis. Because of this we advocate end-to-end anastomosis (see later) into the common carotid artery.

Carotosubclavian bypasses became the standard operation for the correction of subclavian steal syndrome in the 1970s. When it was not deemed advisable to use the carotid as the donor vessel (because it was the only carotid artery patent or because of significant disease in the common carotid artery), the correction of subclavian steal was achieved with bypasses tended between both subclavian or both axillary arteries. These remote subclaviosubclavian and axilloaxillary bypasses became known by the awkward name of extraanatomic operations. Although they have the undisputable advantage of avoiding a thoracotomy and of carrying a lower operative mortality, they do not achieve the same long-term patency rates as axial reconstructions. In the case of axilloaxillary bypasses the graft crosses in front of the sternum, giving a poor cosmetic result and being liable to external compression as well as interfering with a midsternotomy possibly required for coronary revascularization later on.

Most of the cervical bypasses done in the 1970s used saphenous vein as a preferred graft material. There was fear of embolization from the "neointima" of prosthetic tubes and doubts about their patency rates. However, saphenous veins also presented specific problems. They were not always available and there were often gross mismatches in caliber between the vein and the recipient arteries. In addition, the length involved in these remote bypasses brought the possibility of axial rotation and/or of compression or kinking of the vein with rotation of the neck. Because of this many surgeons explored prosthetic substitutes as the preferred material for these remote neck bypasses. The long-term results observed make them preferable to saphenous vein: they provide a good caliber match and their patency rates are excellent,[4] no doubt as a result of the high flow rates usually measured in these vessels.

Anatomic Indications for Cervical Repairs

Innominate Artery Occlusion/Stenosis. A variety of cervical techniques are available for the correction of innominate artery stenosis or occlusion. Subclaviosubclavian and axilloaxillary bypasses can supply the right carotid by retrograde flow in the subclavian or axillary artery. Uncommonly, the needed supply to the right common carotid or right subclavian may be derived through a remote bypass from the left subclavian artery. Carotocarotid bypasses are technically feasible, but for this particular indication they probably represent an unnecessary risk, since both carotid systems are severely hypotensive during insertion of the bypass in the donor left common carotid artery (unless shunted).

If the innominate artery lesion is suspected to be emboligenous or if it presents a grossly irregular surface or large ulcerations, this distal portion should be ligated at the completion of the procedure. This is not always possible using the supraclavicular approach. A complex solution to this need is an end-to-end anastomosis between the proximal subclavian and the proximal right common carotid artery, with ligation of the proximal carotid stump and then revascularization of the middle or distal third of the right subclavian through a remote bypass from the other side of the neck. In general, we prefer to do axial reconstructions in all innominate artery lesions.

Common Carotid Artery Occlusion/Stenosis. The common carotid can be revascularized by means of a subclaviocarotid bypass with the distal anastomosis being end-to-end to avoid embolization from the proximal common carotid artery. Even in those cases in which the entire carotid system on one side is not visualized on the arteriogram one must consider the possibility of the carotid bifurcation being intact, with retrograde flow from the external carotid perfusing the internal carotid artery. Delayed subtracted films may show this late opacification. Duplex imaging and flow recording is another expedient way to show patency of the bifurcation and its branches. In these circumstances there is usually an additional plaque at the origin of the internal carotid artery that will need to be cleared by endarterectomy. After amputation of the distal common carotid artery the carotid bulb is opened posteriorly and the endarterectomy of the internal carotid is done. At the completion of the endarterectomy the bypass from the subclavian artery is anastomosed to this spatulated bulb in an end-to-end fashion, supplying both external and internal carotid arteries.

An alternative method (Fig. 32–1) is to open the bifurcation as is usually done for an endarterectomy, clear the plaque in the distal common and proximal internal carotid arteries, and do an end-to-side anastomosis of the bypass to the arteriotomy as an "on-lay" patch. This end-to-side anastomosis is functionally transformed into an end-to-end junction by ligation of the common carotid artery below the anastomosis, in the soft segment created by endarterectomy of the distal portion of the common carotid artery.

If the common carotid artery is stenosed at its origin and its midportion is free of disease, the transposition of the midportion of the common carotid artery to the subclavian artery is a better procedure than the subclaviocarotid bypass. It requires only one anastomosis and no prosthetics. On occasion a thrombosed common carotid artery with a patent bifurcation can be thrombectomized after dividing its origin and doing an eversion endarterectomy, which is terminated under direct vision through the standard arteriotomy used for internal carotid endarterectomy. Following endarterectomy the common carotid is reimplanted into the second portion of the subclavian. Subclaviocarotid bypasses and transposition of the carotid into the subclavian are easier on the right side, where the subclavian artery is more accessible.

In those cases in which the ipsilateral subclavian artery is not a suitable donor vessel a common carotid artery lesion may be corrected by means of a carotocarotid bypass. This operation is traditionally done by subtending a bypass between both carotids in front of the airway. We prefer to use the shorter retropharyngeal route (see later in this chapter).

Subclavian Artery Occlusion. Most operations are done to correct a symptomatic subclavian steal, and a few for emboligenous lesions of the proximal subclavian. Carotosubclavian bypass is a proven operation to correct these problems. In those cases in which the subclavian lesion is thought to be a source of embolization, the prevertebral subclavian artery must be ligated at the time of the bypass. Our preference for the last 10 years has been to use a direct transposition of the subclavian artery (prevertebral portion) into the common carotid artery. Although the operation is slightly more complex technically, it

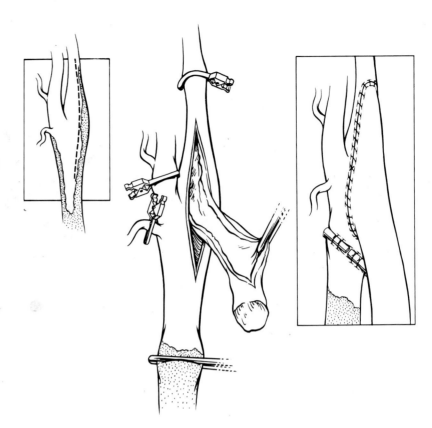

FIGURE 32–1. A method for anastomosing the limb of a graft to an endarterectomized carotid bulb. The occlusion of the common carotid artery immediately below the anastomosis transforms it into a functional end-to-end junction.

involves only one anastomosis and excludes the diseased proximal subclavian as well.

Description of the Techniques for Cervical Repair

Carotosubclavian or Subclaviocarotid Bypass and Carotid (or Subclavian) Transposition. The approach is through a supraclavicular incision dividing the clavicular head of the sternocleidomastoid. The dissection is first lateral to the jugular vein, which is retracted medially. The prescalene fat pad is entered and the scalenus anticus exposed. The subclavian artery may be isolated behind the scalenus anticus (second portion) or lateral to it (third portion). In the first case the phrenic nerve is isolated from the surface of the latter and, after division of the scalenus anticus, the subclavian artery is exposed. The site chosen for anastomosis is usually lateral to the thyrocervical trunk. Alternatively, the subclavian artery may be exposed in the third segment without dividing the scalenus anticus muscle.

The dissection is then moved medial to the jugular vein and the common carotid artery is exposed. A suitable site is selected for the anastomosis of the graft to the carotid artery. In the case of carotosubclavian bypass for subclavian steal, the vein graft or prosthetic tube is anastomosed to the side wall of the carotid artery and then tunneled under the jugular vein into proximity of the subclavian artery (Fig. 32–2). Both anastomoses are end-to-side.

If the bypass is intended to revascularize the common carotid artery, the subclavian artery anastomosis is done first and the graft is then tunneled under the jugular vein and anastomosed end-to-end to the common carotid artery, or to the bifurcation (Fig. 32–3), ligating the proximal carotid stump. Another alternative is to do an end-to-side anastomosis to the

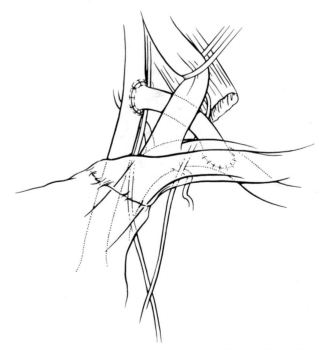

FIGURE 32–2. Carotosubclavian bypass graft tunneled under the jugular vein.

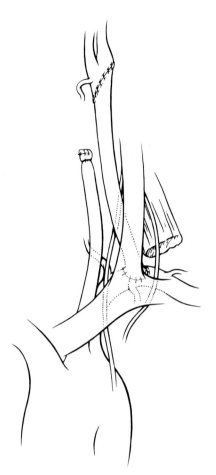

FIGURE 32–3. A bypass from the left subclavian artery to the left carotid bifurcation.

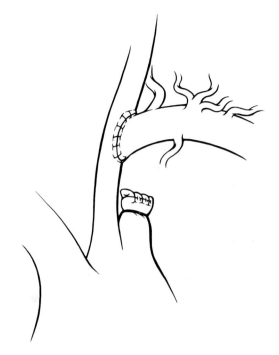

FIGURE 32–4. Transposition of the left subclavian artery to the left common carotid artery.

common carotid artery and ligate the common carotid artery immediately proximal to the anastomosis, which makes it functionally an end-to-end anastomotic junction. This is necessary to avoid proximal embolization from the proximal common carotid artery or extension of the thrombus from the common into the distal carotid artery.

Other than in cases of common carotid artery occlusion we seldom use the bypass technique between the carotid and subclavian arteries. The transposition of one of these vessels into the other (Fig. 32–4) is a better surgical solution in that only one artery-to-artery anastomosis is necessary. The long-term patency rates are superb. The drawbacks are some increased technical difficulty and the possibility of severe mediastinal bleeding from improper handling of the stump of the left subclavian artery. The transposition operation is particularly easy when the common carotid artery is the one being translocated; once freed, the common carotid, which has no branches, moves about the neck with ease. The translocation of the subclavian artery into the common carotid may be difficult on the left side, where the subclavian artery may have a deep location and where the vertebral artery may take a low origin. In cases in which this low origin interferes with good proximal control

of the short first portion of the subclavian, we have divided both the vertebral artery and the subclavian (distal to it) and reimplanted the subclavian artery into the common carotid artery and, separately, the vertebral artery in one of the two vessels. When translocating the subclavian artery care must be taken to assure proper position of the vertebral artery in the planned anastomosis. Excessive length in the vertebral artery once the subclavian artery is freed and moved upward may cause kinking of this vessel and its thrombosis. Although some have advocated division of the left internal mammary artery to facilitate the transposition, we believe this to be unnecessary, and probably unwise, as it negates the possibility of a later myocardial revascularization using the internal mammary artery.

Subclaviosubclavian Bypass. The incision is supraclavicular on both sides and the second or third portions of the subclavian are approached in the manner as described above. The tunnel connecting the two subclavian arteries is made behind the sternocleidomastoid, staying as low as possible to protect the graft behind the upper edge of the manubrium. Care is taken to avoid any axial rotation of the graft when tunneling across the neck.

Axilloaxillary Bypass. The axillary arteries are exposed between the sternal and clavicular heads of the pectoralis major. Removal of part or all of the pectoralis minor from the coracoid process improves exposure of the axillary artery. The graft is tunneled under the sternal part of the pectoralis major and through presternal subcutaneous tissue into the opposite axillary artery (Fig. 32–5). Both anastomoses are end-to-side.

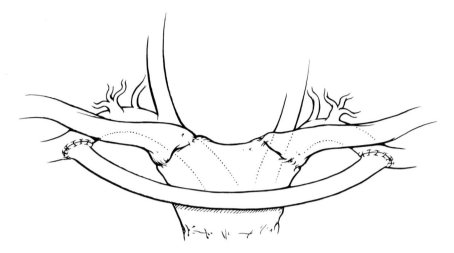

FIGURE 32–5. An axilloaxillary bypass.

Carotocarotid Bypass. This technique is used to revascularize a common carotid artery whose origin in the mediastinum is involved by disease. One carotid acts as donor vessel to the other. Since exposure of the common carotid arteries is a reasonably simple procedure, carotocarotid bypass is a good technique to revascularize one common carotid trunk when the other one is healthy and the ipsilateral subclavian artery is not suitable as a donor vessel. The bypass between both common carotid arteries lies low in the midline, partially hidden by the upper edge of the manubrium. Although these grafts make a rather lengthy loop and take off from the donor site at an oblique angle, their patency rate is excellent provided the donor vessel is free of disease. These bypasses are sometimes cosmetically poor and, as mentioned previously, the grafts run a lengthy trajectory to link two vessels that anatomically are only four finger-breadths apart. We prefer to subtend the bypass between both carotids through the retropharyngeal space (Fig. 32–6), which is a much shorter and therefore better path. The tunnel for the bypass is behind the pharynx and in front of the prevertebral lamina. This space is loose and admits easily a good-sized prosthesis without any pharyngeal compression.[5]

The distance between both carotids in the retropharyngeal space is short enough that it permits the direct reimplantation of one carotid into the other without a graft (Fig. 32–7). This procedure has the disadvantage of requiring clamping of both common carotid arteries simultaneously and because of this it is one of the few instances in which the protection of a shunt may be required to perfuse a clamped (donor) common carotid artery.

Axial Repairs

In reconstruction of the innominate artery endarterectomy was the first technique reported[6]; it was later formally described and perfected by Wylie and his group.[7] Endarterectomy has the appeal of being a true anatomic reconstruction and of avoiding the need for a prosthesis. Its main drawback is the difficulty of clamping the origin of the innominate artery without occluding the left common carotid artery or damaging the plaque that may be present about the ostium of the latter. A common origin for the innominate and left common carotid is present in 17 per cent of individuals. In addition, the left common carotid artery is a branch of the innominate in another 8 per cent of individuals. Additional difficulties may be encountered in terminating satisfactorily the endarterectomy in the aortic wall, where often tacking sutures are required. Finally, about half of the patients we see with symptomatic innominate artery stenosis have severe lesions of either the left common carotid or left subclavian artery. These concomitant lesions cannot be treated by endarterectomy using the transsternal approach.

We prefer currently to use a bypass from the ascending aorta to correct innominate and other associated lesions that may be present. The technique of

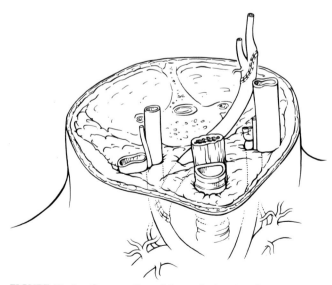

FIGURE 32–6. Cross-section of the neck showing the trajectory of a carotocarotid bypass through the retropharyngeal space.

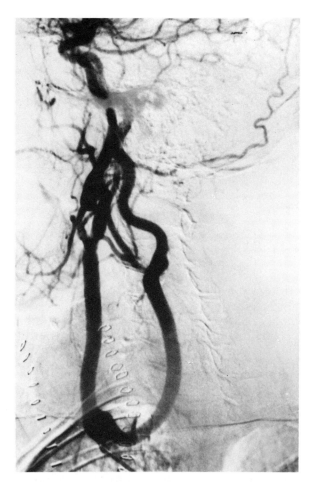

FIGURE 32–7. A direct transposition of the left carotid artery to the right common carotid artery using the retropharyngeal route. (From Berguer R: The short retropharyngeal route for arterial bypasses across the neck. Ann Vasc Surg 1:127–129, 1986.)

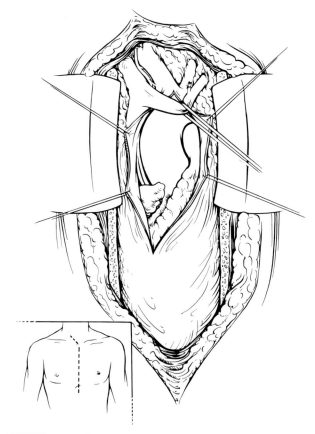

FIGURE 32–8. Exposure of the ascending aorta and anterior SATs.

bypass from the ascending aorta was introduced by DeBakey and his associates.[8] We reserve endarterectomy of the innominate artery for single and discrete lesions involving the distal two thirds of this vessel.

The approach to the vessels in the mediastinum is through a midsternotomy (Fig. 32–8). If either carotid bifurcation needs to be reached the sternotomy is prolonged through a short incision following the anterior edge of the sternocleidomastoid. After dividing the sternum the innominate vein is dissected and the thymic veins are ligated. The thymus is separated through its midline or reflected from one side onto the other. It is important to preserve the thymus to be used as tissue interposed between the graft and the sternum at the time of closure. The ascending aorta is approached below the innominate vein, opening the pericardial sac. The dissection continues over the origin of the innominate artery and onto its bifurcation. During dissection of the innominate bifurcation care is taken not to injure the recurrent nerve near the origin of the right subclavian artery. If the intent is to perform an innominate bypass or

endarterectomy, the origin of the right common carotid artery is also cleared.

Bypass from the Ascending Aorta

If the intent is to replace the innominate artery with a bypass no further neck dissection is necessary. More often, however, one and sometimes both carotid bifurcations need to be exposed to be revascularized. This is done by dissecting anterior to the sternocleidomastoid in the same manner as is done for a carotid endarterectomy. After obtaining control of the right subclavian and common carotid arteries an appropriate prosthetic tube is selected for the pass. We use a 10-mm polytetrafluoroethylene (PTFE) tube: it matches the caliber of the innominate artery, requires only a moderate amount of aortic wall to be excluded, and does not occupy much space in the anterior mediastinum.

The proximal end of the prosthesis is beveled and the patient is prepared for exclusion clamping of the proximal aorta. Secure clamping requires the use of nitroglycerin or nitroprusside and isoflurane to reduce the systemic pressure to about 110 mm Hg systolic. The exclusion clamp is placed on the proximal aorta (Fig. 32–9). With the clamp secured, the aorta is opened and the beveled end of the graft is anastomosed to the ascending aortotomy with a continuous 3-0 polypropylene suture. To avoid air embolization the patient is then placed in the Trendelenburg

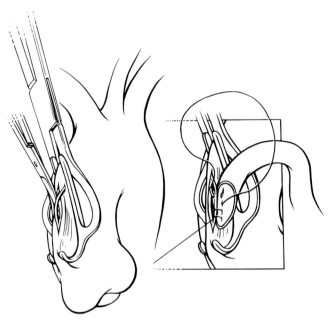

FIGURE 32–9. Exclusion clamping of the ascending aorta and anastomosis of the main prosthesis to the aortotomy.

position and, with the distal end of the graft pinched between the fingers, the proximal anastomosis is vented and tested. If found satisfactory a proximal clamp is placed immediately above the anastomosis and the table is returned to the horizontal position.

The patient is then systemically heparinized. Occluding clamps are placed first in the proximal right carotid and subclavian arteries and then in the midportion of the innominate artery. The innominate artery is divided distal to the proximal clamp and the distal innominate artery, immediately proximal to its bifurcation, is prepared for anastomosis. The bypass graft, which runs over the innominate vein, is cut to appropriate length and is anastomosed to the innominate artery with a continuous 5-0 polypropylene suture. The graft and the distal vessels are back-bled prior to completing the anastomosis, and flow is reestablished first into the right subclavian and then into the right common carotid artery. The proximal stump of the innominate artery is closed with a continuous double running suture and an additional proximal ligature.

In those cases in which additional arteries need to be revascularized (usually the left common carotid), an additional 8-mm PTFE side branch would have been anastomosed at an appropriate angle to the 10-mm PTFE main prosthesis, after the proximal suture line is completed. Adding side branches as needed before the distal anastomosis is done avoids having to reclamp the innominate portion of the bypass after having established flow through it. With the side branch anastomosed and excluded one can maintain perfusion in the right carotid (and vertebral) artery while the left carotid anastomosis is being done (Fig. 32–10).

In multiple replacements of the SATs the main

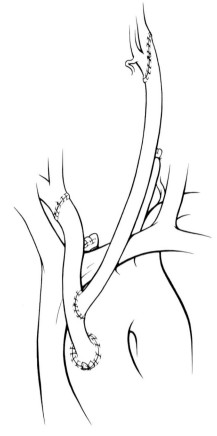

FIGURE 32–10. A common pattern for revascularization of the anterior SATs: the main prosthetic (10-mm PTFE) replaces the innominate artery and an 8-mm PTFE side branch supplies the left carotid system.

bypass is the one supplying the right-sided trunk (innominate or right carotid and right subclavian). From this trunk emerge the branches supplying the left carotid and/or the left subclavian arteries (Fig. 32–11).

Innominate Endarterectomy

The technique of endarterectomy of the innominate artery requires a midsternotomy and the same approach to the ascending aorta described previously. The innominate artery is dissected. The innominate vein crosses the innominate artery and it is retracted either superiorly or inferiorly to provide the best exposure. The patient is systemically heparinized and the carotid and subclavian clamps are placed first. A "J"-clamp is placed about the origin of the innominate artery, taking care not to involve the origin of the left common carotid artery in this exclusion clamping (Fig. 32–12). Enough rim of the aortic wall surrounding the origin of the innominate artery is included in the exclusion clamp to be able to properly terminate the endarterectomy and, as is often necessary, tack the edge of the intima to the aortic wall after removing the plaque. The endarterectomy plane is most obvious in the midportion of the innominate

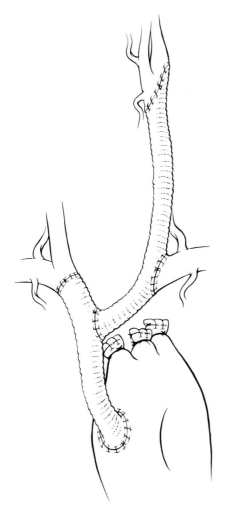

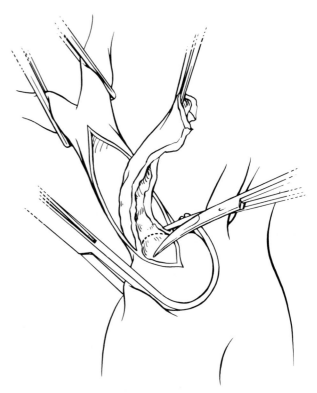

FIGURE 32–12. Endarterectomy of the innominate artery ends proximally at the level of the aortic arch. The intima of the latter is later affixed to the endarterectomized wall of the innominate artery by a continuous monofilament suture to avoid retrograde dissection when flow is reestablished.

FIGURE 32–11. Revascularization of all three SATs completed by transposing the left subclavian to the prosthetic that replaces the left carotid system.

artery and should be at the level of the internal elastic membrane (superficial). Tacking sutures may be needed proximally at the origin of the innominate artery from the aortic arch. Sometimes endarterectomy has to be carried out beyond the bifurcation of the innominate artery and into one of its branches because of ostial lesions at the origin of the subclavian or common carotid arteries.

The closure of the arteriotomy may require a patch. Prior to completing the closure the patient is placed in the Trendelenburg position, the distal and proximal arteries are bled into the wound, and flow is reestablished by removing first the subclavian, then the aortic, and finally the common carotid clamp.

Results and Complications of the Reconstruction of the Supra-Aortic Trunks

Transthoracic reconstructions are generally done in younger individuals with multiple vessel involve-

ment. Cervical repairs are done in older individuals, less likely to tolerate a thoracotomy, who have single-vessel disease.

It is difficult to compare the results of the thoracic and cervical approach in the experience published in the literature because the groups of patients in whom a transthoracic or a cervical repair are advised are different. In addition to age and anatomic extent of disease there are other considerations that weigh in the choice of the approach, such as pulmonary function, previous coronary artery bypass surgery, and life expectancy.

Our experience with reconstruction of the SAT encompasses 199 cases; 128 cervical and 71 transthoracic reconstructions. At the beginning of the experience we favored cervical repairs in patients who carried a high cardiopulmonary risk. In the last 5 years we have favored simultaneous transthoracic repair of the SAT and myocardial revascularization. The most frequent indication for a cervical repair in our practice is previous myocardial revascularization or single-trunk disease (carotid or subclavian artery). Innominate artery lesions are operated through the chest.

Operative mortality for transthoracic repair may range from 3 to 19 per cent,[9,10] with most authors reporting series of 20 to 40 patients and some smaller series reporting no mortality.[11] Increasing experience, refinement in anesthesia and perioperative care, and better patient selection have brought down the mortality of transthoracic repair from 10 to 5 per cent in the reports of the Baylor group[10,12] and from 10 to 4 per cent from the first to the second half of our experience.

In the literature, the mortality for cervical repairs has been considered lower than for thoracic repairs and has been reported between 0 and 4 per cent. In our series, the stroke/TIA morbidity in patients undergoing cervical repair has been higher (10 per cent) and concentrated in the early part of our experience when patients with evidence of intracranial disease were not systematically excluded from surgery. In our series, patients undergoing cervical repair are among the highest risk in the group with cerebrovascular disease. Patients who have had previous myocardial revascularization procedures and those with severe pulmonary disease are more likely to undergo a cervical operation.

The higher morbidity noted in our earlier experience with cervical reconstructions has dropped dramatically. Over the last 10 years we have switched operative techniques and noted a fall in operative complications and an increase in patency rates. While 10 years ago we often did subclaviocarotid and carotosubclavian grafts, today most of these reconstructions are done by direct transposition of one vessel to the other. The improvement in patency rates and the decrease in reoperations has been substantial. The patency rate for transposition procedures has been 100 per cent.

Likewise, the techniques for transthoracic reconstruction have been refined and extended. Endarterectomy of the innominate artery is now a rare operation. We often combine myocardial revascularization with bypass from the ascending aorta. In addition we attempt to revascularize the left subclavian artery in patients who may later be candidates for myocardial revascularization. In our series, the mortality and morbidity for cervical and transthoracic repair has been similar. This may be a reflection of our selection of patients, which has changed during the last decade. Table 32–1 shows the incidence of death and stroke after cervical and transthoracic repair in our entire series.

The most frequent and serious complication reported after either cervical or transthoracic repair of the SATs is myocardial infarction.[4,13] The second most frequent complication is stroke, which may develop during the operation or after 3 to 4 days. The latter may be hemorrhagic and probably related to hyperperfusion and regional hypertension. In our experience stroke has been a more frequent complication than myocardial infarction. Perioperative strokes are more common in patients with multiple intra- and extracranial involvement.[10] Some may be due to technical mishaps resulting in distal embolization. Clamping time ischemia may be the cause of some operative strokes, and the usual cerebral protection methods have been reported by different authors. We do not use shunts in repair of the SATs with the rare exception listed under the description of carotocarotid bypass and in the rare patient with a left carotid arising as a branch of the innominate in whom an endarterectomy of the latter is indicated. In the latter case we use a temporary aorta-left carotid shunt.

Technical problems may cause peri- or postoperative bleeding, which can be severe and life threatening. Suture line bleeding, aortic wall tears from clamp or suture injury, and bleeding from a ligated arterial stump may result in serious operative bleeding or severe mediastinal compression postoperatively.

Postoperative graft thrombosis and infections are rare. The long-term outcome of these patients is largely determined by their atherosclerotic disease. Ten-year survival is less than 50 per cent,[12-14] with myocardial infarction being the most common cause of death. Late stroke is the second ranking cause of long-term mortality.

The long-term patency of these reconstructions is different for transthoracic repair, in which it is excellent,[12] than for traditional cervical bypasses, in which 3- and 5-year patency rates have been reported as 76 and 85 per cent, respectively.[4,14] Transpositions, however, have the best patency rate of all cervical repairs, which has been 100 per cent in our series of cases. Saphenous veins fare worse than synthetics in cervical repairs: axial rotation, caliber mismatch, kinking, and intimal hyperplasia probably account for this.

In conclusion, cervical reconstruction is indicated in patients who have had previous myocardial revascularization and in those with single lesions of the common carotid or subclavian arteries. In this last group, our preference today is to use transposition techniques between the carotid or subclavian or, if the midline needs to be crossed, a retropharyngeal bypass. These techniques using short (retropharyngeal) bypasses or no bypasses at all have outstanding patency rates that contrast with the poor patency rates reported for the conventional "extraanatomic" bypasses. The transthoracic approach is favored for patients with multiple-vessel disease. It may be done in conjunction with coronary artery bypass grafts. This approach should be confined to centers with experience in these techniques where the operative mortality is similar to that obtained in cervical repairs.[12]

RECONSTRUCTION OF THE VERTEBROBASILAR SYSTEM

Two types of vertebral artery reconstructions are done: reconstructions of its proximal segment for

TABLE 32–1. INCIDENCE OF DEATH AND STROKE/TIA FOLLOWING CERVICAL AND TRANSTHORACIC REPAIR

	Number	Stroke/TIA[a]	Death
Cervical repair	128	10%	4%
Transthoracic repair	71	4%	6%

[a]TIA, transient ischemic attack.

stenosing disease of the ostium and distal vertebral reconstructions for compression or thrombosis of the intraspinal portion of this artery.

Reconstruction of the Proximal Vertebral Artery

Although the first reconstructions of the vertebral arteries were endarterectomies,[15-17] this technique is seldom used today. Vertebral artery bypass was advocated in the 1970s.[18] Today most proximal vertebral artery lesions are dealt with by transposition[19] of the artery into the neighboring common carotid artery. The appeal of this operation is that it consists of one anastomosis and does not require a vein graft (needed for bypass) or the dissection of the subclavian artery (needed for endarterectomy) (Fig. 32–13).

The operation is done through a supraclavicular incision. The approach is between the bellies of the sternocleidomastoid muscles. The vertebral artery is isolated below the vertebral vein, dissected from its origin up to the point where it disappears under the longus colli, and freed from the overlying stellate ganglion or crossing sympathetic fibers. After clearing the adventitia of the chosen transposition site in the posterolateral wall of the common carotid artery, the patient is heparinized and the vertebral artery is divided above the stenotic area, suture-ligating its proximal stump. The distal segment of the artery is swung into the common carotid artery (Fig. 32–14). A small arteriostomy is made in the common carotid wall with an aortic punch and the vertebral artery is translocated to this orifice in end-to-side fashion using a 7-0 polypropylene suture and an open-type anastomosis.

In a few instances this technique is not possible. The most common problems are a contralateral common/internal carotid artery occlusion or a short first segment of the vertebral artery entering the cervical spine through the transverse process of C7 rather than that of C6. In this situation, if the artery is too short to be brought easily to the common carotid artery wall, it can be bypassed from the subclavian artery using a saphenous vein graft.[18] The bypass takes origin from the subclavian artery lateral to the thyrocervical trunk and is anastomosed end-to-end to the vertebral artery below the longus colli muscle. This procedure does not require any type of shunting. The most frequent complications are partial Horner's syndrome from manipulation (or injury) of the intermediate or stellate ganglia overlying the vertebral artery and an occasional lymphocele from injury to or inappropriate ligature of the main or accessory thoracic ducts.

Reconstruction of the Distal Vertebral Artery

Regardless of the level below C2 at which the external compression or the occlusive process takes place,

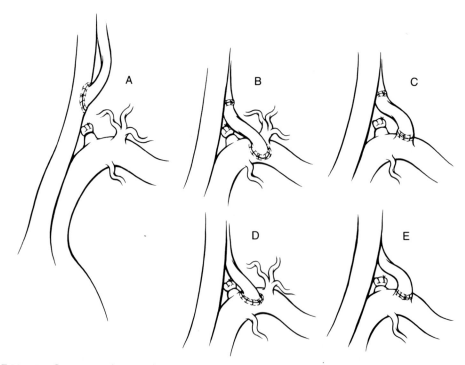

FIGURE 32–13. Common techniques for reconstruction of the proximal vertebral artery. *A,* Transposition of the proximal vertebral artery to the common carotid artery. *B,* Bypass from the subclavian to the proximal vertebral artery. *C,* Subclaviovertebral bypass taking origin in the amputated stump of the thyrocervical trunk. *D,* Transposition of the vertebral artery to another subclavian site. *E,* Transposition of the vertebral artery to the stump of the thyrocervical trunk.

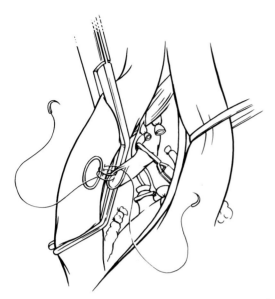

FIGURE 32–14. Technique for transposing the left vertebral artery to the left common carotid artery. The thoracic duct is seen doubly ligated. The proximal vertebral artery stump has been clipped and suture ligated. The sympathetic chain left intact is now seen behind the distal segment of the vertebral artery as the latter is brought to the common carotid artery for its anastomosis.

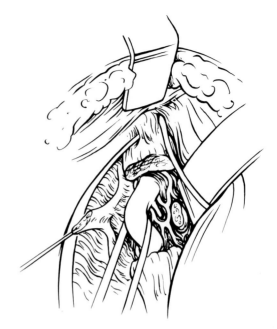

FIGURE 32–15. The vertebral artery is isolated between the transverse process of C1 and C2. The anterior ramus of the C2 nerve has been divided and is pulled out of the field by a stay suture. The artery has been dissected away from the surrounding vertebral plexus, which is now seen behind it.

the distal vertebral artery is reconstructed at the space between the C1 and C2 transverse processes. This is the widest gap between transverse processes in the neck and is also the segment where the vertebral artery is often maintained patent by collaterals from the occipital artery, even though the proximal segment of the artery may be occluded.[20,21]

The operation is done through an incision similar to that used for carotid endarterectomy. Exposure of the vertebral artery at this level requires dissecting posterior to the jugular vein, and identifying the spinal accessory nerve and the levator scapula muscle. The levator is cut and the transverse course of the anterior ramus of the C2 nerve is exposed. The artery lies below the ramus and is perpendicular to it. The ramus is cut and the artery is exposed. Dissection of the vertebral artery is made difficult by the plexus of veins that surrounds it.

Once the artery is isolated (Fig. 32–15) it can be reconstructed in several ways. The classic reconstruction is a bypass from the common carotid artery to the distal vertebral artery immediately below the transverse process of C1 using autogenous vein (Fig. 32–16). This requires dissection of the common carotid below the bifurcation and the availability of a saphenous vein with a size matching that of the vertebral artery.

Another alternative is to use the external carotid artery (or, in rare cases, the occipital artery) to revascularize the distal vertebral artery (Fig. 32–17). The external carotid is skeletonized and transposed below the jugular vein, anastomosing it end-to-end to the distal vertebral artery. The appeal of this procedure is that it does not require clamping the in-

ternal carotid supply and that the caliber match between the distal external carotid artery and the vertebral artery is usually good. This choice obviously requires the external carotid and, for that matter, the carotid bifurcation to be free of atherosclerotic disease. We have used this type of operation most

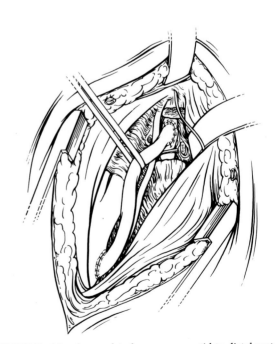

FIGURE 32–16. A completed common carotid to distal vertebral artery bypass graft. A metal clip occludes the distal vertebral artery immediately below the anastomosis, making the latter a functional end-to-end junction.

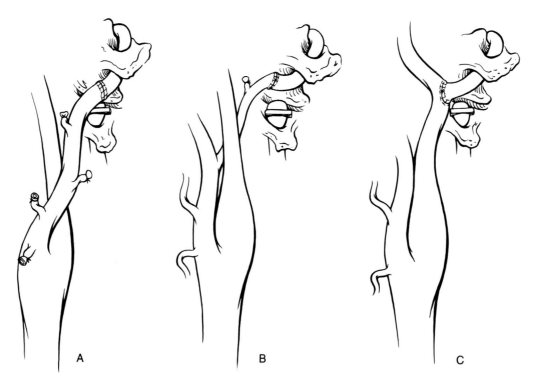

FIGURE 32–17. Alternative methods of reconstruction of the distal vertebral artery. *A,* External carotid transposition to the distal vertebral artery. *B,* Occipital artery transposition to the distal vertebral artery. *C,* Transposition of the distal vertebral artery to the distal cervical internal carotid artery.

often in individuals who have external compression/occlusion of the vertebral artery by osteophytes during neck rotation, who are generally younger and free of disease in the carotid bifurcation.

A third solution is translocation of the distal segment of the vertebral artery into the internal carotid artery by means of an end-to-side anastomosis. This again has the appeal of a limited dissection and the lack of need of a vein graft. The shortcoming is that one needs to clamp the internal carotid artery for the end-to-side anastomosis. This technique should not be used in patients in whom the opposite internal carotid artery is severely diseased or occluded.

Results and Complications of Reconstructions of the Vertebral Arteries

The risks and patency rates of vertebral artery operations are different for proximal and distal repairs. Proximal reconstructions are technically easier. Distal reconstructions are more demanding and lengthier procedures.

It is noteworthy that among patients undergoing isolated proximal or distal vertebral artery reconstruction the 10-year survival rates are 84 and 82 per cent, respectively.

We have done 172 proximal vertebral artery reconstructions, with a 1.1 per cent combined mortality and morbidity. The cumulative secondary patency rate for these proximal reconstructions has been 92 per cent at 10 years.

In 55 distal vertebral artery reconstructions the combined mortality/morbidity has been 3.6 per cent, over three times higher than that found in proximal repairs. Kieffer,[21] in a larger series, has reported a 2.4 per cent mortality.

Postoperative thrombosis of a proximal reconstruction is rare. We have seen this complication in 3 of 140 cases. In all three cases there was a short vertebral artery (entering at C7) that could not be repaired by a subclavian-vertebral bypass because of subclavian artery disease. In one case tension at the anastomotic line and in two others a kink in an interposition vein graft resulted in postoperative thrombosis. All patients were reoperated, underwent thrombectomy, and the technical flaw was corrected. They have remained patent after 3, 5, and 7 years.

Postoperative thrombosis of distal vertebral artery reconstructions has been higher. We have seen it in 4 of 55 distal reconstructions. The causes were faulty anastomoses and/or inadequate vein grafts. Thrombectomy and the insertion of a new graft reestablished patency in two of the four failures.

Other complications of proximal reconstruction have been an occasional lymphocele, a partial Horner's syndrome from manipulation/injury to the lower cervical sympathectics. In one case of distal reconstruction we noted an injury to the spinal accessory nerve.

Clinical symptoms have been relieved in 83 per cent of the patients.[18,21]

REFERENCES

1. Hass WK, Fields WS, North RR, et al: Joint study of extracranial arterial occlusion. II. Arteriography, techniques, sites, and complications. JAMA *203*:159, 1968.
2. Berguer R, Higgins RF, Nelson R: Noninvasive diagnosis of reversal of vertebral flow. N Engl J Med *301*:1349–1351, 1980.
3. Lyons C, Gailbraiter G: Surgical treatment of atherosclerotic occlusion of the internal carotid artery. Ann Surg *146*:487–494, 1957.
4. Criado FJ: Extrathoracic management of aortic arch syndrome. Br J Surg *69*(suppl):545, 1982.
5. Berguer R: The retropharyngeal route for arterial bypasses across the neck. Ann Vasc Surg *1*:155–156, 1986.
6. David JB, Grove WJ, Julian OC: Thrombotic occlusion of the branches of the aortic arch, Martorell's syndrome: Report of a case treated surgically. Ann Surg *144*:124–126, 1956.
7. Carlson RE, Ehrenfeld WK, Stoney RJ, et al: Innominate artery endarterectomy: A 16-year experience. Arch Surg *112*:1389, 1977.
8. DeBakey ME, Morris GC, Jordan GL, et al: Segmental thrombo-obliterative disease of branches of aortic arch. JAMA *166*:988, 1958.
9. Brewster DC, Moncure AC, Darling RC, et al: Innominate artery lesions: Problems encountered and lessons learned. J Vasc Surg *2*:99, 1985.
10. DeBakey ME, Crawford ES, Cooley DA, et al: Surgical considerations of occlusive disease of the innominate, carotid, subclavian and vertebral arteries. Ann Surg *149*:690–710, 1959.
11. Thompson BW, Read RC, Campbell GS: Operative correction of proximal blocks of the subclavian or innominate arteries. J Cardiovasc Surg *21*:125, 1980.
12. Zelenock GB, Cronenwett JL, Graham LM, et al: Brachiocephalic arterial occlusions and stenoses: Manifestations and management of complex lesions. Arch Surg *120*:370–376, 1985.
13. Crawford ES, Stowe CL, Powers RW Jr: Occlusion of the innominate, common carotid, and subclavian arteries: Long term results of surgical treatment. Surgery *94*:781, 1983.
14. Vogt DP, Mertzer NR, O'Hara PJ, et al: Brachiocephalic arterial reconstruction. Ann Surg *196*:541, 1982.
15. Moore WS, Malone JM, Goldstone J: Extrathoracic repair of branch occlusions of the aortic arch. Am J Surg *132*:249, 1976.
16. Cate WR, Scott HW: Cerebral ischemia of central origin: Relief by subclavian vertebral artery thromboendarterectomy. Surgery *45*:19, 1959.
17. Imparato AM, Lin JPT: Vertebral artery reconstruction: Internal plication and vein patch angioplasty. Ann Surg *166*:213, 1967.
18. Natali J, Maraval M, Kieffer E: Surgical treatment of stenosis and occlusion of the carotid and vertebral arteries. J Cardiovasc Surg *13*:4, 1972.
19. Berguer R, Bauer RB: Vertebral artery reconstruction: A successful technique in selected patients. Ann Surg *193*:441, 1981.
20. Roon AJ, Ehrenfeld AJ, Cooke PB, et al: Vertebral artery reconstruction. Am J Surg *138*:29, 1980.
21. Berguer R: Distal vertebral artery bypass: Technique, the "occipital connection" and potential uses. J Vasc Surg *2*:621, 1985.
22. Kieffer E, Rancurel G, Richard T: Reconstruction of the distal cervical vertebral artery. *In* Berguer R, Bauer RB (eds): Vertebrobasilar Arterial Occlusive Disease. New York, Raven Press, 1984, p 265.
23. McNamara MF, Berguer R: Simultaneous carotid-vertebral reconstruction. J Cardiovasc Surg *30*:101–164, 1989.

33

VASCULAR DISEASE OF THE UPPER EXTREMITY AND THE THORACIC OUTLET SYNDROMES

HERBERT I. MACHLEDER

The upper extremities are subject to a variety of unique intrinsic arterial and venous disorders, as well as the peripheral manifestations of systemic collagen vascular diseases. The extensive use of the upper extremities for venous and arterial vascular access additionally results in a host of problems requiring recognition and management by the vascular surgical specialist.

Patients developing arterial insufficiency of the upper extremities will generally demonstrate one of three different clinical patterns: (1) attacks of Raynaud's disease symptoms, (2) digital ischemia and gangrene, or (3) crampy pain with exercise, often referred to (with disregard for the word origin) as claudication. The uniformity of clinical symptoms belies the multiplicity of underlying diseases, which range from relatively simple cases of trauma to complex autoimmune and connective tissue disorders. This complexity of underlying disease requires a methodical approach to ensure expeditious diagnosis and an effective therapeutic plan.

A peculiar blanching and cyanosis of the fingertips characterizes upper extremity vascular insufficiency. Raynaud put it rather succinctly in the introduction to this second treatise on vasospastic syndromes affecting the upper extremity:

In the slight cases the ends of the fingers and toes become cold, cyanosed, and livid, and at the same time more or less painful. In grave cases the area affected by cyanosis extends upwards for several centimeters above the roots of the nails; . . . finally, if this state is prolonged for a certain time, we see gangrenous points appear on the extremities; the gangrene is always dry, and may occupy the superficial layers of the skin from the extent of a pin's head up to the end of a finger, rarely more.[1]

The initial evaluation should enable differentiation of arterial and venous obstruction, the recognition of chronologic elements of the obstructive phenomena (such as repetitive events versus a single isolated and progressive event) and whether or not the ischemic symptom is related to vasospasm or true arterial occlusion. It is also important to recognize at the outset whether the vascular manifestations in the upper extremity are symmetrical, part of a generalized process, or are confined to an isolated event in the affected extremity.

Raynaud's phenomenon, which is characteristic of the early onset of many types of vascular occlusive phenomena, is generally quite evident to the patient and is noticed as a blanching of a single digit, perhaps symmetrically disposed to both upper extremities, usually precipitated by a drop in temperature, which may, however, be quite slight (of only several degrees' magnitude). The blanching becomes cadaveric in appearance and the finger becomes numb, and then within seconds to minutes, and occasionally longer, the blanching is replaced by a mottled, deeply cyanotic, and ruborous appearance. The return of capillary filling is generally accompanied by dysesthesia and occasionally frank burning pain. The symptom may spread to other digits, as time progresses, and in fact may involve the entire hand unilaterally or both hands symmetrically. Occasionally this sequence of events can be seen in traumatic situations, which although not specifically linked to temperature changes, may well be exacerbated by exposure to cold.

VASCULAR EXAMINATION OF THE UPPER EXTREMITY

The initial examination of the upper extremity should begin with *inspection* for color changes; areas of gangrene; discoloration such as blanching, cyanosis, and livido reticularis; or areas of erythema. A note should be made of abnormal distention of veins, particularly related to positional changes of the upper extremity. Ordinarily prominent veins on the dorsum of the

592

hand and antecubital fossa should be flat as the arms reach the cardiac position. Observation of marked collateral vessels, particularly around the shoulder, should be noted, particularly if they are asymmetrical. When venous obstruction is suspected, measurement of recumbent venous pressure in an antecubital vein can be easily done with a spinal manometer filled with saline.

Palpation should follow inspection and should involve palpation of the carotid arteries bilaterally, and for prominent pulsations in the supraclavicular area, as well as assessment of the axillary, brachial, radial, and ulnar pulses. The Allen's test should be performed routinely in assessing the arterial competence of the palmar arch. The test is performed in the following manner, evaluating one hand at a time. With the patient facing the examiner, palmar surface of the hand up, both the radial and ulnar arteries are compressed. The examiner's thumb is placed on the arteries and the remaining digits are placed along the back of the patient's wrist. The arteries are compressed while the patient clenches his fist to evacuate blood from the hand. When the hand is opened, the palm has a pale, mottled appearance. Radial artery compression is released first, whereupon prompt color or even reactive hyperemia should appear on the entire palmar surface of the hand. In the presence of radial artery occlusion, the pallor remains and mottling continues. When there is insufficient collateral flow across the palmar arch, only the radial portion of the hand will be perfused, and the ulnar part of the hand will remain blanched and mottled. When the ulnar artery is then released, color will return to the ulnar aspect of the hand. The examiner next repeats the test by compressing the radial and ulnar artery with the thumbs while the patient clenches his hand, and then opens it, revealing the blanched, mottled appearance. Compression is then released from the ulnar artery, and again, if normal, prompt blushing of the hand or even reactive hyperemia should occur. In the event of ulnar artery occlusion, the hand remains white and mottled; if there is insufficient collateral circulation across the palmar arch, perfusion of only the ulnar aspect of the hand will be apparent. The test is then repeated on the contralateral extremity. When properly performed, this test is extremely accurate, with a high degree of sensitivity and specificity.

Auscultation is an important part of upper extremity examination and should begin in the supraclavicular fossa. Subclavian bruits often begin just lateral to the palpable carotid pulse at the base of the neck and will radiate toward the acromioclavicular joint and below the middle third of the clavicle toward the axilla. Auscultation should be done bilaterally with the arm in the neutral position, and then with Adson's maneuver. Auscultation should then be performed with the diaphragm of the stethoscope placed just beneath the middle third of the clavicle as the arm is gradually brought into the abducted and externally rotated position. This is done while palpating the radial pulse, and if obliteration of the radial pulse occurs, careful auscultation should be then augmented by moving the stethoscope laterally in the infraclavicular area, then medially in the supraclavicular area in an attempt to detect any site of compressive occlusion. Bruits in this area are typically obliterated over a few degrees of the abduction and external rotation arc, and the maneuver must be performed slowly so that the point of maximum bruit can be ascertained. Placing the arm in a full abducted and externally rotated position may totally obliterate the pulse, and the bruit may be overlooked.

The bell and diaphragm of the stethoscope should be used to auscultate over any abnormal group of veins or angiomatous malformation. Arteriovenous fistulas will often be identified in this manner, and this technique is highly accurate in identifying this type of lesion.

VASCULAR LABORATORY DIAGNOSIS

Noninvasive vascular testing can be utilized to further document disorders that may be suggested by symptoms or subtle physical findings. The systolic pressure should be measured at the brachial artery and at the radial or ulnar artery with the patient supine and the arm in the neutral position. This is done by placing the blood pressure cuff around the upper arm in a manner identical to that used in assessing the standard blood pressure using auscultation for Korotkoff's sounds. The vascular examination uses the Doppler flow detector to assess the exact point of initiation of systolic flow. The flow detector is placed over the antecubital brachial artery, and the pressure cuff is inflated until arterial signals are obliterated. Pressure is slowly released, and the pressure is noted at which the initial thumping arterial sound resumes (Fig. 33–1). By doing this first over the brachial artery and then over the radial and ulnar with the cuff moved to the forearm, segmental pressures can be recorded that may further indicate a site of obstruction if this should be the case. If thoracic outlet obstruction is a possibility, the test should be repeated with the patient in the sitting position. It is difficult to elicit vascular compressive signs of

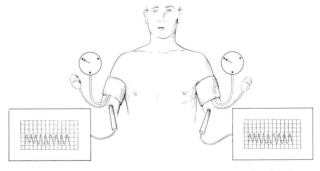

FIGURE 33–1. Use of the Doppler flow detector for the determination of brachial artery pressures.

thoracic outlet compression when the patient is recumbent.

The sensitivity of all tests must be well recognized by the examiner, and it should be specifically understood that reductions of cross-sectional area in an artery less than 75 per cent or reductions of cross-sectional diameter less than 50 per cent will rarely result in a pressure drop unless specific measures are used to reduce peripheral resistance and increase flow rates (such as reactive hyperemia or specific ergometric testing).

A specific and detailed history of positional characteristics that bring on symptoms of arterial or venous obstruction must be documented and these positions utilized when performing a variety of arterial and venous tests. The extensive collateralization of the upper extremity may lead to a paucity of signs and symptoms at rest in the face of severe disability when specific muscle groups are called upon during work or recreational activity.

As in the lower extremity, the more distal the obstruction (especially in the presence of tandem lesions), the more severe will be the pressure drop appreciated peripherally. Occasionally, differences of up to 15 mm Hg between the two upper extremities may be within the normal range and can be accounted for by the extreme sensitivity of the upper extremity vessels to sympathetic innervation and minute changes in peripheral resistance. In general, an occlusion at the level of the subclavian artery will result in a pressure drop of between 30 and 40 mm Hg. When evaluating upper extremity pressures that are symmetrical, particularly in the face of other evidence of vascular insufficiency, an ankle-brachial index should be assessed in an attempt to recognize symmetrical occlusions of the major aortic branches, as occur in some varieties of arteritis. When suspicion is high, oculopneumoplethysmography can also be used in an attempt to assess the true central arterial pressure in the event of symmetrical subclavian occlusive disease (Figs. 33–2 and 33–3).

The presence of an abnormal Allen's test on the initial examination should always be further assessed by measuring segmental pressures with the probe placed over the radial as well as the ulnar artery in an attempt to establish the level of occlusive disease. In more sophisticated testing, small finger cuffs can

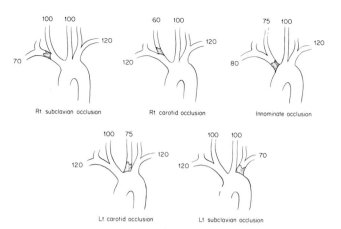

FIGURE 33–3. Representative pressures obtained from oculopneumoplethysmography and Doppler brachial artery pressure measurements in typical occlusive lesion of the brachiocephalic vessels.

be used to assess individual digital artery pressures. This can be done either with a Doppler flow probe or with a mercury strain gauge or digital photoplethysmograph.

The significant reactivity of the digital vessels to sympathetic stimulation should alert the examiner to changes in ambient temperature as well as changes in the patient's apprehension during the examination. Insensitivity to these factors may often give rise to results that in retrospect become difficult to interpret. Many individuals have a dramatic response to smoking, which may last from 1 to 8 hours after even a single cigarette. Before embarking on these sensitive arterial evaluations, the history of recent smoking must be noted.

Digital plethysmography can be useful in differentiating proximal from distal arterial obstructive phenomena, and the effect of reactive hyperemia on the pulse wave pattern will also differentiate primary Raynaud's disease from Raynaud's phenomenon associated with collagen vascular diseases. When vasodilatation is effected either by immersing the hand in warm water or applying a cuff to maintain ischemia for 5 minutes, patients with primary vasospastic syndromes will demonstrate a normal return of pulse volume and curve characteristics. Those with collagen diseases, however, have vascular obstructive phenomena secondary to intimal proliferation or deposition of immune complexes and will have fixed lesions that demonstrate minimal, if any, change after reactive hyperemia. These tests are extremely useful in assessing the potential response to vasodilating or sympatholytic therapies.[2]

In addressing the upper extremity arterial circulation, the examiner should become familiar with the normal and abnormal Doppler signal, which is obtained from peripheral vessels. The ordinary signal is described as triphasic, but can be appreciated only by assiduous listening, to establish a good baseline for recognition. Although tracings can be subjected to more sophisticated analysis, this should rarely be neces-

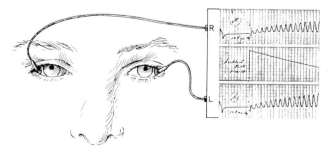

FIGURE 33–2. Use of oculopneumoplethysmography to assess carotid artery pressure as reflected in ophthalmic artery pressure.

sary in all but the most extensive of upper extremity vascular evaluations. The normal high-frequency short burst of systolic flow, followed by a short low-pitched diastolic component, is easily recognized and can be detected in other peripheral vessels that clinically do not seem involved in the disease process. The abnormal flow sound is usually described as monophasic, is of lower frequency and longer duration, and is more undulant in quality. At times it approaches the venous signal, which can be utilized as a reference. Segmental auscultation with the Doppler flowmeter can often reveal the site of obstruction without more sophisticated testing.

The need for sequential performance of these tests cannot be overemphasized, because the Allen test will often identify an obstruction in the radial or ulnar artery, whereas nondirectional Doppler assessment may reveal a relatively normal flow pattern in both vessels. The flow, however, may well be reversed in the obstructed vessel because of the extensive collateralization across the palmar arch. It should be quite obvious that the Allen test, although based on a visual interpretation, can be further documented by performance using the Doppler flow detector to assess signal changes during compression.

Some specific noninvasive assessment procedures aid in the diagnosis of *venous obstruction*. The presence of swelling should be documented by segmental girth measurements. Occasionally, there will be distention of the superficial veins and mild cyanosis. Patient complaints generally are of heaviness and pressure or a distensive feeling with exercise. Although venous collateral vessels develop rapidly and extensively, symptoms abate slowly, if at all, and are particularly exacerbated by exercise (Fig. 33–4). Edema, present from primary lymphatic obstruction, may oc-

casionally be difficult to differentiate from venous obstruction, but often can be clarified by measurement of antecubital vein pressures using the saline-filled manometer.

Flow in the upper extremity is paradoxically related to venous flow in the lower extremity, and these facts must be kept in mind when assessing upper extremity venous outflow. Often, outflow in the upper extremities will be decreased with deep inspiration related to changes in intrathoracic pressure. The upper extremity venous return tends to be more pulsatile than that demonstrated in the lower extremities. Velocity changes in the antecubital and axillary veins can be assessed with the Doppler flowmeter much as they can in the lower extremities when these important differences are kept in mind.

Surgically constructed arteriovenous fistulas will be dealt with in more detail in later chapters. Several characteristics should be appreciated, however, referable to the previously described examinations. The arterial flow distal to a surgically constructed arteriovenous fistula may well be retrograde in the artery distal to the fistula. Additionally, flow in the distal vein of a side-to-side arteriovenous fistula is commonly reversed such that the flow is traveling in a distal direction. Dramatic augmentation of flow will be appreciated in the donor artery to the arteriovenous fistula. Compression of the fistula would generally restore normal flow patterns in the distal, arterial, and venous vessels.[3]

SMALL VESSEL OCCLUSION IN THE UPPER EXTREMITY

Gangrene of the digits of the upper extremity is most often secondary to small arterial occlusive disease. Nevertheless, in somewhat less than half the patients with this presentation, a proximally obstructing or embolizing lesion can be found and must be looked for carefully. A majority of these gangrenous manifestations will be due to occlusions of the proper digital vessels or of major vessels of the palmar arch. In ascertaining the underlying cause of these small arterial occlusions, one must take into account a host of local phenomena as well as a large array of systemic diseases that may have other manifestations but that present primarily with digital gangrene. Digital gangrene is rarely associated with primary Raynaud's disease, and an underlying occlusive process generally will be identified if a meticulous evaluation is undertaken.

The so-called group of *collagen vascular diseases* manifest themselves by deposition of immune complexes in the intimal and subintimal surfaces of small vessels. Additionally, obliterative proliferative processes characterize selective diseases such as scleroderma and diabetes. The fact that digital ischemia may precede systemic manifestations of these diseases adds to the difficulty of the initial diagnosis and emphasizes the need for a logical approach, which may have

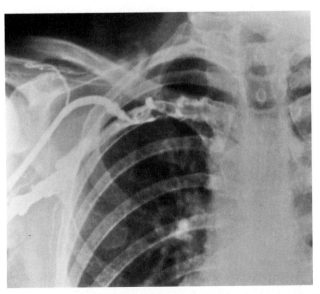

FIGURE 33–4. Axillosubclavian vein thrombosis characteristic of the Paget-Schroetter or effort thrombosis varient of thoracic outlet compression syndrome. Note the collateral vessels and intraluminal thrombus.

to be repeated on occasion during the evolution of a patient's disease.[4,5] Certain patients with digital ischemia may be subject to hypersensitivity associated with increase in circulating catecholamines or release of other humeral elements (prostaglandins, serotonin). These manifestations have been reviewed by Bauer et al.[6] The response to cigarette smoking, particularly in males who have been suspected of suffering from Buerger's disease, is characteristic of this group of patients. The process of gangrene in the fingers is quite different from that of necrosis, which is a wet suppurative process. Fingertip gangrene is more often a process of desiccation and mummification, which was meticulously described by Raynaud.

The presence of digital gangrene in the young patient without evidence of atherosclerosis or aneurysmal disease and particularly in the presence of normal upper extremity segmental pressures should indicate the possibility of a generalized collagen vascular disease as the most likely etiology for the digital ischemic changes. Thoracic outlet arterial compression with poststenotic dilatation and aneurysm formation is uncommon but nevertheless must be suspected. Axillobrachial aneurysms of atherosclerotic origin are extremely uncommon but must also be considered in these types of lesions. Industrial trauma, such as use of vibrating equipment (jackhammers, laboratory tools), or exposure to heavy metals should be investigated. Occupational exposure, such as the particular use of tools and the use of the hand in pounding, will often indicate the source of traumatic occlusion. This is particularly pertinent where the hamate process of the wrist occludes the ulnar artery in a well-described but infrequently recognized hypothenar hammer syndrome.

Many authors have emphasized that the presence of gangrene is unlikely in vasospastic disorders; and, in the vast majority of cases, areas of actual digital occlusive processes will be identified.

Arteriography is useful in excluding proximal lesions, although rarely will it demonstrate specific changes that may be characteristic of certain of the arteritides (Fig. 33–5). The serologic tests that form the basis for the diagnostic work-up in these patients include: serum protein electrophoresis, cold agglutinins, rheumatoid factor, VDRL, Hep-2, antinuclear antibodies, antinative DNA antibodies, total hemolytic complement, extractable nuclear antibody, complement (C3,C4), immunoglobulin electrophoresis, cryoglobulin, cryofibrinogen, direct Coombs' test, HBsAb hepatitis B antibodies, and HBsAg–hepatitis B antigen. In cases in which skin biopsy is performed, immunofluorescence staining is extremely helpful. Collagen vascular diseases may also be documented by plain x-ray films of the hands, which demonstrate distal phalangeal tuft reabsorption and evidence of soft tissue atrophy with particular loss of pulp dimensions on the palmar surface of the distal phalanges. Evidence of skin atrophy and shiny tenseness or calcinosis of the skin is also an extremely valuable

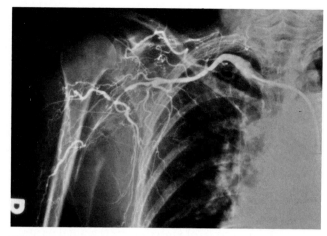

FIGURE 33–5.   Typical pattern of axillosubclavian arterial occlusive disease seen in giant cell arteritis.

diagnostic finding. When a diagnosis can be made early, scleroderma will be the most common entity presenting with digital ischemia.

A pragmatic approach to this problem is justifiable, understanding that the definitive diagnosis may not be made during the early periods of significant symptoms. Medical therapy should be initiated either systemically or locally. The most effective systemic medications have been Aldomet, reserpine, guanethidine, and phenoxybenzamine. More recently, agents such as nifedipine have proven useful in relief of arterial spasm and associated digital ischemia.

Medical management includes avoidance of cold exposure, use of gloves, and discontinuation of tobacco use. Pharmacologic therapy for nonrelated disorders must be reviewed to eliminate medications that may aggravate peripheral vasospasm, such as propranolol, or ergot preparations for migraine. Calcium channel blockers currently form the primary pharmacologic agents for the treatment of digital vasospasm, ischemia, and gangrene. Nifedipine in 10-mg doses may be used up to four to six times per day. Peripheral edema, dizziness, headache, and fatigue often limit the use of this important drug before a sustained digital effect can be achieved. Diltiazem at a dose of 30 mg twice a day, given alone or as a supplement to nifedipine, has been reported to be effective.[7]

When episodes of ischemia or Raynaud's symptoms are infrequent and do not require long-term sustained treatment, sublingual nifedipine is rapid in onset, with fewer side effects. The nongeneric Procardia (Pfizer, Parsippany, NJ) must be used. The 10-mg capsule is perforated with an 18-gauge needle and two or three drops are placed sublingually by the patient.

We avoid the use of topical antibiotics, because the vehicle often leads to maceration of otherwise desiccated tissue. The occasional case of suppuration can be effectively combated with systemic antibiotics. Patients are advised to avoid cold and to use gloves during all possible episodes of exposure. During the winters we have patients carry a camping-type pocket hand warmer for additional protection. Patients who are refractory to these therapeutic measures or whose digital ischemia is exacerbated while on optimum medical therapy for the systemic collagen vascular disease will often respond to dorsal cervical sympathectomy. Periods of spontaneous remission are quite common, and extensive progression of these gangrenous lesions is extremely unusual, although partial digital amputation is occasionally necessary. Sympathectomy, although not demonstrably superior to conservative therapy, has the advantage of avoiding long-term exposure to potent vasodilating drugs and a host of side effects that may be associated with their use. Nevertheless, the frequent effectiveness of conservative therapy must be emphasized.

ARTERIOGRAPHY

Arteriography can be useful in the diagnosis and assessment of vascular disorders of the upper extremity, but it plays a much less prominent role than in vascular disorders of the visceral or lower extremity vessels. The transfemoral route is preferred, particularly to enable visualization of the proximal aortic vessels and to avoid the need to traverse a potentially diseased axillosubclavian vessel. Upper extremity arteriography with meglumine diatrizoate (60 per cent) is generally perceived as painful by most patients, and premedication is useful, as is the addition of lidocaine to the angiographic solution. The use of Priscoline or nitroglycerin will assist in magnification views of the digital vessels, particularly when one is looking for small, clearly occlusive processes.

Proximal arterial aneurysms and atherosclerotic occlusive disease as well as ulcerating plaques are generally well identified radiographically. Thoracic outlet compression is infrequently identified, particularly when the procedure is performed in the supine position. The recent use of digital intravenous angiography, allowing the patient to be radiographed in the sitting position, demonstrates a much higher yield of arterial compression lesions, correlating much more closely with the clinical findings (Fig. 33–6). Proximal subclavian occlusion with subclavian steal phenomena and retrograde flow in the vertebral artery is easily demonstrated angiographically. This lesion should be suspected whenever there is a pressure discrepancy greater than 40 mm Hg in contralateral brachial artery pressure (Fig. 33–3).

Some arteriographic findings that are specific to various collagen vascular diseases have been well documented: in general, the lesions occur bilaterally, and the vessels show evidence of obstruction without evidence of calcium in the vessel wall or in the body of the lesion. Atherosclerotic changes are generally absent. The arterial lumen is smoothly narrowed with a smooth reduction in the caliber of the vessel above the thrombosed segment. Lesions may be totally oc-

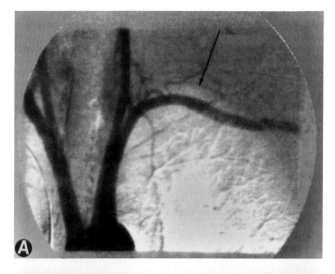

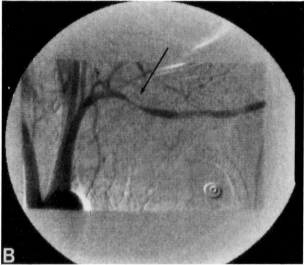

FIGURE 33–6. Digital intravenous axillosubclavian angiogram performed (*A*) in the supine and (*B*) in the sitting position to demonstrate thoracic outlet compressive changes (arrows) seen frequently only in the sitting position.

clusive or may show a stringlike appearance (Fig. 33–5). Multiple segmental occlusive lesions occur predominantly in the forearm and hand, with sites of predilection in the cubital arch, palmar arch, and digital arteries. Collateral circulation is generally less well developed than in arteriosclerotic vascular occlusive disease. This collateralization is primarily through the vasa vasorum of the thrombosed segment, giving a winding corkscrew appearance of the fine vessels that accompany the occluded segment. The small attenuated terminal digital branches have often been described as having the appearance of a "tree root."[8]

Characteristics of Takayasu's arteritis are generally confined to the proximal great vessels of the aortic arch, with solitary or multiple segmental narrowings of a tapered configuration. Linear calcifications in aneurysm formation are also often seen. Giant cell arteritis, on the other hand, generally is manifest by long smooth stenotic segments alternating with areas of relatively normal or dilatated segments. The occlusive process is generally smooth and tapered, with absence of irregular plaques and ulcerations. Distinction between giant cell arteritis and Takayasu's arteritis is often difficult to establish, particularly in the upper extremity.

Magnification views of the hand during arteriography, particularly if augmented by hand cooling, hand warming, or injection of intraarterial vasodilating drugs such as papaverine, can differentiate between Raynaud's phenomenon, which is generally associated with segmental occlusions, and Raynaud's disease, which is generally identifiable only by a vasospastic hypersensitivity. The angiographic characteristics of arterial vasospasm are: marked delay in flow, a threadlike appearance, and tapered areas of occlusion relieved subsequently by injection of vasodilating drugs or hand warming.

Arteriography is extremely useful in the identification and assessment of arteriovenous malformation. When adequate to enable morphologic identification of arteriovenous malformations it requires large volumes of contrast material injected at rapid rates, and often the true extent of the lesion will not be evident unless selective arterial injections are utilized.

Acquired arteriovenous fistulas will often have an associated false aneurysm, and although the fistula itself may not be demonstrable, owing to extremely high flow rates, the immediate filling of the adjacent vein is a reliable diagnostic finding. Ordinarily the proximal artery may be dilated, tortuous, and even aneurysmal and will often show atherosclerotic change. The proximal veins are generally dilated as well. Transcatheter embolization is useful in palliation and occasionally cure of these symptomatic and destructive lesions. A number of critical aspects of transcatheter embolization have been identified, including preservation of the feeding vessels, in contradistinction to the previous practice of feeding vessel obliteration. The feeding vessel offers access to the nidus or central portion of the arteriovenous malformation, which must be extensively occluded, and thrombosis initiated if successful obliteration is to be accomplished. Obliteration of the feeding vessels without prior thrombosis of the central nidus will only lead to rapid reformation of the arteriovenous malformation. A host of embolic materials have been developed, but the essential facet is careful subselective arteriography and central lesion embolization. In general, embolization will be followed by pain, fever, and elevated creatinine phosphokinase. Fibrin split products may be transiently elevated, and such patients require hospitalization, sedation, and parenteral analgesics. Low-grade fever may persist for several weeks, although most symptoms resolve within 3 to 7 days. Embolization may require several staged procedures, and the therapy should always be considered palliative, with the potential for additional therapy necessary over time.

AFFLICTIONS OF THE MAJOR VASCULAR STRUCTURES OF THE UPPER EXTREMITY

In cases of acute arterial insufficiency of the upper extremity, about 50 per cent will be secondary to embolization, and of the remainder, 25 per cent will be the result of primary arterial thrombosis and 25 per cent will be iatrogenic in origin. The vast majority of embolic arterial occlusions in the upper extremity are of cardiac origin, but brachiocephalic aneurysmal disease occasionally will result in embolic episodes.

The diagnosis of upper extremity ischemia is quite straightforward. The triad of symptoms—pain, paresthesias, and pallor—is generally accompanied by a loss of radial and ulnar pulse and diminished segmental pressures on noninvasive testing. Surprisingly, atherosclerotic occlusive disease, which is so prominent in the lower extremities, afflicts the upper extremity less commonly in the occlusive process. The mortality rate in patients with arterial embolization to the upper extremities is about 25 per cent, primarily attributable to recurrence and repetition of the embolic process into other additional arterial distributions, particularly cerebrovascular, renal, and mesenteric.

Diagnostic and therapeutic measures must be prompt in episodes of acute upper extremity embolization. It has been documented that patients successfully treated within 12 hours of the embolic episode have excellent long-term results. After a period of 12 hours, only approximately 25 per cent of the patients will have normal return of function and vascular integrity. The exact 12-hour time period may not be critical, but it does emphasize the problem of delay and the relative ineffectiveness of rapid collateral revascularization.[9,10]

Two modes of therapy may well provide satisfactory results in the treatment of this problem. The most efficacious has been the immediate administration of continuous intravenous heparin with careful monitoring of the thromboplastin time. Intravenous heparin can be discontinued for a short period of time to allow for angiographic investigation, but can be maintained during arterial embolectomy, which is ideally performed through the antecubital fossa. The embolectomy should be carried out promptly and careful observation then instituted for development of compartment syndrome. This compressive hydrostatic change occurs less frequently than in the lower extremities, but nevertheless must be managed promptly by fasciotomy when it is recognized.

Selected cases, particularly patients who represent poor operative risks, may be managed with fibrinolytic therapy. This therapy is best carried out when initiated within 36 hours of the embolic event. A serum fibrinogen level assay is done prior to the start of therapy, and a loading dose of streptokinase of 250,000 units is given intravenously. This is followed by 100,000 units/hr and continued with a minimum of hematologic monitoring. After 4 hours, a fibrinogen assay is repeated, and if there has not been a decline of at least 100 mg/dl, the therapy will not be effective and should be discontinued. Recently, experience has grown with direct intraarterial fibrinolytic therapy, which can immediately follow angiographic diagnosis and localization of the lesion.[11]

Trauma to the brachial vessels generally carries a poor prognosis secondary to the commonly associated nerve injury (Fig. 33-7). Lateral arterial repair and suture, or end-to-end anastomosis, is generally satisfactory in low-velocity missile and stab wounds. As in other areas of the body, high-velocity missile injury generally requires resection of the damaged artery to avoid recurrent thrombosis secondary to more extensive intimal damage. Reversed interposition vein graft is the most satisfactory reconstructive material and should be the graft of choice in the upper extremity.

When signs of ischemia accompany an upper extremity fracture, fracture reduction should be done as a primary maneuver, and reassessment of arterial integrity should be done promptly. In the presence of residual signs of ischemia, abnormal segmental arterial pressures, or incomplete return of pulses, arteriographic investigation is advisable. Although spasm can occur with torsion and traction on upper extremity arteries, there is generally a fairly prompt remission and restitution of normal pulses. We have rarely encountered spasm of a magnitude sufficient to cause a fall in segmental arterial pressures when assessed with the Doppler flowmeter and blood pressure cuff. A pressure drop in the range of 20 to 30 mm Hg lasting more than 30 minutes should be considered an indication of arterial occlusion, and the proper diagnostic and therapeutic steps should be

instituted promptly. The consequence of delaying treatment in this type of ischemia in the upper extremity is a Volkmann's-type ischemic contraction, which may often develop insidiously in the presence of minimal signs of arterial insufficiency. This difficult problem is particularly characteristic in children who have suffered a supracondylar fracture, in whom meticulous attention may not have been paid to concomitant arterial insufficiency.

Humeral fractures and shoulder dislocation are also associated with axillobrachial artery occlusions, and the basic principles of arterial reassessment after fracture reduction is advisable. False aneurysms of the brachial vessels may develop in instances of humeral fracture even in the presence of distal arterial integrity. These generally will present as a pulsatile mass, occasionally associated with extensive hematoma and ecchymosis. In the absence of acute neurovascular compression, delayed repair has been satisfactory in these cases.

With the extensive use of the upper extremity for arterial blood pressure monitoring, sampling of arterial blood gases, and creation of arteriovenous fistula for dialysis, 25 per cent of episodes of upper extremity ischemia arise as a consequence of these diagnostic and therapeutic necessities. The incidence of radial and ulnar artery occlusion after percutaneous arterial cannulation is in the range of 30 per cent.[12] The smallest incidence of complications has been reported with Teflon catheters of 20-gauge size or smaller. Other materials and larger sizes have a significantly higher complication rate.

In general, the more disastrous complications of radial or ulnar artery occlusion occur in patients with an incomplete palmar arch or other anatomic abnormalities that lead to poor perfusion. Although most instances of thrombosis may be totally asymptomatic, it is incumbent upon the physician to perform the Allen test prior to utilizing the radial or ulnar arteries for diagnostic or therapeutic procedures.

Brachial artery catheterization is a well-documented cause of upper extremity ischemia. The absence of a pulse or a persistent drop in segmental pressures lasting more than 30 minutes to an hour should indicate the likelihood of occlusion and should suggest the need for further diagnostic studies and operative therapy. Occlusion at the brachial level may be asymptomatic at rest but will be accompanied by a significant degree of ischemic arm symptoms with exercise and work-related activities.[13]

Axillary cannulation has become a particularly popular method for angiographic study, and it is exceedingly important to be aware of the neurologic complications that occasionally accompany this particular site of access. Postcannulation bleeding tends to be confined to the axillary sheath and will often lead to neurologic impairment. The patient who has a neurologic deficit after axillary artery cannulation, particularly in the distribution of the median nerve, should undergo surgical exploration for decompression of

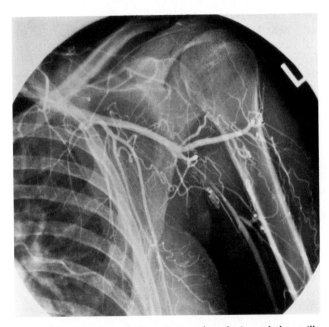

FIGURE 33–7. Intimal dissection and occlusion of the axillobrachial artery at the level of the brachial plexus cords. This lesion is best repaired by reverse vein grafting, care being taken to avoid entrapment of brachial plexus elements.

the hematoma. Failure to decompress this area will often lead to permanent neurologic impairment.

It should be evident that careful arterial assessment of the upper extremity, as outlined earlier in this chapter, should always be undertaken before axillofemoral grafting procedures or other extraanatomic bypasses that utilize the axillosubclavian vessels. This will avoid the uncommon but serious complications of upper extremity ischemia that occasionally result from these increasingly popular reconstructive procedures.[14]

Aneurysms of the axillobrachial vessels are relatively uncommon. Although tortuous subclavian vessels often are suspected of being aneurysmal at the time of clinical assessment, the diagnosis is rarely sustained after angiographic investigation. Nevertheless, when these infrequent abnormalities are encountered, the treatment of choice is excision and interposition vein graft reconstruction.

In episodes of acute embolization or thrombosis with ischemia, we have used intraarterial thrombolytic agents (primarily urokinase) as well as intravenous infusion of prostaglandin E_1. These measures can serve as an effective bridge to subacute and chronic maintenance therapy. Pentoxifylline at 400 mg given three times per day has been effective (by clinical observation) in improving the capillary circulation in some of our patients with upper extremity digital ischemia.

High-dose local infusion of urokinase by a transarterial catheter has been effective in the lysis of intraarterial thrombi. This technique can be used intraoperatively to more effectively remove thrombotic material from the very vasoactive vessels of the upper extremities, thus avoiding the trauma of repetitive passage of a balloon embolectomy catheter. An infusion of 250,000 units of urokinase dissolved in 100 ml of normal saline can be given over a 30-minute period. If the patient is not systemically heparinized, 1000 units of heparin can be added to the infusate. If there is any clinical or radiographic evidence of vasospasm, 30 mg of papaverine can be infused via the same catheter.[15]

VENOUS INSUFFICIENCY OF THE UPPER EXTREMITY

Although thoracic outlet compression can lead to axillosubclavian vein thrombosis, the vast majority of venous occlusive processes result from trauma or iatrogenic injury.

Long-term intravenous alimentation, upper extremity intravenous access for therapy, or procedures such as central venous pressure monitoring and Swan-Ganz monitoring may result in axillosubclavian thrombotic episodes. It is important to recognize that chronic axillosubclavian vein thrombosis may be an indolent and relatively silent process and is infrequently associated with symptoms in the upper extremity. During the course of monitoring and therapy using the upper extremity veins, the more serious

illness for which the patient is being treated or monitored may overshadow subtle signs of progressive axillosubclavian thrombosis. Whenever this problem has been looked at prospectively, however, the incidence of venous thrombosis in the major upper extremity veins approaches 25 per cent and is significant perhaps when repetitive subclavian vein catheterizations might be required in the course of a long or recurrent illness. Heparin therapy rarely leads to lysis but may prevent extension of thrombosis when the problem is recognized and cannulas have been removed. Thrombolytic therapy with streptokinase or urokinase may prove efficacious, but good controlled studies in the upper extremity have not yet been satisfactorily documented. Reports of successful surgical therapy by either thrombectomy or interposition grafting do not demonstrate any superiority over conservative management, and the failure rate is sufficiently high that enthusiastic recommendation of surgical intervention cannot be supported.

Spontaneous, or effort-related, thrombosis of the axillosubclavian vein is a disabling disorder of young, otherwise healthy individuals that was described independently over 100 years ago by Paget in England and Von Schroetter in Germany. In 1949, Hughes analyzed 320 cases of spontaneous upper extremity venous thrombosis collected from the medical literature. He recognized the first two descriptions by naming the entity the "Paget-Schroetter syndrome."[16] Over the course of subsequent investigations, it has come to be understood that, in contrast to the apparent spontaneous nature of the event, there is an underlying chronic venous compressive anomaly at the thoracic outlet (Fig. 33-4). The subclavius muscle tendon can be demonstrated to be the site of obstruction in many cases in which intermittent obstruction is present but has not yet led to thrombosis. Pulmonary embolism from axillosubclavian vein thrombosis has been well documented, and deaths from pulmonary embolism from these sources have also been recorded in the surgical literature.

Recent studies of a relatively large group of patients have shown the value of immediate catheter-directed thrombolytic therapy with urokinase followed by a period of anticoagulation to allow the acute phlebitic process to subside. Patients are then treated by transaxillary first rib resection to relieve the external compression. In patients with long-standing compression of the vein, stricture and fibrosis may result. This can be treated with transvenous balloon angioplasty after the external compressive elements have been removed. With this course of therapy an excellent functional result can be expected.[17-19]

THORACIC OUTLET COMPRESSION

Thoracic outlet compression syndrome can be associated with a constellation of neurologic or vascular symptoms. The vascular compressive phenomena in

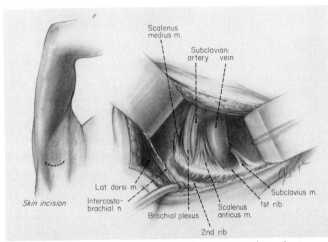

FIGURE 33–8. View of thoracic outlet structures from the transaxillary approach to first rib resection. (From Machleder HI (ed): *In* Vascular Disorders of the Upper Extremity, 2nd ed. Mt. Kisco, NY, Futura Publishing Co, 1989.)

this entity are much more apt to be demonstrable both on clinical and currently available objective tests. The first rib generally forms the floor of the axillary canal, through which the neurovascular structures traverse. The superior portion of this canal is formed by the clavicle and subclavius muscle. Structures that enter the thoracic outlet canal and can cause symptoms of neurovascular compression include the scalenus anticus muscle, which inserts on the first rib between the axillary artery and vein, and the subclavius muscle tendon, which inserts at the medial border of the costochondral junction of the first rib and, as has been mentioned previously, often will compress the subclavian vein. Most laterally, the scalenus medius muscle has insertions to the first rib that are closely associated with the cords of the brachial plexus (Fig. 33–8). A host of fibrocartilaginous congenital bands have been described in this area.

Many are perhaps rudimentary insertions of incompletely formed cervical ribs. Complete cervical ribs often will insert on the first rib and occasionally will be accompanied by an area of hyperostosis or even a fairly well-developed joint structure. Minor trauma, which may upset the rather close tolerances of the thoracic outlet by upsetting the musculoskeletal balance, leads to the thoracic outlet compression syndrome (Figs. 33–9 and 33–10).

Recent studies focusing on careful histochemical and morphometric analysis of the anterior scalene muscle have opened a new area for investigating the causes of neurovascular compression at the thoracic outlet. This research has been particularly useful in demonstrating the changes that occur in posttraumatic neurogenic thoracic outlet compression syndrome and often appear in the absence of obvious structural abnormalities.[20,21]

Vertebrate skeletal muscle is composed of several distinctive muscle fiber types, each having different morphologic, metabolic, and contractile characteristics that are distinguishable by specific histochemical staining methods. Despite a high degree of specialization, these fibers retain the capacity for accommodating changes in demand and patterns of stimulation, responding with alterations in basic biochemical elements.

Human skeletal muscle usually comprises predominantly type 2, quick-reacting fibers that have low oxidative enzyme capacity. A smaller percentage of slow tonic-contracting type 1 fibers, characterized by greater oxidative capacity, complete the complement. These later fibers (type 1) are common to postural muscle groups. Anterior scalene muscle demonstrates type 1 fiber predominance, which indicates that this muscle is, at the outset, uniquely structured in fiber composition to sustain protracted periods of tonic contraction.

Striking increases in type 1 fiber composition and

FIGURE 33–9. Typical hypertrophy of the subclavius tendon and associated exostoses seen at the subclavius and scalenus anticus insertions to the first rib (visualized from the transaxillary surgical approach). The vein is compressed in the most medial area of the thoracic outlet. (From Kunkel JM, Machleder HI: Treatment of Paget-Schroetter syndrome: A staged multidisciplinary approach. Arch Surg *124*:1153–1158, 1989. Copyright 1989 AMA.)

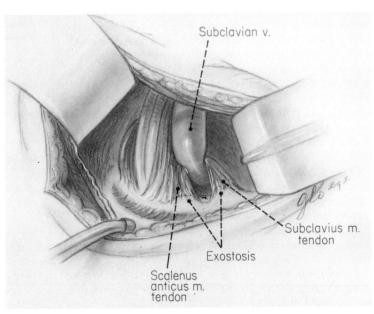

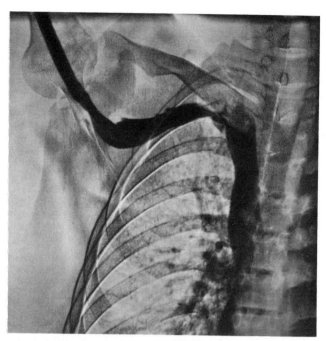

FIGURE 33–10. Typical venographic picture of axillosubclavian compression at the thoracic outlet that eventually leads to thrombosis and the acute clinical presentation.

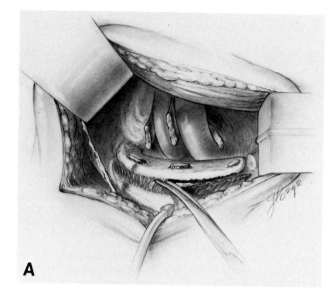

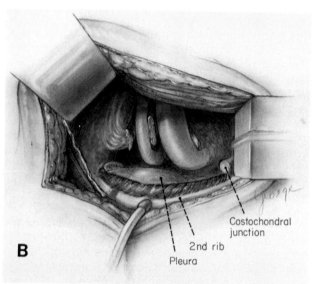

FIGURE 33–11. Steps in transaxillary first rib resection. *A*, Division of subclavius, scalenus anticus, and scalenus medius tendons as well as initial incision of the intercostal muscle. *B*, Relationship of structures after removal of first rib.

selective hypertrophy of the type 1 fiber system occur in patients with posttraumatic thoracic outlet compression syndrome. The anterior scalene muscle in these patients demonstrates an extraordinary adaptive transformation and recruitment response in the type 1 fiber system, possibly reflecting chronic increased tone or motor neuron stimulation. It seems likely that in posttraumatic thoracic outlet syndrome stretch injury to the muscle initiates a response of muscle contraction or denervation and reinnervation, compromising the interscalene triangle (between anterior and middle scalene muscles) and constricting the brachial plexus, to both accentuate and perpetuate the neurovascular compressive phenomenon.

Symptoms may be predominantly ulnar or median in distribution and occasionally will involve both nerve groups. Numbness, weakness, and paresthesias, particularly when the arms are in the abducted and externally rotated position, are characteristic. Common activities such as combing the hair, reaching or working with arms overhead, and even automobile driving when hands are placed on top of the steering wheel will bring on symptoms. Patients will generally seek therapy when symptoms become quite severe or when they occur in association with occupational requirements. Clinical findings are most useful in diagnosis and include reduction or obliteration of radial pulse with thoracic outlet maneuvers such as the costoclavicular, scalenus anticus, Adson's, and the abduction–external rotation (AER) maneuvers. These maneuvers will often reproduce symptoms or result in a subclavian bruit.

Progress has been made in facilitating the objective evaluation of neurogenic thoracic outlet compression by defining the role and usefulness of the somato-

sensory-evoked response.[22,23] The most characteristic abnormality found in patients with neurogenic thoracic outlet compression syndrome is a reduction in the amplitude of the ulnar nerve response at the N9, Erbs point, or brachial plexus recording electrode. This dampening of the N9 amplitude can be accentuated, or the potential completely ablated, by placing the arm in the abducted and externally rotated position, which is the most symptomatic position for patients with thoracic outlet compression syndrome. Criteria for performing and interpreting sensory-evoked potential testing have been established in a recent preoperative and postoperative study of patients undergoing surgical correction of neurovascular compression at the thoracic outlet.[24]

Objective tests are useful for the diagnosis of thoracic outlet compression and can include:

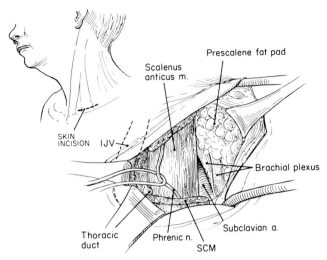

FIGURE 33–12. Transcervical approach to scalenectomy for relief of thoracic outlet compression syndrome. The relationship of major surrounding anatomic structures is depicted. *IJV*, internal jugular vein; *SCM*, sternocleidomastoid muscle. (From Machleder HI, Moll FL: *In* Trout, Giordano, DePalma (eds): Reoperative Vascular Surgery. New York, Marcel Dekker, 1987.)

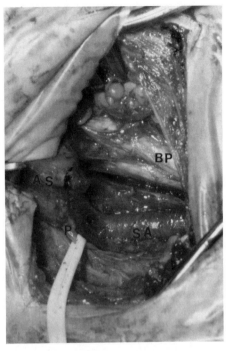

FIGURE 33–13. Operative view of transcervical approach after resection of anterior scalene muscle. *AS*, anterior scalene muscle stump; *SA*, subclavian artery; *BP*, brachial plexus; *P*, phrenic nerve.

1. Cervical spine x-ray films for assessment of arthritic or degenerative changes, and presence of cervical ribs.

2. Chest x-ray film to identify apical lung pathology and superior sulcus tumor.

3. Nerve conduction studies and electromyography to delineate the possible significance of neuroforaminal or cervical disk disease, as well as median nerve compression at the carpal tunnel or ulnar nerve compression at the cubital or Guyon's tunnel. These studies are very helpful in those patients having the "double crush syndrome" where there are multiple sites of peripheral nerve compression.

4. F-wave studies and somatosensory-evoked responses to evaluate the brachial plexus.

5. Venography, which is indispensible in the evaluation of the acutely swollen upper extremity where the possibility of Paget-Schroetter syndrome exists.

6. Angiography, which should generally be reserved for patients who have evidence of ischemia

or embolization. This will identify any arterial damage that may be associated with the compressive syndrome.

Although therapy for this condition undergoes periodic revisions, a number of standard surgical approaches have been successful. Cervical rib resection is the oldest documented therapy in the English literature and is still used as an isolated procedure in selected cases. More often, resection of the first thoracic rib concomitant with cervical rib removal (when present) will result in significant relief of symptoms (Fig. 33–11).[25]

Scalenotomy or scalenectomy, as a single operation or combined with first rib resection, has become an accepted surgical approach to this problem (Figs. 33–12 and 33–13).[26,27]

REFERENCES

1. Raynaud M: New researches on the nature and treatment of local asphyxia of the extremities. Archives Generales de Medecin, January 1874.
2. Burth DE: Digital Plethysmography. New York, Grune & Stratton, 1954.
3. Summer DS: Hemodynamics and pathophysiology of arterial venous fistulas. *In* Rutherford RB (ed): Vascular Surgery. Philadelphia, WB Saunders Company, 1977, pp 737–765.
4. Fan PT, Davis JA, Summer T, et al: A clinical approach to systemic vasculitis. Semin Arthritis Rheum 9:248, 1980.
5. Fauci AS, Hanes BF, Katz P: The spectrum of vasculitis. Ann Intern Med 89:660, 1978.
6. Bauer GM, Porter JM, Bardana EJ, et al: Rapid onset of hand ischemia of unknown etiology. Ann Surg 186:184, 1977.
7. Edwards JM, Harker CT, Taylor LM Jr, Porter JM: Small artery disease of the upper extremity. *In* Machleder HI (ed): Vascular Disorders of the Upper Extremity, 2nd ed. Mt. Kisco, NY, Futura Publishing Co, 1989.
8. Rivera R: Roentgenographic diagnosis of Buerger's disease. Cardiovasc Surg 14:40–46, 1973.
9. Kofoed H, Hansen HJ: Arterial embolism in the upper limb. Acta Chir Scand [Suppl] 47:113–115, 1976.
10. Savelyev BS, Zatevakhin II, Stephanov NV: Arterial embolism of the upper limbs. Surgery 81:367–375, 1977.

11. Chaise LS, Comerota AJ, Sonlen RL, et al: Selective intraarterial streptokinase therapy in the immediate postoperative period. JAMA 247:2397–2400, 1982.
12. Davis FM, Stewart JM: Radial artery cannulation: A prospective study. Br J Anaesth 52:41–47, 1980.
13. Machleder HI, Sweeney JP, Barker WF: The pulseless arm after brachial artery catheterization. Lancet I:407–409, 1972.
14. Quiñones-Baldrich WJ, Freischlag JA, Machleder HI, Busuttil RW, Moore WS: Inflow failure of grafts originating in the axillary artery. Ann Vasc Surg 2:303–308, 1988.
15. Quiñones-Baldrich WJ, Baker JD, Busuttil RW, Machleder HI, Moore WS: Intraoperative infusion of lytic drugs for thrombotic complications of revascularization. J Vasc Surg 10:408–417, 1989.
16. Hughes ESR: Venous obstruction in the upper extremity (Paget-Schroetter's syndrome). Int Abstr Surg 88:89–217, 1949.
17. Kunkel JM, Machleder HI: Treatment of Paget-Schroetter syndrome. A staged multidisciplinary approach. Arch Surg 124:1153–1158, 1989.
18. Machleder HI: Upper extremity venous thrombosis. Semin Vasc Surg 3:219–226, 1990.
19. Machleder HI: Effort thrombosis of the axillosubclavian vein: A disabling vascular disorder. Compr Ther 17:18–24, 1991.
20. Machleder HI, Moll F, Verity MA: The anterior scalene muscle in thoracic outlet compression syndrome: Histochemical and morphometric studies. Arch Surg 121:1141–1144, 1986.
21. Sanders RJ, Pearce WH: The treatment of thoracic outlet syndrome: A comparison of different operations. J Vasc Surg 10:626, 1989.
22. Glover JL, Worth RM, Bendick PJ, Hall PV, Markand OM: Evoked responses in the diagnosis of thoracic outlet syndrome. Surgery 89:86–93, 1981.
23. Siivola J, Pokela R, Sulg I: Somatosensory evoked responses as a diagnostic aid in thoracic outlet syndrome (a postoperative study). Acta Chir Scand 149:147–150, 1983.
24. Machleder HI, Moll F, Nuwer M, Jordan S: Somatosensory evoked potentials in the assessment of thoracic outlet compression syndrome. J Vasc Surg 6:177–184, 1984.
25. Machleder HI: Transaxillary operative management of thoracic outlet syndrome. In Ernst C, Stanley J (eds): Current Therapy in Vascular Surgery, 2nd ed. Philadelphia, BC Dekker, 1991.
26. Dale WA: Thoracic outlet compression syndrome: Critique in 1982. Arch Surg 117:1437–1445, 1982.
27. Roos DB: The place for scalenectomy and 1st rib resection in thoracic outlet syndrome. Surgery 92:1077–1085, 1982.

REVIEW QUESTIONS

1. Allen's test is useful in evaluating:
   (a) thoracic outlet compression
   (b) presence of cervical rib
   (c) integrity of palmar arch
   (d) digital blood flow
   (e) acute effort flow

2. The thoracic outlet is bounded by which of the following structures?
   (a) medial border of sternum
   (b) first thoracic rib
   (c) clavicle
   (d) subclavian artery
   (e) subclavius tendon

3. The thoracic outlet is traversed by which of the following structures?
   (a) subclavian artery
   (b) brachial plexus
   (c) scalenus anticus muscle
   (d) pectoralis major tendon
   (e) scalenus medius muscle

4. Digital gangrene is frequently associated with:
   (a) Raynaud's syndrome
   (b) Swan-Ganz central monitoring
   (c) Raynaud's disease
   (d) thoracic outlet compression
   (e) McLeary's syndrome

5. Digital plethysmographic tracings are most apt to be misinterpreted secondary to:
   (a) cuff malfunction
   (b) transducer malfunction
   (c) segmental arterial occlusions
   (d) changes in sympathetic activity
   (e) poor light

6. A common cause of prominent right-sided supraclavicular pulsation is:
   (a) common carotid aneurysm
   (b) subclavian aneurysm
   (c) subclavian tortuosity or elongation
   (d) innominate artery aneurysm
   (e) mycotic aneurysm

7. Effort thrombosis of the subclavian vein is often associated with:
   (a) straining at bowel movement
   (b) weight lifting
   (c) thoracic outlet compression syndrome
   (d) CRST syndrome or scleroderma
   (e) collagen vascular disease in general

8. When peripheral pulses are absent following fracture dislocation of the humerus:
   (a) arteriography should be done promptly prior to reduction
   (b) arterial exploration should be done at the fracture site as the first step
   (c) fracture reduction should be followed by arterial reevaluation
   (d) sympathetic block should be performed immediately
   (e) pulses should be rechecked in about 1 hour, prior to fracture manipulation

9. Gunshot injuries to the axillobrachial vessels have a poor prognosis owing to:
   (a) particularly poor collateral circulation in these areas
   (b) associated vein injury
   (c) associated nerve injury
   (d) difficulty in maintaining patency in these arteries even after appropriate repair
   (e) forearm compartment syndrome

10. Volkmann's ischemic contracture occurs most commonly:
  (a) in adults
  (b) in children

(c) after radial artery cannulation and thrombosis
(d) following fracture of the humeral neck
(e) in collagen vascular diseases

ANSWERS

| 1. c | 2. b,c,e | 3. a,b | 4. a | 5. d | 6. c | 7. c |
| 8. c | 9. c | 10. b,d | | | | |

34

HEMODIALYSIS AND VASCULAR ACCESS

ROBERT S. BENNION and SAMUEL E. WILSON

Direct access to the vascular system for the delivery of medications and for the removal of life-threatening endogenous or exogenous chemicals from the circulation is one of the foundations of modern clinical practice. In broad terms, vascular access includes any form of cannulation of arteries or veins. This chapter briefly reviews the historical aspects; provides a practical consideration of external cannulation or shunts, autogenous fistulas, and internal bridge fistulas; and discusses the selection of prosthetic materials. The complications and outcome of each type of vascular access will be analyzed.

Temporary access to the venous system for the infusion of drugs and, somewhat surprisingly, considering the outcome, for the transfusion of blood products has been in fairly common practice for over 300 years. Sir Christopher Wren, the great 17th century English architect, is generally credited with the development of an instrument for intravenous therapy in 1656 that was utilized for injecting drugs (opium and crocus metallorum) into the veins of dogs.[1] It consisted of a cannula made from a goose quill with a pointed tip, which permitted penetration of the skin and underlying vein. In 1663, Robert Boyle described and published Wren's experiments and was the first person to extend intravenous infusions to man, using prison inmates in London as subjects.[2]

The development of long-term cannulation of the circulatory system, however, was spurred by the introduction of a practical hemodialysis machine by Willem Kolff in the mid-1950s.[3] Initial enthusiasm for hemodialysis was blunted by the major technical problems associated with the need for repeated vascular access. Having to perform a cutdown on the artery and vein for each dialysis access, and then to ligate these vessels at the termination of each procedure, essentially limited early hemodialysis to short-term therapy for acute renal failure. In 1960, the development of the Scribner arteriovenous shunt[4] afforded long-term, relatively safe access to the circulation, and prolonged use of hemodialysis in the treatment of chronic renal failure became a reality. Although these partially exteriorized arteriovenous shunts have largely been replaced by internal fistulas, they are still used in the management of acute renal failure, drug overdoses, and have occasional, although diminishing, application in the treatment of chronic renal failure.

The number of individuals requiring vascular access for hemodialysis has continued to increase. During the 10 years from 1980 to 1989, the number of patients with renal failure undergoing dialysis has doubled from about 52,000 in 1980 to just under 100,000 in 1989.[5] In addition, nearly 43,000 patients required the initial creation of chronic vascular access for hemodialysis in 1989, while another 23,000 patients underwent at least one operation for revision of their existing access in the same year.[5]

EMERGENCY VASCULAR ACCESS

The external arteriovenous shunt described by Quinton, Dillard, and Scribner in 1960 consisted of a loop of Silastic tubing lying on the volar aspect of the forearm connecting Teflon catheters placed in both the radial artery and nearby wrist vein (Fig. 34-1).[4] Although quickly and widely adopted as a practical means of providing access in chronic renal failure patients, three major disadvantages to long-term use of external shunts became apparent: (1) high infectibility because of the likelihood of bacterial contamination along the Silastic tubing entrance sites into the skin; (2) frequent clotting due to the small diameter of the Silastic and Teflon conduits; and (3) restriction of patients' daily activities by the external appliance, the extra care necessary to prevent dislodgement or infection, and the additional strain the shunt placed on their already heavily burdened tolerance. Consequently, patency rates of external shunts were very low.[6]

Although acute hemodialysis in the past has been carried out primarily with external shunts, these have

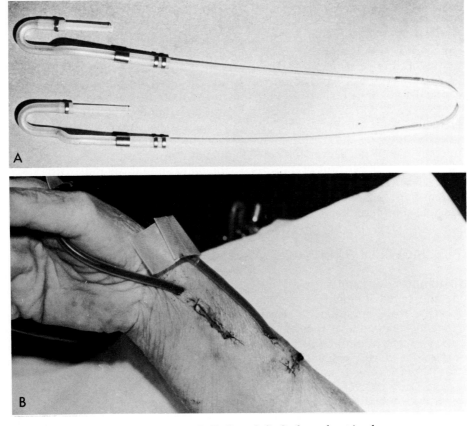

FIGURE 34–1.   *A,* Scribner shunt apparatus. *B,* Radiocephalic Scribner shunt in place.

now been essentially replaced by percutaneously placed central venous catheter hemodialysis.[7] This technique allows important preservation of the vascular sites best suited for later construction of subcutaneous arteriovenous fistulas. The usual indications for hemodialysis by percutaneous venipuncture are: (1) acute renal failure in which it is anticipated that only a short course of dialysis will be required; (2) during the immediate postoperative period following placement of an internal fistula in patients with chronic renal failure; (3) patients with transplantations who have thrombosed arteriovenous fistulas; (4) patients needing urgent transfer from peritoneal dialysis; and (5) treatment of poisonings.

Using this technique, short-term dialysis needs are met through the percutaneous introduction of a catheter with an external diameter of less than 2.0 mm. The catheters are usually introduced by the Seldinger technique over a guidewire, and may be easily left in place for a week or, with care, can last up to several months.[8] The catheters should be changed over a guidewire every 7 days, and the catheter tip cultured, with any drainage from the cutaneous entry site cultured routinely. Depending on the clinical demands, either single-catheter dialysis with pulsatile flow or double-catheter dialysis with continuous flow may be elected, with the latter usually chosen when urgent and aggressive hemodialysis is necessary, since

this is 20 to 30 per cent more efficient than a single-catheter dialysis. Thrombosis is prevented by continuous low-dose heparin infusion, or an intermittent injection of heparin every 12 hours. Stable patients may be given the option of going home with the catheter in place on receiving intermittent heparin injections for outpatient dialysis. Interestingly, it has recently been shown that patients with these catheters in place have a 40 per cent incidence of moderate to severe ipsilateral subclavian vein stenosis on angiography, while no stenoses were found in a control group of patients without a recent history of central venous catheters in the subclavian vein.[9] Although the effect that these stenoses may have on the function of a planned permanent vascular access is not known, it would seem prudent to avoid placing a percutaneous access line ipsilateral to a planned permanent access site.

These catheters are usually placed via the subclavian route into the superior vena cava, and are attended by the usual dangers of a percutaneous subclavian venipuncture.[10] The inferior vena cava may also be used; however, because of the danger of pelvic venous thrombosis, the catheter should not be left in place from one dialysis session to another. Although the incidence of catheter sepsis is generally low, one series reported a 28 per cent incidence of infection in catheters left in position more than 4 weeks.[11]

Long-term use of percutaneous vascular access is becoming a more frequent alternative form of chronic hemodialysis. Using a silicone dual lumen catheter with a Dacron cuff, a 1-year catheter survival rate of 65 per cent and median length of catheter use of 18.5 months has been achieved.[12] Although thrombotic complications occurred in 46 per cent of patients, the use of thrombolytic therapy was successful in restoring catheter function over 95 per cent of the time. Catheter exit site infection in 21 per cent of patients (which almost always resolved with parenteral antibiotics) and bacteremia in 12 per cent of patients were the other principle complications.

AUTOGENOUS ARTERIOVENOUS FISTULA

The autogenous arteriovenous fistula, usually constructed by joining the cephalic vein to the radial artery at the level of the wrist, continues to remain the longest lasting and most dependable type of long-term vascular access. One recent long-term prospective study demonstrated a useful patency rate for first-time fistulas for 90 per cent at 1 year, and over 75 per cent at 4 years.[13] In addition, revision of a failing autogenous arteriovenous fistula can extend its longevity. An autogenous arteriovenous fistula may be unsatisfactory, however, in patients (especially diabetics) with advanced atherosclerotic changes extending into the radial artery, or in patients whose veins are too small, fragile, or thin walled to mature sufficiently for repeated needle punctures.

Brescia-Cimino Arteriovenous Fistula

The subcutaneous autogenous arteriovenous fistula was initially described by Brescia, Cimino, Appel, and Hurwich in 1966.[14] Readily accepted by nephrologists and surgeons, the Brescia-Cimino fistula, constructed of the patient's own vessels, in great part overcomes the disadvantages of infection and early clotting found in external arteriovenous fistulas. Following formation of the fistula, arterial pressure is transmitted directly into the contiguous veins, resulting in dilation and development of a hypertrophied muscular wall (Fig. 34–2). This "arterialization" of the veins may take up to 6 weeks before sufficiently sized and thick-walled vessels have developed that will tolerate repeated venipuncture. Hemodialysis, if necessary during this postoperative period, may be accomplished using a Scribner shunt, subclavian or femoral vein cannulation, or peritoneal dialysis.

Our technique is as follows. Before operation, the veins, preferably in the nondominant arm, are distended and examined using a sphygmomanometer with cuff applied to the upper arm and inflated to below the systolic pressure level to produce venous engorgement. All suitably sized veins are marked with an indelible pen. This is performed so that, should the fistula of choice fail just following construction, these markings can aid the surgeon in identification of other possible fistula sites. The ulnar and radial artery pulses are palpated, and if there is any uncertainty as to adequacy, the systolic pressure in each is measured with the Doppler. It is advantageous to determine beforehand by the Allen test that the ulnar artery can support the circulation of the hand should the radial artery need to be divided or subsequently clot. Digital compression, occluding both arteries at the wrist, is followed by pallor of the elevated hand. Release of compression over the ulnar artery returns a normal appearance to the hand if the blood supply is sufficient.

Local infiltration anesthesia using 0.5 to 1.0 per cent lidocaine is usually satisfactory for construction of autogenous arteriovenous fistulas at the wrist or antecubital fossa. Although general anesthesia may be required in an extremely apprehensive or potentially uncooperative patient, a recent report of the effect of different types of anesthesia on blood flow during creation of a fistula showed that general anesthesia significantly decreased mean arterial blood pressure when compared to local infiltrative anesthesia or brachial plexus block.[15] In addition, it was noted that brachial plexus block (supraclavicular approach) significantly increased brachial artery blood flow when compared to local anesthesia. What the effect of these findings are on either short- or long-term patency of a fistula is not known.

The arm is prepared with povidone-iodine, abducted at a right angle from the body on an arm board, and sterilely draped. An oblique or longitudinal incision is made over the radial artery, proximal to the wrist skinfold. An adjacent 4- to 5-cm length of cephalic vein is dissected free of surrounding subcutaneous tissue. Its tributaries are ligated, freeing it further so that it lies adjacent to the radial artery without kinking or twisting. A comparable length of the radial artery, found under the deep fascia of the forearm, is also isolated from surrounding structures. Adequately mobilized lengths of the two vessels are necessary so that they may rest side by side without tension. In the event that tension exists, the distal cephalic vein may be divided and its proximal segment approximated to the radial artery in an end-to-side fashion.

Four different anastomotic connections of artery and vein are in common use (Fig. 34–3), and each has its advantages and disadvantages:

1. *Side-to-side anastomosis,* with a fistula opening approximately 1 cm long. Technically, this is an easy anastomosis to construct and has the highest fistula blood flow.[16] It is also the most likely fistula to be associated with venous hypertension of the hand.[17] This complication is moderated by the presence of

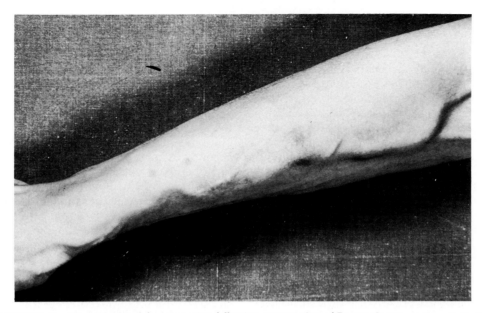

FIGURE 34–2. View of dilated forearm veins following construction of Brescia-Cimino radiocephalic fistula.

venous valves that prevent reversal of venous blood flow in the hand, at least in the early months.

2. *Arterial end–to–vein side anastomosis* minimizes turbulence and distal steal of blood, but results in slightly lower fistula flows and is subject to twisting of the artery during construction.

3. *Vein end–to–arterial side anastomosis* also decreases turbulence if constructed properly, and results in the highest proximal venous flow with minimal distal venous hypertension.[18] It is somewhat

technically more difficult to construct than the side-to-side fistula, and fistula flow overall is somewhat less. Most surgeons prefer this anastomosis because of the absence of vascular complications.

4. *End-to-end anastomosis* produces the least distal arterial steal and venous hypertension, but has the lowest fistula flow of the four configurations.[19]

Proximal and distal control of the two vessels is gained by application of small bulldog clamps or a

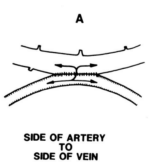

SIDE OF ARTERY
TO
SIDE OF VEIN

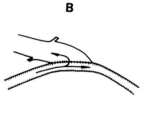

END OF VEIN
TO
SIDE OF ARTERY

FIGURE 34–3. Four anastomotic options for autogenous arteriovenous fistula construction.

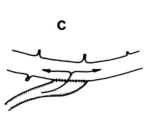

END OF ARTERY
TO
SIDE OF VEIN

END OF VEIN
TO
END OF ARTERY
(SPATULATED)

fine Silastic sling. The vessels are anastomosed in the desired configuration with 6-0 or 7-0 polypropylene suture, with knots placed outside of the lumen. One must be careful that, in approximating the artery and vein, spiral rotation of either vessel does not occur. Before the anastomosis is finally closed, a check is made by gentle passage of a coronary artery or biliary dilator to detect any stenosis. Hydrostatic dilation with heparin-treated saline of a marginally small vein may aid in maintaining early patency.[20] Any bleeding from the anastomotic site should first be controlled by simple pressure with a gauze swab for several minutes. Too hasty a resort to suture repair is liable to produce further bleeding sites and narrowing of the anastomosis.

Upon conclusion, the artery and vein should lie beside each other without twists or kinks. A thrill should be easily felt over the fistula and propagated for a moderate distance along the contiguous venous channels. A transmitted pulse without a thrill suggests an outflow obstruction or a clotted fistula. In this case, the proximal vein may be probed and inflated with a Fogarty catheter (avoiding intimal damage by not inflating the balloon during manipulation of the catheter) or carefully dilated with bougies. If these maneuvers do not produce a strong thrill, and the fistula is technically satisfactory, construction of the fistula at another, more proximal, site should be considered. On occasion, however, the appearance of a bruit and thrill is delayed until the veins dilate and blood flow increases, especially when no outflow obstruction can be demonstrated.

After the operation, the arm is slightly elevated by the patient's side for 24 hours. Avoidance of constricting dressings, sphygmomanometer cuffs, and tight clothing is mandatory. Any swelling present usually resolves over subsequent weeks. At least 4 to 6 weeks should elapse before the fistula is used for hemodialysis. Puncturing the vessels before they are arterialized is often associated with hematoma formation, because the dilated veins are thin walled in the first few weeks.[17] Although exercise of the forearm by squeezing a rubber ball to increase fistula flow and promote maturation of the arterialized veins has been advocated,[20] this has been reported to be of no benefit.[21]

The long-term patency for the Brescia-Cimino fistula as compiled from published results is shown and compared with other forms of vascular access in Figure 34–4.

Reverse Arteriovenous Fistula

The internal reverse arteriovenous fistula[22] (Fig. 34–5) is a method to salvage a failed or failing Brescia-Cimino fistula. This type of access procedure involves a side-to-side brachial artery–to–basilic vein anastomosis, thereby reversing blood flow into the superficial median antecubital and ulnar veins, and provides an additional site for a hemodialysis fistula in patients in whom the forearm vessels have been exhausted surgically. A primary requisite for the procedure is the presence of a 4- to 5-cm segment of antecubital vein.

Three technical points are emphasized in this procedure for reversing flow in the forearm veins. First, the valves in the forearm veins just distal to the level of the anastomosis must be ruptured via a basilic venotomy with a blunt probe; however, because of the previous venous arterialization, these valves are often incompetent and require little instrumentation. Second, in carrying out rupture of the valves, care must be taken not to injure the deep brachial veins, since these eventually will represent the major route of venous return in the arm, and damage to them may result in venous hypertension. Finally, the basilic vein proximal to the anastomosis is plicated to direct arterial inflow distally in the forearm. Plication, rather than ligation, preserves the proximal basilic vein as a future site of vascular access.

Brachiobasilic and Brachiocephalic Arteriovenous Fistulas

Brachiobasilic and brachiocephalic arteriovenous fistulas are another type of secondary upper extremity vascular access procedure that may be performed after failure of a more distal extremity arteriovenous fistula, or because the forearm vessels are inadequate. Patency rates of approximately 70 per cent at 2 years demonstrate the usefulness of this type of vascular access for chronic hemodialysis.[23]

The brachiobasilic fistula (Fig. 34–6C) is constructed by initially identifying the basilic vein just anterior to the medial epicondyle of the humerus, and then mobilizing the vein proximally to the axilla. Care must be taken during mobilization not to injure the cutaneous nerve to the forearm, which lies adjacent to the vein. The vein is divided in the antecubital fossa and relocated in a subcutaneous tunnel running down the anterior aspect of the arm. The proximal end of the vein remains in continuity with the axillary vein. The brachial artery is isolated in the antecubital fossa, and the end of the relocated vein is anastomosed to the anterior aspect of the artery in an end-to-side fashion at this level using a 1-cm arteriotomy. Construction of the brachiocephalic fistula (Fig. 34–6B) is similar, although technically easier. The cephalic vein already lies in a superficial position on the anterolateral aspect of the arm, so there is no need for repositioning; the vein need only be mobilized proximal to the antecubital fossa a sufficient distance to secure a tension-free end-to-side anastomosis.

VASCULAR GRAFTS (BRIDGE FISTULAS)

Successful long-term management of chronic renal failure frequently means that the patient will outlive the usefulness of several serially constructed vascular access routes. When it no longer becomes feasible to reconstruct an autogenous arteriovenous fistula, the use of a prosthetic conduit to form a bridge arterio-

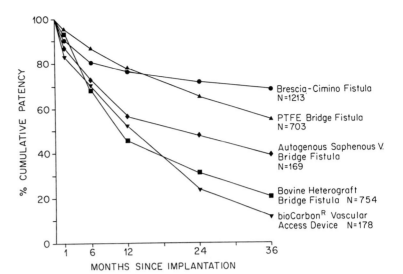

FIGURE 34–4. Patency rates of various types of vascular access for hemodialysis with at least 36-month follow-up (published results).

venous fistula is the best alternative. Bridge fistulas can be placed between almost any suitably sized superficial artery and vein in the body. After implantation, these easily palpable conduits can be readily punctured by needle; however, if possible, this should be avoided for about 2 weeks until there is incorporation of the prosthesis into the patient's tissues. Premature use may result in leaking of blood from the puncture site with formation of a perigraft hematoma.[24]

The prosthetic material used for the conduit in an arteriovenous bridge fistula is anastomosed end-to-side to the recipient artery and vein. If the two anastomoses are situated close by each other, the conduit takes on a "U"-shaped configuration; if separated by some distance, the conduit may lie straight or in a gentle curve. The conduit courses subcutaneously, allowing an adequate length for hemodialysis access.

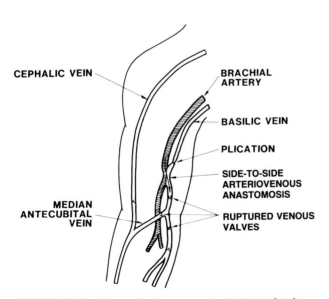

FIGURE 34–5. Reversed autogenous arteriovenous fistula.

Bridge Fistula Sites

Bridge arteriovenous fistulas may be (and have been) constructed at almost every location on the body where suitably sized arteries and veins are surgically accessible. For patient comfort, ease of handling at hemodialysis, and safety, however, the majority are constructed in either the upper extremity or thigh.

In the upper extremity, bridge arteriovenous fistulas may be satisfactorily constructed between the radial artery and an antecubital fossa vein, the brachial artery (in the antecubical fossa prior to its branching) and either the adjacent cephalic or basilic vein ("U"-configuration loop), and the brachial artery and the axillary vein (Fig. 34–7). Construction of an upper extremity bridge fistula is often more technically demanding than a thigh fistula, and its long-term patency is not as high.[25,26] This is generally attributed to the larger vessels and greater blood flow in the thigh. The risk of infection and distal limb ischemia is less in fistulas constructed in the upper extremity,[24] however, and this is the site of preference. Patients with claudication or an ankle arterial pressure less than 80 per cent of that at the wrist are not suitable for thigh fistulas because the proximal steal of blood through the fistula is likely to increase the ischemia in the leg.[27] Therefore, upper extremity fistulas are particularly well suited for elderly patients with significant atherosclerosis in the lower extremities. Obese patients in whom perspiration or dermatitis involving the groin skinfolds may increase the likelihood of infection should have placement of an arm fistula.

In the thigh, the arterial anastomosis should, in the first instance, be to the superficial femoral artery, immediately proximal to either the adductor canal or its more cephalad portion (Fig. 34–8A). If the superficial femoral artery is occluded, the common femoral artery may be used (Fig. 34–8B), with the understanding that if it becomes infected and ligation is subsequently necessary, leg ischemia may ensue. At

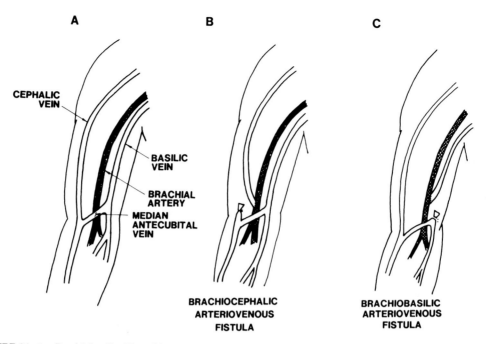

FIGURE 34–6.   Brachiobasilic (*C*) and brachiocephalic (*B*) autogenous arteriovenous fistulas.

times, patency of a short segment, including the origin of the superficial femoral artery, can be reestablished and used for the arterial anastomosis. The venous anastomosis is made to the proximal saphenous, common, or superficial femoral vein.

Traditionally, the site generally selected for initial placement of an arteriovenous bridge fistula was in the upper extremity from the distal radial artery to the cephalic or basilic vein in the antecubital fossa.[28] The graft should be anastomosed in an end-to-side fashion to the distal radial artery, tunneled along the lateral aspect of the forearm, and then anastomosed end-to-side to the largest vein in the antecubital fossa. In positioning the graft, it is most important to ensure that the patient's arm will rest comfortably while on hemodialysis. Actual bridging of the elbow joint should be avoided to aid in the long-term patency of the graft.

Other vascular access sites in the upper extremity for bridge fistulas include brachiocephalic or brachiobasilic loop fistulas in the forearm and brachioaxillary fistula in the upper arm. The loop fistulas placed in the forearm allow a large area of graft to be available for needle puncture, whereas the brachioaxillary fistula, which curves over the lateral aspect of the upper arm, allows a smaller area for needle puncture. These upper extremity loop grafts have also been found to have significantly higher patency rates at all time intervals over straight upper extremity grafts.[29] Upper extremity procedures may be easily performed using an axillary nerve block or local infiltration anesthesia.

Arteriovenous bridge fistulas in the thigh are usually constructed with the patient under a spinal or general anesthetic, although in cooperative patients a local infiltration technique can be used. It is often advisable to place the arterial origin of the conduit just proximal to the adductor canal portion of the superficial femoral artery so that, should a vascular complication cause occlusion of the artery, adequate collateral channels will provide filling of the popliteal segment. The end-to-side arterial anastomosis should be oblique, and the graft should leave the vessel at an acute angle, to minimize turbulence. The venous anastomosis is also performed in an end-to-side fashion, and as obliquely as possible. This is to counteract any pursestring effect of the suture, as well as buildup of fibrin and fibrous tissue at the venous anastomosis, which commonly causes late graft thrombosis. A vascular steal phenomenon, with reversal of flow in the distal superficial femoral artery, is more common in bridge fistulas in the lower extremity and can lead to symptoms of limb ischemia.[30] Fortunately, most patients with steal do not have symptoms, since the activity of the dialysis patient is often limited.

The femorosaphenous bridge fistula is curved subcutaneously over the lateral aspect of the thigh and is anastomosed to the proximal saphenous vein. The caudal portion of the saphenous vein may be ligated to prevent retrograde venous flow, although venous hypertension in the lower extremity is not a problem with a patent iliofemoral system. A less favorable lower extremity access configuration is the loop fistula placed in the groin from the common femoral or very proximal superficial femoral artery to the femoral vein. The high blood flow rate (greater than 700 ml/min) can lead to a significant increase in cardiac output. The possibility of limb loss should infectious complications develop and the increased risk of infection could make this site less desirable.[30]

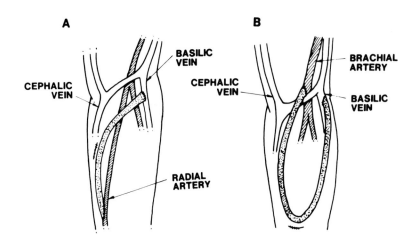

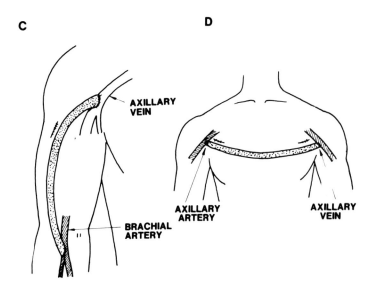

FIGURE 34–7. Upper extremity bridge arteriovenous fistulas.

With the increased survival of chronic hemodialysis patients, the surgeon may be called to evaluate a patient who requires vascular access and find that all extremity access sites have been expended. In this circumstance, a more central location, such as a bridge arteriovenous fistula placed between the axillary artery on one side and the axillary vein on the other side, has been employed successfully (Fig. 34–7D).[31] The grafts are of fairly large diameter, so they are easy to cannulate, flow is reported as excellent, and, despite having the access site on the anterior chest wall, patients are stated to adapt to it very promptly.[22] The major drawback of central access sites is that, when complications occur, they are serious and more difficult to manage.

Bridge Fistula Materials

Both biologic and prosthetic materials have been used in the creation of arteriovenous bridge fistulas for hemodialysis since this modality came into use in 1969.[32] Each material has its own advantages and disadvantages that must be weighed when a fistula

is to be constructed. The long-term patency rates for various types of bridge fistulas are shown and compared with the Brescia-Cimino fistula in Figure 34–4.

Saphenous Vein

The initial conduit for construction of a bridge arteriovenous fistula was a reversed autogenous saphenous vein forearm loop fistula.[32] The vein graft was found to dilate and its walls thicken so that repeated cannulation was successful. A prospective experience of 71 autogenous saphenous vein conduits in Sydney, Australia, demonstrated a cumulative patency rate of 66 per cent at 24 months, although this decreased to 40 per cent at 36 months.[33] In this series, no evidence of graft stenosis or false aneurysm formation was found, although a longer hospital stay was required because of the need to provide closed suction drainage to the leg after excision of the vein. Other reports have indicated a 3-year patency rate of 64 per cent, and a rate of 57 per cent at 5 years.[34,35] Only a 20 per cent patency rate at 24 months was reported in a series from the United States, however, with the accelerated loss attributed to graft fibrosis and stenosis from chronic

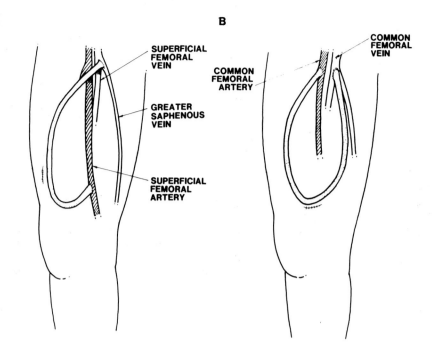

FIGURE 34–8. Lower extremity bridge arteriovenous fistulas.

needle puncture.[36] In addition, the need to preserve the saphenous vein for future coronary artery bypass surgery tends to make this a less desirable material. True aneurysmal dilation has also been reported for autogenous saphenous vein grafts.[37]

Preserved saphenous vein allografts have been proposed as materials for bridge fistulas.[38] Freeze-preservation of veins at −40° to −60°C causes death of all living cells, leaving a collagen conduit which may be used as a vascular graft resistant to rejection due to its very low antigenicity.[39] Following implantation, the endothelium of the patient has been found to quickly colonize the inner surface of the allograft. The allografts were generally acquired from patients undergoing surgical removal of varicose veins and specifically represent the abnormally dilated portion of the greater saphenous vein removed proximal to below-knee varicosities. For best results, the segment should be at least 7 mm in diameter (a diameter of 10 mm being ideal) and devoid of varicosities. A patency rate of approximately 90 per cent at 12 months has been reported, and no evidence of infection was found in over 36 months of use in a multiinstitutional trial.[40,41] Graft occlusion was found to occur at a rate of about 10 per cent per year, and small aneurysms were noted to occur in an allograft that contained varicosities at the time of acquisition.

Bovine Heterografts

Originally developed as a conduit for arterial bypass surgery, heterografts fashioned from bovine carotid arteries have long been employed as conduits for arteriovenous bridge fistulas. The modified bovine heterograft is prepared by enzymatic débridement of fresh bovine carotid arteries, followed by tanning with a dialdehyde starch solution. This yields

a collagen tube, 40 to 50 cm long and 6 to 1 mm in internal diameter. The initial response to the material was quite favorable as a substitute for saphenous vein in patients with failed autogenous fistulas, with 12-month patency rates of approximately 75 per cent being reported.[42,43] In addition, the ready availability of a conduit of constant caliber in almost any desired length, the material's pliability and biocompatibility, and the ease of suturing anastomoses proved definite technical advantages.

With continued experience, however, bovine heterografts used in vascular access began to exhibit several shortcomings that have blunted enthusiasm and led to essentially its abandonment as an access material. Aneurysmal dilation of bovine heterografts was found to occur increasingly with time. Thought to result from progressive degeneration of the graft material itself, one institution with a large experience identified 16 symptomatic aneurysms in 200 grafts (8 per cent), with a mean time to presentation of 16.4 months,[44] whereas another institution reported nonanastomotic aneurysms developing in 50 per cent of patent bovine heterografts followed for more than 1 year.[45] Found most often in grafts in proximal locations, the dilation was thought to be due possibly to increased flow rates. A change in the preservation technique has been reported that appears to obviate these dilation problems by ensuring no loss of vessel wall thickness, thereby making aneurysm formation less likely.[46] Infection of bovine heterografts was also noted to occur relatively frequently, with an incidence as high as 16 per cent noted to occur in one series of 113 bovine heterograft placements, compared to 6 per cent of 86 polytetrafluoroethylene (PTFE) graft placements in the same series.[47] In a compilation of 11 series comprising 560 fistulas, an overall incidence of infection of 7 per cent was found.[48] Outflow stenosis leading to late thrombosis of the graft has also been frequently noted in bovine heterografts.[43,47,49]

Human Umbilical Vein Graft

In an effort to obviate the shortcomings of the bovine heterograft, the human umbilical cord vein has been modified for use as a conduit for vascular access. Prepared from human umbilical cords obtained atraumatically at delivery and tanned with either dialdehyde starch or glutaraldehyde 0.2 per cent, the ordinarily flaccid umbilical vein is converted to a more rigid collagen tube capable of withstanding repeated needle punctures.[50] Scanning electron microscopy demonstrates few defects in the subendothelial lining or internal elastic lamina that can expose substantial amounts of the potentially thrombogenic medial components. The human umbilical vein graft (HUVG) also retains a critical surface tension level similar to an autogenous saphenous vein.[51] Thus, this material is reported to be more resistant to thrombus formation than either synthetic grafts (Dacron, PTFE) or modified bovine heterografts.[52]

Like bovine heterografts, aneurysmal dilatation of HUVGs over time is a problem. Using duplex scanning, one center has found that 33 per cent of HUVGs patent at 3 years were aneurysmal, rising to 45 per cent at 4 years.[53] These aneurysmal grafts, although patent, are at high risk for either rupture or thrombosis, and it has been recommended that all aneurysmal HUVGs be completely resected, since segmental resection of just the diseased portions of the grafts results in metachronous aneurysm recurrence.[54] Also, like bovine heterografts, these shortcomings have led to the abandonment of this material for access usage.

Dacron Velour

Conduits constructed of Dacron velour have been employed in reconstructive vascular surgery for many years and have been used as a material for arteriovenous bridge fistulas since about 1973.[55] It was noted that the material can be punctured, was self-sealing, remained patent, and provided adequate flow for hemodialysis. The high patency, specifically, of the Dacron velour conduit is considered to be due to increased ingrowth of tissue through the relatively large interstices of the material and consequently, more firm adherence of the inner lining, avoiding flap formation and ultimate occlusion. This increased tissue ingrowth is also thought to decrease the infectibility of the graft material (always a concern with prosthetic materials) and, in one study, no infection was found in over 1200 consecutive clinical dialyses.[56]

Cumulative function rates of approximately 80 per cent have been found for bridge fistulas constructed with Dacron velour at 24 months, compared to 60 per cent with bovine heterografts.[34] No evidence of anastomotic intimal hyperplasia, pseudoaneurysm formation, or thrombosis was found in a chronic study

of Dacron velour fistulas placed in dogs subjected to sham dialysis three times per week.[57] These laboratory results were borne out in one clinical comparison of vascular access graft materials,[58] whereas another report noted a 19 per cent incidence of thrombosis, a 5 per cent incidence of pseudoaneurysm formation, and a 5 per cent incidence of graft infection.[59] No true aneurysmal dilation of a Dacron velour hemodialysis fistula has yet been reported. However, Dacron has not gained widespread use for hemodialysis, perhaps because of its increased resistance to needle puncture.

Expanded Polytetrafluoroethylene

Since its initial introduction as an alternative material in the creation of arteriovenous bridge fistulas in 1976,[60] expanded PTFE has become the most commonly used material. Much of its popularity stems from its ease of handling, lack of necessity to preclot, wide availability, long shelf life, and high patency rates. PTFE bridge fistulas are consistently reported to have 24-month patency rates of over 70 per cent,[34,49,61] and, in a large comparative clinical study comprising 187 graft placements, 36-month patency rates of PTFE grafts were found to be significantly greater than bovine heterografts (62 per cent for PTFE versus 24 per cent for bovine heterografts).[36] Forty-eight month patency rates of 43 to 60 per cent have been reported.[62,63] However, multiple procedures for revision are usually required to maintain patency, with one study reporting an average of one operation for revision being required for every 1.1 years of graft (with a range of 1 to 16 revisions per graft).[64]

Thrombosis of the conduit appears to be a relatively common event in PTFE bridge fistulas, with figures ranging from 7 to 55 per cent.[22,34,49] Most, however, are easily dealt with by thrombectomy with good results, with nearly 90 per cent responding to simple Fogarty balloon catheter embolectomy alone.[63] Infection of PTFE fistulas is another fairly frequently encountered event, with one report of 80 fistulas followed for 30 months showing an overall incidence of infection of 19 per cent, with 67 per cent of these infections occurring during the initial 4 months of use.[65] Of the infected fistulas, 73 per cent required excision, and the remainder were treated successfully with antibiotics. Pseudoaneurysm at needle puncture sites have been noted to develop in approximately 5 per cent of fistulas.[47,49]

ATRAUMATIC VASCULAR ACCESS

Repeated percutaneous needle puncture of either primary arteriovenous fistulas or bridge fistulas at the time of hemodialysis is one of the leading causes of fistula failure. Thus, repeated puncture can lead to hematoma formation, bleeding from needle sites requiring excessive pressure (which contributes to thrombosis), graft infection from skin contamination, and pseudoaneurysm formation at puncture sites. In addition, many patients, especially children, tolerate needle punctures poorly. In an attempt to circumvent these problems, skin-level ports have been recently developed, which permit chronic vascular access for hemodialysis without the necessity of percutaneous needle puncture.[66,67]

The no-needle access device consists of a "T"-shaped body lined with a chemically inert, nonreactive, and nonthrombogenic form of carbon, and coated externally with a thin layer of Dacron velour, which provides a surface for ingrowth of surrounding tissue, securely anchoring the device (Fig. 34–9). The device may then be implanted directly into an arterialized vein in this basic configuration, or, with short lengths of PTFE graft material attached to each flange, interposed between an artery and vein. The neck of the device exits the skin. Access to the bloodstream for hemodialysis is obtained through the device employing either a single-cannula[66] or double-cannula[67] access set. The double-cannula access set allows extracorporeal blood flow rates of up to 400 ml/min, with less than 5 per cent recirculation.[68] Short-term patency of the device has been reported as 81 per cent at 12 months.[69]

One multicenter long-term survival study revealed cumulative patency rates at 24 months of 24 per cent and at 36 months of 13 per cent with these devices (Fig. 34–4); however, when their implantation criteria were revised to exclude those patients that they had previously identified as having a high risk for occlusion of any access device, their 24-month patency increased to 66 per cent.[70]

The most frequent complication was thrombosis, which occurred in close to 50 per cent of patients in another multicenter experience with this device, although 78 per cent of these were easily and successfully thrombectomized.[71] In addition, cutaneous exit site infection was noted in 33 per cent of patients, with 26 per cent of these not responding to conservative measures and requiring removal of the device.

Advocates of the use of an atraumatic device as a form of vascular access in chronic hemodialysis report several distinct advantages: (1) elimination of the use of needles, with the associated trauma to the skin, subcutaneous tissues, and graft material; (2) avoidance of pain, persistent bleeding, hematoma, or false aneurysm formation, and infection due to needle contamination; (3) immediate use after implantation; (4) limitation of total fistula flow by the use of small-diameter PTFE grafts, but with retention of adequate flow for dialysis; (5) use of multiple sites; and (6) minimal skill and time required to initiate and terminate hemodialysis. However, the advantages must be weighed against rather high thrombosis and infection rates, and overall patency rates that do not appear to compare favorably with other chronic access methods.

PEDIATRIC VASCULAR ACCESS

Maintenance of chronic vascular access in children is a formidable task for vascular surgeons, since the small vessel size is a major limiting factor. While many of the principles and techniques are the same as for the adult, certain aspects of the placement of long-term central venous catheters for total parenteral nutrition (to be discussed later) and creation of hemodialysis access sites are sufficiently different to warrant discussion.

Dialysis (either hemodialysis or peritoneal dialysis) with subsequent renal transplantation is the preferred therapeutic regimen for end-stage renal disease in children. Transplantation is usually attempted as quickly as possible, because, in general, children tolerate dialysis poorly in that they frequently develop severe growth retardation (not reversible by transplantation), failure of maturation, renal osteodystrophy, and psychosocial problems.[72] In addition, long-term hemodialysis is, at best, difficult in children less than 10 years of age, and is extremely difficult in those under 5 years.

Short-term hemodialysis in children may be performed in a variety of ways with good results. Newborn or premature infants can be dialyzed via direct cannulation of the umbilical vessels using a no. 5 or

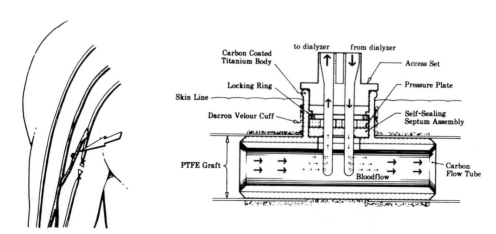

FIGURE 34–9. Diagrammatic representation of atraumatic vascular access device (Hemasite).

8 French catheter. Single-cannula hemodialysis may be employed in older children in whom either the superior or inferior vena cava has been cannulated by either the Seldinger technique or direct venous cutdown.[73] Another method in the older child involves placement of an indwelling brachial artery catheter and a large-bore Silastic central venous catheter placed via the external jugular vein to separate inflow and return, and provide the hemodialysis return with a large-bore egress route.[74]

The preferred method for long-term vascular access for hemodialysis in children weighing under 20 kg is the placement of a central venous Silastic arteriovenous shunt inserted as described previously.[72] In addition, creation of an autogenous arteriovenous fistula between the brachial artery at the elbow and an antecubital vein using microsurgical techniques has been employed in children weighing between 10 kg and 23 kg, with excellent results.[75]

For long-term hemodialysis access in children weighing over 30 kg, an internal form of access, either autogenous fistula or bridge fistula, should be attempted. Children weighing between 20 and 30 kg will have to be individualized as regards the type of access attempted according to the size of their vessels. A Brescia-Cimino autogenous arteriovenous fistula may be created in children weighing over 30 kg without much difficulty, and with patency rates of approximately 80 per cent at 12 months.[72] The use of microsurgical techniques enhances the patency rate, especially in children with small vessels to be anastomosed together.[76] Bridge fistulas of PTFE have also been employed in children with good results and patency rates of 88 per cent at 24 months in one study.[77]

The usual types of complications and their rates for both autogenous and bridge fistulas in children approximate those seen in adults. However, one of the most common complications of hemodialysis in small children is convulsions, occurring in up to 30 per cent of hemodialyzed children.[78] This is probably due to two factors: (1) the use of overly efficient dialysis, and (2) the greater sensitivity of children to changes in osmolality. It can probably be avoided by tight regulation of the efficiency of the dialysis procedure based on the child's body weight.

One major disadvantage of the use of internal vascular access fistulas in children that must be specifically mentioned, however, is the physically and psychologically terrifying pain of needle puncture, which may require much time and counseling to overcome.

VASCULAR ACCESS COMPLICATIONS

Infection

Infection is a devastating complication for the chronic renal failure patient and represents the second most common cause of death among patients on chronic hemodialysis, causing 10 per cent of all deaths in dialysis patients, exceeded only by cardiovascular disease.[79] Many of the systemic infections encountered in these patients are direct complications of an infection established at the site of hemodialysis access. In two large dialysis centers, an incidence of 0.11 septic episodes per patient-dialysis-year related specifically to the vascular access site was found.[80] This represented over 73 per cent of the total number of septic episodes encountered.

The elevated rate of sepsis associated with hemodialysis vascular access sites is partially due to the deficient immune defense mechanisms in chronic renal failure patients and consequent increase in infection risk.[81,82] The bacterial phagocytic and killing ability of polymorphonuclear leukocytes has also been demonstrated to be decreased by nearly 50 per cent in patients with chronic renal failure.[83] Lymphocytes in chronic renal failure have been noted to exhibit suppressed cellular immunity,[84] and inhibition of lymphocyte transformation, which is unaffected by dialysis, has been found.[85] In addition, the serum of uremic animals has been found to contain a nondialyzable inhibitor of the mixed lymphocyte reaction, which is probably a glycoprotein and distinct from either α-macroglobulin or immune complexes.[86] The actual ability of the animal to produce antibodies when antigen stimulated, however, does not appear to be depressed in chronic renal failure.[87]

In addition to alterations in host defense mechanisms, other factors contribute to the increase in the propensity of patients on chronic hemodialysis to develop infection. Poor healing of surgical wounds is a recognized consequence of renal failure,[88] and may result in wound infections. Measurement of the bacterial colonization rate of hemodialysis patients revealed that 62 per cent of these patients carried *Staphylococcus aureus* in their oro- or nasopharynx or on the skin, and 65 per cent of those patients with positive cultures developed infections in their hemodialysis access sites.[89] Furthermore, it was found that 30 per cent of the dialysis staff carried *S. aureus*, whereas only 11 per cent of normal controls had positive cultures. In the same study, it was noted that more than 70 per cent of all infections encountered were due to *S. aureus*. It has been recently shown that the patient's own level of personal hygiene represents the best indicator for *S. aureus* colonization and vascular access site infection risk.[90]

Although infection of an autogenous arteriovenous fistula is unusual, it can occur. Repeated needling of the fistula may result in formation of a hemotoma that can subsequently become infected from skin microflora. In addition, the anastomotic site of the fistula itself may become infected, resulting in an endovasculitis with subsequent septicemia and metastatic abscess formation. Treatment generally consists of therapeutic courses of appropriate antibiotic agents coupled with local measures, such as drainage of a perifistula abscess from an infected hematoma. Rarely, the fistula anastomosis may have to be dismantled and the vessels ligated in the presence of an infection-induced anastomotic pseudoaneurysm.

Bridge fistulas placed for vascular access are susceptible to multiple sources of infection. Contamination may occur during implantation from skin flora, and occurs more frequently when the fistula is placed on the thigh than when it is located in the upper extremity. This is due to the greater difficulty in preparing a sterile surgical field on the medial thigh and inguinal skinfold.[91,92] Direct inoculation of the graft by needle puncture through inadequately prepared skin also occurs, as well as inoculation of hematomas resulting in perigraft abscess formation.

The type of material in bridge fistulas also affects the infection rate, with autogenous saphenous vein fistulas demonstrating few, if any, infections, and biologic conduits (HUVG, bovine heterograft) being particularly susceptible to aggressive infections; synthetic conduits are also susceptible to infection by low-virulence organisms.[57,58,93] The newly implanted prosthesis is particularly susceptible to infection; however, tissue incorporation and neointima formation confer increased resistance to infection.[94] Delay in initiating hemodialysis using bridge fistulas for about 2 weeks after graft implantation will allow tissue incorporation of the prosthesis and development of a neointima. Disruption of an infected bridge fistula anastomosis (Fig. 34–10) may occur at any time during the course of a prosthetic infection and does not appear to be influenced by incorporation.[93]

Treatment of an established infection of a conduit is excision of the prosthetic material. Attempts at in situ sterilization using antibiotics or povidone-iodine irrigation have not proved reliably successful. A possible exception to this would be infection surrounding an autogenous saphenous vein prosthesis, for which treatment with antibiotics has been reported.[95] After excision of the fistula, several days should be allowed to elapse prior to creation of a new access site for control of any associated bacteremia.

Regimens aimed at prevention of this complication should always be practiced, including the use of perioperative antibiotic administration. Randomized, prospective, double-blind studies have consistently shown the protective role of perioperative antibiotics in vascular surgery.[96,97] This has also been confirmed in vascular access surgery, where perioperative use of a cephalosporin in a randomized, double-blind setting resulted in a significant decrease in postoperative wound infection rates, including cellulitis.[98] Vancomycin has also been found to be very effective in the prevention of vascular access graft infections, especially in the pediatric population.[99] In addition, proper care and use of aseptic technique by the dialysis staff and the patient himself is required to prevent infection at the site of hemodialysis access.

Thrombosis

The most frequent complication encountered in vascular access surgery is thrombosis of the fistula or shunt. The likelihood of thrombosis depends upon multiple factors, including the type of shunt or fistula constructed, site of arteriovenous anastomosis, selection of prosthetic material, and adequacy of the patient's vessels. Thrombosis at the access site may occur at any time after construction. Early thrombosis, usually defined as occurring within the first 3 months, is generally due to technical factors, whereas late thrombosis occurring after 3 months is usually caused by continuing trauma to the access site by needle puncture for hemodialysis or outflow stenosis.

Lack of adequate venous runoff is the primary cause of early failure of distal access sites.[100] In the operating room, this can be recognized soon after completion of the final anastomosis by absence of pulse, bruit, or palpable thrill. Ascertaining the patency and adequate diameter of the runoff vessel by use of a Fogarty embolectomy catheter and/or coronary artery

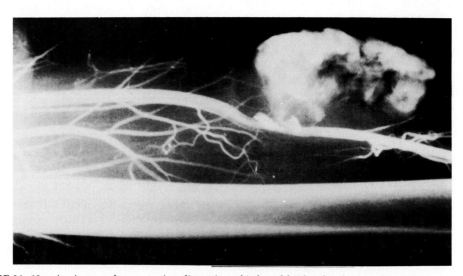

FIGURE 34–10. Angiogram demonstrating disruption of infected bridge fistula anastomosis.

dilators will often guard against this setback. Narrowing of the lumen of the artery or vein during construction or catching the back wall of the vessel while suturing can result in immediate thrombosis. Thrombosis in the early postoperative period may also be due to compression of the fistula by a hematoma. This often results from inadequate hemostasis during the procedure or early puncture of the fistula with subsequent extravasation of blood (Fig. 34–11). Excessive pressure over the needle puncture site following a hemodialysis run may also result in fistula thrombosis. In each of these situations, early reexploration, with evacuation of any hematoma, and thrombectomy of the fistula will often result in salvage of the fistula.[101]

Thrombosis of a vascular access fistula may be due to repeated trauma from needle punctures, with subsequent fibrosis and narrowing. In synthetic bridge fistulas, a needle-induced flap tear of the prosthetic wall can cause late thrombosis.

Outflow obstruction due to stenosis at the site of venous anastomosis is a relatively frequent cause of thrombosis in older bridge fistulas and may be heralded by a gradual increase in the pressure within the fistula. The combination of forceful pulsation throughout the fistula and a loud bruit at the venous end strongly suggests the development of outflow obstruction, which may be confirmed by angiography or duplex scanning (Figs. 34–12 and 34–13). True vessel aneurysmal dilation from repeated needle

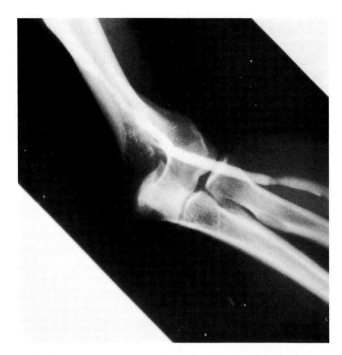

FIGURE 34–12. Angiogram demonstrating stenosis near venous anastomosis.

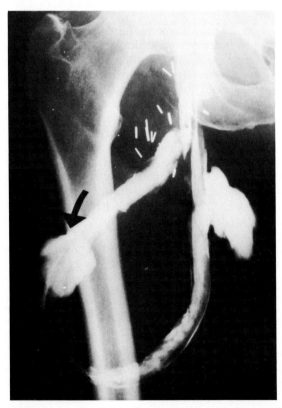

FIGURE 34–11. Angiogram demonstrating extravasation of blood and hematoma formation following too-early use of bridge fistula.

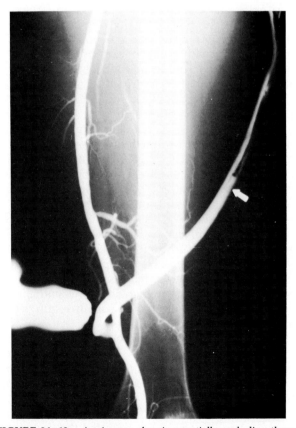

FIGURE 34–13. Angiogram showing partially occluding thrombus in lower extremity bridge fistula.

punctures has also been reported as a major cause of late thrombosis in autogenous fistulas.[100] In addition, cigarette smoking significantly increases the likelihood of thrombosis and late occlusion of arteriovenous fistulas, and is to be avoided if at all possible.[102]

Fistula thromboses were treated successfully by thrombectomy, restoring flow in over 80 per cent of fistulas in one report.[103] This same study, however, indicated that approximately 70 per cent of those fistulas successfully thrombectomized reclotted within 6 months. This was thought to be due to unsuspected anatomic lesions and technical imperfections, which can be demonstrated with angiography.[104] Aggressive fistula revision, directed by angiography at the time of thrombectomy, has resulted in 6-month patency rates of over 70 per cent.[103]

Since elevated venous return pressure during dialysis has been shown to be a very sensitive indicator of significant venous stenosis,[105,106] we strongly recommend some type of radiologic investigation of the fistula as soon as the elevation in venous return pressure is noted. Whereas fistula angiography remains the "gold standard," noninvasive methods of assessing fistula flow have been recently described. By employing Doppler ultrasound examination of the fistula, partial or complete thrombosis, aneurysmal dilation, or perifistula hematoma may be diagnosed with exceptional accuracy.[107,108] Ultrasound imaging should probably be the initial investigative technique in cases of suspected fistula malfunction. If recognized prior to thrombosis, many venous runoff stenoses may be corrected with percutaneous transluminal dilation, with patency rates of 91 per cent at 1 year and 57 per cent at 2 years being reported.[109]

If acute thrombosis has already occurred, the use of fibrinolytic agents has been found to be successful in clearing the fistula of thrombus. In one series employing streptokinase, 52 per cent of thrombosed fistulas were restored to function without surgical intervention, and another 21 per cent had restoration of flow but required surgical correction of an underlying problem thereafter.[110] Another group was successful in restoring function in over 65 per cent of cases using urokinase.[111] The use of fibrinolytic agents in this manner appears to be most successful when the cause of failure is thrombosis secondary to sepsis, hypotension, or excessive compression of fistula puncture sites following dialysis. Fistula failure associated with excessive proliferation of neointima does not respond nearly as well, and usually requires surgical revision.

In an effort to improve upon the thrombogenic tendency of vascular access fistulas, prophylaxis against thrombosis has been attempted with encouraging results. By using low-dose aspirin therapy (160 mg/day), one investigative group reported a highly significant reduction in fistula thrombotic episodes.[112] Another group has reported the successful establishment and maintenance of arteriovenous fistulas in nonuremic individuals by the use of aspirin and low-dose heparin therapy.[113] The use of oral pentoxifylline has also been shown to significantly decrease access thrombosis in patients on chronic hemodialysis.[114]

Hemodynamic Complications

The three principal hemodynamic complications of an arteriovenous fistula are congestive heart failure, peripheral vascular insufficiency or steal phenomenon, and venous hypertension. The physiologic responses of an arteriovenous fistula for hemodialysis have been reported as: a decrease in total systemic vascular resistance; an increase in cardiac output, with increases in both heart rate and, somewhat later, stroke volume; an increase in venous pressure and venous return to the heart; and reversal of flow in the artery distal to the site of the fistula when the diameter of the fistula opening exceeds the diameter of the feeding artery.[18,19,115] In addition, it has recently been found that there is a significant decrease in subcutaneous tissue oxygen tension to levels under 30 mm Hg.[116]

Depending upon the diameter of the arteriovenous communication and the size of the artery feeding it, the venous return to the heart from an arteriovenous fistula increases proportionately. This leads to a variable increase in the cardiac output and work of the heart, which can be significant enough to lead to cardiomegaly and congestive heart failure. Fistula flow as low as 20 to 25 per cent of the resting cardiac output has been demonstrated to result in heart failure.[117] Since the mean blood flow rate through distal (radiocephalic) upper extremity autogenous or bridge fistulas has been measured in one report as 242 ± 89 ml/min, high-output heart failure is unusual, but does occur.[118,119] In the same report, however, resting flow rates from more proximal upper extremity fistulas based on the brachial artery were noted to more than double, averaging as much as 641 ± 111 ml/min. Similarly, bridge fistulas placed in the thigh arising from the superficial femoral artery had resting flow rates of 592 ± 134 ml/min. Therefore, congestive heart failure is much more likely to result from the more proximally located fistula.

Initial blood flow through any type of arteriovenous fistula for hemodialysis is too low to cause heart failure, except in patients with an underlying severely compromised cardiac function.[119] With dilation of the venous outflow system, shunted blood flow through the fistula can increase greatly. One group of investigators, using echocardiographic evaluation of cardiac performance, has suggested that creation of any hemodialysis vascular access fistula causes a significant time-related cardiac decompensation when compared to normal controls.[120] Echocardiographic assessment may also be useful preoperatively in identifying those patients with poor contractility, as manifested by changes in the mean velocity of fiber shortening, and ejection fraction, as well as by left ventricular or septal wall hypertrophy.[121] Abnormal studies may warn the clinician of a propensity toward future development of heart failure and may lead to construction of the smallest, and if possible distal, arteriovenous fistula compatible with adequate access.

When congestive heart failure arises from a high-flow arteriovenous fistula, operative correction is fortunately quite simple. Although revision of the fistula with narrowing of the anastomosis or construction of a completely new fistula may be used to correct the problem, the simplest procedure for correction is banding of the existing fistula by suturing a small cuff (1 cm wide) of synthetic material (Dacron, PTFE) around the prosthesis of a bridge fistula or the main venous outflow tract of an autogenous fistula. An electromagnetic flowmeter is placed around the vein proximal to the fistula and banding cuff, and continuous flow is recorded. When the fistula flow is within the range of 300 to 400 ml/min, the banding cuff is securely sutured.

Patients who can be identified preoperatively as being at risk for the development of access-induced congestive failure (elderly, existing cardiac dysfunction, etc.) and who require a bridge fistula should have either a tapered or stepped graft placed. These grafts are manufactured with the diameter of one end 2.5 to 3.0 mm smaller than the other so that when placed in the patient (it is important to remember that the smaller end is anastomosed to the artery), flow through the graft is somewhat reduced, thereby lessening the risk of the development of congestive failure.

Arterial insufficiency or steal syndrome in vascular access for hemodialysis was originally described as occurring in Brescia-Cimino fistulas with side-to-side anastomoses because of reversed blood flow in the distal radial artery.[122] An area of very low resistance is formed on the venous portion of the anastomosis, so that the blood flow tends to course through the palmar arch from the ulnar to the radial side and steals flow from the muscles and soft tissues of the palm and fingers.[123] The syndrome is characterized by pain on exertion of the musculature of the hand, and the hand often appears cold, clammy, and pale. Severely symptomatic radial artery steal is rare, with one large study reporting only 8 of 444 (1.6 per cent) patients who had had 516 Brescia-Cimino fistulas constructed for hemodialysis developing significant steal symptoms,[124] although as many as 80 per cent of patients with Brescia-Cimino fistulas do have mild, asymptomatic arterial steal as documented by a significant decrease in thumb blood pressure.[125] Steal syndrome has also been recently described in 6.4 per cent of a series of 357 patients with upper extremity bridge fistulas, one third of which required fistula

ligation to preserve the function of the hand, while the other two thirds were successfully managed with surgical narrowing of the arterial side of the fistula.[126] Surgical correction of radial steal from a side-to-side autogenous fistula is most easily accomplished by ligation of the radial artery immediately distal to the fistula, which converts the side-to-side anastomosis to an arterial end-to-side anastomosis.[123]

Arterial insufficiency has also been noted with the use of proximally based bridge fistulas in both the upper extremity[36] and lower extremity[27] as the result of steal from the high-flow fistulas. When steal becomes symptomatic with bridge fistulas, banding of the fistula or venous outflow tract to decrease fistula flow will often cause these patients to become asymptomatic.[25] Very rarely, the entire fistula may have to be dismantled.

Arterialization of the venous system proximal to an arteriovenous fistula results in venous hypertention and, if the venous valves are incompetent, retrograde venous flow. Noted most frequently with side-to-side Brescia-Cimino fistulas and, to a lesser exent, reverse arteriovenous fistulas, retrograde venous hypertension is marked by distal extremity edema, bluish discoloration, and pigmentation of the skin (Fig. 34–14). Ulceration and neuralgias can also occur in long-standing cases.[127,128] Surgical correction is obtained by ligation of the vein immediately distal

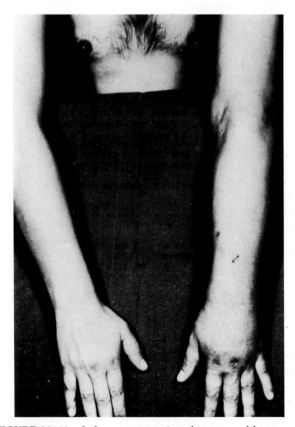

FIGURE 34–14. Left upper extremity edema caused by venous hypertension from Brescia-Cimino fistula.

to the fistula, converting the side-to-side anastomosis of the Brescia-Cimino fistula to a functional venous end-to-side, and converting bridge fistulas to a functional end-to-end anastomosis.

Intimal Hyperplasia

Progressive venous stenosis occurring as a consequence of vascular access fistula placement is a recurring problem leading to thrombosis and multiple revisions or replacement fistulas of patients requiring long-term hemodialysis. Indeed, it is the main drawback associated with prosthetic conduits. While the stenosis may be related to the technical performance of the anastomosis, in the main it can be attributed to chronic changes known to occur in the runoff veins of arteriovenous fistulas. The development of intimal fibromuscular hyperplasia may result from focal endothelial trauma caused by the shearing effect of blood flow at the site of the venous anastomosis.[129,130] In addition, venous hypertension in the runoff vessels of an arteriovenous fistula aggravates venous atherosclerosis and intimal lipid deposition, further compounding the situation.[131] Segmental stenosis of autogenous fistulas and bridge fistulas constructed using biological conduits has also been noted to occur from fibrosis and intimal hyperplasia secondary to the trauma of repeated needle punctures.[132]

Surgical correction of the stenotic area may be accomplished by patch angioplasty if the stenosis is very localized or at the site of an anastomosis, by placing an extension of the graft around a larger stenotic area, by locating the venous anastomosis to a new vein, or by complete resection of the stenotic segment with placement of an interposition conduit. Recently, the use of percutaneous transluminal balloon angioplasty has been advocated for dilation of stenotic segments in failing arteriovenous fistulas and shunts.[109] Using the Seldinger technique to gain access to the fistula, a double-lumen dilation catheter is placed at the site of the stenosis under fluoroscopic control and the stenosis is dilated twice for 30 seconds each time. Prior to catheter removal an angiogram is performed, and the dilation repeated if there is greater than 30 per cent residual stenosis. Using this technique, an initial success rate of 95 per cent has been achieved.[109]

Aneurysm Formation

Aneurysmal dilation of bridge fistula conduits depends upon the material used. True aneurysm formation has been found to occur primarily in biologic materials (saphenous vein, bovine heterograft, HUVG) and has been attributed to degeneration of the graft material itself with time.[37,44,45,54] Early PTFE grafts were also prone to true aneurysm formation from nodal fracture and a gradual stretching of the Teflon fibrils[133]; however, with an increase in the wall thickness of the material, this is no longer a problem. Excessive aneurysmal enlargement of the fistula is best treated with surgical excision of the hemodialysis fistula, with placement of a new conduit of a synthetic material at another site. Pseudoaneurysm formation secondary to trauma at the site of needle punctures can occur with any of the materials used for bridge fistulas (Fig. 34–15). If no infection can be demonstrated to be present, treatment can be occasionally achieved by local suture repair of the defect in the graft material. Somewhat larger defects may require excision of the defect and the interposition of a new small segment of graft material. Recently, aneurysmal dilation of the outflow vein proximal to the bridge fistula has been described.[134] Although rare, once diagnosed the aneurysmal segment should be bypassed and then excluded through ligation.

VASCULAR ACCESS FOR TOTAL PARENTERAL NUTRITION OR CHEMOTHERAPY

The use of surgically created arteriovenous fistulas as a means of vascular access for reasons other than hemodialysis is increasing. Several reports have found that chronic total parenteral nutrition (TPN) can be performed using an arteriovenous fistula with length of patency up to 7 years.[135,136] The advantages were found to be a very low incidence of infection and the longevity of the access site. The primary disadvantage was that the patient must undergo a significant operation to establish the vascular access. In addition, the use of an autogenous arteriovenous fistula for the delivery of chemotherapeutic agents has been advocated.[137,138] Bridge arteriovenous fistulas have also been used; however, one series reported a significantly higher complication rate for bridge fistulas when compared to Silastic right atrial catheters (48 versus 19 per cent, respectively) for chemotherapy use.[139]

Despite these increasing reports regarding the use of arteriovenous fistulas for chemotherapy and TPN, the more general method employed for delivering these therapeutic modalities is a chronic indwelling central venous catheter. For a number of years, the accepted method for central venous cannulation involved percutaneous catheterization with a polyethylene catheter. Recognition of the propensity of percutaneously placed polyethylene catheters toward infection and thrombosis, and the inherent dangers of the technique of placing these catheters, however, has led to the development of specialized large-bore catheters that are less reactive and less thrombogenic.

The Broviac[140] and Hickman[141] central venous catheters are made of soft radiopaque rubber measuring 90 cm in length and have a small Dacron felt cuff 30 cm from the Luer-Lok external end. The Broviac catheter has an internal diameter of 1 mm, and the Hickman modification differs only in that it has an internal diameter of 1.6 mm. Each catheter consists of a rel-

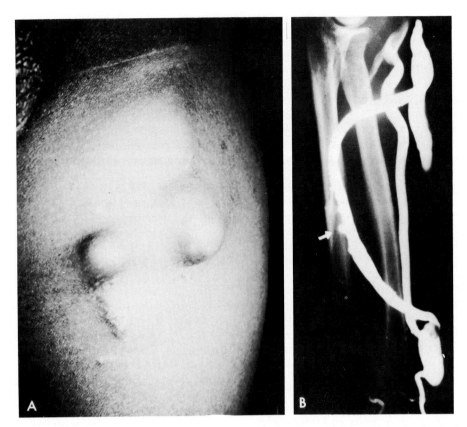

FIGURE 34–15. *A,* Pseudoaneurysm formation at needle puncture sites of hemodialysis fistula. *B,* Angiogram demonstrating multiple pseudoaneurysms at needle puncture sites of bridge fistula.

atively thin-walled intravascular segment, and a thicker walled extravascular portion. A smaller, pediatric-sized Broviac catheter is also available, as are double-lumen catheters in various sizes. These catheters are placed via direct venous cutdown into the cephalic (Fig. 34–16), external jugular, or greater saphenous veins, and the extravascular portion of the catheter is tunneled through the subcutaneous tissue in order to separate the skin exit site from the venotomy site. Fibrous tissue ingrowth into the Dacron cuff located in the subcutaneous tunnel serves to anchor the catheter and has been found to present an effective barrier to the migration of microorganisms from the skin into the venous system along the outer surface of the catheter. For further protection against infection, many of these catheters can also be ordered with an additional cuff (VitaCuff) in place that is impregnated with an antimicrobial agent that is positioned in the subcutaneous tunnel between the Dacron cuff and the skin exit site. As a consequence, the sepsis rate with these catheters is relatively low.[142–144]

Two recent innovations in central venous access have been the introduction of the Groshong catheter and implantable ports. Unlike either the Hickman or Broviac catheters, the Groshong catheter has no clamps, comes without the hub attached, and possesses a unique two-way valve. This valve is designed to remain closed when the catheter is not in use, and opens either outward for fluid infusion or

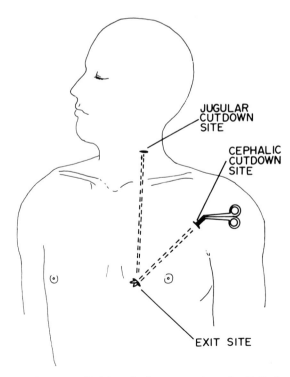

FIGURE 34–16. Position of subcutaneous tunnel exit site for upper body Broviac or Hickman catheter.

inward for blood draws. This design allows for significantly less maintenance by either the patient or the health care worker, with only a single 5-ml saline flush being recommended once a week when the catheter is not in use. One group has even suggested less frequent flushings if a heparinzed saline solution is used.[145]

Implantable ports are central venous access devices that consist of a subcutaneously implantable reservoir containing a self-sealing septum that can withstand over 2000 needle punctures and are connected to a silicone rubber catheter of internal diameters ranging from 1.0 to 1.6 mm. The reservoir body, which can be constructed of either plastic, stainless steel, or titanium, is placed in a subcutaneous pocket over the anterior chest or abdomen in an easily palpable location, and is accessed using a Huber needle for either blood withdrawal or drug delivery. These implantable ports have the advantage of requiring little daily care and therefore interfere less with the patient's normal activities. Also, implantable ports have been found to have a catheter-related sepsis rate of 3 per cent and a 1 per cent incidence of thrombosis, as compared to a 15 per cent rate of catheter-related sepsis and 22 per cent incidence of thrombosis in external central venous catheters.[146] In addition, a prospective comparison demonstrated that external shunts have 0.13 exit site infections and 0.03 bacteremic episodes per 100 catheter-days, compared to 0.06 pocket infections and 0 bacteremic episodes per 100 catheter-days for implantable ports.[147]

The placement of any central venous catheter for TPN or chemotherapy is always considered to be an elective, sterile, operative procedure. Thus, the patient should have hypovolemia and electrolyte abnormalities corrected prior to catheter palcement. Adequate lighting, instruments, assistance, and aseptic techniques are absolute prerequisites for safe insertion of the catheter. A thorough knowledge of the venous anatomy and adequate experience or supervision are likewise mandatory. In theory, the Broviac or Hickman catheter may be placed into any vein accessible by cutdown; but in practice, the cephalic vein in the deltopectoral groove, the external jugular vein in the neck, and the greater saphenous vein at its confluence with the common femoral vein are the preferred sites. If these are unavailable, the internal jugular, the common facial, the large pectoral radial, and the thoracoacromial veins are alternatives.[24] In patients requiring long-term central venous catheterization who have had numerous previous catheters placed, preoperative venography may be required to verify patency of the vena cavae (superior or inferior), the subclavian or iliac veins, or their tributaries.

In most hospitals, Broviac or Hickman catheter insertion is performed in the controlled environment of the operating suite, where radiography or fluoroscopy is available to confirm the proper position of the catheter tip prior to skin closure. The cutdown site is then selected. For the cephalic vein cutdown, the skin incision is made just inferior to the coracoid

process in the area of the deltopectoral groove. For the external jugular vein approach, a transverse mid-cervical incision is made over the vein. When the greater saphenous vein is used, a longitudinal incision over the vein and just distal to the inguinal ligament is employed.

After dissection verifies patency and adequate size of the selected vein, a subcutaneous tunnel is made from the cutdown site to a cutaneous exit either medial to the breast (if a cephalad central vein is chosen) or the anterior abdominal wall if a caudad vein is used. A small stab wound is made at the cutaneous exit site, and the catheter is drawn through the tunnel until the Dacron cuff resides 2 to 4 cm inside the tunnel. The catheter is then shortened so that the tip will just reach the right atrium from the upper body or about the level of the renal veins from the lower body, and filled with heparin-treated saline by syringe. The vein is ligated distally, and the catheter is introduced through a small venotomy, advanced to its full length, and aspirated with the attached syringe. If dark venous blood does not return, the catheter is either kinked or misplaced, and it should be withdrawn and advanced again. A proximal ligature placed around the vein secures the catheter in place. Radiographic verification of proper catheter tip position should always be obtained prior to wound closure (Fig. 34–17). The catheter is fixed to the skin at the exit site with a monofilament suture, which is removed 7 to 14 days later after fibrous ingrowth into the Dacron cuff has occurred. Povidone-iodine ointment and a sterile dressing are applied to the exit site, and the loop of redundant catheter is taped to the body wall. The catheter may either be heparin locked using the Luer-Lok can provided or immediately connected to an intravenous infusion set.

Once properly inserted and positioned, Broviac and Hickman catheters have been left in place for more than 1 year, with an average duration reported of over 2 months.[143,144] Because of the chronic nature of the underlying diseases often seen in patients who require long-term catheterization, multiple insertions were necessary in 13 per cent of patients in one study.[143] The primary complications of Broviac and Hickman catheter use are sepsis, thrombosis, and dislodgement of the catheter, which have been reported in two recent series comprising 199 catheter placements as occurring in 12, 5, and 3.5 per cent of cases, respectively.[143,144] Central vein thrombosis as a result of long-term catheterization has also been noted to occur, although infrequently.

An alternative technique for placement of Broviac and Hickman catheters involving direct venipuncture has been reported.[148] With this technique, two small (less than 1 cm) skin incisions are made at the proposed venous entry site and skin exit site and a subcutaneous tunnel created between them. The catheter is then brought through the tunnel until the Dacron cuff lies 2 to 4 cm within the tunnel. The chosen vein is then punctured through the vein entry incision as if for placement of a central venous pressure (CVP)

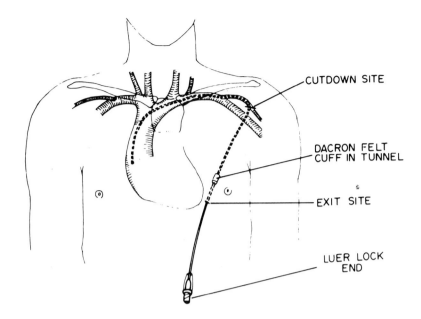

FIGURE 34–17. Correct position of Broviac or Hickman catheter placed via cephalic vein.

line. A guidewire is inserted through the needle, thus allowing the needle to be removed. A vein dilator and peel-away sheath are then placed over the guidewire, and, once in place, the guidewire and dilator are removed. The Broviac or Hickman catheter is then introduced into the vein through the peel-away sheath, the sheath is withdrawn, and peeled apart, leaving the catheter in place. Radiologic verification of catheter position is then achieved, and wound closure and catheter care performed as with standard Broviac or Hickman catheter placement (Fig. 34–18).

Although the only reported complications in 21 catheter insertions using direct venipuncture were three cases of malposition,[148] any of the complications seen with standard CVP placement are possible because of the relatively "blind" nature of the technique. This would include pneumohemothorax, arterial laceration or perforation, arteriovenous fistula formation, brachial plexus or other nerve injury, air or catheter embolism, or lymphatic fistula formation.[10]

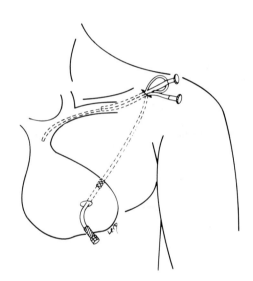

FIGURE 34–18. Placement of a Silastic catheter by percutaneous subclavian venipuncture.

REFERENCES

1. Garrison FH: An Introduction to the History of Medicine, 4th ed. Philadelphia, WB Saunders Company, 1929, p 273.
2. Wheatley HB: The Diary of Samuel Pepys, vol II. New York, Random House, 1966, p 426.
3. Kolff WJ: The first clinical experience with the artificial kidney. Ann Intern Med 62:608–619, 1965.
4. Quinton WE, Dillar D, Scribner BH: Cannulation of blood vessels for prolonged hemodialysis. Trans Am Soc Artif Intern Organs 6:104–113, 1960.
5. Graves EJ: Detailed diagnoses and procedures, National Hospital Discharge Survey, 1989. National Center for Health Statistics. Vital Health Stat 13(108), 1991.
6. Ishihara AM, Meyers CH: Longevity of arteriovenous shunts for hemodialysis. Ann Surg 168:281–286, 1968.
7. Harder F, Landmann J: Trends in access surgery for hemodialysis. Surg Annu 16:135–149, 1984.
8. Dunn J, Nylander W, Richie R: Central venous dialysis access: Experience with a dual-lumen, silicone rubber catheter. Surgery 102:784–789, 1987.
9. Surratt RS, Picus D, Hicks ME, et al: The importance of preoperative evaluation of the subclavian vein in dialysis planning. AJR 156:623–625, 1991.
10. Herbst CA: Indications, management and complications of percutaneous subclavian catheters: An audit. Arch Surg 113:1421–1425, 1978.
11. Giacchino JL, Geis WP, Wittenstein BH, Gandhi VC: Recent trends in vascular access. Am Surg 48:501–504, 1982.
12. Moss AH, Vasilakis BS, Holley JL, et al: Use of a Silicone dual-lumen catheter with a Dacron cuff as a long-term vascular access for hemodialysis patients. Am J Kidney Dis 16:211–215, 1990.
13. Reilly DT, Wood RFM, Bell PRF: Prospective study of di-

alysis fistulas: Problem patients and their treatment. Br J Surg 69:549–553, 1982.

14. Brescia MJ, Cimino JE, Appel K, Hurwich BJ: Chronic hemodialysis using veni-puncture and a surgically created arteriovenous fistula. N Engl J Med 275:1089–1092, 1966.

15. Monquet C, Bitker MO, Bailliart O, et al: Anesthesia for creation of a forearm fistula in patients with endstage renal failure. Anesthesiology 70:909–914, 1989.

16. Johnson G: Local pathophysiology of an arteriovenous fistula. *In* Swam KG (ed): Venous Surgery in the Lower Extremity. St. Louis, Warren H. Greene, 1975, pp 41–50.

17. Bennion RS, Williams RA: The radiocephalic fistula. Contemp Dial 3:12–16, 1982.

18. Anderson CB, Etheridge EE, Harter HR, et al: Local blood flow characteristics of arteriovenous fistulas in the forearm for dialysis. Surg Gynecol Obstet 144:531–533, 1977.

19. Johnson G, Dart CH, Peters RM, Steele F: The importance of venous circulation in arteriovenous fistula. Surg Gynecol Obstet 123:995–1000, 1966.

20. Mindich BP, Levowitz BS: Enhancement of flow through arteriovenous fistula. Arch Surg 111:195–196, 1976.

21. Moran MR, Enriquez AA, Boyero MR, et al: Hand exercise effect in maturation and blood flow of dialysis arteriovenous fistulas. Angiology 35:641–644, 1984.

22. Giacchino JL, Geis WP, Buckingham JM, et al: Vascular access: Long-term results, new techniques. Arch Surg 114:403–409, 1979.

23. Cantelmo NL, LoGerfo FW, Menzoian JO: Brachiobasilic and brachiocephalic fistulas as secondary angioaccess routes. Surg Gynecol Obstet 155:545–548, 1982.

24. Wilson SE, Stabile BE, Williams RA, Owens ML: Current status of vascular access techniques. Surg Clin North Am 62:531–551, 1982.

25. Owens ML, Stabile BE, Gahr JE, Wilson SE: Vascular grafts for hemodialysis: An evaluation of sites and materials. Dial Transplant 8:521–525, 1979.

26. Rohr MS, Browder W, Freutz GD, McDonald JC: Arteriovenous fistulas for long-term dialysis: Factors that influence fistula survival. Arch Surg 113:153–155, 1978.

27. Fee HJ, Golding AL: Lower extremity ischemia after femoral arteriovenous bovine shunts. Ann Surg 183:42–45, 1976.

28. Humphries AL, Nesbit RP, Carnana RJ, et al: Thirty-six recommendations for vascular access operations: Lessons learned from our first thousand operations. Am Surg 47:145–151, 1981.

29. Rizzuti RP, Hale JC, Burkart TE: Extended patency of expanded polytetrafluoroethylene grafts for vascular access using optimal configuration and revisions. Surg Gynecol Obstet 166:23–27, 1988.

30. Wilson SE, Hillman M, Owens ML: Hemodynamic effects of bovine femorosaphenous fistula. Dial Transplant 6:84–89, 1977.

31. Garcia-Rinaldi R, Von Koch L: The axillary artery to axillary vein bovine graft for circulatory access. Am J Surg 135:265–268, 1978.

32. May J, Tiller D, Johnson J, et al: Saphenous-vein arteriovenous fistula in regular dialysis treatment. N Engl J Med 280:770, 1969.

33. May J, Harris J, Fletcher J: Long-term results of saphenous vein graft arteriovenous fistulas. Am J Surg 140:387–390, 1980.

34. Jenkins AM, Buist TAS, Glover SD: Medium-term follow-up of forty autogenous vein and forty polytetrafluoroethylene (Goretex) grafts for vascular access. Surgery 88:667–672, 1980.

35. Lornoy W, Becans I, Gillardin JP, et al: Autogenous saphenous vein AV fistula for haemodialysis: Eight years experience with 30 patients. Proc Eur Dial Transplant Assoc 19:227–233, 1982.

36. Haimov M, Burrows L, Schanzer H, et al: Experience with arterial substitutes in the construction of vascular access for hemodialysis. J Cardiovasc Surg 21:149–154, 1980.

37. Szilagyi DE, Elliot JP, Hageman JJ, et al: Biologic fate of autogenous vein implants as arterial substitutes: Clinical,

angiographic and histopathologic observations in femoral popliteal operations for atherosclerosis. Ann Surg 178:232–246, 1973.

38. Piccone VA, Lee H, Ramos S, et al: Preserved allografts of dilated saphenous vein for vascular access in hemodialysis: An initial experience. Ann Surg 182:727–732, 1975.

39. Baraldi A, Manenti A, Di Felice A, et al: Absence of rejection in cryopreserved saphenous vein allografts for hemodialysis. ASAIO Trans 35:196–199, 1989.

40. Piccone VA, Sika J, Ahmed N, et al: Preserved saphenous vein allografts for vascular access. Surg Gynecol Obstet 147:385–390, 1978.

41. Siegal B: Access operation for chemotherapy and dialysis using freeze-preserved vein allografts. J Cardiovasc Surg 22:543–545, 1981.

42. Hertzer NR, Beven EG: Venous access using the bovine carotid heterograft. Techniques, results, and complications in 75 patients. Arch Surg 113:696–701, 1978.

43. Oakes DD, Spees EK, Light JA, Flye MW: A three year experience using modified bovine arterial heterografts for vascular access in patients requiring hemodialysis. Ann Surg 187:423–429, 1978.

44. Garvin PJ, Casteneda MA, Codd JE: Etiology and management of bovine graft aneurysms. Arch Surg 117:281–284, 1982.

45. Rossi G, Munteau FD, Padula G, et al: Non-anastomotic aneurysms in venous homologous grafts and bovine heterografts in femoropopliteal bypasses Am J Surg 132:358–362, 1976.

46. West NC, Sells R, Korn Y, McVerry BA: A new modified bovine heterograft for vascular access in haemophiliacs. Clin Lab Haematol 6:375–377, 1984.

47. Lilly L, Ngheim D, Mendez-Picon G, Lee HM: Comparison between bovine heterografts and expanded PTFE grafts for dialysis access. Am Surg 46:694–696, 1980.

48. Wilson SE, Hutchinson WB: Infection of newly implanted and well-incorporated bovine heterografts. Dial Transplant 5:38–41, 1976.

49. Butler HG, Baker LD, Johnson JM: Vascular access for chronic hemodialysis: Polytetrafluoroethylene (PTFE) versus bovine heterograft. Am J Surg 134:791–793, 1977.

50. Dardik H, Ibrahim IM, Dardik I: Arteriovenous fistulas constructed with modified human umbilical cord vein graft. Arch Surg 111:60–62, 1976.

51. Baier RE, Akers CK, Perlmutter S: Processed human umbilical cord veins for vascular reconstructive surgery. Trans Am Soc Artif Intern Organs 22:514–526, 1976.

52. Dardik H, Ibrahim IM, Sussman B: Gluteraldehyde-stabilized umbilical vein prosthesis for revascularization of the legs. Am J Surg 138:234–237, 1979.

53. Karkow WS, Cranley JJ, Cranley RD, et al: Extended study of aneurysm formation in umbilical vein grafts. J Vasc Surg 4:486–492, 1986.

54. Hasson JE, Newton WD, Waltman AC, et al: Mural degeneration in the gluteraldehyde-tanned umbilical vein graft: Incidence and implications. J Vasc Surg 4:243–250, 1986.

55. Flores L, Dunn I, Frumkin E, et al: Dacron arteriovenous shunts for vascular access in hemodialysis. Trans Am Soc Artif Intern Organs 19:33–37, 1973.

56. Levowitz BS, Flores L, Dunn I, Frumkin E: Prosthetic arteriovenous fistula for vascular access in hemodialysis. Am J Surg 132:368–372, 1976.

57. Lindenauer SM, Williams R: Dacron velour arteriovenous fistula for hemodialysis access. Ann Surg 193:43–48, 1981.

58. Kester RC: Arteriovenous grafts for vascular access surgery in hemodialysis. Br J Surg 66:23–28, 1979.

59. Jamil Z, O'Donnell JA, Merk EA, Hobson RW: A comparison of knitted Dacron velour and bovine heterograft for hemodialysis access. J Surg Res 26:423–429, 1979.

60. Baker LD, Johnson JM, Goldfarb D: Expanded polytetrafluoroethylene (PTFE) subcutaneous arteriovenous conduit: An improved vascular access for chronic hemodialysis. Trans Am Soc Artif Intern Organs 22:382–387, 1976.

61. Sabanayagam P, Schwartz AB, Soricelli RR, et al: A com-

parative study of 402 bovine heterografts and 225 reinforced expanded PTFE grafts as AVG in the ESRD patient. Trans Am Soc Artif Intern Organs 26:88–92, 1980.

62. Munda R, First MR, Alexander JW, et al: Polytetrafluoroethylene graft survival in hemodialysis. JAMA 249:219–222, 1983.

63. Palder SB, Kirkman RL, Whittemore AD, et al: Vascular access for hemodialysis. Patency rates and results of revisions. Ann Surg 202:235–239, 1985.

64. Schuman ES, Gross GF, Hayes JF, Standage BA: Long-term patency of polytetrafluoroethylene graft fistulas. Am J Surg 155:644–646, 1988.

65. Bhat DJ, Tellis VA, Kohlberg WI, et al: Management of sepsis involving expanded polytetrafluoroethylene grafts for hemodialysis access. Surgery 87:445–450, 1980.

66. Golding AL, Nissenson AR, Raible D: Carbon transcutaneous access device (CTAD). Proc Clin Dial Transplant Forum 9:242–247, 1979.

67. Shapiro FL, Keshavich PR, Carlson LD, et al: Blood access without percutaneous punctures. Proc Clin Dial Transplant Forum 10:130–137, 1980.

68. Collins AJ, Shapiro FL, Keshaviach PR, et al: Blood access without skin puncture. Trans Am Soc Artif Intern Organs 27:308–313, 1981.

69. Carter KH: Clinical experience with atraumatic vascular access for hemodialysis. Contemp Dial 3:24–30, 1982.

70. Kaplan AA, Grant J, Galler M, et al: Regional experience with the Hemasite no-needle access device. Trans Am Soc Artif Intern Organs 29:369–372, 1983.

71. Nissenson AR: The bioCarbon vascular access system (bVAS) no-needle hemodialysis. Trans Am Soc Artif Intern Organs 29:784–789, 1983.

72. Offner G, Aschendorff C, Hoyer PF, et al: End stage renal failure: 14 years' experience of dialysis and renal transplantation. Arch Dis Child 63:120–126, 1988.

73. Gibson TC, Dyer DP, Postlethwaite RJ, Gough DCS: Vascular access for acute hemodialysis. Arch Dis Child 62:141–145, 1987.

74. Hiatt JR, Busuttil RW: A method for vascular access in small children. Surgery 93:343–344, 1983.

75. Kinnaert P, Janssen F, Hall M: Elbow arteriovenous fistula (EAVF) for chronic hemodialysis in small children. J Pediatr Surg 18:116–119, 1983.

76. Bourquelot P, Wolfeler L, Lamy L: Microsurgery for haemodialysis distal arteriovenous fistulae in children weighing less than 10 kg. Proc Eur Dial Transplant Assoc 18:537–541, 1981.

77. Applebaum H, Shashikumar VL, Somers LA, et al: Improved hemodialysis vascular access in children. J Pediatr Surg 15:764–769, 1980.

78. Nevins TE, Kjellstrand CM: Hemodialysis for children: A review. Int J Pediatr Nephrol 4:155–169, 1983.

79. Jacobs C, Brunner SP, Chantler C, et al: Combined report on regular dialysis and transplantation in Europe. Proc Eur Dial Transplant Assoc 14:3–69, 1977.

80. Dobkin JF, Miller MH, Steigbigel NH: Septicemia in patients on chronic hemodialysis. Ann Intern Med 88:28–33, 1978.

81. Martin RR, Eknoyan G, Saenz C, et al: Effects of renal failure on leukotaxis. J Med 10:267–278, 1979.

82. Peresesuschi G, Blum M, Aviram A, Spirer ZH: Impaired neutrophil response to acute bacterial infection in dialyzed patients. Arch Intern Med 141:1301–1302, 1981.

83. Salant DJ, Glover AM, Anderson R, et al: Depressed neutrophil chemotaxis in patients with chronic renal failure on dialysis and after renal transplantation. J Lab Clin Med 88:536–545, 1976.

84. Hanicki Z, Cichocki T, Komerowska Z, et al: Some aspects of cellular immunity in the construction of vascular access for hemodialysis. Nephron 23:273–275, 1979.

85. Hurst KS, Saldhana LF, Steinberg SM, et al: The effects of varying dialysis regimens on lymphocyte transformation. Trans Am Soc Artif Intern Organs 21:329–334, 1975.

86. Raskova J, Morrison AB, Shea SM, Raska K: Humoral inhibitors of the immune response in uremia. II. Further characterization of an immunosuppressive factor in uremic serum. Am J Pathol 97:277–290, 1979.

87. Nelson J, Ormrod DJ, Wilson D, Miller TE: Host immune status in uraemia. III. Humoral response to selected antigens in the rat. Clin Exp Immunol 42:234–240, 1980.

88. Montgomerie JZ, Kalmanson GM, Guze LB: Renal failure and infection. Medicine 47:1–32, 1963.

89. Kirmani N, Tuazon CU, Murry HW, et al: *Staphylococcus aureus* carriage rate of patients receiving long-term hemodialysis. Arch Intern Med 138:1657–1659, 1978.

90. Kaplowitz LG, Comstock JA, Landwehr DM, et al: Prospective study of microbial colonization of the nose and skin and infection of the vascular access site in hemodialysis patients. J Clin Microbiol 26:1257–1262, 1988.

91. Morgan AP, Knight DC, Tilney NL, Lazaris JM: Femoral triangle sepsis in dialysis patients. Frequency, management, and outcome. Ann Surg 191:460–464, 1980.

92. Wilson SE, Van Wagenen P, Passaro S: Arterial infection. Curr Probl Surg 15:1–89, 1978.

93. Bennion RS, Wilson SE, Williams RA: Vascular prosthetic infection. Infect Surg 1:45–55, 1982.

94. Moore WS, Swanson RJ, Compagna G, et al: Pseudointimal development and vascular prosthesis susceptibility to bacteremic infection. Surg Forum 25:250–251, 1974.

95. Ehrenfield WK, Wilbur BG, Olcott CN, Stoney RJ: Autogenous tissue reconstruction in the management of infected prosthetic grafts. Surgery 85:82–92, 1979.

96. Kaiser AB, Clayson DR, Mulherin JL, et al: Antibiotic prophylaxis in vascular surgery. Ann Surg 188:283–289, 1978.

97. Pitt HA, Postier RG, MacGowen WAL, et al: Prophylactic antibiotics in vascular surgery. Ann Surg 192:356–364, 1980.

98. Bennion RS, Hiatt JR, Williams RA, Wilson SE: A randomized, prospective study of perioperative antimicrobial prophylaxis for vascular access surgery. J Cardiovasc Surg 26:270–274, 1985.

99. Fivush BA, Bock GH, Guzzetta PC, et al: Vancomycin prevents polytetrafluoroethylene graft infections in pediatric patients receiving chronic hemodialysis. Am J Kidney Dis 5:120–123, 1985.

100. Raju S: PTFE grafts for hemodialysis access. Techniques for insertion and management of complications. Ann Surg 206:666–673, 1987.

101. Bell DD, Rosental JJ: Arteriovenous graft life in chronic hemodialysis. A need for prolongation. Arch Surg 123:1169–1172, 1988.

102. Griffin PJA, Davies F, Salaman JR, Coles GA: Effects of smoking on long term patency of arteriovenous fistulas. Br Med J 286:685–686, 1983.

103. Bone GE, Pomjzl MJ: Management of dialysis fistula thrombosis. Am J Surg 138:901–906, 1979.

104. Glanz S, Bashist B, Gordon DH, et al: Angiography of upper extremity access fistulas for dialysis. Radiology 143:45–52, 1982.

105. Schwab SJ, Raymond JR, Saeed M, et al: Prevention of hemodialysis fistula thrombosis. Early detection of venous stenoses. Kidney Int 36:707–711, 1989.

106. Gain JS, Fowler PR, Steinberg AW, et al: Use of the fistula assessment monitor to detect stenoses in access fistulae. Am J Kidney Dis 17:303–306, 1991.

107. Rittgers SE, Garcia-Valdez C, McCormick JT, Posner MP: Noninvasive flow measurement in expanded polytetrafluoroethylene grafts for hemodialysis access. J Vasc Surg 3:635–642, 1986.

108. Weber M, Kuhn FP, Quintes W, et al: Sonography of arteriovenous fistulae in hemodialysis patients. Clin Nephrol 22:258–261, 1984.

109. Gmelin E, Winterhoff R, Rinast E: Insufficient hemodialysis access fistulas: Late results in treatment with percutaneous balloon angioplasty. Radiology 171:657–660, 1989.

110. Zeit RM, Cope C: Failed hemodialysis shunts. One year of experience with aggressive treatment. Radiology 154:353–356, 1985.

111. Mangiarotti G, Canavese C, Thea A, et al: Urokinase treat-

ment for arteriovenous fistulae declotting in dialyzed patients. Nephron *36*:60–64, 1984.

112. Harter HR, Burch JW, Majerus PW, et al: Prevention of thrombosis in patients on hemodialysis by low-dose aspirin. N Engl J Med *301*:577–579, 1979.

113. Flye MW, Mundinger GH, Schulz SC, et al: Successful creation of arteriovenous fistulas in nonuremic patients with heparin and aspirin therapy. Am J Surg *142*:759–673, 1981.

114. Radmilovic A, Boric Z, Naumovic T, et al: Shunt thrombosis prevention in hemodialysis patients—a double-blind, randomized study: Pentoxifylline vs placebo. Angiology *38*:499–505, 1987.

115. Johnson G, Blythe WB: Hemodynamic effects of arteriovenous shunts used for hemodialysis. Ann Surg *171*:715–721, 1970.

116. Jensen JA, Goodson WH, Omachi RS, et al: Subcutaneous tissue oxygenation falls during hemodialysis. Surgery *101*:416–421, 1987.

117. Ahern DJ, Maher JF: Heart failure as a complication of hemodialysis arteriovenous fistula. Ann Intern Med *77*:201–204, 1972.

118. Anderson CB, Codd JR, Graff RA, et al: Cardiac failure and upper extremity arteriovenous dialysis fistulas. Arch Intern Med *136*:292–297, 1976.

119. Anderson CB, Etheridge EE, Harter HR, et al: Blood flow measurements in arteriovenous dialysis fistulas. Surgery *81*:459–461, 1977.

120. Riley SM, Blackstone EH, Sterling WA, Diethelm AG: Echocardiographic assessment of cardiac performance in patients with arteriovenous fistulas. Surg Gynecol Obstet *146*:203–208, 1978.

121. Von Bibra H, Castro L, Autenieth G, et al: The effects of arteriovenous shunts on cardiac function in renal dialysis patients: An echocardiographic evaluation. Clin Nephrol *9*:205–209, 1978.

122. Storey BG, George CRP, Stewart JOH, et al: Embolic and ischemic complications after anastomosis of radial artery to cephalic vein. Surgery *66*:325–327, 1969.

123. Bussell JA, Abbott JA, Lim RC: A radial steal syndrome with arteriovenous fistula for hemodialysis. Ann Intern Med *75*:387–394, 1971.

124. Haimov M: Vascular access for hemodialysis. Surg Gynecol Obstet *141*:619–625, 1975.

125. Duncan H, Ferguson L, Faris I: Incidence of the radial steal syndrome in patients with brescia fistula for hemodialysis: Its clinical significance. J Vasc Surg *4*:144–147, 1986.

126. Odland MD, Kelly PH, Ney AL, et al: Management of dialysis-associated steal syndrome complicating upper extremity arteriovenous fistulas: Use of intraoperative digital photoplethysmography. Surgery *110*:664–670, 1991.

127. Knezevic W, Mastaglia FL: Neuropathy associated with Brescia-Cimino arteriovenous fistulas. Arch Neurol *41*:1184–1186, 1984.

128. Wood ML, Reilly GD, Smith GT: Ulceration of the hand secondary to a radial arteriovenous fistula: A model for varicose ulceration. Br Med J *287*:1167–1168, 1983.

129. Bond MG, Hotstetler JR, Karayannocas PE, et al: Intimal changes in arteriovenous bypass grafts. Effects of varying the angle of implantation at the proximal anastomosis and of producing stenosis in the distal runoff artery. J Thorac Cardiovasc Surg *71*:907–916, 1976.

130. Telles D, Weinstein P: Intimal cellular response to microvascular anastomosis. Scan Electron Microsc *3*:227–234, 1980.

131. Stehbens WE, Karmody AM: Venous atherosclerosis associated with arteriovenous fistulas for hemodialysis. Arch Surg *110*:176–180, 1975.

132. Mennes PA, Gilula LA, Anderson CB, et al: Complications associated with arteriovenous fistulas in patients undergoing chronic hemodialysis. Arch Intern Med *138*:1117–1121, 1978.

133. Owens ML, Shinaberger JH, Wilson SE, Wang SMS: Aneurysmal enlargement of e-PTFE fistulas. Dial Transplant *7*:692–694, 1978.

135. Engels JGL, Skotincki SH, Buskens FGM, van Tougeren JHM: Home parenteral nutrition via arteriovenous fistulae. JPEN *7*:412–414, 1983.

136. Havill JH, Blair RD: Home parenteral nutrition using shunts. JPEN *8*:321–324, 1984.

137. Wobbes T, Slooff MJH, Lichtendahl DHE, et al: The radiocephalic fistula as vascular access for chemotherapy. World J Surg *7*:532–535, 1983.

138. Wobbes T, Slooff MJH, Sleijfer DT, et al: Five years' experience in access surgery for polychemotherapy. An analysis of results in 100 consecutive patients. Cancer *52*:978–982, 1983.

139. Raaf JH: Results from use of 826 vascular access devices in cancer patients. Cancer *55*:1312–1321, 1985.

140. Broviac JW, Cole JJ, Scribner BH: A silicone rubber atrial catheter for prolonged parenteral alimentation. Surg Gynecol Obstet *136*:602–606, 1973.

141. Hickman RO, Buckner CD, Clift RA, et al: A modified right atrial catheter for access to the venous system in bone marrow transplant recipients. Surg Gynecol Obstet *148*:871–875, 1979.

142. Reilla MC, Scribner BH: Five years' experience with a right catheter for prolonged parenteral nutrition at home. Surg Gynecol Obstet *143*:205–208, 1976.

143. Thomas JH, MacArthur RI, Pierce GE, Hermreck AS: Hickman-Broviac catheters. Indications and results. Am J Surg *140*:791–796, 1980.

144. Weber TR, West KW, Grosfeld JL: Broviac central venous catheterization in infants and children. Am J Surg *145*:791–796, 1983.

145. Bedini AV, Tavecchio L, Bonalumi MG, et al: Reliability of prolonged infusion in cancer chemotherapy with the Groshong central venous catheter. Reg Cancer Treat *3*:232–234, 1990.

146. Greene FL, Moore W, Strickland G, McFarland J: Comparison of a totally implantable device for chemotherapy (Port-A-Cath) and long-term percutaneous catheterization (Broviac). South Med J *81*:580–585, 1988.

147. Ross MN, Haase GM, Poole MA, et al: Comparison of totally implanted reservoirs with external catheters as venous access devices in pediatric oncologic patients. Surg Gynecol Obstet *167*:141–144, 1988.

148. Stellato WE, Gauderer MW, Cohen AM: Direct central vein puncture for silicone rubber catheter insertion. An alternative technique for Broviac catheter placement. Surgery *90*:896–899, 1981.

REVIEW QUESTIONS

1. Following creation of a radiocephalic autogenous fistula, the configuration that is associated with the lowest incidence of venous hypertension is:

   (a) arterial side–to–vein side anastomosis
   (b) vein end–to–arterial side anastomosis
   (c) arterial end–to–vein side anastomosis
   (d) arterial end–to–vein end anastomosis
   (e) none of the above

2. The highest 3-year patency rate in vascular access procedures has been achieved with:

   (a) PTFE bridge fistulas
   (b) autogenous saphenous vein bridge fistulas
   (c) Scribner shunts
   (d) autogenous radiocephalic fistulas
   (e) percutaneous double-lumen Silastic catheters

3. Postoperative hemodynamic changes that may be encountered following the construction of a proximally located bridge fistula for hemodialysis includes all the following except:
   (a) increased stroke volume
   (b) reversal of flow in the distal artery when the fistula opening exceeds the diameter of the feeding artery
   (c) increased cardiac output
   (d) increased heart rate
   (e) decreased total systemic resistance

4. Which of the following is not a complication of percutaneous subclavian central venous catheterization?
   (a) hemopneumothorax
   (b) catheter embolism
   (c) brachial plexus injury
   (d) lymphatic fistula formation
   (e) none of the above

5. Correction of localized venous runoff stenosis can be accomplished by all of the following except:
   (a) patch angioplasty of the outflow anastomosis
   (b) extension bypass graft to a more proximal vein
   (c) percutaneous transluminal dilatation
   (d) relocation of venous anastomosis to adjacent vein
   (e) replacement with new conduit

6. Characteristics of venous runoff stenosis include all of the following except:
   (a) may be related to the shearing effect of blood flow at the anastomotic site
   (b) rarely develops before 2 years after fistula creation
   (c) most often seen following construction of bridge fistulas
   (d) manifests as an increase in venous return pressure while on dialysis
   (e) may be due to compliance mismatch

7. The potential benefits of implantable ports over external central venous catheters for the delivery of chemotherapy include all the following except:
   (a) lower catheter-related sepsis rates
   (b) lower incidence of thrombosis
   (c) does not require constant heparinization
   (d) requires little daily care
   (e) interferes less with the patient's normal activities

8. Vascular access in children weighing less than 10 kg may be most reliably accomplished by each of the following except:
   (a) percutaneous central vein catheterization
   (b) forearm PTFE bridge fistula
   (c) creation of brachial artery–antecubital vein autogenous fistula
   (d) direct cannulation of umbilical vessels if a newborn
   (e) placement of external arteriovenous shunt

9. The increased risk of infection of a prosthetic bridge fistula for hemodialysis can be related to all of the following except:
   (a) use of the graft prior to tissue incorporation and pseudointimal formation
   (b) high colonization rate of dialysis patients and dialysis staff with *S. auerus*
   (c) decreased chemotactic responses of PMNs in uremia
   (d) decreased bacterial phagocytosis in uremic patients
   (e) all of the above

10. Limitations in the use of the Scribner shunt include all of the following except:
    (a) long-term patency unlikely
    (b) high risk of infection
    (c) easily dislodged
    (d) cannot be used in acutely ill patients
    (e) high rate of thrombosis

ANSWERS

1. d	2. d	3. a	4. e	5. e	6. b	7. c
8. b	9. e	10. d				

35

VASCULAR TRAUMA

MALCOLM O. PERRY

Trauma is the fourth leading cause of death in the United States. Over 140,000 deaths occur each year from accidents.[1] Many of the patients have multiple injuries, but wounds of major vascular structures are the sole cause or major contributing cause in many of the deaths, and even those patients who survive may experience severe disability as a result of vascular injuries that lead to amputation of limbs or impaired function.

In most situations, there is little difficulty in ascertaining that the patient has a serious injury, but patients who have multiple wounds present a severe test of the discipline and training of a young surgeon. A careful assessment of all injuries and the establishment of priorities in treatment are essential to a successful outcome.

ETIOLOGY

Major vascular wounds may occur in any environment, but the greatest incidence is seen in urban areas, where violence is endemic. Penetrating trauma is much more common than blunt trauma; most of the penetrating wounds are caused by knives and bullets, although accidental wounds may occur as a result of injuries inflicted by shards of glass or metal projections during motor vehicle accidents or industrial mishaps (Table 35–1).

Stab wounds are much more common than gunshot wounds, but since such injuries are not as deep nor usually as widespread, they are less likely to produce severe vascular wounds and often can be treated with relatively minor procedures. Deeper structures are often spared because small knives are commonly used, and in certain segments of society, knife wounds are meant to punish, but not to maim or kill, and the point is extended in such a fashion that only a small cut will result. Gunshot wounds usually penetrate deeply, often involving the trunk or thorax as well as the extremities, and therefore are likely to produce more serious wounds, including major arteries and veins. The vessels of the extremities are most often involved, since they are longer and located more superficially. Also, the victim may attempt to defend himself with his arms or legs and thus invite injuries to his extremities (Table 35–2).

MECHANISMS OF INJURY

Most penetrating injuries are caused by stabbing or bullets traveling at a low velocity, and the damage is mainly confined to the wound tract. Punctures, lacerations, and contusions may be encountered. Knife wounds usually cause lacerations, but bullets inflict direct damage to the neurovascular structures in the path, and complete vessel transection is likely. The concussive effects caused by higher velocity missiles produce widespread damage. The cavitation effect of a high-velocity bullet (1500 to 3000 feet/sec) may even damage a vessel remote from the wound tract, and when the blast cavity collapses, a suction effect is generated that can draw surface structures such as bits of skin, clothing, or dirt into the wound, thus contributing to the possibility of infection.

A high-velocity bullet or metal fragment can produce a great deal of tissue damage, and if it strikes bone and all of the bullet's energy is dissipated in the target, widespread destruction often occurs. Such destructive effects may not be suspected from initial inspection of the skin and surface, where, in some cases, there may be only a small entrance and exit wound, yet the interior damage is extensive, and wide débridement is required if invasive sepsis is to be avoided.

Special problems are encountered as a result of a close-range shotgun blast, although the muzzle velocity of a shotgun pellet is similar to that produced

TABLE 35–1. VASCULAR TRAUMA ETIOLOGY
(665 CASES)

	Percentage
Gunshot	55
Edged instruments	36
Blunt trauma	9

TABLE 35–2.   ARTERIAL INJURIES DISTRIBUTION

Extremity	501
Visceral	37
Cervical	96
Aorta	31
Total	665

by the familiar 22-caliber rifle bullet (approximately 1200 feet/sec). Damage inflicted by multiple pellets is usually widespread, and the shotshell wadding and bits of clothing carried into the wound greatly enhance the possibility of infection. As with high-velocity wounds, close-range shotgun blasts often cause a great deal more damage to the interior structures than is apparent from inspection of the entry sites in the skin.

Motor vehicle accidents continue to increase in frequency and seriousness as traffic density increases and the size of the automobile decreases. These accident victims commonly have multiple injuries that frequently include fractures and dislocations. Direct injury of major vessels may occur, but in many cases the major vascular wounds are the results of these fractures; this is especially likely to occur with fractures near the joints where the vessels are relatively fixed and therefore more vulnerable to shear forces. Posterior dislocations of the knee, for example, are particularly likely to injure the popliteal artery and vein.[2,3]

The bending and sudden breaking of large heavy bones such as the femur or the tibia release tremendous forces. The damage to soft tissue and neurovascular structures is frequently extensive, and the effects on these tissues are quite similar to those produced by the cavitation associated with high-velocity bullet wounds (Fig. 35–1). Remote vascular injuries can occur, but after the bones fall back into a near-normal position, the magnitude of the injuring forces may not be appreciated, and the severity of damage is often underestimated. Examination of these patients is particularly difficult because there is extensive soft tissue and bony deformity.

GENERAL PRINCIPLES

Diagnosis

Clinical Features

Injuries of large arteries in the extremities usually can be readily identified because of severe hemorrhage, but wounds of deeper vessels may not be evident. Table 35–3 lists the indications for operative exploration of a suspected vascular wound; often a combination of these clinical features is present. Hemorrhage, hematoma, and pulse deficits are the usual findings, and these features, in the presence of a penetrating wound, are often sufficient to establish the diagnosis. Ischemia of the extremity is

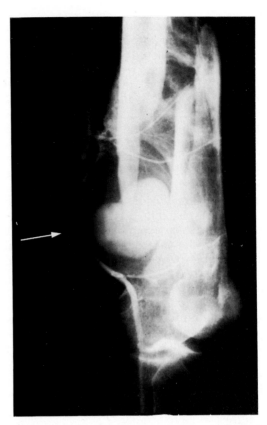

FIGURE 35–1.   This spiral fracture of the femur caused extensive damage to the soft tissues of the thigh and punctured the superficial femoral artery.

TABLE 35–3.   INDICATIONS FOR EXPLORATION

Diminished or absent pulse
Major hemorrhage with hypotension
Large or expanding hematoma
Bruit at or distal to injury
Anatomically related neurologic defect
Ischemia

uncommon with isolated vascular injuries, except with a wound causing occlusion of the popliteal or common femoral artery. When present, ischemia is an important finding, but its absence does not rule out significant vascular wounds.

Although weak or absent pulses beyond the suspected vascular wound is a fairly common finding, pulses may be normal in up to 20 per cent of operatively proven arterial injuries.[4] The pulse wave is a pressure wave that attains velocities of 7 to 13 m/sec, and this pressure wave may be transmitted beyond intimal flaps, through limited areas of fresh soft clot, or via the collateral vessels and thus be detectable distal to a significant arterial injury. The flow wave of blood has a velocity of 40 to 50 cm/sec, and it is distinct from the pulse wave; the physical examination must take this fact into account. Wounds of arteries crossing the shoulder or the pelvis, areas with rich collateral circulation, are therefore likely to be associated with intact distal pulses. Moreover, injuries of arteries such as a profunda femoris or deep brachial would not disturb distal pulses. Major venous wounds, of course, will not be exposed by examination of the pulses; the only finding in these patients may be hematomas or persistent bleeding.

The detection of Doppler signals and the measurement of distal arterial systolic blood pressure by this or other techniques are helpful, but the specificity of these tests is influenced by the same hemodynamic features that govern distal pulses. Subtle abnormalities in these measurements are common, but relatively normal values are also seen, thus compromising the reliability of these methods for the exclusion of vascular wounds. They are useful adjuncts and serve as an extension of the physical examination, but they may be misleading from time to time.

Wounds of the profunda femoral or profunda brachial artery will not alter distal pulses or distal limb blood pressure measurements. An injury of a single tibial artery also may not change the ankle-brachial index. In questionable cases duplex ultrasound tests may expose the injury, or may detect false aneurysms or arteriovenous fistulas. In the absence of other indications for surgical exploration these adjunctive methods can offer helpful information regarding possible injuries to large arteries.[5,6]

Injuries of the heart and great vessels present special diagnostic problems because of their inaccessibility to a direct clinical examination. Table 35–4 lists those clinical features that suggest the presence of significant intrathoracic vascular injuries. Hemopneumothorax or mediastinal bleeding is common with penetrating injuries of the chest even without injury of a major artery. The patients may be initially stable and thought to have only minor parenchymal lung damage until sudden hemodynamic collapse occurs. Preoperative identification of such severe injuries is important, permitting the surgeon to prepare for the possibility of major vascular reconstruction of the heart or great vessels. Many of these patients will benefit from preoperative arteriography if they are sufficiently stable to permit the delay required for such studies.

A computed tomographic (CT) scan has proven to be very useful in the initial evaluations of patients with multiple injuries, especially those caused by blunt trauma. Injuries to parenchymal intraabdominal organs, hematomas, and displacement of other structures may be seen clearly by careful CT scanning, thus validating the need for operative exploration.

Negative studies, of course, are of less value in ruling out injuries, but a positive study gives compelling reasons for proceeding with surgery. Magnetic resonance imaging (MRI) promises to be of more value than CT scanning, since the delineation of structures is much clearer, and the detection of even minor abnormalities should be possible with this innovative method.

Arteriography

In the management of trauma preoperative arteriography is used mainly for three reasons: to exclude the need for surgery, to expose a suspected injury not otherwise detectable, and to plan the operation. In Table 35–5 some indications for preoperative arteriography are listed. In a study of 183 patients with penetrating injuries of the extremities, the validity and usefulness of arteriography was established.[7] In this group of patients with penetrating injuries of the arms and legs, all had arteriograms and were operated upon for the listed indications regardless of the arteriographic findings. One false-negative examination was encountered, and there were 28 false-positive examinations; therefore, it was concluded from this study that high-grade biplane arteriography offers reliable but not infallible evidence as to the presence or absence of arterial injuries. Particular problems are encountered with preoperative arteriography in the assessment of injuries of the great vessels near the arch of the aorta; it is difficult to obtain good biplane films of this area because of overlapping images.

Recent studies have shown that when arteriograms are performed because the wound is thought to be near a major artery, there will be a low yield (3 to 5 per cent). A careful physical examination will usually determine the need for arteriograms.[8] In patients who are hemodynamically stable and who have no indications for surgical exploration, it often is acceptable to delay arteriography, rather than obtain emergency studies in the middle of the night. Careful observation is required until the tests are completed and precise treatment initiated. Noninvasive tests may help separate these patients from those who require expedient surgery.

It is also clear that when firm indications for operation are present, arteriograms may be unnecessary; any untoward delay is undesirable, and in some situations dangerous. If the patient is unstable, further evaluation is best performed in the operating room, utilizing the routine commonly employed for the management of patients with leaking abdominal

TABLE 35–4.   CLINICAL FEATURES SUGGESTING INJURIES OF THE GREAT VESSELS

Cardiac arrest
Persistent shock
Cardiac tamponade
Wide mediastinum
Recurring hemothorax

TABLE 35–5.   INDICATIONS FOR PREOPERATIVE ARTERIOGRAPHY

Blunt trauma, fractures
Penetrating injuries to chest
Cervical injuries—base of skull
Assessment of multiple pellet wounds
Injuries to forearm, leg

aortic aneurysms. The patients are taken directly to the operating room, and further assessment is performed while preparations for surgery are underway. If sudden cardiovascular collapse does occur, immediate operation can be undertaken, and control of bleeding can be achieved rapidly. These patients should not be sent to the radiology department for study nor admitted to an intensive care unit if they are unstable; an emergency operation may be required at any time.

Priorities and Resuscitation

The management of trauma patients requires a rapid yet thorough evaluation. Many of these patients have associated injuries, as shown in Table 35–6, and certain priorities must be set if a successful conclusion is to be gained. Initial attention to the airway and control of bleeding must always be the first priority, and it is usually obvious what is required. A more dangerous situation exists when the patient has achieved a degree of cardiopulmonary stability via compensatory mechanisms, and then suddenly the internal adjustments required to maintain this state deteriorate: collapse is sudden, and irreversible shock may occur. The initial evaluation and work-up must be concluded expeditiously in patients who are hemodynamically unstable.

Once an airway is secured and control of external bleeding has been obtained, the vital signs are assessed, an overall evaluation is made, and proper priorities are set. Baseline studies are recorded and a rapid physical examination performed to be certain that all injuries are identified and emergency measures completed (such as closed thoracostomy, stabilization of cervical spine injuries and other fractures, insertion of catheters and access lines).

Fluid and blood requirements in the injured patient are often impressive, and adequate intravenous access lines are needed. Large catheters are placed into an uninjured upper and lower extremity and carefully secured. During the selection of veins for the administration of intravenous fluids, the possibility of injury to the vein proximal to the site of insertion of the line must be considered, since it may be necessary to clamp that vein to control bleeding. One line is committed only for fluid replacement; it is not used for drug administration or anesthetic manipulations because, if hemorrhage is severe, large vol-

umes of blood must be infused rapidly. There may be a need for venous autografts for vascular repair, and it is often prudent to preserve the saphenous or cephalic vein in an uninjured extremity, but the treatment of shock must take priority, and these veins may be needed for resuscitation.

The combination of a balanced salt solution, such as lactated Ringer's solution, and whole blood is chosen for resuscitation. As described by Shires and his colleagues, trauma and shock cause internal shifts of interstitial fluid; this is best treated with balanced salt solutions and whole blood.[9] Blood loss is subsequently replaced with blood, but it is wise not to overtransfuse these patients, especially if chest trauma or cardiac disease is present. A whole blood hematocrit of approximately 30 per cent is optimum; further increases in hemoglobin during this stage are unnecessary, and may increase the possibility of cardiac overload.

Often, arterial lines and Swan-Ganz catheters are extremely helpful in these patients, especially if they are hemodynamically unstable. A radial artery catheter inserted in a patient who has a normal Allen's test (which demonstrates connection of the radial and ulnar artery through the palmar arch) is a safe and useful technique. This line should not be irrigated with large amounts of fluid, since a thrombus in the catheter can be dislodged and multiple emboli scattered throughout the arm. The line is kept open with a continuous infusion of minute amounts of heparinized saline. The brachial artery should not be chosen for continuous in-line monitoring if other sites are accessible because brachial artery lines are associated with the highest complication rate of all arterial entries.

A central line can be inserted from a peripheral vein rather than a direct subclavian puncture if there is thought to be an injury on that side of the chest, or in the root of the neck. Difficult subclavian vein punctures may produce an additional vascular injury, complicating the evaluation and care of the patient, and it is best to insert these lines with a great deal of care.

Wound Protection

During the initial treatment of patients with serious injuries, there may be a tendency to overlook the problem of wound care. Because the incidence of infection and subsequent complications may be directly related to contamination of these wounds at the time of resuscitation, such injuries should be protected, and all undamaged tissue should be conserved to be utilized in covering repaired vessels. When multiple wounds are present, the use of several incisions may be required, especially if there are fractures and other injuries. If these are poorly placed, intervening tissue may be devitalized, important collateral vessels may be divided unnecessarily, and final cover of the vessels may be difficult to arrange.

TABLE 35–6. ASSOCIATED INJURIES IN TRAUMA PATIENTS

	Percentage
Significant vein	34
Major nerve	18
Separate artery	7
Lung, abdominal viscera	39
Shock	36

Wound care is an extremely important part of the initial measures in the care of these patients, especially if there is extensive soft tissue damage, as may be seen in close-range shotgun wounds and with motor vehicle accidents. Remote bypass grafts to restore flow may be required because of heavy contamination of the initial wounds, and exploratory incisions should be placed so as to preserve areas for the use of subcutaneous grafts. Meticulous care in opening and handling these incisions is essential to avoid secondary infections.

Most trauma surgeons employ prophylactic antibiotic administration in these situations. Second-generation cephalosporins are often chosen and are begun when the patient is initially seen. Customarily, they are continued while central lines are in place, or as long as there are specific indications for antibiotic therapy.

Anticoagulation

Although during the course of many vascular operations regional or systemic anticoagulation may be employed while major arteries and veins are temporarily occluded during repair, it is generally best not to administer systemic heparin to these patients unless they have an isolated vascular injury. Distal clot propagation is a problem in such patients, especially if they are hypotensive, and thrombosis can convert an initially reasonable situation into one with risk of tissue loss. Nevertheless, systemic anticoagulation in patients with multiple injuries (especially in those with injuries of the central nervous system, eyes, and bones) carries an unacceptably high risk. Expeditious surgery rather than systemic ganticoagulation is preferred.[4,10]

OPERATIVE MANAGEMENT

Anesthesia

During the preparation for surgery, the selection of the anesthetic agent may be important, especially in those patients who are already hypotensive. A careful assessment of the mild cardiodepressant action of anesthetic agents should be kept in mind as the operation begins. Certain standard precautions should be observed as well. Careful positioning of the neck during induction of anesthesia is necessary to avoid dislodging clots in injured vessels in the neck. Moreover, care is necessary to avoid damage in patients who may have cervical spine injuries. The patients generally are positioned supine in the anatomic position, thus affording access to the chest, the abdomen, and all four extremities. If the surgeon needs only to enter the left chest for repair of a single injury of the subclavian artery other positions may be chosen.

Vertical exploratory incisions are preferred because they may be easily extended and, in the extremities, they are parallel to the neurovascular structures. Midline abdominal incisions can be easily extended into the chest as a median sternal splitting incision, and vertical incisions along the anterior sternocleidomastoid muscle to expose the carotid and jugular vessels also may be extended into a median sternal incision if there are injuries in the root of the neck.[11] Transverse incisions in these areas limit flexibility and are not recommended.

Control of Bleeding

Most external bleeding can be controlled with direct digital pressure. If the wound is not bleeding, it is best not to disturb it during the early resuscitation, and no attempt should be made to remove foreign bodies or to evacuate clots until surgical control is possible. Penetrating objects that are still in the wound must be protected during transportation, but they should not be removed until the patient is in the operating room and it is possible to gain proximal and distal control of major arteries in that area. No attempt should be made to blindly clamp vessels prior to taking the patient into the operating room. In cases in which fatal hemorrhage appears imminent, the wound can be extended and vascular clamps can be applied under direct vision.

In some situations, in emergency rooms staffed by experienced people, thoracotomy can be done rapidly and safely in serious situations when patients are in shock. Closed-chest cardiac massage in patients in hypovolemic shock may not be effective, and open massage is often required. An aggressive approach is warranted in these infrequent situations, but a team of experienced surgeons is required if these maneuvers are to be successful.[12]

Once the surgical plan has been established, the wounds are approached directly through vertical incisions. If the hematoma is large, it is often best to expose the vessels proximally and gain control in an area in which the artery and vein may be clearly visualized. In extremities with multiple distal wounds and large hematomas, exposure of the vessels can be difficult, and it may be prudent to place an orthopedic tourniquet around the extremity proximal to the injury. If severe bleeding is encountered prior to direct control of the artery, the orthopedic tourniquet can be quickly inflated, thus arresting the hemorrhage while precise identification and control is obtained.

In other areas, proximal control of the artery may be attained utilizing soft vascular tapes, latex tubing, or vascular clamps. These measures, combined with adequate suction and direct pressure with fingers or sponge sticks, will usually be satisfactory to control hemorrhage while all the injuries are identified and vascular clamps are put in place.

Once the injury has been exposed, the clot should be evacuated carefully and the extent of the injury examined. Every effort should be made to avoid fragmenting and dislodging clots or extending the damage to the vessel, a problem especially in patients who have atherosclerosis and fragile arteries. In some cases it may be necessary to insert a Foley catheter, or a Fogarty catheter with an attached three-way stopcock, to control hemorrhage. The catheters are inserted into the wound, inflated, and gently retracted until bleeding is stopped, and then left in place while more precise proximal and distal control is obtained. Repairs are not begun until all hemorrhage is arrested and the extent of associated injuries assessed. It is wise to pause at this point in the resuscitation and be certain that there is no persistent bleeding. Resuscitation should be well in hand before definitive repair of noncritical structures is begun. Certain organs (kidney, liver) are more susceptible to hypoxia than others, and repair of major vessels supplying these organs should be undertaken first while less vulnerable organs are placed lower on the priority list.

Basic Techniques

The selection of suture materials for repair of major vessels is largely the choice of the operating surgeon, but there has been a tendency over recent years to select a less reactive plastic suture rather than the braided cardiovascular silk sutures popular in the past. Silk sutures handle well, and although they are not permanent sutures (most of their tensile strength is gone in 6 months or so), this is not a major drawback in primary repairs, since one expects the reunited vessels to heal. The smallest sized practical sutures should be employed in most of these cases, since healing of autogenous tissues is expected, and suture line integrity does not depend indefinitely upon the suture material.

The nonreactive monofilament plastic sutures are less likely to harbor bacteria than braided sutures and therefore may reduce the risk of postoperative infection. They are often chosen by vascular surgeons despite their relative stiffness and lack of pliability. Satisfactory results are obtained with all of these suture materials, but polypropylene and Dacron are more popular than others.

The vessels are repaired by the usual vascular techniques; continuous over-and-over sutures are quite effective and can be used in almost all vessels. It may be prudent in small vessels (less than 4 mm in diameter) to use interrupted sutures in order to ensure intima-to-intima coaptation, although with magnification it has been clearly demonstrated that continuous sutures, even in small arteries, are equally effective when properly inserted. Small vessels may be sewn end to end more easily if they are transected obliquely, or spatulated to obtain a larger suture line, which also has less chance of subsequent stenosis.

Tangential lacerations of larger vessels can be successfully treated by lateral suture repair utilizing standard vascular surgical techniques, but débridement is as important in the management of vascular injuries as it is in other injuries, and it is best not to make a firm decision as to the type of repair until the débridement has been concluded. Most civilian vascular wounds are inflicted by knives or low-velocity missiles, and wide débridement is generally not required. With the usual bullet wound, it is necessary to débride only that amount of vessel that can be seen to be injured. In high-velocity gunshot wounds, the injury often extends beyond that which is immediately visible to the naked eye, an it is advisable to remove approximately 5 mm of vessel beyond the apparent damage.

Smaller vessels can rarely be repaired by lateral suture techniques and require either patch graft angioplasty or, more commonly, resection and end-to-end anastomosis. The most commonly injured vessels (femoral, brachial) can usually be mobilized to permit resection of 1 cm or so and still allow a satisfactory end-to-end anastomosis. If the extent of the injury is so wide that end-to-end anastomosis cannot be accomplished without tension, it is best to interpose a suitable autograft rather than to accept an improper repair. The saphenous vein is usually chosen for such autografts in medium and small vessels of the extremities, but the hypogastric artery, external iliac, and other arterial autografts may be employed if necessary. An arterial autograft apparently is more resistant to the invasive problems associated with subsequent infection than other types of prosthetic grafts.[13] In situations in which heavy bacterial contamination has occurred, such arterial autografts are favored.

Recent studies suggest that the disruption caused by infection is not unfavorably influenced by the presence of plastic prostheses, particularly polytetrafluoroethylene (PTFE) grafts, and that these plastic substitutes may be used even when bacterial contamination is present. This opinion is not shared by all vascular surgeons, and most prefer that autogenous tissues be used if they are available in appropriate sizes.[10] In the aortoiliac system, plastic prostheses are used when there is extensive damage, because large autografts are not available. If bacterial contamination is heavy, as it may be with combined aortic and colon injuries, it may be best to oversew the major vascular injuries and construct remote subcutaneous bypass grafts on a temporary basis until healing is complete. Axillofemoral and femorofemoral grafts are often selected in these circumstances to avoid placing the repaired arteries in heavily contaminated areas.

Assessment of Repair in the Operating Room

In most cases, vascular repair is followed by the immediate return of pulsatile flow. In patients who are incompletely resuscitated, hypotensive, cold, and vasoconstricted, it can be difficult to determine clinically if the repair is satisfactory. Other measures are required. A sterile Doppler probe is useful in documenting distal patency in such circumstances. If there is a question as to the patency or the adequacy of the repair, an operative arteriogram is required.

In the postoperative period, if there is any question as to the adequacy of flow, an arteriogram is needed. The sine qua non for viability of the extremity is continued perception of light touch and adequate intrinsic motor function. Any deterioration in these modalities is a compelling reason to perform an arteriogram, regardless of skin color, temperature, presence or absence of pulses, or limb blood pressure.[4]

MANAGEMENT OF SPECIFIC PROBLEMS

Brachiocephalic Arterial Injuries

Most wounds of the cervical vessels are caused by penetrating trauma, and the common carotid artery is usually involved, the left more often than the right. There are special problems encountered in these patients when there is a vascular injury and a neurologic deficit. There also may be associated wounds of the pharynx, esophagus, and trachea, thus increasing the likelihood of bacterial contamination. The neurologic deficit associated with some of these injuries presents a unique and often perplexing problem. It appears that the outcome in most patients is directly related to the extent of the initial neurologic damage, unless a technical misadventure occurs during resuscitation and repair.[14,15]

Carotid Injuries

It may be helpful to divide carotid injuries into three groups for evaluation. The first and largest group contains those patients with common or internal carotid artery wounds, but who have no neurologic deficit. Group 2 includes those patients who have a mild deficit, and group 3 those with a severe neurologic deficit (coma, hemiplegia).[15]

The results of several large studies strongly support surgical repair of all carotid artery injuries in patients who have either no neurologic deficit or have only a mild deficit. Thus, all of the patients in groups 1 and 2 would undergo repair of isolated carotid artery injuries. This decision is easy to reach when the arterial injury is bleeding actively, but it may be more difficult when there is complete carotid artery occlusion and no neurologic symptoms.[16] In such a situation, technical problems encountered during surgery could conceivably produce brain damage, although in the reported experience this has been rare.[17] The risk does exist, however, and careful neurologic and arteriographic studies are required before operation is undertaken in these patients in order to accurately assess the danger.

Even an artery depicted as being completely blocked by arteriography may at operation be open. It is clear that new techniques such as MRI can be of great assistance in determining if indeed the artery is occluded or not. This may be helpful in patients suspected of having a hyperextension injury of the internal carotid artery. In this situation, the artery is forcibly stretched over the transverse process of C3 and the body of C2, a mechanism of injury that predisposes to thromboembolic events. Until a neurologic problem appears, there usually is little evidence of carotid artery injury (Fig. 35–2).

Preoperative Evaluation

The basic management of penetrating trauma to the neck is straightforward: wounds that pierce the platysma muscle require some form of surgical exploration. It may be helpful to divide penetrating wounds of the neck into three zones, as suggested by Monson et al.[18] Zone III extends from the base of the skull to the angle of the mandible, zone II from the angle of the mandible to 1 cm above the head of the clavicle, and zone I from 1 cm below the head of the clavicle to include the rest of the thoracic outlet. By clinical examination, it may be difficult to ascertain if injuries in zones I and III actually include damage to major vascular structures, and in these patients, if they are hemodynamically stable, preoperative arteriography is extremely important. Patients with penetrating injuries in zone II who have no neurologic deficit but require surgery may be operated upon without arteriography, although preoperative arteriography is helpful in these patients also.

Signs and symptoms suggesting arterial injury in the extremities apply equally to the neck, but unfortunately these arteries may not be accessible for examination, especially after blunt trauma (Fig. 35–3). In Table 35–7 the clinical features of blunt trauma to the carotid artery as suggested by Jernigan and Gardner are listed.[19] There may be few signs of injury, because less than half of the patients will have local evidence of blunt trauma in these situations. Arteriography should be used liberally in patients who have blunt and penetrating trauma to the neck and thoracic outlet.

Operative Management

Patients who have carotid artery injuries and continued prograde flow are candidates for surgical repair. A patient who has complete occlusion of the internal carotid artery as a result of blunt trauma, who is not bleeding, and who has a severe neurologic deficit manifested by coma and hemiplegia is probably best treated by nonoperative techniques, or by ligation of the internal carotid artery if operation is required for other reasons.[17] Complete removal of thrombus in these situations is often difficult, and residual clot may embolize and extend the neurologic damage.[20]

Vascular control and repair are performed as described in the preceding sections. Standard techniques are used, and every effort is made to avoid

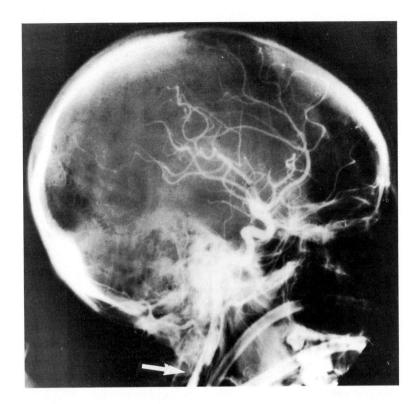

FIGURE 35–2. The arrow points to the area of the internal carotid artery damaged by hyperextension trauma.

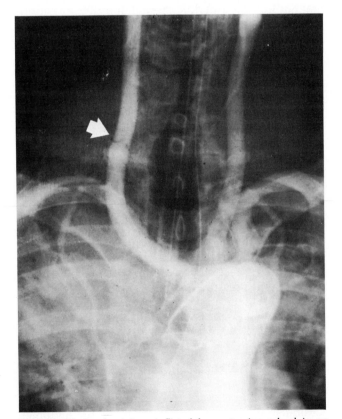

FIGURE 35–3. An injury inflicted by a steering wheel in an automobile accident caused pulmonary contusions and a fracture of the right common carotid artery. A graft was required to replace this section of the vessel.

thromboembolic complications; precise suture and graft techniques are essential. As shown in Figure 35–4, the external carotid artery may be used to repair the internal carotid artery in certain circumstances. If lateral repair is not possible, interposition of a saphenous vein graft or an arterial autograft may be employed, as shown in Figure 35–5. If the back-pressure from the internal carotid artery is below 70 mm Hg, or if there is scanty back-bleeding, the use of an intraluminal shunt is a satisfactory method to maintain cerebral blood flow while repairs are completed.

Postoperative Care

Although any vascular repair can be susceptible to bleeding, it is unusual in these patients unless there are multiple injuries or coagulation defects. Drains are not usually employed in isolated vascular wounds, but in selected patients with cervical injuries, they may be used for 12 hours or so to prevent the accumulation of blood, which may cause a compressing hematoma beneath the relatively rigid cervical fascia. Patients are carefully monitored for the appearance of neurologic problems. Neurologic symptoms usu-

TABLE 35–7. CLINICAL FEATURES OF BLUNT TRAUMA TO CAROTID ARTERIES[a]

Hematoma of lateral neck
Horner's syndrome
Transient ischemic attack
Lucid interval
Limb paresis in an alert patient

[a]From Jernigan WR, Gardner WC: Carotid artery injuries due to closed cervical trauma. Trauma 11:429, 1971.

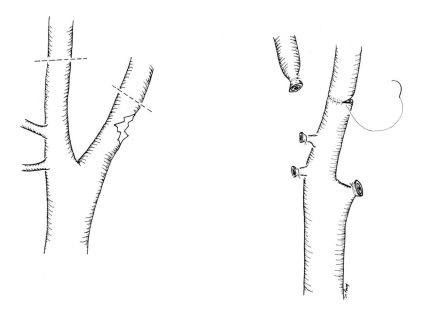

FIGURE 35–4. If the internal carotid artery cannot be repaired directly, the external carotid can be mobilized and used as a substitute graft.

ally require arteriography to evaluate the status of the repair and to assess the possibility of cerebral thromboembolism. Postoperative carotid artery occlusion rarely occurs, but if it does, the patient should be returned immediately to the operating room for thrombectomy, correction of any technical errors, and reestablishment of flow. In these situations, it is best not to delay for arteriography; thrombosis and the emergence of a stroke require immediate surgery. Expeditious restoration of flow is often successful in preventing permanent neurologic problems.

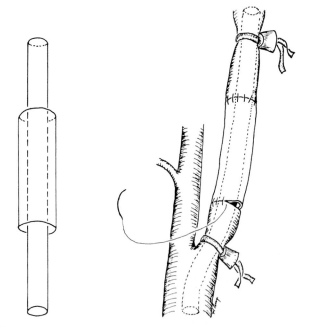

FIGURE 35–5. When injuries of the internal carotid artery are associated with low back-pressures (less than 70 mm Hg) or scanty back-bleeding, a saphenous vein graft can be placed over the temporary inlying shunt as the repair is completed.

Injuries of Vessels of the Root of the Neck

Injuries of vessels in zone I, at the thoracic outlet, may be particularly difficult to evaluate because the injury may be obscure, and yet operative exposure of the wound without proximal control can lead to fatal hemorrhage. If the penetrating wound in zone I is thought to have injured the great vessels, proximal control via a middle sternal splitting incision is recommended before exposing the wound. Similarly, if during the course of cervical exploration through an incision along the anterior sternocleidomastoid muscle border, bleeding, hematoma, or blood staining of the carotid sheath in the depths of the wound at the root of the neck are encountered, an immediate sternal splitting incision should be made to control the great vessels of the arch.[11] All the vessels of the arch with the exception of the left subclavian can be reached easily through the incision, and if necessary the incision may be extended into the second or third interspace, or a separate left thoracotomy incision may be opened to control the left subclavian artery.

Repairs of these arteries are performed in the same fashion as described in the preceding sections. In most cases, the back-pressures in the innominate or left common carotid exceed 70 mm Hg, and temporary shunting techniques are not required if the patient's blood pressure is maintained within a normal range. Prosthetic grafts will be needed more often for repair of the great vessels of the arch, since autografts of this size are usually not available (Fig. 35–6).

Injuries of the Abdominal Aorta and its Branches

Almost all major vascular injuries in the abdomen are caused by penetrating trauma, usually gunshot wounds, and frequently there are other serious in-

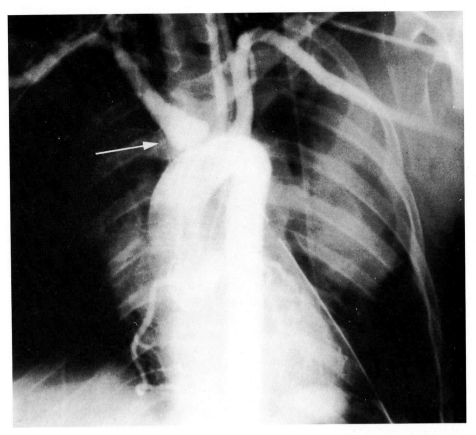

FIGURE 35–6.   A load of lumber fell on this young man and produced lung contusions and a wide mediastinum, which prompted the arteriogram. The arrow points to the nearly avulsed innominate artery.

juries. This is a lethal combination, especially if there are multiple vascular wounds, and less than half of the patients survive.[12,21]

Diagnosis

A penetrating wound of the abdomen in a patient in shock is the common picture. The usual signs and symptoms of vascular injuries can be suggested, but since the arteries are inaccessible for examination, indirect evidence of injury assumes more importance; this generally means detecting bleeding.

Although abdominal distention from the accumulation of blood can occur, massive retroperitoneal bleeding can be hidden, and there may be little blood in the peritoneal cavity. This is especially true with knife wounds that enter from the back, particularly if the blade passes between two of the lower ribs. Such a wound may appear benign. Moreover, pulse deficits, if present, and limb ischemia are difficult to interpret in hypotensive patients. Because of the severity of most of these injuries, there usually is little time for protracted examination and diagnostic studies. The need for surgical exploration is obvious.

Plain x-ray studies, CT scans, intravenous urograms, and arteriography all may be useful, and even if a vascular wound is not seen, such studies can expose other problems that require surgical correc-

tion. Abdominal paracentesis or lavage can document intraperitoneal bleeding, but false-negative results do occur.[22]

A special case exists in patients who have renovascular injuries, especially when caused by blunt trauma. Hematuria, or suspected kidney trauma, is an indication for further studies; these include an intravenous urogram and CT scan. If the kidney functions normally, and there is no parenchymal or collecting system dysfunction, hospitalization and observation are acceptable. If kidney function is impaired or absent, or if there is parenchymal disruption, renal arteriography is indicated. If major renal vascular architecture is intact, observation is sufficient, with repeated studies. If vascular wounds or collecting system disruption are diagnosed, surgical correction is required.[4]

Arteriography can be very helpful in managing these patients, particularly those who have sustained blunt trauma and those in whom no other indication for exploration exists.

A flush aortogram presents useful information about the vascular system and can be used to evaluate the liver, spleen, and kidney as well. False-negative results do occur, and if firm indications for exploration exist, expeditious surgery is recommended rather than waiting for other studies.

Operative Management

Hemodynamically unstable patients are taken immediately to the operating room; preparations for surgery are completed as necessary diagnostic maneuvers are finished and interpreted. The operating team is scrubbed and ready to intervene if sudden collapse occurs.[12]

The abdomen is opened through the usual long midline incision, a rapid exploration is performed, and attention is directed toward the major vessels. If a bleeding wound can be seen and exposed easily, it is controlled with vascular clamps. This is often the case with isolated wounds of the branches of the visceral arteries. Injuries of the aorta, especially the supraceliac aorta and that part containing the origins of the visceral branches (zones I and II as described by Lim et al.) usually require a supraceliac clamp to control bleeding.[21] This part of the aorta is approached through the gastrohepatic ligament, and the aorta is freed from the left crus of the diaphragm with finger dissection. Only the front and sides are mobilized to permit placing a long straight or slightly curved vascular clamp directly across the aorta in an anterior-posterior plane. Temporary aortic occlusion at this level allows more rapid and precise exposure of wounds of the lower aorta and its branches.

Infrarenal aortic wounds (Lim et al.'s zone III) usually can be approached directly through the root of the mesentery in the usual method employed in elective aortic operations. Wounds in the center of the mesenteric root often involve the pancreas and duodenum and can damage the major veins located here. A combination of aortic and major venous wounds is often lethal, and control of large venous injuries in this area is difficult to achieve.

When exposure of midaortic wounds is difficult because of obscuring hematomas, brisk bleeding, and multiple organ damage, reflection of the left colon, spleen, and pancreas can allow the surgeon to reach the aorta and its branches. Reflection of the ascending colon and duodenum will expose the vena cava and aorta from the right side.

Once the vascular wounds are controlled, priorities of repair are set. Blood flow should be restored to the kidneys and liver first, because these organs are more sensitive to hypoxia. The intestine and the lower extremities can tolerate longer periods of ischemia. Repairs rarely require more than an hour, however.

The methods of vascular reconstruction are dictated by the nature of the wounds. Usually, resection and end-to-end anastomosis are adequate for the aortic branches, unless tissue loss is extensive and interposition grafts are needed. Aortic wounds caused by knives and low-velocity gunshot wounds occasionally can be repaired by simple suture; more extensive damage mandates patch angioplasty or grafting. Plastic prostheses are customarily needed to reconstruct the aortoiliac tree.

As described in the section concerned with general principles, large bowel penetration resulting in heavy bacterial soilage in association with aortic wounds presents special problems. Autogenous tissue repairs may succeed in some of these cases, but occasionally even arteries that are simply oversewn break down later because of infection. Severe contamination is an indication of the need to restore blood flow to the lower extremities via a remote bypass rather than by aortoiliac grafting. Axillofemoral and femorofemoral subcutaneous grafts are favored. It may be possible to sew the two common iliac arteries together and thus use one axillofemoral graft to perfuse both legs. This avoids placing a prosthetic graft into an abdominal cavity with heavy bacterial contamination. Careful closure of oversewn arterial stumps (aortic and iliac especially) is essential, and the closed ends are protected by covering them with pedicle flaps of the greater omentum. Antibiotics are continued until all wounds are healed, and all intravenous lines are removed. Once healing is complete, restoration of normal vascular architecture can be considered.

Injuries of the Arteries of the Extremities

Femoral arteries are among the most frequently injured vessels, comprising approximately 20 per cent of all arterial injuries. Acute ligation of the common femoral artery results in an amputation rate of approximately 50 per cent, only slightly less than that noted following acute occlusion of the popliteal artery. Large veins and important nerves are found within the femoral triangle, and associated injuries of these structures are common.

Popliteal artery injuries are especially difficult problems, and failure to repair them results in limb loss in almost two thirds of the patients.[23] Penetrating wounds are usually easily diagnosed; these patients almost invariably have pulse deficits and frequently have ischemia of the lower extremity. Patients with blunt trauma often present more difficult problems in evaluation. Posterior dislocations of the knee, for example, are very likely to injure the popliteal artery. As Lefrac, Dart, and others have indicated, these patients should have preoperative arteriography.[2,3] Lefrac reported that of 152 patients with knee dislocations, 28 per cent sustained popliteal artery injuries; half of these eventually lost the limb.[3] It is very easy to miss an unstable knee during the examination of a patient who has multiple injuries. Although popliteal artery injuries caused by fracture dislocations are usually easily identified because of a pulse deficit, and in most cases ischemia, inexperienced examiners may assume that spasm is at fault. This can be a serious error, one that can result in loss of limb. Preoperative arteriography, therefore, is an important adjunctive measure in these patients and may be the only way of ascertaining the extent of the injury.

Preoperative Preparation

Many of these patients have suffered a great deal of blood loss at the time they are initially seen, and the resuscitation should proceed in an aggressive manner prior to surgery. Stabilization of fractures should be performed early. This is easier if the patients are taken directly to the operating room, especially if they are hemodynamically unstable. Many surgeons favor the use of external techniques for bone stabilization so as to avoid introducing foreign bodies into the area of potential vascular repair, but there is no unanimity of opinion in this regard, and both internal and external fixation have been used successfully. Some type of temporary stabilization is essential during the early care of these patients to prevent further damage.

Operative Management

As with other vascular wounds, the patient is usually operated upon under general anesthesia. The opposite extremity is prepared so that if vascular autografts are required, the contralateral saphenous vein will be available. If there are concomitant femoral or popliteal vein injuries, one may wish to preserve the ipsilateral saphenous veins in the event more serious vein injuries cannot be repaired. It is especially important to repair concomitant popliteal vein injuries if the saphenous vein is also damaged.[23]

Rich and his colleagues present compelling reasons for repair of the popliteal vein as well as the artery, pointing out that the incidence of thromboembolic events is approximately 13 per cent after vein repair, but more than 50 per cent after ligation.[24] Rich and Snyder also suggest that continued popliteal artery patency is enhanced by simultaneous repair of popliteal vein injuries.[23,24]

In most situations, the wounds are approached through the medial vertical incisions commonly used for elective surgery. Proximal and distal control can be difficult to obtain when the patient is prone and the vessels are approached posteriorly through the popliteal space.

The basic techniques of repair are those used in vascular surgery elsewhere. Damaged tissue is resected, and an end-to-end anastomosis with careful intimal coaptation is constructed. Popliteal arteries are especially vulnerable to injury by a vascular clamp, and soft noncrushing instruments are suitable for temporary occlusion. If the injury is in an atherosclerotic artery, it may be more suitable to control bleeding by inserting an intraluminal catheter, thus avoiding wall damage that might predispose to immediate thrombosis or enhance the subsequent progress of the atheromatous disease.

In patients who have sustained blunt trauma and who also have multiple fractures, often it is necessary to repair the popliteal artery and vein first, and then the vascular surgeon remains in attendance while final stabilization of the fractures is obtained by either internal or external fixation. In those situations in which there is no severe ischemia, such as with a superficial femoral artery occlusion, it may be practical to first complete the orthopedic repairs; once the bone is stabilized, it is easier to construct an arterial repair of the proper length and tension. If the foot is ischemic and extensive orthopedic repairs are required, temporary inlaying shunts can be placed in the popliteal artery and vein. These decisions should be made, in consultation, by the vascular surgeon and the orthopedic surgeon; both should be in attendance during the repair of the bones to avoid disruption of the vascular suture lines.

Postoperatively, patency of the repair is usually apparent by the immediate reappearance of pedal pulses. If there is any question as to the adequacy of the repair, or if the possibility of distal thromboembolism appears likely, operative arteriography is indicated, because failure to restore pulses is most often a technical problem; it is rarely caused by persistent spasm.

Tibial Artery Injuries

Injuries to the tibial arteries present a difficult problem because, in most cases, they do not result in severe ischemia unless two of the three arteries are damaged. In patients who have penetrating trauma but who otherwise would not require operative exploration, if only one tibial artery is occluded and there is no bleeding, such an injury can be accepted without repair. Arteriographic survey of these patients is essential in order to determine if indeed there is a significant problem. In the absence of other indications, surgical exploration of a tibial artery customarily would be performed only if it were bleeding, or if by arteriogram there was an arteriovenous fistula or false aneurysm seen.

False Aneurysms and Arteriovenous Fistulas

Complications of vascular injuries such as thrombosis, delayed bleeding, arteriovenous (AV) fistulas, and false aneurysms are more likely to occur and much more difficult to manage if the injury is not treated promptly. False aneurysms and AV fistulas can occur immediately after the injury; bleeding occurs into a tract that is confined by surrounding tissue and a hematoma (sometimes false aneurysms are called pulsating hematomas). Although spontaneous cure of AV fistulas and false aneurysms can occur, the studies of Shumacker and Wayson have demonstrated that this is an unlikely event.[25] Less than 3 per cent of AV fistulas and less than 6 per cent of false aneurysms heal spontaneously.

These lesions resolve only when they thrombose, and it is obvious that, in many situations, thrombosis of major arteries will not be tolerated without unacceptable ischemic symptoms. Because spontaneous cure is an unlikely event, and since most AV fistulas and false aneurysms increase in size and complexity with the passage of time, operative repair becomes much more difficult if surgery is delayed. Increasing edema, inflammation, and expansion of the lesion slowly encroach upon and involve surrounding neurovascular structures, and thus the difficulty of repair progressively increases (Fig. 35–7). Repair will be necessary in most cases and there is no reason to procrastinate: arterial injuries should be treated by immediate surgery.

A false aneurysm is a result of an incomplete injury that permits continued bleeding from a laceration. Transection of an artery is customarily followed by retraction and clotting, and, in the case of small vessels, cessation of bleeding. Contiguous tangential wounds of arteries and veins may develop into AV fistulas, even acutely.

The most obvious clinical feature of a false aneurysm is a pulsatile mass that is associated either with an acute or a chronic penetrating wound. There may be a murmur over the mass because the tangential laceration of the artery permits the escape of blood into the surrounding tissues, then forming a tamponading clot. Although the physical diagnosis is usually easy when these are located in the extremities, arteriography is important in ascertaining the exact number and location of the involved vessels in order to properly plan the operative repair.

An AV fistula may be associated with a false aneurysm, or there may be a clean endothelial channel formed in a chronic AV fistula. In some cases, there may be very little inflammation about the lesion, although the presence of high-pressure arterial blood flow entering the veins will produce varicosities and thin-walled veins that are very fragile. Occasionally, false aneurysms and AV fistulas are combined.

The Nicolodani-Branham sign can be elicited in some of the patients with an AV fistula. Occlusion of the fistula may result in a slowing of the heart rate (reduction in flow into the right atrium). Most of these patients will have a continuous, machinery-type murmur over the fistula, and there may be evidence of venous hypertension and varicosities in the area. When the shunt is quite large, there may be ischemia of the distal extremity as a result of shunting of large amounts of arterial blood into the low-pressure venous system. On rare occasions, large traumatic AV fistulas between the aorta and the vena cava cause florid heart failure as a result of the recirculation of enormous amounts of blood. Emergency operations may be required to treat congestive heart failure.

Large AV fistulas produce a relentless enlargement of the feeding vessels and an increase in the number and complexity of the veins in the drainage system. The arteries become elongated and tortuous and the walls thinner. Spontaneous rupture is unusual, but trauma can lead to dangerous bleeding.

Mural thrombosis within the system can occur; thrombosis is a risk, although not a frequent problem. Intravascular coagulation can cause bleeding tendencies as clotting factors are depleted. Such complications should be identified and corrected before surgical repair is undertaken.

The initial surgical treatment of all identified arterial injuries is indicated; the incidence of traumatic AV fistulas and false aneurysms will be almost completely eliminated by this policy. Only those injuries that were missed on the initial examination and not immediately apparent will subsequently become large enough to develop symptoms. These clearly are few in number when appropriate repair is undertaken following the initial trauma.

Preoperative arteriographic survey of AV fistulas and false aneurysms is an important step for the planning of the operation because the lesion may be much more extensive than it appears clinically. This is especially true of deep-seated lesions involving the root of the neck, the cervical vessels, or the abdominal vessels. Even in the extremities, these lesions can be formidable, however, and prior to opening them, proximal and distal control of major arteries and veins must be achieved. In the extremities, this may be facilitated by the use of a proximal pneumatic orthopedic tourniquet, but in other areas it requires a careful dissection remote to the area of the AV fistula in order to gain control before the lesion is entered (Fig. 35–8).

In the case of nonessential small vessels involved with a false aneurysm or AV fistula, ligation may be

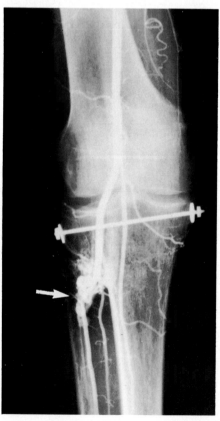

FIGURE 35–7. An arteriovenous fistula of the anterior tibial artery and vein is marked by the arrow. Orthopedic repairs were completed previously, without knowledge of the vascular wound.

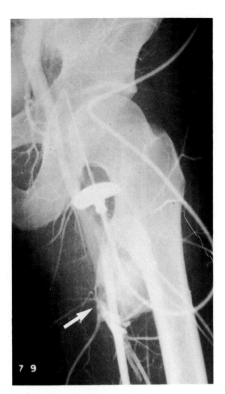

FIGURE 35–8. This large false aneurysm of the profunda femoral artery (arrow) was diagnosed only by arteriography.

TABLE 35–9.   ETIOLOGY OF INFERIOR VENA CAVA INJURIES

	No.	Died	Mortality (%)
Bullet	74	24	32
Shotgun pellets	8	6	75
Stab wound	15	2	13
Blunt trauma	13	11	85
Total	110	43	39

permit the vessel to retract and clot. If lateral repair is not possible without undue narrowing, patch graft angioplasty may be performed, or resection and anastomosis, or appropriate graft interposition as described in the preceding section.

The postoperative care of these patients is similar to that following repair of other arterial lesions. Not only must the pulses be followed, but neuromuscular function of the extremity is tested to ascertain if the repair remains adequate.

Injuries of the Inferior Vena Cava

Wounds of the inferior vena cava are among the most lethal of vascular injuries.[26] It has been reported that 1 in every 50 gunshot wounds and 1 in every 300 knife wounds of the abdomen will injure the vena cava. Because of these serious injuries, one third of the patients die before they reach the hospital, and half of the remainder die during their hospitalization. Most of the deaths during treatment occur from bleeding because of the difficulties in controlling injuries of large veins, but many of the patients also have associated injuries. As described by Perry, 79 per cent of the patients with penetrating trauma causing inferior vena cava wounds had injuries of other retroperitoneal structures.[4] This often can be an adverse influence on survival rates. The renal or portal vein, aorta, and its branches are also vulnerable to these same injuries and of course so are the colon, liver, pancreas, and duodenum. Table 35–8 shows those injuries often associated with vena cava wounds, in the author's experience.

The etiology of vena cava injuries has a bearing on the mortality, as can be seen in Table 35–9. Patients who have blunt trauma and shotgun injuries are more likely to have a fatal outcome than those who have stab wounds, especially if the injury is located in the upper part of the vena cava (Table 35–10).

a satisfactory procedure, but in major muscular arteries, repair is indicated. This is performed in the usual fashion once the vessels are controlled and identified. With large false aneurysms, the most expedient method generally involves obtaining proximal and distal control without entering the immediate area of the pseudoaneurysm, and then once the vessels are clamped, the aneurysm is opened and feeding branches are controlled from within the aneurysm sac by using intraluminal occlusion catheters, such as a Fogarty catheter with an attached three-way stopcock, or special balloon occlusion catheters designed for this purpose. Repair is then completed in the usual fashion, which in many cases will require only a lateral arteriorrhaphy, since most false aneurysms result not from complete transection of the artery, but from a tangential laceration that does not

TABLE 35–8.   INJURIES ASSOCIATED WITH 110 INFERIOR VENA CAVA INJURIES

	Number
Aorta, iliac artery	13
Major splanchnic vessel	26
Renal artery or vein	20
Liver	46
Duodenum	27
Kidney	21
Pancreas	18
Spleen	10
Colon	27
Other	21

TABLE 35–10.   MORTALITY FROM INFERIOR VENA CAVA INJURIES BY LOCATION

	No.	Died	Mortality (%)
Above renal veins	20	11	55
At renal veins	22	13	59
Below renal veins	52	15	29
Bifurcation	16	4	25

Most of these patients, when initially seen, obviously have a serious injury; hypotension is frequent, and occasionally there is abdominal distention. There are few laboratory data of much diagnostic value, except perhaps for the presence of hematuria or gastrointestinal bleeding, suggesting the presence of other injuries. Routine x-ray studies of the chest and abdomen are recommended if the patient is stable, but except for inferior venacavography these tests are rarely specific.

Operative Management

Most of these wounds can be managed with the usual midline abdominal incision from the xiphoid to the pubis, but in some instances thoracotomy may be required if the patient has a suprarenal caval injury. The chest should be prepared in case the incision must be extended into the thorax.

A rapid abdominal exploration usually exposes major vascular injuries; then the surgeon can establish priorities of repair as described in the preceding sections. It is preferable to initially control the bleeding, complete the resuscitation, and assign priorities for repair, but control of retroperitoneal bleeding may require direct pressure with fingers or sponge sticks while the vein is exposed and vascular clamps put in place. This exposure is likely to cause injuries to other veins if it is performed hastily or roughly.

It has been suggested that some retroperitoneal injuries do not need to be explored unless they are

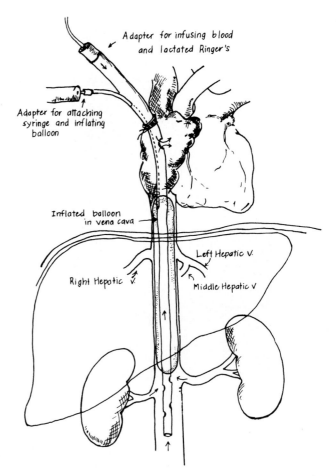

FIGURE 35–10. The Madding-Kennedy intracaval shunt. (Redrawn from Madding GF, Kennedy PA: Trauma to the Liver. Philadelphia, WB Saunders Company, 1971.)

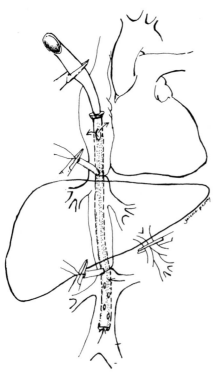

FIGURE 35–9. A transatrial intracaval shunt in place. (Redrawn from Schrock T, Blaisdell FW, Mathewson C Jr: Management of blunt trauma to the liver and hepatic veins. Arch Surg *96*:698, 1986.)

expanding or pulsatile, but this has not been the author's experience. In a study of 110 patients with penetrating caval injuries, the size of the hematoma did not predict the injury.[4] Moreover, three fourths of the patients had an associated injury of some kind. In contrast, pelvic hematomas caused by fractures are not opened unless specific injuries have been identified by arteriography or other studies. Bleeding from cancellous pelvic bones is often profuse and difficult to control.

Simple lacerations or punctures are usually seen, and these can be repaired by venorrhaphy and tangential repair. If the wound is large, a partially occluding clamp may be placed about it and the lesion oversewn with a continuous suture. In patients who have anterior and posterior injuries of the vena cava,

TABLE 35–11. MORTALITY WITH BLEEDING INFERIOR VENA CAVA INJURIES

	No.	Died	Mortality (%)
Active bleeding	45	34	78
Tamponade	62	9	16
Not specified	3	0	0

repair of the posterior wound may be obtained by rotation of the cava (perhaps requiring ligation of lumbar veins) and direct suture. In some instances, the anterior caval wound can be enlarged and the posterior wall laceration repaired from the inside under direct vision.[22]

Transections of the vena cava usually can be repaired by end-to-end vascular techniques, although mobilization of the cava does not permit loss of a long segment. If the cava is severely lacerated or if there are multiple wounds that require complicated grafts, or if repair poses a prohibitive risk in a patient with multiple injuries, ligation of the infrarenal cava is acceptable. This is rarely necessary, however.

Wounds at or above the renal veins are difficult to expose and carry a higher mortality; over half of the patients die.[26] If bleeding from behind the liver is encountered and cannot be easily identified as coming from a laceration of the anterior cava below the caudate lobe, other maneuvers may be needed. Division of the supporting ligaments permits the liver to be displaced medially a considerable distance, and in some people, adequate exposure can be obtained for primary repair of the cava.[10,27] Sudden interruption of the inferior vena cava blood flow returning to the heart may result in cardiac arrest; temporary caval occlusion should be approached cautiously with careful monitoring of the blood pressure and heart rate. If there are extensive suprarenal caval injuries seen after mobilization of the liver, or if two or three hepatic veins are involved in the injury, it may be necessary to employ an intracaval shunt as described by Schrock and others[28] (Fig. 35–9). A no. 38-French tygon shunt with appropriate openings can be inserted by the transatrial technique as shown in the accompanying figures, although McClelland and others have described a method using an infrarenal caval shunt.[22] In most situations this technique is not required, since adequate mobilization often permits temporary occlusion and repair. If an intracaval shunt is used, the balloon shunt described by Madding and Kennedy[27] may be the simplest for these procedures (Fig. 35–10).

Concomitant repair of hepatic vein injuries is easier in these situations if an intracaval shunt is in place, but one of the hepatic veins may be safely ligated if repair is not possible.

These caval repairs usually can be completed within 30 minutes, a period of ischemia that is well tolerated by the normothermic liver. Some hypothermia occurs almost inevitably with these injuries, since there is an infusion of large amounts of blood and electrolyte solutions, but further regional hypothermia for liver protection may be induced by irrigating the liver directly with a saline solution at 4°C. This will offer additional protection if there is to be prolonged liver ischemia during caval repair (and especially if temporary hepatic artery occlusion is required).

Results

In patients with isolated wounds of the inferior vena cava below the renal veins, direct suture is usually effective and complications are few; the operative mortality is approximately 11 per cent. In the author's experience, 67 per cent of the patients who had a vena caval injury associated with one or more major vessel injuries had a fatal outcome. All of the patients with inferior vena caval wounds at or above the renal veins had associated injuries, usually to the liver or bowel, and occasionally to the pancreas, stomach, and colon. The mortality is very high in this group of patients regardless of the etiology, but especially if the vena cava is injured as a result of blunt trauma or shotgun blast, and if it is actively bleeding at the time of surgery (Table 35–11).

Late thromboembolic phenomena are uncommon, and although few studies have described serial inferior venacavograms, most of the patients who had isolated caval wounds have not had recurrent thrombosis or thromboembolic phenomena. These data strongly suggest that repair of the vena cava is an effective procedure and will be associated with fewer problems than ligation.

REFERENCES

1. Shires GT: Trauma. *In* Schwartz SI (ed): Principles of Surgery. New York, McGraw-Hill, 1989.
2. Dart CH, Braitman HE: Popliteal artery injury following fracture or dislocation at the knee. Arch Surg 112:969, 1977.
3. Lefrac EA: Knee dislocation. Arch Surg 111:1021, 1976.
4. Perry MO: Management of Acute Vascular Injuries. Baltimore, Williams & Wilkins, 1981.
5. Lynch J, Johansen KH: Can Doppler pressure measurement replace "exclusion" arteriography in the diagnosis of arterial trauma? Ann Surg 214:737–741, 1991.
6. Bynoe RP, Miles WS, Bell RM, et al: Noninvasive diagnosis of vascular trauma by duplex ultrasonography. J Vasc Surg 14:346–352, 1991.
7. Snyder WH III, Thal ER, Bridges RA, et al: The validity of normal arteriography in penetrating trauma. Arch Surg 113:424, 1978.
8. Reid JDS, Weigelt JA, Thal ER, et al: Assessment of proximity of a wound to major vascular structures as an indication for arteriography. Arch Surg 128:942, 1988.
9. Shires GT, Canizaro PC, Carrico CJ: Shock. *In* Schwartz SI (ed): Principles of Surgery. New York, McGraw-Hill, 1989.
10. Rich N, Spencer F: Vascular Trauma. Philadelphia, WB Saunders Company, 1978.
11. Flint LM, Snyder WH, Perry MO, Shires GT: Management of major vascular injuries in the base of the neck. Arch Surg 106:407, 1973.
12. Mattox KL, McCollum WB, Beal AC, et al: Management of penetrating injuries of the suprarenal aorta. J Trauma 15:808, 1975.
13. Ehrenfeld WK, Wilbur BC, Olcott CN, Stoney RJ: Autogenous tissue reconstruction in the management of infected prosthetic grafts. Surgery 85:82, 1979.
14. Bradley EE: Management of penetrating carotid injuries: An alternate approach. J Trauma 13:248, 1973.

15. Thal ER, Snyder WH, Hyas RJ, Perry MO: Management of carotid artery injuries. Surgery 76:955, 1974.
16. Yamada S, Kindt GW, Youmas JR: Carotid artery occlusion due to nonpenetrating injury. J Trauma 7:333, 1967.
17. Liekweg WG, Greenfield LJ: Management of penetrating carotid injury. Ann Surg 188:587, 1978.
18. Monson DO, Saletta JD, Freeark RJ: Carotid-vertebral trauma. J Trauma 9:987, 1969.
19. Jernigan WR, Gardner WC: Carotid artery injuries due to closed cervical trauma. Trauma 11:429, 1971.
20. Perry MO: Carotid artery injuries caused by blunt trauma. Ann Surg 192:74, 1980.
21. Lim RC, Trunkey DD, Blaisdell FW: Acute abdominal aortic injury. Arch Surg 109:706, 1974.
22. McClelland RM, Canizaro PC, Shires GT: Repair of hepatic venous, intrahepatic vena caval and portal venous injuries. Major Prob Clin Surg 3:146, 1971.
23. Synder WH, Watkins WL, Bone GE: Civilian popliteal artery trauma: An eleven year experience with 83 injuries. Surgery 85:101, 1979.
24. Rich N, Spencer F: Venous injuries. *In* Vascular Trauma. Philadelphia, WB Saunders Company, 1978.
25. Shumacker HB, Wayson EE: Spontaneous care of aneurysms and arteriovenous fistulas with some notes on intravascular thrombosis. Am J Surg 79:532, 1950.
26. Graham JM, Mattox KL, Beall AC, DeBakey ME: Traumatic injuries of the inferior vena cava. Arch Surg 113:413, 1978.
27. Madding GF, Kennedy PA: Trauma to the Liver. Philadelphia, WB Saunders Company, 1971.
28. Schrock T, Blaisdell FW, Mathewson C Jr: Management of blunt trauma to the liver and hepatic veins. Arch Surg 96:698, 1968.

REVIEW QUESTIONS

1. A 20-year-old man had a stab wound of the right groin near the common femoral artery. There was arterial bleeding initially, but now there is only a 2 × 2-cm hematoma overlying the vessels. Which of the following protocols is preferred?
   (a) immediate exploration in the operating room
   (b) arteriogram with runoff films
   (c) B mode sonogram
   (d) hospitalization and observation for a few days

2. Arterial injuries as a result of blunt trauma are especially likely with which of the following injuries?
   (a) shoulder dislocation
   (b) posterior knee dislocation
   (c) midfemoral shaft fracture
   (d) clavicle fracture

3. A 25-year-old man is admitted because of a bullet wound of the right flank. He is not in shock, and has no hematuria or gastrointestinal bleeding. At exploration there is a moderate collection of blood overlying the aorta and inferior vena cava above the bifurcation. What should be done now?
   (a) if the colon and small bowel are intact, nothing
   (b) exposure and exploration of the right kidney
   (c) arteriogram on the table
   (d) exploration of midline hematoma

4. A 30-year-old woman was in a motor vehicle accident and was unconscious for a few minutes. Admission examination reveals a left Horner's syndrome but there is no external evidence of a neck injury. The preferred management includes which of the following?
   (a) exploratory burr holes
   (b) admission to neurology for tests and observations
   (c) duplex ultrasonography of cervical arteries
   (d) intravenous arteriogram

5. A 17-year-old man experienced a penetrating wound of his left medial thigh during a motor vehicle accident. When examined he had no ischemia but there was moderate swelling surrounding the wound. A continuous murmur was heard in this area. Which of the following clinical features are inappropriate?

   (a) Nicolodani-Branham sign
   (b) tachycardia
   (c) empty veins
   (d) decreased ankle blood pressure

6. The patient in question number 5 should:
   (a) be admitted for observation awaiting resolution
   (b) have observation and measurements of the ABI every 4 hours
   (c) be scheduled for MRI of legs
   (d) be admitted for arteriography

7. Patients who have experienced blunt trauma to the carotid artery:
   (a) have a cervical hematoma
   (b) usually are disoriented
   (c) often are paraplegic
   (d) have only limb paresis

8. Following successful repair of a penetrating wound of the left common carotid artery the patient is neurologically intact, but 2 hours later develops aphasia. Which of the following is preferable?
   (a) CT scan of head
   (b) digital intravenous arteriogram
   (c) immediate reexploration
   (d) carotid arteriogram

9. A young man in a motor vehicle accident was noted on admission to have a bruise on his anterior chest. He was awake and had normal limb pulses and blood pressures. Arteriography is indicated if:
   (a) mediastinum is wider than 8 cm in the second interspace
   (b) second and third rib are shattered
   (c) left clavicle is shattered and left acromioclavicular joint is disrupted
   (d) there is a fracture of T3 and T4

10. Concomitant tibial bone fractures causing transection of the popliteal vein and artery should be treated by:
    (a) immediate external fixation and stabilization of the tibia

(b) initial traction and internal fixation with arterial
    repair
(c) repair of vein and artery and internal fixation of
    bones
(d) exploration and repair of artery

ANSWERS

1. a   2. b   3. d   4. c   5. c   6. d   7. d
8. d   9. a   10. c

36

ACUTE ARTERIAL AND GRAFT OCCLUSION

WILLIAM J. QUIÑONES-BALDRICH

The clinical presentation of an acute arterial occlusion ranges from subtle to dramatic. It is therefore critical for vascular surgeons to be familiar with the wide range of clinical symptoms that may be produced by acute occlusion of the main blood supply of an organ. Clearly, prompt diagnosis and management remain most important in achieving a successful outcome. Delays in treatment invariably lead to increased morbidity and mortality.

The pathophysiology of acute ischemia and reperfusion has generated increasing interest within the vascular research community. Although controversy still exists, there seems to be a general consensus that significant injury occurs during the early phases of reperfusion. Knowledge of the operating mechanisms during this important interval will help vascular surgeons restore circulation to the affected area and at the same time minimize the possible deleterious effects of reperfusion. Emerging from this research effort is an understanding that differing mechanisms may be operating in different tissues and that various mechanisms may acquire importance at different times during the reperfusion phase.

Equally important developments have occurred in the overall management of patients following revascularization of acutely ischemic tissue. Systemic effects secondary to reperfusion of a major body part have been well recognized and documented. The source and effect of these systemic changes may be ameliorated by newer medical treatments. Anticipation of these changes is perhaps the most important of all actions taken during the management of these difficult cases.

This chapter will concentrate on the etiology, pathophysiology, clinical manifestations, and medical and surgical management of the patient with an acutely ischemic extremity. In modern vascular practice, patients presenting with acute extremity ischemia can be divided into those that have native artery occlusion either from embolism or thrombosis, and patients that have failure of a previously performed

vascular reconstruction. Although these patients will frequently have similar clinical manifestations, their etiology and management differs significantly, so that they are best considered separately. Both groups will be discussed in detail in this chapter. Patients with acute brain or visceral ischemia will frequently share etiologic and pathophysiologic mechanisms discussed in this chapter. Nevertheless, their specific clinical manifestations and management are discussed in other chapters within this book specifically dealing with those organs.

PATHOPHYSIOLOGY

The ultimate effect of a period of ischemia in a particular tissue will, in general, depend on a balance between supply and metabolic demand. Supply may be defined as the adequate delivery of nutrients and oxygen with elimination of metabolic waste. The metabolic demands of various tissues vary widely and, even within the same tissue, depend on their state of metabolic activity. For example, myocardium is relatively sensitive to ischemia, given that it must continue to function in order to assure survival of the organism. Efforts at reducing ischemic infarct size concentrate on reducing metabolic demand by unloading the heart during the critical recovery phase. The brain, on the other hand, is exquisitely sensitive to ischemia, because it is incapable of significantly reducing its metabolic demand. Efforts to artificially reduce its demand, as with pentobarbital coma, will significantly prolong the tolerance of central nervous tissue to ischemia during surgical manipulation. In an extremity, tissues differ in their ability to tolerate ischemia based on their metabolic demands. Skin and subcutaneous tissue appear to be relatively resistant to prolonged ischemia. Peripheral nerve, traditionally considered resistant to ischemia, has recently been shown to be exquisitely sensitive to both ischemia and reperfusion, with prolonged functional deficit demonstrated after 3 hours of ischemia.[1] The impres-

648

sion that peripheral nerves are resistant to ischemia may be secondary to the subtleness of the morphologic injury demonstrable by microscopy. Nevertheless, the pathophysiologic impairment of its function underscores the importance of adequate nutrient flow to maintain cellular membrane gradients.

Skeletal muscle comprises the bulk of tissue in an extremity. In recent years, increasing attention has been focused on the study of ischemia and reperfusion of skeletal muscle. The relative tolerance of skeletal muscle to ischemia, in large part, is due to its slow metabolic rate at rest, its large stores of glycogen and high-energy phosphate bonds in the form of creatine, and its ability to maintain basic cellular functions through anaerobic glycolysis.

In the clinical situation, the supply side of this equation is variable and largely depends on the location of the vascular occlusion, the rapidity with which such occlusion has developed, and the presence of collateral circulation prior to the occlusion. Thus, a specific ischemic interval will have variable effects, depending on all of the above parameters. The concept of a safe period of ischemia beyond which the viability of the tissue is unlikely, cannot be substantiated. Thus, other parameters must be utilized in the assessment of the ischemic extremity. In the experimental animal, measurement of contractile function has been shown to be much more reliable than time as a predictor of ischemic injury.[2]

Although the rate at which changes occur within the cell with interruption of nutrient blood flow varies among tissues, similar mechanisms appear to be common to all tissues. As the supply of energy diminishes, the cell is capable of maintaining vital functions by use of stored energy supply in the form of adenosine triphosphate (ATP). If the metabolic demands can be reduced, as occurs in skeletal muscle, these energy stores may be replenished at the same rate of utilization, through anaerobic glycolysis or stored energy sources such as creatine. With time, however, these stores become inadequate and ATP is metabolized to adenosine diphosphate (ADP), and further to adenosine monophosphate (AMP). Gradients across the membrane can no longer be maintained and there is a general influx of calcium into the cell. This forms the rationale for the potential role of calcium channel blockers during reperfusion.[3] The influx of calcium into the intracellular space has detrimental effects on delicate enzyme systems. Experimental studies in heart, intestine, and kidney have shown that specifically, the enzyme xanthine dehydrogenase is changed to xanthine oxidase as the intracellular milieu changes. As AMP is further metabolized to xanthine and hypoxanthine, accumulation of hypoxanthine occurs.[4] These metabolites are lipid soluble and may leak across the membrane; thus, further loss of substrate occurs. The metabolic alternatives for adenine nucleotide synthesis through salvage pathways or de novo synthesis are very slow and energy dependent in and of themselves.[5] Thus the inability to replenish the energy stores immedi-

ately upon reperfusion further limits the cell's capability to recover from ischemic injury. Eventually, the respiratory system of the mitochondria is impaired, membrane integrity cannot be maintained, and cell death occurs.

Experimental studies looking at ischemia and reperfusion have fairly well established the fact that in addition to ischemic injury, cells may undergo lethal changes during the early periods of reperfusion. The latter has been termed "reperfusion injury," and efforts in controlling it have inspired many investigators to alter their methods and content of the reperfusate in order to ameliorate these deleterious changes. In tissues with a relatively high content of xanthine dehydrogenase, accumulation of xanthine and the progressive change of xanthine dehydrogenase to xanthine oxidase leads to an undesirable environment in which the introduction of molecular oxygen can lead to the rapid production of oxygen radical species capable of permanently destroying delicate cellular membranes by lipid peroxidation. Oxygen radical injury has been demonstrated in most tissues subjected to ischemia and reperfusion.[4,6–9] Specifically, malondialdehyde, a product of lipid peroxidation, has been shown to increase upon reperfusion of ischemic cells.[10,11] The sources of these radicals, however, remain uncertain. Initially, it was thought that the xanthine oxidase pathway was an important source of these toxic radicals. However, not all tissues contain the same amount of xanthine oxidase and in skeletal muscle specifically, this pathway is of questionable significance.[12] Nevertheless, experimental data support the role of oxygen and hydroxy radicals in the injury that occurs upon reperfusion. Administration of oxygen and hydroxy radical scavengers during the early periods of reperfusion has been suggested as beneficial in retrieving ischemic skeletal muscle.[7,9,13] Potential sources of these radicals are present in other cellular components and, specifically, in white blood cells that may be resident in tissues during the ischemic period or introduced during the early phases of reperfusion. Cellular receptors specific for white blood cells appear to be necessary to induce this radical injury.[14] These receptors may be exposed as the result of ischemia and represent a conformational change or up-regulation of neutrophil adhesion receptors CD11/CD18 complex. Increased expression of endothelial leukocyte adhesion molecule (ELAM) has also been observed.[15] White cell accumulation in reperfused skeletal muscle has been demonstrated experimentally.[16] Once adhesion has occurred, activation may proceed with release of cytotoxic enzymes, as well as free oxygen radicals.[17] Progressive sequestration of white blood cells has also been observed following the first few hours of reperfusion.[18]

Other processes during the ischemic interval and/or early reperfusion phase may impair adequate reperfusion of the tissue because of progressive microcirculatory obstruction. This process, termed the "no-reflow" phenomenon, tends to occur with progressive ischemic intervals and, because it prevents adequate nutrient flow in spite of axial blood flow restoration, may prolong the ischemic phase. In our laboratory, we have observed this process of no reflow to acquire importance as the ischemic interval is lengthened. Whereas muscles that are made ischemic from 1 to 3 hours are easily reperfused without evidence of no reflow, muscles subjected to 5 hours of ischemia demonstrate this phenomenon in up to 40 to 50 per cent of the preparations.[19]

The cause of the no-reflow phenomenon is not well established. Blood is a nonnewtonian fluid whose particular rheology requires consideration. The energy required to reestablish movement of blood after it has been stagnant is proportional to the third power of the red cell mass and the second power of the fibrogen content.[20] Thus, the concept of opening pressure may be important in the early phases of reperfusion. More energy is required to restart flow than to maintain patency of the circulation. This concept is parallel to that of airway opening pressure when there is collapse in the bronchial tree.

When muscles subjected to 5 hours of ischemia, in which no reflow is seen, are evaluated under the microscope, large amounts of sludging of red cells are seen in the microcirculation. Experimentally, this process can be significantly reduced by the administration of fibrinolytic agents during the early periods of reperfusion.[21] This suggests a significant role for fibrin in the no-reflow phenomenon. This process appears to occur mostly during the early phases of reperfusion, as muscles that are subjected to ischemia only do not show the typical fibrin strands and red cell sludging seen in reperfused specimens (unpublished data). Clearly, if this microcirculatory sludging occurs during the early phases of reperfusion, the cellular elements of blood would be undesirable in the initial reperfusate. Clearing the microcirculation prior to introduction of the red cell mass may be a desirable goal in the early phases of reperfusion. This may be accomplished with the use of agents capable of lysing fibrin. The use of an acellular reperfusate with oxygen-carrying capacities may achieve some of these objectives. This is currently under investigation.

Other important changes during ischemia may contribute to the no-reflow phenomenon. Cellular swelling may lead to capillary obstruction and plugging of white cells during the early phases of reperfusion.[22–25] The administration of hyperosmotic agents such as mannitol may be beneficial in this regard. In addition, mannitol is a hydroxy radical scavenger, which may have additional benefits.[26] The contribution of white blood cells to the no-reflow phenomenon is questionable. Elimination of white blood cells from the initial reperfusate was of no advantage in an experimental model of ischemia and reperfusion of skeletal muscle.[21] It may be, however, that the contribution of the white blood cell to the reperfusion injury can be modified by either inhibition of white blood cell mechanisms responsible for oxygen radical production or elimination of these cells from the initial reperfusate.[27]

Thus, there appear to be two major components responsible for reperfusion injury. First, cellular injury occurs by the untimely introduction of oxygen without adequate preparation of the cell to handle it properly. Thus, efforts to control this part of the reperfusion process have centered around control of oxygen radical injury by oxygen radical scavengers,[7,9,13] elimination of white blood cells from the reperfusate,[27] administration of important intermediate metabolites,[28] and control of the rate of reperfusion.[29] The second major component of reperfusion injury appears to be the no-reflow phenomenon. Although both of these major mechanisms may occur in a continuum, understanding them and perhaps even addressing their management is best accomplished by considering them separately. The no-reflow phenomenon acquires importance as the ischemic interval is lengthened. The deposition of fibrin in the microcirculation appears to be a significant factor in its establishment, and thus fibrinolytic agents may find a role to ameliorate this process.[21] Endothelial cell swelling, rheology of stagnant blood, and the rate at which tissues are reperfused appear to be significant factors that may require control in order to optimize reperfusion.

Following acute occlusion of an artery, the clinical outcome will depend in large part on the presence or absence of collateral circulation. This, in turn, will depend on the preexistence of occlusive arterial disease and the site of occlusion. Following the initial event, ischemia may be aggravated by proximal and/or distal thrombus propagation. This impairs collateral circulation, and thus worsens the ischemia. Fragmentation of the embolus may occur with subsequent distal or discontinuous occlusion, further aggravating the process. This fragmentation, on the other hand, may produce intermittent changes of improvement and worsening depending on its severity and location. Venous thrombosis may accompany acute extremity ischemia, usually as a secondary event due to the low flow and thrombogenicity of the system. This further aggravates the ischemic process and may complicate revascularization.

In addition to the local injury that occurs during reperfusion, the significant systemic effects of revascularization of an ischemic extremity must be considered. The end result in the most severe cases has been termed the "myonephropathic metabolic syndrome."[30] As blood flow is reestablished in an ischemic extremity, acidic blood is returned to the systemic circulation, capable of causing an abrupt and rapid metabolic acidosis. This can be anticipated, and judicious use of bicarbonate during the early phases of reperfusion is highly recommended. Leakage of the major intracellular cation (potassium) during cell death will lead to hyperkalemia during the acute reperfusion phase. This may be aggravated by acute renal failure secondary to myoglobin precipitation in the collecting tubules. Both of these processes require careful attention during the early reperfusion phase. Administration of glucose and insulin will drive potassium into cells, and thus control hyperkalemia. Maintaining a high urine output with an alkaline urine is best to control the myoglobinuria and potential renal failure. This can be achieved by the systemic administration of mannitol to promote an osmotic diuresis and bicarbonate or acetazolamide to maintain an alkaline urine.

The pathophysiologic changes that occur during acute ischemia and reperfusion of an extremity are not yet fully understood. Nevertheless, accumulating experimental and clinical evidence has helped elucidate some of the mechanisms that may be important to address during reperfusion. Emerging from this literature is an increasing understanding that the retrievability of ischemic tissue will largely depend on the method and content of the initial reperfusate. Thus, it is likely that in the future the method of reperfusion will be aimed at control of important factors during this phase of therapy.

ETIOLOGY

Acute Arterial Occlusion

Table 36–1 summarizes the possible etiologies of acute ischemia of an organ. Acute occlusion of an artery secondary to emboli is by far the leading cause of acute ischemia, accounting for over 80 per cent of cases.[31–33] Its incidence appears to be increasing, in large part as a result of better diagnosis, increasing age of the population, and improved survival in patients with cardiac disease.[33] Of these cases, most are caused by emboli originating in the heart. The etiology of these clots originating in the heart has changed, as the incidence of rheumatic valvular heart disease has decreased. Complications of atherosclerotic heart disease account for approximately 60 to 70 per cent of emboli originating in the heart.[31–35] Most commonly, it follows an acute myocardial infarction from ventricular mural thrombi formed in an area of hypokinesia or dyskinesia. Mural thrombi can occur within hours to weeks following myocardial infarction and are seen in up to 40 per cent of autopsy specimens.[36] Anterior myocardial transmural infarcts are the leading cause of ventricular thrombi. Patients who develop a ventricular aneurysm secondary to a myocardial infarction may embolize long after the myocardial event. In contrast, peripheral embolization may be the initial manifestation of an otherwise silent myocardial infarction. In addition, arrhythmias secondary to coronary artery disease or valvular heart disease account for a significant number of patients presenting with peripheral emboli. Most of these are secondary to atrial arrhythmias, which predispose to the formation of atrial clot. Almost 75 per cent of patients seen with embolic occlusion of an extremity will have a history of either an acute myocardial infarction and/or atrial fibrillation within the preceding weeks.[31,34,37]

Emboli originating from the heart will most com-

TABLE 36–1. ETIOLOGY OF ACUTE ARTERIAL ISCHEMIA

EMBOLIC	TRAUMATIC
Heart	Penetrating trauma
Atherosclerotic heart disease	Direct vessel injury
Coronary artery disease	Indirect injury
Acute myocardial infarction	Missile emboli
Arrhythmia	Proximity
Valvular heart disease	Blunt trauma
Rheumatic	Intimal flap
Degenerative	Spasm
Congenital	Iatrogenic
Bacterial	Intimal flap
Prosthetic	Dissection
Artery-to-artery	Presence of medical device
Aneurysm	Space-occupying thrombosis
Atherosclerotic plaque	Clot propagation
Idiopathic	External compression
Paradoxical embolus	Drug abuse
	Intraarterial administration
	Drug toxicity
	Contaminant
	Microembolization
THROMBOSIS	OUTFLOW VENOUS OCCLUSION
Atherosclerosis	Compartment syndrome
Low-flow states	Phlegmasia
Congestive heart failure	
Hypovolemia	LOW-FLOW STATES
Hypotension	Cardiogenic shock
Hypercoagulable states	Hypovolemic shock
Vascular grafts	Drug effect
Progression of disease	Mesenteric—digoxin
Intimal hyperplasia	—H_2 blockers
Mechanical	

monly travel to the extremities. The upper extremities are less frequently affected, accounting for approximately 15 per cent of all emboli. The lower extremities are most frequently affected and account for 60 to 70 per cent of all recognized embolism.[33,37] The location of the embolus within the extremity is usually at a branching site, such that femoral emboli are most common at the bifurcation of the common femoral artery, iliac emboli at the bifurcation of the common iliac artery, and popliteal emboli at the level of the trifurcation. Visceral embolism is probably underrecognized and accounts for 7 to 10 per cent of all recognized emboli. The cerebral circulation is involved in approximately 15 to 20 per cent of instances. It is somewhat fortunate that embolism tends to occur more commonly in the extremities, because these are easier to recognize and their treatment is familiar to most vascular specialists.

Although rheumatic disease has significantly decreased as a source of emboli, prosthetic valve embolization is acquiring importance, as more patients with prosthetic heart valves are living longer. In spite of the use of tissue valves, antithrombotic therapy is highly recommended, specifically for patients with mitral valve replacement and those with prosthetic mechanical aortic valves. In the absence of chronic anticoagulation, peripheral embolization is a major risk in these patients. Mechanical failure with embolization of parts of the prosthesis is rare.[38] Bacterial endocarditis has seen an increased incidence within the last 10 years secondary to increased intravenous drug abuse. It remains an important cause of embolization in young individuals without other risk factors. Intracardiac tumors, such as myxomas, are rare but may present as peripheral embolization of either parts of the tumor or clot formed because of the tumor.[39] Gross and microscopic examination of the material removed during surgical intervention may lead to the correct diagnosis.

Paradoxical embolization can occur in spite of the absence of a clinically detectable atrial septal defect. Patients with deep vein thrombosis developing an acute arterial occlusion should be suspect. This is especially true if the patient has had a pulmonary embolus with concomitant rise in right-sided heart pressures, which may open a patent foramen ovale. Other rare causes of embolization from a central origin include tumor invasion of the intrathoracic vessels, or direct arterial invasion with concomitant tumor and/or thrombi embolization.[40,41] Malignancies may, in addition, be associated with a hypercoagulable state.

Artery-to-artery embolization is well recognized when an aneurysm is identified proximal to the acute occlusion. The most common are abdominal aortic and popliteal aneurysms, which cause acute extremity ischemia. Less well recognized is the potential for atherosclerotic plaques to serve as a source of microembolization to the lower extremities.[42] Although the syndrome of transient ischemic attacks is well recognized in the carotid distribution secondary to an atherosclerotic plaque in the carotid bifurcation, microemboli may have less obvious clinical manifestations in the lower extremities. In its most dramatic presentation, a microembolus can produce acute ischemia of a toe, leading to gangrene of a single or adjacent digits. This is referred to as the blue-toe syndrome. The source of emboli may be a proximal plaque in the system or, less commonly, a thrombus within the aorta[43] (Fig. 36-1). In fact, it is remarkable that more clinically evident ischemic episodes are not seen, considering the frequency of ulcerated plaques in the aortoiliac and femoral systems in patients with peripheral arterial disease. In fact, several tibial diseases may be, in part, the result of multiple subclinical emboli.[44] This certainly should be suspected in patients with marked asymmetry in their distal disease pattern, or those with rapid progression of distal disease with evidence of ulcerated plaques in the proximal segments. It may also be a consideration in patients with repeated failures of infrainguinal reconstructions of otherwise unexplained cause.

Thrombosis of an underlying stenotic artery can lead to mild to moderate acute symptoms secondary to its gradual development and the presence of collateral circulation. Nevertheless, propagation of the thrombus may lead to rapid, progressive ischemia requiring immediate medical attention. Differentia-

tion of this process from an acute embolus is of utmost importance, considering that therapy is very different for the two entities (see section, Management, later in this chapter). Low-flow states, such as congestive heart failure, hypovolemia, or hypotension of any cause, may contribute to thrombosis of a diseased arterial segment. Ischemia is thus compounded by the low-flow state. This is most commonly seen in elderly individuals in an intensive care unit being supported for their primary disease. Improving the hemodynamics remains the primary goal, with priorities established once this has been accomplished.

Thrombosis may be secondary to hypercoagulable conditions. These comprise a long list of factors that predispose to thrombosis in an otherwise unaffected arterial segment. Heparin-induced thrombosis is an important cause, usually recognized by a significant drop in the platelet count during heparin therapy and occurrence of a thrombotic event. When not recognized in a timely fashion, this may lead to limb- or life-threatening complications.[45,46] Most other hypercoagulable states are properly treated with heparin (with concomitant administration of fresh-frozen plasma for antithrombin III deficiency), with intervention indicated by the severity of the ischemia. Malignancy is an important underlying etiology in elderly individuals presenting with a hypercoagulable condition.[47] Chemotherapy may actually temporarily aggravate the process and lead to arterial embolism or thrombosis.[48]

Traumatic injury of an axial artery may lead to immediate thrombosis, disruption, or embolization. Penetrating trauma may disrupt an artery, thus causing acute extremity ischemia. Embolization of a missile has been reported and must be kept in mind in a patient with a remote penetrating injury developing acute extremity ischemia.[49] Injuries due to proximity are usually seen with high-velocity missiles and are secondary to intimal disruption of the adjacent artery. Blunt trauma may cause acute arterial obstruction secondary to intimal disruption of the adjacent artery, intimal flap or, on occasion, spasm due to a large expanding hematoma. Blunt trauma to an extremity may cause fractures with associated arterial injury. This is most commonly seen with supracondylar fractures of the upper extremity, where the brachial artery is in intimate relationship with the humerus. In the lower extremity, fractures of the distal femur and posterior knee dislocations, with or without tibial plateau fractures, are most commonly associated with arterial injury. These may range from complete disruption of the artery to intimal tears and fractures, leading to secondary thrombosis (Fig. 36-2). Ascribing severe distal extremity ischemia to spasm without appropriate arteriographic evaluation is to be condemned and may lead to unnecessary tissue loss. Comparing distal pressures obtained by Doppler of the involved extremity with that of an uninvolved extremity, has been suggested as an accurate means to determine which patients need arteriog-

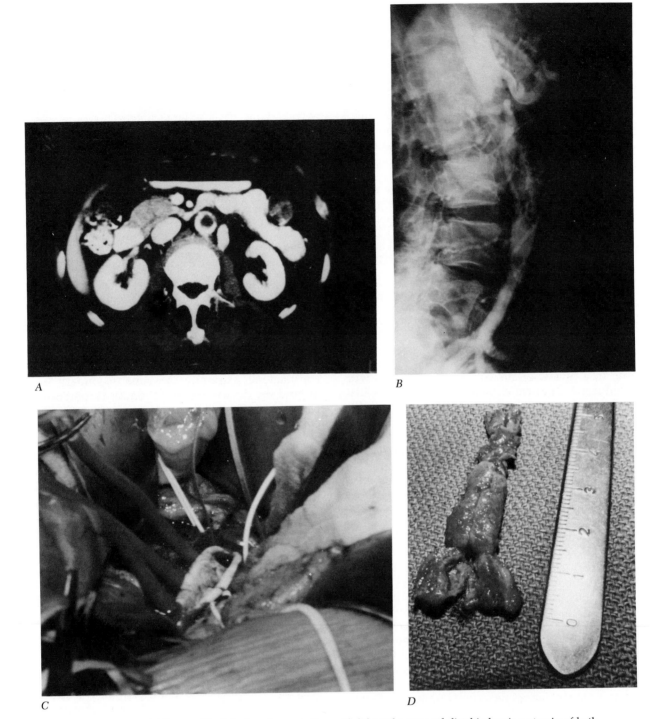

FIGURE 36–1. A 72-year-old white female presenting with bilateral acute and distal ischemic rest pain of both lower extremities secondary to microembolization. *A,* Computed tomography scan with intravenous contrast shows intraluminal defect in abdominal aorta. *B,* Lateral aortogram demonstrates intraluminal defect starting at the level of the superior mesenteric artery. *C,* Operative view of infrarenal aorta with temporary control of lumbar arteries, bilateral renal artery control with vessel loops, and supraceliac aortic cross-clamping. *D,* Operative specimen after complete abdominal aortic thrombectomy. Angioscopy was helpful in assessing the completeness of the suprarenal portion of the embolectomy.

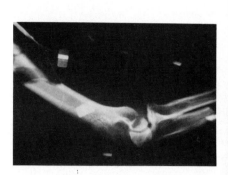 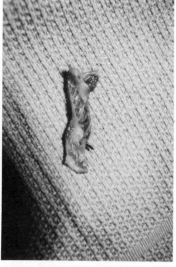 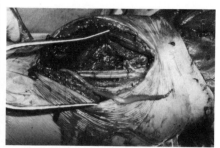

FIGURE 36–2. A 27-year-old patient involved in a motorcycle accident presenting with fracture of the left humerus. *Left,* Arteriogram shows complete occlusion of the midbrachial artery and fracture of the distal third of the humerus. *Middle,* Operative specimen showing spiral disruption of the intima with thrombosis. *Right,* Operative appearance of segmental vein interposition repair. Note that complete transection of median nerve accompanied this injury and was major cause of morbidity.

raphy. In a review of 509 consecutive patients with isolated upper or lower extremity penetrating injury, Weaver et al. found that only pulse deficit and/or ankle-brachial index less than 1.0 were predictors of significant arterial injury.[50]

Acute aortic dissection may occasionally present with acute limb ischemia. Patients are usually hypertensive and complain of severe chest and back pain. Arteriography prior to intervention is of utmost importance to establish the diagnosis and assess for visceral ischemia. On occasion, a patient taken to the operating room, misdiagnosed as having an embolic occlusion to a limb, may be suspect for aortic dissection when passage of the Fogarty catheter fails to go beyond the occlusion or does not retrieve clot or induce blood flow. The artery itself may appear friable, with easy separation of the intima through the medial plane. The inner layers of the vessel may be retrieved by the Fogarty catheter, thus compounding the problem. Failure to establish the proper diagnosis may prove fatal.

With the increased use of percutaneous endovascular techniques, iatrogenic arterial trauma is acquiring importance as an etiology of acute extremity ischemia. These are usually secondary to intimal flaps, dissection, and/or thrombosis, and frequently require operative therapy. Treatment may prove difficult in the patient with preexisting peripheral vascular disease. Although arteriography may be omitted in the young patient without occlusive disease, it is highly recommended in those instances in which preexisting disease may mandate an involved vascular reconstruction to reestablish circulation. The presence of a medical device, in and of itself, within the arterial system may cause significant extremity ischemia. Intraaortic balloon pumps may lead to ipsilateral or contralateral extremity ischemia secondary to clot around the device, embolization, or thrombosis. The clinical manifestations are aggravated usually because of the low-flow state requiring the device. Temporarizing with heparinization is a reasonable alternative, if it is anticipated that the intraaortic balloon will be removed within the next few hours. Otherwise, construction of an extraanatomic bypass distal to the balloon insertion site may be limb saving.

Hand ischemia secondary to a radial artery line is usually the result of inadequate preinsertion evaluation. The performance of the Allen test to document the integrity of the palmar arch is an underemphasized maneuver prior to the insertion of an arterial line in the upper extremity. Failure to do so will inevitably result in patients experiencing hand ischemia because of interruption of radial artery flow. Removal of the radial artery cannula may result in improvement, with an occasional patient requiring operative intervention.

External compression secondary to either tourniquet or cast application to an extremity is an important preventable cause of acute extremity ischemia. Patients with peripheral vascular disease undergoing orthopedic procedures should be managed with caution, because subcutaneous collateral vessels serving to irrigate the distal extremity are most susceptible to external compression and, because of the rheology of stagnant blood, may require higher pressures to spontaneously open once they are collapsed. Emergency reconstructions in these patients may prove difficult because of the orthopedic device and preexisting peripheral vascular process. These patients are best evaluated prior to the orthopedic intervention so that appropriate recommendations can be made, the tourniquet avoided altogether, and intervention facilitated if a complication were to occur.

Accidental intraarterial administration of illicit drugs can lead to devastating extremity ischemia secondary to toxicity of the drug itself, or contaminant microembolization. Treatment is usually supportive, and tissue loss is common with this entity.

Occlusion of venous outflow of an extremity may be secondary to the compartment syndrome. The latter may be seen after revascularization following prolonged ischemia, trauma, or any other process that may increase compartmental pressures. As the pressure in a fascial compartment increases, venous outflow is impeded, thus producing further increase in the compartmental pressures. If this process is left unchecked, arterial inflow is restricted, leading to nerve and muscle ischemia. Early fasciotomy can be limb saving. Outflow occlusion secondary to venous thrombosis is rare but should be recognized in the markedly swollen and painful extremity. As the venous thrombotic process progresses, arterial inflow is impeded, leading to limb-threatening ischemia (phlegmasia). Treatment alternatives include heparinization, thrombolytic therapy, and/or venous thrombectomy.

Extreme low-flow states usually seen in patients with cardiogenic or hypovolemic shock can lead to extremity ischemia, especially in those patients with preexisting peripheral vascular disease. This process is aggravated by vasoactive drugs, which are frequently needed to support the patient. Correction of the hemodynamic derangement is the primary goal, with intervention reserved for those patients with persistent ischemia. Heparinization may be of benefit, preventing thrombosis in these poorly perfused extremities.

Vascular Graft Failure

Early and late failures of arterial reconstructions clearly can be caused by processes that have been discussed before in the section, Acute Arterial Occlusion. In addition, processes specifically involving the graft, and either the inflow and outflow vascular bed, will influence the performance of these reconstructions.

For the purposes of discussion, it is convenient to divide the causes of graft failure into those affecting prosthetic reconstructions separate from those affecting autogenous reconstructions. It is also preferable to discuss reconstructions involving the aortofemoral segment separate from infrainguinal reconstructions. We will limit the scope of these discussions to lower extremity bypasses. The reader is referred to specific chapters dealing with other areas where failure of vascular reconstructions may be affected by similar or alternate mechanisms. Infection is an important cause of vascular graft failure and is discussed at length in Chapter 38. Suffice it to say that autogenous reconstructions are more resistant to infection and, in fact, may be utilized as an alter-

native to a prosthetic implant in the presence of infection.[51] Acute infection of an autogenous graft will usually require graft replacement through uninvolved tissue. Chronic late occurring infections of prosthetic grafts may be appropriately treated with autogenous reconstruction in the same bed. Exceptions to this will be organisms causing necrotizing infections, such as *Pseudomonas* and *Salmonella*.

Autogenous reconstruction of the lower extremities is usually seen in infrainguinal bypasses where either reversed, nonreversed, or in situ saphenous vein is used. Early failures of such reconstructions are usually secondary to technical defects that are best avoided by the liberal use of angiography, duplex scanning, or another modality at the completion of the original operation to document the technical success of the repair. Early failure may also be secondary to a defect in the graft, usually the result of previous episodes of superficial phlebitis, which may have led to sclerotic changes in a segment of the vein.[52] Additionally, injury may be caused at the time of harvest or preparation. Preservation of endothelial function should be the goal and is best accomplished by careful technique, avoiding trauma to the vein. Distention of the graft should be accomplished gently, preferably using heparinized blood. Alternatively, distention may be accomplished by the arterial pressure itself, after connecting the graft in its proximal anastomosis. One of the potential advantages of the in situ technique is that it minimizes the degree of ischemia suffered by the vein graft. Other causes of early failure include external compression or kinks, the latter avoided by assuring no twists in the vein (either in situ or reversed). Marking the proximal and distal ends of the veins prior to mobilization may help accomplish this with minimal effort. Tunnels performed anatomically for autogenous grafts may produce external compression on the vein. This can be identified on completion angiography by the effacement of the contrast during injection. Subcutaneous tunnels may have an advantage in this regard, with the additional benefit of being readily accessible if revision becomes necessary.

In situ saphenous vein bypasses, in addition, may fail acutely secondary to residual arteriovenous (AV) fistulas, or inadequate valve lysis. Residual AV fistulas do not lead to clinical symptoms in most instances. On occasion, however, they will manifest with limb edema out of proportion to the expected swelling. They can be readily diagnosed on physical examination by the presence of a murmur over the fistula. Inadequate valve lysis can manifest as an early or late failure, due to stenosis of the segment. The use of angioscopy has been suggested by some as a means of assuring complete valve lysis in preparation of the in situ graft. Alternatively, these may be identified on continuous-wave Doppler examination by a change in signal quality, implying high velocities through that segment. Completion angiography will also detect these defects and avoid early failure.[53]

Intimal hyperplasia of either the proximal or distal

anastomosis, or of the vein graft itself, continues to be the most frequent cause of late failure of autogenous infrainguinal reconstruction.[54] These lesions tend to occur within the first year after implantation and are rare beyond 2 years. In a series of 109 primary femoropopliteal bypasses, failures within the first 30 days resulted primarily from technical or judgmental errors. Stenotic lesions developing within the vein graft were noted to be the most common cause of failure within the first year. Progression of distal disease was the leading cause of failure after 2 years.[55] Thus, the point in time when failure occurs will aid in determination of the etiologic mechanism.

Other lesions may affect autogenous vein grafts in their long-term performance. Aneurysmal dilatation is rare. When it occurs, it threatens the patency of the bypass, usually by either thrombosis or distal embolization. Stenotic lesions may develop at the inflow or outflow portion of the aneurysm, usually secondary to a kink. Rupture is rare. Repair is indicated when the lesion threatens patency of the reconstruction.

Failure of prosthetic vascular reconstructions differs from autogenous grafts in that intrinsic graft problems are extremely unusual. With the exception of the umbilical vein graft, aneurysmal dilatation is not seen. Prosthetic graft stenoses are usually the result of external compression, or twists during implantation. Externally supported grafts may avoid some of these problems. Kinking of the outflow popliteal artery in above-knee femoropopliteal bypass has been described and may account for some failures of above-knee reconstructions.[56] By far the most common cause of failure within the first 2 years after implantation of a prosthetic infrainguinal reconstruction is progression of distal disease. In a review of 111 failures of PTFE infrainguinal bypasses over a 10-year interval, 64 per cent of failures occurred within the first year. Fifty-six per cent were either due to severity or progression of the distal disease. Progression of inflow disease occurred in 25 per cent of instances and was most commonly seen as progression of iliac disease in patients operated upon to relieve claudication and thrombosis of an inflow reconstruction in limb salvage patients. Only 8 per cent of cases had isolated intimal hyperplasia as a cause of failure, although half of patients in whom progression of distal disease was seen had some degree of intimal hyperplasia at the distal anastomosis.[57]

Infection is a rare but important cause of failure of infrainguinal prosthetic reconstructions. When it occurs, graft excision with alternative revascularization, when indicated, is the preferred treatment.

If after a thorough search for the cause of early failure, none is identified, a hypercoagulable condition should be suspected. History of superficial or deep thrombophlebitis, prior bypass failure, or other thrombotic events in the past would suggest this etiology. Identification of the specific abnormality is important in directing management. From a clinical standpoint, however, heparin is the treatment of choice, with the exception of heparin-induced thrombosis and the need for supplementation of antithrombin III in deficient patients. Identification of heparin-induced thrombosis is of paramount importance to avoid continued thrombotic events. Serial platelet counts during heparin therapy will be most helpful, with confirmation of the diagnosis by in vitro platelet aggregation studies. Although most commonly seen in the early postoperative period, hypercoagulable conditions may play a role in early failures during the first few months after surgery. Specifically in prosthetic grafts, due to their initial thrombogenicity, some patients will present with acute thrombosis in whom no identifiable cause for failure can be determined. These patients may benefit from long-term anticoagulation.[58]

CLINICAL MANIFESTATIONS

Acute Arterial Occlusion

The clinical manifestations of acute extremity ischemia will vary depending on the level and severity of the obstruction and, most importantly, the adequacy of collateral circulation. The latter is mostly dependent on the presence or absence of concomitant arterial occlusive disease and, to a lesser degree, location of the occlusion. In obtaining a history, it is therefore important to determine the functional status of the extremity prior to the event. Patients with no history of claudication or previous vascular reconstruction are most likely affected by peripheral embolization.

Acute occlusion of an otherwise normal, noncollateralized artery will lead to the classic manifestations of acute extremity ischemia: pulselessness, pain, pallor, paresthesia, and paralysis (the five "P"'s). Certainly, the disappearance of a previously palpable pulse or the absence of a pulse in a patient with these symptoms and normal pulses in the opposite extremity is pathognomonic of an acute arterial occlusion. The presence and/or severity of these manifestations will depend on the severity of the ischemia.

In addition to the disappearance of the pulse, an arterial occlusion may cause tenderness over the affected artery. This is usually proximal to the ischemic changes. The ischemic manifestations will usually be most severe one joint distal to the level of obstruction. The classic example is the patient presenting with foot ischemia with a relatively well-perfused calf secondary to an embolus to the level of the trifurcation of the popliteal artery.

Pain is the most common manifestation of an acute arterial occlusion. Characteristically, it is severe and progressive, with the most distal part of the extremity affected early. As the ischemia progresses, however, sensory deficits may ensue that may mask the pain, confusing the inexperienced clinician. The pain is slowly replaced by a feeling of numbness, which denotes progression of the ischemic progress and demands immediate attention.

Pallor is one of the initial manifestations of acute ischemia. The extremity rapidly develops a waxy appearance secondary to complete emptying and vasospasm of the arterial circulation. With progression, however, this is replaced by mottling, secondary vasodilation, and stagnant circulation in the capillary bed. Blanching of these mottled areas with application of digital pressure denotes a retrievable capillary bed. Once the mottled areas become nonblanching, a manifestation of capillary sludging, early gangrene, is likely. This represents advanced ischemia. Without revascularization, this will lead to blistering of the skin with further discoloration established; as water is lost, dessication occurs with changes typical of dry gangrene.

Paralysis and sensory deficits are usually late manifestations of severe ischemia. Because of lack of nutrient flow, skeletal muscle and nerve dysfunction lead to decreasing ability of the patient to move the extremity. As the energy stores within the muscle decrease, inability to relax the muscles leads to rigor, a sign of far advanced ischemia. Large sensory nerve fibers are responsible for pressure, deep pain, and temperature sensations that may be maintained until ischemia is advanced. Proprioception and light touch are usually lost early. Careful sensory examination may help the clinician estimate the severity of ischemia. Palpation of the muscle groups may denote tenderness initially, but, as the ischemia progresses, the muscles may become hard (rigor), a sign of skeletal muscle death. Even with prompt revascularization, functional impairment is likely, limb loss often occurs, and systemic effects of revascularization are a major risk. Revascularization at this late stage is likely to fail, with systemic manifestations of such an undertaking profound and sometimes lethal. This has led some authors to suggest that ischemia of this severity and duration is best treated with systemic anticoagulation, allowing for demarcation of the extremity, and early amputation.[59]

Physical examination of the patient with an acutely ischemic extremity is of utmost importance in planning appropriate management. Examination of the contralateral extremity may provide clues as to the preischemic status of the involved extremity. The exact location of the embolus or thrombosis may be determined by the level of clinical manifestations of the ischemic process. Pain and temperature changes are usually seen one joint below the level of obstruction. Tenderness over an arterial segment usually implies the presence of thrombus within its lumen. A pale, waxy extremity implies early ischemia. Mottling of the skin that blanches with elevation or digital pressure implies a retrievable capillary bed with prompt revascularization. Nonblanching represents advanced ischemia. Retrievability may require prompt revascularization and adjunctive measures, such as fibrinolytic therapy. Paralysis may occur early. If the muscle mass is hard, with marked resistance to passive motion (rigor), ischemia is far advanced. Appropriate planning for therapy may be guided by these findings.

Vascular Graft Occlusion

The clinical manifestations of vascular graft occlusion also vary widely and deserve special emphasis. The indication of the original intervention will influence the presentation, with patients operated upon for disabling claudication usually manifesting recurrent symptoms, and patients operated upon for limb salvage presenting with limb-threatening ischemia. In the former group, however, when late occlusions occur, the patient may present with limb-threatening ischemia. The cause of failure will influence clinical presentation. When we analyzed the pattern and causes of primary failure of PTFE grafts in a series of patients operated on for claudication, when failure was due to progression of proximal or distal disease, most commonly patients presented with limb-threatening ischemia.[57] Of 14 patients initially operated on for severe claudication whose graft failed because of progression of distal occlusive disease, 12 manifested severe limb-threatening ischemia after failure of the reconstruction. Similarly, 50 per cent of patients operated on for claudication whose graft failed due to progression of disease in the inflow arterial segment manifested limb-threatening ischemia, whereas the rest manifested recurrent claudication. Thus, whereas most patients operated upon for limb salvage will manifest limb-threatening ischemia upon failure of the reconstruction, patients with claudication will manifest recurrent claudication unless there is significant progression of disease in the inflow or outflow segments.

When the cause of failure is graft related, which most commonly occurs in autogenous grafts, clinical manifestations are usually similar to the original presentation and indication for the reconstruction. This is particularly the case within the first 12 to 18 months after reconstruction. Beyond that time, other factors, mainly progression of disease, will influence the clinical presentation of the failed vascular graft.

A small number of patients whose initial indication for reconstruction is limb-threatening ischemia (specifically, those with tissue loss) may present after healing of their affected areas with failure of the reconstruction and perhaps symptoms of claudication without clinical symptoms of severe ischemia. This is evident in most series of infrainguinal reconstructions where limb salvage figures are almost universally higher than primary patency rates. Most of these patients do not require intervention, as their symptoms may be managed conservatively with control of risk factors and exercise.

More recently, the concept of the failing vascular graft has been emphasized with several series documenting improved results when intervention is directed at the time when the graft still is patent. Clinical manifestations of failing grafts include diminished pulses, recurrent symptoms of claudication, or failure of areas of tissue loss in the foot to heal completely after an initial period of rapid healing. Most commonly, however, failing grafts may have no clinical manifestations, and therefore it behooves the physician caring for the patient to identify these by noninvasive means. Serial ankle-arm indices have not been found sensitive enough to predictably detect the failing graft.[60] The most important mode of identification is with duplex scanning by uncinating the entire graft, identifying areas of stenosis that will lead to increased velocities in that segment. In addition, average velocity throughout the graft may decrease over time, again suggesting that the graft may be failing. Although cutoff points for velocities have been proposed, to date, these have not been sensitive enough to be completely reliable. Whereas most grafts with velocities higher than 45 cm/sec will continue to demonstrate long-term patency, grafts below this cutoff point will not necessarily fail nor will a demonstrable lesion be present on arteriography. Additional duplex scan criteria to detect failing grafts has been proposed and includes diameter reduction, and peak and end-systolic velocities.[61–63] This is specifically evident in very distal reconstructions at the ankle, where the outflow bed may not allow for velocities in this range throughout the graft. Nevertheless, experience has shown excellent long-term results without the need for further interventions. Perhaps a more sensitive way to follow these grafts is to obtain velocity measurements early in the postoperative period using these values as baseline for that particular reconstruction. On follow-up, decreasing velocities would suggest further evaluation with arteriography. Identification of the failing graft is perhaps the most important factor in assuring excellent long-term results in patients with infrainguinal reconstructions.

MANAGEMENT

Initial Evaluation

Acute Arterial Occlusion

The morbidity and mortality of an acute arterial occlusion will largely depend on the overall medical condition of the patient, degree of ischemia of the extremity at presentation, and promptness in management. It is critical that all three of these aspects be carefully evaluated and documented. In general, prompt revascularization should be the goal after stabilization and control of coexistent medical conditions in patients presenting with an acute, ischemic extremity. Few patients with far-advanced ischemia, however, are best treated medically (see later), an option more likely to result in loss of the limb.

The majority of patients presenting with acute arterial occlusion of an extremity will have atherosclerotic heart disease, which must be addressed prior

to any intervention. An acute myocardial infarction must be excluded by appropriate clinical and laboratory evaluation. Although its presence does not preclude surgical intervention, it mandates appropriate maneuvers, such as placement of Swan-Ganz catheters and/or arterial lines, to minimize morbidity and mortality associated with surgical intervention. Stabilization of hemodynamics is of primary importance including correction of arrhythmias, replenishment of circulating volume, and establishment of an adequate urine output.

The history prior to the event will give the clinician clues as to the status of the extremity prior to the acute arterial occlusion. Patients without history of claudication or previous vascular reconstructions are more likely victims of embolization. Patients with history of peripheral vascular disease, claudication, or previous vascular reconstructions are more likely affected by an arterial thrombosis. The importance of attempting to differentiate between these two processes is evident when one considers their management. Whereas patients with embolization are appropriately managed by thromboembolectomy, patients with preexisting vascular disease usually require a much more involved vascular reconstruction. Careful preoperative planning may make the difference in their outcome. Therefore, a patient with an identifiable source for an embolus, without claudication, and with a normal contralateral extremity is a classic presentation for an embolus. Patients without an identifiable source of emboli, with history of claudication, and with physical findings specifically in the opposite limb suggestive of the presence of peripheral vascular disease, are more likely suffering from an arterial thrombosis. History of a previous embolic event will be seen in up to one third of patients presenting with an embolus, and history of atrial fibrillation in up to 74 per cent of these patients. In contrast, patients with an acute thrombotic occlusion will have atrial fibrillation by history in only 4 per cent of instances.[64] Symptoms tend to be much more acute in patients with an embolic occlusion, with a fairly well-established area of demarcation. Patients with a thrombotic occlusion are likely to present with less severe symptoms and a larger area of transition.

Heparinization of patients presenting with an acutely ischemic extremity is well established. In general, at least 10,000 units of intravenous heparin are recommended to establish immediate and complete anticoagulation. The goals of immediate anticoagulation are prevention of proximal and distal thrombus propagation, prevention of distal thrombosis, and prevention of venous thrombosis. In general, patients will experience an almost immediate improvement in their symptoms, likely secondary to the nonanticoagulant effects of heparin. Clearly, patients with a history of heparin-induced thrombosis should be excluded from this recommendation. Patients with associated traumatic injuries or other systemic diseases that may present an unacceptable bleeding risk, who are not candidates for systemic heparinization, may receive local instillation of a dilute heparin solution in the vascular bed during operative therapy.

Once the patient has been stabilized and adequate anticoagulation accomplished, a decision regarding preoperative arteriography should be made. The desirability of arteriography is increased in patients with preexisting vascular disease or reconstruction. Arteriography should be avoided, however, if it is going to significantly delay revascularization. Alternatively, operative arteriograms can be obtained at the time of intervention. Nevertheless, if the patient can tolerate the ischemia, preoperative arteriography may be extremely helpful in elucidating the etiology and planning the proper surgical approach. A patient whose history and physical examination is suggestive of an embolus may be properly handled without arteriography. If arteriography is undertaken, typically the outflow vascular bed is not well visualized and the increased time necessary for this study prolongs the ischemia without adding useful information. When the differentiation between embolic and thrombotic event cannot be made, or in cases in which the etiology is uncertain, arteriography is appropriate. A sharp cutoff with a crescent-shaped (meniscus sign) occlusion in an otherwise normal artery is suggestive of an embolus. Multiple filling defects are also suggestive of an embolic occlusion. The location of the occlusion may also be helpful, with emboli tending to lodge in areas of bifurcations (Fig. 36–3). Clot propagation, following either an embolic or thrombotic event, may make this distinction difficult.

Doppler examination of the extremity can be most helpful in determining patency of the distal outflow tract. In patients with an embolic occlusion, its presence is reassuring, because it implies an open distal tree and, therefore, a retrievable situation. In a patient with preexisting vascular disease, Doppler examination may help identify the most suitable distal bed for bypass reconstruction. Doppler examination of the venous system may disclose an otherwise unsuspected venous thrombosis.

Patients with concomitant injuries, such as fractures or dislocations, should have prompt restitution of blood volume and restoration of adequate blood pressure. Stabilization of the extremity is essential in preventing further injury and, on occasion, restoring distal circulation. Life-threatening injuries should take precedence over limb-threatening injuries. The use of temporary arterial shunts in these circumstances may help in preservation of the limb.

Vascular Graft Occlusion

Initial evaluation of a patient presenting with vascular graft occlusion will be influenced by the clinical presentation. Patients presenting with recurrent claudication may be evaluated electively. Anticoagulation is not indicated in these patients. Intervention is indicated only in those patients whose claudication is disabling. Patients presenting with limb-threatening ischemia, on the other hand, are best evaluated on

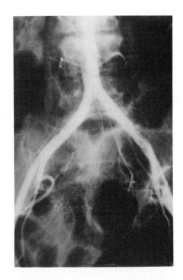

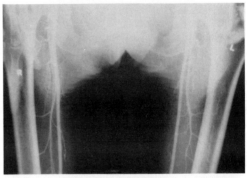

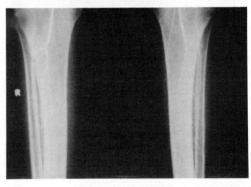

FIGURE 36–3. Arteriogram of 67-year-old female presenting with acute left lower extremity ischemia. *Top,* Left iliac filling defect at the level of the bifurcation typical of an embolus. Some fragmentation has occurred, with filling defects also involving the distal external iliac and proximal common femoral. The patient had flow around this embolus to produce a normal femoral pulse. *Middle,* Open superficial femoral and profunda system without evidence of significant atherosclerotic disease. *Bottom,* Evidence of distal fragmentation of the embolus with occlusion of the posterior tibial and peroneal arteries. Successful embolectomy was carried out through a combined transfemoral and infrapopliteal approach.

an urgent basis, considering that some of the nonoperative means of management (including thrombolytic therapy) may be most effective within a short time after thrombosis. In most instances, the initial management is similar to patients presenting with acute ischemia secondary to native vessel occlusion.

Patients presenting with indications for intervention (disabling claudication or limb-threatening ischemia) due to failure of a previous vascular reconstruction are best evaluated with thorough arteriography. This study should include both inflow and outflow systems, with an attempt to establish the cause of failure. Herein lies one of the main advantages of thrombolytic therapy in the initial management of the failed infrainguinal reconstruction. Although both early and long-term results remain unclear when compared to surgical intervention, thrombolytic therapy in most instances will identify the cause of failure, allowing directed intervention.

Examination of the patient should include not only the presence or absence and quality of pulses in the involved extremity, but also alternative inflow sites that may be necessary and, most importantly, availability of autogenous tissue for secondary reconstruction. Experience within the last 10 years suggests that patients requiring secondary bypasses after failure of an infrainguinal reconstruction are best managed with a new autogenous reconstruction. In addition to physical examination, duplex scanning of the remaining venous segments may be of benefit, if properly performed. This examination should be performed either with application of a proximal tourniquet to distend the vein, or with the patient semierect. Failure to do so will usually result in an underestimate of the size and quality of available veins.

Surgical Management

In a review of 682 cases at the Massachusetts General Hospital, a trend toward increasing use of surgical management in patients with acute extremity ischemia was noted.[31] With the introduction of the Fogarty catheter in 1963, surgical intervention in patients with peripheral emboli has been greatly simplified. Nevertheless, the systemic effects of this very effective intervention must be appropriately managed to minimize mortality. In addition, the principles of embolectomy must be adhered to, avoiding common pitfalls that may lead to failure.

The surgical approach will be greatly influenced by the results of the initial evaluation. Decisions regarding patients with significant peripheral vascular disease suspected of having a thrombotic occlusion will be guided by the results of arteriography. In any event, wide prepping and draping is highly recommended to avoid unnecessary delays if a change in operative plan is required. The choice of anesthetics will be influenced by the general condition of the patient and the planned operative procedure. By and large, femoral and brachial embolectomies can be adequately performed under local anesthesia with careful cardiac monitoring. Similarly, patients requiring femorofemoral reconstruction for a thrombotic iliac occlusion may be operated on under local anesthesia with the understanding that if a more involved procedure is required, general anesthesia may be necessary. A general anesthetic is recommended for more difficult embolectomies, such as popliteal or axillary, and in instances in which involved vascular procedures such as endarterectomy or bypass are required. Patients operated upon because of a failed bypass graft frequently will require a relatively involved procedure, and thus general anesthesia is preferred. If a simple thrombectomy is anticipated, local anesthesia is appropriate, provided it can be converted to general anesthesia if the need arises. Because of the general medical condition of these patients and the expected effects of reperfusion, adequate monitoring with arterial lines and Swan-Ganz catheters is recommended. These adjunctive maneuvers, however, should not delay revascularization. Regional anesthesia is usually not feasible, because these patients are most likely fully anticoagulated by the time they reach the operating room.

Embolectomy

Prior to 1963, an embolus to an arterial segment was usually retrieved by direct exposure, by passage of suction catheters, or with the use of rigid instruments that were very traumatic and ineffective.[65-67] With the introduction of the Fogarty catheter, the surgical technique was markedly simplified, allowing exposure remote to the level of occlusion with retrieval of the embolus by the use of the balloon catheter.

Femoral embolectomy is perhaps the most common operation done for lower extremity emboli. A vertical groin incision is made over the femoral pulse and exposure of the artery is carried out in standard fashion (Fig. 36–4). Control of the common, profunda, and superficial femoral arteries is obtained. The arteriotomy should allow visualization of the profunda and superficial femoral artery orifices. If the artery is normal to palpation, a transverse arteriotomy may be made over the profunda orifice. In diseased arteries, however, a longitudinal arteriotomy is preferable, because it allows better manipulation of the catheter and, if necessary, endarterectomy or bypass. Otherwise, closure with a patch is frequently necessary to avoid narrowing of the artery (its only disadvantage). The size of the Fogarty catheter selected should be appropriate for the artery. For the superficial femoral and popliteal arteries, a no. 4 Fogarty catheter is appropriate. For the iliac system, a no. 4 or 5 Fogarty catheter is best. For more distal insertion and for the profunda system, a no. 3 Fogarty catheter is utilized. Insertion into the profunda should not be beyond 25 cm. The catheter is gently inflated with saline as traction is maintained, avoiding overinflation, without movement of the catheter. This will help determine when appropriate balloon inflation has been obtained, avoiding forceful traction. The catheter is handled by a single operator, because both maneuvers must be coordinated to avoid arterial injury. Inability to pass the catheter beyond the point of obstruction is usually the result of occlusive disease, rather than embolus. Nevertheless, well-organized embolic material may prevent passage

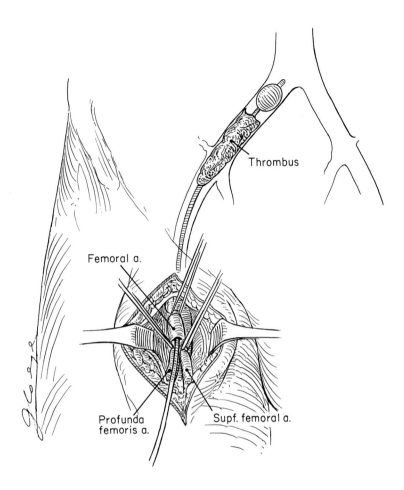

FIGURE 36–4. Illustration of the operative technique for femoral embolectomy. Note control of common, superficial, and profunda femoral arteries with slings, which allow passage of the Fogarty catheter without undue blood loss from backbleeding. The arteriotomy is placed over the profunda orifice. A transverse arteriotomy is preferred, if the artery is normal and without evidence of significant atherosclerotic disease. Proximal passage of the Fogarty catheter should not be beyond the midinfrarenal aorta, to avoid inadvertent cannulation of visceral vessels, overdistention of the balloon, and potential vessel injury.

of the catheter, requiring more distal or direct exploration. From the femoral approach, almost 90 per cent of distal insertions will pass the catheter into the peroneal artery.[68] Several maneuvers may be helpful in orienting the catheter toward either the anterior tibial or posterior tibial artery. Bending the tip of the catheter to the appropriate side with rotation during insertion may allow cannulation of the desired artery. Use of fluoroscopy may be helpful, especially if a second small catheter is placed in the peroneal artery with the balloon gently inflated to promote passage of the catheter to the remaining vessels. More recently, endoscopy has been useful in direct visualization and cannulation of the tibial arteries. Palpation of the posterior tibial artery at the ankle or the dorsalis pedis artery in the foot during retrieval of a distally placed catheter may help identify which vessel is being maneuvered.

The establishment of adequate inflow is usually not difficult to assess. Completeness of the distal embolectomy, however, can prove difficult to determine, because there are no reliable clinical guidelines. The presence or adequacy of back-bleeding following embolectomy is an unreliable parameter of the completeness of the distal embolectomy. Operative arteriography is mandatory, unless the patient's critical condition dictates otherwise. In fact, when operative arteriograms are reviewed after embolectomy, up to

30 per cent of cases will show residual thrombi.[69] In these instances, repassage of the embolectomy catheter, more distal exploration, or infusion of intraoperative fibrinolytic agents may help in resolution of these distal thrombi.[70-77] Evaluation of the distal circulation by Doppler ultrasound can be extremely helpful, especially in instances in which complete retrieval of all occlusive material cannot be accomplished.

Popliteal embolectomy is best carried out through an infrageniculate incision. Although a suprageniculate incision is technically easier, it offers little advantage, because tibial branches are not readily accessible. Figure 36–5 illustrates the preferred approach for transpopliteal embolectomy. The goal is individual cannulation of all three tibial branches, so that distal emboli can be retrieved. It is the author's preference to use this approach when there is radiographic evidence of infrapopliteal embolism, or when there is clinical evidence that the embolus is distal (i.e., palpable popliteal pulse). The popliteal artery is exposed through a standard infrageniculate incision. The origin of the soleus muscle usually requires proximal division to expose the tibial-peroneal trunk. The anterior tibial artery is exposed after careful ligation of the anterior tibial vein to allow encircling the origin of the anterior tibial with vessel loops for control. Dissection beyond the tibial-peroneal trunk is rarely necessary, because digital compression of

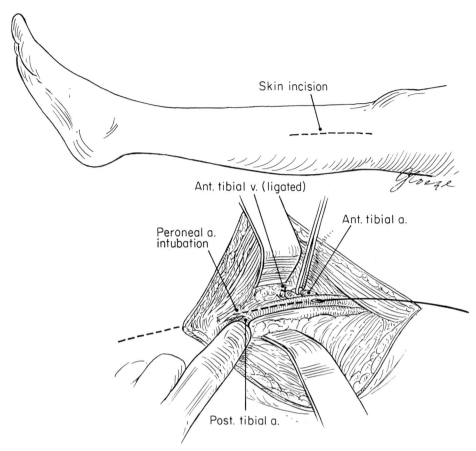

Skin incision

Ant. tibial v. (ligated)

Ant. tibial a.

Peroneal a.
intubation

Post. tibial a.

FIGURE 36–5. Illustration of operative technique for popliteal embolectomy. An infrageniculate incision is preferred, because it will allow individual cannulation of the anterior tibial, posterior tibial, and peroneal arteries. The arteriotomy is performed over the orifice of the anterior tibial artery, with selective passage into the peroneal or posterior tibial artery facilitated by digital compression of one while cannulating the other. Care must be taken during ligation of the anterior tibial vein, a critical maneuver in obtaining adequate control of the anterior tibial artery at its origin. Closure usually requires an autogenous patch to avoid narrowing.

each branch will allow selective cannulation of either the posterior tibial or peroneal trunks. A longitudinal arteriotomy is preferred, because it permits better visualization of the origin of the anterior tibial artery and manipulation of the catheter. In addition, if a bypass is required, extension of the arteriotomy can be performed for distal anastomosis. Otherwise, patch closure is preferred.

Evidence of persistent ischemia after popliteal embolectomy, or the presence of residual thrombus inaccessible to the thromboembolectomy catheter from this approach, are indications for more distal exploration or, alternatively, intraoperative fibrinolytic therapy (see Chapter 41). Exploration of the tibial vessels at the ankle and foot may allow retrieval of thrombi not accessible through the transpopliteal approach.[77] A cutdown is performed over the appropriate distal vessel (posterior tibial and/or dorsalis pedis) and proximal and distal control is obtained with vessel loops. If the artery has no evidence of calcification or atherosclerosis, a transverse arteriotomy is preferable, because it allows easier closure with interrupted, fine monofilament vascular su-

tures. If the vessel is diseased, a longitudinal arteriotomy is preferred, with either patch closure or distal bypass.

Upper extremity emboli are usually approached through a cutdown in the brachial artery, just above the elbow. A transverse arteriotomy is usually preferred, because this vessel is rarely involved with significant atherosclerotic changes. A no. 3 Fogarty catheter can be directed into the radial and ulnar artery, recognizing that reestablishing patency to one or the other is usually sufficient. Care should be taken to protect the median nerve, which runs adjacent to the artery. More proximal emboli may be approached through an infraclavicular incision similar to the one used for axillofemoral reconstructions. Preservation of branches of the axillary artery is recommended, because they serve as an important collateral pathway.

Intraoperative assessment of the adequacy of the embolectomy cannot be overemphasized. Doppler examination of the distal part of the extremity is useful, but unreliable in terms of the completeness of the procedure. Intraoperative arteriography remains the best method to assure complete removal of all embolic material. It is the author's preference to drape the distal extremity with a transparent sterile bag so that clinical assessment of skin perfusion can be readily made. Instillation of fluid into the bag and sterile petroleum jelly on the outside of the bag allow for Doppler examination of the various sites. The rest of the draping should reflect appropriate planning for the approach. Alternative inflow and outflow sites should be included in the operative field so that delays in revascularization are minimized.

Spasm of the runoff arteries, specifically tibial vessels in younger individuals and/or upper extremity vessels at all ages, is frequent following embolectomy. Intraarterial administration of papaverine or other vasodilators is recommended, although not infrequently it results in little resolution of this spastic process. This may be secondary to unrecognized residual thrombus with release of platelet vasoactive substances, specifically thromboxane. Intravenous administration of prostaglandin E_1 may be helpful, although it is of unproven value. Repeated mechanical dilatations are to be avoided, because the spasm not only quickly returns but it may lead to further intimal injury. If the presence of residual occlusive material can be excluded by adequate arteriography, it is preferable to maintain the patient fully anticoagulated with administration of a mixture of dextran (40 mg) and papaverine (300 mg in 500 ml at 50 ml/hr) to maintain patency of the circulation while the spasm spontaneously resolves. This may prove most difficult in the upper extremities in younger individuals, where very reactive distal vessels are present. Provided that no residual occlusive material is present and that flow through the vessel can be maintained with appropriate antithrombotic regimens, resolution usually occurs within the first 12 hours.

A large embolus to the aortic bifurcation (saddle embolus) can produce severe ischemia and major systemic changes upon revascularization. The transfemoral approach is still preferable, with bilateral groin incisions and simultaneous passage of no. 5 or 6 Fogarty catheters to avoid spillage of material to the contralateral side. Concomitant atherosclerotic disease may prevent reestablishment of flow to one or both sides. If adequate inflow is established to one side, a femorofemoral reconstruction may suffice to preserve both limbs. Transperitoneal exploration is indicated when there is failure to establish inflow on at least one side, or suspicion of visceral embolization. It is important to maintain adequate intravascular volume, because blood loss from flushing is considerable and the systemic effects of reperfusion are amplified because of bilateral lower extremity involvement.

It is critical for the surgeon involved in revascularization of acutely ischemic limbs to be familiar with the systemic effects of such intervention. Initiation of management of systemic effects of revascularization should be carried out in the operating room and maintained throughout the initial postoperative period. These effects are discussed in detail later in this chapter.

Bypass Graft Thrombectomy

The principles of Fogarty catheter embolectomy are applicable to thrombectomy of bypass grafts. The technique is similar, with care taken specifically in autogenous reconstructions not to overinflate the balloon, which will likely lead to intimal disruption and occasionally tears in a fibrotic segment of the vein graft. In this regard, vein graft thrombectomy is much more demanding than prosthetic graft thrombectomy.

Surgical thrombectomy of a prosthetic graft is a relatively simple and straightforward procedure. Proper planning, however, will eliminate unnecessary delay and incisions. It is our practice to approach a failed infrainguinal prosthetic bypass at its distal anastomosis. This allows evaluation of the outflow system and identification and correction of the most common site for intimal hyperplasia. Unless a lesion away from this area has been demonstrated by preoperative evaluation, distal exploration is preferred. If a lesion limited to the first one or two centimeters of the distal anastomosis is identified, patch angioplasty to include the distal portion of the graft is a very reasonable alternative. If, on the other hand, the problem is distal to this site, extensions with prosthetic or autogenous graft material have had limited long-term results, with patency of 30 to 40 per cent at 3 years.[57] In this instance, we prefer to construct an entirely new graft, preferably with autogenous tissue.

Graft thrombectomy of autogenous vein grafts is usually best for early failures, or in patients where a hypercoagulable condition may have led to failure of the bypass. Late failures, however, are usually complicated not only by progression of the disease proximal and distal to the reconstruction, but also by a fibrotic thickened graft, which is difficult to repair after graftotomy. In addition, the compliance of the graft is such that balloon embolectomy usually leads to significant intimal injury. Long-term results of saphenous vein graft thrombectomies have been notoriously poor.

Bypass Graft Revision or Replacement

Perhaps the most important element in assuring a successful secondary reconstruction after failure of an infrainguinal bypass is identification of the cause of failure. This may allow directed intervention. Such is the case with the identification of a stenotic lesion in the midportion of a vein graft. When the lesions are short (less than 5 cm), they may be appropriately treated with balloon angioplasty. The 24-month patency rate for lesions less than 1.5 cm in vein grafts greater than 3 mm in diameter has been excellent, with a significant lower patency demonstrated in longer lesions in smaller grafts.[78] Recurrent stenosis, on the other hand, or lesions that are not suitable for balloon angioplasty, are best treated either with surgical vein patch angioplasty or interposition graft replacement, as the situation may dictate. If the graft is placed deep in the thigh or leg, revision will require a more extensive operative dissection. With most grafts in the subcutaneous tissue, however, surgical intervention can be both simple and effective.

Similarly, identification of residual AV fistulas may be treated with a simple incision and ligation. This may be done under local anesthesia on an outpatient basis. Presence of an incompletely lysed valve usually will require patch angioplasty with autogenous tissue. Lesions at the proximal or distal anastomosis of an otherwise good vein graft can also be treated with patch angioplasty quite effectively. As already mentioned, this is best done while the graft has maintained patency. Otherwise, when graft thrombectomy is necessary to the angioplasty, the results are significantly affected.

The surgical management of a failed infrainguinal prosthetic graft will also depend on the cause of failure. Patch angioplasty may be appropriate for lesions that are limited to the first 1 to 2 cm at the proximal or distal anastomosis. It has been our practice to transect the stenotic lesion and not to attempt an endarterectomy of the area, unless one is dealing with a late failure where atherosclerotic changes are present. A patch is then placed across the lesion to allow relief of the stenosis. Other alternatives include a new prosthetic bypass to a more distal site, extension of the failed bypass with prosthetic or vein graft, or a new vein graft to a more distal site. The technical aspects of these reconstructions are covered elsewhere. But suffice it to say that the results of a new bypass with autogenous saphenous vein are superior to any of the other alternatives.[57]

Fasciotomy

One of the most common manifestations of reperfusion injury after prolonged ischemia is marked swelling of skeletal muscle. Because these muscles are enveloped in fascial compartments, increased pressure within the compartment can cause poor capillary perfusion, increased venous resistance, and a vicious cycle leading to further ischemia. Normal tissue pressure within the compartment is approximately zero. As pressure within the compartment rises, tissue perfusion declines progressively and at a level of about 20 mm Hg becomes impaired. When the pressure is within 30 mm Hg of the diastolic blood pressure, flow is significantly decreased unless adequate decompression can be carried out.[79]

The decision to proceed with fasciotomy is usually based on clinical findings. Palpation of the specific compartment may reveal a very tense muscle group with tenderness. Pain on passive motion implies significant increase in tissue pressure. Numbness in the distribution of the nerves within the compartment implies nerve ischemia. The presence of these findings indicates the need for fasciotomy. Compartment pressure may be measured by use of a slit catheter,

with commercial kits available that can be connected to pressure transducers.

Fasciotomy may be achieved in a semiclosed manner when the indication is the anticipation of increased compartmental pressures following revascularization. This is performed through a small incision in the proximal portion of the compartment, incising the fascia using either long scissors or a menisectomy knife. For a fully established compartment syndrome, this method will likely result in inadequate decompression, mainly because of difficulty in assessing the completeness of the fasciotomy. In addition, the skin may become the limiting factor, with continued elevated compartmental pressure until complete skin incision is performed. Thus, semiclosed fasciotomies should be reserved for very mild cases, or as a prophylactic maneuver. Selection mainly relies on the experience of the operator.

Open fasciotomy can be limb saving following revascularization after prolonged ischemia when muscle swelling rapidly develops. Figure 36–6 illustrates one method of achieving decompression of all four compartments through a single incision. A longitudinal incision is made over the fibula and anterior and posterior flaps are developed. The fascia is incised to allow identification of the four specific compartments and placement of the fasciotomy incisions. The disadvantage of this approach is the creation of fairly extensive skin flaps in potentially compromised skin. In the anterior compartment, care must be taken not to injure the superficial branch of the peroneal nerve. Alternatively, medial and lateral incisions may be made that avoid the creation of skin flaps (Fig. 36–7), while achieving complete decompression. A third approach involves complete fibulectomy. Although the latter achieves complete four-compartment decompression, it is fairly morbid, with injury to the peroneal artery, vein, and nerve being common complications. It also may interrupt important collateral circulation. The medial and lateral incision technique is preferred by the author.

Most recently, foot fasciotomy has been advocated in patients with persistent foot ischemia after more proximal fasciotomy and revascularization.[80] Although it may improve foot salvage in selected cases, it is rarely necessary.

Complications after fasciotomy are usually related to wound infection. In the semiclosed method, bleeding may be a problem, mainly because these patients are thoroughly anticoagulated. Nerve injury, specifically of the superficial branch of the peroneal nerve, is a risk with this method. Maintaining the incision in the fascia, close to the tibia, will minimize the risk of peroneal nerve injury.

Postoperative management of open fasciotomy incisions is critical to reduce morbidity. Sterile techniques should be used for dressing changes until adequate granulation tissue has developed. As the swelling decreases, the use of Steri-Strips for pro-

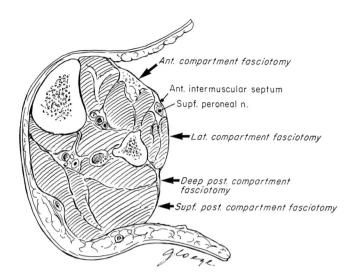

FIGURE 36-6. Technique of four-compartment fasciotomy using a single lateral incision. Creation of anterior and posterior flaps is necessary, which may be undesirable after revascularization for acute ischemia. Care must be taken to avoid injury to the superficial peroneal nerve, which runs just anterior to the fibula.

gressive closure of the incision will usually result in almost complete closure in most cases. Skin grafting may be necessary if this cannot be accomplished. Blistering of the skin secondary to the Steri-Strip application can be minimized by alternating site of placement.

Controversy exists as to the need for or role of fasciotomy following limb revascularization. Some authors have suggested that a significant tradeoff occurs between its usefulness and the increased risk of infection following fasciotomy.[81] The argument has been made that swelling occurring after revascularization is indicative of cell death, and thus little is gained by decompression. The majority of the reported experience, however, would support fasciotomy in selected patients. In the author's experience, timely fasciotomy can be limb saving.

Delayed Embolectomy

A small but significant group of patients may experience mild to moderate symptoms following an acute arterial embolus, with gradual improvement over the subsequent weeks. This is followed by either symptoms of claudication or, more importantly, progressive ischemia because of clot propagation. Delayed arterial embolectomy can be safely performed in these cases.[82,83] Usually the procedure can be planned electively, with appropriate arteriographic evaluation. Embolectomy will be guided by arteriographic and clinical findings.

The technique is similar to acute embolectomy, recognizing that direct exposure of the occluded segment is necessary. Passage of the catheter from a remote exposure may be difficult, because the material is organized and rubbery. The surgeon must be familiar with the appearance of a thrombosed arterial segment and carefully develop a plane between the thrombus and the intima. Failure to do so may result in significant intimal injury and early rethrombosis. Heparinization in the immediate postoperative period is indicated, with chronic anticoagulation based on the clinical risk factors leading to the embolism. The thrombogenicity of the chronically embolectomized segment would dictate an aggressive use of anticoagulants. Long-term results are variable, with some patients experiencing early reocclusion due to throm-

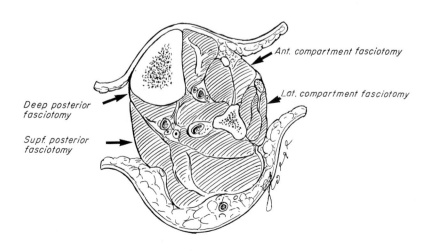

FIGURE 36-7. Preferred technique for four-compartment fasciotomy of the lower extremity using a medial and lateral incision. Note that the lateral incision is placed along the fibula to allow fasciotomy of the anterior and lateral compartments. The superficial and deep posterior compartment decompression may be facilitated by an initial transverse incision in the fascia to properly identify the compartments. Care must be taken during anterior compartment fasciotomy to avoid injury to the superficial peroneal nerve.

bosis and/or marked intimal hyperplasia. The latter may be secondary to intimal injury from the procedure or the presence of the chronic thrombus.

Nonoperative Management

Because of the high mortality noted with revascularization of acutely ischemic limbs in most surgical series, some authors have advocated routine high-dose heparinization in patients presenting with an acutely ischemic limb. The rationale is to select out those patients with nonviable extremities, proceeding with elective planned revascularizations in those who maintain viability of the extremity after this initial treatment. Using this approach, Blaisdel et al. found a decrease in mortality to 7.5 per cent with limb salvage of 67 per cent, in 59 patients.[84] Very high doses of heparin were used, with an initial bolus of 20,000 units followed by 2000 to 4000 units/hr. This report has been criticized, since these results were compared to historical controls.

Controversy exists as to the appropriateness of nonoperative treatment in severely ischemic extremities. Clearly, extremities that are nonviable at the time of presentation are best treated nonoperatively. This approach is aimed at reduction in mortality. More recent series have documented an improvement in limb salvage, without an increase in operative mortality, with modern techniques of revascularization. Thus, it is appropriate to consider surgical intervention in most patients. With adequate medical support, this will result in both limb and life preservation.

Thrombolytic Therapy

An attractive alternative in patients presenting with acute limb ischemia is the use of thrombolytic therapy. This modality, however, should be reserved for patients with clearly viable extremities and should be performed in centers that are familiar with the use and complications of thrombolytic agents. In patients with prior multiple vascular reconstructions, thrombolytic therapy may facilitate recognition of the causative lesion, with either percutaneous or surgical correction done in a timely fashion. When ischemia is severe, however, thrombolytic therapy, especially when carried out by inexperienced clinicians, may delay revascularization and increase tissue loss.

In a recent series reported by McNamara et al., 53 patients with acute severe ischemia were treated with thrombolytic therapy with a respectable reduction in mortality compared to historical controls, and no significant increase in limb loss compared to surgical series.[85] It is important to recognize that the time needed for complete resolution of these thrombotic events was significantly shortened by use of high-dose urokinase. This modality, when used by experts, may achieve timely revascularization. Interestingly, reperfusion occurs gradually, which may prove to be of additional benefit. Nevertheless, the routine use of thrombolytic therapy for severely ischemic limbs cannot be supported and should be individualized. Surgical intervention remains the main form of therapy in patients with acutely ischemic limbs. Fibrinolytic therapy may serve as an important adjunct in specific circumstances. In patients with failed infrainguinal grafts, initial therapy with thrombolytic agents will usually identify the cause of failure, thus simplifying management.

Percutaneous Thromboembolectomy

A catheter-guided system has been developed specifically for the aspiration of thrombotic material from the pulmonary vasculature.[86] Initially used for the treatment of iatrogenic emboli secondary to balloon angioplasty, this technique has now been reported in primary embolism, with a carefully selected group of patients achieving limb salvage in 40 of 42 instances. At this point, however, this procedure should be considered experimental and should be performed only by those experienced in its development.

COMPLICATIONS

Complications seen after revascularization of an acutely ischemic extremity can be divided into those related to the surgical intervention, those secondary to limb reperfusion, and those secondary to the primary cause of the event. Discussion of the latter is beyond the scope of this chapter, because it relates to management of the primary disease, such as cardiac or peripheral vascular disease. Suffice it to say that patients with emboli originating from the heart or sources that are not surgically correctable will require long-term anticoagulation to prevent further events. This particular aspect is discussed further.

Recurrent Embolization

The reported incidence of recurrent emboli following an embolic event to an extremity or viscera ranges between 6 and 45 per cent. Prevention of recurrent emboli is of utmost importance in the management of these patients. Chronic long-term anticoagulation is indicated in patients following an embolic event when the source of emboli cannot be surgically corrected. Anticoagulation should be started immediately following operation. In a series by Green et al., only 9 per cent of patients developed recurrent emboli when adequately anticoagulated, in contrast to 31 per cent of those not receiving anticoagulants.[66] This difference has been noted by others.[33,37,87-89] Recurrent embolization carries significantly higher morbidity and mortality than the initial event. The random distribution of emboli from the heart places these patients at risk of stroke or visceral embolization, a major cause of morbidity and mortality. Thus, chronic anticoagulation is of utmost importance in their long-term management.

Rethrombosis

Following successful revascularization, recurrent limb ischemia may occur secondary to a second embolus or rethrombosis of the manipulated arterial segment. The latter is more common, because recurrent emboli to the same site are unlikely, especially when the source is the heart. Rethrombosis may occur secondary to (1) residual thrombus in the extremity not recognized at the time of the initial intervention, (2) proximal thrombus that may have been left behind, or (3) inadequate anticoagulation.

When recurrent ischemia occurs, prompt reoperation is indicated unless the patient's general condition dictates otherwise. The secondary procedure may be planned according to the clinical manifestations of the recurrent event. Reexploration of the initial operative site is indicated, with liberal use of operative arteriography and/or endoscopy. Reoperation may be necessary in up to 21 per cent of patients following balloon embolectomy and is usually successful in assuring limb salvage.[90] In patients with a previously failed vascular graft, rethrombosis of the thrombectomized or revised graft usually mandates consideration for placement of a new bypass graft, preferably with autogenous tissue. The liberal use of anticoagulants (including heparin, dextran, and Coumadin) in the postoperative period may benefit patients who experience this complications.

Arterial Injuries Secondary to the Balloon Catheter

Although the surgical technique for arterial embolectomy is familiar to vascular surgeons, complications of such intervention are perhaps more common than actually recognized.[91,92] Manifestations may be delayed and present as distal arterial occlusions secondary to intimal hyperplasia incited by aggressive embolectomy. Perforation is uncommon and usually self-limited, if it occurs in a small branch of the artery. Because these patients are usually fully anticoagulated, however, they may manifest as having compartment syndromes secondary to an expanding hematoma. Alternatively, the injury may present at a later date as a pseudoaneurysm. Perforation into an adjacent vein can occur, as illustrated in Figure 36–8. Clinical presentation can be subtle, with a decrease in palpable distal pulses and/or mild ischemic symptoms. Diagnosis may be established by the astute clinician with auscultation of a bruit over the fistula site. Treatment may involve direct repair, with percutaneous embolization successful in some instances.

Myonephropathic Metabolic Syndrome

One of the most dramatic and often lethal complications of revascularization of an acute severely

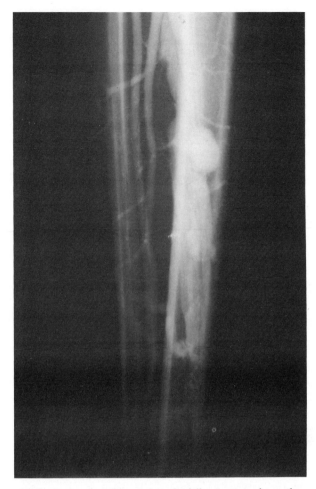

FIGURE 36–8.   Arteriogram 6 weeks following transfemoral embolectomy showing posterior tibial artery and vein AV fistula. Patient developed persistent swelling in the extremity with decreasing distal arterial perfusion. Careful auscultation of the calf suggested the presence of the AV fistula. The fistula was treated successfully by percutaneous embolization.

ischemic extremity is a series of systemic processes that have been termed the "myonephropathic metabolic syndrome."[93] This is the end result of the outpouring of metabolites and cellular debris into the venous circulation following revascularization. Its severity will depend on the amount of tissue involved, the degree of ischemia at revascularization, and the completeness of revascularization. Patients with clearly nonviable extremities at presentation are best treated with heparinization and early amputation to avoid this devastating syndrome. Table 36–2 summarizes drugs of potential benefit in the management of these patients.

With reestablishment of blood flow to the extremity, there is a general outpouring of acidic blood into the systemic circulation, capable of causing a rapid, progressive metabolic acidosis that may lead to poor cardiac function, further acidosis, arrhythmias, and death. Judicious but aggressive use of sodium bicarbonate just prior to and during the initial minutes of reperfusion is advisable, with frequent evaluation of

TABLE 36–2. DRUGS OF POTENTIAL BENEFIT IN THE MEDICAL MANAGEMENT OF PATIENTS WITH ACUTE LIMB ISCHEMIA

Drug	Indication	Contraindication	Dose	Effect	Remarks
Heparin	Acute limb ischemia	Heparin-induced thrombosis; contraindication to anticoagulation	5000–10,000 units IV constant infusion to maintain PTT[a] 1.5–2.0 × control	Potentiate antithrombin III	
Coumadin	Reduce risk of recurrent emboli	Contraindication to anticoagulation	To maintain PTT at 1.5–2.0 × control	Decrease factors II, VII, IX, and X	
Sodium bicarbonate	Metabolic acidosis	Lactic acidosis; metabolic alkalosis; fluid overload; hypernatremia	Guided by blood pH, ½ body weight × base deficit	Reduce H^+	Do not correct deficit with single dose; monitor pH
Mannitol	Maintenance of urine output Reperfusion	Congestive heart failure; anuria and established renal failure	12.5–25 gm IV	Osmotic diuresis	Hydroxy radical scavenger
Insulin & glucose	Hyperkalemia	Diabetic ketoacidosis; hypoglycemia; hypokalemia	12.5–25 gm glucose, 5–10 units insulin	Intracellular shift	
Prostaglandin E_1	Improve renal perfusion	Severe hypotension; hypoxemia	0.005 µg/kg/min; increase q 15 min to reach 0.15–0.2 µg/kg/min	Vasodilator	Unproven value
Acetazolamide	Prevention of myoglobin precipitation in urine	Hypokalemia; severe, uncorrected acidosis	500 mg IV	Alkalinization of urine; increased K^+ excretion	Not effective if HCO_3^- less than 18

[a]*PTT*, partial thromboplastin time.

pH and arterial blood gases. If areas of the extremity remain ischemic, acidosis may persist, requiring continued monitoring and correction.

Hyperkalemia following revascularization of an acutely ischemic extremity can be dramatic and can lead to arrhythmias and cardiac standstill. Administration of glucose and insulin can be life saving by the reintroduction of potassium into cells. Hyperkalemia may be aggravated by concomitant renal failure. Following this initial phase, the use of ion exchange resins, brisk diuresis, or, in some cases, hemodialysis may be necessary.

Myoglobin leakage into the venous circulation may eventually lead to renal failure by precipitation of the myoglobin in the collecting tubules. This is best prevented by maintaining a brisk diuresis with the use of mannitol, adequate hydration, and general hemodynamic support. Alkalinization of the urine may be achieved by the use of acetazolamide, with increased urinary excretion of potassium a secondary benefit. Myoglobinuria may continue for 24 to 48 hours following revascularization, and thus it is of utmost importance that this aggressive support and maintenance of the urine output be continued until the urine is clear. Acute renal failure may be sudden and progressive, with poor chance of recovery. Most recently, we have been impressed with the use of pros-

taglandin E_1 to improve renal perfusion during this acute phase. Although the experience is anecdotal, the results have been encouraging.

The effects of the venous effluent from the revascularized extremity on the pulmonary circulation can be dramatic and can lead to early respiratory failure.[84] It is prudent to maintain these patients with respiratory support, avoiding early extubation. The chest x-ray may disclose a pattern typical of the adult respiratory distress syndrome, a sign of nonspecific pulmonary injury. The exact cause of this lung injury is not clear. Experiments carried out by Blaisdell suggest a relationship between the venous effluent of the extremity and the lung injury, because experimental animals in which the venous effluent from the revascularized extremity was prevented from reaching the lungs did not show the injury (F. W. Blaisdell, personal communication, 1989). Treatment is supportive, avoiding fluid overload.

RESULTS OF THERAPY

Acute Arterial Occlusion

Since the introduction of the Fogarty catheter for the management of acute extremity ischemia, significant improvements have occurred in the morbidity and mortality of patients with this condition. Initially, improved limb salvage was noted in spite of intervention in previously untreatable ischemic limbs. In the 1960s and early 1970s, limb salvage rates averaged 50 to 60 per cent,[6,94–102] with further improvement noted in the decade of the 1970s, when average limb salvage rates ranged between 70 and 80 per cent.[34,66,87,103,104] Mortality, however, remained high, averaging 20 to 30 per cent during these two decades.

With improved recognition, surgical technique, and medical management, the decade of the 1980s has seen improvement in both morbidity and mortality, with limb salvage rates routinely in the 85 to 95 per cent range and mortality decreased to 10 to 15 per cent.[31–33,88,90,105,106] Clearly, aggressive and early management of recognized complications of reperfusion have had a significant impact on the overall mortality of these patients. It is of utmost importance for the clinician to recognize those patients with nonviable extremities who are best treated with early amputation, leading to improved survival. The majority of patients, however, can be managed properly by timely surgical intervention, which can achieve excellent survival and limb salvage.

The presence of atherosclerotic disease negatively influences the outcome. Mortality and limb salvage are lower in patients with nonatherosclerotic causes of acute limb ischemia, whereas patients with atherosclerotic heart disease or severe peripheral vascular disease are at a higher risk for limb loss and death.[6,93] The overall results are likely influenced by underlying cardiac disease and the severity of the ischemia at the time of presentation. Advancing age in this population is likely to stall further improvement in the overall results.

Vascular Graft Occlusion

The results of treatment following occlusion of an infrainguinal reconstruction vary depending on the specific intervention carried out as secondary revascularization. By and large, the best results are obtained with a new autogenous vein graft to a more distal site. In our own series of PTFE infrainguinal bypass comparing the alternatives for treatment of the failed reconstruction, a new bypass at the first reintervention with vein had an 88 per cent primary patency at 30 months. This compares favorably to interventions involving extension with vein or prosthetic material, a new bypass with prosthetic material, and thrombectomy with or without patch angioplasty with patency rates at 30 months ranging between 30 and 33 per cent. Limb salvage rates vary also with the intervention, with the best limb salvage rate obtained with a new bypass with vein at the first reoperation.

In analyzing secondary femoropopliteal recon-structions for failed autogenous infrainguinal revascularization, no correlation was found between the mode of failure and the results of secondary popliteal-tibial reconstruction. An overall 50 per cent 5-year cumulative salvage rate was obtained, with the highest long-term patency achieved when frequent postoperative follow-up allowed recognition of graft failure prior to total occlusion. In the management of the failing vein graft, a simple vein patch angioplasty yielded an 85 per cent 5-year graft patency. When thrombosis occurred, however, the highest 5-year patency rate was accomplished when reconstruction was performed using a new vein graft. When prosthetic material was used for secondary reconstruction, no graft remained patent beyond 3 years.[55]

Based on the reported experience, it is clear that secondary reconstructions, even with a new autogenous vein bypass to a more distal site, carry a lower patency rate than primary reconstructions. Nevertheless, the limb salvage rate is respectable. The 5-year primary patency rate in a series reported by Edwards et al. was 80 per cent for primary grafts, whereas it was 57 per cent for secondary reconstructions with autogenous tissue. Limb salvage rates for failed bypass were excellent and no different than those achieved with the initial intervention.

Prevention of recurrent graft thrombosis is the greatest challenge for vascular disease specialists following patients after intervention. Whereas antiplatelet agents have been suggested as important in the prevention of recurrent graft thrombosis, to date, no prospective randomized study has established this concept. It is routine, however, to maintain patients on aspirin following reconstructions, as some experimental evidence does suggest a decreased incidence of recurrent thrombosis. Coumadin therapy, with long-term anticoagulation, on the other hand, has been shown to significantly reduce the incidence of graft thrombosis in patients following saphenous vein femoropopliteal bypass. This study showed a significant reduction in graft occlusions of 18 per cent in patients treated with Coumadin versus 37 per cent among controls at a mean follow-up of 30 months.[107] The increased complication rate associated with Coumadin therapy, however, suggests a selective approach in patients with infrainguinal reconstruction. It has been our practice to consider Coumadin therapy in patients with no significant contraindication, who have suffered a graft thrombosis and required reintervention, or patients after prosthetic graft failure in whom no cause of thrombosis could be identified.

The overall results of secondary revascularizations after failed infrainguinal reconstructions have steadily improved. This is likely secondary to the ability to perform reconstructions to very distal arteries in the extremity, the use of thrombolytic therapy to specifically identify the cause of failure, and overall improved patient care and surgical technique.

REFERENCES

1. Chervu A, Homsher E, Moore WS, Quiñones-Baldrich WJ: Differential recovery of skeletal muscle and peripheral nerve function after ischemia and reperfusion. J Surg Res 47:12–19, 1989.

2. Colburn MD, Quiñones-Baldrich WJ, Gelabert HA, Nowara H, Moore WS: Standardization of skeletal muscle ischemic injury. J Surg Res 52:309–313, 1992.

3. Fitzpatrick DB, Karmazyn M: Comparative effects of calcium channel blocking agents and varying extra cellular calcium concentration on hypoxia-reoxygenization ischemia-reperfusion-induced cardiac injury. J Pharmacol Exp Ther 228:761, 1984.

4. McCord JM: Oxygen derived free radicals in post ischemic tissue injury. N Engl J Med 312:159, 1985.

5. Tullson P, John-Adler H, Hood D, et al: De novo synthesis of adenine nucleotides in different skeletal muscle fiber types. Am Physiol Soc 255:C271–C277, 1988.

6. Freund U, Romanoff H, Floman Y: Mortality rate following lower limb arterial embolectomy: Causative factors. Surgery 77:201, 1975.

7. Lee KR, Cronenwett JL, Shalafer M, Corpron C, Zelenock GB: Effect of superoxide dismutase plus catalase on calcium transport in ischemic and reperfused skeletal muscle. J Surg Res 42:24–32, 1987.

8. McCord JM, Roy S: The pathophysiology of superoxide: Roles in inflammation and ischemia. Can J Physiol Pharmacol 60:1346, 1982.

9. Perry MO, Fantini G: Ischemia: Profile of an enemy. Reperfusion injury of skeletal muscle. J Vasc Surg 6:231–234, 1987.

10. Rao PS, Mueller HS: Lipid peroxidation in acute myocardial ischemia. Adv Exp Med Biol 161:347–363, 1983.

11. Yoshida S, Inoh S, Asano T, Sano K, Kubota M, Shimazaki H, Ueta N: Effect of transient ischemia on free fatty acids and phospholipids in the gerbil brain: Lipid peroxidation as a possible cause of post ischemic injury. J Neurosurg 53:323–331, 1980.

12. Roy S, McCord JM: Superoxide and ischemia: Conversion of xanthine dehydrogenase to xanthine oxidase. In Greenwald RG (ed): Oxy Radicals and Their Scavenger Systems. Cellular and Molecular Aspects, Vol 2. New York, Elsevier Science, 1983, pp 145–153.

13. Walker PM, Lindsay TF, Labbe R, Mickle DA, Romaschin AD: Salvage of skeletal muscle with free radical scavengers. J Vasc Surg 5:68–75, 1987.

14. Harlan JM: Neutrophil mediated vascular injury. Acta Med Scand [Suppl] 715:123–129, 1987.

15. Simpson P, Fantone J, Mickelson J, et al: Identification of a time window for therapy to reduce experimental canine myocardial injury; suppression of neutrophil activation during 72 hours of reperfusion. Circ Res 63:1070–1079, 1988.

16. Rubin B, Smith A, Liauw K, et al: Skeletal muscle ischemia stimulates an immune system mediated injury. Surg Forum 40:297–300, 1989.

17. Linas S, Shanley P, Whittenberg D, et al: Neutrophils accentuate ischemia/reperfusion injury in isolated perfused rat kidneys. Am J Physiol 255(24):F728–F735, 1988.

18. Walker PM: Ischemia/reperfusion injury in skeletal muscle. Ann Vasc Surg 5(4):399–402, 1991.

19. Quiñones-Baldrich WJ: The role of fibrinolysis during reperfusion of ischemic skeletal muscle. Microcirc Endothelium Lymphatics 5:299–314, 1989.

20. Merril EW: Rheology of blood. Physiol Rev 49:863, 1969.

21. Quiñones-Baldrich WJ, Chervu A, Hernandez JJ, Colburn MD, Moore WS: Skeletal muscle function after ischemia: "No reflow" versus reperfusion injury. J Surg Res 5(1):5–12, 1991.

22. Bagge U, Maundson B, Lauritzen C: White blood cell deformability and plugging of skeletal muscle capillaries in hemorrhagic shock. Acta Physiol Scand 180:159–163, 1980.

23. Chait LA, May JW, O'Brien BM, Hurley JV: The effects of the perfusion of various solutions on the no reflow phenomenon in experimental free flaps. Plast Reconstr Surg 61:421–430, 1978.

24. Leaf A: Cell swelling: A factor in ischemic tissue injury. Circulation 8:455, 1963.

25. Strock PE, Majno G: Microvascular changes in experimental tourniquet ischemia. Surg Gynecol Obstet 129:1213–1223, 1969.

26. Magovern GJ Jr, Bolling SF, Casale AS, Bulkley BH, Gardner TJ: The mechanism of mannitol in reducing ischemic injury: Hyperosmolarity or hydroxyl scavenger? Circulation 70(suppl I):I–91, 1984.

27. Belkin M, LaMorte WL, Wright JG, Hobson RW: The role of leukocytes in the pathophysiology of skeletal muscle ischemic injury. J Vasc Surg 10:14–19, 1989.

28. Beyersdorf F, Matheis G, Kruger S, Hanselmann A, Freisleben HG, Zimmer G, Satter P: Avoiding reperfusion injury after limb revascularization: Experimental observations and recommendations for clinical application. J Vasc Surg 9:757–755, 1989.

29. Wright JG, Fox D, Kerr JC, Valeri CR, Hobson RW: Rate of reperfusion blood flow modulates reperfusion injury in skeletal muscle. J Surg Res 44:754–764, 1988.

30. Haimovici H: Muscular, renal and metabolic complications of acute arterial occlusions. Myonephropathic-metabolic syndrome. Surgery 85:461, 1979.

31. Abbott WM, Maloney RD, McCabe CC, Lee CE, Wirthlin LS: Arterial embolism: A 44 year perspective. Am J Surg 143:460–464, 1982.

32. Connett MC, Murray DH Jr, Wenneker WW: Peripheral arterial emboli. Am J Surg 148:14, 1984.

33. Elliott JP Jr, Hageman JH, Szilagyi DE, Ramakrishnan V, Bravo JJ, Smith RF: Arterial embolization: Problems of source, multiplicity, recurrence, and delayed treatment. Surgery 99:833–845, 1980.

34. Fogarty TJ, Daily PO, Shumway NE, Krippaehne W: Experience with balloon catheter technique for arterial embolectomy. Am J Surg 122:231–237, 1971.

35. Sheiner NM, Zeltzer J, MacIntosh E: Arterial embolectomy in the modern era. Can J Surg 25:373, 1982.

36. Hellerstein HK, Martin JW: Incidence of thromboembolic lesions accompanying myocardial infarction. Am Heart J 33:443, 1947.

37. Darling RC, Austen WG, Linton RR: Arterial embolism. Surg Gynecol Obstet 124:106, 1967.

38. Schwarcz TH, Coffin LH, Pilcher DB: Renal failure after embolization of a prosthetic mitral valve disc and review of systemic disc embolization. J Vasc Surg 2:697, 1985.

39. Brewster DC: How can you best identify and treat arterial embolism? J Cardiovasc Med 7:354, 1982.

40. Harris RW, Andros G, Dulawa LB, Oblath RW: Malignant melanoma embolus as a cause of acute aortic occlusion: Report of a case. J Vasc Surg 3:550–553, 1986.

41. Prioleau PG, Katzenstein AA: Major peripheral arterial occlusion due to malignant tumor embolism: Histologic recognition and surgical management. Cancer 42:2009, 1978.

42. Kempzinski RF: Lower extremity arterial emboli from ulcerating atherosclerotic plaques. JAMA 241:807–810, 1979.

43. Machleder HI, Takiff H, Lois JF, Holburt E: Aortic mural thrombus: An occult source of arterial thromboembolism. J Vasc Surg 4:473–478, 1986.

44. Gelabert HA, Quiñones-Baldrich WJ: Progressive atheromatous disease. Semin Vasc Surg 3(1):29–34, 1990.

45. Becker PS, Miller VT: Heparin induced thrombocytopenia. Stroke 20:1449–1459, 1989.

46. Laster J, Cikrit D, Walker N, Silver D: The heparin induced thrombocytopenia syndrome: An update. Surgery 102:763–770, 1987.

47. Bick RL: Alterations of hemostasis associated with malignancies. Semin Thromb Hemost 5:1–26, 1978.

48. Levine MN, Gent M, Hirsh J, Arnold A, Goodyear MD, Hryniuk W, DePauw S: The thrombogenic effect of anti-

cancer drug therapy in women with stage II breast cancer. N Engl J Med *318*:404–407, 1988.

49. Symbas PN, Harlaftis N: Bullet emboli in the pulmonary and systemic arteries. Ann Surg *185*:318, 1977.

50. Weaver FA, Schwartz MR, Yellin AE, Bauer M: Refining the indications for arteriography in penetrating extremity trauma: A prospective analysis. Abstract presented at the 46th Annual Meeting of the Society for Vascular Surgery, Chicago, IL, June 8, 1992.

51. Quiñones-Baldrich WJ, Gelabert HA: Autogenous tissue reconstruction in the management of aortoiliofemoral graft infection. Ann Vasc Surg *4(3)*:223–228, 1990.

52. Panetta TF, Marin ML, Veith FJ, Goldsmith J, et al: Unsuspected preexisting saphenous vein disease: An unrecognized cause of vein bypass failure. J Vasc Surg *15*:102–112, 1992.

53. Gilbertson JJ, Walsh DB, Zwolak RM, Waters MA, et al: A blinded comparison of angiography, angioscopy, and duplex scanning in the intraoperative evaluation of in situ saphenous vein bypass grafts. J Vasc Surg *15*:121–129, 1992.

54. Donaldson MC, Mannick JA, Whittemore AD: Causes of primary graft failure after in situ saphenous vein bypass grafting. J Vasc Surg *15*:113–120, 1992.

55. Barboriak JJ, Pintar K, VanHorn DL, et al: Pathologic findings in the aortocoronary vein grafts. Atherosclerosis *29*:69–80, 1978.

56. Matsubara J, Nagasue M, Tsuchishima S, Nakatani B, Shimizu T: Clinical results of femoropopliteal bypass using externally supported (EXS) Dacron grafts: With a comparison of above- and below-knee anastomosis. J Cardiovasc Surg *31*:731–734, 1990.

57. Quiñones-Baldrich WJ, Prego A, Ucelay-Gomez R, Vescera CL, Moore WS: Failure of PTFE infrainguinal revascularization: Patterns, management alternatives, and outcome. Ann Vasc Surg *5(2)*:163–169, 1991.

58. Quiñones-Baldrich WJ, Busuttil RW, Baker JD, et al: Is the preferential use of PTFE grafts for femoral-popliteal bypass justified? J Vasc Surg *8*:219–228, 1988.

59. Blaisdell FW, Steele M, Allen RE: Management of acute lower extremity arterial ischemia due to embolism and thrombosis. Surgery *84*:822, 1978.

60. Barnes RW, Thompson BW, MacDonald CM, et al: Serial noninvasive studies do not herald postoperative failure of femoropopliteal or femorotibial bypass grafts. Ann Surg *210*:486–494, 1989.

61. Bandyk DF, Cato RF, Towne JB: A low flow velocity predicts failure of femoropopliteal and femorotibial bypass grafts. Surgery *98*:799–809, 1985.

62. Sladen JG, Reid JDS, Cooperberg PL, et al: Color flow duplex screening of infrainguinal grafts combining low- and high-velocity criteria. Am J Surg *158*:107–112, 1989.

63. Buth J, Disselhoff B, Sommeling C, Stam L: Color-flow duplex criteria for grading stenosis in infrainguinal vein grafts. J Vasc Surg *14*:716–728, 1991.

64. Cambria RP, Abbott WM: Acute arterial thrombosis of the lower extremity. Arch Surg *119*:784, 1984.

65. Dale WA: Endovascular suction catheters. J Thorac Cardiovasc Surg *44*:557, 1962.

66. Green RM, De Weese JA, Rob CG: Arterial embolectomy before and after the Fogarty catheter. Surgery *77*:24, 1975.

67. Lerman J, Miller FR, Lund CC: Arterial embolism and embolectomy. JAMA *94*:1128–1133, 1930.

68. Short D, Vaughn GD III, Jachimczyk J, Gallagher MW, Garcia-Rinaldi R: The anatomic basis for the occasional failure of transfemoral balloon catheter thromboembolectomy. Ann Surg *190*:555–556, 1979.

69. Plecha FR, Pories WJ: Intraoperative angiography in the immediate assessment of arterial reconstruction. Arch Surg *105*:802, 1972.

70. Cohen LH, Kaplan M, Bernhard VM: Intraoperative streptokinase: An adjunct to mechanical thrombectomy in the management of acute ischemia. Arch Surg *121*:708, 1986.

71. Comerota AJ, White JV, Grosh JD: Intraoperative intraarterial thrombolytic therapy for salvage of limbs in patients with distal arterial thrombosis. Surg Gynecol Obstet *169*:283, 1989.

72. Greep JM, Aleman PJ, Jarrett F, Bast TJ: A combined technique for peripheral arterial embolectomy. Arch Surg *105*:869–874, 1972.

73. Gupta SK, Samson RH, Veith FJ: Embolectomy of the distal part of the popliteal artery. Surg Gynecol Obstet *153*:254–256, 1981.

74. Norem RS, Short DH, Kerstein MD: Role of intraoperative fibrinolytic therapy in acute arterial occlusion. Surg Gynecol Obstet *167*:87–91, 1988.

75. Parent FN III, Bernhard VM, Pabst TS III, McIntyre KE, Hunter GC, Malone JM: Fibrinolytic treatment of residual thrombus after catheter embolectomy for severe lower limb ischemia. J Vasc Surg *9*:153–160, 1989.

76. Quiñones-Baldrich WJ, Baker JD, Busuttil RW, Machleder HI, Moore WS: Intraoperative infusion of lytic drugs for thrombotic complications of revascularization. J Vasc Surg *10*:408–417, 1989.

77. Youkey JR, Clagett GP, Cabellon S, Eddleman WL, Salander JM, Rich NM: Thromboembolectomy of arteries explored at the ankle. Ann Surg *199*:367–371, 1984.

78. Sanchez LA, Gupta SK, Veith FJ, Goldsmith J, et al: A ten-year experience with one hundred fifty failing or threatened vein and polytetrafluoroethylene arterial bypass grafts. J Vasc Surg *14*:729–738, 1991.

79. Whitesides TE, Haney TC, Harada H, Holmes HE, Morimoto K: A simple method for tissue pressure determination. Arch Surg *110*:1311–1313, 1975.

80. Ascer E, Strauch B, Calligaro KD, Gupta SK, Veith FJ: Ankle and foot fasciotomy: An adjunctive technique to optimize limb salvage after revascularization for acute ischemia. J Vasc Surg *9*:594–597, 1989.

81. Blaisdell FW: Is there a reason for controversy regarding fasciotomy? J Vasc Surg *9*:828, 1989.

82. Jarrett F, Dacumos GC, Crummy AB, Detmer DE, Belzer FO: Late appearance of arterial emboli: Diagnosis and management. Surgery *86*:898–905, 1979.

83. Levin BH, Giordano JM: Delayed arterial embolectomy. Surg Gynecol Obstet *155*:549–551, 1982.

84. Blaisdell FW, Lim RC, Amberg JR, Choy SH, Hall AD, Thomas AN: Pulmonary microembolism: A cause of morbidity and death after major vascular surgery. Arch Surg *93*:776–786, 1966.

85. McNamara TO, Bomberger RA, Merchant RF: Intraarterial urokinase therapy for acutely ischemic limbs. Paper presented at the Fourth Annual Meeting of the Western Vascular Society, Kauai, Hawaii, January 18–22, 1989.

86. Greenfield LJ, Kimmell GO, McCurdy WC III: Transvenous removal of pulmonary emboli by vacuum-cup catheter technique. J Surg Res *9*:347, 1969.

87. Hight DW, Tilney NL, Couch NP: Changing clinical trends in patients with peripheral arterial emboli. Surgery *79*:172, 1976.

88. Silvers LW, Royster TS, Mulcare RJ: Peripheral arterial emboli and factors in their recurrence rate. Ann Surg *192*:232, 1980.

89. Tawes RL Jr, Beare JP, Scribner RG, Sydorak GR, Brown WH, Harris EJ: Value of postoperative heparin therapy in peripheral arterial thromboembolism. Am J Surg *146*:213–215, 1983.

90. Tawes RL Jr, Harris EJ, Brown WH, Shoor PM, Zimmerman JJ, Sydorak GR, Beare JP, Scribner RG, Fogarty TJ: Arterial thromboembolism: A 20-year perspective. Arch Surg *120*:595–599, 1985.

91. Dainko EA: Complications of the use of the Fogarty balloon catheter. Arch Surg *105*:79–82, 1972.

92. Dobrin PB: Mechanisms and prevention of arterial injuries caused by balloon embolection. Surgery *106*:457–465, 1989.

93. Haimovici H, Moss CM, Veith FJ: Arterial embolectomy revisited. Surgery *78*:409, 1975.

94. Barker CF, Rosato FE, Roberts B: Peripheral arterial embolism. Surg Gynecol Obstet *123*:22, 1966.

95. Billig DM, Hallman GI, Cooley DA: Arterial embolism: Surgical treatment and results. Arch Surg 95:1, 1967.

96. Buxton B, Morris P: Arterial embolism of the lower limbs: Experience with the use of the Fogarty embolectomy balloon catheter. Aust NZ Surg 39:179, 1969.

97. Cranley JJ, Krause RJ, Strasser ES, Hafner CD, Fogarty TJ: Peripheral arterial embolism: Changing concepts. Surgery 55:57–63, 1964.

98. Edwards EA, Tilney NL, Lindquist RR: Causes of peripheral embolism and their significance. JAMA 196:133, 1966.

99. Fogarty TJ, Cranley JJ: Catheter technique for arterial embolectomy. Ann Surg 161:325, 1965.

100. Karageorgis BP: Experience with the catheter technique in arterial embolectomy. J Cardiovasc Surg 8:375, 1967.

101. McMahon JW, Sako Y: Arterial embolism and embolectomy. Geriatrics 23:132, 1968.

102. Tarnay TJ: Arterial embolism of the extremities: Experience with 62 patients. Arch Surg 99:615, 1969.

103. Satiani B, Gross WS, Evans WE: Improved limb salvage after arterial embolectomy. Ann Surg 188:153, 1978.

104. Thompson JE, Sigler L, Raut PS, et al: Arterial embolectomy: A 20-year experience. Surgery 67:212, 1970.

105. Dale WA: Differential management of acute peripheral arterial ischemia. J Vasc Surg 1:269, 1984.

106. Kendrick J, Thompson BW, Read RC, Campbell GS, Walls RC, Casali RE: Arterial embolectomy in the leg: Results in a referral hospital. Am J Surg 142:739–743, 1981.

107. Kretschmer G, Wenzl E, Piza F, Polterauer P, Ehringer H, Minar E, Schemper M: The influence of anticoagulant treatment on the probability of function in femoropopliteal vein bypass surgery: Analysis of a clinical series (1970 to 1985) and interim evaluation of a controlled clinical trial. Surgery 102:453–459, 1987.

37

MYOINTIMAL HYPERPLASIA

MICHAEL D. COLBURN and WESLEY S. MOORE

Since its conception, vascular reconstructive surgery has been plagued by the problems of graft occlusion and recurrent arterial stenosis. If one reviews all of the published series describing the clinical results of infrainguinal bypass procedures since 1981, and if one includes all grafts extending to all levels, the average primary patency rate at 5 years is 60 to 70 per cent.[1] Therefore, at this time interval, approximately 30 to 40 per cent of all grafts have failed. Long-term results of carotid endarterectomies have been equally concerning.[2] In one study of 301 patients at risk following carotid artery surgery, 26 per cent developed restenosis at 7 years.[3] In addition, of those patients with recurrent hemodynamically significant lesions, 14 per cent developed symptoms of cerebral ischemia. Several studies using duplex scanning have confirmed that the rate of recurrent carotid stenosis following endarterectomy approaches 20 per cent.[4]

On investigating the pathologic mechanisms of both graft failure and recurrent arterial stenosis, a distinctive lesion can be identified. Intimal hyperplasia is the characteristic fibromuscular cellular response of the vascular system to injury. In one series, 50 per cent of late failures identified in 5000 arterial reconstructions, including both endarterectomy and bypass operations, were due to this exuberant hyperplastic intimal response.[5] The purpose of this chapter is to survey the current literature regarding the pathology, pathophysiology, and clinical manifestations as well as the management of intimal hyperplasia. In addition, a completed review of the experimental basis for the pharmacologic control of this process is provided.

PATHOLOGY

Intimal hyperplasia can be described as the abnormal continued proliferation of cells and connective tissue elements that occurs at sites of endothelial injury. As early as 1910, it was noted that "within a few days after the operation, the stitches placed in making the anastomosis became covered with a glis-

tening substance similar in appearance to the normal endothelium."[6] This early description of arterial healing probably represents the normal response of an artery to injury. Intimal hyperplasia, alternatively, is more likely to be the result of the inability to control, or the continued stimulation of, this normal regenerative process. Grossly, when operations are repeated for stenosis or graft failure, a pale, firm, homogeneous lesion is uniformly encountered. The area is smooth, shiny, and appears subendothelial. It has been suggested that, in fact, a true new intima does not form on the surface of the injured lumen. Rather, these investigators prefer the term "myointimal hyperplasia," highlighting the origin of the proliferating tissue as the medial smooth muscle cell. Histologic examination of the lesion shows features consisting of many stellate cells surrounded by a clear fibromyxomatous-appearing stroma and connective tissue. The characteristic morphology (external lamina, dense bodies, and myofilaments), immunocytology (positive staining for smooth muscle cell–specific actin chains), and histochemistry (positive staining for sulfated glycosaminoglycans) of these stellate cells have identified them as smooth muscle cells.[7,8] It is probable, but not definite, that these cells originate in the media as differentiated smooth muscle cells. In response to injury, these smooth muscle cells undergo a series of distinct changes, the earliest of which is replication. This is followed by migration from the media, across the internal elastic lamina, into the intima. Once in the intima, they proliferate and ultimately synthesize and secrete extracellular matrix.[9] This cellular proliferation, as well as the deposition of connective tissue elements, forms the basis of the observed intimal changes in the lumen of a traumatized vessel (Fig. 37–1).

Since the cellular component of intimal hyperplasia is derived from smooth muscle cells, an understanding of the normal physiology of these cells and their role in the healing response of a vascular wound is crucial to our understanding of intimal hyperplasia. The normal arterial wall consists primarily of three layers: the intima, media, and adventitia. Normally, smooth muscle cells are located within the media

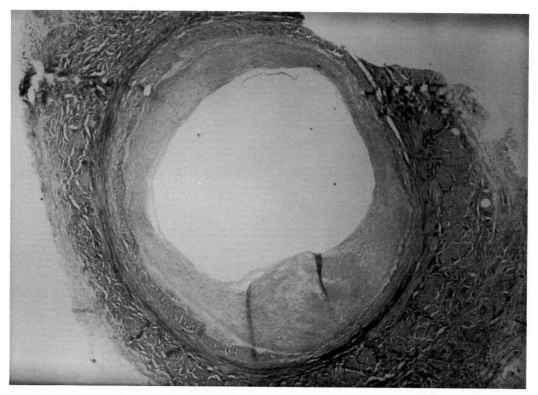

FIGURE 37–1.   Photomicrograph of a failed infrainguinal autologous vein bypass graft showing a large amount of hyperplastic intimal proliferation (Verhoeff van Geison's stain; original magnification X20).

along with a connective tissue mixture of collagen, elastin, and possibly some fibroblasts. The smooth muscle cells are responsible for maintaining the configuration and tone of the vascular wall. The intima is generally considered to consist of a single layer of endothelial cells, on the luminal surface, and a thin basal lamina. One striking characteristic of the normal healthy vessel wall is the slow growth rate of both the intimal endothelial cells and their underlying medial smooth muscle cells. Damage to the vascular endothelium somehow triggers a complex series of events by which these cells undergo a transformation from this resting state to one of great activity. This leads to the migration of smooth muscle cells into the intima and ultimately to intimal hyperplasia.

PATHOPHYSIOLOGY

The precise pathophysiologic pathways leading to the development of intimal hyperplasia have not been characterized. The initiating event is thought to be damage to the vascular endothelium. Subsequent exposure of the subendothelial arterial wall elements triggers the activation of a myriad of cellular and enzymatic events that ultimately lead to the migration and proliferation of medial smooth muscle cells.[9] The response of the medial smooth muscle cell to vascular injury can be divided into four distinct stages: (1) an initial medial proliferative response, (2) migra-

tion from the media across the external elastic lamina and into the intima, (3) subsequent proliferation within the neointima, and (4) synthesis and deposition of extracellular matrix. The end result of this complex process is intraluminal thickening and reduction of the luminal diameter. Traditionally, several theories have attempted to characterize the precise mechanisms responsible for controlling each of these four stages. Among those most often cited have been hemodynamic factors such as turbulence and compliance mismatch, as well as complex interaction between endothelial and smooth muscle cells and circulating factors such as platelets and components of the inflammatory system.[10] More recently, a much more complex view has emerged that involves the synergistic action of several biological pathways. The remainder of this section will review, separately, the experimental basis for the hypothesized involvement of each of these systems.

Hemodynamic Factors

A wide variety of hemodynamic factors including high- and low-flow velocities,[11] high and low wall shear stress,[12] and mechanical compliance mismatch[13] have all been implicated in the formation of intimal hyperplasia. The common pathway, shared by all of these forces, is likely to be the resulting damage to the endothelial cell layer.

The effects of flow velocity on the subsequent development of intimal hyperplasia has been studied in a variety of models. In a high-flow renal artery–to–vena caval anastomosis, significant intimal thickening was documented by electron microscopic examination 3 months after formation.[14] Similar intimal lesions have also been noted in arteriovenous (AV) fistulas constructed for hemodialysis access.[15] However, in a canine carotid vein interposition model, it was found that segments with low flow velocities developed significantly thicker intimal layers.[16] Furthermore, others have found that 6 months after construction of an AV fistula in monkey iliac vessels, no increase in intimal thickening was seen on the experimental side.[17] In this study, while flow rate and velocity were found to be increased markedly on the side of the AV fistula, the calculated wall shear stress was equal on both sides. This equality of shear stress, despite a significant difference in flow velocities, was found to be the result of a twofold increase in diameter of the vessel lumen. This finding has been confirmed by data from other researchers. Together, these findings support the concept that flow velocity may not be a major determinant of intimal hyperplasia. Rather, tangential or wall shear stress may be the essential hemodynamic factor leading to the development of this lesion.

In an ideal tube, the flow pattern is defined as being laminar or having a parabolic wave profile. The layer of fluid adjacent to the wall is known as the boundary layer and is usually a region of low shear stress. In the human arterial tree, blood flow tends to be turbulent, with sudden changes in geometric configuration. This causes areas with complex flow patterns involving the cessation or reversal of flow in the boundary layer. The flow separation that occurs in these areas leads to the generation of shear stress forces. Confusingly, it has been postulated that both high and low wall shear stress may contribute, adversely, to the development of intimal hyperplasia. It is likely, however, that the mechanism by which each end of the shear stress spectrum stimulates this response is very different. Regions of low wall shear stress may increase intimal proliferation, possibly by increasing the time for lipid transport.[11,16] The results of postmortem studies have shown that early atherosclerotic lesions occurred more commonly in areas of low wall shear stress.[18] Conversely, it has also been shown that extremely high shear stress will cause endothelial injury, which may lead to development of intimal lesions.[19]

A model incorporating the effects of both high and low wall shear stress has been suggested.[20] In a model of the human carotid artery bifurcation, dye injected into the central high-velocity flow lines of the common carotid segment is noted to strike the vessel wall near the bifurcation (a high shear stress region) and then, with loss of momentum, traverse circumferentially along the carotid sinus wall to enter the adjacent boundary layer area. This is a low shear stress area and corresponds to the region, across from the external carotid origin, where most atherosclerotic plaques are known to occur. It has been hypothesized that there may be platelet activation, from intimal damage, in the region of high shear stress and that these same activated platelets may then enter the area of boundary layer separation, causing further intimal damage by virtue of the increased exposure time afforded by the low shear stress forces. This hypothesis is strongly supported by the spectral analysis of pulsed Doppler velocity waveforms in carotid artery bifurcations of young healthy individuals. These studies demonstrate similar zones of flow separation.[21]

Compliance mismatch has also been reported to be an important hemodynamic factor in the production of anastomotic intimal hyperplasia. Compliance is defined as the percentage of radial change per unit pressure and is a useful index of vessel wall distensibility to a pressure force. While experimental and clinical studies have shown that grafts with compliance values approaching the native artery demonstrate increased patency, in none of these studies did the design control for differences in graft surfaces. An intriguing experiment was recently reported that attempted to control for the vessels' flow surfaces.[22] In this study, autografts were made from one carotid artery and after preparation, bilateral femoropopliteal grafts were constructed. The compliant graft was infused with 0.025 per cent glutaraldehyde and externally bathed with saline solution for 30 minutes. The stiff graft was infused with a similar concentration of glutaraldehyde, but was bathed in 10 per cent glutaraldehyde for 60 minutes. At explant, only 43 per cent of stiff grafts were patent compared with 86 per cent of compliant grafts. While these results did demonstrate increased patency with more compliant grafts, no effect on intimal hyperplasia was demonstrated. The authors concluded that the role of compliance mismatch, in the development of intimal hyperplasia, is questionable. The compliance of a vein graft, at the time of implantation, is similar to a native artery and, according to the results of one study, the compliance values remain within the normal range for a median follow-up of 33 months.[23] Textile and fabric prostheses, on the other hand, are relatively noncompliant. Furthermore, 4 months after implantation, a significant loss of compliance is noted in both Dacron and polytetrafluoroethylene (PTFE) grafts.[24] For this reason, some authors have suggested imposing a short cuff of autologous vein between native artery and prosthetic grafts.[25]

In summary, when taken together, operative manipulation and hemodynamic factors may contribute, in part, to the development of intimal hyperplasia. Clinically, overaggressive dissection while harvesting vein grafts may lead to injury of the vasa vasorum and disruption of the endothelial layer.[26] Mechanical distention of a vein segment above 200 mm Hg has been shown to lead to endothelial cellular damage.[27] It is likely, however, that these factors are only facilitative and that numerous other contributing elements are necessary for the development of the full hyperplastic response.

Alterations in Lipid Metabolism

Histologic examination of hyperplastic intimal lesions reveals an architecture that is strikingly similar to that seen in specimens of atherosclerosis. Both contain abundant lipid and connective tissue elements, as well as proliferating smooth muscle cells. This observation has led to the hypothesis that intimal hyperplasia may in fact be another variant within the spectrum of atherogenesis. In this theory, atherosclerosis and intimal hyperplasia share a common pathophysiologic pathway but differ in the kinetics of the lesion formation.

Atherosclerotic plaques are a diverse group of lesions that differ in composition depending on their age, anatomic location, and the physiologic status of each individual in which they form. The lesions consist of a matrix of connective tissue proteins in which smooth muscle cells and varying amounts of extracellular lipid are embedded. Early lesions are called fatty streaks and consist primarily of lipid-saturated cells and cholesterol deposits. Fibrous plaques are more advanced lesions that are characterized by a necrotic lipid core surrounded by proliferating smooth muscle cells and a connective tissue matrix. Ultimately, the variant of atherosclerosis that is expressed by each person is determined by the relative proportions of these components.

Atherosclerosis forms over decades and appears somehow connected to the slow accumulation of lipids. The association of atherogenesis and high levels of plasma low-density lipoprotein (LDL) has long been recognized. Population studies measuring the plasma concentration of LDL among Eskimos have shown much lower levels in this group compared to age-matched Danes.[28] This difference may be related to the very low incidence of atherosclerotic heart disease in the Eskimo population. Lipids are essential components of all cells and are involved in a number of cellular structures (particularly membranes) and functions. Furthermore, they play an important carrier function—delivering cholesterol for cellular use. Normally, the vascular smooth muscle cell regulates the accumulation of lipid and cholesterol at the level of a surface membrane high-affinity LDL receptor.[29,30] These receptors bind LDL and internalize the bound compounds by endocytosis. The lipids are incorporated by the cellular membranes and the cholesterol is transported to the liposomes, where it is degraded and processed for use by the cell. In atherosclerosis, many years of oversaturation with high concentrations of plasma LDL may lead to increased storage of intracellular cholesterol esters and the development of foam cells. Later, necrosis of these cells, liberation of their lipid contents, and finally calcification may lead to the necrotic, lipid-rich extracellular debris seen in mature atherosclerosis. Intimal hyperplasia, on the other hand, is characterized by a higher proportion of smooth muscle cell proliferation and less lipid-laden necrosis. This may be the result of a sudden loss of endothelial integrity immediately exposing the underlying smooth muscle cells to large amounts of plasma-bound LDL. The smooth muscle cells respond by both upregulating production of LDL receptors and initiating cellular replication. LDL has been shown to be a potent smooth muscle cell mitogen.[31] Thus, in this theory, both intimal hyperplasia and atherogenesis are related to alterations in lipid metabolism. However, the rapid kinetics of intimal hyperplasia formation leads to a predominantly cellular lesion with moderate amounts of extracellular matrix, whereas atherosclerosis develops slowly over many decades leading to necrotic, lipid-laden lesions with a relatively sparse cellular component.

Platelets

Platelets play an important role in the reaction of the vessel wall to injury. To date, most research in this area has focused on the activation of platelets by the injured endothelium as the major factor in the development of intimal hyperplasia. Unfortunately, extensive work using antiplatelet agents (aspirin, dipyridamole, ibuprofen), in an attempt to reduce this response, has yielded mixed results.

Denudation of the arterial wall exposes the subendothelial matrix, which leads to adherence of platelets. This adherence requires the interaction of subendothelial collagen, a platelet membrane glycoprotein receptor GPIb, plasma von Willebrand factor, and fibronectin. The activated platelet subsequently releases adenosine diphosphate (ADP) and activates the arachidonic acid pathway to release thromboxane (TxA$_2$). Both of these factors lead to platelet recruitment. Recruitment of platelets requires the rapid expression of the platelet membrane receptor complex GPIIb and GPIIIa, which functions as the fibrinogen receptor. Blocking GPIIb and GPIIIa with a murine monoclonal antibody (LJ-CP8) has decreased platelet aggregation in response to collagen and ADP.[32] However, this antibody does not significantly decrease deposition of platelets on Dacron or PTFE grafts in an arteriovenous shunt model.[33] Once platelet aggregation is initiated by the pathways mentioned above, its further formation is limited by an intact endothelium. Thus, a damaged endothelium not only initiates platelet activation but also impairs its inhibition.

With activation of platelets there is secretion of a platelet-derived growth factor (PDGF) along with other granule constituents including platelet factor 4, thromboglobulin, and thrombospondin. PDGF consists of two subunits (A and B) and is a cationic protein with a molecular weight of 28,000 to 31,000. It is a chemoattractant as well as a mitogen for smooth muscle cells and fibroblasts.[34] It binds with high affinity to smooth muscle cells, but not to endothelium.

Thus, it may attract the smooth muscle cells from the media into the intima, bind to them, and cause their proliferation. Interestingly, the platelet may not be the only source of this protein. PDGF (A and B subunits) has been demonstrated to be produced by human umbilical vein and saphenous vein endothelial cells.[35] In fact, injured endothelial cells show a large increase in PDGF production. Both A-chain and B-chain messenger ribonucleic acid (mRNA) have also been noted in fresh endarterectomy specimens obtained at carotid surgery.[36] Also, smooth muscle cells themselves produce PDGF-like activity in response to arterial injury,[37] and it has been shown that smooth muscle cells from human atheroma contain mRNA for the PDGF A-chain.[38] In combination, these findings may explain how intimal proliferation continues after reendothelialization occurs. PDGF may be released by both platelets and endothelial cells, causing migration and proliferation of smooth muscle cells, which can then autoregulate themselves.

While platelet release of PDGF may play a role in the early response to vessel injury, attempts to modify intimal hyperplasia, by interfering with these activation pathways, have yielded disappointing results. This work is discussed below in the section, Experimental Basis for Pharmacologic Control.

Inflammatory Cell Pathways

Unlike the platelet, the role of inflammatory cells in the development of intimal hyperplasia is not universally accepted. It has long been appreciated, however, that the biological responses of inflammation and cellular proliferation are closely related. These processes often occur together as a normal physiologic reaction to injury. In the case of vascular injury, this association has been demonstrated by a number of investigators.

At any time, a significant portion of the intravascular pool of polymorphonuclear leukocytes are adherent to the vascular endothelium. These cells are available and released to the systemic circulation by a number of stimuli. Electron microscopic studies, following a balloon catheter intimal injury, have shown that leukocytes attach to the deendothelialized surface of an arterial lumen.[39,40] Both monocytes and lymphoctyes have also been shown to adhere to damaged endothelium and, in some instances, even penetrate through it.[41] In one study, monocytes were demonstrated to enter the arterial media 42 days after a denuding injury, with labeled cells seen deep within the hyperplastic lesions.[40] Furthermore, in an in vivo model of vasculitis, an interesting phenomenon was observed.[42] In this study, endotoxin-soaked thread was used to produce an inflammatory response on one half of a rat femoral artery. This method consistently resulted in a profound leukocyte infiltration that occurred exclusively on the treated side of the vessel. After 14 days, histologic examination demonstrated marked eccentric intimal lesions, composed primarily of proliferating smooth muscle cells, which were located exclusively on the side of the lumen adjacent to the treated half of the arterial wall. Again, this finding suggests an association between the inflammatory and proliferative processes.

Questions still exist, however, as to the mechanism of this leukocyte deposition and its possible role in intimal hyperplasia. One possibility involves the exposure of medial smooth muscle cells that follows an endothelial injury. It has been shown that serum, containing media that has been conditioned with smooth muscle cells, significantly enhances white blood cell migration. More importantly, others have shown that smooth muscle cells and macrophages secreted potent chemotactic factors for leukocytes, suggesting that, once present, these cells could sustain continued leukocyte recruitment.[43] Other chemotactic agents for leukocytes include PDGF and, in some reports, factors released by fibroblasts.

Once deposited, the mechanism by which leukocytes contribute to the development of intimal hyperplasia remains unknown. After a denuding endothelial injury with deposition of inflammatory cells, a number of inflammatory products may be elaborated. These include chemotactic factors, growth factors, complement components, and enzymes. One of the most important products is monocyte- and macrophage-derived growth factor (MDGF). MDGF is a well-known stimulator of smooth muscle cell and fibroblast proliferation.[44] This growth factor may be similar, if not identical, to PDGF.[45] Thus, one mechanism by which inflammatory cells play a role in the formation of hyperplastic lesions is by the stimulation of smooth muscle cell proliferation.

A second mechanism involves the production of degradation enzymes. Activated leukocytes elaborate several potent proteases capable of degrading collagen and other matrix structural proteins. Infiltration of these cells into the wall of an injured vessel may serve to "loosen" the extracellular matrix. Therefore, migration of smooth muscle cells from the medial layer toward the lumen is facilitated.

Lastly, leukocytes may also act at sites of endothelial injury through a more destructive mechanism. Neutrophils are activated by components of the complement system, immune complexes, and endotoxin. Within 60 seconds of activation, degranulation and oxidative metabolism begin. These processes lead to release of toxic products, including serine proteases and oxygen free radicals. Neutrophils, exposed to activated complement, induce endothelial cell damage mediated primarily through oxygen radicals.[46] For maximal cell injury, close approximation of the neutrophil and endothelial cells is necessary. The importance of these findings may be the role that neutrophils play in denuding arterial injuries. With neutrophil activation, the marginally adherent endothelial cells bordering a lesion may be detached, increasing the magnitude of the injury to the vessel. This further exposure of the subendothelial layer will allow increased platelet cell adherence, aggregation, and activation, as well as the recruitment of more white blood cell mediators and therefore the stimulation of a continued cycle of inflammatory injury.

Role of the Renin-Angiotensin System

The classical view of the regulatory function of the renin-angiotensin system is that it is primarily an endocrine-based system designed for the homeostatic control of hemodynamic and electrolyte balance. This mechanism can be simplified conceptually as follows. In response to low perfusion pressures, renin is released by renal tissue and circulates in the plasma, where it cleaves angiotensinogen, produced by the liver, into angiotensin I. Angiotensin I is converted into active angiotensin II by angiotensin-converting enzyme (ACE) located in the pulmonary vasculature. Finally, angiotensin II exerts its homeostatic hemodynamic effects via specific angiotensin II receptors located in peripheral vascular arterial beds. Recently, this traditional view of the renin-angiotensin system has been revised, and a much more complex concept has emerged. In this new description, the primary site of angiotensin II production is not the pulmonary vasculature, but locally within the affected tissues themselves. This portion of the entire renin-angiotensin axis has been referred to as the "tissue renin-angiotensin system."

The concept that active angiotensin II in the vascular wall is synthesized locally and not delivered via the systemic circulation was originally suggested by Swales and Thurston.[47] In this report, the authors noted that the amount of angiotensin antiserum required to inhibit endogenous angiotensin effects in sodium-loaded rats could not be explained solely on the basis of systemic production. In addition, several investigators had noticed residual reninlike activity in animal studies following bilateral nephrectomy.[48] More convincing evidence for the existence of a locally active vascular renin-angiotensin system, operating independently of the classical systemic circuit, has been recently provided by several studies. First, angiotensinogen mRNA, the only known precursor of the angiotensin peptides, has recently been detected in several extrahepatic vascular tissues, including the aorta.[49,50] Second, using monoclonal antirenin antibodies, immunohistochemical studies have stained positively for the presence of renin in cells located throughout the vascular wall.[51] To specifically identify the cells in the arterial wall responsible for this renin production, tissue culture techniques have been utilized. These studies have demonstrated that both vascular smooth muscle and endothelial cells can synthesize renin in vitro.[52,53] Also, mRNA coding for renin has been identified in human vascular smooth muscle cells.[48,54] Finally, it is widely known that ACE is primarily located on the luminal surface of vascular endothelial cells.[55] Thus, the normally functioning vascular wall possesses all of the necessary components for the independent local production of angiotensin II.

The physiologic function of locally produced angiotensin II is an area of continued controversy. Angiotensin II receptors have been identified on vascular endothelial cells,[48] smooth muscle cells,[56,57] as well as on circulating platelets.[58] Angiotensin II stimulation of endothelial cell–bound receptors leads to the secretion of prostacyclin (PGI_2) and possibly endothelial-derived relaxant factor (EDRF).[59,60] Both these substances have been shown to cause medial smooth muscle cell quiescence and relaxation. On the other hand, activation of the angiotensin receptors located directly on the smooth muscle cells themselves causes the opposite effect. Campbell-Boswell and Robertson reported that angiotensin II stimulated the proliferation of human vascular smooth muscle cells in vitro.[61] Also, Geisterfer and associates found that the protein content of these smooth muscle cells increased by 20 per cent when stimulated by angiotensin II for 4 days.[62] Furthermore, this stimulation was abolished by the angiotensin receptor antagonist saralazin. Finally, the *mas* proto-oncogene, located on the surface of medial smooth muscle cells, increases mitogenic activity when stimulated and has recently been identified as a functional angiotensin II receptor.[63] Therefore, one possibility for the physiologic function of a locally active renin-angiotensin system seems to be the autocrine balance of vascular wall metabolic activity and tone.

This view has led many investigators to study the effect of the local production of angiotensin II on the subsequent development of intimal hyperplasia. In this hypothesis, denudation of the arterial endothelium disrupts the balance of the local renin-angiotensin system and allows the anabolic and mitogenic effects of angiotensin II on the medial smooth muscle cells to proceed unchecked. Another possible mechanism for the promotion of hyperplastic neointimal growth by the local production of angiotensin II involves the activation of platelet metabolic pathways. As mentioned previously, human platelets possess specific binding sites for angiotensin II,[58] and it has been postulated that platelet activation and the subsequent release of PDGF may play a role in the development of intimal hyperplasia. In a recent study by Swartz and Moore, it was demonstrated that angiotensin II enhanced both collagen-induced platelet aggregation as well as the production of TxA_2.[64] Finally, the expression of PDGF, by activated smooth muscle cells, has been shown to be upregulated in the presence of angiotensin II.[65]

Role of Peptide Growth Factors

A universal theme recurring in all the postulated mechanisms of intimal hyperplasia is the promotion of vascular smooth muscle cell growth by peptide mitogens. Examples include PDGF and MDGF. Likewise, intimal hyperplasia can be seen as a hemodynamic response of the vessel wall to the endogenous trophic actions of angiotensin II, another peptide mitogen. Emerging from this idea is the concept of the vascular wall as a complex integrated organ complete with its own endogenous local autocrine system. In this model, intimal hyperplasia can be viewed as the result of an imbalance of these local hormonal systems. This may be due to an excess of trophic peptides or, alternatively, the smooth muscle cell proliferation could be the result of the absence or reduction of the suppressive effects of inhibitory hormones. The sources and effects of the above-mentioned mitogens have already been discussed. This section will highlight the role of another potent promoter of cellular growth: basic fibroblast growth factor (bFGF).

Basic fibroblast growth factor is a known active stimulator of angiogenesis.[66] This protein has become a focus of research in the area of intimal hyperplasia for several reasons. First, recent reports have shown that smooth muscle proliferation, following a balloon catheter injury, occurs even in the absence of platelets.[67] This work suggests that the elaboration of PDGF, in this setting, may not play a major role in the subsequent stimulation of smooth muscle replication. More importantly, the response of an arterial wall to injury has been shown to vary depending on the method of injury.[9,68-70] Specifically, balloon catheterization significantly damages the medial smooth muscle cells as well as denuding the endothelium.[68] On the other hand, wire denudation that also damages the endothelium does not injure the medial cells.[69] Since the latter technique is a much less potent inducer of medial smooth muscle proliferation,[69] it has been suggested that direct smooth muscle cell damage may be an important stimulus for their subsequent activation. In this view, damaged smooth muscle cells might release an endogenous intracellular growth factor that locally autoregulates the adjacent undamaged medial cells. Several pieces of experimental evidence suggest that bFGF may be this factor. It is known to be synthesized by smooth muscle cells,[71,72] and the expression of bFGF mRNA in these cells in increased following injury.[73] Also, bFGF is a potent growth stimulator of smooth muscles cells.[74-76]

To test the hypothesis that bFGF plays an important role in the development of vascular lesions following injury, several in vivo investigations have been undertaken. In one study by Lindner and associates, arteries denuded with a balloon catheter were studied following the systemic administration of bFGF.[77] In this model, bFGF was found to increase the degree of smooth muscle cell replication from 11.5 per cent in controls to 54.8 per cent. Furthermore, a similar increase was seen in arteries denuded by the wire loop technique, suggesting the ability of exogenously administered bFGF to upregulate undamaged medial cells. Interestingly, when the bFGF was given to normal nondenuded vessels, no effect on smooth muscle replication was observed. Finally, prolonged administration of the growth factor was shown to cause a twofold increase in the resulting intimal thickness

compared to control arteries. In a related study, Cuevas et al. demonstrated that the direct local infusion of bFGF into either normal adventitia or injured media results in the proliferation of both vasa vasorum and vascular smooth muscle cells.[76]

In summary, it seems probable that bFGF plays an important role in the development of hyperplastic intimal lesions and that the initial stimulus for this effect is likely to be direct damage to the medial smooth muscle cell.

Role of Plasmin

The establishment of a mature intimal lesion following an arterial insult requires the combination of several biologic pathways. From the perspective of the medial smooth muscle cell, many steps in the proper sequence must be coordinated in order for these lesions to progress. Specifically, smooth muscle cell activation within the media is followed by migration across the internal elastic lamina and finally by replication within the neointimal lining. The regulation of smooth muscle cell activation and proliferation has been extensively studied and is described thoroughly in the preceding sections. Conversely, little information regarding the mechanisms regulating smooth muscle cell migration is available. As mentioned, PDGF is a potent chemoattractant for these medial cells[34]; however, how these cells pass through the physical barrier imposed by the thick medial collagenous extracellular matrix remains a perplexing and unresolved issue. One theory proposed to explain these phenomena involves the vascular thrombolytic system.

The active end-product of the tissue plasminogen-plasmin system is the proteolytic enzyme plasmin. Other important components of this system include the precursor plasminogen and its main endogenous activators: urokinase-type plasminogen activator (u-PA) and tissue-type plasminogen activator (t-PA). The catalytic action of these proteases are inhibited in vivo by the plasmin inhibitors α_2-antiplasmin and α_2-macroglobulin, as well as a group of related plasminogen activator inhibitory proteins (PAI). In recent years, increased knowledge regarding the interaction of all these components at the cellular level has been accumulated.

The hypothesis that the protease plasmin is involved in smooth muscle cell migration following an arterial injury is built on several related observations. First, circulating plasminogen is a relatively large protein that is normally prevented from entering the medial layer by an intact endothelium. However, following endothelial damage this protein can readily diffuse into this area.[78] Once present in the extracellular medial layer, conversion of plasminogen into plasmin can directly degrade several matrix proteins as well as activate other potent collagenases.[79] The key to this conversion depends on the local presence of specific plasminogen activators. Smooth muscle cells have been found to express plasminogen activator activity in tissue culture.[80,81] Finally, in an in vivo model of arterial repair, Clowes and associates have demonstrated that vascular smooth muscle cells contain increased levels of both u-PA and t-PA.[82] Furthermore, these two plasminogen activators appear to act synergistically, and their secretion depends on the functional state of the smooth muscle cells. During cellular proliferation, u-PA is the major product; whereas during migration, t-PA expression predominates. The combination of these experimental observations suggests the following hypothesis. Injury to the endothelium may allow for the local penetration of plasminogen and chemotactic substances (elaborated from activated platelets and leukocyte) into the arterial wall. The conversion of extracellular plasminogen into plasmin by medial smooth muscle cells degrades the structural matrix proteins. This process may be enhanced by the presence of leukocyte-derived enzymes. Finally, activation of smooth muscle cells by the elaborated growth and chemotactic factors initiates migration of these cells through the weakened arterial wall. The direction of migration is determined automatically by the gradient of plasminogen and mitogenic activity that is highest adjacent to the endothelial defect. Precise characterization of the role of local plasminogen-plasmin pathways in the development of intimal hyperplasia requires further research.

CLINICAL MANIFESTATIONS AND CURRENT MANAGEMENT

The number of procedures performed annually for occlusive vascular disease continues to increase. Currently, approximately 500,000 patients undergo reconstructive vascular surgery each year—half are coronary bypass procedures; the remainder includes various operations on the peripheral vascular tree. These peripheral interventions encompass a wide assortment of procedures including autologous and prosthetic bypass grafts, endarterectomies, and a variety of new endovascular procedures.

Most established vascular procedures, as well as the new technologies and applications, have proven to be both technically feasible and safe. The value of any surgical procedure, however, must be measured not only by the success with which it can be initially performed, but also in terms of the durability of the results. Although the in-hospital success rates are excellent, the long-term durability of most of these procedures has been disappointing. Furthermore, the common culprit accounting for much of the poor long-term success rate following these procedures is intimal hyperplasia. Clearly, this process is a significant cause of morbidity in patients undergoing procedures on the vascular system and investigation into methods to prevent or reverse this process is of great importance.

Restenosis Following Peripheral Bypass

The 3-year primary patency rate for infrainguinal bypass grafts ranges from 40 to 60 per cent with prosthetic conduits, to 60 to 80 per cent when an autologous graft is utilized.[1] Of those grafts that fail between 6 months and 2 years, most are due to intimal hyperplasia.[5,83] In prosthetic grafts, the area most affected by hyperplastic change is the distal anastomosis. Although this location is also the likely point of obstruction in autologous tissue grafts, focal lesions throughout the entire length of the graft are also common.

Treatment options for a failed or failing peripheral bypass graft due to intimal hyperplasia are limited. Chronically thrombosed vein grafts can rarely be salvaged and invariably need to be replaced. Often, when this is not technically possible and the patient is suffering from severe ischemia, an amputation will be required. Thrombosed grafts that are recognized early can frequently be reopened using thrombolytic therapy. After reestablishing flow through the graft, the lesion responsible for the occlusion is sometimes visualized. Even though it is possible to treat some of these hyperplastic lesions percutaneously with balloon dilation or atherectomy devices, results of these techniques are usually less than satisfactory. Immediate patency is usually excellent; however, because of the fibrous character and progressive growth of these lesions, the recurrence rates are unacceptably high. Therefore, reoperation for distal anastomotic graft stenoses is generally recommended. Reconstruction will usually require implantation of a new graft, construction of a jump graft, or patch angioplasty of the existing bypass.

Restenosis Following Carotid Endarterectomy

The mean incidence of asymptomatic carotid restenoses ranges between 7 and 15 per cent, and between 1 and 5 per cent develop restenoses associated with recurrent symptoms.[84–94] In those rare instances in which a recurrent lesion becomes symptomatic, the management algorithm is straightforward: most surgeons consider this an indication for angiography and reoperation. Unfortunately, like primary carotid lesions, there is little information regarding the natural history of recurrent carotid stenoses in asymptomatic patients and therefore the appropriate management of these individuals remains unclear. The risk of subsequent stroke or ischemic events in these patients is clearly different from primary atherosclerotic lesions. Smooth fibrous intimal hyperplastic lesions, even of the same or greater degree of stenosis than the original atherosclerotic plaque, are well tolerated by most patients. This is likely due to the low risk of embolic events related to these lesions relative to the soft necrotic atherosclerotic plaques originally found in these patients. It follows that the majority of patients who become symptomatic due to a recurrent carotid stenosis do so on the basis of a hemodynamic flow–related mechanism or have a mixed plaque recurrence with a significant atherosclerotic component. This may explain the observation that patients with symptomatic recurrences are often found to have tight stenoses or occlusions of the contralateral carotid artery.[85,87] In general, the decision to operate on an asymptomatic patient with a recurrent carotid stenosis should be individualized and is based on several factors including (1) the degree and rate of progression of the stenosis, (2) the histological character of the lesion, (3) the condition of the remainder of the cerebral circulation, and (4) the age and overall general medical condition of the patient.

The incision and principles of exposure when managing a recurrent carotid lesion are the same as for a standard endarterectomy. The dissection is invariably more difficult due to the scarring from the previous procedure, and extra care must be taken to avoid injury to the cranial nerves. The hypoglossal nerve is particularly vulnerable, as it can be draped over the bifurcation by the scar tissue. Once completely dissected, the common, external, and internal carotid vessels are clamped, and the bifurcation opened using a longitudinal arteriotomy. The histologic property of carotid bifurcation atherosclerotic lesions that allows for the performance of a standard endarterectomy is the ease with which a plane of dissection can be developed between the plaque and the circular medial fibers of the arterial wall. Unfortunately, recurrent carotid lesions composed of hyperplastic intimal tissue do not share this property. Thus, it is not possible to form a precise plane of dissection that allows for the removal of the luminal narrowing disease without dangerously thinning the remaining arterial wall. The surgical approach to recurrent carotid lesions, therefore, is patch angioplasty rather than endarterectomy. On the other hand, when the recurrent lesion is found to be composed of ordinary atheroma, a standard endarterectomy can be performed.

The choice of patch material varies amongst surgeons treating this disease. Some use prosthetic material as their first choice, whereas others prefer the use of autologous vein. There is a theoretical argument that prosthetic material may contribute to the hyperplastic intimal process, but this has not been proven experimentally. In fact, it has been suggested that autologous vein, with its intact endothelium elaborating humoral growth factors, may be a greater stimulus to a continued hyperplastic reaction in the patched arterial segment. When vein is chosen, saphenous vein is most frequently used. Experience has shown that vein segments taken from the neck are ordinarily too thin and should be avoided. Regardless of the material chosen, the patch should always be constructed in such a way as to reapproximate the native size of the carotid bulb. Large patulous repairs increase the luminal diameter of the reconstructed carotid bulb and, by the application of the law of Laplace, lead to abnormally increased tangential wall tension. This could result in a blowout of the patch suture line. Alternatively, sacular patch repairs may lead to the accumulation of laminar thrombus and result in distal embolization. Occasionally, the recurrent disease is so advanced and patch angioplasty is not feasible. In these rare cases, reconstruction can be accomplished by the use of an interposition graft.

Restenosis Following Endovascular Surgery

Endovascular surgery is a relatively new field that originated with the development of percutaneous transluminal balloon angioplasty (PTA) and has evolved to include angioscopy, laser and mechanical atherectomy, and intravascular stents. Together, these techniques have managed impressive initial success rates. However, with the test of time, complications such as dissections, perforations, and especially restenosis have limited their application. Recent advances such as over-catheter systems and "smart" laser technology have reduced the incidence of these early technical complications. Unfortunately, the problem of restenosis remains the "Achilles heel" of endovascular interventions and threatens to limit their ultimate usefulness.

Results following PTA in the lower extremity have been published by several authors. The combined failure rate after 1-year follow-up ranges from 2 to 40 per cent.[95] Some of these recurrences are no doubt due to either a progression of atherosclerosis, or other mechanisms such as intraplaque hemorrhage. However, the majority are the result of intimal hyperplasia. Likewise, long-term results following laser-assisted angioplasty have not been encouraging. In one representative study, White et al. reported their results of laser-assisted balloon angioplasty for advanced lesions of the lower extremity.[96] In this study, several different technologies were utilized, including argon, Nd:YAG, and metal hot-tipped systems. Although the initial recanalization rate was 67 per cent, only 11 per cent remained patent at 1 year. Results from other investigators have been similar. The results of peripheral atherectomy vary depending on the device used and the anatomic location of the lesion. At UCLA we have had experience treating arterial occlusions with the Auth Rotablator (Biophysics International, Bellevue, WA).[97] Initial success was achieved in 92 per cent of the cases and the primary patency was 67 per cent at 6 months. However, follow-up at 24 months noted only a 9.5 per cent patency rate. Unfortunately, the long-term outcomes of other devices have not reported any significant improvement over these results. Again, the majority of these failures can be attributed to intimal hyperplasia.

The treatment for restenotic lesions following endovascular surgery depends on the site affected, degree of symptoms, and overall condition of the patient. In general, "redo" endovascular procedures are possible but uniformly suffer a similar fate as the original intervention. Most frequently, in this setting, conventional vascular surgical techniques have been employed, including formal bypass grafts or limited endarterectomies. Of course, as described above, these methods also possess a small but definite risk of failure due to intimal hyperplasia and therefore do not guarantee long-term success.

EXPERIMENTAL BASIS FOR PHARMACOLOGIC CONTROL

The ability of various pharmacologic agents to suppress the development of intimal hyperplasia has been well documented. Particularly striking is the large variety of medications that have been effective in limiting this response. At least five different classes of drugs have been studied and shown to be at least partially successful in this regard (Table 37–1): lipid metabolites,[98–100] antiplatelet agents,[101–103] antiinflammatory agents,[104,105] antihypertensive agents,[106–109] and anticoagulants.[110] In addition, many other substances that interfere with normal cellular growth have also shown some promise.[77,111–115] This clearly attests to the complexity of the pathways leading to the development of this lesion and implies that no one agent will likely be totally effective in its elimination. Unfortunately, the nonuniformity of the models of intimal hyperplasia studied and the doses and duration of the agents investigated make comparison of the results of these trials unreliable. Therefore, the clinical usefulness of pharmacologic therapy, in this setting, remains undetermined. Nevertheless, if effective pharmacologic therapy to suppress the growth of intimal hyperplasia and prevent the associated recurrent arterial stenoses could be developed, this would have a major impact on the durability of vascular procedures and lower their associated morbidity, mortality, and cost. Also, in addition to suppressing the development of intimal hyperplasia, one or more of these medications may prove to be effective in reducing established hyperplastic lesions. This would be an alternative therapy for the patient with a failing previous vascular procedure and would represent a significant advance in the management of this highly morbid and potentially lethal complication of peripheral vascular surgery.

Experimental Models

Several models have been employed in an attempt to elucidate the pathophysiologic mechanisms leading to the development of intimal hyperplasia. These include both in vitro and animal replica of this lesion. Smooth muscle as well as endothelial cells have been grown in tissue culture. Although these studies have been helpful in determining isolated effects of various mitogens, growth factors, and hormones on the growth patterns of these vascular cells, it is clear that these investigations suffer greatly from the abnormal cellular relationships inherent in their preparation. Conventional anatomic descriptions of the vascular wall depict the endothelial cell as being separated from the underlying smooth muscle cells by a continuous elastic lamina. This concept of two independently functioning and autonomous cell layers has more recently been replaced by a more complex description portraying mechanisms of mutual regulation between the two cell systems.

The possibility of endothelial–smooth muscle cell interaction was first suggested by electron microscopic evidence of smooth muscle cell cytoplasmic extensions traversing holes in the elastic lamina and projecting into the overlying endothelial cell cytoplasm.[116] The subsequent description of several endothelial cell–derived substances that either promote or inhibit the growth and activation of the medial smooth muscle cell lends further support to the concept of the vascular wall functioning as an interrelated organ system. In addition, contact of the endothelial cell layer with the cellular and serum components of flowing blood further complicates the normal functioning environment of these vascular elements. It is therefore very difficult to make useful conclusions based on data collected within in vitro systems in which the processes being studied clearly exist in an artificial environment. For these reasons, in an attempt to study the pathophysiology of this lesion in a setting in which the normal regulatory interrelationships have not been disturbed, most in-

TABLE 37–1. PHARMACOLOGIC AGENTS REPORTED TO BE EFFECTIVE IN SUPPRESSING THE FORMATION OF INTIMAL HYPERPLASIA

Lipid metabolites
    Omega-3 polyunsaturated fatty acids (EPA)[a]
Antiplatelet agents
    Aspirin
    Dipyridamole
    Thromboxane synthetase inhibitors
Antiinflammatory agents
    Dehydroepiandrosterone
    Dexamethasone
    Cyclosporin
Antihypertensive agents
    ACE[b] inhibitors
        Cilazapril, captopril, enalaprilat
    Calcium channel blockers
        Verapamil, nimodipine
    α_1-Adrenergic inhibitors
        Prazosin
Growth factor inhibitors
    Angiopeptin
    bFGF[c]-saporin
    Ornithine decarboxylase inhibitors
Anticoagulant agents
    Heparins and heparinoids

[a]EPA, eicosapentaenoic acid.
[b]ACE, angiotensin-converting enzyme.
[c]bFGF, basic fibroblast growth factor.

vestigators have turned to animal models of intimal hyperplasia.

The classic animal model of smooth muscle cell intimal hyperplasia is a balloon catheter arterial injury model. The induction of smooth muscle cell growth following a balloon catheter denuding injury was first described by Baumgartner over 20 years ago.[117] Since that time several modifications of this procedure have been utilized. The basic concepts of the model, however, remain the same. A segment of artery to be studied is isolated and a balloon catheter is introduced into the lumen. By inflating the balloon and withdrawing the catheter, complete denudation of the endothelial layer can be achieved. Following this injury, a lesion is formed that is histologically identical to that which is observed clinically. The advantages of this model are its ease and reproducibility. In addition, the anatomic injury produced mimics the cleavage plain that occurs clinically in the endarterectomized vessel. Criticisms of this model include the vessel distention that occurs at the time of injury, as well as its failure to address the intimal hyperplasia that occurs at graft anastomotic sites. A second type of injury model employs hydrostatically stretching the vessel without deliberately denuding the endothelial surface.[118] This model attempts to isolate and define the role of vascular distention as a contributing factor in the development of these lesions. This mode of injury does produce an increase in medial smooth muscle cell activity and lends support to the mechanical theories of hyperplasia. A third type of arterial injury model that has been utilized is the denudation of the intimal layer by a loop of fine nylon wire.[9] This model differs from the balloon injury in that the wire removes the endothelium without the complicating effects of distention. This model suffers, however, from the difficulty in standardizing the degree of vessel injury and its lack of a true anatomical correlate in clinical situations. Finally, to study the development of intimal hyperplasia at anastomotic sites, several animal models utilizing bypass grafts of both autologous and prosthetic material have been successful in reproducing the lesions seen clinically in humans.[12,105]

Agents Studied

Lipid Metabolites

As mentioned previously, Eskimos have extremely low plasma levels of LDL; this may explain their low incidence of atherosclerotic heart disease.[28] Further characterization of Eskimo plasma lipid composition has demonstrated low levels of circulating arachidonic acid and unusually high concentrations of eicosapentaenoic acid (EPA).[119] EPA is an omega-3 polyunsaturated fatty acid that is present in large amounts in fish but cannot be synthesized de novo by humans. Following ingestion, EPA enters the prostaglandin synthesis pathway and competes directly with arachidonic acid. In contrast to arachidonic acid metabolism, which leads to the formation of TxA_2 (a potent stimulator of platelet aggregation), EPA is converted into TxA_3, which has no effect on platelet function.

Several studies have tested the hypothesis that high levels of EPA present at the time of an endothelial injury may inhibit the production of intimal hyperplasia. Both Cahill et al. and Landymore et al. have reported the ability of small doses of marine oils to reduce intimal thickening in vein graft models.[98,99] Most recently, O-hara et al. have reported a marked suppression of intimal hyperplasia following treatment with EPA in a rabbit PTFE graft model.[100]

Further investigation is needed to establish both the precise mechanism by which EPA prevents intimal hyperplasia, as well as the dose and duration of exposure at which this effect is optimal.

Antiplatelet Agents

Excitement about the possibility of limiting intimal hyperplasia by inhibiting platelet pathways began with the work of Friedman et al., who reported reduced hyperplasia after an aortic balloon catheter injury in thrombocytopenic rabbits.[120] Unfortunately, inhibition of intimal hyperplasia using a number of different antiplatelet drugs has yielded mixed results. Antiplatelet drugs inhibit the synthesis of prostaglandins by blocking arachidonic acid metabolic pathways. Aspirin irreversibly acetylates platelet cell cyclooxygenase. Dipyridamole increases platelet cyclic adenosine monophosphate (AMP) and inhibits the precursors TxA_1 and TxB_2. Thus, both aspirin and dipyridamole inhibit platelet adherence, as well as aggregation, by interfering with the production of prostaglandin metabolites.

Clinically, and in experimental models, aspirin has been shown to decrease platelet adherence to prosthetic vascular grafts.[121–123] The addition of dipyridamole may or may not enhance this effect. Findings from other studies, however, have demonstrated that although antiplatelet agents may decrease subsequent platelet aggregation and thrombus formation, they have no effect on the initial platelet deposition.[124] The effect of these agents on patency and the development of intimal hyperplasia has also been inconsistent. In one study, bilateral vein bypass grafts were placed to ligated iliac arteries in rhesus monkeys.[125] These monkeys were given aspirin (165 mg administered twice daily) and dipyridamole (25 mg administered twice daily) beginning 3 weeks before the surgical procedure. Sixteen weeks after the procedure, at sacrifice, the intimal area was compared and found to be significantly reduced in the experimental group. On the other hand, in a follow-up study using a balloon catheter injury model in rabbits, no significant difference between the two groups in tritiated thymidine incorporation, nuclear proliferation, or progression of intimal hyperplasia was established.[103] In a similar study performed in rabbits, aspirin significantly increased the patency of an end-to-side iliac anastomosis but had no effect on the development of intimal hyperplasia.[101]

Thromboxane synthetase converts cyclic endoperoxide precursors from the arachidonic acid pathways into TxA_2. TxA_2 is synthesized and stored in the developing platelet. It is a powerful mediator of both platelet aggregation and vascular constriction. Inhibitors of thromboxane synthetase block this conversion of intermediate endoperoxide precursors into TxA_2. Furthermore, in doing so, the intracellular prostaglandin metabolic pathways are shifted toward the production of PGI_2. Thus, theoretically, thromboxane synthetase inhibitors can block platelet-derived TxA_2 while actually enhancing the production of endothelial cell–derived PGI_2. It is postulated that these agents may therefore be more specific inhibitors of platelet function. In a recent report, the efficacy of thromboxane synthetase inhibition in the prevention of distal anastomotic intimal hyperplasia was investigated and compared to aspirin.[126] A bilateral aortoiliac bypass graft model was used and two different types of grafts were evaluated: thin-walled PTFE and PTFE seeded with autologous endothelial cells. Treatment groups consisted of antiplatelet therapy with either aspirin or the thromboxane synthetase inhibitor U-63,577A. Interestingly, in both types of grafts, aspirin was significantly more effective in maintaining patency and inhibiting intimal hyperplasia. Within the thromboxane synthetase inhibitor group, however, the agent was more effective when the bypass grafts were seeded. Also, both types of graft were improved when compared to no therapy at all. In conclusion, in combination with other antiplatelet drugs, these agents could prove to be potent inhibitors of platelet function. However, no clinical trials are yet available.

To summarize, at the present time antiplatelet drugs would seem to increase the patency of vein and prosthetic bypass grafts, but probably do not significantly alter the development of intimal hyperplasia. More work is necessary to determine the role of newer agents in complementing or enhancing these effects.

Antiinflammatory Agents

In inflammatory states, neutrophils adhere to endothelial linings and penetrate the vascular wall.[127] Histologically, leukocyte infiltration has also been noted as a consistent feature occurring in hyperplastic intimal lesions. For these reasons, it has been suggested that modification of leukocyte function may be effective in the prevention of intimal hyperplasia.

The first suggestion that glucocorticoids may have a role in preventing intimal proliferation following a vascular injury came from a report by Gordon and associates in 1988.[128] In this study, the administration of the endogenous steroid dehydroepiandrosterone caused a reduction of atherogenesis in hypercholesterolemic rabbits. Prior to this report, Hoepp et al. found no significant differences in patency or the hyperplastic response between steroid-treated and control groups in a canine femoropopliteal Dacron

bypass graft model.[105] In this experiment, however, the animals were treated with a relatively low dose of the short-acting steroid methylprednisolone, and the drug was given only after the completion of the procedure rather than preoperatively. More recently, a large, randomized, double-blind clinical study (M-HEART project) assessed whether or not a single large dose of methylprednisolone (1 gm) given intravenously prior to angioplasty could alter the incidence of restenosis.[129] The results could not demonstrate a significant difference between the steroid- and placebo-treated groups. However, again in this study, a relatively short-acting steroid was given as a single one-time dose. It should be recognized that it has been demonstrated that the period of maximal intimal proliferation following an arterial injury is between 2 and 4 weeks.[68] Also, the results of several experiments have suggested that starting steroid treatment prior to the arterial injury may be important. Finally, in a balloon catheter injury model performed in rabbits, dexamethasone (0.10 mg/kg given intramuscularly) was reported to produce a marked reduction of intimal hyperplasia.[104] In this study, the steroid was begun 2 days prior to the carotid endothelial injury and was continued for a period of 8 weeks. Furthermore, in a follow-up study, this response to dexamethasone treatment was found to be dose dependent (Figs. 37–2 and 37–3).[130]

The mechanism for this observed effect by glucocorticoids is unclear. One possibility is the well-known effect of these agents on fibroblast growth and wound healing. Several investigators have demonstrated the

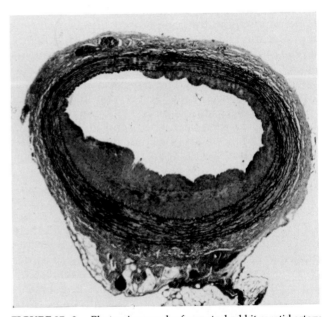

FIGURE 37–2. Photomicrograph of a control rabbit carotid artery 12 weeks following a balloon catheter endothelial injury, demonstrating a large amount of intimal hyperplasia (Verhoeff van Geison's stain; original magnification X20). (From Colburn MD, Moore WS, Gelabert HA, Quiñones-Baldrich WJ: Dose responsive suppression of myointimal hyperplasia by dexamethasone. J Vasc Surg 15:510–518, 1992.)

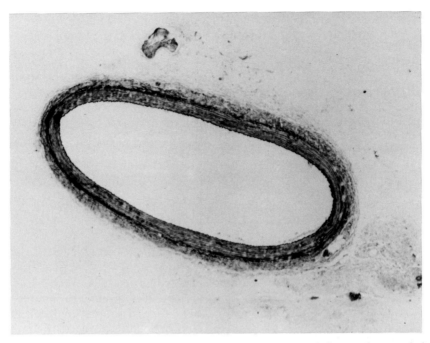

FIGURE 37–3. Photomicrograph of a carotid artery 12 weeks following a balloon catheter endothelial injury, demonstrating an absence of significant intimal hyperplasia after treatment for 8 weeks with dexamethasone 0.125 mg/kg (Verhoeff van Geison's stain; original magnification X20). (From Colburn MD, Moore WS, Gelabert HA, Quiñones-Baldrich WJ: Dose responsive suppression of myointimal hyperplasia by dexamethasone. J Vasc Surg *15*:510–518, 1992.)

ability of glucocorticoids to inhibit the growth of cultured fibroblast cell lines.[131,132] Likewise, considerable information regarding the effect of steroids on leukocyte function is available. In in vitro studies, steroids have been reported to decrease leukocyte aggregation to several chemotactic factors.[133–136] Some steroids have also been shown to alter the C^3 receptor on human white blood cells, which plays a role in phagocytosis.[137] In addition, they have been demonstrated to decrease leukocyte-to-endothelial cell adhesion.[138,139] Finally, steroids have been related to an inhibition of white blood cell cytotoxic function. This observation is manifested primarily by the impaired release of zymogen granules and a decrease in the production of superoxide anions.[140] In an in vivo study, high-dose methylprednisolone was shown to prevent subendothelial and transmural accumulation of leukocytes, as well as endothelial sloughing in vein grafts.[141] This effect on endothelial sloughing may decrease the stimuli for the development of intimal hyperplasia.

The role of the immune system in the evolution of intimal hyperplasia is not clear. Atherosclerotic plaques have been found to contain activated lymphocytes and smooth muscle cells that express class II major histocompatibility antigens.[142] Interaction of these antigens and immune cells may propagate an immune response and result in the release of other inflammatory mediators and cytokines. The effect of treatment with cyclosporin was studied in a rat common iliac artery injury model.[143] Prior to undergoing the arterial injury, rats were administered parenteral cyclosporin at a dose of 5 mg/kg/day that was continued for 2 and 6 weeks. The results showed that those arteries treated with cyclosporin demonstrated significantly less medial thickening at each time interval. These data provide further evidence that immunologic mechanisms may be important in the development of intimal hyperplasia.

Antihypertensive Agents

Angiotensin-converting enzyme inhibitors, calcium channel blockers, and α_1-adrenergic antagonists are all agents used clinically in the treatment of systemic hypertension. Each of these categories of antihypertensive drugs has also been reported to be effective in suppressing intimal hyperplasia.

The first study that reported the ability of an ACE inhibitor to reduce myointimal proliferation after a vascular injury appeared in a paper by Powell and associates in 1989.[107] In this study, rats were subjected to an endothelial denudation injury using a balloon catheter. Experimental animals received 10 mg/kg of cilazapril, mixed with their normal chow, beginning 6 days before the endothelial injury. Therapy was continued daily for 14 days. The results showed a significant inhibition of intimal hyperplasia in the treated group, and this effect was independent of any changes in blood pressure. In a follow-up study, the same investigators observed a reversal of this effect following the intravenous infusion of angiotensin II.[70] Recently, O'Donohoe and associates have reported the inhibition of intimal hyperplasia in experimental vein grafts by the long-term administration of an ACE inhibitor.[144] For this study, a carotid interposition vein graft model was utilized. Experimental animals received oral doses consisting of 10 mg/kg of captopril daily. The drug was started 1 week before grafting and continued until sacrifice at 28 days. Results documented a 40 per cent reduction in intimal thickness compared to control animals. Lastly, captopril has also been reported to cause a significant decrease in aortic atherosclerosis in a heritable hyperlipidemic rabbit model.[145]

Unfortunately, all of these previous in vivo studies relied on the oral consumption of the pharmacologic agent. This route of drug administration in any animal model makes the interpretation of the observed results difficult and unreliable. Both captopril and enalapril are available in an injectable form, whereas cilazapril is not. Enalaprilat is an active free metabolite of enalapril and is the form of the drug that is administered parenterally. Enalaprilat is more potent and much longer acting than the injectable form of captopril, and is therefore better suited for animal studies in which once-a-day dosing is better tolerated and more practical.[146] Also, the in vivo mechanism of action of captopril is complicated by the fact that, unlike other ACE inhibitors, it contains a sulfhydryl (—SH) group. The —SH group can act as a free radical scavenger,[147] and one postulated mechanism for the development of intimal hyperplasia at sites of endothelial injury is the production of free radicals by activated neutrophils.[46] At least one study investigating the ability of parenterally administered enalaprilat to inhibit intimal hyperplasia has been completed. This report does suggest that this agent is effective in this regard.[148]

Calcium channel antagonists are effective agents used in a variety of cardiovascular disorders. In general, the common mechanism of action of all these agents is an interruption of membrane calcium channels, thereby reducing the availability of this cation for a variety of intercellular processes. Calcium has been implicated in a number of events involved in the development of intimal hyperplasia including platelet activation, release of PDGF, medial smooth muscle cell proliferation, and the formation of extracellular matrix. Treatment with calcium antagonists has been shown to significantly reduce the development of intimal hyperplasia after a mechanical arterial injury.[149] In addition, both verapamil and nimodipine have been effective in reducing intimal hyperplasia in vein bypass graft models.[108,109]

Another important mediator of vascular tone is the α_1-adrenergic receptor. These receptors are found on vascular smooth muscle cells and, when stimulated, result in profound contraction. Experimental studies have demonstrated that endothelial denudation is accompanied by a selective increase in the sensitivity of the α_1-adrenergic receptor.[150] Also, the cytoplasmic secondary messenger system for this receptor response has recently been reported to involve an increase in the turnover of the intracellular phosphatidylinositol cycle.[151] It is interesting that PDGF function has also been linked to an up-regulation of the intracellular phosphatidylinositol cycle. Intermediates of this cycle stimulate protein kinase C to initiate a series of phosphorylating reactions which ultimately lead to cellular mitosis.[152] Therefore, the intracellular mechanisms of smooth muscle cell proliferation, and contraction are connected through a common cytoplasmic pathway: the phosphatidylinositol cycle. Prazosin is a selective α_1-adrenergic receptor blocker and has been studied for its ability to prevent intimal hyperplasia. In a balloon catheter injury model in the rabbit aorta, prazosin was shown to produce a statistically significant reduction in the development of intimal hyperplastic lesions.[106] No clinical trials utilizing this agent have been reported.

Growth Factor Inhibitors

Somatostatin is a widely occurring peptide hormone that acts as a modulator of a diverse class of endogenous growth promoters. It has been postulated that, if intimal hyperplasia is the result of an imbalance in local vascular autocrine systems following an endothelial injury, somatostatin may be effective in limiting this response. Unfortunately, because of storage instability and a very short half-life, somatostatin is unsuitable for use in in vivo models. Angiopeptin is a stable octapeptide somatostatin analog that has been shown to be an effective long-acting somatostatin receptor agonist. This analog has been extensively studied as a potential inhibitor of intimal hyperplasia.

Several authors have reported the success of angiopeptin in suppressing the development of intimal hyperplasia in animal models.[111–113] In one publication, angiopeptin was also shown to significantly reduce the degree of posttransplant coronary artery intimal hyperplasia in rabbits.[114] This study was complicated, however, by the fact that these rabbits also received cyclosporin immunosuppression which, as discussed above, has also been reported to affect the development of hyperplastic lesions. Whether or not angiopeptin is actually antagonizing the trophic effects of growth promoters in this setting is not clear. In vitro work has also demonstrated the ability of angiopeptin to directly inhibit the proliferation of smooth muscle cells.[153] This suggests that the action of angiopeptin may not be related to an inhibition of the somatostatin receptor. This is further supported by the fact that some somatostatin analogs have not been successful in limiting the intimal hyperplastic response.[113] Nonetheless, the concept of the vascular tree functioning as a complex local hormonal system, and the possibility of altering and controlling this balance with pharmacologic therapy, remains an exciting area of investigation.

Another approach to inhibiting the effects of peptide mitogens involves the use of conjugated toxins. This concept relies on the competitive inhibition of a mitogenic receptor by a "mitotoxin" comprised of a specific growth factor that has been bound to a cytotoxin. A potent cellular growth inhibitor has recently been described that competes for the bFGF receptor.[154] This compound is formed by conjugating bFGF to the ribosome-inactivating protein saporin. In one in vivo study, bFGF-saporin caused a marked reduction in the number of replicating smooth muscle cells found in an arterial wall following a denuding injury.[77] Whether this or other conjugated mitotoxins will be effective in reducing the degree of intimal hyperplasia following arterial injury requires further investigation.

Finally, rather than inhibiting the effects of peptide growth factors at the level of their membrane-bound receptors, attempts have also been made to inhibit cellular growth by interfering with cellular proliferative pathways at the cytoplasmic level. Polyamines are felt to be important compounds in the regulation of cell growth and differentiation.[155] Because polyamines are synthesized from ornithine by the action of ornithine decarboxylase (ODC), and since this enzyme constitutes the rate-limiting step in this reaction, ODC inhibition has been postulated as a possible method of preventing cellular proliferation. This concept is supported by the fact that ODC activity is known to increase in tissues undergoing active cell division.[156] The ability of ODC inhibition to reduce the amount of intimal hyperplasia following an arterial injury has been studied in an animal model.[115] In this study, animals treated with the ODC inhibitor α-difluoromethylornithine developed significantly less intimal hyperplasia then similarly injured controls.

Anticoagulants

Heparin is a naturally occurring polymer containing chains of sulfonated mucopolysaccharides. In vivo, it is concentrated in mast cells and found in several different tissues, including the endothelium. The length, and thus molecular weight, of heparin polymers is highly variable. Furthermore, different size polymers have different anticoagulant potency.[157] Because of this variability, heparin has unpredictable biological activity and is therefore quantified in international units rather than by weight.

Heparin works through its inhibition of the plasma-bound proteolytic clotting cascade. Antithrombin III is a potent naturally occurring anticoagulant that inhibits several of the activated coagulant proteins. Certain size heparin polymers combine with antithrombin III. This binding greatly enhances the enzymatic action of antithrombin III. Also, because these bound cofactors are not consumed by the inhibition reaction, only a small amount of heparin is required when the plasma load of activated coagulant proteins is moderate. This forms the basis of low-dose heparin therapy for prophylaxis.

Clinically, heparin has been used most frequently in the prophylaxis and treatment of venous thrombosis and pulmonary emboli. A few studies have concluded that perioperative high-dose heparin can prevent early thrombosis in peripheral bypass grafts.[158] This action is presumably due to the drug's ability to shift the balance of the coagulation cascade and counteract the thrombotic forces of low-flow states and thrombogenic surfaces. Recently, heparin has also been shown to prevent smooth muscle cell migration and proliferation both in vitro and in vivo.[110,159–163] The mechanism of this action has not yet been established. One theory is that the heparin inhibits bFGF that is released by damaged medial smooth muscle cells.[70] Alternatively, Clowes and associates have postulated that heparin inhibits smooth muscle cell migration by interfering with the degradation of their surrounding extracellular matrix. Evidence supporting this view comes from the demonstration that heparin decreases the expression of both t-PA and collagenase in the arterial media.[70] Finally, available data indicate that both anticoagulant and nonanticoagulant fractions of heparin possess this antiproliferative activity.[110] Low molecular weight (LMW) heparin is a combination of short-chain heparin polymers with significantly lower anticoagulant activity than standard heparin preparations. Interest in this heparin derivative stems from its potential in modulating intimal hyperplasia without affecting the coagulation system. At least one recent study has shown that LMW heparin may be effective in this regard.[110]

FUTURE DIRECTIONS

Photodynamic Therapy

Another way to view the intimal hyperplastic response is as a process akin to that of a benign neoplastic lesion. In this scheme, the proliferating intimal smooth muscle cell is pictured as an undifferentiated pluripotent medial myofibroblast whose growth continues in the absence of normal cellular controls. The resulting lesion can be considered a form of "vascular keloid." Recently, photodynamic therapy has been shown to be safe and effective in the treatment of several rapidly growing benign neoplasms. In photodynamic therapy, a chemosensitizing agent is administered to living tissue. Differential absorption and clearance favor selective concentration of the agent in rapidly dividing cells.[164] Following exposure to light of a specific wavelength, "photoactivation" results. Once photoactivated, the chemosensitizing agent injures the tissue exposed to the light.

The mechanism by which photodynamic therapy induces cellular toxicity is still being elucidated. Photoactivation of hematoporphyrin derivatives has been hypothesized to result in the formation of oxygen species and other free radicals. These in turn induce several changes, including oxidation of membrane components, alteration of surface charges, and ultimately loss of cell membrane integrity.[165] The initial site of drug accumulation appears to be the cell membrane, but other intracellular organisms such as lysosomes, mitochondria, and nuclei are also affected.[166] Boegheim et al. reported that photodynamic therapy inactivates cytosolic, mitochondria, and lysosomal enzymes; decreases cellular adenosine triphosphate; and reduces glutathione concentration in murine fibroblasts.[167] Enzymes involved in transport across the cell membrane and related to deoxynucleic acid regulation are also inactivated after exposure to light.[167]

Because intimal hyperplasia also involves cells exhibiting increased mitotic activity, photodynamic therapy has been proposed as a means to modulate this hyperplastic response. In 1988, Neave et al. reported the destruction of fibrocellular atheroma in the aorta of rabbits treated with dihematoporphyrin ether porphyrin II.[168] Mackie et al. and Spear et al. have reported that atherosclerotic plaque preferentially absorbs hematoporphyrin II (photofrin) and that photodynamic therapy leads to ablation of only the fibrous portion of the atherosclerotic lesion.[169–171] These investigators were discouraged that the atherosclerotic plaque could not be ablated completely due to the remaining calcified noncellular material. Nevertheless, these experiments showed that photodynamic therapy could ablate a fibrosclerotic plaque.

The potential for using photodynamic therapy for intimal hyperplasia (rather than atherosclerosis) was perhaps most convincingly suggested by Dartsch et al., who showed that human-derived intimal hyperplasia smooth muscle cells preferentially absorbed photofrin II and that subsequent exposure to light significantly inhibited growth of the photofrin II–bound cells.[172–174] Meanwhile, cells derived from normal arteries remained uninhibited in vitro. The ability of human intimal hyperplastic lesions to selectively absorb porphyrin compounds in vivo has not been demonstrated. However, photodynamic therapy remains an intriguing area of investigation in the treatment of intimal hyperplasia.

Modulation of the Immune System

The contribution of inflammatory mediators in the pathophysiology of intimal hyperplasia has already been discussed. It is possible that these same pathways could be manipulated to control these very same processes. Immunotherapy for a variety of neoplastic conditions has emerged as an exciting new area of research. The basic idea of programming the body's own immune defenses against specific antigens located on the surface of offending tumor cells is likely to be applicable to other conditions as well.

Activated T lymphocytes have already been detected in atherosclerotic plaques.[142] These lymphocytes produce gamma interferon and various interleukins that promote expression of class II major histocompatibility antigens and perpetuate the immune response. Future work in directing this response against specific smooth muscle cell antigens expressed within intimal hyperplastic lesions may provide an exciting new research direction.

In Vivo Gene Transfer

The development of the technology to transfer genetic material into human vascular cells has opened up new frontiers in the treatment of vascular disorders. Gene transfer methods are yielding important information regarding the biology of several types of vascular cells, and treatment strategies for problems such as thrombosis, atherosclerosis, vasculitis, and restenosis are already being devised.

The basic technique involves the introduction of new genetic material into the genome of various vascular cells. These genetically engineered cells subsequently express specific proteins or traits for which they have been programmed that ultimately alter the local biology of the vessel wall. The endothelial cell is often proposed as the ideal recipient for human gene therapy. This is largely due to its accessibility to recombinant vectors as well as the possibility for any produced products to be secreted directly into the bloodstream. Furthermore, endothelial seeding of vascular grafts and stents is an area of research that is currently in relatively advanced stages of development. Gene transfer into vascular endothelial cells has primarily been accomplished by one of two different methods. The first method involves the introduction of genes into cultured endothelial cells in vitro. Later these "engineered" cells are reintroduced into the vessel wall of the recipient. Alternatively, in vivo gene transfer into the vessel wall has been performed by injecting the genetic material directly into the lumen of the host vessel. This method requires either a retroviral or plasmid vector in order to successfully transfer new genes.

Several in vitro experiments have documented the ability to transfer specific genes into cultured endothelial cells.[175–177] In these studies, genes coding for neomycin resistance,[175,177] β-galactosidase,[176,177] growth hormone,[175] prostacyclin,[177] and t-PA[176] have all been successfully expressed. Furthermore, transduced endothelial cells have been shown to grow on both vascular prostheses[175] and stainless steel stents.[176]

Recently, recombinant gene expression by transduced endothelial cells has also been achieved in vivo. In a series of experiments, Nabel and associates have successfully transferred the genes responsible for β-galactosidase production into iliofemoral arterial segments of pigs.[178,179] These investigators have documented detectable levels of the transduced gene in this model for as long as 5 months.[179] The ability of a vascular graft lined with genetically modified endothelial cells to maintain activity of the transduced gene has also recently been demonstrated.[180] In this study, grafts continued to express the β-galactosidase gene for up to 5 weeks following implantation. Furthermore, this activity was documented in both the seeded cells and their progeny.

The potential of genetically vascular cells to modify the vessel wall and impact the development of vascular disorders is clear and research in this area is rapidly progressing. However, several problems with this technology must still be overcome and, as with any new area of research, perplexing questions are as frequent as are new advances. For example, the use of retroviral vectors limits the size of the gene that can be transduced. Also, transduction rates using these methods remain quite low and alternative methods to improve the efficiency of this process are needed. Issues requiring further investigation include the effect of transduced genes on the function of host cells, the duration of activity of these genes within the host cells, and the potential of foreign genetic material to induce a host immunologic response. Nonetheless, the potential exists for this technology to someday play a role in altering the complex pathways leading to the development of intimal hyperplasia.

REFERENCES

1. Dalman RL, Taylor LM Jr: Basic data related to infrainguinal revascularization procedures. Ann Vasc Surg 3(3):309–312, 1990.
2. Healy DA, Clowes AW, Zierler RE, Nicholls SC, Bergelin RO, Primozich JF, Strandness DE: Immediate and long-term results of carotid endarterectomy. Stroke 20:1138–1142, 1989.
3. Healy DA, Zierler RE, Nicholls SC, et al: Long-term follow-up and clinical outcome of carotid restenosis. J Vasc Surg 10:662–669, 1989.
4. Bernstein EF, Torem S, Dilley RB: Does carotid restenosis predict an increased risk of late symptoms, stroke, or death? Ann Surg 212(5):629–636, 1990.
5. Imparato AM, Bracco A, Kim GE, Zeff RZ: Intimal and neointimal fibrous proliferation causing failure of arterial reconstructions. Surgery 72:1107–1117, 1972.
6. Carrel A, Guthrie CC: Anastomosis of blood vessels by the patching method and transplantation of the kidney. JAMA 47:1648–1651, 1906.
7. Spaet TH, Stemerman MB, Veith FJ, Lejnieks I: Intimal injury and regrowth in the rabbit aorta: Medial smooth muscle cells as a source of neointima. Circ Res 36:58–70, 1975.
8. Clowes AW, Schwartz SM: Significance of quiescent smooth muscle migration in the injured rat carotid artery. Circ Res 56:139–145, 1985.
9. Clowes AW, Clowes MM, Fingerle J, Reidy MA: Regulation of smooth muscle cell growth in injured artery. J Cardiovasc Pharmacol 14(suppl 6):S12–S15, 1989.
10. Chervu A, Moore WS: An overview of intimal hyperplasia. Surg Gynecol Obstet 171:433–447, 1990.
11. Rittgers SE, Karayannacos PE, Guy JF, et al: Velocity distribution and intimal proliferation in autologous vein grafts in dogs. Circ Res 42:792–801, 1978.
12. Morinaga K, Okadome K, Kuroki M, et al: Effect of wall shear stress on intimal thickening of arterially transplanted autogenous veins in dogs. J Vasc Surg 2:430–433, 1985.
13. Sottiurai VS, Kollros P, Glagov S, et al: Morphological alteration of cultured arterial smooth muscle cells by cyclic stretching. J Surg Res 35:490–497, 1983.
14. Imparato AM, Baumann FG, Pearson J, et al: Electron microscopic studies of experimentally produced fibromuscular arterial lesions. Surg Gynecol Obstet 139:497–504, 1974.
15. Bond MG, Hostetler JR, Karayannacos PE, et al: Intimal changes in arteriovenous bypass grafts: Effects of varying the angle of implantation at the proximal anastomosis and of producing stenosis in the distal runoff artery. J Thorac Cardiovasc Surg 71:907–916, 1976.
16. Berguer R, Higgins RF, Reddy DJ: Intimal hyperplasia: An experimental study. Arch Surg 115:332–335, 1980.
17. Zarins CK, Zatina MA, Giddens DP, et al: Shear stress regulation of artery lumen diameter in experimental atherogenesis. J Vasc Surg 5:413–420, 1987.
18. Caro CG, Fitz-Gerald JM, Schroter RC: Arterial wall shear: Observation, correlation and proposal of a shear dependent mass transfer mechanism for atherogenesis. Proc R Soc Lond 177:109–159, 1971.
19. Fry DL: Acute vascular endothelial changes associated with increased blood velocity gradients. Circ Res 22:165–167, 1968.
20. LoGerfo FW, Nowak MD, Quist WC, et al: Flow studies in a model carotid bifurcation. Atherosclerosis 1:235–241, 1981.
21. Phillips DJ, Greene FM, Langlois Y, et al: Flow velocity patterns in the carotid bifurcations of young, presumed normal subjects. Ultrasound Med Biol 9:39–49, 1983.
22. Abbott WM, Megerman J, Hasson JE, et al: Effect of compliance mismatch on vascular graft patency. J Vasc Surg 5:376–382, 1987.
23. Lye CR, Sumner DS, Strandness DE: The transcutaneous measurement of the elastic properties of the human saphenous vein femoropopliteal bypass graft. Surg Gynecol Obstet 141:891–895, 1975.
24. Hokanson DE, Strandness DE: Stress-strain characteristics of various arterial grafts. Surg Gynecol Obstet 127:57–60, 1968.
25. Miller JH, Foreman RK, Ferguson L, Faris A: Interposition vein cuff for anastomosis of prosthesis to small artery. Aust NZ J Surg 54:283–285, 1984.
26. Corson JD, Leather RP, Balko A, et al: Relationship between vasa vasorum and blood flow to vein bypass endothelial morphology. Arch Surg 120:386–388, 1985.
27. Abbott WM, Weiland S, Austen WG: Structural changes during preparation of autogenous venous grafts. Surgery 76:1031–1040, 1974.
28. Bang HO, Dyerberg J, Nielsen A: Plasma lipid and lipoprotein pattern in greenlandic west-coast Eskimos. Lancet 1:1143–1145, 1971.
29. Brown MS, Faust JR, Goldstein JL: Role of the low density lipoprotein receptor in regulating the content of free and esterified cholesterol in human fibroblasts. J Clin Invest 55:783, 1975.
30. Goldstein JL, Brown MS: The low-density lipoprotein pathway and its relation to atherosclerosis. Ann Rev Biochem 46:879, 1977.
31. Wissler RW: Biochemistry of Atherosclerosis, Vol 7. New York, Marcel Dekker, 1979, p 345.
32. Hanson S, Pareti F, Ruggeri Z, et al: Antibody-induced platelet inhibition reduces thrombus formation in vivo. Clin Res 34:658, 1986.
33. Torem S, Schneide P, Hanson S: Monoclonal antibody-induced inhibition of platelet function: Effects on hemostasis and vascular graft thrombosis in baboons. J Vasc Surg 7:172–180, 1988.
34. Grotendorst G, Chang T, Seppa H, et al: Platelet derived growth factor is a chemoattractant for vascular smooth muscle cells. J Cell Physiol 113:261–266, 1982.
35. Collins T, Ginsburg D, Boss J, et al: Cultured human endothelial cells express platelet-derived growth factor B chain: cDNA cloning and structural analysis. Nature 316:748–750, 1985.
36. Barrett T, Benditt E: Platelet-derived growth factor gene expression in human atherosclerotic plaques and in nor-

mal artery wall. Proc Natl Acad Sci USA 85:2810–2814, 1988.

37. Majesky M, Reidy M, Benditt EP, Schwartz S: Expression of platelet-derived growth factor (PDGF) A- and B-chain gene in smooth muscle during repair of arterial injury. J Mol Cell Cardiol 19(suppl IV):S3, 1987.

38. Libby P, Warner S, Salomon R, Birinyi L: Production of platelet-derived growth factor-like mitogen by smooth muscle cells from human atheroma. N Engl J Med 318:1493–1498, 1988.

39. Cole C, Lucas J, Mikat E, et al: Adherence of polymorphonuclear leukocytes to injured rabbit aorta. Surg Forum 35:440–442, 1984.

40. Lucas J, Makhoul R, Cole C, et al: Mononuclear cells adhere to sites of vascular balloon catheter injury. Curr Surg 43:112–115, 1986.

41. Joris I, Stetz E, Majno G: Lymphocytes and monocytes in the aortic intima: An electron-microscopic study in the rat. Atherosclerosis 34:221–231, 1979.

42. Prescott MF, McBride CK, Venturini CM, Gerhardt SC: Leukocyte stimulation of intimal lesion formation is inhibited by treatment with diclofenac sodium and dexamethasone. J Cardiovasc Pharmacol 14(suppl 6):S76–S84, 1989.

43. Mazzone T, Jensen M, Chait A: Human arterial wall cells secrete factors that are chemotactic for monocytes. Proc Natl Acad Sci USA 80:5094–5097, 1983.

44. Leibovich S, Ross R: A macrophage-dependent factor that stimulates the proliferation of fibroblasts in vitro. Am J Pathol 84:501–513, 1976.

45. Shimokado K, Raines E, Madtes D, et al: A significant part of macrophage-derived growth factor consists of at least two forms of PDGF. Cell 43:277–286, 1988.

46. Sacks T, Moldow C, Craddock P, Bowers T: Oxygen radicals mediate endothelial cell damage by complement-stimulated granulocytes: An in vitro model of immune vascular damage. J Clin Invest 61:1161–1167, 1978.

47. Swales JD, Thurston H: Generation of angiotensin II of peripheral vascular level: Studies using angiotensin II antisera. Clin Sci Mol Med 45:691–700, 1973.

48. Dzau VJ: Vascular angiotensin pathways: A new therapeutic target. J Cardiovasc Pharmacol 10(suppl 7):S9–S16, 1987.

49. Campbell DJ, Habener JF: Angiotensin gene is expressed and differentially regulated in multiple tissues of the rat. J Clin Invest 78:31–39, 1986.

50. Campbell DJ: Tissue renin-angiotensin system: Sites of angiotensin formation. J Cardiovasc Pharmacol 10(suppl 7):S1–S8, 1987.

51. Molteni A, Dzau VJ, Fallon JT, Haber E: Monoclonal antibodies as probes of renin gene expression. Circulation 70(suppl II):II-196, 1984.

52. Re R, Fallon JT, Dzau VJ, Ouay SC, Haber E: Renin synthesis by canine aortic smooth muscle cells in culture. Life Sci 30:99–106, 1982.

53. Lilly LS, Pratt RE, Alexander RW, et al: Renin expression by vascular endothelial cells in culture. Circ Res 57:312–318, 1985.

54. Ohashi H, Matsunaga N, Pak CH, Kawai C: Serial change in renin release by the cultured human vascular smooth muscle cells. J Hypertens 4(suppl 6):S472–S473, 1986.

55. Drouet L, Baudin B, Baumann FC, Caen JP: Serum angiotensin-converting enzyme: An endothelial cell marker. J Lab Clin Med 112:450–457, 1988.

56. Penit J, Faure M, Jard S: Vasopressin and angiotensin II receptors in rat aortic smooth muscle cells in culture. Am J Physiol 244:E72–E82, 1983.

57. Griendling K, Tsuda T, Berk BC, Alexander RW: Angiotensin II stimulation of vascular smooth muscle. J Cardiovasc Pharmacol 14(suppl 6):S27–S33, 1989.

58. Moore T, Williams G: Angiotensin II receptors on human platelets. Circ Res 51:314–320, 1982.

59. Gimbrone M, Alexander RW: Angiotensin II stimulation of prostaglandin production in cultured human vascular endothelium. Science 189:219–220, 1975.

60. Toda N: Endothelium-dependent relaxation induced by an-

giotensin II and histamine in isolated arteries of dog. Br J Pharmacol 81:301–307, 1984.

61. Campbell-Boswell M, Robertson AL: Effects of angiotensin II and vasopressin on human smooth muscle cells in vitro. Exp Mol Pathol 35:265, 1981.

62. Geisterfer AA, Peach MJ, Owens JK: Angiotensin II induces hypertrophy, not hyperplasia, of cultured rat aortic smooth muscle cells. Circ Res 62:749–756, 1988.

63. Jackson TR, Blair LAC, Marshall J, Goedert M, Hanley MR: The *mas* oncogene encodes an angiotensin receptor. Nature 335:437–440, 1988.

64. Swartz S, Moore T: Effect of angiotensin II on collagen-induced platelet activation in normotensive subjects. Thromb Haemost 63(1):87–90, 1990.

65. Naftilan AJ, Pratt RE, Dzau VJ: Induction of platelet-derived growth factor A-chain and *c-myc* gene expressions by angiotensin II in cultured rat vascular smooth muscle cells. J Clin Invest 83:1419–1424, 1989.

66. Folkman J, Klagsbrun M: Angiogenic factors. Science 235:442–447, 1987.

67. Fingerle J, Johnson R, Clowes AW, Majesky MW, Reidy MA: Role of platelets in smooth muscle proliferation and migration after vascular injury in rat carotid artery. Proc Natl Acad Sci USA 86:8412–8416, 1989.

68. Clowes AW, Reidy MA, Clowes MM: Kinetics of cellular proliferation after arterial injury. I. Smooth muscle growth in the absence of endothelium. Lab Invest 49:327–333, 1983.

69. Fingerle J, Au YPT, Clowes AW, Reidy MA: Intimal lesion formation in the rat carotid arteries after endothelial denudation in the absence of medial injury. Arteriosclerosis 10:1082–1087, 1990.

70. Clowes AW, Reidy MA: Prevention of stenosis after vascular reconstruction: Pharmacologic control of intimal hyperplasia—a review. J Vasc Surg 13(6):885–891, 1991.

71. Gospodarowicz D, Ferrara N, Haaparanta T, Neufeld G: Basic fibroblast growth factor: Expression in cultured bovine vascular smooth muscle cells. Eur J Cell Biol 46:144–151, 1988.

72. Weich HA, Iberg N, Klagsbrun M, Folkman J: Expression of acidic and basic fibroblast growth factors in human and bovine vascular smooth muscle cells. Growth Factors 2:313–320, 1990.

73. McNeil PL, Muthukrishnan L, Warder E, D'Amore PA: Growth factors are released by mechanically wounded endothelial cells. J Cell Biol 109:811–822, 1989.

74. Gospodarowicz D, Ferrara N, Schweigerer L, Neufeld G: Structural characterization and biological functions of fibroblast growth factor. Endocr Rev 8:95–114, 1987.

75. Baird A, Walicke PA: Fibroblast growth factors. Br Med J 45:438–452, 1989.

76. Cuevas P, Gonzalez AM, Carceller F, Baird A: Vascular response to basic fibroblast growth factor when infused onto the normal adventitia or into the injured media of the rat carotid artery. Circ Res 69:360–369, 1991.

77. Lindner V, Lappi DA, Baird A, Majack RA, Reidy MA: Role of basic fibroblast growth factor in vascular lesion formation. Circ Res 68:106–113, 1991.

78. Clowes AW, Collazzo RE, Karnovsky MJ: A morphologic and permeability study of luminal smooth muscle cells after arterial injury in the rat. Lab Invest 39:141–150, 1978.

79. Werb Z, Mainardi C, Vater CA, Harris ED: Endogenous activation of latent collagenase by rheumatoid synovial cells: Evidence for a role of plasminogen activator. N Engl J Med 296:1017–1023, 1977.

80. Levin EG, Loskutoff DJ: Comparative studies of the fibrinolytic activity of cultured vascular cells. Thromb Res 15:869–878, 1979.

81. Goldsmith GH, Ziats NP, Robertson AL: Studies on plasminogen activator and other proteases in subcultured human vascular cells. Exp Mol Pathol 35:257–264, 1981.

82. Clowes AW, Clowes MM, Au YPT, Reidy MA, Belin D: Smooth muscle cells express urokinase during mitogenesis and tissue-type plasminogen activator during mi-

gration in injured rat carotid artery. Circ Res *67*:61–67, 1990.

83. Szilagyi DE, Elliott JP, Hageman JH, et al: Biologic fate of autologous vein implants as arterial substitutes: Clinical, angiographic and histologic observations in femoropopliteal operations for atherosclerosis. Ann Surg *178*:232–246, 1973.

84. Stoney RJ, String ST: Recurrent carotid stenosis. Surgery *80*:705–710, 1976.

85. Cossman D, Callow AD, Stein A, Matsumoto G: Early restenosis after carotid endarterectomy. Arch Surg *113*:275–278, 1978.

86. Kremen JE, Gee W, Kaupp HA, McDonald KM: Restenosis or occlusion after carotid endarterectomy. Arch Surg *114*:608–610, 1979.

87. Hertzer NR, Martinez BD, Benjamin SP, Beven EG: Recurrent stenosis after carotid endarterectomy. Surg Gynecol Obstet *149*:360–364, 1979.

88. Cossman DV, Treiman RL, Foran RF, Levin PM, Cohen DL: Surgical approach to recurrent carotid stenosis. Am J Surg *140*:209–211, 1980.

89. Catelmo NL, Cutler BS, Wheeler HB, Herrmann JB, Cardullo PA: Noninvasive detection of carotid stenosis following endarterectomy. Arch Surg *116*:1005–1008, 1981.

90. Zierler RE, Bandyk DF, Thiele BL, Strandness DE: Carotid artery stenosis following endarterectomy. Arch Surg *117*:1408–1415, 1982.

91. Baker WH, Hayes AC, Mahler D, Littooy FN: Durability of carotid endarterectomy. Surgery *94*:112–115, 1983.

92. Salvian A, Baker JD, Machleder HI, Busuttil RW, Barker WF, Moore WS: Cause and noninvasive detection of restenosis after carotid endarterectomy. Am J Surg *146*:29–34, 1983.

93. Pierce GE, Iliopoulus JI, Holcomb MA, Rieder CF, Hermreck AS, Thomas JH: Incidence of recurrent stenosis after carotid endarterectomy determined by digital subtraction angiography. Am J Surg *148*:848–854, 1984.

94. O'Donnell TF, Callow AD, Scott G, Shepard AD, Heggerick P, Mackey WC: Ultrasound characteristics of recurrent carotid disease: Hypothesis explaining the low incidence of symptomatic recurrence. J Vasc Surg *2*:26–41, 1985.

95. Wilson SE, Sheppard B: Results of percutaneous transluminal angioplasty for peripheral vascular occlusive disease. Ann Vasc Surg *4*(1):94–97, 1990.

96. White RA, White GH, Mehringer MC: A clinical trial of laser thermal angioplasty in patients with advanced peripheral vascular disease. Ann Surg *211*:257–265, 1990.

97. Ahn SS, Eton D, Mehigan JT: Preliminary clinical results of rotary atherectomy. *In* Yao JST, Pearce WH (eds): Technologies in Vascular Surgery. Philadelphia, WB Saunders Company, 1992, pp 388–401.

98. Cahill PD, Sarris GE, Cooper AD, et al: Inhibition of vein graft intimal thickening by eicosapentaenoic acid: Reduced thromboxane production without change in lipoprotein levels or low-density lipoprotein receptor density. J Vasc Surg *7*:108–117, 1988.

99. Landymore RW, Manku MS, Tan M, MacAulay MA, Sheridan B: Effects of low-dose marine oils on intimal hyperplasia in autologous vein grafts. J Thorac Cardiovasc Surg *98*:788–791, 1989.

100. O-hara M, Esato K, Harada M, Kouchi Y, Akimoto F, Nakamura T, Wakamatsu T, Zempo N: Eicosapentaenoic acid suppresses intimal hyperplasia after expanded polytetrafluoroethylene grafting in rabbits fed a high cholesterol diet. J Vasc Surg *13*:480–486, 1991.

101. Quiñones-Baldrich W, Ziomek S, Henderson T, Moore W: Patency and intimal hyperplasia: The effect of aspirin on small arterial anastomosis. Ann Vasc Surg *2*(1):50–56, 1988.

102. Landymore RW, Karmazyn M, MacAulay MA, Sheridan B, Cameron CA: Correlation between the effects of aspirin and dipyridamole on platelet function and prevention of intimal hyperplasia in autologous vein grafts. Can J Cardiol *4*(1):56–59, 1988.

103. Radic ZS, O'Malley MK, Mikat EM, Makhoul RG, McCann RL, Cole CW, Hagen PO: The role of aspirin and dipyridamole on vascular DNA synthesis and intimal hyperplasia following deendothelialization. J Surg Res *41*(1):84–91, 1986.

104. Chervu A, Moore WS, Quiñones-Baldrich WJ, Henderson T: Efficacy of corticosteroids in suppression of intimal hyperplasia. J Vasc Surg *10*:129–134, 1989.

105. Hoepp LM, Elbadawi A, Cohn M, et al: Steroids and immunosuppression: Effect on anastomotic intimal hyperplasia in femoral arterial Dacron bypass grafts. Arch Surg *114*:273–276, 1979.

106. O'Malley MK, McDermott EW, Mehigan D, O'Higgins NJ: Role for prazosin in reducing the development of rabbit intimal hyperplasia after endothelial denudation. Br J Surg *76*(9):936–938, 1989.

107. Powell JS, Clozel JP, Müller RK, Kuhn H, Hefti F, Hosang M, Baumgartner HR: Inhibitors of angiotensin-converting enzyme prevent myointimal proliferation after vascular injury. Science *245*:186–188, 1989.

108. El-Sanadiki MN, Cross KS, Murray JJ, Schuman RW, Mikat E, McCann RL, Hagen P: Reduction of intimal hyperplasia and enhanced reactivity of experimental vein bypass grafts with verapamil. Ann Surg *212*(1):87–96, 1990.

109. Guyotat J, Pelissou-Guyotat I, Lievre M, Chignier E: Inhibition of subintimal hyperplasia or autologous vein bypass grafts by nimodipine in rats: A placebo-controlled study. Neurosurgery *29*:850–855, 1991.

110. Dryjski M, Mikat E, Bjornsson TD: Inhibition of intimal hyperplasia after arterial injury by heparins and heparinoid. J Vasc Surg *8*(5):623–633, 1988.

111. Calcagno D, Conte JV, Howell MH, Foegh ML: Peptide inhibition of neointimal hyperplasia in vein grafts. J Vasc Surg *13*:475–479, 1991.

112. Conte JV, Foegh ML, Calcagno D, Wallace RB, Ramwell PW: Peptide inhibition of myointimal proliferation following angioplasty in rabbits. Transplant Proc *21*:3686–3688.

113. Lundergan C, Foegh ML, Vargas R, et al: Inhibition of myointimal proliferation of the rat carotid artery by the peptides, angiopeptin and BIM 23034. Atherosclerosis *80*:49–55, 1989.

114. Foegh ML, Khirabadi BS, Chambers E, Amamoo S, Ramwell PW: Inhibition of coronary artery transplant atherosclerosis in rabbits with angiopeptin, an octapeptide. Atherosclerosis *78*(2-3):229–236, 1989.

115. Endean ED, Kispert JF, Martin KW, O'Connor W: Intimal hyperplasia is reduced by ornithine decarboxylase inhibition. J Surg Res *50*:634–637, 1991.

116. Ryan US, Whitaker C, Hart MA, et al: Structural interaction between endothelial and smooth muscle cells. J Cell Biol *79*:207a, 1979.

117. Baumgartner HR: Eine neue methode zur erzeugung von thromben durch gezielte uberdehnung der gefasswand. Z Gesamte Exp Med *137*:227, 1963.

118. Clowes AW, Clowes MM, Reidy MA: Role of acute distention in the induction of smooth muscle proliferation after arterial denudation (abstr). Fed Proc *46*:270, 1987.

119. Dyerberg J, Bang HO, Stoffersen E, Moncada S, Vane JR: Eicosapentaenoic acid and prevention of thrombosis and atherosclerosis. Lancet *2*:117–119, 1978.

120. Friedman RJ, Stemerman MB, Wenz B, Moore S, Gauldie J: The effect of thrombocytopenia on experimental arteriosclerotic lesion formation in rabbits: Smooth muscle cell proliferation and re-endothelialization. J Clin Invest *60*:1191–1201, 1977.

121. McCollum C, Crow M, Rajah S, Kester R: Anti-thrombotic therapy for vascular prosthesis. An experimental model testing platelet inhibitory drugs. Surgery *87*:668–676, 1980.

122. Oblath R, Buckley F, Green R, et al: Prevention of platelet aggregation to prosthetic vascular grafts by aspirin and dipyridamole. Surgery *84*:37–44, 1978.

123. Zammit M, Kaplan S, Sauvage L, et al: Aspirin therapy in small-caliber arterial prostheses: Long-term experimental observations. J Vasc Surg *1*:839–851, 1984.

124. Plate G, Stanson A, Hollier L, Dewanjee M: Drug effects

on platelet deposition after endothelial injury of the rabbit aorta. J Surg Res 39:258–266, 1985.

125. McCann R, Hagen P-O, Fuchs J: Aspirin and dipyridamole decrease intimal hyperplasia in experimental vein grafts. Ann Surg 191:238–243, 1980.

126. Graham LM, Brothers TE, Darvishian D, Harrell KA, Vincent CK, Burkel WE, Stanley JC: Effects of thromboxane synthetase inhibition on patency and anastomotic hyperplasia of vascular grafts. J Surg Res 46:611–615, 1989.

127. Atherton A, Born G: Quantitative investigations of the adhesiveness of circulating polymorphonuclear leukocytes to blood vessels. J Physiol 222:447–474, 1972.

128. Gordon GB, Bush DE, Weisman HF: Reduction of atherosclerosis by administration of dehydroepiandrosterone. J Clin Invest 82:712–720, 1988.

129. Pepine C, Hirshfeld JW, Macdonald RG, et al: A controlled trial of corticosteroids to prevent restenosis after coronary angioplasty. Circulation 81:1753–1761, 1990.

130. Colburn MD, Moore WS, Gelabert HA, Quiñones-Baldrich WJ: Dose responsive suppression of myointimal hyperplasia by dexamethasone. J Vasc Surg 15:510–518, 1992.

131. Ruhmann AG, Berliner DL: Effects of steroids on growth of mouse fibroblasts in vitro. Endocrinology 76:916–927, 1965.

132. Pratt WB: The mechanism of glucocorticoid effects in fibroblasts. J Invest Dermatol 71(1):24–35, 1978.

133. Majeski JA, Alexander JW: The steroid effect on the in vitro human neutrophil chemotactic response. J Surg Res 21:265–271, 1976.

134. Hammerschmidt D, White J, Craddock P, Jacob H: Corticosteroids inhibit complement-induced granulocyte aggregation: A possible mechanism for their efficacy in shock states. J Clin Invest 63:798–803, 1979.

135. Kurihara A, Ohuchi K, Tsurufuji S: Reduction by dexamethasone of chemotactic activity in inflammatory exudates. Eur J Pharmacol 101:11–16, 1984.

136. Oseas R, Allen J, Yang H-H, et al: Mechanism of dexamethasone inhibition of chemotactic factor induced granulocyte aggregation. Blood 59:265–269, 1982.

137. Boxer LA, Richardson SB, Bachner RL: Effects of surface-active agents on neutrophil receptors. Infect Immun 21:28, 1978.

138. Mishler J: The effects of corticosteroids on mobilization and function of neutrophils. Exp Hematol 5:15–32, 1977.

139. MacGregor R, Spagnuolo P, Lentnek A: Inhibition of granulocyte adherence by ethanol, prednisone, and aspirin measured with a new assay system. N Engl J Med 29(81):642–646, 1974.

140. Goldstein I, Roos D, Weissmann G, Kaplan H: Influence of corticosteroids on human polymorphonuclear leukocyte function in vitro enzyme release and superoxide production. Inflammation 1:305–315, 1976.

141. Pearce J, Dujovny M, Ho K, et al: Acute inflammation and endothelial injury in vein grafts. Neurosurgery 17:626–634, 1985.

142. Hansson GK, Holm J, Jonasson L: Detection of activated T lymphocytes in the human atherosclerotic plaque. Am J Pathol 135:169–175, 1989.

143. Wengrovitz M, Selassie LG, Gifford RRM, Thiele BL: Cyclosporine inhibits the development of medial thickening after experimental arterial injury. J Vasc Surg 12(1):1–7, 1990.

144. O'Donohoe MK, Schwartz LB, Radic ZS, Mikat EM, McCann RL, Hagen P-O: Chronic ACE inhibition reduces intimal hyperplasia in experimental vein grafts. Ann Surg 214:727–732, 1991.

145. Chobanian AV, Haudenschild CC, Nickerson C, Drago R: Antiatherogenic effect of captopril in the watanabe heritable hyperlipidemic rabbit. Hypertension 15:327–331, 1990.

146. Cushman DW, Ondetti MA, Gordon EM, Natarajan S, Karanewsky DS, Krapcho J, Petrillo EW: Rational design and biochemical utility of specific inhibitors of angiotensin-converting enzyme. J Cardiovasc Pharmacol 10(suppl 7):S17–S30, 1987.

147. Chopra M, Scott N, McMurray J, et al: Captopril: a free radical scavenger. Br J Clin Pharmacol 27:396–399, 1989.

148. Colburn MD, Hajjar G, Gelabert HA, Quiñones-Baldrich WJ, Moore WS: Enalaprilat, but not dimethylsulfoxide (DMSO), inhibits intimal hyperplasia in injured rabbit carotid arteries. Submitted, 1993.

149. El-Sanadiki M, Cross K, Mikat E, Hagen P-O: Verapamil therapy reduces intimal hyperplasia in balloon injured rabbit aorta. Circulation 76(suppl):314, 1987.

150. O'Malley MK, Mikat EM, McCann RL, Hagen P-O: Increased vascular sensitivity to norepinephrine following injury. Surg Forum 35:445–447, 1984.

151. O'Malley M, Cotecchia S, Hagen P-O: Receptor mediated noradrenaline supersensitivity in rabbit aortic intimal hyperplasia. Eur Surg Res 18:43, 1986.

152. Mark J: The polyphosphoinositides revisited. Science 228:312–313, 1985.

153. Vargas R, Bormes GW, Wroblewska B, Foegh ML, Kot PA, Ramwell PW: Angiopeptin inhibits thymidine incorporation in rat carotid artery in vitro. Transplant Proc 21:3702–3704, 1989.

154. Lappi DA, Martineau D, Baird A: Biological and chemical characterization of basic FGF-saporin mitotoxin. Biochem Biophys Res Commun 160:917–923, 1989.

155. Pegg AE, McCann PP: Polyamine metabolism and function. Am J Physiol 243:C212, 1982.

156. Heby O, Gray JW, Lindl PA, Marton LJ, Wilson CB: Changes in l-ornithine decarboxylase activity during the cell cycle. Biochem Biophys Res Commun 71:99, 1976.

157. Cifonelli J: The relationship of molecular weight, and sulfate content and distribution to anticoagulant activity of heparin preparations. Carbohydr Res 37:145, 1974.

158. Schweiger H, Klein P, Ruf St, Meister R: Avoiding early failure of tibial prosthetic bypass grafts. Thorac Cardiovasc Surg 35:148–150, 1987.

159. Hoover RL, Rosenberg R, Haering W, Karnovsky MJ: Inhibition of rat arterial smooth muscle cell proliferation by heparin. II. In vitro studies. Circ Res 47:578–583, 1980.

160. Majack RA, Clowes AW: Inhibition of vascular smooth muscle cell migration by heparin-like glycosaminoglycans. J Cell Physiol 118:253–256, 1984.

161. Clowes AW, Clowes MM: Kinetics of cellular proliferation after arterial injury. II. Inhibition of smooth muscle growth by heparin. Lab Invest 52:611–616, 1985.

162. Clowes AW, Clowes MM: Kinetics of cellular proliferation after arterial injury. IV. Heparin inhibits rat smooth muscle mitogenesis and migration. Circ Res 58:839–845, 1986.

163. Majesky MW, Schwartz SM, Clowes MM, Clowes AW: Heparin regulates smooth muscle S phase entry in the injured rat carotid artery. Circ Res 61:296–300, 1987.

164. Figge F, Wieland G, Manganiello L: Cancer detection and therapy. Affinity of neoplastic, embryonic, and traumatized tissue for porphyrins and metalloporphyrins. Proc Soc Exp Biol Med 68:640–641, 1948.

165. Weishaupt KR, Gomer CJ, Dougherty TJ: Identification of singlet oxygen as the cytotoxic agent in photo-inactivation of a murine tumor. Cancer Res 36:2326–2329, 1976.

166. Kessel D: Porphyrin localization: A new modality for detection and therapy of tumors. Biochem Pharmacol 33:1389–1393, 1984.

167. Boegheim JPJ, Scholte H, Dubbleman TMAR: Photodynamic effects of hematoporphyrin derivative on enzyme activities of murine L929 fibroblasts. J Photochem Photobiol 1:61–73, 1987.

168. Neave V, Giannotta S, Hyman S, Schneider J: Hematoporphyrin uptake in atherosclerotic plaques: Therapeutic potentials. Neurosurgery 23:307–312, 1988.

169. Mackie RW, Vincent GM, Fox J, Orme EC, Hammond EH, Chang-Zong C, Johnson MD: In vivo canine coronary artery laser irradiation: Photodynamic therapy using dihematoporphyrin ether and 632nm laser. A safety and dose-response relationship study. Lasers Surg Med 11:535–544, 1991.

170. Hundley RF, Weinstein R, Spears JR: Photodynamic cyto-

lysis of rat arterial smooth muscle cells with hematopor-phyrin derivative in vitro. Lasers Life Sci 2:19–27, 1988.

171. Spears JR, Serur J, Shopshire D, et al: Fluorescence of experimental atheromatous plaques with hematoporphyrin derivative. J Clin Invest 71:395–399, 1983.

172. Dartsch PC, Ischinger T, Betz E: Differential effect of photofrin II on growth of human smooth muscle cells from nonatherosclerotic arteries and atheromatous plaques in vitro. Arteriosclerosis 10:616–624, 1990.

173. Dartsch PC, Ischinger T, Betz E: Responses of cultured smooth muscle cells from human nonatherosclerotic arteries and primary stenosing lesions after photoradiation: Implications for photodynamic therapy of vascular stenoses. J Am Coll Cardiol 15:1545–1550, 1990.

174. Dartsch PC, Betz E, Ischinger T: Effect of dihematoporphyrin derivatives on cultivated human smooth muscle cells from normal and atherosclerotic vascular segments. Overview of results and implications for photodynamic therapy. Z Kardiol 80:6–14, 1991.

175. Zwiebel JA, Freeman SM, Kantoff PW, Cornetta K, Ryan

US, Anderson WF: High-level recombinant gene expression in rabbit endothelial cells transduced by retroviral vectors. Science 243:220–222, 1989.

176. Dichek DA, Neville RF, Zwiebel JA, Freeman SM, Leon MB, Anderson WF: Seeding of intravascular stents with genetically engineered endothelial cells. Circulation 80:1347–1353, 1989.

177. Brothers TE, Stanley JC: Impact of genetic engineering on vascular disease and biology. *In* Veith FJ (ed): Current Critical Problems in Vascular Surgery. St. Louis, Quality Medical Publishers, 1990, pp 42–50.

178. Nabel EG, Plautz G, Boyce FM, Stanley JC, Nabel GJ: Recombinant gene expression in vivo within endothelial cells of the arterial wall. Science 244:1342–1344, 1989.

179. Nabel EG, Plautz G, Nabel GJ: Site-specific gene expression in vivo by direct gene transfer into the arterial wall. Science 249:1285–1288, 1990.

180. Wilson JM, Birinyi LK, Salomon RN, Libby P, Callow AD, Mulligan RC: Implantation of vascular grafts lined with genetically modified endothelial cells. Science 244:1344–1346, 1989.

38

INFECTION IN PROSTHETIC VASCULAR GRAFTS

WESLEY S. MOORE and DAVID H. DEATON

The development of prosthetic materials for use as vascular substitutes has made possible many of the reconstructive procedures presently employed in the management of vascular disorders. Despite a relatively low incidence, the profound consequences of infection make sepsis the major catastrophe associated with the use of vascular grafts. This chapter deals with current methods of diagnosis and management of this grave complication and reviews techniques that may help to prevent its occurrence.

INCIDENCE

Vascular graft infection is rare and may occur at any time after implantation. There are no published prospective series to document the true incidence of vascular graft infection following reconstructive surgery, but a reasonable approximation can be made by reviewing large retrospective series that have follow-up data that extend for longer than 5 years. Table 38-1 summarizes several such series.[1-6] The incidence of graft infection ranged from 1.34 per cent when the study was confined to aortic prostheses to as high as 6 per cent when the series included grafts in the femoropopliteal position. The data in this table serve to emphasize the serious implications of prosthetic graft infection: The mortality rate is as high as 75 per cent when an infected aortic prosthesis is involved, and as many as 75 per cent of the patients who undergo successful treatment eventually lose a limb.

ETIOLOGY

While there are several potential sources for bacterial contamination, probably the most common cause of vascular sepsis is bacterial contamination at the time of implantation. The origin of bacterial inoculation may be the graft itself, or surgical instruments, as a result of inadequate sterilization practices. These sources are unusual. Graft contamination at the time of implantation may result from bacteria originating with the surgical team or with the host. Breaks in surgical technique that allow the prosthesis to come in contact with exposed skin or the edge of the wound are an important and frequently overlooked cause of bacterial seeding. Unlike tissues that have the potential to handle contamination with normal host defense mechanisms, a prosthetic graft is inert and will harbor bacteria indefinitely, since it is a multifibered foreign body. The risk of skin contamination is enhanced by placement of the prosthesis in a superficial position, such as a subcutaneous femoropopliteal graft.[7] Another source of bacterial contamination of prosthetic grafts is from infected lymph. Lymph channels that drain compromised tissues, such as a gangrenous lower extremity, are a potential source of direct contamination of prosthetic grafts.[8] This is particularly true of groin incisions, where lymph nodes or open lymphatics may contain bacteria with the potential to contaminate the field where a graft is positioned. A less well understood source of sepsis is the diseased vessel itself. Bacteria may be harbored by atherosclerotic vessels themselves or in associated thrombus such as is found lining the lumen of an aneurysm.[9] A recent prospective study of patients undergoing peripheral arterial bypass surgery revealed an incidence of positive arterial wall cultures of 41 per cent. Of the positive cultures, 68 per cent were coagulase-negative *Staphylococcus*, of which half were slime producers.[10]

While direct contamination at the time of implantation is the most common mode of contamination, the prosthesis may also be seeded by hematogenous transfer of organisms from remote sites. In experimental animals the infusion of 10^7 organisms of *Staphylococcus aureus* immediately following implantation of a prosthetic graft in the abdominal aorta resulted in a 100 per cent incidence of graft infection.[11,12] Later studies carried out at intervals following implantation show a lesser rate of graft sepsis

TABLE 38–1.   ANALYSIS OF INFECTED GRAFT SERIES

Series	Incidence (%)	Mortality (%)	Limb Loss (%)	Predominating Organisms	No. of Patients	Graft Location	No. of Patients
Hoffert et al.[4]	6 (12 patients)	25 (3 patients)	75 (9 patients)	S. aureus	7	Femoropopliteal	7
Fry and Lindenauer[2]	1.34	75 (9 patients)	8 (1 patient)	S. aureus	8	Aortoiliac and aortofemoral	12
Conn et al.[1] (1970)	5 (22 patients)	46 (9 patients)	38 (5/13 patients)	Gram-negative	15	Femoropopliteal	9
				S. aureus	8	Aortoiliac	5
						Aortofemoral	5
						Autogenous	2
						Carotid-subclavian	1
Szilagyi et al.[6]	1.5 (40/2145 patients)	37.5 (15 patients) Aortoiliac 40 Aortofemoral 58	9	S. aureus	13	Aortofemoral	20
				S. albus	6	Femoropopliteal	8
				E. coli	9	Aortoiliac	3
Goldstone and Moore[3]	20 (27 patients)	37 (10 patients)	37 (10 patients)	S. aureus	11	Aortofemoral	15
				S. albus	7	Aortoiliac	5
				E. coli	4	Axillofemoral	3
				Pseudomonas	2	Femoropoliteal	4
				Providencia	1		
				Unknown	2		
Reilly et al.[5]		40 (14/32)	25			Aortoenteric fistula	32
		14 (8/57)	25			Perigraft infection	57

that correlates with the incorporation of the prosthesis into a fibrous capsule and the development of a pseudointima.[13,14] Nevertheless, the vulnerability of prosthetic grafts to infection following a standard challenge of hematogenously distributed bacteria probably persists indefinitely and has been shown to last at least 1 year following implantation. Data have been published showing that 30 per cent of aortic grafts challenged by a single bacterial infusion 1 year after implantation became infected. It was of interest that the anatomic difference between noninfected and infected grafts was the presence of a complete neointimal lining.[11] The potential for transient bacteremia to colonize Dacron grafts has been recently reconfirmed in an elegant study by Leport et al.[15] The authors produced transient bacteremia in a group of dogs with thoracoabdominal grafts by an intravenous infusion of 6×10^8 organisms of S. aureus. Two hours later, the grafts were harvested and colony-forming units of S. aureus were counted with scanning electron microscopy. Graft implantation times prior to bacteremia included 2 hours, 8 days, 1 month, 2 months, and 6 months. The number of colony-forming units precipitously dropped as a function of prior implantation time, further corroborating the importance of neointimal healing in providing a protective insulation against bacteremic seeding.[11,13,14] The authors also pointed out that the bacterial entrapment was related to the amount of fibrin deposits, unorganized thrombotic matrix, and presence of bare polyester filaments.

The significance of remote contamination in the clinical realm is unknown, but it does suggest that transient bacteremia associated with such things as dental procedures, insertion of urinary catheters, and septic phlebitis from intravenous lines have the potential to cause graft infection and may account for some of the clinical occurrences of this phenomenon, sometimes many years following graft implantation.

Graft infection has been reported to occur as late as 7 years following the surgical procedure; it seems unlikely that contamination at the time of implantation would take this time to develop to a clinically recognizable degree. Pseudointima that is incompletely developed, or becomes injured in any way, could expose the prosthesis to bacterial seeding during a period of bacteremia and may account for many of these late occurrences of graft sepsis.[11,12]

BACTERIOLOGY

Staphylococcus aureus, Staphylococcus epidermidis, and *Escherichia coli* are the causative organisms in approximately 80 per cent of graft infections. Other organisms such as *Klebsiella, Proteus, Enterobacter, Pseudomonas, Bacteroides,* and nonhemolytic streptococci account for the remainder.[7,16]

Staphylococcus epidermidis has emerged as a particularly difficult organism. It secretes a biofilm made up of a glycocalyx that insulates the bacteria and prevents its growth using standard bacteriology techniques. The graft infection that is produced has unusual characteristics that include a sterile exudate, absence of graft incorporation, and a normal leukocyte count.[17] The difficulty in obtaining a positive culture has often led to delay in diagnosis. Surgeons have explained such findings as an "allergic" reaction to the prosthesis.[18] Recently, Bergamini and colleagues have advocated the use of high-frequency sonication as a way to "shake loose" the bacteria from their protective biofilm and permit culture in broth. They demonstrated that the bacterial recovery was only 30 per cent when plated on agar media. This rose to 72 per cent in broth media, and rose further to 83 per cent with a combination of sonication and broth media.[19]

As a part of the effort to preserve infected grafts

or to replace them in situ, a number of investigators have tried to differentiate the pathogenicity of various organisms responsible for graft infections. A recent study in dogs demonstrated the relative virulence of *Pseudomonas aeruginosa* as opposed to the indolent nature of *Staphylococcus epidermidis* with respect to graft thrombosis, aneurysmal degeneration, and rupture.[20]

NATURAL HISTORY OF A GRAFT INFECTION

The natural history of prosthetic graft infection has been demonstrated by failed attempts at conservative management and by the observation of cases in which the correct diagnosis was not reached before disastrous consequences occurred. Infection in a prosthetic graft may begin at any site along its course, at the site of an anastomosis or in its midportion. If the infectious process has a path of drainage it may remain localized to that portion of the graft, but if confined, will extend along the potential space between the fibrous capsule and the wall of the graft until the entire prosthesis is involved.

If the infectious process remains localized and away from an anastomosis, the only immediate consequence is continued low-grade sepsis. The only exception is that of exposed vein grafts in suppurating wounds, which have a very significant incidence of rupture and life-threatening hemorrhage if not recognized and treated immediately with débridement and soft tissue coverage. More extensive destruction will occur if an anastomosis becomes involved. Infection at the site of an anastomosis will lead to destruction of the host artery with disruption of the anastomosis and the development of an infected false aneurysm or thrombosis. Subsequent events will be determined by the site of this process. For example, if the infection involves an anastomosis in the abdomen, erosion into the adjacent bowel may occur. This may present clinically with gastrointestinal bleeding from an aortoenteric fistula (Fig. 38–1). When an affected anastomosis is in the groin or midextremity, its enlargement and compression of adjacent structures will be more apparent to the patient and his physician. Bleeding in the latter instance will be confined to the soft tissue spaces of the limb, whereas in aortoenteric fistula there may be exsanguinating hemorrhage. Regardless of the location, infection that involves an anastomosis ultimately results in disruption and hemorrhage.

CLINICAL MANIFESTATIONS

The diagnosis of a prosthetic graft infection is often difficult, particularly when the graft is confined to the abdomen. The possibility of infection should be considered in any patient with a prosthesis in whom an otherwise unexplained illness develops. It is the

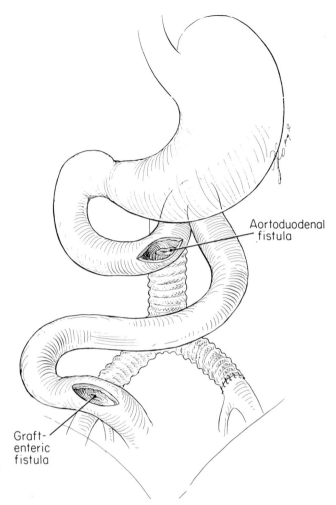

FIGURE 38–1. A communication may develop between the bowel lumen and the graft. Hemorrhage may be due to a direct communication between the aorta and the bowel (aortoenteric fistula) or from vessels in the bowel wall that have been eroded by the prosthetic graft (enteroparaprosthetic fistula).

responsibility of the clinician to prove that a graft infection is not present under these circumstances.

Acute graft infection in the immediate postoperative period is rare, and the diagnosis is usually obvious, since it frequently follows wound sepsis. Relatively superficial grafts, such as those in the femoral or popliteal artery, are vulnerable to infection from direct extension of a wound infection.[7] If the graft is visible after a purulent collection in the wound is drained, prosthetic infection is an obvious diagnosis. Acute infection can also occur in an abdominal graft and should be suspected if abdominal signs persist longer than the usual period of postoperative ileus.

Infection in a prosthetic graft usually occurs months to years following implantation.

Systemic Findings

Prosthetic graft infection may be caused by organisms of low virulence and the usual systemic manifestations of sepsis may be absent. Fever, for example, is not always present in patients with prosthetic graft infection. However, graft infection must be suspected when fever of unexplained origin is present in a patient with a prosthetic graft in place. An *increase in the erythrocyte sedimentation rate* is one of the most constant features of graft sepsis. This has been verified in experimental studies,[11] but the lack of specificity limits its usefulness unless other information is available to confirm the diagnosis. *Septic embolization*, while rare, is one of the classic signs of vascular sepsis and is strong presumptive evidence of graft infection in this clinical setting. Septic emboli present as clusters of petechiae on the skin of the extremity downstream from the infected prosthesis. Another rare but important observation is that hypertrophic osteoarthropathy may develop in limbs distal to an infected graft and should lead the clinician to suspect graft infection as the underlying cause.[21] *Leukocytosis*, frequently accompanied by a left shift, may be present. However, the absence of leukocytosis does not rule out graft infection. Indeed, infection with *Staphylococcus epidermidis* rarely demonstrates any of these systemic signs and is now thought to be one of the most common infecting organisms.[10]

Sepsis in Specific Graft Sites

Aortoiliac Graft Infection

Graft sepsis in this location is associated with abdominal or back signs and symptoms. Vague abdominal or back pain may be the early manifestation of graft infection. As the inflammatory phlegmon surrounding the infected graft enlarges, it may then compress adjacent structures such as the duodenum, small bowel, ureter, or iliac vein and produce symptoms of compression of these structures. Erosion into the duodenum or small bowel by an expanding false aneurysm may present as gastrointestinal hemorrhage. Free rupture of a false aneurysm into the abdominal cavity or the retroperitoneum will result in hemorrhagic shock.

Aortofemoral Graft Sepsis

Evidence of sepsis will usually present at one or both femoral anastomoses. When this happens, infection may be confined to the presenting portion of the involved graft, or it may be a manifestation of infection involving the entire prosthesis. Rarely will the initial presentation of an infected aortofemoral graft be within the abdomen, but it may occur and will then mimic the findings of an infected aortoiliac graft.

A false aneurysm in one or both groins is the most common presentation of an infected aortofemoral graft. This must be distinguished from a sterile or disruptive aneurysm. This distinction has become increasingly difficult given the recent recognition of *Staphylococcus epidermidis* as an occult pathogen in many collections and pseudoaneurysms that had previously been considered "sterile."[22,23] Graft sepsis may also present as a wound infection or abscess. Once this is drained, the persistence of purulent drainage from the site usually heralds the presence of an infected graft, and exploration of the tract will often disclose the true nature of the problem.

Femoropopliteal Graft Infection

The clinical presentation of a femoropopliteal graft infection is usually more obvious than sepsis in an aortic graft. It often presents as sepsis involving either the femoral or popliteal wound. Persistent drainage of an abscess or cellulitis is usually evidence of an underlying graft infection. Failure of the inflammatory process to respond to antibiotic therapy suggests a more serious infection and the need for more detailed investigation. Organisms of low virulence will slowly destroy the host artery at the site of an anastomosis and will lead to the formation of a femoral or popliteal false aneurysm.

Hemoaccess Grafts

Infections involving prosthetic renal dialysis access grafts are often related to the frequent punctures to which these grafts are subjected. These infections are usually localized processes involving the midportion of the graft where it is punctured for dialysis access. Graft exposure and aneurysmal degeneration are common and thus make rupture and uncontrolled hemorrhage a significant risk. The bacteriology of these infections is related to skin flora, in that the majority of the infections are a result of *Staphylococcus aureus*. In a recent series, approximately 50 per cent of these infections were successfully managed with partial graft excision and interposition with new graft through virgin tissue while the other grafts required complete excision.[24]

DIAGNOSTIC EVALUATION

History

Fever of unknown origin, septicemia, abdominal pain, or the development of a pulsatile mass should alert the clinician to the possibility of a graft infection. Unexplained gastrointestinal bleeding in a patient with an abdominal graft must be considered an aortoenteric fistula until proved otherwise. Recognition of the relatively nonspecific manner in which graft sepsis may present is essential if the diagnosis is to be made early, before uncontrolled bleeding occurs and the situation demands emergency rather than elective operative management. A review of the patient's previous operative notes and hospital course may provide some clues to support the presumptive diagnosis. Specifically, one should be alerted to the presence of preoperative or postoperative sepsis in the extremities or in any of the incisions. Finally, it is important to obtain a detailed history of any recent illness or invasive procedure that may have been accompanied by transient bacteremia.

Physical Examination

A careful physical examination should be directed toward identification of a tender or pulsatile mass in the area of anastomosis. The extremities should be inspected for evidence of petechiae occurring in clusters distal to prosthetic grafts as evidence of septic embolization. Cellulitis, abscesses, and a draining sinus in a scar overlying the graft are some of the more obvious manifestations of graft sepsis.

Laboratory Studies

Routine laboratory studies, including white blood cell count, erythrocyte sedimentation rate, and blood cultures, should be obtained.

Special Studies

Angiography is often helpful in evaluating a suspected graft infection. The specific finding on the angiogram is a false aneurysm at one or more anastomotic sites (Fig. 38–2).

Computed tomography (CT) can be helpful in making the diagnosis of graft sepsis. Evidence of anastomotic breakdown, false aneurysm formation, or visualiza-

tion of a fluid collection around the prosthesis is presumptive evidence of sepsis.

The value of *magnetic resonance imaging* (MRI) in the diagnosis of vascular graft infection was recently reported by Olofsson et al.[25] They reported their experience with 18 patients with presumed aortic graft sepsis who underwent preoperative MRI scanning. Twelve patients also had CT scans performed. Of the 16 patients with infection proven at operation, 14 were currently identified by MRI because of persistent perigraft fluid or the suggestion, by increased signal intensity of adjacent muscle on T_2-weighted images, of the presence of local inflammation. Conversely, CT scans in 12 patients enabled the correct diagnosis to be made in only five patients. Others have documented the appearance of uninfected grafts immediately after implantation and at 1 month postoperatively, establishing a baseline from which to compare grafts suspected of infection. These studies reveal that T_2-weighted images are only mildly enhancing in grafts undergoing the normal process of incorporation as opposed to the marked increased signal intensity of perigraft tissue in the presence of active infection.[26] The difficult diagnosis of *Staphylococcus epidermidis* infection has also been shown to be enhanced using MRI. Peter et al. have shown that dogs bearing polytetrafluoroethylene (PTFE) grafts intentionally infected with *Staphylococcus epidermidis* were correctly diagnosed by MRI, while angiography missed anastamotic disruption in three of six dogs.[27] Magnetic resonance imaging is also helpful in delineating the extent of the infection, as it is sensitive for the inflammatory process and will therefore allow

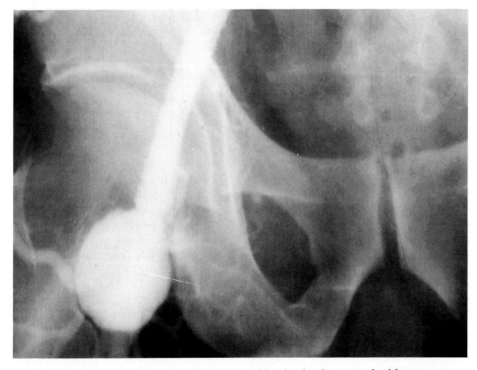

FIGURE 38–2. Graft infection was first manifested by the development of a false aneurysm.

better preoperative planning when graft preservation is a consideration. As experience with this modality grows, its utility and role in the diagnosis of prosthetic graft infection will become more defined and, quite likely, more prominent.

Scanning with ^{62}Ga- *or* ^{111}In-*labeled white blood cells* (WBCs) is highly specific for graft sepsis when positive. The absence of nonspecific bowel uptake and higher target-to-background ratio in comparison to ^{67}Ga makes scanning with ^{111}In-labeled WBCs one of the most helpful means of establishing the diagnosis of graft infection, particularly when the graft is within the abdominal cavity.[28] LaMuraglia et al. reported their clinical experience with the new technique of *scanning with* ^{111}In-*labeled human immunoglobulin G* in 25 patients with suspected vascular infection. In 10 of 10 patients with positive scans, infection was confirmed at the involved site. In 14 of 15 patients with a negative scan, no infection has been found. There was one false-negative in a patient with aortoduodenal fistula.[29] A number of other nuclear scans using radioactive antigranulocyte antibodies[30] and labels other than ^{111}In, such as ^{99m}Tc-*hexametazine*[31] for leukocytes have shown nearly identical sensitivity and specificity for graft infections but offer no significant advantages over ^{111}In-*labeled leukocyte scans*.

Aspiration of the perigraft space may provide material that will confirm the presence of sepsis. If any material is recovered from the space around the graft it should be examined by Gram staining to determine if bacteria are present. The presence of organisms is diagnostic of graft sepsis. Cultures of this material should be taken to specifically identify the organism and its antibiotic sensitivities.

The limits of a draining sinus suspected of communicating with a prosthetic graft may be determined with an *x-ray sinogram*. This examination is especially useful, since localization of the perigraft sepsis to a well-defined area may allow for salvage of the noninfected portion of the graft. Care must be exercised in performing this procedure so that forceful injection of contaminated contrast material into a clean graft area is avoided (Fig. 38–3).

Endoscopy, as part of the investigation of gastrointestinal bleeding, must be carried out cautiously in patients with intraabdominal arterial prostheses.[32] Visualization of the prosthetic graft, of course, confirms the diagnosis. When blood clot is seen in the duodenum, it may be tempting to dislodge it in an attempt to see the graft. When an aortic prosthesis is in place the endoscopist must resist this temptation, since the clot may be all that prevents torrential bleeding from an aortoduodenal fistula. When in doubt, intraoperative endoscopy may be employed if alternative diagnoses are being entertained.

Once identified, an aneurysm at the site of an anastomosis must be differentiated from a sterile disruption of the suture line. A presumptive clinical diagnosis supported by these investigations justifies exploration.

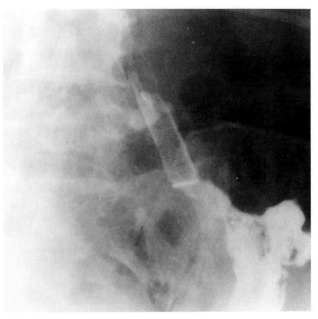

FIGURE 38–3. A sinogram demonstrates the extent of the septic process. (Note the corrugated folds of the prosthetic graft.)

MANAGEMENT OF GRAFT INFECTION

General Principles

Removal of Entire Infected Graft

This is an absolute principle when a suture line is involved. Conservative management of graft infection using drainage, débridement, systemic and topical antibiotic therapy, and the variable use of coverage with vascularized muscle flaps has been described in a number of centers. In general, these efforts are successful in managing perigraft infection limited to the groin or more distal extremity sites. Thorough débridement and coverage with a muscle pedicle, either a rotational flap or a free flap, are the central themes of this therapy.[33–36] PTFE grafts are recognized by some groups as more amenable to this form of salvage. While graft anastamoses involved in the infection represent a higher risk group, these infections have been treated successfully with débridement and vascularized soft tissue coverage. *Pseudomonas aeruginosa* infections represent a group for which graft salvage is a poor option and the risk of rupture and life-threatening hemorrhage is significantly higher. In general, the "gold standard" for graft infection remains complete excision and reconstruction, preferably with autogenous tissue, through uninfected tissue. Failure to control infection involving a prosthetic graft inevitably leads to extension to all anastomotic sites and eventual rupture and hemorrhage.

Use of Monofilament Suture

The use of braided, multifibered suture may provide the nidus for continued bacterial contamination and should be avoided when closing the arteriotomy after removal of the graft.[37] Continued sepsis in the arterial wall will lead to disruption of the arterial closure and secondary hemorrhage.

Débridement and Drainage

Even after the affected graft has been removed, sepsis in the region of the proximal aortic stump remains a threat. Blowout and late hemorrhage from the proximal aortic stump is the mode of death in many patients despite successful excision of the infected aortic graft. Every effort must be made to ensure that the aortic tissue and the surrounding structures are not involved with the infectious process. The need for radical débridement and drainage after removal of an infected graft will depend largely on the virulence of the causative organisms. When the process is caused by organisms of low virulence, little more than removal of the foreign body will be necessary. However, if the organisms are of a more virulent nature, the bed of the graft should be débrided and as much of the affected tissue as possible removed. Drainage should be provided when necessary.

Antibiotic Therapy

Large doses of specific systemic antibiotics should be administered preoperatively when the sensitivity of the organisms is known. Otherwise, broad-spectrum bactericidal antibiotics that achieve high vascular tissue levels as well as high circulating blood levels, such as penicillin or cephalosporin, should be given.[38] All traumatized tissue beds as well as superficial wounds should be generously irrigated with a topical antibiotic solution, such as a combination of bacitracin and kanamycin, prior to closure of the incisions.[39] Long-term antibiotics, given orally, should be continued for 3 to 6 months. While this may not be necessary in every case, it is probably safer and will yield the best results when applied uniformly. Malone and colleagues reviewed their clinical experience and noted a striking correlation between the presence of positive cultures from remaining arterial wall and subsequent blowout of the proximal arterial closure. This complication was prevented in patients with positive arterial wall cultures who received long-term antibiotics.[40]

Revascularization by Extraanatomic Bypass

Almost all cases of graft sepsis will require some procedure to revascularize the bed previously supplied by the infected graft.[41] This may be carried out prior to removal of the infected prosthesis or afterward. Either method may be selected in specific circumstances, but our preference is to provide for revascularization before removal of the infected graft. The wisdom of this approach has been demonstrated by Trout et al. in a study of patients with graft enteric erosions or fistulas.[42] They found an overall mortality rate of 53 per cent (40 of 75) if the infected graft removal preceded remote bypass and 17 per cent (5 of 29) if it was performed first. In performing the clean bypass procedure, care must be taken to isolate the area of infection from the operative field. Once the fresh graft is in place, the patient must be redraped so that the fresh incisions are protected before the infected graft is removed. The use of the plastic adherent dressing Op-site is a convenient way to protect fresh, clean incisions before proceeding with removal of the infected graft. This sequence also allows for the removal of the infected graft without the need for anticoagulation. The patient harboring an infected graft poses the continuous threat of transient bacteremia in spite of systemic antibiotic therapy. Experimental data suggest that fewer bacteria are seeded on PTFE grafts than other prosthetic materials when exposed to an acute bacteremic challenge.[43] These experimental implications have been shown to hold in the clinical arena in a recent retrospective comparison of Dacron and PTFE axillobifemoral grafts in which the PTFE group had a lower infection rate.[44] Our current practice is to use PTFE for bypass grafts for extraanatomic repair in situations in which there is a significant risk of bacteremia and autogenous tissue is unavailable or is an inappropriate arterial substitute.

Aortoiliac Bifurcation Graft

Extraanatomic Bypass

If the graft was a replacement for an abdominal aortic aneurysm, or if the proximal anastomosis was end to end, it is highly likely that an extraanatomic bypass will be required. Assuming that the diagnosis of graft sepsis is reasonably secure, it is advisable to proceed initially with placement of an axillobifemoral bypass graft (Fig. 38–4). A recent randomized prospective trial has shown a markedly improved patency rate for axillobifemoral grafts that utilize a flow splitter similar to that found in aortic bifurcated grafts rather than a near 90-degree takeoff for the contralateral femoral limb of the graft that is most commonly used in clinical practice. The patency rate at 2 years was approximately 84 per cent for the grafts with a flow splitter versus approximately 38 per cent for the more typical configuration.[45] After closure of the skin incisions, they may be protected with an adhesive plastic dressing before proceeding with laparotomy and removal of the aortic graft.

Remove the Entire Graft. Even if only one portion of the graft is involved it is not possible to excise that portion without contaminating the rest of the graft. Once the abdomen is open, the aorta proximal to the graft anastomosis and the iliac arteries distal to anastomotic sites should be mobilized so that the inflow and outflow are controlled prior to graft excision.

Close Arteriotomy Sites with Monofilament Sutures. After removal of the infected graft the arteriotomy should be closed with monofilament sutures such as Prolene to prevent residual infection within a suture line.

Irrigate Retroperitoneal Tissues with Antibiotic So-

Aortofemoral Bifurcation Graft

Effective management depends upon the site of the infection and the extent of the process. If the entire graft is involved it must be removed. However, if the infected part can be isolated from the remainder of the graft through a clean tissue plane, it may be possible to remove only the affected limb of the graft and thus preserve circulation to the opposite leg.[3] If the infection involves the intraabdominal portion as well as the femoral anastomotic site, it is impossible to develop a clean tissue barrier to prevent contamination of the body of the prosthesis and the entire graft must be removed.

In graft infection suspected of being limited to the femoral region, the critical decision can be made by exploring the retroperitoneum proximal to the infected site. This is carried out through a suprainguinal oblique incision. If the graft limb is found to be unaffected at this level, a segment of sterile graft is removed and the remaining proximal and distal graft oversewn. The surrounding tissues are allowed to fill the space that will act as a biologic tissue barrier between the infected graft below and the sterile graft above. Cultures of the segment of graft that was removed must confirm the absence of a septic process in this part of the graft. The distal infected segment can be removed in a second stage or at the same operation if circumstances demand immediate attention. The arteriotomy in the femoral artery is then oversewn with monofilament suture and the wound packed open with iodoform gauze and allowed to heal by secondary intention (Fig. 38–5).

If the proximal graft culture is positive, or if infection initially presented bilaterally, the entire graft must be removed. The same steps described for management of infection in an aortoiliac prosthesis are followed.

When the indication for graft placement was occlusive disease and the graft was placed end to side on the aorta, it may be possible to close the aorta after removal of the graft and to restore blood flow to the lower extremities through native vessels. Even though the blood flow through the native vessels is compromised by the occlusive process, it may be sufficient to obviate the need for immediate revascularization. This determination can be made by assessing the viability of the lower extremities after the graft has been removed.

If revascularization of one or both extremities appears to be required after removal of the aortofemoral graft, anastomosis in the usual site on the femoral artery may be precluded by infection in that area. When the superficial femoral artery is patent extraanatomic bypass can be employed,[46] passing the graft wide of the infected groin and making the distal anastomosis in the midthigh (Fig. 38–6). Another technique is to bypass the infected groin by passing the graft through the obturator canal and the ad-

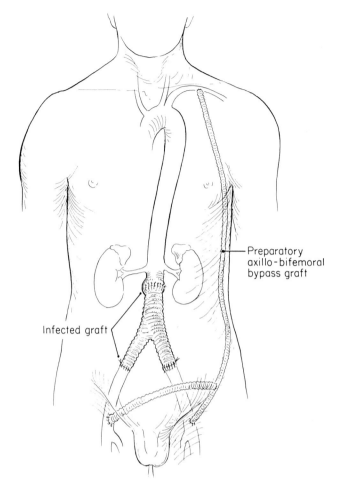

FIGURE 38–4. Before removing an infected intraabdominal prosthetic graft, perfusion of the lower extremities is established by an axillobifemoral bypass graft. This technique provides for uninterrupted perfusion of the lower limbs and reduces the morbidity associated with ischemic changes that occur when reconstitution of flow is delayed until after the aortic graft has been removed.

lution. The retroperitoneal space should be treated as an infected bed and all necrotic material should be débrided and the area copiously irrigated with a suitable antibiotic solution. A mixture of bacitracin and kanamycin in saline is a suitable topical antibiotic combination. If there is extensive purulence and necrotic tissue in the retroperitoneum following removal of the graft, the area should be débrided and drained. The drains should be brought out through stab wounds in both flanks to allow for dependent drainage. The peritoneum must be closed over the space to prevent loops of bowel from becoming adherent to the inflamed area. If sufficient tissue is unavailable to accomplish this, a pedicle of omentum should be used to cover the anastomotic region.

Administer High-Dosage Systemic Antibiotics. The choice of antibiotics should be based upon known sensitivities of the organism(s); alternatively, broad-spectrum bactericidal drugs should be employed empirically. It is recommended that long-term antibiotics be combined orally from 3 to 6 months.

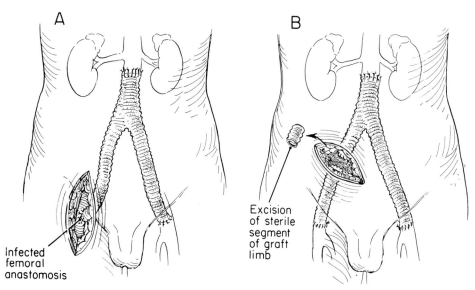

FIGURE 38–5. Through a retroperitoneal approach the sterility of the proximal portion of the graft limb is determined. The sterile graft above is isolated from the area of infection at the groin by excision of a segment of graft and obliteration of the communicating tissue planes between the two areas. The distal portion of the graft limb is then removed from below after the clean procedure has been carried out in the retroperitoneal space and the wound has been closed.

ductor compartment to the superficial femoral artery in the midthigh.[47] This should only be attempted when the infection is confined to the groin and the retroperitoneal portion of the graft is found to be incorporated in an unaffected fibrous capsule.

When the superficial femoral artery is occluded but the popliteal arteries are patent, bilateral axillopopliteal bypass may be performed. These grafts pass lateral to infected femoral wounds, then wind medial to insert into the popliteal segment. Our preference is to use ring-reinforced PTFE grafts to help prevent external compression (Fig. 38–7).

Alternative techniques involve the use of autogenous conduits into the infected field. These include saphenous veins or endarterectomized superficial femoral arteries placed from the aorta to the femoral artery.[48,49] The use of autogenous tissue to perform reconstruction in an infected field carries the risk of hemorrhage as a result of destruction of an anastomosis by the septic process. An attempt to salvage a patient's limb should never be made when reconstruction must be done in a grossly contaminated area. However, when the area can be adequately débrided of necrotic material and autogenous tissue is available, experimental data[50] would support reconstruction in a field with minimal contamination where autogenous vascular replacement can be expected to heal and function, with clearing of the infectious process by conventional antibiotic therapy.[51]

Femoropopliteal Bypass Graft

Management of an infected femoropopliteal bypass graft can be accomplished in the following manner:

1. Remove the graft in its entirety. The same gen-

eral principle applies with regard to infection of any multifibered foreign body. While arterial flow is occluded the patient should be adequately anticoagulated with heparin.

2. Oversew arteriotomies with monofilament suture.

3. Administer systemic and topical antibiotics.

4. Observe the limb for viability.

A limb that is not viable following removal of an infected femoropopliteal graft must be managed by revascularization or amputation. If the saphenous vein is available in either leg, it may be used to achieve revascularization provided the septic process can be appropriately managed by débridement and the anastomoses will not be created in an area of gross infection. Another option is to use the superficial femoral artery after closed thromboendarterectomy. In either case, the principles outlined above for the use of autogenous tissue in an infected field must be scrupulously adhered to.

If it is decided not to revascularize the limb, amputation should be delayed if possible as long as the patient can tolerate the ischemia, to allow maximum development of collaterals. The delay may allow sufficient collateral channels to develop to permit amputation below the knee rather than at a higher level, which is associated with much greater disability.

New Frontiers in Management of Graft Infection

In an attempt to more effectively manage the proximal aortic stump following removal of an infected

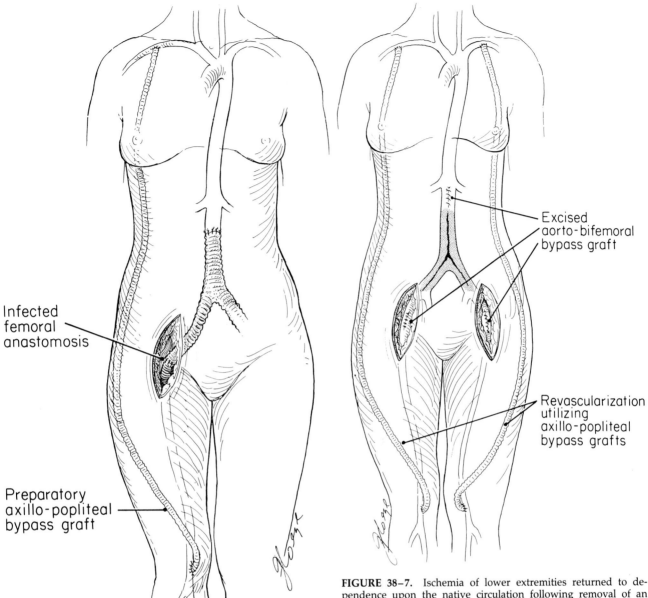

FIGURE 38–6. Perfusion of an ischemic extremity in the presence of sepsis in the ipsilateral groin is achieved with an axillopopliteal bypass graft. Care is taken to bring the graft wide of the groin through unaffected tissue planes.

FIGURE 38–7. Ischemia of lower extremities returned to dependence upon the native circulation following removal of an infected aortic graft may be successfully managed by bilateral axillopopliteal bypass grafts.

aortic graft, an experimental model has been developed to test the efficacy of highly vascular tissue pedicles in preventing late disruption.[52] In experiments in which segments of jejunum stripped of mucosa were applied to the proximal aortic stump, no evidence of sepsis was found in the stump on histologic sections at 3 weeks. These efforts are justified in light of the considerable risk entailed in graft resection and extraanatomic reconstruction. Quiñones-Baldrich et al. reported a recent series of patients with aortic graft sepsis managed with graft excision in which perioperative mortality was 24 per cent, the 5-year limb loss rate was 33 per cent, and the 3-year

graft thrombosis rate was 35 per cent.[53] This series represents one of the more favorable experiences with the standard management of aortic graft infections in a large university practice of vascular surgery and should therefore be considered the best outcome this form of therapy has to offer.

Alternative management schemes directed at graft conservation or in situ replacement have been investigated in recent years. Coverage with muscle flaps or omentum has become the most favored method of providing vascularized coverage for the freshly débrided and drained septic field when graft salvage or in situ prosthetic replacement is contemplated.[34–36] The implantation of gentamycin beads, more commonly used by orthopedic surgeons in the management of osteomyelitis, to control localized perigraft sepsis has been reported by several groups.[54,55]

While these procedures must continue to be described as experimental, their use is becoming more common and represents a viable alternative to the more conservative methods of prosthetic graft infection management that still entail considerable morbidity and mortality.

PREVENTION OF GRAFT INFECTION

Many graft infections arise as a result of preventable breaks in technique. Careful attention to important details in each step of the preoperative, operative, and postoperative care of the vascular surgical patient is the first line of prevention of graft sepsis. Once a vascular prosthesis is in place the patient and his physician must be made aware of circumstances that may be associated with transient bacteremia, which will put the graft at risk of becoming infected.

As is true in other surgical disciplines, patients undergoing vascular reconstructive procedures tend to have a higher incidence of wound complications when their immune and nutritional statuses are compromised.[56] Nutritional support is an important adjunct in the management of patients with graft sepsis.[57]

Preoperative Prophylaxis

Foci of infection are frequently present preoperatively in the candidate for vascular reconstruction. Whenever possible these should be eradicated before surgery. Patients with open or infected lesions of the feet or toes may have bacteria within the lymphatics and lymph glands in the inguinal region.[8,58] This condition will increase the risk of graft infection, particularly if a bypass graft to the femoral artery is necessary. Every effort should be made to prepare the patient with specific antibiotic therapy prior to operation, so as to sterilize the tissues adjacent to a proposed graft site. If reconstruction is required under these circumstances, careful thought should be given to the use of autogenous repair such as aortofemoral thromboendarterectomy, if it is technically possible.

Preoperative administration of prophylactic antibiotics, even in the absence of an intercurrent infection, should be carried out, particularly when prosthetic material will be used for the bypass. This policy is borne out by data from trials in other clinical conditions, as well as by randomized experimental studies demonstrating a lowered incidence of infection in grafts challenged by a transient bacteremia when prophylactic antibiotics were employed.[59–62] Even in patients without overt evidence of a septic focus, the insertion of urinary catheters and endotracheal and nasogastric tubes, which are an integral part of the operative procedure in most instances, pose the potential for brief and transient bacteremia in all patients, which should be anticipated. Our present policy in this regard is to administer a cephalosporin the night before and immediately before an operation in which a prosthetic graft is to be employed.

Intraoperative Precautions

1. Continue prophylactic antibiotic therapy by intravenous administration during the conduct of the operations.

2. Carefully ligate and divide any lymphatics that appear in the wound during the dissection. This is particularly important in inguinal incisions, where lymphatic channels are abundant and may harbor bacteria that originate in infected lesions of the feet or toes. In an experimental model of foot sepsis, ligation and division of the lymphatic channels resulted in fewer graft infections in the inguinal region than either careful preservation or simple transection.[62]

3. Avoid bringing the graft into contact with the skin by using the following precautions. Use a plastic drape to cover the exposed skin adjacent to the operative field. Prevent graft contact with superficial wound edges by covering the skin edges with sponges soaked in bacitracin-kanamycin solution. Make the operating team aware of the importance of protecting the graft from any contaminating contact.

4. Irrigate the graft and adjacent wounds with a bacitracin-kanamycin solution prior to closure.

5. Recognize that the superficial placement of a graft such as a femoral anastomosis increases the risk of graft infection, particularly if a complication of wound healing occurs. We close the femoral subcutaneous tissue in three layers, and use polyglycolic acid sutures because they seem to produce less tissue reaction. Finally, use skin staples or a subcuticular closure, rather than transcutaneous sutures. Comparative observation suggests that subcuticular sutures produce considerably less skin reaction than transcutaneous sutures.

6. A variety of investigators have explored the use of grafts to which an antibiotic has been chemically bound. The primary challenge has been to find an antibiotic with appropriate specificity that can be bound to the graft in a manner sufficient to produce locally effective tissue concentrations for a sufficient length of time. Chervu et al. have employed a collagen/rifampin bonded Dacron graft that shows excellent activity against *Staphylococcus epidermidis* for up to 7 days after implantation in a model of aortic graft infection in the dog.[63] Another interesting experience with graft impregnation has been the use of ciprofloxacin and silver incorporated into a PTFE graft that has shown significant activity against *Staphylococcus epidermidis* at both 7 and 14 days.[64] The efficacy of these novel grafts in the prevention of clinical graft infection will remain unknown until they are available for clinical use in a sufficient number of centers.

7. The choice of prosthetic material may be im-

portant in some circumstances, particularly when unavoidable bacteremia is probable. In an experimental in vitro model, adherence of *S. aureus* to PTFE was much less than adherence to either Dacron or human umbilical vein. The addition of a suture line in the PTFE doubled the bacterial adherence.[13] However, it has also been shown in an experimental dog model in which grafts have been allowed to heal for 10 to 12 months that endothelial seeding offered no advantage over the normal healing process. Each was equally effective in resisting infection from bacteremic challenge.[65]

Early Postoperative Prophylaxis

Ideally, systemic antibiotic prophylaxis should last for 48 hours. However, systemic prophylactic antibiotic therapy may be continued until major vascular lines are removed. This may extend administration 5 to 7 days.

Late Postoperative Prophylaxis

Experimentally, seeding of bacteria on prosthetic grafts after a standard challenge persists until the material becomes incorporated into a fibrous capsule and the luminal surface becomes covered with pseudointima. This process may take as long as a year to complete and even then may not entirely cover the graft.[11] These data suggest that prosthetic grafts have a significant risk of becoming infected even long after implantation and may never be completely eliminated. This has been convincingly shown in a recent study that examined the susceptibility of prosthetic grafts to infection as a result of late bacteremic challenge and confirmed the need for prophylactic antibiotic coverage in any patient with an arterial prosthesis undergoing an invasive procedure (e.g., dental work, colonoscopy, etc.).[66] While it is probably neither reasonable nor wise to continue prophylactic antibiotic therapy throughout the lifetime of the graft, it is important for the patient and physician to recognize the potential for transient bacteremic episodes to cause graft infection. Patients with prosthetic grafts in place should be given broad-spectrum prophylactic antibiotics when bacteremia is likely, such as during urinary tract manipulation and dental extraction (two examples of common procedures with the potential to cause bacteremia). While the incidence of graft infection remains low, its consequences are profound and justify this meticulous approach toward prevention.

REFERENCES

1. Conn JH, Hardy JD, Chavez CM, et al: Infected arterial grafts: Experience in 22 cases with emphasis on unusual bacteria and technics. Ann Surg *171*:704, 1970.
2. Fry WJ, Lindenauer SM: Infection complicating the use of plastic arterial implants. Arch Surg *94*:600, 1967.
3. Goldstone J, Moore WS: Infection in vascular prostheses: Clinical manifestations and surgical management. Am J Surg *128*:225, 1974.
4. Hoffert PWK, Gensler S, Haimovici H: Infection complicating arterial grafts. Personal experience with 12 cases and review of the literature. Arch Surg *90*:427, 1965.
5. Reilly LM, Altman H, Lusby RJ, et al: Late results following surgical management of vascular graft infection. J Vasc Surg *1*:36, 1984.
6. Szilagyi DE, Smith RF, Elliott JP, et al: Infection in arterial reconstruction with synthetic grafts. Ann Surg *175*:321, 1972.
7. Liekwig WJ Jr, Greenfield LJ: Vascular prosthetic infections: Collected experience and results of treatments. Surgery *81*:335, 1977.
8. Papa MA, Haiperan Z, Adar R: Infections in vascular operations. Isr J Med Sci *17*:257, 1981.
9. Macbeth GA, Rubin JR, McIntyre EE, et al: The relevance of arterial wall microbiology to the treatment of prosthetic graft infections: Graft infection vs. arterial infection. Vasc Surg *1*:750, 1984.
10. Lalka SG, Malone JM, Fisher DF Jr, Bernhard VM, Sullivan D, Stoeckelmann D, Bergstrom RF: Efficacy of prophylactic antibiotics in vascular surgery: An arterial wall microbiologic and pharmacokinetic perspective. J Vasc Surg *10*(5):501–510, 1989.
11. Malone JM, Moore WS, Campagna G, et al: Bacteremic infectibility of vascular grafts: The influence of pseudointimal integrity and duration of graft function. Surgery *78*:211, 1975.
12. Moore WS, Rosson CT, Hall AD, et al: Transient bacteremia—

a cause of infection in prosthetic vascular grafts. Am J Surg *117*:342, 1969.
13. Moore WS, Malone JM, Keown K: Prosthetic arterial graft material: Influence on neointimal healing and bacteric infectibility. Arch Surg *115*:1379, 1980.
14. Moore WS, Swanson RJ, Campagna G, et al: Pseudointimal development and vascular prosthesis susceptibility to bacteremic infection. Surg Forum *15*:250, 1974.
15. LePort C, Goéau-Brissonnière D, LeBrault C, et al: Experimental colonization of a polyester vascular graft with *Staphylococcus aureus*: A quantitative and morphologic study. J Vasc Surg *8*:1–9, 1988.
16. Moore WS, Malone JM: Vascular infection. *In* RJ Howard, RL Simmons (eds): Surgical Infectious Diseases. New York, Appleton-Century-Crofts, 1982, pp 777–793.
17. Bergamini TM, Bandyk DF, Govostis D, et al: Infection of vascular prostheses caused by bacterial biofilms. J Vasc Surg *7*:21–30, 1988.
18. Bellenot F, Chatenet T, Kantelip B, Tissandier P, Ribal JP, Glanddier G: Aseptic periprosthetic fluid collection: A late complication of Dacron arterial bypass. Ann Vasc Surg *2*(3):220–224, 1988.
19. Bergamini TM, Bandyk DF, Govostis D, et al: Identification of *Staphylococcus epidermidis* vascular graft infections: A comparison of culture techniques. J Vasc Surg *9*:665–670, 1989.
20. Geary KJ, Tomkiewicz ZM, Harrison HN, Fiore WM, Geary JE, Green RM, DeWeese JA, Ouriel K: Differential effects of a gram-negative and a gram-positive infection on autogenous and prosthetic grafts. J Vasc Surg *11*(2):339–347, 1990.
21. Dalinka MK, Reginato AJ, Berkowitz HD, et al: Hypertrophic osteoarthropathy as an indication of aortic graft infection and aortoenteric fistula. Arch Surg *117*:1355, 1982.
22. Seabrook GR, Schmitt DD, Bandyk DF, Edmiston CE, Krepel

CJ, Towne JB: Anastomotic femoral pseudoaneurysm: An investigation of occult infection as an etiologic factor. J Vasc Surg 11(5):629–634, 1990.

23. Downs AR, Guzman R, Formichi M, Courbier R, Jausseran JM, Branchereau A, Juhan C, Chakfe N, King M, Guidoin R: Etiology of prosthetic anastomotic false aneurysms: Pathologic and structural evaluation in 26 cases. Can J Surg 34(1):53–58, 1991.

24. Padberg FT Jr, Lee BC, Curl GR: Hemoaccess site infection. Surg Gynecol Obstet 174(2):103–108, 1992.

25. Olofsson PA, Auffermann W, Higgins CB, et al: Diagnosis of prosthetic aortic graft infection by magnetic resonance imaging. J Vasc Surg 8:99–105, 1988.

26. Auffermann W, Olofsson PA, Rabahie GN, Tavares NJ, Stoney RJ, Higgins CB: Incorporation versus infection of retroperitoneal aortic grafts: MR imaging features. Radiology 172(2):359–362, 1989.

27. Peter AO, Spangler S, Martin LF: Evaluation of three techniques for documenting *Staphylococcus epidermidis* vascular prosthetic graft infections. Am Surg 57(2):80–85, 1991.

28. Lawrence PF, Dries DJ, Alazraki N, et al: Indium[111]-labeled leukocyte scanning for detection of prosthetic vascular graft infection. J Vasc Surg 2:165, 1985.

29. LaMuraglia GM, Fischman AJ, Strauss HW, et al: Utility of the indium 111-labeled human immunoglobulin G scan for the detection of focal vascular graft infection. J Vasc Surg 10:20–28, 1989.

30. Cordes M, Hepp W, Langer R, Pannhorst J, Hierholzer J, Felix R: Vascular graft infection: Detection by ^{123}I-labeled antigranulocyte antibody (anti-NCA95) scintigraphy. Nuklearmedizin 30(5):173–177, 1991.

31. Insall RL, Jones NA, Chamberlain J, Lambert D, Keavey PM: New isotopic technique for detecting prosthetic arterial graft infection: 99mTc-hexametazime-labelled leucocyte imaging. Br J Surg 77(11):1295–1298, 1990.

32. Champion MC, Sullivan SN, Coles JC, et al: Aortoenteric fistula: Incidence, presentation, recognition, and management. Ann Surg 195:314, 1982.

33. Kwaan JWM, Connolly JE: Successful management of prosthetic graft infection with continuous povidone-iodine irrigation. Arch Surg 116:716, 1981.

34. Samson RH, Veith FJ, Janko GS, Gupta SK, Scher LA: A modified classification and approach to the management of infections involving peripheral arterial prosthetic grafts. J Vasc Surg 8(2):147–153, 1988.

35. Perler BA, Vander Kolk CA, Dufresne CR, Williams GM: Can infected prosthetic grafts be salvaged with rotational muscle flaps? Surgery 110(1):30–34, 1991.

36. Calligaro KD, Westcott CJ, Buckley RM, Savarese RP, DeLaurentis DA: Infrainguinal anastomotic arterial graft infections treated by selective graft preservation. Ann Surg 216(1):74–79, 1992.

37. Gonzaigz LL, Boyd AD, Altemeier WA: Susceptibility of vascular sutures to infection in experimental bacteremia. Surg Forum 15:68, 1964.

38. Mutch D, Richards G, Brown RA, et al: Bioactive antibiotic levels in the human aorta. Surgery 92:1068, 1982.

39. DiGiglia JD, Leonard GL, Ochsner JL: Local irrigation with an antibiotic solution in the prevention of infection in vascular prostheses. Surgery 67:836, 1970.

40. Malone JM, Lalka SG, McIntyre KE, et al: The necessity for long-term antibiotic therapy with positive arterial wall cultures. J Vasc Surg 8:262–267, 1988.

41. Ehrenfeld WK, Lord RSA, Stoney RJ, et al: Subcutaneous arterial bypass grafts in the management of fistulae between the bowel and plastic arterial prostheses. Ann Surg 168:29, 1968.

42. Trout HH, Kozioff L, Giordano JM: Priority of revascularization in patients with graft enteric fistulas, infected arteries or infected arterial prostheses. Ann Surg 199:669, 1984.

43. Rosenman JE, Pearce WH, Kempczinski RF: Bacterial adherence to vascular grafts after in vitro bacteremia. J Surg Res 38:648, 1985.

44. Bacourt F, Koskas F: Axillobifemoral bypass and aortic exclusion for vascular septic lesions: A multicenter retrospective study of 98 cases. Ann Vasc Surg 6(2):119–126, 1992.

45. Wittens CH, van Houtte HJ, van Urk H: Winner of the ESVS prize 1991. European prospective randomised multi-centre axillo-bifemoral trial. Eur J Vasc Surg 6(2):115–123, 1992.

46. Blaisdell FW, Hali AD: Axillary-femoral bypass for lower extremity ischemia. Surgery 54:563, 1963.

47. Pearce WH, Ricco J-P, Yao JST, et al: Modified technique of obturator bypass in failed or infected grafts. Ann Surg 97:344, 1983.

48. Ehrenfeld WK, Wilbur BG, Olcott CN IV, et al: Autogenous tissue reconstruction in the management of infected prosthetic grafts. Surgery 85:62, 1979.

49. Wylie EJ: Vascular replacement with arterial autografts. Surgery 157:14, 1965.

50. Moore WS, Blaisdeli FW, Gardner M, et al: Effect of infection on autogenous vein arterial substitutes. Surg Forum 13:235, 1962.

51. Moore WS, Swanson RJ, Campagna G, et al: The use of fresh tissue arterial substitutes in infected fields. J Surg Res 18:299, 1975.

52. Buchbinder D, Leather R, Shah D, et al: Pathologic interactions between prosthetic aortic grafts and the gastrointestinal tract. Am J Surg 140:192, 1980.

53. Quiñones-Baldrich WJ, Hernandez JJ, Moore WS: Long-term results following surgical management of aortic graft infection. Arch Surg 126(4):507–511, 1991.

54. Nielsen OM, Noer HH, Jorgensen LG, Lorentzen JE: Gentamycin beads in the treatment of localised vascular graft infection—long term results in 17 cases. Eur J Vasc Surg 5(3):283–285, 1991.

55. Reilly DT, Grigg MJ, Mansfield AO: Intraperitoneal placement of gentamicin beads in the management of prosthetic graft sepsis. J R Coll Surg Edinb 34(6):314–315, 1989.

56. Casey J, Flinn WR, Yao JST, et al: Correlation of immune and nutritional status with wound complications in patients undergoing vascular operations. Surgery 93:822, 1983.

57. Kwaan JHM, Dahl RK, Connolly J: Immunocompetence in patients with prosthetic graft infection. J Vasc Surg 1:45, 1984.

58. Rubin JR, Malone JM, Goldstone J: The role of the lymphatic system in acute arterial prosthetic graft infections. J Vasc Surg 2:92, 1985.

59. Kaiser AB, Clayson RR, Mulherin JL, et al: Antibiotic prophylaxis in vascular surgery. Ann Surg 188:283, 1978.

60. Lindenauer SM, Fry WJ, Schaub G, et al: The use of antibiotics in the prevention of vascular graft infection. Surgery 62:487, 1967.

61. Moore WS, Rosson CT, Hall AD: Effect of prophylactic antibiotics in preventing bacteremic infection of vascular prostheses. Surgery 69:825, 1971.

62. Pitt HA, Postier RG, MacGowan WA, et al: Prophylactic antibiotics in vascular surgery. Topical, systemic, or both? Ann Surg 192:356, 1980.

63. Chervu A, Moore WS, Gelabert HA, Colburn MD, Chvapil M: Prevention of graft infection by use of prostheses bonded with a rifampin/collagen release system. J Vasc Surg 14(4):521–525, 1991.

64. Kinney EV, Bandyk DF, Seabrook GA, Kelly HM, Towne JB: Antibiotic-bonded PTFE vascular grafts: The effect of silver antibiotic on bioactivity following implantation. J Surg Res 50(5):430–435, 1991.

65. Keller JD, Falk J, Bjornson HS, et al: Bacterial infectibility of chronically implanted endothelial cell-seeded expanded polytetrafluoroethylene vascular grafts. J Vasc Surg 7:524–530, 1988.

66. Goeau-Brissonniere O, Leport C, Lebrault C, Renier FJ, Bacourt F, Vilde JL, Pechere JC: Antibiotic prophylaxis of late bacteremic vascular graft infection in a dog model (comments). Ann Vasc Surg 4(6):528–532, 1990.

39

NONINFECTIOUS COMPLICATIONS IN VASCULAR SURGERY

GLENN C. HUNTER, DAVID A. BULL, and VICTOR M. BERNHARD

Complications following aortoiliac and peripheral arterial reconstruction often develop and progress rapidly to produce disastrous consequences related to life, limb, and major organ failure. They may be the result of technical errors, the extent of the pathologic process, or one or more of a group of frequently associated diseases. A time-worn surgical principle applies especially to vascular surgery: "A complication not anticipated is sure to be experienced."

The primary problems to be reviewed are those of operative bleeding, thrombosis, operative embolization, iatrogenic injury, major organ failure, graft deterioration, progressing atherosclerotic disease, chylous ascites, anastomotic false aneurysm, and postoperative lower extremity edema. To be concise and avoid repetition, a given problem will be discussed generically in relation to its most prominent area of occurrence or severity and then reviewed briefly to highlight details and bring out differences in other circumstances.

AORTOILIAC SURGERY

Complications of aortoiliac arterial reconstruction are similar whether the procedure is for abdominal aortic aneurysmal or occlusive disease.

Operative Bleeding

Operative bleeding is most commonly due to venous injury because of the close anatomic relationship of the aorta and iliac arteries to the inferior vena cava, and the inferior mesenteric, left renal, left gonadal, lumbar, and iliac veins[1] (Fig. 39–1). Careful operative dissection, a thorough understanding of the anatomy, and familiarity with the characteristics of major venous anomalies are essential to avoid this complication.[2] The most vulnerable point is the area of tight adherence of the right posterolateral surface

of the aorta and common iliac artery to the adjacent wall of the vena cava and right iliac vein at the level of the aortic bifurcation. Complete separation of these structures by circumferential dissection is usually unnecessary, since temporary occlusion can usually be achieved without this maneuver by clamp control or by use of intraluminal balloon catheters. If one of these veins is inadvertently lacerated, bleeding should be controlled by gentle finger tamponade and the venous laceration closed with a few stitches of fine monofilament suture. Application of clamps is hazardous and may enlarge the rent in the vein.

The left renal vein should be routinely identified early during dissection of the aorta above an aneurysm or proximal to the area of major aortic occlusive disease. Its caudal border should be clearly defined so that this structure can be easily retracted out of harm's way. Failure to find the left renal vein in its usual position suggests its aberrant location behind the aorta (Fig. 39–2). This anomaly occurs in approximately 2 per cent of patients, and, when present, the vein is somewhat more caudal in position and may be readily injured during circumferential dissection of the infrarenal aorta preparatory to application of an occluding clamp.[1,2]

An arteriovenous (AV) fistula involving the aorta or iliac arteries is an uncommon complication of spontaneous aneurysm rupture into an adjacent vein (about 80 per cent) or of retroperitoneal injury to these major vessels. The incidence of this complication is quite low, occurring in less than 1 per cent of all aneurysms and only 3 to 4 per cent of ruptured aneurysms.[3-6] The presence of an AV fistula is suggested by a continuous bruit over the aneurysm associated with the sudden onset of lower extremity venous hypertension, oliguria, hematuria, and congestive heart failure. If suspected, the diagnosis of aortocaval or iliac AV fistula can be confirmed by color Doppler imaging, computed tomography (CT) scanning, or angiography. In the series reported by Brewster et al., the presence of an AV fistula was

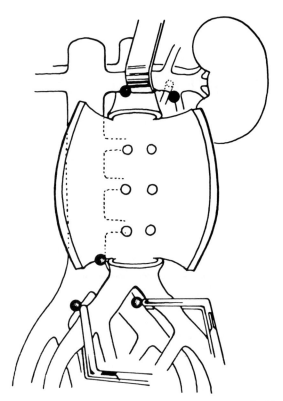

FIGURE 39–1. Sites of venous injury. (From Downs A: Problems in resection of aortoiliac and femoral aneurysms. *In* Bernhard VM, Towne JB (eds): Complications in Vascular Surgery. New York, Grune & Stratton, 1980, p 68.)

unsuspected in 25 per cent of the patients at the time of aortic aneurysm surgery.[5] Occasionally, the fistula may be unsuspected intraoperatively because of its small size or obscuration by the laminated thrombus within the aneurysm only to become apparent when sudden massive venous hemorrhage occurs within the lumen of the aorta during evacuation of the lam-

inated thrombus from the aneurysmal sac.[7] In this case, direct finger pressure over the fistula followed by proximal and distal caval compression with sponge sticks will usually control bleeding so that the venous defect can be visualized and closed with a running suture from within the aortic sac (Fig. 39–3). No attempt should be made to separate the aneurysm wall from the cava at the fistula site. In all patients undergoing aortic aneurysm repair, it is wise to palpate the inferior vena cava for the presence of a thrill, indicating an aortocaval fistula in the otherwise unsuspected case. If a fistula is suspected, the inferior vena cava should then be occluded with a sponge stick or a clamp adjacent to the neck of the aneurysm before opening the aneurysm to prevent embolism of clot or air to the lungs.[4]

Intraoperative bleeding from iliac AV fistulae is often more difficult to control because of their location deep within the pelvis, the size of the defect, and the intimate relationship between the vein and artery. Elective placement of occlusion balloon catheters above and below the aneurysm via the femoral vein prior to entering the aneurysm may control venous bleeding and permit closure of the defect without massive blood loss. Autotransfusion is a useful adjunct in the management of aortocaval and iliac fistulae.[3]

Arterial bleeding usually arises from the lumbar or the inferior mesenteric arteries during circumferential aortic dissection or after the aorta has been opened.[1] Lumbar vessel injury can be avoided in aneurysm surgery by limiting the dissection to its anterior surface and suture ligature of the lumbar orifices from within the sac after the aneurysm has been opened.[8] A tear in a fragile aortic wall may occur from suture placement during anastomosis. Additional sutures, frequently with Teflon pledgets, may be required to control these bleeding points.[1] The aorta should be clamped briefly while additional repair sutures are

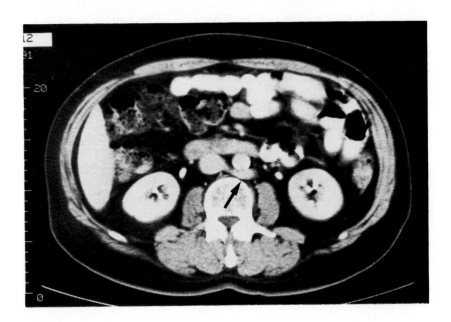

FIGURE 39–2. Retroaortic renal vein. Computed tomography scan demonstrating a retroaortic left renal vein (arrow).

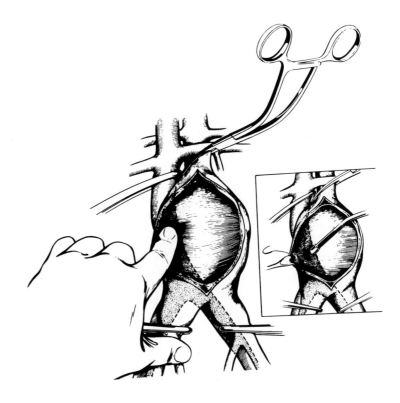

FIGURE 39-3. Aortocaval fistula. The fistula orifice is exposed through the aneurysm and controlled by simple digital occlusion of the hole into the inferior vena cava. The fistula is closed with a simple over-and-over suture from within the aneurysmal sac. A clear and unencumbered field is provided by rapid aspiration and autotransfusion of blood pouring into the aneurysmal sac from the cava. (From Bernhard VM: Aortocaval fistulas. *In* Haimovici H (ed): Vascular Emergencies. New York, Appleton-Century-Crofts, 1982, p 357.)

being placed and tied in order to avoid further tears in the aortic wall.

Bleeding in the immediate postoperative period usually comes from suture lines or inadequately ligated lumbar vessels. This is manifested by a continuing need for blood replacement and the development of a retroperitoneal hematoma. This can be identified by palpating the flank, usually the left, which loses its normal soft concavity and becomes distended and tense. When aortic or iliac suture line bleeding is rapid, shock is more obvious and the patient complains of severe backache similar to the pain of a ruptured aortic aneurysm.

Postoperative hemorrhage is treated by immediate return to the operating room for identification and control of the bleeding site under fully monitored general anesthesia. Prevention of this complication requires thorough inspection of the intraabdominal anastomoses and the periaortic area, with special attention to the orifices of the lumbar vessels, the inferior mesenteric artery, and the ligated or oversewn stumps of the aorta or the iliac vessels. This search for the potential bleeding site should be done when blood volume and pressure are at the patient's normal level before closing the retroperitoneum over the aortoiliac reconstruction.

Bleeding due to unrecognized coagulopathy usually can be prevented by careful preoperative history and evaluation of the platelet count, bleeding time, prothrombin time, and partial thromboplastin time.[9] These preliminary screening studies will reliably identify the need to search for precise factor deficiencies and direct their replacement prior to and during surgery. Intraoperative monitoring of the activated clotting time before and after heparin administration is the most effective means of identifying variations in the individual response to intraoperatively administered heparin and to determine the adequacy of its reversal before closing the incision.[9] Transfusion reaction and disseminated intravascular coagulopathy (DIC) are rare causes of operative or early postoperative bleeding; however, consumption coagulopathy secondary to massive blood loss and replacement is more common and will require the judicious use of fresh-frozen plasma and platelets. Proper management of bleeding due to congenital or acquired deficiencies requires repeated monitoring of pertinent coagulation parameters during and immediately after the operative procedure.

Thrombosis

Graft thrombosis in the early postoperative period is almost invariably due to technical problems (Fig. 39-4), which usually occur at the distal anastomoses.[1,10-12] These include an elevated intimal flap; narrowing of the artery at the anastomotic suture line; failure to remove clot adherent to the inner wall of the graft prior to completion of the anastomosis; twisting or kinking in the retroperitoneal tunnel; compression of the femoral limb of the graft by the inguinal ligament; unrecognized inflow disease; or inadequate runoff secondary to unappreciated iliac, profunda, superficial femoral, or infrapopliteal disease. Rarely, thrombosis following aortofemoral bypass or aneurysm replacement is due to hypercoagulability from antithrombin III deficiency, protein

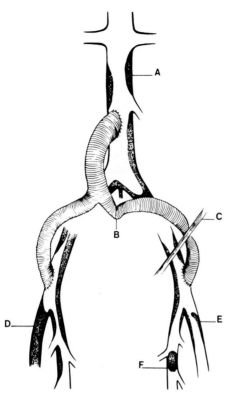

FIGURE 39–4. Mechanical factors that may cause early thrombosis of aortofemoral graft. *A*, Aortic anastomosis distal to obstructing atherosclerosis at subrenal level. *B*, Kinking of graft limb due to placement of the proximal anastomosis low on the aorta with too long an aortic graft segment. *C*, Compression by the inguinal ligament. *D*, Inadequate runoff due to occlusion of the superficial femoral artery and severe stenosis of the profunda. *E*, Elevation of distal intima. *F*, Peripheral embolization or thrombosis. (From Bernhard VM: The failed arterial graft: Lost pulses and gangrene. *In* Condon RE, DeCosse JJ (eds): Surgical Care. Philadelphia, Lea & Febiger, 1980, p 155.)

C or S deficiency, anticardiolipin antibodies or heparin-induced platelet aggregation, or stasis due to reduced cardiac output.[13–16]

The adequacy of pulsatile blood flow through the graft or endarterectomy should be evaluated in the operating room before the wounds are closed, not only by palpation of the graft itself and the arteries immediately distal to anastomoses, but also by palpation of distal pulses and direct inspection of the pedal circulation beneath the drapes. If necessary, noninvasive measurements such as Doppler flow, ankle pressure, or pulse volume recorder (PVR) tracings can be obtained intraoperatively.[10,11,17–19] Intraoperative completion angiograms should be obtained in all patients who have had extensive reconstructive procedures of the common femoral, superficial femoral, or profunda femoris arteries to ensure the adequacy of the repair. Noninvasive studies should be performed routinely in the recovery room when pulses cannot be felt distal to the repair or when the anticipated improvement in circulation has not occurred. Objective information obtained from these easily performed studies is particularly valuable in the imme-

diate postoperative period when patients are frequently hypothermic and peripherally vasoconstricted. Detection of unsatisfactory graft function mandates immediate direct evaluation of involved anastomoses before wound closure or by prompt return to the operating room if graft flow deteriorates subsequently.

Treatment of immediate postreconstructive thrombosis consists of thorough inspection of the intraluminal aspect of the involved anastomosis. This is best accomplished through an incision in the distal end of the graft or by takedown of the anastomosis in order to directly view the intima and the runoff vessels adjacent to the arteriotomy. Effective revision may require stabilization of an elevated plaque, extension of an iliac limb to the common femoral artery, or patch angioplasty of a profunda or proximal superficial femoral stenosis. Infrequently, complementary bypass from the femoral to the popliteal of the infrapopliteal vessels may be required when adequate runoff cannot be achieved through the profunda.[20,21] The lie of the graft should always be inspected throughout its length to ensure that there is no kinking, twisting, or external compression within the retroperitoneal tunnel.

Prevention of early graft thrombosis depends on an accurate evaluation of the distal runoff bed by preoperative arteriography, noninvasive hemodynamic testing, and by direct palpation of the iliac artery throughout its length before selecting this vessel, rather than the femoral, as the site for distal anastomosis. The orifices of the runoff vessels should be inspected and calibrated. Special attention should be given to the profunda orifice, which often requires angioplasty when the distal anastomosis is performed at the common femoral level. Finally, technical perfection in the performance of anastomoses is mandatory to avoid narrowing of the runoff vessels. Tacking sutures may be required to prevent distal intimal dissection.

Thrombosis is the most frequent late complication of aortoiliac and aortofemoral procedures[22,23] and usually presents as unilateral limb ischemia[24–26] (Fig. 39–4D). Impaired outflow through the external iliac artery or the major branches of the common femoral is the most common etiology and is due to progressive downstream atherosclerosis or anastomotic fibrointimal hyperplasia. Anastomotic fibrointimal hyperplasia causes stenosis, usually at the distal anastomoses, by the circumferential development of fibrous tissue at the distal graft-artery interface; occlusion occurs when flow diminishes sufficiently to result in stasis thrombosis.[29] The majority of patients initially managed with aortofemoral bypass will have occlusion of the superficial femoral artery at the time of the primary procedure. Therefore, an adequate lumen at the origin of the deep femoral artery is the most significant factor in assuring long-term patency of these grafts.[18,23,25,28,30] Underestimating the severity of outflow disease at the time of primary reconstruction is an important cofactor of progressing atherosclerosis that increases susceptibility to late graft limb occlusion.[31] In spite of an adequate primary procedure, progression of femoral or infrapopliteal atherosclerotic disease is more likely to occur in patients with continued exposure to atherogenic risk factors, particularly those who continue to smoke.[24,31]

Impaired inflow is the second most common cause of late postrevascularization thrombosis. Although it is four to nine times less frequent than impaired outflow,[31] it is the most common cause of simultaneous bilateral postreconstructive lower limb ischemia following aortoiliac or femoral surgery.[23,26] The most common mechanism is obstruction from progressive infrarenal aortic atherosclerosis proximal to the site of previous repair (Fig. 39–4A). This is usually the consequence of placing the proximal anastomosis too low on the aorta (i.e., at or below the inferior mesenteric artery) (Fig. 39–5). The area between this site and the renal arteries is an active site of progressive atherosclerosis.[18] Likewise, following aortoiliac endarterectomy, late occlusion is more likely if the proximal infrarenal aorta is not included in the endarterectomy.[32] The use of an end-to-end rather than an end-to-side aortic anastomosis may be

associated with fewer thrombotic failures, although this has not been clearly defined. Superior hemodynamic flow characteristics, the absence of competitive flow, less chance of embolization from the host aorta, and less angulation of the limbs as they arise from the body graft[18,32] have been cited as the advantages of the end-to-end aortic anastomosis.

Angulation of the graft limb at the bifurcation may produce kinking due to failure to pull the graft limb out to full length before the distal anastomoses are performed or excessive length of the graft body resulting in too wide a bifurcation angle (Fig. 39–4B). Inadequate retroperitoneal tunneling of the graft limbs may promote thrombosis as a consequence of extrinsic compression from the mesentery of the sigmoid colon or the recurrent portion of the inguinal ligament[31] (Fig. 39–4C).

Less frequent causes of late thrombosis of aortoiliac and femoral reconstructions include accumulation of mural thrombus and false aneurysm. Mural thrombus develops when the graft diameter is significantly larger than the outflow artery. The flow pattern of the larger graft adjusts itself to the smaller outflow artery, leaving a peripheral layer of slowly moving blood that clots to form the mural thrombus. The normal, smooth, firmly adherent fibrous neointima becomes lined with a thick, gelatinous, loosely adherent mural thrombus that reduces the functioning lumen to the diameter of the outflow vessel. Fragmentation with distal embolization or progressive narrowing of the graft lumen with secondary acute thrombotic occlusion may then occur.[29] Anastomotic false aneurysms, although relatively rare causes of late limb ischemia, may also produce peripheral embolization or thrombosis of the aneurysm and the adjacent vessel lumen.[31] Finally, an aortoiliac reconstruction can progress suddenly to thrombosis in the presence of cardiac embolization or decreased cardiac output secondary to myocardial infarction or congestive failure. Rarely, no apparent cause for late thrombosis can be identified, implicating thrombogenicity of the graft surface or degeneration and disruption of the neointima.

The diagnosis of late thrombosis is suggested by the sudden or progressive recurrence of symptoms, a decrease or loss of previously present distal pulses, and a concomitant reduction in ankle pressure, Doppler flow, or PVR waveform. The degree of ischemia following thrombosis of a reconstruction is usually more severe than prior to the primary revascularization procedure.[23,26] The frequency of late thrombosis increases from 5 to 10 per cent in the first 5 years to 20 to 30 per cent at 10 years.[18,30,33–35] Therefore, routine and long-term follow-up of these patients at regular intervals is required to monitor the adequacy of graft function. If significant stenosis can be demonstrated prior to complete thrombosis, surgical correction is simplified. When either abrupt or gradual change is apparent, prompt aortography should be performed to determine the status of the

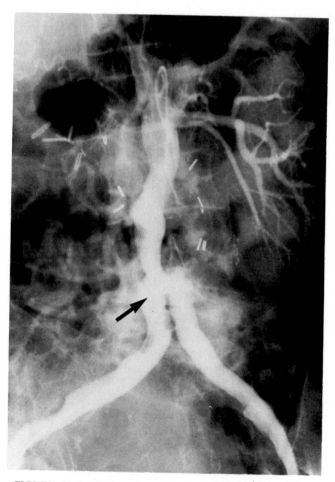

FIGURE 39–5. Progressive inflow obstruction. An aortogram demonstrating progressive atherosclerosis proximal to an incorrectly placed bifurcation graft (arrow).

graft, the anastomoses, the inflow, and the runoff bed.[17,36]

The severity of recurrent ischemia, which may range from minimal to severe claudication, rest pain, or pregangrene, depends upon the extent of compensating collaterals and the vigor of the patient's normal activity. Arteriography is required to determine whether further surgery is feasible and to guide the surgeon in the selection of the most appropriate reoperative procedure, considering the patient's age, state of health, and general level of activity.[24,31]

Correction of late thrombosis requires operative determination of the underlying mechanical problem followed by appropriate corrective maneuvers.[31,37] The occlusion of one limb of an aortoiliac bifurcation graft is usually due to overlooked or progressing disease in the external iliac and femoral arteries. Retroperitoneal exposure of the occluded limb, balloon catheter thrombectomy, and graft extension to the femoral level is a reliable solution. Femoral-to-femoral bypass is the alternative if the donor iliofemoral inflow is satisfactory, especially in the higher risk patient. Axillofemoral bypass may be required if neither of the preceding methods is feasible.[2,20]

The most commonly encountered situation is a thrombosed aortofemoral graft limb with impaired outflow. Inflow can usually be restored by graft thrombectomy using a balloon thromboembolectomy catheter[37] (Fig. 39–6). A thromboendarterectomy stripper is often required to complete the extraction of adherent clot and old pseudointima. The Fogarty catheter is passed through the ring of the stripper into the patent aortic portion of the graft and its balloon fully inflated and pulled down to occlude the proximal end of the limb to control bleeding and prevent crossover embolization. The stripper is passed back and forth around the catheter within the occluded graft limb up to the distended balloon to scrape thrombus from the graft wall. Thereafter, the balloon is deflated just enough to permit its tight withdrawal through the graft limb en masse with the stripper and detached thrombus (Fig. 39–6). The patient is systemically heparinized (100 to 125 units/kg) during all of these maneuvers.

Thrombectomy is usually combined with a profundaplasty of varying extent to provide outflow. However, femoropopliteal or femoral distal bypass may be required, depending on the extent and location of outflow disease.[20,21,37,38] If an occluded graft limb cannot be reopened by thrombectomy, a femorofemoral graft can be inserted. Replacement of the graft limb is another alternative but is technically more difficult.

If an entire bifurcation graft is thrombosed, a problem at the proximal anastomosis such as low placement of the graft with proximal disease, kinking, or anastomotic aneurysm is a likely cause. A CT scan will be required to identify the latter. If no proximal problem can be demonstrated, balloon thrombectomy can be attempted but is usually not successful. The alternatives are replacing the original prosthesis or inserting an axillobifemoral bypass. The latter procedure is less technically demanding, less hazardous, and is the reoperation of choice in the physiologically compromised patient.[37]

When groin scarring is especially intense, bypass to the midprofunda simplifies the outflow repair of the reoperative procedure by avoiding a tedious and hazardous dissection in the area of a previous femoral anastomosis.[39] In certain circumstances, intraarterial thrombolytic therapy can be a helpful adjunct in the management of occluded aortoiliac reconstructions.[40]

An aggressive attitude toward reoperation after thrombotic failure of aortoiliac reconstruction is warranted, especially if the patient will derive sustained benefit from long-term patency and improved limb function,[37] since operative morbidity and mortality rates are low. Reoperative mortality rates of 3 per cent with cumulative 3-year patency rates of 68 to 75 per cent have been reported.[23,37] Judicious use of extraabdominal approaches has contributed significantly to reduced reoperative morbidity and mortality.[31]

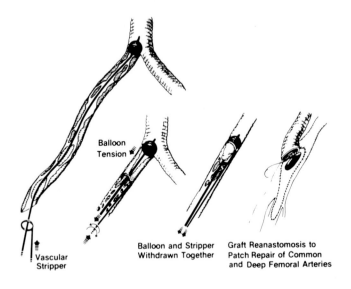

Balloon
Tension

Vascular
Stripper

Balloon and Stripper
Withdrawn Together

Graft Reanastomosis to
Patch Repair of Common
and Deep Femoral Arteries

FIGURE 39–6. A ring endarterectomy stripper is used in conjunction with a balloon catheter to remove thrombus and pseudointima adherent to the wall of an occluded limb of an aortofemoral graft. The cleared graft limb is thereafter sutured to the common or profunda femoral outflow after patch angioplasty. (From Bernhard VM: Late vascular graft thrombosis. *In* Bernhard VM, Towne JB (eds): Complications in Vascular Surgery, 2nd ed. Orlando, FL, Grune & Stratton, 1985, p 193.)

Lytic Therapy for Graft Thrombosis

While thrombectomy until recently has been the treatment of choice in the management of occluded aortofemoral and femoropopliteal bypass grafts, incomplete removal of thrombotic material and the difficulties associated with reoperation have led to the evaluation of direct intraarterial infusion of thrombolytic agents either preoperatively or intraoperatively for the management of this problem. The potential benefits of lytic therapy include: delineation of the cause of the graft thrombosis (most commonly distal occlusion due to neointimal fibrous hyperplasia or progression of disease) and as a consequence, a shorter operation; reduced blood loss; and the ease of extraction of any residual thrombus. Potential disadvantages and complications of thrombolytic therapy include the need for monitoring in an intensive care unit, delay in surgical intervention, and the risks of bleeding or renal impairment from the contrast load requisite to frequent arteriographic evaluations.

Furthermore, mechanical thrombectomy for aortofemoral graft limb occlusion is at least as effective as clot lysis while adding little to the operative procedure required to restore outflow. Successful lysis, which does not appear to be affected by the duration and cause of the graft thrombosis, can be achieved in 50 to 90 per cent of occluded prosthetic graft limb, 50 to 77 per cent of saphenous veins, and 38 to 71 per cent of prosthetic grafts.[41–48] In a recent series, Gardiner et al. reported an overall success rate of 69 per cent of the patients, with an 84 per cent success rate when urokinase was used compared to 48 per cent in those receiving streptokinase.[49] Presently, although both agents are effective in dissolving thrombus, urokinase appears to have some advantage over streptokinase due to its more predictable response, fewer bleeding complications, and shorter infusion time. In addition, infusion with streptokinase often cannot be repeated due to the development of antibodies. Although the cost of streptokinase is considerably less than urokinase, the shorter infusion time and lower complication rates negate the benefits of the initial lower cost of the former.[50]

For effective therapy, the catheter is usually imbedded within the thrombus. Most radiologists initially "lace" the thrombus with a bolus dose of 150,000 to 250,000 units of urokinase distributed through the length of the graft thrombus and continue with an hourly infusion of 20,000 to 40,000 units.[42,44,45] Either low-dose heparin or the lytic agent is infused into the sheath surrounding the infusion catheter to prevent pericatheter thrombosis. There are no useful laboratory tests available to evaluate the efficacy of lytic therapy, although titration of the lytic infusion to maintain a serum fibrinogen level of greater than 100 mg/dl is used by most investigators to monitor therapy. The duration of therapy ranges from 18 to 48 hours.

Bleeding, the major complication of lytic therapy, occurs following 7 to 48 per cent of infusions.[45,50] The most common sources of bleeding are arteriography or venous puncture sites, the interstices of prosthetic grafts, and systemic bleeding from remote sites. Central nervous system bleeding is rare with urokinase.

The most important determinant of long-term success in the study by Gardiner et al. was the presence of a lesion correctable by surgical revision or balloon catheter dilatation. Such lesions responsible for the occlusion can be identified in approximately 50 per cent of patients. Gardiner et al. reported an 84 per cent 1-year patency in 25 grafts with underlying stenotic lesions, compared to 37 per cent of a similar number of grafts without detectable lesions.[49]

To date, no prospective randomized study comparing thrombectomy versus lytic therapy has been undertaken to determine which form of therapy is the most beneficial in restoring patency to occluded grafts. The relatively low incidence of complications, improved technique of administration, and the efficacy of thrombolytic agents have reduced the need for urgent thrombectomy in patients with noncritical limb ischemia. Successful lytic therapy readily identifies the cause of the graft limb occlusion and may allow a less extensive repair. In addition, lytic therapy may reduce the risk of wound and graft complications associated with extensive redo procedures.

Lytic therapy should be regarded as complementary to surgical therapy for the treatment of graft thrombosis.

Operative Embolization

Atherothrombotic debris is present to some degree in most atherosclerotic arteries and especially in the distal aorta. Variable amounts of this material may be dislodged and carried into the downstream arterial territory as a consequence of manipulation during arterial dissection.[17,51,52] It may also occur upon reestablishment of circulation due to the accumulation of fresh thrombus in the temporarily static blood column above or below the clamps that is not carefully evacuated before circulation is restored.

Larger emboli lodging in major vessels can usually be retrieved with a balloon thrombectomy catheter. Smaller embolic particles that cannot be retrieved will be flushed into end arteries of the foot or toes, leading to the "trash foot" syndrome.[1,17,51,52] The end result is the appearance of patchy areas of painful skin gangrene at these sites (Fig. 39–7). This may be a minor and self-limited problem, or it may produce extensive gangrene of all of the digits and the forefoot.

Prevention is the key issue, since it is frequently difficult or impossible to treat this complication. A variety of technical maneuvers have been employed to prevent operative embolization.[1] Unnecessary and overly vigorous handling of vessels prior to the application of clamps should be avoided. Effective preclamping heparinization, preferably monitored by intraoperative measurement of the activated clotting

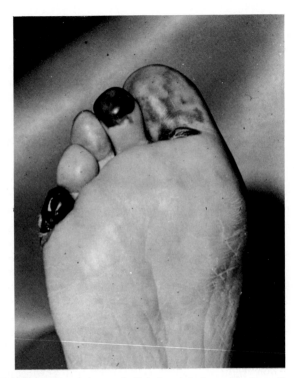

FIGURE 39–7. Atheroembolic ischemic lesions of the toes. (From Eastcott HHG: Complication of aortoiliac reconstruction for occlusive disease. *In* Bernhard VM, Towne JB (eds): Complications in Vascular Surgery. New York, Grune & Stratton, 1980, p 59.)

time, will reduce stasis thrombus formation above the proximal clamp and in the sluggish circulation distally. In patients with suspected or demonstrable atheromatous debris within the aorta on CT scans, the distal clamps should be applied to the common femoral or iliac arteries prior to proximal occlusion to avoid downstream displacement of debris when the aortic clamp is placed. The lumen of the aortic prosthesis should be thoroughly aspirated to remove blood and debris after testing the proximal suture line and efforts should be made to prevent the accumulation of blood within the prosthesis while distal iliac or femoral anastomoses are being performed. Vigorous prograde flushing of the proximal vessel and retrograde flushing from the distal arteries as the last few stitches are being placed in an anastomosis before restoration of circulation is the most reliable maneuver for ensuring that retained debris and clot are effectively removed.[52]

Treatment depends upon the severity of embolization. Minor patchy areas of cyanosis or necrosis can be observed since spontaneous recovery can be anticipated. More extensive involvement with threatened viability of the distal foot requires attempted removal of embolic material with small Fogarty catheters passed into the distal vessels through the patent popliteal artery accompanied by distal intraarterial infusion of urokinase.

Declamping Hypotension

A sudden decrease in blood pressure should be anticipated following removal of the aortic clamp to restore flow to one or both extremities after aortoiliac reconstruction.[53–56] The cause is hypovolemia due to incompletely replaced blood loss and fluid sequestration during surgery, compounded by a variable degree of preoperative dehydration that is usually present.[8] Contributing factors are peripheral vasodilatation secondary to limb ischemia during the period of aortic occlusion and a decrease in cardiac output caused by a sudden return of acidic blood and other vasoactive metabolites to the central circulation upon restoration of limb perfusion. The major consequences are significant reduction in coronary perfusion, which may promote myocardial injury, especially in patients with significant coronary artery disease, and temporary renal ischemia, which may contribute to renal failure. Prevention is preferable to treatment after a hypotensive insult has occurred, and depends upon adequate hydration and effective restoration of intravascular volume during the procedure and especially prior to clamp release.[55,57] Effective volume replacement requires careful monitoring of blood loss and accurate estimation of the extracellular fluid shifts due to sequestration and loss from evaporation. The extent of intravascular depletion is directly related to the duration of intraperitoneal and retroperitoneal exposure during surgery.

The most reliable guide for ensuring adequate volume replacement without circulatory overload is the use of the Swan-Ganz catheter to monitor left heart filling pressures and myocardial performance.[57] Cooperation between the surgeon and the anesthesiologist is essential during the critical moments prior to clamp release. Left atrial filling pressures should be optimized prior to release of the clamps. The arterial pressure must be continuously observed while blood flow is slowly restored to the extremities by gradual release of the clamp until full flow can be tolerated without hypotension. Finally, when a bifurcation graft is inserted, it is best to complete the anastomosis to one limb and restore its circulation immediately so that lower body perfusion can be resumed with the least amount of delay to avoid washout acidosis and reduce declamping hypotension.

Renal Failure

Acute renal failure (ARF) accompanying aortic surgery has a major impact on operative mortality. The reported incidence of ARF following elective aortic aneurysmectomy is 1 to 8 per cent, with a mortality rate of 40 per cent. However, if the aneurysmectomy is emergent, the reported incidence of ARF is 8 to 46 per cent, with a mortality of 57 to 95 per cent.[58,59] The major cause is reduced renal perfusion due to decreased cardiac output, decreased blood volume, and dehydration. A contributing factor is renal cortical vasospasm produced by subrenal application of the aortic clamp, which stimulates the renin angiotensin mechanism.[60,61] Other promoting factors include suprarenal aortic cross-clamping, which totally eliminates renal perfusion, ligation of the left renal vein, and intraoperative renal arterial embolization.[62] The latter may originate from debris and clot accumulating proximal to the aortic clamp or from manipulation of the juxtarenal aorta.[59,63] Renal artery obstruction may be produced by displacement of large atherosclerotic plaques at the orifices of the renal arteries when an aortic clamp is applied. Preoperative angiography may produce a mild to moderate degree of renal dysfunction, which may be compounded by hypotension and dehydration during the operative procedure.[59] Myoglobinemia can occur following restoration of circulation to limbs that have been severely ischemic for an extended period of time. Finally, nephrotoxic antibiotics employed perioperatively must be considered.

The critical issue is prevention, which is primarily related to the maintenance of an effective circulating blood volume and adequate hydration in the immediate perioperative period.[59,64] It is essential that the patient be well hydrated, with a good urinary output at the commencement of surgery. Any significant extracellular fluid volume deficits should be restored the evening before surgery, especially if angiography has been recently performed. The creatinine level should be measured following angiography, and if a decrease in renal function is identified, surgery should be delayed if possible. Central filling pressures should be monitored perioperatively to ensure that volume replacement is optimal in relation to cardiac output and myocardial performance.[57] It is appropriate to give mannitol and commence an infusion of renal dose dopamine just prior to cross-clamping the aorta to promote an osmotic diuresis and reduce the effects of renal cortical vasospasm.[60] Bicarbonate is given to alkalinize the urine if there is any question of significant myoglobin washout from renewed perfusion of limbs that have undergone prolonged ischemia.

During dissection required to gain proximal control of large infrarenal or juxtarenal aneurysms, the left renal vein is vulnerable to injury. Access to this portion of the aorta is facilitated by division of the left renal vein.[65] In the past, this maneuver has been viewed as one of little long-term consequence. However, recently, Huber et al.[66] and AbuRahma et al.[67] have demonstrated increased serum creatinine concentrations in patients who have had renal vein ligation. Whether the renal dysfunction following renal vein ligation is a consequence solely of the resultant increased venous pressure or develops because of a combination of venous hypertension and transient ischemia from intraoperative suprarenal clamp placement (which is required more frequently in these

patients) is not yet clear. Nonetheless, it would appear prudent to repair the renal vein when possible as advocated by Szilagyi et al.[65]

Renal arteries should be dissected free and temporarily clamped in patients with total aortic occlusion in which thrombus extends up to the renal orifices. The quality of the renal pulses must be evaluated and blood flow assessed by Doppler after restoration of circulation through the aorta in any patient who has had significant juxtarenal aortic manipulation or if urine output should suddenly diminish. Immediate renal repair is required if renal artery occlusion is identified.

Postoperatively, the continued retroperitoneal and intraperitoneal sequestration of extracellular fluid will require replacement with Ringer's lactate solution, within the limits imposed by left heart filling pressures, in order to ensure adequate renal output.[8] Volume replacement should be reduced after the second postoperative day to prevent fluid overload from the mobilization of large volumes of sequestered extravascular fluid. The urinary output is monitored continuously and should be maintained at or above 0.5 ml/kg/hr. The specific gravity is determined frequently, and the blood urea nitrogen and creatinine measured daily for 2 or 3 days to determine the quality of renal function. Diuretics should not be given until intravascular volume has been fully restored. If ARF is diagnosed, fluid replacement should be restricted to maintain central filling pressure in the normal range. Dialysis is used aggressively to control excess volume and relieve azotemia and hyperkalemia.[59,68]

The liberal use of aortography before surgery is recommended to identify renal anomalies, renal artery stenoses, or suprarenal extension of an aneurysm so that appropriate alterations in operative management can be planned. This may include the use of temporary renal perfusion with cold lactated Ringer's solution containing heparin, mannitol, and methylprednisolone.[59] Postoperatively, aortography should be performed immediately if total renal shutdown appears, since this suggests a renal artery occlusion. This will require immediate reoperation to restore kidney circulation.

Intestinal Ischemia

Intestinal ischemia may complicate aortic bypass or endarterectomy for occlusive disease, but the majority of cases follow aneurysmectomy.[69,70] Almost all reported instances of intestinal ischemia following aortic surgery are a result of arterial obstruction; venous ischemia is extremely rare.[71] Small bowel ischemia occurs in 0.15 per cent of cases.[69] The clinical presentation of ischemic colitis occurs in 0.2 to 10 per cent of aortic procedures and most commonly involves the rectosigmoid area.[72] However, if routine colonoscopy is performed, a much higher incidence of intestinal ischemia is noted because of the identification of subclinical ischemic colitis. Hagihara, Ernst, and Griffen[73] found a 6 per cent incidence in patients undergoing elective or urgent reconstruction of the abdominal aorta for aneurysmal or occlusive disease, whereas the incidence of ischemic colitis was 60 per cent following repair of ruptured aneurysm. The overall mortality rate for patients with colon ischemia is approximately 50 per cent and approaches 90 per cent for transmural colon involvement.

The cause of bowel ischemia is operative atheroembolization or interruption of the primary or collateral arteries to the bowel wall.[69,70] There are two sets of vessels that are critical to colon perfusion: (1) the superior rectal branch of the inferior mesenteric artery that connects with the middle and inferior rectal branches of the hypogastric vessels, thus connecting the visceral with the systemic circulation; and (2) the inferior mesenteric artery and its left colic branch that connects with the superior mesenteric through the arch of Riolan and to a lesser extent the marginal artery of Drummond.[72] The former connection is referred to as the "meandering mesenteric artery," especially when it becomes enlarged as a collateral to compensate for superior or inferior mesenteric artery obstruction.[74] This vessel is present in about two thirds of normal individuals and can be seen on angiography in 27 to 35 per cent of patients who have aneurysmal or occlusive disease.[75] Areas of deficiency in this normal anatomic relationship are at Griffith's point at the splenic flexure and in the collateral vessels of the rectosigmoid (Fig. 39–8).

Obstruction of the primary arteries supplying the viscera makes viability of the bowel dependent upon this collateral circulation. Occlusion of the orifice of the inferior mesenteric artery is frequently associated with aneurysmal disease and obstructive aortic atherosclerosis, thus placing the burden of bowel circulation upon collaterals from the superior mesenteric artery and the hypogastric vessels. Severe obstruction or occlusion of the superior mesenteric artery is compensated for by branches from the celiac and retrograde flow from the inferior mesenteric artery through the left colic and middle colic. Hypogastric obstruction requires collateral flow from branches of the inferior mesenteric artery. When this source is also impaired, colon circulation must depend upon more tenuous connections between the arch of Riolan and the marginal artery and the distal branches of the hypogastric, which in turn derive their blood supply from the parietal circulation.

A critical loss of blood flow to an intestinal tract that is dependent upon this extensive collateral network may occur if a patent inferior mesenteric artery is ligated during aortic surgery. Collateral flow may be further compromised by ligating the inferior mesenteric artery peripherally rather than flush with the aortic wall, since this may occlude the connection between the left colic and the superior rectal arteries. Failure to ensure perfusion through at least one hypogastric may promote colon ischemia if this is the primary supply in the absence of the inferior mesenteric artery or effective collateral flow from the meandering artery. Loss of the inferior mesenteric artery or the meandering artery will produce right colon and small bowel ischemia when these viscera depend upon retrograde flow because of superior mesenteric arterial occlusion (Fig. 39–9). The large hematoma associated with a ruptured aneurysm may compress significant collateral vessels, which may explain the high incidence of colon ischemia in this circumstance.[69] Furthermore, angiography is almost never available prior to repair of a ruptured aneurysm, and the surgeon does not have precise information regarding intestinal circulation in order to design an operative procedure that will conserve or augment colon perfusion.

Depending on the severity of ischemia and the thickness of bowel wall involved, three forms of ischemic colitis are recognized. Type I is mucosal ischemia, which is transient and mild. Type II, with mucosal and muscularis involvement, reflects more severe ischemia that may result in healing with fibrosis, scarring, and stricture. Type III is transmural ischemia that produces irreparable damage with gangrene and bowel perforation.[76]

The clinical manifestations of intestinal ischemia immediately after aortic surgery are often masked by incisional discomfort and other problems that may explain abdominal pain, tenderness, fever, an elevated white blood cell count, and fluid sequestration. Findings that suggest the presence of intestinal ischemia and progressing infarction of the colon include progressive distention, sepsis, increasing peritoneal signs, and unexplained metabolic acidosis. The most common clinical presentation is diarrhea, either brown liquid or bloody, which occurs in 65 to 76 per cent of patients with intestinal ischemia.[72,77] Although the onset may occur as long as 14 days after operation, diarrhea usually appears within 24 to 48 hours after surgery.[72] Bloody diarrhea has been reported to be a more ominous prognostic sign than nonbloody diarrhea[78]; however, some investigators have noted no correlation between extent of ischemic injury and presence of bloody diarrhea.[79]

Postoperative *Clostridium difficile* colitis may mimic ischemic colitis. Therefore, in critically ill patients who develop fever, abdominal distention, diarrhea, and leukocytosis following emergency aortic procedures, stool specimens for culture and for *C. difficile* toxin should be obtained and endoscopic evaluation of the colon performed. Appropriate antibiotic therapy (metronidazole or vancomycin) should be instituted if the diagnosis of *C. difficile* is confirmed.[80,81]

Early diagnosis of ischemia is the key to effective management of ischemic colitis. The diagnosis depends upon a high index of suspicion and the prompt performance of endoscopy with the flexible sigmoidoscope or colonoscope. Occurrence of ischemic colitis without left colon involvement is rare enough that endoscopy to 40 cm is usually sufficient to establish the diagnosis.[69] Once detected, endoscopy should be

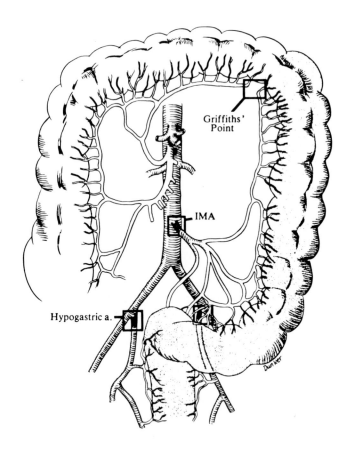

FIGURE 39–8. Lack of marginal artery continuity at splenic flexure (Griffith's point) with inferior mesenteric (IMA) and hypogastric arterial occlusions predisposing to left colon ischemia. (From Ernst CB: Colon ischemia following abdominal aortic reconstruction. *In* Bernhard VM, Towne JB (eds): Complications in Vascular Surgery. New York, Grune & Stratton, 1980, p 383.)

terminated to avoid perforation. Mild changes of ischemic colitis consist of submucosal hemorrhage and edema that is usually circumferential. Pseudomembranes, erosions, and ulcers indicate more advanced ischemia. A yellowish green, necrotic, noncontractile surface indicates gangrene.[72] Repeated endoscopy,

every other day by the same individual, is required to document resolution or progression of the process.

Patients under observation for intestinal ischemia are managed by frequent reexamination; serial endoscopy; monitoring of blood gases, urine output and fluid requirements; institution of broad-spectrum

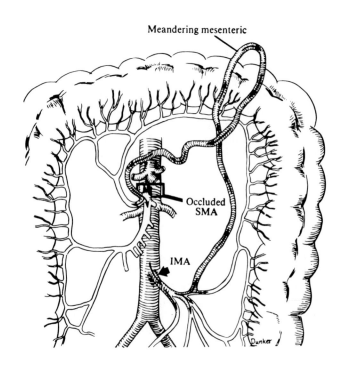

FIGURE 39–9. When superior mesenteric artery (*SMA*) is occluded, meandering mesenteric blood flow is from inferior mesenteric artery (*IMA*) to SMA. Meandering mesenteric sacrifice under these conditions predisposes to small bowel as well as colonic ischemia. (From Ernst CB: Colon ischemia following abdominal aortic reconstruction. *In* Bernhard VM, Towne JB (eds): Complications in Vascular Surgery. New York, Grune & Stratton, 1980, p 385.)

antibiotic coverage; and bowel rest with nasogastric suction. If the colon appears distended, either clinically or radiographically, it should be decompressed by the gentle insertion of a rectal tube, since increased intraluminal pressure may further compromise colon blood flow.[72]

Improvement of the patient as evidenced by diminishing diarrhea, improvement in vital signs, clinical exam, lab parameters, and resolution of the ischemia documented by endoscopy permits continuation of nonoperative management.[69] Reversible ischemic lesions should improve within 7 to 10 days.[76,82] Continuing clinical evidence of ischemia beyond 2 weeks requires operative intervention because this usually reflects a walled-off perforation with local peritonitis.[72] Finally, progression of the intestinal ischemia during the period of observation, identified by deteriorating clinical signs and symptoms, requires prompt celiotomy. Surgery for transmural ischemic colitis requires resection of nonviable bowel, end-colostomy, and formation of a Hartmann's pouch or resection of the rectum, if involved.[83]

Prevention of intestinal ischemia depends upon an appreciation of the potential for this complication and the institution of appropriate steps to either avoid injury to the collateral circulation of the colon or augment circulation to the bowel as part of the aortic reconstructive procedure.[84] Routine preoperative aortography will identify a patent inferior mesenteric artery with retrograde flow through a large meandering artery that is functioning as a collateral pathway for an obstructed superior mesenteric artery.[85] In this circumstance, flow through the inferior mesenteric must be preserved by sparing this orifice through construction of an end-to-side aortic anastomosis or by reimplantation of the inferior mesenteric onto the side of an aortic graft using a variation of the Carrel patch technique.[69] In a prospective study of 100 patients undergoing aortic reconstructive procedures, Zelenock et al. observed a 3 per cent incidence of endoscopic colonic ischemia. Adjunctive procedures were utilized in 12 per cent of the patients, compared to 4 per cent in earlier studies from their institution.[86] Bypass to the superior mesenteric should also be considered.[84] A large meandering artery with flow from the superior mesenteric toward the sigmoid and rectum in the presence of inferior mesenteric artery occlusion is strong evidence for adequate collateral supply to the bowel.[75] Ischemic colitis is unlikely under these circumstances if this collateral is not impaired by surgery. The status of the hypogastric vessels should be identified on the aortogram so that arterial reconstruction can be designed to maintain flow through at least one of these arteries by direct revascularization or by retrograde perfusion from a femoral anastomosis, especially if a patent inferior mesenteric artery must be ligated.[82]

Measurement of the inferior mesenteric artery back-pressure during aortic reconstruction may be a useful guide to the need for restoration of flow to the inferior mesenteric artery.[82] A mean pressure greater than 40 mm Hg and an inferior mesenteric artery–systemic pressure ratio of greater than 0.4 indicate satisfactory collateral circulation without the need for mesenteric arterial repair.

Thorough mechanical preparation of the bowel prior to aortic surgery will reduce the fecal burden to which the potentially ischemic bowel is exposed.[69] During aortic surgery, every effort should be made to prevent injury to the mesenteric vessels. Undue traction on the left colon mesentery should be avoided. When inferior mesenteric ligation is required, this should be carried out by suture ligature within the aortic lumen or immediately adjacent to the aortic wall to avoid injury to its ascending and descending branches.[69] Finally, the presence of Doppler flow signals over the base of the bowel mesentery and the serosal surface of the colon suggests that adequate collateral circulation is present.[77] Absence of a flow signal after reconstruction suggests the need to restore perfusion through the inferior mesenteric artery or through some other major collateral vessel.

Spinal Cord Ischemia

This problem occurs most frequently during repair of thoracic and thoracoabdominal aneurysms, but is occasionally encountered during resection of an abdominal aortic aneurysm and rarely following aortoiliac bypass for ischemia.[62,87,88] The overall incidence of this complication for abdominal aortic surgery has been reported to be 0.23 per cent and is 10 times higher following the repair of ruptured abdominal aortic aneurysms than following elective aneurysm resection.[88,89] The incidence of spinal cord ischemia following thoracic aortic reconstruction is in the range of 1 to 10 per cent, depending upon the extent of the lesion repaired.

The upper level of the neurologic deficit was found to be T10 to L2 in 88.6 per cent of 44 cases reviewed at the Henry Ford Hospital.[89] Postoperative mortality was directly related to the severity of paraplegia. When the neurologic deficit initially was complete, involving both sensory and motor function, 76 per cent of the patients expired; there were only two complete neurologic recoveries and one partial. By contrast, when the initial loss was only partial motor and/or sensory loss, 24 per cent expired and some degree of recovery was noted in all but one case.[88,90,91]

The major cause of spinal cord ischemia is interruption of flow through the great radicular artery of Adamkiewicz, which is the major source of supply to the anterior spinal artery at the lower end of the cord.[87,92] The great radicular artery is a major branch of the posterior division of one of the intercostal vessels arising between T8 and L1. On occasion, it may originate from a lumbar branch of the infrarenal aorta. The anterior spinal artery itself is long and has rather poor collateral contributions from the posterior spinal arteries or from the radicular arteries derived from more proximal intercostal vessels. Since the spinal cord is only tenuously supplied in its lower portion by vessels other than the great radicular, any injury to this vessel during aortic reconstruction may lead to some degree of cord infarction. The effectiveness of collateral pathways may be further compromised by hypotension, especially in patients with ruptured aneurysm. The placement of a high aortic clamp for temporary control of a ruptured aneurysm, however, does not clearly correlate with the incidence or severity of cord ischemia.[88]

Williams et al. and Kieffer et al. have recently reported successful angiographic visualization of the origin of the artery of Adamkiewicz in 49 and 69 per cent of patients with thoracoabdominal aneurysms, respectively. The very low incidence of spinal cord ischemia following operations on the *infrarenal* aorta and the risks associated with preoperative or operative angiographic demonstration of the major blood supply to the lower spinal cord render visualization impractical and potentially dangerous.[67,92–94] Moreover, the occurrence of this complication has been unpredictable and may be unpreventable in association with infrarenal aortic reconstruction. Monitoring of somatosensory-evoked potentials during thoracic surgery has been shown to correlate with cord ischemia.[95] These abnormal findings have been reversed by temporary shunting and implantation of intercostal vessels into the thoracic aortic graft. Practical application of this technique to abdominal aortic surgery is undergoing continued investigation.[95–98]

Although there are no data to identify specific preventive measures, it would seem prudent to avoid high aortic clamping unless absolutely necessary, to maintain cord perfusion pressure by avoiding systemic hypotension, and to prevent stasis thrombosis in collateral vessels by effective heparinization. Suturing a patch of posterior aortic wall with its intercostal vessel orifices into a window cut out of the graft has been recommended for thoracoabdominal aneurysms.[62] Finally, it is important to ensure pelvic perfusion through one or both hypogastric arteries to maximize collateral contribution to the spinal cord.[99]

When ischemic injury to the spinal cord occurs, treatment is palliative and supportive.[88]

Ureteral Injury

The ureters are immediately adjacent to the operative field and may be easily injured during dissection and arterial repair.[100] This is especially important in patients with large iliac and hypogastric aneurysms or when there is increased adherence to vascular structures in the presence of an "inflammatory" aneurysm or retroperitoneal fibrosis.[101] A thorough knowledge of the anatomic relationships of the ureters at the level of the iliac bifurcation is essential. Occasionally, multiple ureters may be present or they may be in an aberrant position owing to congenital anomalies. These variations may be defined by a preoperative intravenous pyelogram or a pyelographic film during the preoperative aortogram or CT scan. A preoperative intravenous pyelogram (IVP) or contrast-enhanced CT scan is especially indicated in reoperative aortoiliac surgery to identify postoperative changes in the ureteral anatomy or demonstrate possible injury incurred during the initial surgery.

Direct injury to the ureter can best be avoided by keeping the dissection close to the iliac artery at the point at which the ureter normally crosses the common iliac bifurcation in transit to the bladder. This is especially important during the blind development of the retroperitoneal tunnel for aortofemoral bypass. The ureter should be elevated away from the iliac vessels so that the graft will lie dorsal to it. Inadvertent passage of the graft ventral to the ureter may cause it to be compressed between the graft limb and the underlying iliac artery, producing hydronephrosis. The incidence of ureteral obstruction after aortic grafting in a recent prospective study was 2 per cent.[102] The ureter may be entrapped in perigraft scar, however, even though placed in its proper position ventral to the prosthesis.[100]

Both ureters should be demonstrated before closing the retroperitoneum. The right ureter must be carefully protected during retroperitoneal closure, since this structure can easily be caught up in the suture line. Iatrogenic ureteral injuries sustained during placement or revision of a vascular graft should be repaired primarily. Although renal salvage is possible when the diagnosis is delayed, nephrectomy is often necessary if there has been extensive contamination of the graft.[103]

Wright et al. have recently reported a 35-year experience with 58 ureteral complications in patients undergoing aortoiliac reconstructions.[104] Two of the six patients who had ureteric obstruction treated prior to or in conjunction with repair of their aneurysms developed graft complications (one graft limb thrombosis and one graft infection). The remaining 44 patients had 46 complications including: hydronephrosis (42), ureteric leaks (3), and ureteric necrosis (1). Twenty-four patients had 36 graft complications including: anastomotic aneurysms (19), graft limb thrombosis (8), graft infections (6), and aortoenteric fistulae (3). Twenty-nine of the 44 patients underwent graft or ureteral operations, or both, with a mortality rate of 21 per cent.[104]

Patients in whom hydronephrosis is recognized preoperatively may benefit from ureteral stent placement in order to decompress the obstruction and facilitate ureteral identification during repair. Postoperative hydronephrosis detected on ultrasonography, CT scans, or IVP may initially be followed expectantly, as it will often resolve. Only 12 of the 58 patients reported by Wright et al. required surgical intervention for progressive hydronephrosis.[104] The selective use of stents and antibiotics in conjunction with operative repair is essential if the high incidence of graft complications is to be reduced.

Impotence

The loss of ability to achieve or maintain an erection adequate for satisfactory coitus may be due to vasculogenic, psychogenic, neurogenic, endocrinogenic, or medication-related factors.[105–109] Eighty per cent of patients who present with aortoiliac occlusive disease will have significant erectile dysfunction.[105] Nearly 25 per cent of patients undergoing direct aortic reconstruction will suffer iatrogenic erectile dysfunction if appropriate technical modifications are not employed. Therefore, careful evaluation of penile erectile function by history, noninvasive techniques, and angiography should be included in the preoperative evaluation before elective aortic surgery.[109,110] This will determine whether there is normal sexual function that should be preserved or whether there is already an established pattern of impotence that may possibly be relieved by altering pelvic blood flow. This information may also provide valuable insights into the psychogenic and cultural factors contributing to an existing problem and will provide the surgeon with an estimate of the importance of sexual function to the patient. Such preoperative information might alter the type of aortic operation previously planned.

Preoperative evaluation of erectile function includes nocturnal tumescence studies. The absence of tumescence during an adequate sleep study is strong evidence of organic impotence. Documentation of normal erections during rapid eye movement (REM) sleep establishes the psychogenic basis of the patient's erectile dysfunction. Unfortunately, the failure of erection is often qualitative rather than complete, making tumescence studies less discriminating between organic and psychogenic impotence.[105,110]

If organic impotence is suspected, the next step is noninvasive vascular testing. At present, the most reliable measurement is the penile systolic pressure and the penile-brachial ratio (penile-brachial index or PBI).[105] Kempczinski found that age had a deleterious effect on the PBI that was independent of sexual potency.[110] Patients under the age of 40 had a mean PBI of 0.99 compared to a PBI of 0.74 for equally potent males over 40. This difference was statistically significant. By contrast, impotent males over the age of 40 had a mean PBI of 0.58, also a statistically significant difference. Despite the significant differences in PBI in these three groups, there is a failure of correlation between PBI and the degree of erectile dysfunction.[110,111] Although a low PBI is not sufficient to establish the diagnosis of vasculogenic impotence, the finding of a PBI greater than 0.8 confirms the adequacy of penile blood flow and suggests that a vasculogenic etiology is extremely unlikely.[105]

Neurogenic impotence is commonly a result of neuropathy secondary to diabetes mellitus or may follow autonomic nerve injury from genitourinary or abdominopelvic surgery. This diagnosis is often one of exclusion, but abnormal pudendal nerve velocity studies (sacral latency testing) and abnormal cystometrography (the anatomic pathways in micturition and erection being similar) can implicate this etiology.[105,112]

The diagnosis of endocrinologic impotency requires measurement of thyroid function and serum levels of testosterone and other associated hormones. Finally, a thorough medication history is required.[112]

Preoperative angiography is useful in identifying the patency of the hypogastric vessels and their contribution to pelvic perfusion. Unfortunately, angiographic findings correlate poorly with the patient's erectile function.[105] Selective injections to identify the flow through the pudendal vessels into the penis may be required to more accurately assess patients being evaluated primarily for vasculogenic impotence.[105]

Careful preservation of the sympathetic-parasympathetic plexus overlying the aorta and its bifurcation and maintenance of blood flow through the hypogastric and pudendal arteries are the important factors to be considered in order to prevent impotence in men undergoing elective aortic surgery.[107,109,113] Dissection should be carried down to the aortic wall on its right anterolateral surface and the paraaortic structures gently retracted to the left to avoid trauma to the nerves contained within these tissues (Fig. 39–10A and B). During aneurysm resection, the inferior mesenteric artery should not be dissected free but should be controlled by suture ligature from inside the aorta after the aneurysm has been opened to avoid disruption of nerve fibers at the junction of the inferior mesenteric artery with the aorta (Fig. 39–10B and C). There should be minimal division of the longitudinal periaortic tissues to the left of the infrarenal aorta, and the nerve plexuses that cross the left common iliac artery should be spared.[105,113] The limbs of bifurcation grafts should be placed within the lumina of common iliac aneurysms to avoid external dissection and minimize the injury to perivascular nerve fibers.

Although the findings on preoperative angiograms correlate poorly with erectile function, preservation of adequate perfusion into at least one hypogastric artery appears to be a vital component in minimizing iatrogenic impotence.[105] When possible, direct antegrade perfusion of the internal iliac artery should be assured. This may require thromboendarterectomy of the hypogastric orifice. If both external iliac arteries are occluded or stenotic and bypass into the common femoral arteries is anticipated, precluding retrograde iliac flow, the proximal aortic anastomosis should be constructed end-to-side when feasible in order to preserve pelvic blood flow. When proximal aortic disease is extensive, requiring an end-to-end proximal anastomosis, and impaired penile perfusion has been diagnosed by preoperative noninvasive testing, it may be necessary to reimplant the hypogastric artery into one limb of an aortobifemoral graft or add a jump graft to one hypogastric artery to improve pelvic inflow.[105,112] Finally, careful flushing of the graft in both directions before completion of the final suture line

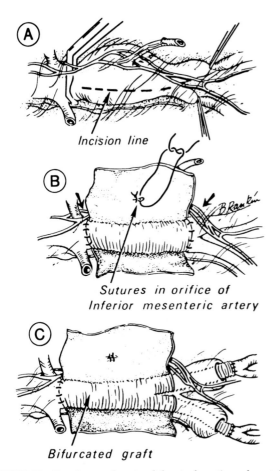

Incision line

Sutures in orifice of Inferior mesenteric artery

Bifurcated graft

FIGURE 39–10. Approaches to abdominal aortic and aortoiliac aneurysm. Sac is left intact and sutured over inlay graft. (From DePalma RG: Impotence as a complication of aortic reconstruction. *In* Bernhard VM, Towne JB (eds): Complications in Vascular Surgery. New York, Grune & Stratton, 1980, p 437.)

is important to prevent embolization of small particles into the pelvic arteries.

Anastomotic False Aneurysm

False aneurysms can develop at any anastomotic site. They are almost invariably associated with prosthetic rather than autogenous tissue suture lines.[114–120] The most common sites of occurrence are femoral anastomoses following placement of aortofemoral bypass grafts.[115,117,120] Pathologically, there is a partial separation of the graft from the arterial wall.[114,118,120] The perianastomotic fibrous tissue prevents immediate hemorrhage and forms a capsule around the hematoma that gradually expands owing to the pressure transmitted from the arterial lumen. The fibrous capsule may rupture, with rapid painful enlargement of the mass, or erode the overlying skin to produce infection and external hemorrhage. In the abdomen, false aneurysms are prone to erode into adjacent bowel, forming aortoenteric fistulas.[120–122] Since blood flow within the pseudoaneurysm is static, its lumen becomes partially filled with thrombus, which may

embolize.[114,120] The luminal distortion produced by the pseudoaneurysm and its thrombus may also cause occlusion of a graft.[120]

In the immediate postoperative period, all vascular anastomoses are entirely dependent on suture material alone. With time, a prosthetic-artery junction is maintained by the integrity of the suture material and also by external fibrous bonding caused by scarring.[123] The important factors involved in the development of an anastomotic false aneurysm include arterial wall weakness,[119] endarterectomy at the anastomotic site,[124] compliance mismatch between the graft and host artery,[125,126] dilatation of the graft material,[122,127] prosthetic deterioration or an actual flaw in the graft material,[128] increased tension at the anastomotic site due to insufficient length of the prosthesis,[128] deterioration of suture material,[129] and uneven tension on the anastomosis as a result of beveling of the end of the graft.[123]

Pseudoaneurysm is occasionally due to underlying infection, although this is infrequently identified.[117,120] When infection is the causative factor, a purulent perigraft exudate is usually, but not necessarily, present. Therefore, during repair of any pseudoaneurysm, its wall and contents should be routinely cultured by aerobic and anaerobic techniques.

The incidence of false aneurysm formation ranges between 1.4 and 4 per cent.[118] Recognition is usually quite simple at groin anastomoses, where a large, pulsatile, and sometimes tender mass becomes apparent to both the patient and the examining physician. False aneurysms developing in the retroperitoneum at an aortic or iliac anastomosis rarely become palpable and will go unnoticed until rupture produces pain and shock or erosion occurs into an adjacent loop of bowel, with gastrointestinal hemorrhage.[130] Occasionally, false aneurysms are identified during routine arteriography for some other vascular problem. Ultrasonography and CT are reliable methods for evaluating grafts and anastomoses for dilatation and pseudoaneurysm formation.[131] Diagnosis of a pseudoaneurysm is usually confirmed by arteriography, which demonstrates widening at the anastomosis and an extraluminal accumulation of dye at the point of anastomotic disruption. Since the false aneurysm is partially filled with thrombus, the extent of extraluminal dye accumulation only partially outlines the full extent of the process. A more accurate measure of the true size of the defect can be obtained by ultrasonography or CT scanning.[131]

Retroperitoneal false aneurysms should be repaired as soon as they are identified to avoid rupture or bowel erosion.[118,121,130] Unfortunately, this complication is frequently the first indication that a false aneurysm is present. When there is no evidence of infection, the suture line defect can be dissected free and repaired either directly or by the interposition of fresh graft material. When infection or visceral erosion has taken place, the graft must be removed entirely and the aorta and iliac vessels closed. Management of this problem is discussed in detail elsewhere in this text.

Generally, peripheral false aneurysms should be repaired as soon as they are identified. However, false aneurysms that are small, stable, and asymptomatic may be observed, especially if the patient is at increased risk for reoperation.[117,119,120] If surgery is delayed, reexamination at frequent intervals is mandatory so that repair can be carried out when expansion is evident but before complications develop.

Surgical repair of a false aneurysm is usually carried out through the site of the original incision. Dissection is carried down to the graft wall proximally so that it can be controlled with a circumferential tape. Further dissection is then carried distally along the graft to define the anastomosis, the aneurysmal bulge, and the branches of the common femoral artery. It is usually difficult and tedious to dissect out the major branches of the artery at the anastomotic site. When extensive scarring is encountered, further dissection may be abandoned and the patient is given intravenous heparin. The graft is then clamped and disconnected from the aneurysm and branch control is achieved by the insertion of balloon occlusion catheters into the lumina of the major branches.[118] The anastomotic site is carefully surveyed to identify the cause of the psuedoaneurysm. The distal frayed end of the graft at the anastomosis is resected, and the edges of the artery are trimmed back to healthy tissue. In order to avoid tension at the new anastomosis, a short piece of new graft material is usually required to connect the proximal end of the old prosthesis with the freshened arterial orifice. The diameter of the interposed graft segment should usually not exceed 8 mm to more closely approximate the size of the outflow tract rather than the larger inflow prosthetic limb.[127] Unless retrograde flow up the external iliac must be preserved, it is best to convert the femoral anastomosis from end to side to end to end.[118] Prior to repairing the anastomosis, the orifices of the superficial femoral and profunda should be inspected so that significant stenoses can be repaired by endarterectomy and/or patch angioplasty to ensure adequate runoff.

Overall mortality for repair of anastomotic femoral false aneurysms was 3.5 per cent and the amputation rate was 2.8 per cent in a recent review.[123] Results are distinctly better if this lesion is repaired electively rather than as an emergency.[119,120] The recurrence rate of anastomotic femoral false aneurysms after initial repair has been reported to be 5.7 per cent; these are amenable to secondary repair.[123,127]

Recurrent Anastomotic Aneurysm

Femoral anastomotic aneurysms (FAA) develop in approximately 3 per cent of all femoral anastomoses and in 6 per cent of patients undergoing aortofemoral bypass. Repair of FAA remains durable in approximately 80 per cent of patients; however, a small percentage of patients develop recurrent anastomotic aneurysms (RFAA). In a series of 43 FAAs, Ernst reported a 19 per cent incidence of this complication.[132]

Factors predisposing to RFAA include graft dilatation, local wound complications, and females who previously had repair of an FAA.[127,132] Although there appears to be an inverse relationship between atherosclerotic heart disease and RFAA, the significance of this observation is difficult to explain. Furthermore, factors that have been implicated in the development of FAA (e.g., hypertension, smoking, diabetes, suture material, type of graft, and performance of an endarterectomy) have not been related to the development of RFAA.

Recurrent femoral anastomotic aneurysms are subject to the same complications as primary FAA such as rupture, thrombus, or peripheral embolization.

Repair is indicated in good-risk patients with RFAAs greater than 2 cm in size. Management includes careful follow-up for anastomotic aneurysms less than 2 cm in size, especially if coexisting medical problems make surgical intervention risky. The principles of repair are similar to those for primary FAAs and include careful dissection of the distal outflow vessels, use of graft material approximately the size of the outflow vessel, and conversion from end-to-side to end-to-end anastomosis.[127,132]

Chylous Ascites

Chylous ascites, issuing from a damaged cisterna chyli and its tributaries at the root of the mesentery, is a rare complication of aortic reconstruction. Interruption of the lymphatics and chylous ascites are not invariably related, since the lymphatics are often interrupted during aortic operations without apparent sequelae.[133]

Patients with chylous ascites present usually within 2 or 3 weeks of aortic repair with anorexia and progressive abdominal distention. Ascites is usually evident on physical examination and can be confirmed by abdominal radiographs, ultrasound, or CT scans. The fluid obtained by abdominal paracentesis is milky, with a high lymphocyte count and lipid content, and is bacteriologically sterile. An additional complication is leakage of ascites to the outside through a defect in the incision; this increases the fluid and protein loss and heightens the risk of infection. Such a leak should be repaired under sterile conditions and prophylactic antibiotic coverage.

The management of chylous ascites includes abdominal paracentesis, a low-fat diet rich in medium-chain triglycerides, and total parenteral nutrition (TPN). However, repeated paracentesis may result in the loss of large amounts of protein and lipid that cannot readily be replaced. An additional risk is that of line-related sepsis. In patients who do not respond to repeated paracentesis, a peritoneal venous shunt, in addition to diet control or TPN, may relieve the ascites. Operative ligation may be necessary in resistant cases.[133]

INFRAINGUINAL ARTERIAL RECONSTRUCTION

Femoropopliteal and femoroinfrapopliteal bypasses are the most commonly performed procedures for revascularization of the lower extremity below the inguinal ligament. Specific problems related to endarterectomy of either the superficial femoral, popliteal, or profunda femoris arteries will be reviewed in discussion of these procedures. The basic principles of infrainguinal bypass are similar to those for aortoiliac reconstruction, with the following significant differences: the vessels involved are smaller and the length of the bypass conduit is greater, with a consequent increase in the incidence of early and late thrombosis; vein grafts are used rather than prostheses for the majority of procedures; and there is a tendency for less severe systemic complications owing to the more peripheral and less traumatic nature of the operative procedure.

Bleeding

Major blood loss or hemorrhage is not a frequent complication during this surgery but may become a problem in the immediate postoperative period. The most common sources are the anastomoses, insecure ligatures on branches of a vein graft, laceration of the vein wall by instruments in the in situ technique, blind disruption of small vessels encountered during blunt dissection of thigh and leg tunnels, inadequate hemostasis during the dissection of the major vessels, incomplete reversal of heparin anticoagulation, and oozing from antiplatelet medication.[134] In the immediate postoperative period, bleeding usually appears as wound swelling of the extremity and the severity of hypotension, if present, mirrors the extent and rapidity of hemorrhage. Prompt return to the operating room is required to control the source of bleeding and to evacuate the hematoma, which may interfere with healing and promote infection. Long-term graft patency has been shown to be significantly reduced in patients who develop wound hemorrhage in the immediate postoperative period.[134] Wound hemorrhage that occurs after 48 to 72 hours is frequently due to infection involving the graft at an anastomosis and is less likely to be caused by mechanical factors.[134] However, hemorrhage may occur later in the immediate postoperative period in patients who have been maintained on anticoagulants or in whom fibrinolytic agents have been infused for graft thrombosis within 10 days to 2 weeks of surgery.[135]

Thrombosis

The most common significant complication of infrainguinal bypass or endarterectomy is thrombosis of the reconstruction. In the early postoperative period (less than 30 days), thrombosis is usually related to technical factors[17,37,136,137] (Fig. 39–11). The most common of these is imprecise construction of the suture line resulting in stenosis or elevation of a distal intimal flap that obstructs flow; this is especially important at a distal anastomosis to a small-caliber tibial or peroneal vessel. A prosthetic or reversed saphenous vein graft may become twisted when drawn through the thigh tunnel. Kinking or entrapment may occur owing to compression by nerve trunks or other tissues crossing the tunnel or by tracking the graft inappropriately in relation to the adductor muscles of the thigh or the medial head of the gastrocnemius. Vein graft stenosis may be produced by a branch ligature placed too close to the main saphenous trunk.

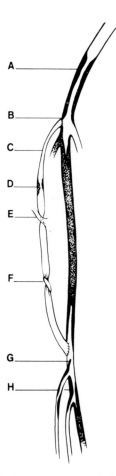

FIGURE 39–11. Mechanical factors underlying early thrombosis of femoropopliteal and femorotibial grafts. *A,* Stenosis of iliac inflow. *B,* Stenosis of proximal anastomosis produced by suturing a small vein to a thick-walled femoral artery. *C,* Proximal vein graft less than 4 mm in diameter. *D,* Recanalized saphenous phlebitis. *E,* External compression tissue bands in tunnel. *F,* Graft twist. *G,* Elevation of distal intima. *H,* Inadequate runoff. (From Bernhard VM: The failed arterial graft: Lost pulses and gangrene. *In* Condon RE, DeCosse JJ (eds): Surgical Care. Philadelphia, Lea & Febiger, 1980, p 156.)

For reversed saphenous vein grafts, factors leading to early thrombosis are vein diameter less than 3.5 to 4 mm, thick-walled vein, marked varicosities, and evidence of previous phlebitis.[138,139] In the in situ saphenous vein bypass, technical factors causing early thrombosis are platelet deposition at sites of endothelial damage from improper intraluminal instrumentation, missed valves or incomplete cusp lysis, diversion of the flow by significant fistulas, venospasm, and torsion or kinking of the proximal or distal free segments of the vein. Atherosclerotic disease in the inflow or outflow arteries inadequately evaluated prior to surgery is another significant cause for graft thrombosis. Other, technical errors include inadequate heparinization, improper flushing of the arterial system prior to restoration of graft flow, and clamp injury to the inflow or outflow vessels or the bypass conduit.[37,140] Nonmechanical causes of early thrombosis are decreased cardiac output, arterial vasospasm, and hypercoagulability.[37,141]

Thrombosis that occurs after 1 month and up to 1 year is most frequently due to degenerative changes in the graft itself or at an anastomosis.[136,137,142,143] In reversed saphenous vein bypass, thrombosis is usually caused by fibrosis of a valve or fibrotic changes in the vein graft wall due to injury during harvest and preparation before insertion.[37,137,144] These intrinsic vein graft defects are more common in the narrow proximal portion of reversed vein grafts.[137] In in situ saphenous vein bypass grafts, stenoses of the conduit have been reported at the mobilized upper or lower ends of the graft due to fibrous dysplastic lesions and in the midportion as the result of thickening around a valve cusp.[145] For all types of arterial bypasses, intimal fibroplasia at or just beyond the distal anastomosis may be produced by turbulent flow secondary to alteration of the arterial stream at the junction of graft and artery,[29,146–148] a compliance mismatch,[125,149] and the interplay of platelets and other blood factors at anastomoses.[150] Fibrointimal hyperplasia may also be a consequence of clamp injury to the graft or artery incurred at the time of surgery.[137]

Thrombosis occurring after 1 to 2 years is most frequently due to progressive atherosclerosis in the arteries proximal or distal to the arterial repair.[137,142,151,152] Arterialized venous conduits in the atherosclerotic patient also tend to become atherosclerotic themselves[152]; this appears to apply only to reversed, but not in situ, vein bypass grafts.[139,145]

There is a higher incidence of thrombosis when prosthetic conduits are employed, especially when they are carried below the knee to the distal popliteal or to the infrapopliteal vessels.[153–158] Thrombosis following vein grafting appears to level off between 1 and 2 years, whereas it is continuously progressive in prosthetic grafts.[137,156] The specific causes for prosthetic thromboses are the absence of a true intima with its antithrombotic characteristics; the tendency to develop progressive fibrointimal hyperplasia usually at the distal anastomosis due to the complex interactions between the more rigid prosthetic graft and the arterial wall; and the greater likelihood of kinking of prosthetic materials as they cross the knee joint. Thrombosis may also occur as a consequence of false aneurysm formation, which is more frequent with prostheses than with vein grafts.

Thrombosis in a bypass graft may involve only the graft itself without loss of flow in the segments of the vessel proximal and distal to the points of anastomosis. Under these circumstances, the leg will return to its previous degree of ischemia, assuming that there has been no significant change in the inflow or outflow vessels and collateral pathways. If thrombosis extends beyond the anastomosis into the popliteal and infrapopliteal arteries, however, ischemia will invariably be more severe and the limb may become acutely nonviable unless circulation can be restored.[17]

When a reversed vein graft becomes thrombosed in the immediate postoperative period, the intima and muscularis suffer prolonged anoxic injury due to loss of nutritive blood flow from the lumen in addition to the absence of normal graft wall perfusion through the vaso vasora that were disrupted during vein graft harvest.[53] The vein thus becomes a less satisfactory conduit, even though flow can be restored within a few hours. This is reflected in the reduced long-term patency of those vein grafts that have undergone thrombosis and initially successful thrombectomy.[113]

In the case of late or neglected thrombosis of a vein conduit, either reversed or in situ, the vein tends to undergo changes that make retrieval irreversible. The vein wall becomes thick and edematous and the lumen becomes stringlike. Thrombus usually cannot be removed by any means and dilatation of the vein by a balloon catheter may result in splitting of the wall.[145]

In the immediate postoperative period, peripheral vasospasm may make clinical evaluation unreliable. However, noninvasive tests will permit identification of thrombosis at the earliest possible moment.[19,159,160] Therefore, quality of graft flow and overall limb circulation should be evaluated by noninvasive hemodynamic techniques as well as clinical observation intraoperatively, immediately after completion of the reconstruction, and at frequent intervals in the early postoperative period.[35,161] Doppler waveform analysis, ankle pressures, and PVRs provide reliable objective information. Surgical reintervention should be carried out immediately in the event of obstructed graft flow to limit propagation of thrombus into distal vessels and minimize the period of ischemia to the limb and the wall of a vein graft.

Beyond the immediate postoperative period, patients with infrainguinal arterial reconstruction, especially with vein grafts, should continue to be examined at regular intervals at least every 3 to 4 months for 12 to 18 months and every 6 months thereafter. A history of increasing claudication, the recognition of reduced distal pulses, and the development of new bruits over the graft or its anastomoses are important findings that should be documented at each visit. In addition, noninvasive hemodynamic tests including duplex scanning (which provide quantitative and objective information) should be carried out, since they identify impending thrombosis in the absence of symptoms or clinical findings.[79,160–162] Any evidence of decreasing graft function signals the need for prompt angiography to identify the problem before thrombosis occurs.

Correction of abnormalities within the graft or in the vessels adjacent to a failing graft should be carried out as soon as reduced perfusion has been identified.[160] When possible, intervention should occur before thrombosis has taken place or in the early postthrombotic period, when mechanical disobliteration or lytic therapy is most effective. Delay of an aggressive surgical approach may be required in patients who are poor operative risks. Anticoagulants may prevent thrombosis in the presence of progressing stenosis if surgery must be delayed. However, once occlusion has occurred, the longer the thrombus has been present, the less effective recanalization attempts will be.

Areas of isolated stenosis within the graft, at an anastomosis or in the inflow or outflow arteries, may be successfully managed by percutaneous balloon angioplasty.[135] If this technique cannot be satisfactorily employed, a direct surgical approach at the site of the stenosis is indicated.[17,137] Vein patch angioplasty can usually be accomplished with relative ease to relieve stenosis of the graft itself or at an anastomosis (Fig. 39–12). If the proximal segment of a reversed saphenous vein graft is too narrow, it can be widened (Fig. 39–13). Progressive disease in the inflow vessels will require a jump graft from the lower end of the original graft to a patent distal popliteal or an infrapopliteal artery to bypass the obstruction.[137]

When thrombosis has already occurred and is recent, the graft lumen may be restored by mechanical extraction of thrombus with a balloon thromboembolectomy catheter; prosthetic grafts are more amenable to this procedure than vein grafts.[17,137,163] Thrombectomy of a fresh reversed saphenous vein graft usually requires exposure of both anastomoses. A transverse incision is made at the distal wider end of the graft so that thrombus at that level can be removed and the internal aspect of the distal anastomosis viewed directly (Fig. 39–12). A second incision over the proximal anastomotic vein hood or partial takedown of the proximal suture line is required for passage of balloon thromboembolectomy catheters and for vigorous forward flushing, since retrograde manipulations will be impeded by valves (Fig. 39–14). Prosthetic graft declotting can sometimes be accomplished through a single distal graft opening if thrombosis has been recent. The thoroughness of thrombus removal is determined by the vigor of flow through the graft from the proximal to the distal end, which also suggests that there is no inflow obstruction. Operative arteriography is re-

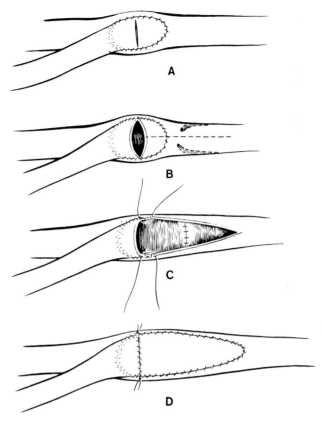

FIGURE 39–12. Technical sequence for inspection and repair of distal anastomosis of femoropopliteal or femorotibial graft. *A,* Transverse incision in wide "cobra head" overlying the distal anastomosis facilitates thrombus extraction, visualization of internal aspect of suture line, and closure without stenosis. *B* and *C,* When distal intima is elevated, arteriotomy is extended beyond area of injury, redundant intima is removed, and cut edge secured with tacking sutures. *D,* Closure of defect with vein patch. (From Bernhard VM: The failed arterial graft: Lost pulses and gangrene. *In* Condon RE, DeCosse JJ (eds): Surgical Care. Philadelphia, Lea & Febiger, 1980, p 160.)

quired after declotting of either venous or prosthetic grafts to confirm that thrombus has been completely extracted, to view both anastomoses, to evaluate the entire length of the intervening graft in order to identify areas of stenosis that need to be repaired, and to reevaluate the inflow and the runoff bed.

The direct intraarterial infusion of thrombolytic agents is an alternative to balloon catheter thrombectomy in the patient who does not have sensory or motor deficits or signs of impending muscle necrosis.[45,135,145,164,165] Thrombolytic therapy has been successfully applied to vein grafts, prostheses, and endarterectomized segments at all levels of the lower extremity arterial system. The endothelial lining of vein grafts and of small runoff vessels is spared the trauma of mechanical thrombectomy, which may be an important factor in restored vein graft function over the long term. Although effective lysis can be accomplished several weeks after an occlusion has occurred,[40,166] best results with this form of therapy are usually achieved within hours or days of throm-

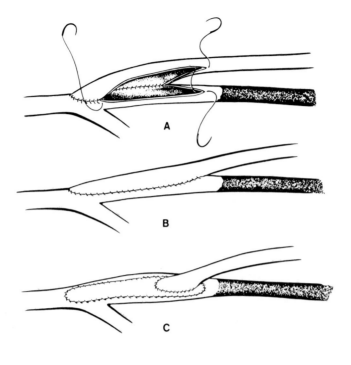

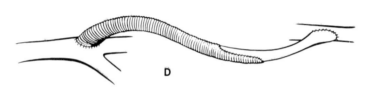

FIGURE 39–13. Techniques for revision of the femoral anastomosis to avoid stenosis caused by narrow vein and thick intima of artery. *A,* Proximal superficial femoral artery is incised to match long incision in vein graft; the vein graft incision is carried distally until vein diameter is at least 4 mm. *B,* Completion of anastomosis. *C,* Alternate technique using vein patch to increase diameter of artery; vein graft is then anastomosed to the patch. *D,* Composite vein–Dacron graft is another alternative solution when available saphenous vein is too short. (From Bernhard VM: The failed arterial graft: Lost pulses and gangrene. *In* Condon RE, DeCosse JJ (eds): Surgical Care. Philadelphia, Lea & Febiger, 1980, p 165.)

bosis.[167] The technique of percutaneous intraarterial thrombolytic therapy is discussed elsewhere in this book.

As soon as the clot has been effectively cleared from the graft by lytic therapy, angiographic investigation of the entire length of the graft, both anastomoses, the inflow, and the runoff bed is required to identify the cause of graft failure that must be corrected in order to avoid reocclusion. In the interim between lytic recanalization and correction of the causes of graft thrombosis, patients must be effectively anticoagulated to forestall rethrombosis.[40] It is important to recognize that although lytic recanalization of occluded grafts can be achieved, thrombolytic therapy alone will suffice in only the minority of patients. Graft stenoses or deterioration of inflow or runoff vessels must be identified and corrected in order to achieve long-term patency and limb salvage.[45,160,166,168]

Recent reports[169–171] indicate that intraoperative fibrinolytic therapy is an effective adjunct to catheter thrombectomy in select cases when residual clot remaining in the distal artery threatens the success of thrombectomy. The use of intraoperative fibrinolytic agents has not been associated with significant bleeding complications.[169,170]

Graft thrombosis that is old or that cannot be reopened by mechanical and/or lytic therapy will re-

quire a secondary bypass procedure if the limb is in jeopardy or claudication is truly incapacitating. Autogenous vein is preferable to prosthetic material, especially for bypasses to the infrapopliteal arteries. When the saphenous vein is not available for reoperation, arm veins and lesser saphenous veins when available are preferable to prosthetic conduits. The long-term results with prosthetic material are poor when employed for secondary bypass, whereas arm veins have recently been shown to have long-term patency rates that may be nearly equal to the saphenous vein.[172]

It is important to emphasize the need to search for nonmechanical reasons for decreased graft flow, such as diminished cardiac output or hypercoagulability, especially when no other causes of thrombosis can be identified. Failure to identify and correct the reason for graft occlusion usually suggests a poor prognosis, since the underlying cause has not been removed.[38] However, thrombosis in polytetrafluoroethylene (PTFE) grafts may occur for no apparent reason other than presumed platelet adherence to a relatively thrombogenic surface. For this reason, antiplatelet therapy in the immediate postoperative period is indicated.[150,173] Long-term anticoagulation with Coumadin (Hoechst) should be considered in patients who have recurrent thrombosis for no apparent reason.

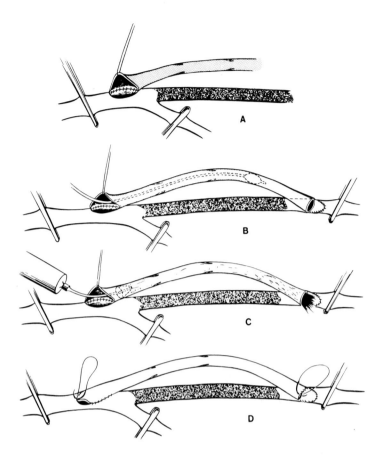

FIGURE 39–14. Partial detachment of the proximal anastomosis and graft thrombectomy. *A*, Partial takedown of proximal suture line. *B*, Passage of Fogarty catheter to distal end of graft and retrograde extraction of clot. *C*, Vigorous flushing of thrombectomized graft with heparinized Ringer's lactate solution. *D*, Resuture of proximal anastomosis and distal transverse venotomy. (From Bernhard VM: The failed arterial graft: Lost pulses and gangrene. *In* Condon RE, DeCosse JJ (eds): Surgical Care. Philadelphia, Lea & Febiger, 1980, p 161.)

Reoperation to maintain extremity circulation is worthwhile, since prolonged limb salvage can be achieved in 40 to 60 per cent of patients undergoing as many as four or more reoperative procedures.[137] The best results after reoperation for failure of an infrainguinal reconstruction are achieved in patients who only require a vein patch to relieve a stenosis that is repaired before thrombosis takes place.[79,137] For example, Whittmore et al.[137] achieved a 19 per cent 5-year patency after thrombectomy and patch angioplasty of thrombosed femoropopliteal vein grafts, a 36 per cent patency at 5 years following secondary autogenous vein bypass, and an overall 50 per cent long-term limb salvage. However, vein patch angioplasty of a stenotic graft or anastomotic lesion prior to thrombosis yielded an 86 per cent 5-year patency. For 72 early and late occlusions of polytetrafluoroethylene (PTFE) femoropopliteal grafts that placed the limb in jeopardy, Veith et al.[174] reported a 5-year graft patency rate of 37 per cent and a 5-year limb salvage rate of 56 per cent in patients undergoing reoperation. PTFE femoropopliteal bypasses appear to be unusual in that thrombectomy alone, even when delayed up to 30 days after thrombosis, can sometimes restore long-term patency. The success rate for reoperation for thrombosis of PTFE grafts to infrapopliteal arteries is considerably less than that for femoropopliteal bypasses.

Whether the long-term use of anticoagulants can prevent thrombosis of autogenous and prosthetic infrainguinal grafts as suggested by the studies of Kretschmer et al. needs further evaluation.[175,176]

Wound Complications

Major wound complications following lower extremity bypass grafting to the tibial or pedal vessels are not often reported but may jeopardize the success of these procedures.

The reported incidence of significant wound complications following autogenous infrainguinal bypass grafting ranges from 7.5 to 11 per cent.[177–179] Predisposing factors are said to include diabetes mellitus, renal failure, anemia, steroid therapy, ipsilateral limb ulceration or infection, and the severity of ischemia. Technical factors, including the length and placement of the incision, location of the distal anastomosis, and the technique of wound closure, may all influence the ultimate healing of these incisions.[177–179]

The use of a continuous incision increases the risk of wound hematoma and/or seroma and, if not positioned directly over the saphenous vein, may necessitate a large posterior flap. The two parallel incisions required to mobilize the artery and vein for in situ grafting to the dorsalis pedis artery risks necrosis of the intervening skin bridge. Wound complications range from erythema and superficial necrosis of the margins to infection of the deeper layers with exposure of the graft. Gram-positive cocci and mixed bacterial flora are frequently cultured from these wounds.[177-179]

Several steps help prevent wound complications following infrainguinal bypass procedures. Preoperative mapping of the course of the saphenous vein with duplex scanning minimizes the likelihood of creating a large posterior flap. Isolation of necrotic or ulcerative skin lesions of the foot prior to preparation of the skin, careful placement of incisions, meticulous hemostasis, and careful skin closure also reduce the incidence of wound complications. Once a wound complication has occurred, however, the treatment should be tailored to the severity of infection. Wound erythema with minimal necrosis of the wound margins usually responds to appropriate antibiotics and local wound care. More extensive wound infection and necrosis require extensive débridement and often skin grafting, muscle transfers, or myocutaneous free flaps.

Rarely, an exposed vein graft ruptures, requiring removal of the graft and placement of a new conduit routed through uninvolved sites. If this is not feasible, amputation may be necessary.

GRAFT SURVEILLANCE

Vein Grafts

The recent resurgence in the technique of in situ vein bypass grafting and the more extensive use of arm veins have increased the number of bypass procedures performed to revascularize ischemic limbs. This increase in frequency of autogenous vein bypass procedures has increased the number of grafts at risk for the late changes including fibrosis, valvular stenosis, dilatation, aneurysm formation, and atherosclerosis as described by Szilagyi et al.[152]

When implanted in the arterial system, vein grafts undergo a series of morphological changes that include thickening of the wall, fibrosis, and myointimal cellular proliferation as an adaptive response to arterial blood pressure. There is also experimental evidence to suggest that vein grafts produce more prostacyclin than normal veins, although the amount produced is still considerably less than that produced by normal arteries.[180] The recent popularity of the in situ saphenous vein bypass graft as an alternative to the reversed technique has increased vein utilization to over 90 per cent; however, the in situ technique may entail more manipulation and damage to the intima from the use of valvulotomes.

Graft failure within the first 30 days is usually due to fibrin platelet thrombus, retained valves, twists, unrecognized AV fistulae or technical problems with the anastomoses, and occurs in up to 3 to 10 per cent of grafts.[181,182] Careful intraoperative assessment of the entire length of the graft with Doppler spectral analysis, angiography, or endoscopy is essential if these early complications are to be avoided. Woelfe et al., in a series of 20 in situ grafts evaluated endoscopically, found eight partially divided valves that were readily corrected at the time of surgery.[183] Bush et al. have reported a 10 per cent incidence of competent valves in the presence of "normal" operative arteriograms.[184] Bandyk et al. performed intraoperative arteriography and pulse Doppler evaluation on 50 in situ vein grafts. Severe flow disturbances were present in 14 per cent of the distal anastomoses, 5 per cent of valve incision sites, and 2 per cent of proximal anastomoses.[185]

Platelet thrombi occur at the sites of valve incision or splits in the intima along the length of the vein. Exploration of these sites, with careful removal of any thrombotic material and repair by patch angioplasty or replacement of the damaged vein segment, is often necessary.

Beyond the initial postoperative period, there is a tendency for vein grafts to develop stenoses that may predispose to thrombosis. Reoperation to correct such defects prior to graft occlusion permits salvage of the grafts and prevention of recurrent ischemia. Unfortunately, between 20 and 40 per cent of grafts occlude without prior warning or with recently recorded normal ankle pressure indices.[186]

Because of the propensity of these grafts to fail, every attempt should be made to detect obstructive changes within the graft, at anastomoses, or in the inflow or runoff vessels prior to occlusion. Indications for impending failure include diminution or absence of previously palpable pulses, fall in the ankle-brachial index of more than 0.15, or reduction in peak velocity to less than 45 cm/sec. If any of these changes are detected, immediate arteriography is indicated. Postoperatively, the patient is seen at 1 month, every 3 months for the first year, then every 6 months.

Although some of the focal lesions observed angiographically during late follow-up appear suitable for balloon catheter dilatation, the recurrence rate is high; patch angioplasty or replacement of a segment of vein offers superior long-term results.

An interesting complication of infrainguinal bypass grafts is functional failure in spite of continued graft patency and is manifest by extension of necrosis or failure to control the infective processes in the foot.[187] The incidence of this complication ranges from 2 to 4 per cent for reversed vein grafts, up to 7.5 per cent for in situ vein grafts, and 8.1 to 9.5 per cent for PTFE grafts.[188,189] Amputation may be required unless graft extension to an additional tibial or pedal vessel is possible. An alternative may be microvascular free flap transfer of healthy muscle to cover a persistent defect that usually involves exposed tendons, bones, or joints.

Prosthetic Graft Dilation

With the continued increase in life expectancy of patients undergoing aortofemoral and femoropopliteal bypass grafting, the need for continued surveillance to detect deterioration in the graft material or complications resulting from implantation of prosthetic devices is becoming increasingly apparent.

Although florid rupture of Dacron grafts and dilatation of PTFE grafts have been eliminated by improvement in graft manufacture of the former and by increasing wall thickness or the application of an external wrap around the latter, deterioration in prosthetic grafts continues to occur.

Dacron Grafts

The true incidence of dilatation is unknown, since patients with apparently well-functioning grafts as evidenced by palpable distal pulses or normal ankle pressure indices on follow-up examinations are seldom evaluated unless some problem, such as an anastomotic aneurysm or acute occlusion of a graft limb, supervenes.

Textile grafts initially dilate approximately 15 to 20 per cent after implantation. This is believed to be due to yarn slippage and is accompanied by a small decrease in tensile strength, which then stabilizes, but may continue throughout the life span of the graft. Three factors are believed to contribute to dilatation of Dacron grafts. These include (1) a flattening of the crimp when the graft is subjected to arterial pressure, (2) an increase in diameter and decrease in length due to rearrangement of textile structure (i.e., the lighter the graft fiber, the greater the porosity and the more likely it is to dilate), and (3) an increase in diameter and length due to deformation of the graft material.[122,190-193]

Dilatation is most likely to occur in knitted rather than woven grafts, as documented in a study by Nunn et al., who evaluated 95 Dacron grafts implanted for a mean of 33 months using Doppler ultrasound. The mean dilatation was 17.6 per cent and was somewhat more severe in hypertensive patients (21 per cent) than their normotensive counterparts (15 per cent). However, some grafts enlarged by more than 100 per cent.[192]

Prosthetic rupture and anastomotic aneurysm formation have been reported in patients with dilated grafts; however, the natural history of such grafts left in place is presently unknown.[122,127,193,194] Nevertheless, removal of a grossly dilated graft may be prudent in an asymptomatic patient without significant cardiorespiratory problems that increase operative risk. In practice, dilated segments of grafts associated with anastomotic aneurysms are replaced. Care should be taken to use a graft corresponding to the diameter of the outflow vessel, and no attempt should be made to match the diameter of the interposition graft to that of the dilated implanted graft.

Umbilical Veins

Umbilical veins have been used as a substitute for saphenous veins, with a 5-year patency of approximately 45 per cent. Dardik, in a series of 756 glutar-

aldehyde-stabilized umbilical vein grafts (UVGs) implanted over a 7-year period, identified aneurysmal change in seven (1 per cent) in the entire series. The incidence of such aneurysms has increased over time from 1.2 per cent at 4 to 6 years to 7.7 per cent at 6 to 8 years.[195-197] It should be noted that this incidence may be underestimated, as follow-up arteriography was performed only in one third of the patients at risk. The mechanisms for UVG dilatation include mechanical fatigue, reversal of crosslinking, and immunologic factors. Julien et al., in a study of 80 UVG segments removed from 70 patients studied by light and electron microscopy, found aneurysmal dilatation in 4 of 80 specimens, bacterial colonization in the absence of overt infection in 26 per cent, and irregular wall thickness with folds on the intraluminal surface in one third of the grafts. Anastomotic thrombus is often associated with this problem.[198]

Because of the small but definite risk of continued deterioration of these grafts, Dardik has recommended that an arteriogram be performed at 3 to 4 years after implantation in addition to noninvasive surveillance.

PTFE

When first introduced, PTFE grafts were manufactured without an external wrap. This was associated with aneurysmal dilatation of the grafts. No further aneurysms have been reported since the application of the wrap (Gortex) or by increasing the thickness of the graft wall (Impra). Furthermore, PTFE does not dilate significantly over time, which makes it the material of choice for repair of anastomotic aneurysms and possibly for aortofemoral bypass.[199-200]

Edema

Some degree of lower extremity edema accompanies the majority of successful infrainguinal arterial reconstructions. The reported incidence is as high as 70 to 100 per cent.[72] The most important factor in the development of this edema appears to be lymphatic interruption, probably at the inguinal, thigh, and popliteal areas during the lower extremity arterial reconstruction. Microcirculatory derangements that exist in the ischemic limb, such as loss of arteriolar autoregulation, loss of the orthostatic vasoconstrictor reflex, capillary recruitment, and focal capillary endothelial injury, all apparently contribute to this lymph-related edema by increasing the net flux of interstitial fluid into the lymphatic system[202] (Fig. 39-15). Venous thrombosis has been shown to be a very infrequent cause of postreconstructive edema.[203,204] The severity of the edema increases in relation to the severity of prebypass ischemia. Furthermore, it is less frequent after aortoiliofemoral reconstruction, presumably because there is less limb lymphatic disruption.[202]

Technical modifications to minimize inguinal and

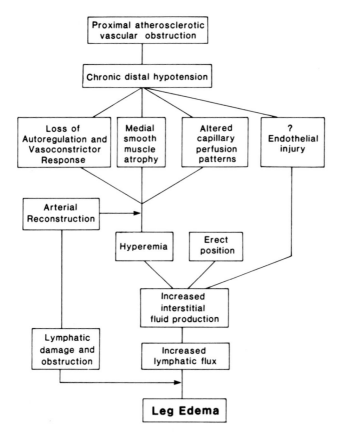

FIGURE 39–15. Schematic overview of the factors involved in postoperative lower extremity edema after femorodistal reconstruction. (From Schubart PJ, Porter JM: Leg edema following femorodistal bypass. *In* Bergan JJ, Yao JST (eds): Reoperative Arterial Surgery. Orlando, FL, Grune & Stratton, 1986, p 328.)

popliteal lymphatic injury during infrainguinal arterial reconstruction may reduce the incidence of postoperative edema.[205] Once this complication occurs, bed rest, elevation, and the use of elastic support stockings will control edema by shifting capillary dy-

namics in favor of fluid reabsorption.[202] Fortunately, in most instances, postreconstructive edema is self-limited and improves or disappears during the first few postoperative months.[38]

Lymph Leak

Drainage of lymphatic fluid from the groin incision is a relatively infrequent complication of arterial reconstruction. It appears as a persistent, clear, watery drainage through the wound after the first few postoperative days, or as an onset of drainage as the patient resumes ambulation.[38] This complication may lead to graft infection and anastomotic disruption if improperly managed.[206]

Lymphatic leakage results from transected and unligated lymphatic channels and lymph nodes in the groin incision. Possible contributing factors include poor wound edge and tissue layer approximation and subcutaneous fat necrosis.[38]

Nonoperative treatment of lymphorrhea includes bed rest and leg elevation to reduce lymph flow while allowing the lymphatics to heal. Wound care must be meticulous and systemic prophylactic antibiotics should be administered in order to reduce the risk of secondary infection.[38]

Nonoperative management of lymphorrhea often takes considerable time. Therefore, Kwann, Connolly, and associates[206] recommend early groin reexploration and direct suture of points of lymph leakage. This reported experience with early wound reexploration suggests shortened hospitalization and reduction in the incidence of graft infection. Since the site of lymphatic disruption may not be recognized on reexploration of the wound, manual massage of the thigh or staining of the lymphatic system by injection of a vital dye in the foot several hours before surgery is recommended to aid in identifying the leak site.

REFERENCES

1. Downs AR: Complications of abdominal aortic surgery. *In* Bernhard VM, Towne JB (Eds): Complications in Vascular Surgery. Orlando, FL, Grune & Stratton, 1985, pp 25–36.
2. Brener BJ, Darling RC, Frederick PL, et al: Major venous anomalies complicating abdominal aortic surgery. Arch Surg 108:159–169, 1974.
3. Bernhard VM: Aortocaval fistulas. *In* Haimovici H (ed): Vascular Emergencies. New York, Appleton-Century-Crofts, 1982, pp 353–363.
4. Duppler DW, Herbert WE, Dillihunt RC, et al: Primary arteriovenous fistulas of the abdomen. Arch Surg 120:786–790, 1985.
5. Brewster DC, Cambria RP, Moncure AC, Darling RC, LaMuragila GM, Geller SC, Abbott WM: Aortocaval and iliac arteriovenous fistulas: Recognition and treatment. J Vasc Surg 13:253–265, 1991.
6. Calligaro KD, Savarese RP, DeLaurentis DA: Unusual aspects of aortovenous fistulas associated with ruptured abdominal aortic aneurysms. J Vasc Surg 12:586–590, 1990.

7. Dardik H, Dardik I, Strom MG: Intravenous rupture of arteriosclerotic aneurysms of the abdominal aorta. Surgery 80:647–653, 1976.
8. Thompson JE, Hollier LH, Patman RD, et al: Surgical management of abdominal aortic aneurysms: Factors influencing mortality and morbidity. A 20 year experience. Ann Surg 181:654–688, 1975.
9. Effeney DJ, Goldstone J, Chin D, et al: Intraoperative anticoagulation in cardiovascular surgery. Surgery 90:1068–1074, 1981.
10. Crawford ES, Manning LG, Kelly FT: "Redo" surgery after operations for aneurysm and occlusion of the abdominal aorta. Surgery 81:41–52, 1977.
11. O'Hara PJ, Brewster DC, Darling RC, et al: The value of intraoperative monitoring using the pulse volume recorder during peripheral vascular reconstructive operations. Surg Gynecol Obstet 152:275–281, 1981.
12. Strom JA, Bernhard VM, Towne JB: Acute limb ischemia following aortic reconstruction: A preventable cause of increased mortality. Arch Surg 119:470–473, 1984.

13. Kapsch DN, Adelstein EH, Rhodes GR, et al: Heparin-induced thrombocytopenia, thrombosis, and hemorrhage. Surgery 86:148–154, 1979.

14. Towne JB: Hypercoagulable states and unexplained vascular thrombosis. *In* Bernhard VM, Towne JB (eds): Complications in Vascular Surgery. Orlando, FL, Grune & Stratton, 1985, pp 381–404.

15. Towne JB, Bernhard VM, Hussey C, et al: Antithrombin III deficiency: A cause of unexplained thrombosis in vascular surgery. Surgery 89:735–747, 1981.

16. Towne JB, Bernhard VM, Hussey C, et al: White clot syndrome: Peripheral vascular complications of heparin therapy. Arch Surg 114:373–379, 1979.

17. Bernhard VM: The failed arterial graft: Lost pulses and gangrene. *In* Condon RE, DeCosse J (eds): Surgical Care: A Physiologic Approach to Clinical Management. Philadelphia, Lea & Febiger, 1980, pp 153–167.

18. Brewster DC, Darling RC: Optimal methods of aorto-iliac reconstruction. Surgery 84:739–748, 1978.

19. O'Mara CS, Flinn WR, Johnson ND, et al: Recognition and surgical management of patent but hemodynamically failed arterial grafts. Ann Surg 193:467–476, 1981.

20. Baird RJ, Feldman P, Miles JT, et al: Subsequent downstream repair with aortoiliac and aortofemoral bypass operations. Surgery 82:785, 1977.

21. Baird RJ: Downstream revascularization after aortofemoral bypass grafting. *In* Bergan JJ, Yao JST (eds): Reoperative Arterial Surgery. Orlando, FL, Grune & Stratton, 1986, pp 223–230.

22. Mulcare RJ, Royster TS, Lynn RA, et al: Long-term results of operative therapy for aortoiliac disease. Arch Surg 113:601–604, 1978.

23. Nevelsteen A, Suy R, Daenen W, et al: Aorto-femoral grafting: Factors influencing late results. Surgery 88:642–653, 1980.

24. Charlesworth D: The occluded aortic and aorto-femoral graft. *In* Bergan JJ, Yao JST (eds): Reoperative Arterial Surgery. Orlando, FL, Grune & Stratton, 1986, pp 271–278.

25. Fulenwider JT, Smith RB III, Johnson RW, et al: Reoperative abdominal arterial surgery. A ten year experience. Surgery 93:20–27, 1983.

26. Robbs JV, Wylie EJ: Factors contributing to recurrent lower limb ischemia following bypass surgery for aorto-iliac occlusive disease and their management. Ann Surg 193:346–352, 1981.

27. Frisch N, Bour P, Berg P, Fieve G, Frisch R: Long term results of thrombectomy for late occlusions of aortofemoral bypass. Ann Vasc Surg 5:16–20, 1991.

28. Nevelsteen A, Suy R: Graft occlusion following aortofemoral Dacron bypass. Ann Vasc Surg 5:32–37, 1991.

29. LoGerfo FW, Quist WC, Nowak MD, et al: Downstream anastomotic hyperplasia. Ann Surg 197:479–483, 1983.

30. Malone JM, Moore WS, Goldstone J: The natural history of bilateral aortofemoral grafts for ischemia of the lower extremities. Arch Surg 110:1300–1306, 1975.

31. Rhodes RS, Hutton MC, Lalka SG: Reoperation for intraabdominal vascular disease. *In* Fry DE (ed): Reoperative Surgery of the Abdomen. New York, Marcel Dekker, 1986, pp 153–174.

32. Wylie EJ, Olcott C: Aortoiliac thromboendarterectomy. *In* Varco RL, Delaney JP (eds): Controversy in Surgery. Philadelphia, WB Saunders Company, 1976, pp 437–450.

33. Crawford ES, Bomberger RA, Glaeser DH, et al: Aorto-iliac occlusive disease: Factors influencing survival and function following reconstructive operation over a twenty-five year period. Surgery 90:1055–1067, 1981.

34. Satiani B, Liapis CD, Evans WE: Aortofemoral bypass for severe limb ischemia: Long-term survival and limb salvage. Am J Surg 141:252–256, 1981.

35. Yao JST, McCarthy WJ: Surgical correction of hemodynamic failure of bypass grafts. *In* Bergan JJ, Yao JST (eds): Reoperative Arterial Surgery. Orlando, FL, Grune & Stratton, 1986, pp 257–270.

36. Bernhard VM: Late vascular graft thrombosis. *In* Bernhard VM, Towne JB (eds): Complications in Vascular Surgery. Orlando, FL, Grune & Stratton, 1985, pp 187–204.

37. Bernhard VM, Ray LI, Towne JB: The reoperation of choice for aorto-femoral graft occlusion. Surgery 82:867–876, 1977.

38. Brewster DC: Early complications of vascular repair below the inguinal ligament. *In* Bernhard VM, Towne JB (eds): Complications in Vascular Surgery. Orlando, FL, Grune & Stratton, 1985, pp 37–53.

39. DePalma RG, Malgieri JJ, Rhodes RS, et al: Profunda femoris bypass for secondary revascularization. Surg Gynecol Obstet 151:387–390, 1980.

40. Van Breda A, Robison JC, Feldman L, et al: Local thrombolysis in the treatment of arterial graft occlusions. J Vasc Surg 1:103–110, 1984.

41. Battey PM, Fulenwider JT, Smith RB, Martin LG, Stewart MT, Perdue GD: Intraarterial thrombolysis for acute limb ischemia: A three-year experience. South Med J 80:479–482, 1987.

42. Gardiner GA, Koltun W, Kandarpa K, et al: Thrombolysis of occluded femoropopliteal grafts. AJR 147:621–626, 1986.

43. Katzen BT, Edwards KC, Albert AS, et al: Low dose direct fibrinolysis in peripheral vascular disease. J Vasc Surg 1:718–722, 1984.

44. McNamara TO, Bomberger RA: Factors affecting initial and 6 month patency rates after intra-arterial thrombolysis with high dose urokinase. Am J Surg 152:709–712, 1986.

45. McNamara TO, Fischer JR: Thrombolysis of peripheral arterial and graft occlusions: Improved results using high-dose urokinase. AJR 144:769–775, 1985.

46. Sicard GA, Schier JJ, Totty WG, et al: Thrombolytic therapy for acute arterial occlusion. J Vasc Surg 2:65–78, 1985.

47. Traughber PD, Cook PS, Micklos TJ, Miller FJ: Intra-arterial fibrinolytic therapy for popliteal and tibial artery obstruction: Comparison of streptokinase and urokinase. AJR 149:453–456, 1987.

48. Van Breda A, Katzen BT, Deutsch AS: Urokinase versus streptokinase in local thrombolysis. Radiology 165:109–111, 1987.

49. Gardiner GA, Harrington DP, Kolun W, Whittemore A, Mannick JA, Levin DC: Salvage of occluded arterial bypass grafts by means of thrombolysis. J Vasc Surg 9:426–431, 1989.

50. Belkin M, Belkin B, Bucknam CA, Straub J, Lowe R: Intraarterial fibrinolytic therapy. Arch Surg 121:769–773, 1986.

51. Kazmier PJ, Sheps SG, Bernatz PE, et al: Livedo reticularis and digital infarcts: A syndrome due to cholesterol infarcts arising from abdominal aortic aneurysms. Vasc Dis 3:12–22, 1966.

52. Starr DS, Lawrie GM, Morris GC: Prevention of distal embolism during arterial reconstruction. Am J Surg 138:764–771, 1979.

53. Attia RR, Murphy JD, Snider M, et al: Myocardial ischemia due to infrarenal aortic cross-clamping during aortic surgery in patients with severe coronary artery disease. Circulation 53:961–965, 1976.

54. Bush HL, LoGerfo FW, Weisel RD, et al: Assessment of myocardial performance and optimal volume loading during elective abdominal aortic aneurysm resection. Arch Surg 112:1301–1306, 1977.

55. Dauchot PJ, DePalma R, Grum D, et al: Detection and prevention of cardiac dysfunction during aortic surgery. J Surg Res 26:574–580, 1979.

56. Silverstein PR, Caldera DL, Cullen DJ, et al: Avoiding the hemodynamic consequences of aortic cross-clamping and unclamping. Anesthesiology 50:462–466, 1979.

57. Whittemore AD, Clowes AW, Hechtman HB, et al: Aortic aneurysm repair: Reduced operative mortality associated with maintenance of optimal cardiac performance. Ann Surg 192:414–421, 1980.

58. Abbott WM, Abel RM, Beck CH, et al: Renal failure after ruptured aneurysm. Arch Surg 110:1110, 1975.

59. Castonuovo JJ, Flanigan DP: Renal failure complicating vascular surgery. *In* Bernhard VM, Towne JB (eds): Compli-

cations in Vascular Surgery. Orlando FL, Grune & Stratton, 1985, pp 258–274.

60. Abbott WM, Austen WG: The reversal of renal cortical ischemia during aortic occlusion by mannitol. J Surg Res 16:482–486, 1974.

61. Berkowitz HD, Shetty S: Renin release and renal cortical ischemia following aortic cross clamping. Arch Surg 109:612–618, 1974.

62. Crawford ES, Synder DM, Cho GC, et al: Progress in treatment of thoraco-abdominal and abdominal aortic aneurysms involving the celiac, superior mesenteric and renal arteries. Ann Surg 188:404–422, 1978.

63. Iliopoulos JI, Zdon MJ, Crawford BG, et al: Renal microembolization syndrome. Am J Surg 146:779–783, 1983.

64. Bush HL, Huse JB, Johnson WC, et al: Prevention of renal insufficiency after abdominal aortic aneurysm reaction by optimal volume loading. Arch Surg 116:1517–1522, 1981.

65. Szilagyi DE, Smith RF, Elliot JP: Temporary transection of the left renal vein: A technical aid to aortic surgery. Surgery 65:32–40, 1969.

66. Huber D, Harris JP, Walker PJ, May J, Tyrer P: Does division of the left renal vein during aortic surgery adversely affect renal function? Ann Vasc Surg 5:74–79, 1991.

67. AbuRahama AF, Robinson PA, Boland JP, Lucente FC: The risk of ligation of the left renal vein in resection of the abdominal aortic aneurysm. Surg Gynecol Obstet 173:33–36, 1991.

68. Olsen PS, Schroeder T, Perko M, Roder OC, Agerskov K, Sorensen S, Lorentzen JE: Renal failure after operation for abdominal aortic aneurysm. Ann Vasc Surg 4:580–583, 1990.

69. Ernst CB: Postoperative intestinal ischemia. In Haimovici H (ed): Vascular Emergencies. New York, Appleton-Century-Crofts, 1982, pp 493–513.

70. Johnson WC, Nasbeth DC: Visceral infarction following aortic surgery. Ann Surg 180:312–321, 1974.

71. Ottinger LW, Darling RC, Nathan MJ, et al: Left colon ischemia complicating aorto-iliac reconstruction. Arch Surg 105:481, 1972.

72. Ernst CB: Intestinal ischemia following abdominal aortic reconstruction. In Bernhard VM, Towne JB (eds): Complications in Vascular Surgery. Orlando, FL, Grune & Stratton, 1985, pp 325–350.

73. Hagihara PF, Ernst CB, Griffen WO: Incidence of ischemic colitis following abdominal aortic reconstruction. Surg Gynecol Obstet 149:571–573, 1979.

74. Moskowitz M, Zimmerman H, Felson B: The meandering mesenteric artery of the colon. Am J Roentgenol 92:1088, 1964.

75. Ernst CB, Hagihara PF, Daugherty ME, et al: Ischemis colitis incidence following abdominal aortic reconstruction: A prospective study. Surgery 80:417–423, 1976.

76. Boley SJ, Brandt LF, Veith FJ: Ischemic disorders of the intestines. Curr Probl Surg 15:1–85, 1978.

77. Hobson RW, Wright CB, O'Donnell JA, et al: Determination of intestinal viability by Doppler ultrasound. Arch Surg 114:165–168, 1979.

78. Bicks RO, Bale GF, Howard H, et al: Acute and delayed colon ischemia after aortic aneurysm surgery. Arch Intern Med 122:249, 1968.

79. Painton JF, Avellone JC, Plecha FR: Effectiveness of reoperation after late failure of femoro-popliteal reconstruction. Am J Surg 135:235–241, 1978.

80. Yee J, Dixon CM, McLean APH, Meakins JL: *Clostridium difficile* disease in a department of surgery: The significance of prophylactic antibiotics. Arch Surg 126:241–246, 1991.

81. Teasley DG, Gerding DN, Olson MM, Peterson LR, Gebhard RL, Schwartz MJ, Lee JT: Prospective randomized trial of metronidazole versus vancomycin for *Clostridium-difficile*-associated diarrhoea and colitis. Lancet 2:1043–1046, 1983.

82. Ernst CB, Hagihara PF, Daugherty ME, et al: Inferior mesenteric artery stump pressure: A reliable index for safe IMA ligation during abdominal aortic aneurysmectomy. Arch Surg 187:641–649, 1978.

83. Welling RE, Roedersheimer R, Arbaugh JJ, et al: Ischemic colitis following repair of ruptured abdominal aortic aneurysms. Arch Surg 120:1368–1370, 1985.

84. Connolly JE, Kwann JHM: Prophylactic revascularization of the gut. Ann Surg 190:514–522, 1985.

85. Brewster DC, Retana A, Waltman AC, et al: Angiography in the management of aneurysms of the abdominal aorta. N Engl J Med 292:822–825, 1975.

86. Zelenock GB, Strodel WE, Knol JA, Messina LM, Wakefield TW, Lindenauer SM, Eckhauser FE, Greenfield LJ, Stanley JC: A prospective study of clinically and endoscopically documented colonic ischemia in 100 patients undergoing aortic reconstructive surgery with aggressive colonic and direct pelvic revascularization, compared with historic controls. Surgery 106:771–780, 1989.

87. DiChiro G, Doppman JL: Paraplegia after resection of aneurysm. N Engl J Med 281:799–803, 1969.

88. Elliot JP, Szilagyi DE, Hageman JH, et al: Spinal cord ischemia: Secondary to surgery of the abdominal aorta. In Bernhard VM, Towne JB (eds): Complications in Vascular Surgery. Orlando, FL, Grune & Stratton, 1985, pp 291–310.

89. Szilagyi ED, Hageman JH, Smith RF, et al: Spinal cord damage in surgery of the abdominal aorta. Surgery 83:38, 1978.

90. Ferguson LRJ, Bergan JJ, Conn J Jr, et al: Spinal ischemia following abdominal aortic surgery. Ann Surg 181:267, 1975.

91. Grace RR, Mattox KL: Anterior spinal artery syndrome following abdominal aortic aneurysmectomy. Arch Surg 112:813, 1977.

92. DiChiro G, Wener L: Angioplasty of the spinal cord. J Neurosurg 39:1–11, 1973.

93. Williams GM, Perler BA, Burdick JF, Osterman FA, Mitchell S, Merine D, Drenger B, Parker SD, Beattie C, Reitz BA: Angiographic localization of spinal cord blood and its relationship to postoperative paraplegia. J Vasc Surg 13:23–35, 1991.

94. Kieffer E, Richard T, Chiras J, Godet G, Cormier E: Preoperative spinal cord arteriography in aneurysmal disease of the descending thoracic and thoracoabdominal aorta: Preliminary results in 45 patients. Ann Vasc Surg 3:34–46, 1989.

95. Cunningham NJ Jr, Laschinger JC, Merkin HA, et al: Measurement of spinal cord ischemia during operations upon the thoracic aorta. Initial experience. Ann Surg 196:285–296, 1982.

96. Coles JG, Wilson GJ, Sima AF, et al: Intraoperative detection of spinal cord ischemia using somotosensory cortical evoked potentials during thoracic aortic occlusion. Ann Thorac Surg 34:299, 1982.

97. Laschinger JC, Cunningham JN, Nathan IM, et al: Detection and prevention of intraoperative spinal cord ischemia after cross-clamping the thoracic aorta: Use of somatosensory evoked potentials. Surgery 92:1109, 1982.

98. Laschinger JC, Cunningham JN, Nathan IM, et al: Experimental and clinical assessment of the adequacy of partial bypass in the maintenance of spinal cord flow during operations on the thoracic aorta. Ann Thorac Surg 36:417, 1983.

99. Picone AL, Green RM, Ricotta JR, May AG, DeWeese JA: Spinal cord ischemia following operations on the abdominal aorta. J Vasc Surg 3:94–103, 1986.

100. Lambardini MM, Ratliff RK: The abdominal aortic aneurysm and the ureter. J Urol 98:590–601, 1967.

101. Goldstone J, Malone JM, Moore WS: Inflammatory aneurysm of the abdominal aorta. Surgery 83:425–435, 1978.

102. Egeblad K, Brochner-Mortensen J, Krarup T, Holstein PE, Bartholdy NJ: Incidence of ureteral obstruction after aortic grafting: A prospective analysis. Surgery 103(4):411–414, 1988.

103. Spirnak JP, Nehemia H, Resnick MI: Ureteral injuries com-

plicating vascular surgery: Is repair indicated? J Urol *141*:13–14, 1989.

104. Wright DJ, Ernst CB, Evans JR, Smith RF, Reddy DJ, Shepard AD, Elliot JP: Ureteral complications and aortoiliac reconstruction. J Vasc Surg *11*:29–37, 1990.

105. Kempczinski RF, Birinyi LK: Impotence following aortic surgery. *In* Bernhard VM, Towne JB (eds): Complications in Vascular Surgery. Orlando, FL, Grune & Stratton, 1985, pp 311–324.

106. Merchant RF, DePalma RG: Effects of femoro-femoral grafts on postoperative sexual function: Correlation with penile pulse volume recordings. Surgery *90*:962–970, 1981.

107. Ohshiro T, Kosaki G: Sexual function after aorto-iliac vascular reconstruction: Which is more important, the internal iliac artery or hypogastric nerve? J Cardiovasc Surg *25*:47–50, 1984.

108. Queral LA, Flinn WR, Bergan JJ, et al: Sexual function and aortic surgery. *In* Bergan JJ, Yao JST (eds): Surgery of the Aorta and its Body Branches. Orlando, FL, Grune & Stratton, 1979, pp 263–276.

109. Queral LA, Whitehouse WM, Flinn WR, et al: Pelvic hemodynamics after aortoiliac reconstruction. Surgery *86*:799–809, 1979.

110. Kempczinski RF: Role of the vascular diagnostic laboratory in the evaluation of male impotence. Am J Surg *138*:278, 1979.

111. Nath RL, Menzoian JO, Kaplan KH, et al: The multidisciplinary approach to vasculogenic impotence. Surgery *89*:124, 1981.

112. Flanigan DP, Sobinsky KR, Schuler JJ, et al: Internal iliac artery revascularization in the treatment of vasculogenic impotence. Arch Surg *120*:271–274, 1985.

113. DePalma RG: Impotence in vascular disease: Relationship to vascular surgery. Br J Surg *69*:514, 1982.

114. Chavez CM: False aneurysm of the femoral artery: A challenge in management. Ann Surg *183*:694–700, 1976.

115. Gardner TJ, Brawley RK, Gott VL: Anastomotic false aneurysms. Surgery *72*:474–483, 1972.

116. Knox WG: Peripheral vascular anastomotic aneurysm: A fifteen year experience. Ann Surg *183*:694–703, 1976.

117. Read RC, Thompson BW: Uninfected anastomotic false aneurysms following arterial reconstruction with prosthetic grafts. J Cardiovasc Surg *16*:558–567, 1975.

118. Satiani B, Kazmers M, Evans WE: Anastomotic arterial aneurysms: A continuing challenge. Ann Surg *192*:674–682, 1980.

119. Szilagyi DE, Smith FR, Elliot JP, et al: Anastomotic aneurysms after vascular reconstruction: Problems of incidence, etiology and treatment. Surgery *178*:800–816, 1975.

120. Satiani B: False aneurysms following arterial reconstruction. Surg Gynecol Obstet *152*:357–363, 1981.

121. Bernhard VM: Aortoduodenal and other aortoenteric fistulas. *In* Veith FJ (ed): Critical Problems in Vascular Surgery. New York, Appleton-Century-Crofts, 1982, pp 399–410.

122. Kim GE, Imparato AM, Nathan I, et al: Dilatation of synthetic grafts and junctional aneurysms. Arch Surg *114*:1296–1303, 1979.

123. Evans WE, Hayes JP, Vermilion B: Anastomotic femoral false aneurysms. *In* Bernhard VM, Towne JB (eds): Complications in Vascular Surgery. Orlando, FL, Grune & Stratton, 1985, pp 205–212.

124. Moore WS: Anastomotic aneurysms. *In* Rutherford RB (ed): Vascular Surgery. Philadelphia, WB Saunders Company, 1984, pp 821–827.

125. Clark RE, Apostolou S, Kardos JL: Mismatch of mechanical properties as a cause of arterial prosthesis thrombosis. Surg Forum *27*:208–210, 1978.

126. Mehigan DG, Fitzpatrick B, Browne JL, et al: Is compliance mismatch the major cause of anastomotic arterial aneurysms? J Cardiovasc Surg *26*:147–150, 1985.

127. Carson SN, Hunter GC, Palmaz J, Guernsey JM: Recurrence of femoral anastomotic aneurysms. Am J Surg *146*:774–778, 1983.

128. Courbier R, Larranaga J: Natural history and management

129. of anastomotic aneurysms. *In* Bergan JJ, Yao JST (eds): Aneurysms: Diagnosis and Treatment. Orlando, FL, Grune & Stratton, 1982, pp 567–580.

129. Starr DS, Weatherford SC, Lawrie GM, et al: Suture material as a factor in occurrence of anastomotic aneurysms: An analysis of 26 cases. Arch Surg *114*:412–415, 1979.

130. Perdue GD, Smith RB, Anoley JD, et al: Impending aortoenteric hemorrhage: The effects of early recognition on improved outcomes. Ann Surg *192*:237–243, 1980.

131. Gooding GAW, Effeney DJ, Goldstone J: The aortofemoral graft: Detection and identification of healing complications by ultrasonography. Surgery *89*:94–101, 1981.

132. Ernst CB, Elliot JP, Ryan CJ, et al: Recurrent femoral anastomotic aneurysms. Ann Surg *208*:401–409, 1988.

133. Williams RA, Vetto J, Quiñones-Baldrich W, Bongard FS, Wilson SE: Chylous ascites following abdominal aortic surgery. Ann Vasc Surg *5*:247–252, 1991.

134. Craver JM, Ottinger LW, Darling RC, et al: Hemorrhage and thrombosis as early complications of femoral popliteal bypass grafts: Causes, treatment and prognostic implications. Surgery *74*:839–846, 1973.

135. Hargrove WC, Barker CF, Berkowtiz HD, et al: Treatment of acute peripheral arterial and graft thromboses with low-dose streptokinase. Surgery *92*:981–993, 1982.

136. LiCalzi LK, Stansel HC: Failure of autogenous reversed saphenous vein femoro-popliteal grafting: Pathophysiology and prevention. Surgery *91*:352–358, 1982.

137. Whittemore AD, Clowes AW, Couch NP, et al: Secondary femoropopliteal reconstruction. Ann Surg *193*:35–42, 1981.

138. Buxton B, Lambert RP, Pitt TTE: The significance of vein wall thickness and diameter in relation to the patency of femoropopliteal saphenous vein bypass grafts. Surgery *87*:425–431, 1980.

139. Corson JD, Shah DM, Leather RP, et al: Reversed autogenous saphenous vein bypass grafts: Complications of their use in the lower extremity. *In* Bernhard VM, Towne JB (eds): Complications in Vascular Surgery. Orlando, FL, Grune & Stratton, 1985, pp 589–610.

140. Bunt TJ, Manship L, Moore W: Iatrogenic vascular injury during peripheral revascularization. J Vasc Surg *2*:491–498, 1985.

141. Samson RH, Gupta SK, Scher LA, et al: Arterial spasm complicating distal vascular bypass procedures. Arch Surg *117*:973–975, 1982.

142. Fuchs CA, Mitchener JS III, Hagen PO: Postoperative changes in autologous vein grafts. Ann Surg *188*:1–11, 1978.

143. LiCalzi LK, Stansel HC: The closure index: Prediction of long term patency of femoro-popliteal vein grafts. Surgery *91*:413–418, 1982.

144. Gundry SR, Jones M, Ishihara T, et al: Optimal preparation techniques for human saphenous vein grafts. Surgery *88*:785–794, 1980.

145. Karmody AM, Leather RP, Shah DM, et al: The in situ saphenous vein arterial bypass: Current problems and solutions. *In* Bernhard VM, Towne JB (eds): Complications in Vascular Surgery. Orlando, FL, Grune & Stratton, 1985, pp 561–588.

146. Brewster DC, LaSalle AJ, Robison JG, et al: Factors affecting patency of femoropopliteal bypass grafts. Surg Gynecol Obstet *157*:437–442, 1983.

147. DeWeese JA: Anastomotic neointimal fibrous hyperplasia. *In* Bernhard VM, Towne JB (eds): Complications in Vascular Surgery. Orlando, FL, Grune & Stratton, 1985, pp 157–170.

148. Green RM, Thomas M, Luka N, et al: A comparison of rapid healing prosthetic arterial grafts and autogenous veins. Arch Surg *114*:944–947, 1979.

149. Echave V, Kovenick AR, Haimov M, et al: Intimal hyperplasia as a complication of the use of polytetrafluoroethylene graft for femoral-popliteal bypass. Surgery *86*:791–800, 1979.

150. Harker LA: Platelet mechanisms in the genesis and prevention of graft related vascular injury reactions and thromboembolism. Nature of the vascular interface. *In* Sawyer

PN, Kaplitt HJ (eds): Vascular Grafts. New York, Appleton-Century-Crofts, 1978.

151. Schuler JJ, Flanigan DP: Alternate inflow for repeated failure of femorodistal grafts. *In* Bergan JJ, Yao JST (eds): Reoperative Arterial Surgery. Orlando, FL, Grune & Stratton, 1986, pp 393–406.

152. Szilagyi DE, Elliot JP, Hageman JG, et al: Biologic fate of autogenous vein implants as arterial substitute. Ann Surg 178:232–251, 1973.

153. Bergan JJ, Veith FJ, Bernhard VM, et al: Radomization of autogenous vein and polytetrafluoroethylene grafts in femoral-distal reconstruction. Surgery 92:921–930, 1982.

154. Corson JD, Johnson WC, LoGerfo FW, et al: Doppler ankle systolic pressure: Prognostic value in vein bypass grafts of the lower extremity. Arch Surg 113:932–935, 1977.

155. Kempczinski RF: Infrainguinal arterial bypass using prosthetic grafts. *In* Kempczinski RF (ed): The Ischemic Leg. Chicago, Year Book Medical Publishers, 1985, pp 437–454.

156. O'Donnell TF, Farber SP, Richmind DM, et al: Above-knee polytetrafluoroethylene femoro-popliteal bypass graft: Is it a reasonable alternative to the below-knee reversed autogenous vein graft? Surgery 94:26, 1983.

157. Robison JG, Brewster DC, Abbott WM, et al: Femoro-popliteal and tibioperoneal artery reconstruction using human umbilical vein. Arch Surg 118:1039, 1983.

158. Rosenthal D, Levine K, Stanton PE, et al: Femoropopliteal bypass: The preferred site for distal anastomosis. Surgery 93:1, 1983.

159. Marinelli MR, Beach KW, Glass MJ, et al: Non-invasive testing versus clinical evaluation of arterial disease: A prospective study. JAMA 241:2031–2034, 1979.

160. Yao JST: Postoperative evaluation of graft failure. *In* Bernhard VM, Towne JB (eds): Complications in Vascular Surgery. Orlando, FL, Grune & Stratton, 1985, pp 1–24.

161. Berkowitz HD, Hobbs CL, Roberts B, et al: Value of routine vascular laboratory studies to identify vein graft stenosis. Surgery 90: 971–979, 1981.

162. Bandyk DF: Postoperative surveillance of femoro-distal grafts: The application of echo-Doppler (duplex) ultrasonic scanning. *In* Bergan JJ, Yao JST (eds): Reoperative Arterial Surgery. Orlando, FL, Grune & Stratton, 1986, pp 59–80.

163. Baker WH, Hadcock MM, Littooy FN: Management of polytetrafluoroethylene graft occlusion. Arch Surg 115:508–513, 1980.

164. Goldberg L, Ricci MT, Sauvage LR, et al: Thrombolytic therapy for delayed occlusion of knitted Dacron bypass grafts in the axillo-femoral, femoropopliteal and femorotibial positions. Surg Gynecol Obstet 160:491–498, 1985.

165. Graor RA, Risius B, Denny KM, et al: Local thrombolysis in the treatment of thrombosed arteries, bypass grafts, and arteriovenous fistulas. J Vasc Surg 2:406–414, 1985.

166. Hargrove WC, Berkowitz HD, Freiman DB, et al: Recanalization of totally occluded femoropopliteal vein grafts with low-dose streptokinase infusion. Surgery 92:890–895, 1982.

167. Dardik H, Sussman BC, Kahn M, et al: Lysis of arterial clot by intravenous or intraarterial administration of streptokinase. Surg Gynecol Obstet 158:137–140, 1984.

168. Husson JM, Fiessinger JN, Aiach M, et al: Streptokinase after late failure reconstructive surgery for peripheral arteriosclerosis. J Cardiovasc Surg 22:145–152, 1981.

169. Quiñones-Baldrich WJ, Zierlar RE, Hiatt JC: Intraoperative fibrinolytic therapy: An adjunct to catheter thromboembolectomy. J Vasc Surg 2:319–326, 1985.

170. Parent FN, Bernhard VM, Pabst TS, McIntyre KE, Hunter GC, Malone JM: Fibrinolytic treatment of residual thrombus after catheter embolectomy for severe limb ischemia. J Vasc Surg 9:1953–160, 1989.

171. Cohen L, Kaplan M, Bernhard VM: Intraoperative streptokinase: An adjunct to mechanical thrombectomy in the management of acute ischemia. Arch Surg 121: 708–716, 1986.

172. Andros G, Harris RW, Salles-Cunha SX, et al: Arm veins

173. Harker LA, Slichter SJ, Sauvage LR: Platelet consumption by arterial prostheses: The effects of endothelialization and pharmacologic inhibition of platelet function. Ann Surg 186:594–601, 1977.

174. Veith FJ, Gupta SK, Ascer E, et al: Reoperations and other reinterventions for thrombosed and failing polytetrafluoroethylene grafts. *In* Bergan JJ, Yao JST (eds): Reoperative Arterial Surgery. Orlando, FL, Grune & Stratton, 1986, pp 377–392.

175. Kretschmer G, Wenzl E, Piza F, et al: The influence of anticoagulant treatment on the probability of function in femoropopliteal vein bypass surgery: Analysis of a clinical series (1970 to 1985) and interim evaluation of a controlled clinical trial. Surgery 102:453–459, 1987.

176. Kretschmer G, Wenzl E, Schemper M, et al: Influence of postoperative anticoagulant treatment on patient survival after femoropopliteal vein bypass surgery. Lancet 1:797–798, 1988.

177. Wengrovitz M, Atnip RG, Gifford RRM, Neumyer MM, Heitjan DF, Thiele BL: Wound complications of autogenous subcutaneous infrainguinal arterial bypass surgery: Predisposing factors and management. J Vasc Surg 11:156–163, 1990.

178. Johnson JA, Cogbill TH, Strutt PJ, Gundersen AL: Wound complications after infrainguinal bypass: Classification, predisposing factors, and management. Arch Surg 123:859–862, 1988.

179. Schwartz ME, Harrington EB, Schanzer H: Wound complications after in situ bypass. J Vasc Surg 7:802–807, 1988.

180. Henderson VJ, Mitchell RS, Kosek JC, Cohen RG, Miller DC: Biochemical (functional) adaptation of "arterialized" vein graft. Ann Surg 203:339–345, 1986.

181. Bandyk DF, Kaebnick HW, Stewart GW, Towne JB: Durability of the in situ saphenous vein arterial bypass: A comparison of primary and secondary patency. J Vasc Surg 5:256–268, 1987.

182. Levine AW, Bandyk DF, Bonier PH, Towne JB: Lessons learned in adopting the in situ saphenous vein bypass. J Vasc Surg 2:145–153, 1985.

183. Woelfle KD, Loeprecht H, Weber H, Zinkl K: Intraoperative assessment of in situ saphenous vein bypass grafts by vascular endoscopy. Eur J Vasc Surg 2:257–262, 1988.

184. Bush HL, Corey CA, Nasbeth DC: Distal in situ saphenous vein grafts for limb salvage. Increased operative blood flow and postoperative patency. Am J Surg 145:542–548, 1983.

185. Bandyk DF, Jorgensen RA, Towne JB: Intraoperative assessment of in situ saphenous vein arterial grafts using pulsed Doppler spectral analysis. Arch Surg 121:292–299, 1986.

186. Bandyk DF, Cato RF, Towne JB: A low flow velocity predicts failure of femoropopliteal and femorotibial bypass grafts. Surgery 98:799–809, 1985.

187. Fowl RJ, Patterson RB, Bodenham RJ, Kempczinski RF: Functional failure of patent femorodistal in situ grafts. Ann Vasc Surg 3:200–204, 1989.

188. Taylor LM, Phinney ES, Porter JM: Present status of reversed vein bypass for lower extremity revascularization. J Vasc Surg 3:288–297, 1986.

189. Veith FJ, Gupta SK, Daly VD: Femoropopiteal bypass to the isolated popliteal segment: Is a polytetrafluoroethylene graft acceptable? Surgery 89:296–303, 1981.

190. Berger K, Sauvage LR: Late fiber deterioration in Dacron arterial grafts. Ann Surg 193:477–491, 1980.

191. Clagett GP, Salander JM, Eddleman WL, et al: Dilatation of knitted Dacron aortic prostheses and anastomotic false aneurysms: Etiologic considerations. Surgery 93:9–16, 1983.

192. Nunn DB, Freeman MH, Hudgins PC: Postoperative alterations in the size of Dacron grafts. Ann Surg 189:741–744, 1979.

193. Pourdeyhimi B, Wagner D: On the correlation between the failure of vascular grafts and their structural and material

properties: A critical analysis. J Biomed Mater Res *20*:375–409, 1986.

194. Cooke PA, Nobis PA, Stoney RJ: Dacron aortic graft failure. Arch Surg *108*:101–103, 1974.

195. Cranley JJ, Karkow WS, Hafner CO, Flanagan LD: Aneurysmal dilatation in umbilical vein grafts. *In* Bergan JJ, Yao JST (eds): Reoperative Arterial Surgery. Orlando, FL, Grune & Stratton, 1986, pp 343–358.

196. Dardik H, Ibrahim IM, Sussman B, et al: Biodegradation and aneurysm formation in umbilical vein graft. Ann Surg *199*:61–68, 1984.

197. Dardik H: Reoperative surgery for complications following femorodistal bypass with umbilical vein grafts. *In* Bergan JJ, Yao JST (eds): Reoperative Arterial Surgery. Orlando, FL, Grune & Stratton, 1986, pp 331–342.

198. Julien S, Gill F, Guidoin R, et al: Biologic and structural evaluation of 80 surgically excised human umbilical vein grafts. Can Soc Vasc Surg *32*:101–107, 1989.

199. Roberts AK, Johnson N: Aneurysm formation in an expanded microporous polytetrafluoroethylene graft. Arch Surg *113*:211–213, 1978.

200. Selman SH, Rhodes RS, Anderson JM, DePalma RG, Clowes AW: Atheromatous changes in expanded polytetrafluoroethylene grafts. Surgery *87*:630–637, 1980.

201. Eickhoff JF, Engell HC: Local regulation of blood flow and the occurrence of edema after arterial reconstruction of the lower limbs. Ann Surg *195*:474–478, 1982.

202. Schubart PJ, Porter JM: Leg edema following femorodistal bypass. *In* Bergan JJ, Yao JST (eds): Reoperative Arterial Surgery. Orlando, FL, Grune & Stratton, 1986, pp 311–330.

203. Husni EA: The edema of arterial reconstruction. Circulation *35*(suppl I):I-169–I-173, 1967.

204. Storen EJ, Myhre HO, Stiris G: Lymphangiographic findings in patients with leg edema after arterial reconstruction. Acta Clin Scand *140*:385–387, 1974.

205. Porter JM, Lindell TD, Lakin PC: Leg edema following femoropopliteal autogenous vein bypass. Arch Surg *105*:883–888, 1972.

206. Kwann JHM, Bernstein JM, Connolly JE: Management of lymph fistula in the groin after arterial reconstruction. Arch Surg *114*:1416–1418, 1979.

40

PORTAL HYPERTENSION

HUGH A. GELABERT and RONALD W. BUSUTTIL

Portal hypertension is a condition in which the circulation of blood in the portal venous system is impeded and results in an increase in portal venous pressure. The elevation of the portal venous blood pressure results in a series of physiological developments that are commonly encountered as the "complications" of portal hypertension and includes ascites, hypersplenism, and variceal hemorrhage. The natural history of patients with portal hypertension differs depending on the cause of the condition. Furthermore, the patient's ability to withstand the stress of hemorrhage or surgery will largely depend on the functional hepatic reserve.

The current care of patients with portal hypertension has become considerably more complex. Recent developments, including the expanded role of hepatic transplantation and the introduction of percutaneous portosystemic shunting, have created considerable confusion in what was already a complex field. For the vascular surgeon caring for patients with portal hypertension and variceal bleeding, knowledge concerning the current management of these patients is essential. This chapter will review the pathophysiology, diagnosis, and management of these patients, with special attention to the recent developments in the field.

PATHOGENESIS

The pathogenesis of portal hypertension results from an aberration in the splanchnic blood flow, which causes either an increase in the portal blood flow (rare), or an obstruction to the outflow of blood from the portal circulation (most common). The obstructions to the portal circulation have been classified anatomically by referring to their location with regard to the hepatic sinusoids. Accordingly, the obstructions may be presinusoidal, sinusoidal, or postsinusoidal. The presinusoidal and postsinusoidal have been further subclassified as intrahepatic or extrahepatic (Table 40–1).

Extrahepatic Presinusoidal Obstruction

Presinusoidal extrahepatic obstruction is most commonly due to thrombosis of the portal vein. While less common than other forms of obstructive portal hypertension, portal vein thrombosis occurs in a significant number of children. It may occur in adults, but the causes are remarkably different between children and adults.

Portal vein thrombosis in children occurs as a complication of an infectious process. Omphalitis and appendicitis are the most common causes. In adults, the most common cause of portal vein thrombosis is a gradual and relentless decrease in the portal blood flow secondary to the high resistance in the hepatic circulation caused by cirrhosis. Other causes in adults include pancreatitis, hypercoagulable states or tumor thrombus, and mechanical obstruction of portal venous flow. The latter may be the result of malignant invasion, lymphadenopathy, or caudate lobe compression. Hypercoagulable conditions may result from polycythemia, cancer, and hypovolemia. Sepsis may lead to portal vein thrombosis by several mechanisms: low-flow states, hypovolemia, and perhaps activation of the coagulation system.

The most common presentation of portal vein thrombosis is variceal hemorrhage and ascites. In children, this is often seen in association with minor infections such as upper respiratory infections. The diagnosis of portal vein thrombosis is usually established by Doppler ultrasound, or the lack of visualization of the portal vein on the venous phase of a celiac or mesenteric angiogram. Wedged hepatic venous pressure is usually normal, as is the hepatic synthetic function. Because of the preservation of hepatic function, patients are able to tolerate episodes of bleeding without much decompensation. In instances of repeated hemorrhage, decompression may be advocated in order to prevent multiple repeated transfusions and the attendant risks of hepatitis, acquired immunodeficiency syndrome (AIDS), cytomegaloviral infections, and hemochromatosis.

TABLE 40–1. ETIOLOGY OF PORTAL HYPERTENSION

Presinusoidal	Postsinusoidal
Extrahepatic: portal vein thrombosis	Intrahepatic
Omphalitis	Cirrhosis
Pancreatitis	Postnecrotic
Trauma	Portal
Malignancy	Hemochromatosis
Polycythemia	Venoocclusive disease
Periportal lymphadenopathy	
Intrahepatic	Extrahepatic
Biliary artresia	Budd-Chiari syndrome
Schistosomiasis	Hepatic vein webs
Sarcoidosis	Malignant obstruction
Arsenic toxicity	Oral contraceptives
Congenital hepatic fibrosis	Pregnancy
Myeloproliferative disorders	Plant alkaloids
	Cardiac causes
	Congestive heart failure
Primary biliary cirrhosis	Constructive pericarditis
Hepatoportal sclerosis	Increased blood flow:
Sinusoidal	Arteriovenous fistulas
Cirrhosis	Splenic artery to splenic vein
Toxic hepatitis	Hepatic artery to portal vein
Fatty metamorphosis	

Intrahepatic Presinusoidal Obstruction

Most causes of intrahepatic presinusoidal obstructive portal hypertension relate to fibrosis and compression of the portal venules, with subsequent restriction of portal flow. Included amongst these diseases are congenital hepatic fibrosis, sarcoidosis, chronic arsenic exposure, Wilson's disease, hepatoportal sclerosis, primary biliary cirrhosis, schistosomiasis, and myeloproliferative disorders.

Schistosomiasis is the most common cause of portal hypertension in Third World countries. Deposition of ova in the portal venule walls results in a granulomatous inflammatory reaction that in turn results in fibrosis and portal flow restriction. Hepatic function is preserved in the early stages, but later stages of this disease are characterized by advanced cirrhosis and loss of hepatic function.[1] Myeloproliferative disorders such as myelosclerosis and myeloid leukemia will occasionally lead to presinusoidal hypertension by virtue of the deposition of primitive cellular material infiltrating the portal zones.[2] Sarcoidosis causes portal hypertension by two mechanisms: first, sarcoid granulomas within the portal vein will lead to obstruction; and second, there is increased portal blood flow.

Hepatic function is usually preserved in the early stages of these diseases. In later stages, significant hepatic impairment may result from progressive cirrhosis. Hemodynamic characteristics are similar to those of extrahepatic portal vein obstruction: low hepatic wedge pressure and elevated portal venous pressure.

Intrahepatic Sinusoidal and Postsinusoidal Obstruction

Sinusoidal portal hypertension may be the sequela of alcoholic hepatitis or toxic hepatitis. Pure sinusoidal obstruction is a rare cause of portal hypertension. It occurs most frequently as a sequela of acute alcoholic hepatitis or toxic hepatitis.

While pure sinusoidal obstruction is relatively rare, it frequently is present as part of a combined sinusoidal and postsinusoidal obstructive picture. Postsinusoidal obstruction is seen most commonly in cases of alcoholic liver disease, postnecrotic cirrhosis, or hemochromatosis. As would be expected in these diseases, the hepatic function is usually significantly impaired.

In the United States, this is the most common type of portal hypertension, and is estimated to be the 10th leading cause of death. Two mechanisms account for the portal hypertension in these patients. The first is the mechanical obstruction of the portal blood flow by the regenerating hepatic nodules and cirrhotic bands within the damaged liver. These changes may extend beyond the confines of the hepatic sinusoids, accounting for the presence of presinusoidal, sinusoidal, and postsinusoidal distortion of the hepatic architecture. The second element is an increase in the splanchnic perfusion, in part attributed to the genesis of multiple arteriovenous (AV) shunts and collateral channels. One third of portal blood flow may bypass functional hepatocytes through these channels.[3] The clinical correlate of this increased blood flow is the hyperdynamic state that typifies cirrhotics: elevated cardiac output and a diminished systemic resistance.[4]

The portal hemodynamic characteristics of these diseases are usually those of elevated hepatic wedge pressure along with elevated portal vein pressure. Since most of these diseases directly affect hepatocytes, hepatic function is frequently impaired even in the early stages of these diseases. These patients will frequently have poor hepatic reserve, and will decompensate with each bleeding episode. Selection and timing of interventions becomes an important step in their management.

Extrahepatic Postsinusoidal Obstruction

Postsinusoidal hepatic vein obstruction is usually the result of thrombosis in the hepatic veins. While the cause of most cases is unknown, a series of associated diseases have been identified. Membranous webs of the hepatic veins, malignancies (hepatomas, renal carcinomas, adrenal carcinomas), trauma, pregnancy, contraceptives, acute alcoholic hepatitis, venoocclusive disease, and *Senecio* toxicity may all result in hepatic vein thrombosis.[5] Constrictive pericarditis and chronic congestive heart failure may also cause postsinusoidal obstruction.

Budd-Chiari syndrome is the result of hepatic venous occlusive disease and is characterized by massive ascites, esophageal varices, variceal hemorrhage, hepatic failure, and death. Chiari's disease is due to primary hepatic vein ostial occlusion. The clinical progression following hepatic vein occlusion may be fulminant or gradual. Hepatic failure is the result of chronic congestion and ischemia from impaired hepatic blood flow. The factors that determine the rate of progression are not well understood. Angiography is essential in establishing the diagnosis: it will identify the presence of thrombus and its location.[6,7]

The fulminant course is marked by rapid development of ascites, fatigue, and jaundice. Additionally, elevation of liver enzymes and prothrombin times indicates hepatocellular damage. Patients who do not improve with anticoagulation should be considered for either shunting or liver transplantation.

The more gradual presentation may have many similar features such as ascites and chronic fatigue, but hepatic function will be preserved to a greater degree. Hypersplenism and variceal hemorrhage may be a more prominent feature in these patients.

An initial trial of anticoagulation may allow endogenous fibrinolysis to resolve the venous thrombosis. Patients whose course is gradually progressive and who have intact hepatocellular function should be considered for portal decompression by either a portacaval, mesocaval, or mesoatrial shunt. The selection of shunt is dependent on the patient's anatomy as defined by angiography. When the Budd-Chiari syndrome leads to deterioration of hepatic function as demonstrated by abnormalities of liver function tests, hepatic transplantation is the procedure of choice.[8]

ARTERIOVENOUS FISTULAS

As a cause of portal hypertension, AV fistulas are relatively rare. Most fistulas are either traumatic or splenic. Traumatic AV fistulas may occur as a consequence of transhepatic biliary manipulations, or as a result of penetrating trauma. Splenic fistulas may be associated with splenic artery aneurysms, sarcoidosis, Gaucher's disease, myeloid metaplasia, or tropical splenomegaly. As with splenic artery aneurysms, women of childbearing age are at greatest risk. The portal hypertension results initially from increased flow in the portal circulation. At later stages, fibrosis and secondary obstruction of the presinusoidal spaces exacerbates the portal hypertension.

DIAGNOSIS

If portal hypertension is defined as elevated portal venous pressure, then the diagnosis of portal hypertension rests upon demonstrating the increased portal venous pressure. In practical terms, the diagnosis of portal hypertension is made by identifying signs of the elevation of portal venous pressure and a history that would support these findings.

The signs of elevated portal venous pressure include the presence of esophageal varices, splenomegaly, ascites, or abdominal wall collaterals. Of these, ascites, splenomegaly, and abdominal wall collateralization may be apparent on physical examination. Esophagogastric endoscopy is currently considered the most reliable means of identifying gastroesophageal varices.

Signs of underlying hepatic disease include spider angiomata, palmar erythema, gynecomastia, muscle wasting, loss of pubertal hair growth, and testicular atrophy. Encephalopathy, asterixis, fetor hepatis, and fatigue may also be noted in chronic hepatic insufficiency. The presence of liver disease does not conclusively signify that the patient has significant portal hypertension.

Historical support for the diagnosis of portal hypertension includes identification of any of the diseases that are known to lead to portal hypertension (e.g., alcohol ingestion, hepatitis, hepatotoxins). Not only the presence, but also the duration of these problems is important in substantiating the diagnosis of portal hypertension. Both alcoholic toxicity and viral hepatitis will lead to cirrhosis and usually portal hypertension, but the time course between the onset of these insults and the development of the hypertension may be as long as 10 or more years.

Adjunctive means of demonstrating portal hypertension include angiography and hemodynamic measurements. Neither is essential in making the diagnosis; both are supportive. Angiography may reveal both splenomegaly and collateralization of the portal region and the gastroesophageal axis. Additionally, angiography may characterize the direction of portal blood flow as either hepatopetal or hepatofugal.

Hemodynamic measurement of the portal circulation is most commonly accomplished by venous catheterization and measurement of the wedged hepatic vein pressure (WHVP).[9] This technique is able to record the pressure in the hepatic veins and the hepatic sinusoids (Fig. 40–1). Elevations of the WHVP reflect elevations in the portal venous pressure. False-negative results may be encountered in patients with presinusoidal obstruction, and in instances of catheter malfunction. Normal hepatic venous pressure is essentially the same as the right atrial pressure (0 to 5 mm Hg); portal venous pressure is about 2 to 6 mm Hg higher than the hepatic venous pressure. A gradient greater than 10 mm Hg is considered abnormal.

Other methods of measuring portal venous pressure have been developed, but have largely been abandoned because of increased risk associated with them. Included in this group are direct cannulation of the portal vein (requires surgical exposure), percutaneous transhepatic portal venous catheterization, transjugular portal vein catheterization, and percutaneous splenic pulp pressure measurement.[10]

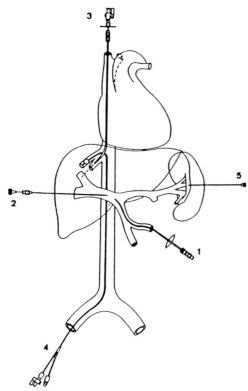

FIGURE 40–1. Schematic representation of the techniques used for the measurement of portal pressure. *1*, Surgical catheterization of the portal vein; *2*, percutaneous transhepatic puncture and catheterization of the portal vein; *3*, transjugular portal vein catheterization; *4*, hepatic vein catheterization (balloon catheter); *5*, splenic pulp puncture. (From Bosch J, Mastai R, Kravetz D, et al: Hemodynamic evaluation of the patients with portal hypertension. Semin Liver Dis 6:309–317, 1986.)

The most recent development in assessing the portal circulation is the application of noninvasive ultrasonography. Duplex scanning has been used to measure the direction and velocity of portal blood flow. Information gathered from this technique will detect portal vein thrombosis, hepatopetal and hepatofugal flow, and portal hypertension.[9–12] Bolondi and associates have used indirect measurements to identify the presence of portal hypertension, with high sensitivity and specificity.[13]

DIAGNOSTIC EVALUATION

Laboratory Testing

While the diagnosis of portal hypertension rests on the combination of physical findings and the historical account, a number of diagnostic tests are helpful in confirming the clinical diagnosis and in planning therapy. The initial point of departure in evaluating most patients is to assess their serum chemistries. Specific attention should be placed on the liver enzymes (serum glutamic-oxaloacetic acid transaminase [SGOT], serum glutamic-pyrovic transaminase [SGPT], lactate dehydrogenase [LDH], al-

kaline phosphatase), and tests of hepatic synthetic function (prothrombin time, serum albumin). Information from these two sets of tests will identify those patients who are suffering acute hepatocellular damage, and those who have had damage sufficient to reduce the liver's ability to synthesize essential proteins. This represents two distinct gradations of the hepatic dysfunction. The first, indicative of an acute insult; the second, representing the degree of hepatic dysfunction. The presence and degree of abnormalities in liver function tests will correlate with the outcome of patients: the more abnormal the tests, the worse the prognosis.[14,15]

Abnormalities of liver function tests combined with physical findings and historical data form the basis of Child's classification of portal hypertensive patients. The Child's classification and the more recent Child-Pugh classification serve as prognosticators of survival in cirrhotic patients who undergo both emergent and elective surgery (Table 40–2).[16]

Additional laboratory investigation should include a determination of serum ammonia and complete blood count (CBC), which includes white blood cells (WBCs), red blood cells (RBCs), and platelets. Serum ammonia may be elevated in instances of severe hepatic dysfunction and coma. It correlates loosely with mentation, but may serve as an indicator for a treatable cause of encephalopathy: hyperammonemia.[17]

The CBC will serve to detect the presence of anemia and hypersplenism. Anemia in cirrhotic patients may result from a number of causes other than hemorrhage. Chronic malnutrition is a particularly important cause of anemia in these patients.

While splenomegaly is present in virtually all portal hypertensive patients, hypersplenism may not develop until later in the course of their disease. The size of the spleen does not correlate directly with either the degree of portal hypertension or the severity of hypersplenism, but an enlarged spleen is found in virtually all patients with portal hypertension and hypersplenism.[18] Hypersplenism is defined principally in terms of splenic sequestration and destruction of formed elements of the blood (platelets in particular, but also WBCs) leading to significant depressions in the platelet and WBC counts. Platelet counts below 50,000 and WBC counts below 2000 support this diagnosis.

Upper Gastrointestinal Endoscopy

Endoscopy plays a pivotal role in management of portal hypertensive patients. Both for diagnostic and therapeutic reasons, endoscopy should be one of the first tests performed. Endoscopy will not only define the presence of varices, but will also identify the source of bleeding in patients who present with hemorrhage.

The diagnosis of portal hypertension may be established by noting the presence of varices. The size, appearance, and location of the varices may signifi-

TABLE 40–2. CHILD'S CLASSIFICATION OF CIRRHOTIC PATIENTS

Criteria	Risk		
	Good	Moderate	Poor
	A	B	C
Bilirubin (mg/100 ml)	Below 2.0	2.0–3.0	Over 3.0
Albumin (gm/100 ml)	Over 3.5	3.0–3.5	Below 3.0
Ascites	Absent	Easily controlled	Poorly controlled
Encephalopathy	Absent	Minimal	Advanced
Nutrition	Excellent	Good	Poor

cantly alter the management of the patient. Endoscopy will also serve to note the presence of other sources of bleeding in portal hypertensive patients such as hypertensive gastropathy, gastritis, gastric ulceration, duodenal ulceration, gastric mucosal lacerations (Mallory-Weiss tears), or esophageal ulcerations. Because of the variety of possible bleeding lesions and significant difference in the management of these lesions, patients admitted for hemorrhage must undergo upper gastrointestinal (GI) endoscopy on each admission. As many as 40 to 60 per cent of patients with documented varices have associated gastritis or peptic ulcer disease.[19] In patients with esophageal and gastric varices, the gastric varices have been documented as the site of bleeding in as many as 18 per cent.[20]

Liver Biopsy

The role of liver biopsy in the preoperative evaluation of portal hypertensive patients has been the focus of controversy. The goal of liver biopsy in this setting is to identify those patients who have active hepatitis. In alcoholic patients this is most commonly denoted by the presence of Mallory bodies, which signify acute hyaline necrosis. Mallory bodies may also be seen in patients with Wilson's disease, cholestasis, and primary biliary cirrhosis. The reason for identifying patients with acute hepatic necrosis is that these patients are thought to be at increased risk of dying in the course of shunt surgery.

The principal body of evidence to support this contention is that of Mikkelsen and associates, who noted operative mortality of 69 per cent in elective shunt cases and 83 per cent in emergent cases in the presence of acute hyaline necrosis.[20,21] Other authors have contested the point of whether acute alcoholic hepatitis alters survival.[14,22] A final item that should be noted is that the Mallory bodies will disappear as patients abstain from alcohol and liver recovers from its insult.[23]

The current recommendation is that patients suspected of having acute hepatitis and who are candidates for elective shunt surgery should undergo percutaneous liver biopsy. If Mallory bodies are identified, then consideration should be given to postponing the elective operation for a period of time to allow for the liver to recover. This must be carefully balanced against the risk of recurrent hemorrhage and the likelihood of the patient's compliance.

Duplex Scanning

Duplex scanning is finding increased application in the evaluation of portal hypertensive patients. In patients who are to be considered for portacaval shunting or for hepatic transplantation, the duplex scan is frequently sufficient to document portal vein patency. Duplex scanning will determine both the patency of the portal vein and the direction of portal venous blood flow. This is the minimum anatomical information required to proceed with the abovementioned operations. The combination of color-flow imaging with duplex scanning has resulted in improved accuracy and extended the range of diagnostic abilities of the duplex scanners.[11]

Angiography

Preoperative anatomical definition is essential for optimal surgical management, particularly when peripheral shunts are being considered. Angiography should be performed on all patients who are to undergo elective shunting procedures. Techniques primarily of historical interest include splenoportography (percutaneous needle into the spleen),[24] umbilical vein catheterization, and transhepatic percutaneous portal venography.[21–30]

Currently, the vast majority of portal angiography is performed by selective cannulation of the celiac and superior mesenteric arteries, and observation of the venous phase of these angiograms. Additional studies that should be obtained include an injection of the renal veins, and a hepatic wedge angiogram and pressure recording. The combination of these studies is commonly referred to as a "liver package."

The goal of these studies is to delineate the major portal tributaries: the splenic vein, the superior mesenteric vein, the portal vein itself, and their relation to the renal vein. An additional goal of the liver package study is to measure the hepatic wedge pressure and visualize the hepatic sinusoidal circulation. These latter two elements are helpful in confirming the presence of portal hypertension, estimating the severity of the hypertension, and determining the etiology of the elevated pressure. Low hepatic wedge pressure (less than 10 to 12 mm Hg) in a patient with variceal hemorrhage should prompt a careful search for evidence of portal vein thrombosis.[31] The wedged hepatic vein catheter allows the determination of the morphology of the sinusoids, as well as the direction of blood flow (Fig. 40–2). Wedge hepatic venogram in cirrhotics demonstrates irregular sinusoids with multiple scattered filling defects. Retrograde portal vein filling indicates hepatofugal flow.[24]

The delineation of the portal tributary anatomy is essential in planning an elective portal decompressive procedure, since the choice of procedure is limited by the patient's anatomy. The angiographic findings correlate with the degree of cirrhosis. In early cirrhosis, no definite angiographic abnormalities are present. As cirrhosis becomes more severe one sees the development of collateral pathways, dilatation of the hepatic artery, and pruning of intrahepatic portal vein branches (Fig. 40–3). In advanced cirrhosis, reversal of flow in the portal vein may be detected.

COMPLICATIONS OF PORTAL HYPERTENSION

Esophageal Varices

Esophageal varices develop in about 30 per cent of cirrhotics. Of cirrhotics who present with upper GI bleeding, about 30 per cent will bleed from their varices. The other 70 per cent bleed from chemical

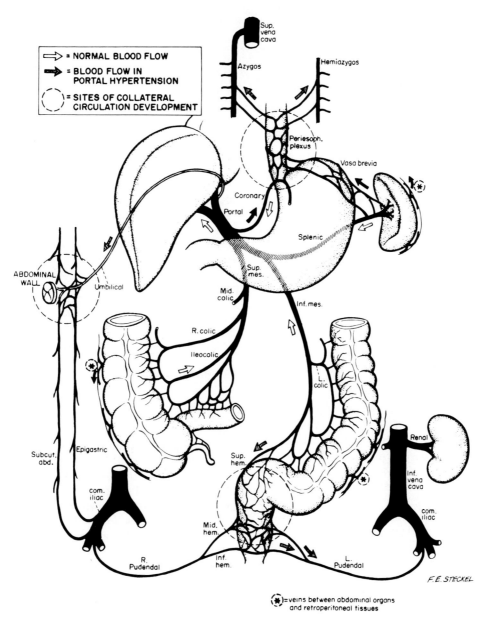

FIGURE 40–2. Abnormal wedged hepatic venogram demonstrating a coarse, mottled parenchymal pattern consistent with cirrhosis.

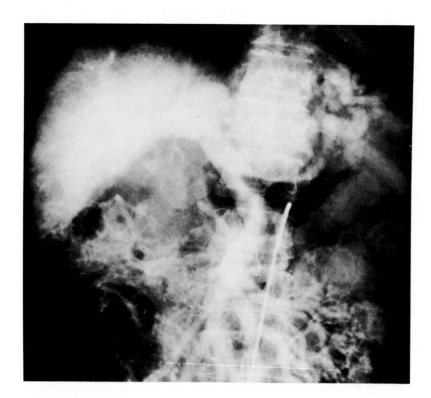

FIGURE 40–3. Venous phase superior mesenteric angiogram demonstrating superior mesenteric, portal, and dilated coronary vein.

gastritis, hypertensive gastritis, ulceration, erosions, mucosal tears, and neoplastic growth. Of the cirrhotic patients who bleed from esophageal varices, about 5 to 15 per cent will have massive hemorrhage that will be difficult to control. The mortality of these patients—bleeding to death from the esophageal varices—is about 30 to 50 per cent.

The pathogenesis of esophageal varices centers around the development of collateral circulatory pathways for blood exiting the portal circulation. The impetus for the development of these collaterals is the difference in pressure between the portal system and the systemic venous circulation. Several major collateral networks have been described in cirrhotics: the coronary-esophageal veins, the umbilical vein, the hemorrhoidal veins, and the retroperitoneal veins (veins of Retzius). Each of these venous systems may develop into significant collateral networks.

Any blood vessel that is attenuated and distended under supranormal pressures is at risk of disruption and bleeding. The addition of mechanical trauma or chemical irritation may further serve to induce bleeding. Consequently, any of the collaterals that develop because of portal hypertension may bleed. Hemorrhoidal vessels, intestinal varices, and stomal varices have all been documented as bleeding sites in cirrhotic patients. The mechanical and chemical irritants that bathe the gastroesophageal region result in esophagitis, attenuation of the mucosal layers, and disruption of the varices. In combination with the increased blood pressure within the varices and periodic exacerbations of this pressure by activities that increase the intraabdominal and intrathoracic pressure (such as coughing or retching), the risk of bleeding from esophageal varices is significantly increased. The elevation of portal pressures results in dilation of all these collateral pathways (Fig. 40–4).

Several attempts have been made to prognosticate the risk of hemorrhage from esophageal varices. Characterization of the severity of portal hypertension on the basis of corrected sinusoidal pressure has not correlated with subsequent hemorrhage. Factors that do predict the risk of bleeding include the size of the varices, the Child's class of the patient, and the presence of erosions on the varices (red-dot signs).[32–36]

Encephalopathy

While not usually considered a life-threatening complication of hepatic failure, encephalopathy may have a profoundly disabling effect on patients. The clinical manifestations of encephalopathy are varied and range from mild inattention to frank coma. The most commonly used system of staging encephalopathy classifies patients on a scale from stage I through stage IV. The progression begins with mild personality alterations, occasionally with asterixis or clonus in stage I. Stage II may be characterized by drowsiness, sometimes with mild confusion. Stage II is typified by stupor and obtundation. Coma is the hallmark of stage IV. Electroencephalography is not specifically diagnostic, characteristically showing only slow-wave activity primarily in the frontal regions.[37]

The mechanism by which liver failure leads to coma

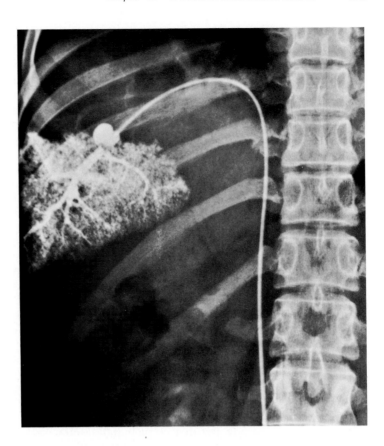

FIGURE 40–4. Schematic diagram of collateral venous pathways. (From Sedgwick CE, et al: Portal Hypertension. Boston, Little, Brown, 1967.)

is not clearly understood. Several agents have been postulated as encephalopathic, especially in the presence of a diseased liver. Ammonia, nitrogenous amines, increased false neurotransmitters, decreased true neurotransmitters, and an increased ratio of aromatic to branch-chain amino acids are the most likely candidates.

Elevated ammonia levels have several significant repercussions. First, they elevate glucagon levels. This in turn stimulates gluconeogenesis, which produces more ammonia. Additionally, the gluconeogenesis leads to elevated insulin levels. The elevated insulin will promote catabolism of branch-chain amino acids. This ultimately leads to increased levels of straight-chain amino acids such as phenylalanine, tyrosine, and methionine. An elevated ratio of straight-chain to branch-chain amino acids drives neutral amino acids past the blood-brain barrier. The cerebral uptake of these neutral amino acids is possible because ammonia stimulates brain glutamine synthesis, allowing rapid equilibration of brain glutamine for straight-chain neutral amino acids. These same neutral amino acids may act as false neurotransmitters, and are thought to produce encephalopathy.[38]

The treatment of encephalopathy is based on reduction of the ammonia levels and supplementation of branched-chain amino acids. Lactulose and neomycin will reduce ammonia uptake from the gut by altering the intestinal pH, reducing the number of intestinal bacteria, and reducing intestinal transit of protein. Other agents such as L-dopa have been used with mixed results in improving encephalopathy.[39]

Ascites

Ascites is a common symptom of portal hypertensive patients. As many as 80 per cent of these patients may have some degree of ascites. The mechanism by which ascites develops is a combination of hemodynamic, physiologic, and metabolic factors. The hemodynamics of the portal circulatory system in the face of cirrhosis is primarily driven by the increased portal venous pressure. In such a state, the Starling forces will tend to drive fluids out of the vessels and into the interstitial space. Compounding this problem is the low oncotic pressure that characterizes many cirrhotics by virtue of their hypoalbuminemia. Finally, many of these patients chronically register relatively low effective intravascular volume, which in turn triggers the renal aldosterone-renin-angiotensin system, and perhaps an additional natriuretic hormone. These then produce a state in which the patients retain free water and salt, both of which aggravate the ascites. The net effect is the translocation of fluid from the intravascular space to the interstitial space and the abdominal cavity.

The compensatory mechanism that normally counteracts the accumulation of interstitial and peritoneal fluid is primarily the lymphatic system. In the cirrhotic patients, the lymph flow is frequently increased. Ascites will accumulate when the ability of the lymphatics to reabsorb this fluid is overwhelmed.

The cornerstone to the management of ascites is the restriction of salt intake and the judicious use of diuretics. These measures will control the vast majority of ascitic patients. In only 5 per cent of cases can ascites be considered to be intractable; in these cases, other means of addressing the ascites are required.

MEDICAL THERAPY

General Medical Care

Medical care of cirrhotic patients may be readily classified as (1) health maintenance care, (2) the management of acute complications, and (3) the postoperative care of the cirrhotic patient. The maintenance care is based on evaluating and defining the cause of the liver disease and addressing any factors related to the cause of the liver disease that are amenable to change (e.g., cessation of alcohol consumption). The second element is the establishment of the patient's current state of health and hepatic function (i.e., defining the presence of portal hypertension, splenomegaly, ascites, or varices). An assessment of the hepatic disease and the degree of hepatic deterioration will help prognosticate the eventual course of the patient.

The next step involves maintenance of nutrition, supplementation of vitamins and minerals, and avoidance of salt (especially in ascitic patients).

Management of Acute Complications

The management of acute complications is a very specialized area in the care of these patients. The most common problem that requires urgent care is hemorrhage. The significance of hemorrhage in these patients is difficult to overstate. Up to 70 per cent mortality may be associated with hemorrhage, depending on the cause and severity of the liver disease and the degree of decompensation of the patient at the time of presentation. Furthermore, the risk of a second bleed within 1 year may be as high as 60 per cent.[16]

The essential steps in caring for a cirrhotic patient with an upper GI hemorrhage include establishing peripheral venous access, volume-resuscitating the patient, and determining the source of bleeding. This is best accomplished by upper GI endoscopy. As mentioned previously, between 40 and 60 per cent of cirrhotics with known varices who present with an upper GI bleed will not be bleeding from their varices.[40]

If the patient is bleeding from an esophageal varix or hypertensive gastritis, then several specific steps should be promptly taken. First, an assessment must be made of the rate of bleeding. Second, the patient

must be adequately resuscitated. Third, the patient must be prepared for a possible therapeutic intervention.

Assessing the rate of bleeding is essential, since it will determine the rate at which the patient must be resuscitated and the substance that should be employed. It will also determine the timing of interventions and, at times, the choice of which interventions are possible. The assessment is largely based on the progressive change in the patient's vital signs, mentation, and perfusion in the course of resuscitation. A nasogastric tube will also provide information as to continued bleeding. Emergency endoscopy may provide insight as to whether the patient is suffering a massive hemorrhage or is bleeding at a moderate rate. The change in the patient's hematocrit is not necessarily the best indicator of bleeding, since there may be a significant lag between the bleeding episode and the subsequent drop in hematocrit.

Patients with relatively minor bleeding episodes will frequently stop bleeding spontaneously. The few patients who are actively bleeding at the time of admission will almost always respond to an infusion of vasopressin. The key to managing these patients is to avoid overloading them with fluid and salts, since this may precipitate a rebleed, with further decompensation.

Patients with moderate bleeding rates stand a reasonable chance of stopping their bleeding without surgical intervention. These patients will frequently respond to infusions of vasopressin (Pitressin), emergency sclerotherapy, or balloon tamponade.

Patients who bleed massively will often require some form of more advanced intervention. This is often in addition to the vasopressin and balloon tamponade. Emergent endoscopy is frequently impaired by the massive bleeding. Subsequent steps include angiographic embolization, percutaneous attempts at creating an intrahepatic shunt (see section, Nonsurgical Shunt Procedures: TIPSS, later in chapter), or emergency surgical shunting.

The resuscitation of a cirrhotic patient who presents with an episode of upper GI hemorrhage is a delicate balance between supplementing the circulatory system with sufficient volume so as to allow perfusion of the vital organs, and the overinfusion of salt solutions, which will eventually further push the patient into a decompensated state. The fluids used in resuscitation will vary with the severity of the hemorrhage. In minor bleeds, the patients may be resuscitated with intravenous crystalloid solutions. In patients with more severe hemorrhages, it may be necessary to supplement this with infusions of albumin. In the severe hemorrhages, it is necessary to infuse both packed red blood cells (PRBCs), and fresh-frozen plasma (FFP). Occasionally, infusions of other blood components will be required such as platelets or cryoprecipitate, yet these instances are relatively rare. The goal of resuscitation is to maintain the patient at a level where they are able to perfuse vital organs while the bleeding source is addressed. The indicators of a successful resuscitation include the ability of the patient to mentate, to produce urine, and to maintain acid-base balance.

The preparation of these patients for possible therapeutic interventions includes the cleansing of the GI tract, the stabilization of the blood volume, the identification of the bleeding source, and the administration of blood components as needed to allow the proposed interventions.

SPECIFIC MEASURES FOR THE CONTROL OF ACUTE HEMORRHAGE

Protein/Gut Lavage

Hemorrhage into the GI tract poses a significant risk of developing encephalopathy, particularly in patients with bleeding varices. The combination of a large protein load in the intestinal tract along with poor hepatic function frequently results in encephalopathy. The intestinal tract must be cleansed of the blood and any other nitrogenous substances by a combination of enemas and oral cathartics.

Cleansing of the GI tract is important, since it will allow visualization of the bleeding source and reduce the subsequent morbidity of having an intestine full of blood. The upper GI tract should be lavaged with the aid of a large-bore tube (e.g., Ewald tube) in order to remove the clotted blood from the stomach. The rest of the GI tract is cleansed at the appropriate time by the administration of lactulose by mouth. The lactulose will frequently lead to rapid transiting of the intestinal content in addition to altering the intestinal pH so as to inhibit the absorption of ammonia. Finally, neomycin is administered along with the lactulose to reduce ammonia production by reducing the urease-producing bacteria inside the gut.

Neomycin and lactulose are given to alter the intestinal absorption of ammonia. Neomycin is a relatively nonabsorbable antibiotic that destroys urease-producing bacteria and thereby decreases ammonia production. Lactulose is converted by lactulase-containing intestinal bacteria into lactic acid and acetic acid, and thus decreases the intraluminal intestinal pH. The lower pH ionizes ammonia into ammonium (NH_4^+), which is less able to diffuse through the colonic mucosa. Lactulose will also promote diarrhea, cleansing the intestine of its contents.[17,41,42]

Vasopressin

Vasopressin has become the first-line therapy in the management of active bleeding varices. Its use is specifically directed at slowing and stopping the variceal hemorrhage. It has been recognized for its vasoconstrictive effects and its ability to decrease portal pressure since 1917.[43] Vasopressin is a naturally occurring nonapeptide that demonstrates a general vasoconstrictive effect with particular efficacy in the splanchnic bed. This splanchnic vasoconstriction leads

to decreasing portal flow. Vasopressin is also known to diminish cardiac output by an average of 14 per cent and heart rate by 11 per cent. This in turn reduces hepatic blood flow by approximately 44 per cent, and WHVP is decreased by 11 per cent. As much as a 23 per cent reduction in the gradient between the hepatic venous and WHVP has been documented.[44]

The first use of vasopressin (then called Pituitrin) in the control of variceal hemorrhage was reported by Kehne et al. in 1956.[45] Subsequently, considerable work has been done in determining the optimal dose and route of administration for this drug. The principal focus of this work has been on the relative merit of intravenous and intraarterial infusions.[46,47] The current opinion firmly supports intravenous infusions as being safer and as effective as the intraarterial vasopressin.[48]

A consequent side effect of the vasoconstrictive effects of vasopressin is the potential exacerbation of cardiac ischemia. In order to counter these ischemic effects, a number of pharmacologic agents have been used in conjunction with vasopressin.[44,49,50] These include isoproterenol and nitroglycerin. Isoproterenol, when administered with intravenous vasopressin, resulted in equivalent reduction of portal vein pressure but maintenance of cardiac output.[50] Sublingual nitroglycerin plus vasopressin has been shown to reduce the deleterious effects of vasopressin alone while preserving the decrease in portal vein pressure.[44,51] In the course of a controlled trial, Gimson and associates noted that nitroglycerin may reverse some of the cardiac suppressive effects of vasopressin as well as enhance the portal hypotensive effects.[52]

Use of Vasopressin

Vasopressin is effective in reducing and halting variceal hemorrhage in 80 per cent of cases. Intravenous vasopressin should be used prior to balloon tamponade. It will stop variceal bleeding in at least 80 per cent of cases. The initial dosage is 0.2 to 0.4 unit/min. If bleeding does not cease with the initial dose, the dosage may be increased up to 1.0 unit/min. The infusion should be continued over a 3-day period. After this period, the drug should be gradually discontinued.[49]

Somatostatin

Somatostatin is a tetradecapeptide derived from the hypothalamus that has demonstrated an ability to decrease splanchnic blood. The mechanism of this action is unclear. It has been demonstrated to be as effective as vasopressin for control of acute bleeding, yet with fewer complications.[53] Hemodynamic studies have indicated that somatostatin does decrease the portal venous pressure gradient.[42,54] While these studies indicate somatostatin to be a promising agent in controlling portal hypertension, it still remains to be demonstrated as the agent of choice—a role currently reserved for vasopressin.

Propranolol

Propranolol, a β-blocking drug, is an agent that has been found to be useful in chronically controlling portal hypertension and reducing the risk of recurrent bleeding from esophageal varices. Its action is thought to be mediated on the basis of reduced cardiac output, reduced systemic pressure and the subsequent reduction in portal venous pressure.

Evidence of its efficacy in the reduction of recurrent bleeding has been mixed. Burroughs and colleagues compared propranolol to placebo and found no significant difference in rebleeding or survival.[55] Fleig et al. randomized 70 patients to sclerotherapy or propranolol and found no difference in rebleeding rate or survival. The propranolol did decrease the size of the varices significantly after 3 months of treatment.[56] In a prospective controlled randomized study of 79 patients, Lebrec and associates noted that 2.6 per cent of patients maintained on propranolol had recurrent GI tract bleeding, compared to 66 per cent maintained on a placebo drug, after 3 months.[56-58] Similar findings have been reported by others.[59] Poynard et al. analyzed 127 patients treated with propranolol and found five factors that were associated with rebleeding: (1) hepatocellular carcinoma, (2) lack of persistent decrease in heart rate, (3) lack of abstinence from alcohol, (4) lack of compliance, and (5) prior history of rebleeding.[60]

Propranolol has been specifically used as maintenance therapy to decrease the risk of recurrent esophageal variceal bleeding in patients with portal hypertension. Its use in acute bleeding episodes has not been studied.

Balloon Tamponade

Balloon tamponade is the technique that employs compression to stem the bleeding of esophageal and gastroesophageal varices. The techniques date to the early 1950s; Linton, Nachlas, Sengstaken, and Blakemoore developed the tubes that came to bear their respective names.

All of these tubes work on the same principle: tamponade of varices. The design variations include the presence of one or two balloons for compression of the stomach alone or of the esophagus and stomach (Linton-Nachlas versus Sengstaken tubes), and the presence of adjunctive ports for aspiration of the stomach and the esophageal secretions (Sengstaken-Blakemore versus Edlich modification or Minnesota tubes).[61,62] The Sengstaken-Blakemore tube is probably more commonly used, since it is able to compress both esophageal and gastric varices, whereas the Linton-Nachlas tube is able to compress only the gastric varices.

Use of the Sengstaken-Blakemore Tube

These tubes may be passed through either the mouth or nose. Passage of these tubes must be performed in a careful, precise manner to prevent associated complications. The manufacturers recommend that the gastric balloon be inflated with a low volume of air (250 ml) and an abdominal x-ray then taken to ensure that the gastric balloon is in the stomach prior to full inflation (with 750 ml of air). This is intended to avoid the problem of fully inflating the gastric balloon in the esophagus, where it could tear open the esophageal wall.

Once the gastric balloon is inflated, it is taped to the face guard of a football helmet with approximately 1 kg of pressure. The gastric and esophageal ports are connected to intermittent low Gompco suction. The position of the gastric balloon is checked periodically to ensure that migration into the esophagus has not occurred. If bleeding does not cease with gastric balloon inflation and tension, the esophageal balloon is inflated to 24 to 45 mm Hg pressure. If bleeding ceases with the Sengstaken-Blakemore tube insertion, it is left inflated for 24 hours. After this period, the esophageal balloon should be deflated. Twenty-four hours later, the gastric balloon is deflated. If bleeding does not recur, the tube is deflated and left in place. It should be removed after an additional day.[63] Esophageal variceal tamponade will result in cessation of hemorrhage in 45 to 92 per cent of cases.[63-66] Bleeding recurs shortly after the Sengstaken-Blakemore tube is deflated in 24 to 42 per cent of cases, however, and cannot be controlled in 33 to 37 per cent of cases.[63,65] The incidence of recurrent bleeding after a second period of balloon control is 40 per cent.[65]

Complications

These tubes have been associated with significant complications: gastroesophageal tears, ulceration, and perforation. Pulmonary complications include aspiration pneumonia, and asphyxia from tracheal intubation. Conn and Simpson reported a complication rate of 41 per cent and mortality rate of 20 per cent.[67] The more commonly encountered incidence of major complications is in the range of 4 to 9 per cent.[63-65]

SURGICAL CORRECTION OF PORTAL HYPERTENSION

Shunt Nomenclature

The nomenclature of shunts has changed as different operations were devised at various periods. Many of these terms remain in use, and an understanding of these is necessary. Two basic sets of nomenclature prevail: the anatomic-based descriptive names, and the taxonomic names.

The anatomic naming of shunts is based on the participant elements of the shunt. Thus the principal shunts are portacaval, mesocaval, and splenorenal.

The first portion of the name denotes the donor vessel, and the second portion of the name denotes the recipient vessel. Because of some ambiguity associated with these names, modifiers are applied. A portacaval shunt may be either a side-to-side portacaval shunt or an end-to-side portacaval shunt. Similarly, a splenorenal shunt may be either a proximal or a distal splenorenal shunt. The principal advantage of this system is that it allows a clear descriptive means of labeling an operation. This is probably the most widely used shunt nomenclature.

The second set of shunt names are derived from physiologic and anatomic considerations. These names, which we refer to as a taxonomic nomenclature, are older and not as frequently employed. Nevertheless, they are traditional and should be understood. The two principal sets of names are central/remote, and selective/nonselective. A central shunt is one that is constructed in the region of the porta hepatis, or at the center of the portal confluence. Included amongst these are the various portacaval shunts. The term is used to distinguish those shunts that involve the portal vein itself from those shunts that are remote from the portal vein, such as the splenorenal and mesocaval shunts. The distinction has regained some usefulness in the context of distinguishing shunts that are recommended for patients who are considered potential liver transplant candidates.

Selective and nonselective shunts are the second set of taxonomic names. Selectivity of a shunt refers to the effect of the shunt on the portal venous blood flow. Essentially, selective shunts preserve, for a period of time, the flow of mesenteric blood through the portal vein to the liver. Nonselective shunts drain the portal blood flow into the vena cava. This has formed the cornerstone of the controversy concerning the superiority of one shunt over another. Selective shunts such as the distal splenorenal shunt are thought to preserve hepatic function to a greater extent than the nonselective shunts. The selective shunts include the distal splenorenal (Warren) shunt and the coronary-caval (Inokuchi) shunt. Nonselective shunts include end-to-side portacaval shunt, side-to-side portacaval shunt, mesocaval shunt, and proximal splenorenal shunt. Currently, the term "selective" is used almost as a synonym for a distal splenorenal shunt.

The last set of shunt names are the eponyms. Many shunts have been associated with the name of a proponent. These names are still frequently used. Included amongst these are the following: the Warren shunt (distal splenorenal), the Linton shunt (proximal splenorenal), the Clatworthy shunt (mesocaval shunt using the inferior vena cava), the Drapanas shunt (mesocaval shunt using a Dacron interposition graft), the Inokuchi shunt (coronary-caval), and the Sarfeh shunt (portacaval polytetrafluoroethylene [PTFE] interposition graft).

Development Of Shunting

Eck, in 1877, performed the first portal systemic shunt in a dog. He demonstrated that not only could the portal vein be anastomosed to the inferior vena cava, but that the animal could survive with total diversion of the portal vein blood flow.[68] Pavlov, in 1893, was the first to recognize the development of a severe neuropsychiatric disorder when a widely patent portacaval shunt was present, and that protein ingestion exacerbated the syndrome. Furthermore, he described the portaprival syndrome, consisting of gross liver atrophy with fatty infiltration following shunts.[69] It was not until 1945, however, that Whipple, as well as Blakemore and Lord, presented their results on the systematic application of portal systemic bypasses for complications of portal hypertension.[70,71] The end-to-side portacaval shunt was the first to be used clinically for the control of variceal hemorrhage, and the initial results with this procedure formed the basis for the enthusiasm for shunting patients with variceal bleeding.[18] With the initial reports demonstrating overall recurrence of variceal hemorrhage of only 2.8 per cent, little attention was directed toward the quality or length of life.[72]

Prophylactic Shunting

While it seemed apparent that portosystemic shunts would reduce the risk of bleeding from esophageal varices, the ultimate role of these shunts in patients who had not yet experienced a variceal hemorrhage was not clear. In the late 1950s attention was directed toward the question of whether a prophylactic portal systemic shunt improved the quality of life. Four prospective controlled studies addressed this question.[19,21,73,74]

These four early studies were similar in design. The patients were divided between medical or surgical treatment. They were then followed, with attention to the incidence of recurrent bleeding, development of encephalopathy, and survival.

The Boston Interhospital Liver Group (BILG) allocated 45 patients to the medical group and 48 to the surgical group. At 1-, 3-, and 5-year intervals, there was no difference in survival; at 5 years the survival rate was 50 per cent. Encephalopathy was likewise equal (21 per cent).[75]

The VA study demonstrated an incidence of encephalopathy of 45 per cent after shunting, almost twice that of medical therapies. Most disconcerting was that the 5-year survival after shunting (51 per cent) was less than for medical therapy (64 per cent).[19] The experience in the Yale group demonstrated again decreased survival after shunting, with an increased incidence of encephalopathy.[73,74]

The indications for prophylactic variceal decompression have been reviewed by the Cooperative Study Group of Portal Hypertension in Japan. By performing only nondecompressive transection procedures or selective shunts, this group found no difference in survival rates at 2 years, and suggested that in certain patients, prophylactic procedures may be indicated.[21] It should, however, be noted that these patients were primarily nonalcoholic, and the applicability of these results has been widely debated in the United States.

These studies have demonstrated that prophylactic shunts should not be undertaken: they do not benefit patients with asymptomatic varices. Although the incidence of variceal hemorrhage is virtually eliminated, these patients tend to suffer from hepatic encephalopathy and die of hepatic failure.

The studies of prophylactic shunt surgery indicate that encephalopathy is increased following portacaval shunting, and long-term survival may in fact be decreased by a shunt procedure. The results are not surprising, in that only 30 per cent of patients who have varices will bleed and that the decreased incidence of death from bleeding may be offset by the operative mortality of a shunt procedure, as well as by the effects of subsequent hepatic encephalopathy.

Therapeutic Shunting

Whereas the notion that portosystemic shunting would prove an effective therapeutic intervention for patients with variceal hemorrhage seems to be self-apparent, on a strictly scientific basis this idea had not been proven. Four prospective randomized clinical trials were performed in the United States and France in an effort to answer the fundamental question of whether therapeutic shunts prolong survival and maintain the quality of life, as compared to conventional medical therapy.[76–79]

The VA study, begun in 1961, followed the survival of 155 selected patients over a 5.5-year period. While 78 patients were randomized into the surgical group, only in 67 were shunts actually performed. Of the 77 patients randomized into the medical group, 26 required a shunt procedure at a later date because of recurrence of variceal bleeding. The majority of shunts performed were end-to-side portacaval. The operative mortality following therapeutic portacaval shunts was 8 per cent. The incidence of recurrence of variceal bleeding was 7 per cent in the surgical group and 65 per cent in the medical group. Encephalopathy occurred with approximately equal frequency in both groups, but was more severe in the shunted group. The long-term survival rate was 57 per cent at 5 years in the shunted group and 36 per cent in the medical group. The increase in long-term survival rates was not, however, statistically significant.[76]

The VA study was followed by the BILG study.[77] In this study, 25 patients underwent an end-to-side portacaval shunt and 21 underwent a side-to-side portacaval shunt; 25 were initially treated with medical therapy. Again, the long-term survival was greater in the shunted group than in the medically treated group, but as in the VA study, the difference was not statistically significant. Seventy per cent of patients in the medical group suffered recurrent hemorrhage, whereas only 9 per cent in the shunted group rebled. Encephalopathy occurred in 48 per cent of shunted patients and 52 per cent of those treated medically. Encephalopathy tended to be more severe in the shunted group.

On the basis of both the VA and BILG studies, Conn concluded that therapeutic portacaval shunts prolong the mean duration of life of cirrhotic patients who have suffered from variceal hemorrhage despite lack of statistical significance.[80]

The University of Southern California group published a 12-year follow-up of a prospective randomized study comparing end-to-side portacaval shunts to medical therapy. Fifty-five patients were randomized to surgery, although only 41 ultimately underwent a portacaval shunt procedure. Forty-four patients were randomized to medical therapy, although seven eventually required a portacaval shunt for unremitting variceal bleeding. Recurrent variceal bleeding was much less common in the shunt group. One hundred ninety episodes of bleeding occurred with medical therapy compared to 11 in the surgical group. Encephalopathy of a moderate to severe degree occurred in 35 per cent of shunted patients. A 5-year life-table analysis of survival revealed a 44 per cent shunt survival and 24 per cent medical therapy survival. This difference is not, however, statistically significant.[21]

Rueff and associates, in a study at the Hospital Beaujon, compared therapeutic end-to-side portacaval shunts to medical therapy.[79] Of the 40 patients assigned to the shunt group, 31 were shunted. Forty-nine were assigned to the medical therapy arm. The long-term survival was 47 per cent in the shunt group and 56 per cent in the medical group. The diminished long-term survival in the shunted group is unique to this study and may be due to their high operative mortality: 19 per cent, compared to 13 per cent for the BILG study and 8 per cent for the VA study. Encephalopathy was equally common in both medical and surgical groups, with an incidence of 40 per cent. As in the other studies, it tended to be more severe and chronic in the shunted groups. Recurrence of bleeding occurred in 8 per cent of the shunt group and in 72 per cent of the medical group.

A number of conclusions may be drawn from these studies. All studies failed to demonstrate a clear-cut survival advantage. Portacaval shunts were clearly superior in preventing recurrent variceal bleeding. Recurrent variceal bleeding occurred in about 9 per cent of shunted patients compared to 70 per cent of medically treated patients. Encephalopathy, the most significant factor involved in the analysis of quality of life, is no more common in patients undergoing a portacaval shunt, but tends to be more severe and chronic. Long-term survival is improved with portacaval shunts, although not to a statistically significant degree.

Several factors limit the significance of these results. First, the portacaval shunt was the only type of shunt used; selective shunts, such as the Warren shunt, have not been compared to a medical regimen. Second, alcoholic cirrhosis was the most common cause of portal hypertension in all of these studies. Because of the tendency of these patients to continue drinking, portal hypertension in these patients may be more severe and lethal. Thus, the results may not apply to a wider population of patients with portal hypertension of other causes. This notion is disputed by other investigators who have suggested that regardless of the cause of cirrhosis, therapeutic portacaval shunts do not improve survival.[81] Third, all four of these studies allowed crossover of the medically treated patients into the surgical treatment arm. They were analyzed on an intent-to-treat basis, therefore favoring the medical arm by virtue of the analytic method. Fourth, the studies were carried out at a time when few patients underwent diagnostic endoscopy. Thus, endoscopic confirmation of bleeding was not universally available. Some patients may have been included as variceal bleeders, whereas in fact they were bleeding from another source. Finally, all patients in these studies were relatively good surgical candidates, the equivalents of Child's class A or B, as evidenced by the excellent 1-year survival of 70 to 80 per cent. Further study is necessary to more completely evaluate the efficacy of shunt procedures.

Emergency Portacaval Shunting

The emergency portacaval shunt is no longer widely used because of the reported high mortality, despite its ability to stop bleeding and prevent further recurrent bleeding.[82] Orloff et al. have continued to advocate the portacaval shunt in the acute setting, and have a 4-year actuarial survival of 69 per cent.[83] Villeneuve and others have also supported the use of this shunt in acutely bleeding patients, if the patients have mild to moderate liver disease and other forms of treatment have failed.[84] In general, emergency surgical intervention is being performed less frequently, as nonsurgical options have become more effective.

Most Common Portasystemic Shunts

Nonselective Shunts: Portacaval Shunts

Both end-to-side and side-to-side portacaval shunts are nonselective and cause diversion of portal flow into the systemic circulation. The only specific indication for portacaval shunts is esophageal variceal hemorrhage. Whereas previously intractable ascites was often treated with a side-to-side portacaval shunt, this technique has now been discarded in favor of peritoneovenous shunting.[85,86]

The question of whether an end-to-side or side-to-side portacaval shunt is a more effective procedure is still debatable. Each has its specific advantages and contraindications. An end-to-side portacaval shunt is certainly not indicated in the presence of the Budd-Chiari syndrome, because the portal vein serves as a decompressive outflow tract for intrahepatic portal blood. Uncontrolled studies comparing end-to-side to side-to-side shunts indicate that the side-to-side shunt is associated with a lower surgical mortality in patients with poor hepatic functions.[87] Others find the side-to-side portacaval shunt to be more technically demanding, however, than the end-to-side portacaval shunt. Encephalopathy has been shown to be somewhat more common in side-to-side than in end-to-side portacaval shunts.[88] Investigators have previously found that in addition to the side-to-side shunt allowing total diversion of portal venous flow, a siphon effect may also exist, permitting egress of hepatic arterial blood through the portal vein rather than the hepatic vein. This may be an explanation for the increased incidence of encephalopathy with side-to-side portacaval shunts.

There are certain technical considerations that preclude a portacaval shunt. First, the portal vein must be patent and free of thrombus. The portal vein diameter should also be at least 1 to 1.5 cm (in adults) and should not have previously undergone thrombosis with recanalization. Thrombectomy of a recanalized portal vein is contraindicated, since it does not result in long-term shunt patency. Previous surgery in the right upper quadrant is a relative contraindication to a portacaval shunt procedure because of the numerous well-vascularized adhesions, which always result in excessive bleeding.

Technique: End-to-Side Portacaval Shunt

Two approaches have been described: the midline incision, and the right subcostal incision. A long right subcostal incision is generally used, although if there is a question as to the patency of the portal vein, a midline incision may be preferable. The major objective is to expose only those structures necessary for the anastomosis. After the abdomen has been entered and explored, the duodenum is mobilized medially to expose the inferior vena cava. The dissection is carried up along the inferior vena cava to the level of the first hepatic vein under the liver. The exposure includes the entire anterior surface of the vena cava. The objective at this point is to expose a very limited portion of the portal vein. The portal vein should then be exposed by carefully rotating the bile duct and hepatic artery using a vein retractor or peanut sponges. The portal vein is then encircled with a vascular tape and dissection is performed up to the bifurcation of the right and left hepatic branches. The division of the portal vein should be done after it has been securely clamped (proximally and distally) and the hepatic portion of the vein suture ligated. Once the portal vein is divided, it can be gently mobilized with traction to expose any medial branches that will preclude an optimal lie to the portal vein.

A Satinsky clamp is placed at the appropriate point

on the vena cava, and an ellipse of cava is removed to allow for an unimpeded anastomosis. Prior to completing the anastomosis, the portal vein should be allowed to bleed in order to evacuate any portal thrombi that may have formed. The vena cava clamp is removed first, followed by the portal clamp. Pressure in the portal vein should be measured in order to document the adequacy of the decompression and detect any unobserved technical problems. A 50 per cent reduction in portal venous pressures should be expected after the shunt is completed.[89,90]

Arterialization of End-to-Side Portacaval Shunts

In an attempt to reduce the morbidity of end-to-side portacaval shunts, a variety of measures have been employed in the effort to maintain portal perfusion of the liver. Portal vein arterialization refers to the anastomosis of an arterialized conduit to the hepatic end of the portal vein. Various arteries have been used for this purpose including the right gastroepiploic artery, splenic artery, and saphenous vein grafts from the hypogastric artery or aorta.

While a number of studies have indicated that there is no increase in morbidity or mortality, and encephalopathy may be reduced, the procedure has not been universally adopted. Maillard's group divided the splenic artery close to the spleen and anastomosed it to the hepatic stump of the portal vein. They found that total hepatic blood flow with arterialization is equal to or slightly greater than that prior to the shunt. Immediate postoperative complications were fewer, and the incidence of encephalopathy was less than with the portacaval shunt alone as well. As this group points out, however, the fistula is not likely to remain open after 1 year.[91] Otte and associates have reported a retrospective study in which the 5-year survival was 48 per cent in arterialized patients compared to 44 per cent in other series. Encephalopathy occurred in 27 per cent of the arterialized patients compared to 40 per cent without.[92] No definitive conclusions may be drawn as to the benefit of arterialization of a portacaval shunt in prolonging life or decreasing encephalopathy. Because of the added time and technical difficulty in performing arterialization, it is unlikely that this technique will gain widespread use.

Technique: Side-to-Side Portacaval Shunt

The side-to-side portacaval shunt is technically more difficult than the end-to-side shunt. It requires more extensive mobilization of both the portal vein and inferior vena cava in order to allow approximation of these vessels. While the initial approach is similar to the end-to-side shunt, a longer segment of the vena cava is exposed and circumferentially dissected so as to lift it out of its bed. The portal vein must also be exposed for a greater length, since a 4-cm segment is necessary for the anastomosis. Portal pressures are measured prior to performing the shunt. After applying the vascular clamps, an elliptical segment measuring approximately 2 cm is then excised from the inferior vena cava and portal vein directly opposite each other. Again, prior to completing the anastomosis, the portal vein is vented to allow any thrombus to be flushed out. Mesenteric pressure measurements should reflect a 50 per cent reduction in portal vein pressure.[89]

Portacaval H graft

An alternative to the side-to-side portacaval shunt is the portacaval H graft. Technically easier than the side-to-side, the large-diameter H grafts (16 to 20 mm) effectively prevent variceal rebleeding, but encephalopathy occurs frequently. Building on this experience, Sarfeh et al. systematically reduced portacaval H graft diameters, and found that an 8-mm PTFE graft combined with portal collateral ablation effectively prevented rebleeding, maintained hepatic perfusion, and reduced encephalopathy. The 5-year cumulative late patency rate was 97 per cent.[93]

Nonselective Shunts: Mesocaval Shunts

In 1955, Clatworthy devised a new portasystemic shunt procedure involving division of the inferior vena cava above its bifurcation and anastomosis of the proximal cava to the side of the superior mesenteric vein.

It has been particularly successful in children with extrahepatic portal vein thrombosis. In adults, massive lower extremity edema has limited its usefulness. Because of the extensive dissection necessary to expose the vena cava, a number of alternative graft materials have been utilized, including cadaveric inferior vena cava, iliac vein, PTFE, and Dacron, which is currently in favor.[94–99]

There has been considerable debate as to whether portal perfusion (hepatopetal flow) is maintained by mesocaval shunts. Drapanas and colleagues documented continued hepatopetal flow in 44 per cent of their patients.[100] Others have noted, however, that portal perfusion can persist only if there is partial or total H graft occlusion.[101] Misinterpretation of angiographic studies may also be attributable to the phenomenon of portal pseudoperfusion as explained by Fulenwider.[102] Currently, H graft mesocaval shunts are considered nonselective shunts.

Clinical Role of Mesocaval Shunts

The primary use of the interposition H graft mesocaval shunt has been for the urgent control of massive variceal hemorrhage. This graft is technically easier to perform than a portacaval or a selective shunt and is frequently indicated in the emergency management of variceal hemorrhage.[103] In the case of previous surgery in the right upper quadrant, a portacaval shunt of any type is especially challenging and is usually contraindicated. If a selective shunt is contraindicated, a mesocaval shunt may be a good alternative. This is true in patients with significant ascites. Other factors that favor mesocaval shunting include extensive periportal fibrosis, a large overriding caudate lobe, an obliterated portal vein, extreme obesity, and Budd-Chiari syndrome.[104]

Technique: Interposition Mesocaval H Graft

The operation as described by Drapanas et al. is essentially unchanged.[100] The abdomen is explored through a midline incision. The transverse mesocolon is elevated superiorly and the small intestine retracted inferiorly. At the root of the small intestine mesentery the peritoneum is opened transversely to expose the superior mesenteric vessels. Anatomically, the superior mesenteric vein lies anterior and to the right of the superior mesenteric artery. During isolation of the vein, only one or two small tributaries need to be divided. An important goal is to preserve as many branches of the superior mesenteric vein to preserve intestinal venous flow. After the superior mesenteric vein is isolated, the anterior surface of the vena cava is exposed through the right transverse mesocolon. This direct route to the vena cava is quicker and incurs less blood loss than exposure by mobilizing the right colon. Only sufficient dissection to permit use of a Satinsky clamp on the vena cava is required. Once the vena cava is partially isolated, the third and fourth portions of the duodenum must usually be mobilized to allow the duodenum to ride above the graft. Failure to do this may cause obstruction of the occasional low-lying duodenum or occlusion of the interposed graft.

The vena cava anastomosis is performed first because it lies in the depth of the field and is potentially more hazardous. A partially occluding vascular clamp is placed on the inferior vena cava, a small ellipse of vein is excised, and a 14- to 18-mm knitted Dacron graft is anastomosed. Construction of the superior mesenteric vein anastomosis is particularly demanding. The superior mesenteric vein lies anteriorly and courses at a 20- to 30-degree angle counterclockwise to the vena cava. Because of this angulation, it is advisable to rotate the graft 20 to 30 degrees clockwise before constructing the superior mesenteric vein anastomosis. The graft length should be only 3 to 6 cm, in order to minimize kinking of the prosthesis. Anastomosis is performed in the posterior surface of the vein with a continuous suture of 5-0 Prolene. With the clamps removed, the graft should balloon out quickly. In most instances, a palpable thrill should be present. Postshunt pressures are then measured in the superior mesenteric vein; if the shunt is functioning properly, there should be at least a 50 per cent reduction of pressure with the shunt open.

A notable variation on this shunt is the "C" loop graft as reported by Cameron and coworkers.[105,106] In their procedure, a longer graft was used, and this had the configuration of a "C." To accomplish this, the superior mesenteric vein anastomosis is placed at the point where the superior mesenteric vein disappears under the neck of the pancreas. The proposed advantage of this variation is that the superior mesenteric vein diameter is greater at a more proximal anastomosis, and this allows for improved shunt flow. The obvious drawback is a longer length of prosthetic material. Despite this theoretical advantage, there is the distinct disadvantage of a more difficult dissection, particularly in patients who have had pancreatitis.

Clinical Results. Sarr et al. published a series of 33 patients who had received the mesocaval C shunt. There was a 24 per cent operative mortality (all Child's class C nonelective cases), 8 per cent rebleed rate, and 46 per cent incidence of encephalopathy. However, there were no graft thromboses.

The average incidence of encephalopathy following a mesocaval graft is about 25 per cent.[103,107] The reported incidence of encephalopathy ranges from 9 to 45 per cent (Table 40–3).[101,105] Late graft occlusion is caused by excessive layering of thrombus, possibly aggravated by perigraft scarring, leading to kinking and constriction.[101] The incidence of shunt occlusions ranges from 4 to 24 per cent.[100,101,106,108–110] Rebleeding occurs in approximately 14 per cent of mesocaval shunts (range: 12 to 16 per cent). A third of these may be related to occlusion of the graft.[103] Overall, the mortality is approximately 15 per cent. The cumulative long-term mortality rate ranges from 28 to 57 per cent. The long-term mortality is probably dependent on the state of liver function rather than the type of shunt.

Mortality related to H mesocaval shunts is not significantly different from that for other types of shunts and is dependent on the Child's classification of the patient. Initial hospital mortality is related to the urgency of surgery, significant elevation of SGOT or bilirubin, or the presence of encephalopathy.[101]

Nonselective Shunts: Proximal Splenorenal Shunts

The nonselective splenorenal shunt, or Linton shunt, was first developed by Blakemore and Lord in 1945, utilizing a vitallium tube.[71] Linton et al. advocated this shunt in years to follow and considered it the operative procedure of choice for correction of portal hypertension.[111] Early reports of noncontrolled studies suggested a decreased incidence of encephalopathy with this shunt compared to the portacaval shunt.[112] This finding, however, has not been substantiated. Other investigators have failed to demonstrate significant differences between central splenorenal and portacaval shunts in regard to encephalopathy or long-term survival. In fact, some reports have noted an increased incidence of thrombosis associated with the central splenorenal shunt.[1,113] The group at Massachusetts General Hospital reported a 10 per cent incidence of recurrent variceal hemorrhage, 19 per cent hepatic encephalopathy, and 18 per cent terminal hepatic failure. Overall operative mortality was 12 per cent.[114] Unlike the distal splenorenal shunt, the central splenorenal shunt functions hemodynamically as a side-to-side portal systemic shunt. Hepatic blood flow as well as portal vein pressures are markedly diminished and angiography does not demonstrate persistent hepatopetal

TABLE 40–3.   INTERPOSITION SHUNT SERIES

Study	Number of Patients	Operative Mortality	Hepatic Encephalopathy	Shunt Occlusion	Overall Mortality
Cameron et al.[105]	44	23%	9%	9%	57%
Reichle et al.[108]	28	18%	—	7%	36%
Thompson et al.[109]	54	11%	10%	7%	36%
Drapanas et al.[100]	80	9%	11%	4%	28%
Busuttil et al.[121]					
(collected review)	409	12%	25%	10%	—
Smith et al.[101]	79	13%	45%	24%	48%

flow in the presence of a patent shunt.[111] Thus, it is generally accepted that a central splenorenal shunt has no distinct advantage over portacaval or mesocaval shunts, except possibly in the instance of severely symptomatic hypersplenism. In this latter instance, the central splenorenal shunt may be combined with splenectomy.

Selective Shunts: Splenorenal Shunts

A significant concern noted with the portacaval shunts is that no study has shown a statistical prolongation of survival. This is thought to occur, in part, because of the progressive hepatic failure that followed portal systemic shunting. The mesocaval, central splenorenal, and portacaval shunts all divert the flow of portal blood away from the liver, regardless of the size or location of the shunt. The total diversion of portal blood away from the liver prevents its perfusion with hepatotrophic substances that may be necessary for its continued function. The detrimental effect of acute loss of portal blood flow to the liver is reflected in increased hepatocellular damage and leads to an increased incidence of postshunt encephalopathy. In an attempt to avoid the complications of total diversion of portal flow, the distal splenorenal (DSRS), or Warren shunt, was developed in the late 1960s.[69,115]

This operation is based on the principle of compartmentalization as discussed by Malt: the portal azygous system and the portal splanchnic system may be surgically separated into parallel and independent hemodynamic units. Decompression of the portal azygous system may thus be accomplished without reducing the portal splanchnic system perfusion pressure or blood flow.[1,104] Hence, one should be able to decompress esophageal varices and prevent hemorrhage without diverting the hepatopetal flow of the portal splanchnic blood. In principle, this is accomplished in two steps. First, by disrupting the coronary vein and right gastroepiploic vein, blood flow into the esophageal variceal system is reduced. Second, by anastomosing the distal splenic to the left renal vein without performing a splenectomy, blood is able to freely drain from the esophageal varices through the short gastrics into the lower pressure systemic circulation (Fig. 40–5).

The promised benefits of the Warren shunt include preservation of hepatic perfusion and function with consequent prolongation of survival and lower risk of disabling encephalopathy, which may accompany the nonselective shunts. The search for evidence of this promise has led to the creation of several randomized trials. Five trials pitted the Warren shunt against portacaval shunts. Three trials have compared the Warren shunt to best nonsurgical management and sclerotherapy.

DSRS Compared to Other Shunts.   Three prospective randomized clinical trials comparing the efficacy of the selective shunt (DSRS) to the end-to-side portacaval shunt have been published: in Toronto, in the Boston–New Haven trial, and at USC.[116–118] Similarly, the DSRS has been compared to mesentericsystemic shunts in two randomized trials: in Atlanta, and in Philadelphia.[108,119,120]

The DSRS has been compared to the end-to-side portacaval shunt in three randomized studies: by Langer in Toronto, Resnick in the Boston–New Haven trial, and Harley at USC[116–118] (Fig. 40–6). Langer's group in Toronto reported an incidence of postshunt encephalopathy of only 14 per cent in the selectively shunted patients, but 50 per cent in the end-to-side portacaval group. There was no difference in the long-term survival.[116] Preliminary data from Resnick and the Boston–New Haven group do not indicate any substantial difference between the two operations with regard to either encephalopathy or long-term survival. It should be noted, however, that their follow-up period is relatively short.[118] Harley and associates at the USC Medical Center randomized 54 patients between the two shunts and failed to demonstrate any superiority of one shunt over the other with respect to encephalopathy or survival. They did experience an unusually high rate of rebleed with the DSRS (27 per cent).[117]

The Atlanta study compared the DSRS to nonselective shunts, most commonly interposition mesorenal shunts.[119,120] The operative mortality was similar for the two groups: 12 per cent for distal splenorenal, and 10 per cent for nonselective shunts. Early postoperative angiography demonstrated persistent hepatopetal flow in 88 per cent of the distal splenorenal shunt patients, but in only 5 per cent of the nonselective shunt patients. Corresponding to this were quantitative measurements of hepatic function, maximal rate of urea synthesis, and Child's score, which were similar to the preoperative values in the

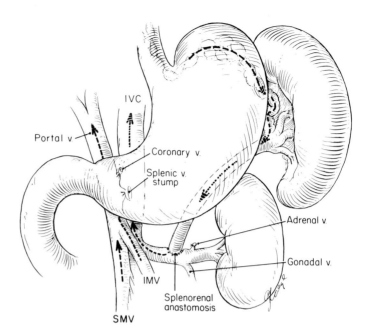

FIGURE 40–5. Diagrammatic illustration of the selective distal splenorenal shunt. *IVC,* inferior vena cava; *IMV,* inferior mesenteric vein; *SMV,* superior mesenteric vein.

distal splenorenal group but greatly decreased in the nonselective group. The incidence of encephalopathy correlated with preservation of hepatopetal blood flow. Patients with hepatopetal flow suffered no encephalopathy and patients with hepatofugal flow experienced a 45 per cent incidence of encephalopathy. Overall, encephalopathy occurred in 27 per cent in the DSRS group and 52 per cent in the nonselective group ($p < .001$). Recurrent variceal hemorrhage occurred in 4 per cent of selective and 8 per cent of nonselective shunts. While survival was similar for the two groups, it appears that the quality of survival was improved in the DSRS group.

These results have been reproduced by others in Philadelphia and Toronto.[108,116] The Philadelphia study compared the DSRS to the H mesocaval shunt. Again, for elective shunts, the operative mortality was similar, 7 per cent. Encephalopathy was significantly much less common with distal splenorenal shunts, consistent with continued hepatopetal flow in 86 per cent of selective but no nonselective shunts. Hemorrhage did not recur in either group undergoing elective surgery. The long-term survival rate of 62 per cent was comparable to that in the Atlanta study.[108] Rebleeding in emergency cases was 2 per cent.

Nonrandomized Studies. Two nonrandomized comparative studies have also indicated excellent results with the DSRS.[81,121–123] In a matched controlled study comparing the DSRS to the portacaval shunt, Busuttil and associates demonstrated an incidence of significant encephalopathy of 85 per cent in the portacaval group and only 7.6 per cent in the DSRS group. Furthermore, this group demonstrated a statistically significant increase in the number of late deaths. There were no recurrent variceal hemorrhages in either group.[121]

Zeppa's group demonstrated that the 5-year survival of patients with nonalcoholic cirrhosis after distal splenorenal shunting was 89 per cent compared to 39 per cent in the alcoholic cirrhotic group.[81] It should be noted that improved survival in nonalcoholic cirrhotics was also suggested by Warren, but other investigators have contended this point.[19,120] In addition, a number of other unmatched studies have demonstrated excellent results from the DSRS.[124–132] A combined review of the literature comparing H mesocaval grafts to distal splenorenal shunts unequivocally demonstrated the DSRS to be superior in decreasing incidence of both encephalopathy and recurrent hemorrhage.[103]

FIGURE 40–6. Combined experience of the distal splenorenal shunt versus the portacaval shunt (data from randomized trials by Rikkers, Langer, and Reichle, Boston-New Haven). *PCS,* portacaval shunt; *DSRS,* distal splenorenal shunt; *PSE,* portasystemic encephalopathy.

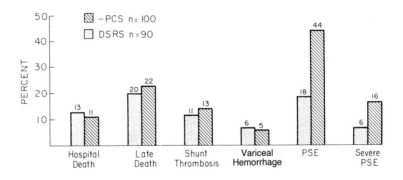

DSRS and Sclerotherapy. Warren and colleagues presented the results of their randomized study of esophageal variceal bleeders who were randomized between DSRS and sclerotherapy (with salvage DSRS) (Table 40–7). A total of 71 patients were entered over a 4-year period. There was a significant difference between the two groups with regard to the preservation of portal perfusion, the maintenance of hepatic function, the rate of rebleeding, and the patients' survival. While the sclerotherapy patients had a significantly higher rate of rebleeding (53 versus 3 per cent), only one of these patients died of uncontrollable hemorrhage. The 2-year survival of the group treated with sclerotherapy (and salvage surgery) was 84 per cent (versus 59 per cent for those undergoing surgery alone). The study clearly demonstrated that the optimal management of these patients involved the use of sclerotherapy as the initial means of controlling their bleeding. Surgery appears to work best when used to manage those patients who are not controllable with sclerotherapy. This study is important because it set the basis for the current method of managing portal hypertensive patients with esophageal variceal hemorrhage.

Splenopancreatic Disconnection. Because of the results of trials which indicated that with the passage of time the DSRS gradually became a nonselective shunt, Warren modified the operation. In 1986, he proposed that the DSRS should include complete dissection of the splenic vein and division of the splenocolic ligament (splenopancreatic disconnection). In theory, this should reduce the pancreatic sump or siphon effect: the tendency of pancreatic branches of the splenic vein to progressively enlarge and serve as an outflow collateral for the portal mesenteric circulatory system. This modification is intended to prolong and preserve the selective quality of the DSRS. Clinically, Warren's group found that this modification did preserve postoperative portal perfusion in alcoholic cirrhotics better than distal splenorenal shunt alone. It also considerably extended the magnitude of the operation.[128]

Indications for DSRS. The principal indication for a DSRS, much like any portal systemic shunt, is to prevent recurrent variceal hemorrhage that is not controllable with sclerotherapy. The specific strengths of the DSRS include its lower incidence of encephalopathy and its anatomical remoteness from the porta hepatis. For these reasons it is considered the shunt of choice in elective patients who require shunting and who do not present a specific contraindication to the DSRS. The most important specific contraindication to DSRS is the presence of significant ascites. In practice, this means ascites that is difficult to control by the administration of diuretics. Additionally, patients should have an adequate sized splenic vein that is patent. Some authors consider the presence of hepatofugal portal blood flow to be a contraindication to the DSRS. This is principally based on the notion that the benefit of preserving portal perfusion is not possible in such situations. Others debate this

point, since the primary goal of any shunt is to decompress the esophageal and gastric varices, and this goal is achieved by the DSRS despite hepatofugal flow. Similarly, in instances of portal hypertension due to extrahepatic portal vein thrombosis, the DSRS has been demonstrated to be effective in preventing recurrent hemorrhage.[133] Finally, while the distal splenorenal shunt has been performed as an emergency procedure, it is not widely considered the shunt of choice in these circumstances because of the relative difficulty of the operation. It should further be noted that numerous studies have demonstrated the advantages of optimizing the patient's general condition prior to surgical intervention if at all possible.

Technique: DSRS

The technique used for the DSRS is essentially the method described by Warren and Millikan.[134] The first goal of this operation is to anastomose the distal splenic vein to the left renal vein. The second goal is to disconnect the portoazygous system from the splanchnic venous system. A bilateral subcostal incision provides optimal exposure. Dividing the umbilical vein and the falciform ligament is an initial maneuver. The splenic vein may be approached either through the lesser sac, or from below the transverse mesocolon. Most surgeons use the lesser sac approach. As part of this approach, the right gastroepiploic vein is divided, but the short gastric veins are carefully preserved. The pancreas is identified, and the peritoneum covering its inferior border is incised. Careful blunt dissection of the retroperitoneal tissue allows the pancreas to be rotated anteriorly and exposes the splenic vein. The splenic vein dissection is the most delicate portion of this operation. It should be carried out to the point of confluence with the superior mesenteric vein. The left renal vein is located by incising the posterior parietal peritoneum in the lesser sac just superior to the fourth position of the duodenum. Often, the ligament of Treitz must be incised and the duodenum reflected inferiorly to locate the vein. Dividing the adrenal vein may allow better mobilization of the renal vein. To prepare the anastomosis, the splenic vein is occluded with vascular clamps and transected close to its junction with the superior mesenteric vein. The stump is ligated with a suture ligature to decrease the incidence of portal vein thrombosis secondary to traumatic manipulation of the splenic vein stump.[95,121] A partial occluding clamp is placed on the left renal vein, and the anastomosis is performed.

After completing the devascularization and the splenorenal anastomosis, measurements may be made of the superior mesenteric, renal, and splenic veins. Superior mesenteric (portal) pressures should not be altered if a total portoazygous disconnection has been performed. Splenic vein pressure will be decreased by 60 to 70 per cent. If this pressure fails to fall, then intraoperative angiography should be employed to demonstrate a technically sound anastomosis.[33]

Graft Interposition. In instances in which complete mobilization of the splenic vein cannot be accomplished because of pancreatic encasement or fibrosis, shunting may be accomplished by the interposition of a 14- to 16-mm Dacron graft between the side of the splenic vein and the side of the renal vein. Following this anastomosis, the portal end of the splenic vein must be ligated if the selective nature of the shunt is to be maintained.

Portoazygous Disconnection. Once the anastomosis is completed and the clamps are removed, attention is focused on completing the portoazygous disconnection. This requires interrupting all collaterals between the portomesenteric and portoazygous systems. Dividing the umbilical vein and the falciform ligament completes the first step of the portoazygous disconnection. Division of the right gastroepiploic vein constitutes the second portion of the portoazygous disconnection. Finally, division of the coronary vein completes the portoazygous disconnection.

Results: DSRS—Patency and Portal Perfusion

The maintenance of portal perfusion in the early postoperative period has been documented in greater than 90 per cent of patients.[103,108,119,132] The principal question regarding this operation, however, is one of durability: How long does the benefit of the Warren shunt last? It has been shown that the incidence of early partial portal vein thrombosis may be as high as 22 per cent, and that the incidence of complete portal vein occlusion is 6 per cent. When followed over a 6-month period, most nonocclusive portal vein thromboses resolve spontaneously.[135] A 10-year follow-up by Warren of his DSRS group revealed that 75 per cent have persistent portal perfusion at 10 years. Patients who were demonstrated to have portal perfusion at 3 years maintained this until the conclusion of the study at 7 years.[69,120,126]

The DSRS has several advantages over other nonselective shunts: it preserves portal flow to the liver; it maintains hepatotrophic perfusion; it permits the metabolism of toxic metabolites; and it maintains a high portal perfusion pressure in the intestinal venous bed, decreasing the absorption of toxic substances.[69] It is the best procedure to perform in a patient with hepatopetal flow under elective conditions. Child's classes A and B patients under emergent conditions will also benefit from selective shunts. It should be noted that the DSRS has not been clearly demonstrated to improve survival by itself, but when used in conjunction with judicious sclerotherapy, appears to provide the best survival to these patients.

NONSHUNT SURGICAL PROCEDURES

Emergency portal systemic shunting will result in an operative mortality of approximately 47 per cent.[15] Furthermore, in the presence of certain clinical laboratory tests, including an SGOT greater than 300, as well as the presence of ascites or other determi-

nants of a Child's C-minus classification (i.e., a bilirubin greater than 6, hyaline necrosis, and severe muscle wasting), a portal systemic shunt is almost sure to result in death. Because of this, numerous nonshunting surgical procedures have been developed.

Splenectomy

Based on Banti's theory that the diseased spleen caused portal hypertension and ascites, splenectomy was one of the first operations proposed for the treatment of Banti's syndrome (splenomegaly, hypersplenism, ascites, often accompanied by esophageal varices).

The use of splenectomy in this setting was in great part due to its advocacy by Osler, a great admirer of Banti's work. It was not until 1936, when Rouselot reviewed the experience at Columbia University in New York, that the failings of this operation were noted: a significant incidence of recurrent hemorrhage following splenectomy and the consequent loss of the splenic and portal veins that would preclude possible shunt surgery.[136] In 1940, Thompson was able to demonstrate statistically that splenectomy was of value only to those patients with isolated splenic vein thrombosis.[137] Finally, in 1945, Pemberton and Kieman reported a 54 per cent incidence of recurrent variceal hemorrhage with splenectomy alone.[138]

Collateralization

Development of collateral pathways between the portal circulation and the systemic circulation was the goal of several procedures. Omentopexy, introduced by Talma in 1898, produces collateral pathways by suturing the omentum to the peritoneum.[139] It was thought to be particularly beneficial in the resolution of ascites. It was sometimes used in conjunction with splenectomy for the relief of ascites associated with splenomegaly and decreased WBC counts.

Another collateral-promoting operation was the transposition of the spleen into the thorax.[140,141] Like omentopexy, its goal was to allow the development of large venous collateral pathways between the portal venous system and the systemic venous circulation. Unfortunately, these collateral pathways were never able to adequately decompress esophageal varices. Thus the patients were doomed to repeated hemorrhage.

Ablation

Ablative procedures to remove the source of bleeding were first advocated by Phemister in 1944, who recommended total gastrectomy.[20] Peters and Womack later encouraged splenectomy with obliteration of both the intraluminal and extraluminal vasculature of the distal variceal-bearing esophagus and proximal stomach.[142] Keagy et al. reviewed the long-term results of the "Womack" procedure and found the risk to be prohibitively high, with a 54 per cent incidence of rebleed and a 35 per cent operative mortality. They concluded that this procedure should be used only in highly selected patients who do not have suitable anatomy for a shunt.[143]

A variation of the Womack procedure was the transthoracic ligation of the esophageal varices without the splenectomy. This operation was introduced in 1949 by Boerema[144] and in 1950 by Crile.[145] Wirthlin and his associates reported on 55 patients who underwent transesophageal ligation of varices, with a 29 per cent operative mortality and a 33 per cent incidence of recurrent hemorrhage resulting in an additional 23 per cent mortality.[146]

Despite these results, the procedure was not abandoned. Technological innovation in the form of the EEA stapler allowed transection and reanastomosis of the distal esophagus with greater facility. The innovation resulted in reduced operative mortality and improved reduction of postoperative hemorrhage. Wexler reported that of six Child's class C patients undergoing this procedure, none had recurrent bleeding.[147] Cooperman and his associates reported five patients with severe hepatic dysfunction and massive variceal bleeding who underwent transabdominal EEA variceal stapling, none of whom developed recurrent bleeding up to 2 years postoperatively.[148]

In a logical extension of these devascularization procedures, other surgeons proposed more extensive operations. Delaney promulgated a devascularization procedure performed through a left thoracotomy, which involves devascularization of the upper half of the stomach and proximally to the level of the left inferior pulmonary vein as well as splenectomy, staple interruption of intramural gastroesophageal collateral vessels, truncal vagotomy with pyloroplasty, and fundoplication. The major disadvantage of this procedure is that the splenectomy will preclude performance of selective shunts at a later time. Delaney reported, however, that none of his four patients had recurrent variceal bleeding.[149]

Perhaps the most successful devascularization procedure was developed by Suguira et al. in Japan.[139,150,151] Because of the significant risk of encephalopathy, shunt procedures were abandoned in favor of an extensive periesophagogastric devascularization accompanied by esophageal transection. The procedure is performed via separate thoracic and abdominal incisions; in poor-risk patients, a two-stage procedure is indicated. The esophagus is devascularized from the gastroesophageal junction to the left inferior pulmonary vein. The vagus nerve is carefully preserved. At the level of the diaphragm, the esophagus is partially transected, leaving only the posterior muscular layer intact. Esophageal varices are occluded, not ligated, by oversewing each with interrupted sutures. The esophageal muscle is closed, but the mucosa is not sutured. The abdominal operation is performed through a separate midline incision and includes splenectomy, devascularization of the abdominal esophagus and proximal stomach, and a pyloroplasty and fundoplication.

The early results of this operation as reported by Suguira and colleagues are excellent. His group has reported an overall operative mortality of 4.6 per cent. Their emergency operative mortality is 20 per cent. Varices were eradicated in 97 per cent of patients, and recurrent bleeding occurred in only 2.5 per cent. Their long-term survival was 84 per cent.[139] A follow-up report by this group on 276 patients indicated equally good survival rates, with excellent control of variceal bleeding and no encephalopathy.[150] In a later report they analyzed their results according to the patients' Child's classification. They found that in class C patients, both operative mortality and long-term survival were discouraging. For the class A and B patients, the results were very good, with combined (A, B, and C) 15-year survivals as high as 72 per cent.[152]

Reports by Suguira's group have been confirmed by others in Japan as well as by selected investigators in this country.[153,154] A number of recent reports have suggested esophageal transection procedures in the management of selected patients with poor hepatic reserves (the Child's class C patient). The EEA stapler has made this a relatively simple procedure, but the possibility of esophageal perforation and leakage still make the procedure one of considerable risk.[155] Overall, these studies demonstrate that esophageal transection should be considered a reasonable option in the management of acute hemorrhage in the debilitated patient with both gastric and esophageal varices.[156–158]

POSTOPERATIVE CARE

The most common problem in the postoperative period is the development of significant ascites. Fluid management is the key to minimizing this problem. Postoperative fluids should be restricted to free water and salt-poor albumin or fresh-frozen plasma. These should be given to maintain adequate intravascular volume, yet avoiding overexpansion of the patient's intravascular space. A diuretic should be started as soon as the patient is begun on oral fluids. Spironolactone is frequently used because of its potassium-sparing characteristics. Its use should be cautioned by the potential complication of metabolic alkalosis. Sodium intake should be restricted to less than 90 mg/day. Prophylactic antibiotics, which should be started 12 hours prior to surgery, are continued for only 1 to 2 days. Chylous ascites may develop in the immediate postoperative period as a result of interruption of retroperitoneal lymphatics, and a 30-gm/day fat restriction should be maintained for 4 weeks to minimize the risk of this problem.[134]

Recurrent Bleeding

If variceal hemorrhage occurs within the immediate postoperative period, angiography should immediately be performed to accurately define the anatomy and patency of the shunt. If a patent collateral such as the coronary vein is identified, one should consider percutaneous transhepatic embolization. If other collateral pathways are present, reexploration may be indicated in order to ligate them. If the shunt is occluded and the patient is bleeding, then reexploration should be undertaken to repair the shunt or to perform another shunt.

NONSURGICAL SHUNT PROCEDURES

Transjugular Intrahepatic Portosystemic Shunt (TIPSS)

Perhaps the most impressive new development in the management of portal hypertensive patients with variceal hemorrhage has been the introduction of the TIPSS. These shunts are the combination of several procedures and technologies that have developed in parallel over the course of the past several years. The TIPSS has borrowed conceptually from the small-diameter Sarfeh portacaval interposition shunts, balloon angioplasty techniques, and the Palmas balloon expandable stents.

The essence of the TIPSS is the creation of a fistula between a hepatic vein and a branch of the portal vein. This fistula is created by passing a needle-directing guidewire through the jugular vein into a hepatic vein, and then into a branch of the portal vein. Once this connection has been established, balloon dilatation is used to enlarge the tract to a size adequate for the decompression of the portal hypertension. Because of the fibrotic nature of the end-stage liver, the tract must be stented open in order to ensure its patency. This is accomplished by placing a Palmaz-type stent at the time of the balloon dilatation.

The attraction of the TIPSS is that it may be a minimally invasive procedure that may effectively reduce portal hypertension. In optimal circumstances, the TIPSS may be placed in a relatively short period of time, using only local anesthetic techniques. It thus avoids a major surgical procedure and a general anesthetic in a debilitated patient. Additional advantages include the preservation of the patient's normal intraabdominal anatomy. This latter is of particular importance to patients who are considered potential candidates for hepatic transplantation, since it will avoid the scarring, neovascularization, and alteration of portal perfusion that is associated with shunt operations.

A final advantage is that the successful TIPSS would be expected to maintain patency of the portal vein as long as the shunt itself is patent. This is of particular importance in patients who may be at risk of portal vein thrombosis, such as those with sluggish hepatopetal or hepatofugal portal flow. The sequela of portal vein thrombosis range from asymptomatic to massive ascites, hepatic failure, and death. The surgical consequence of portal vein thrombosis is that it may preclude further surgery for the patient. In patients who are to be considered for transplantation, portal vein thrombosis may affect both operability and survival.

The principal disadvantage of the TIPSS is that it is a new and as of yet untested procedure. Only a few centers have any experience with this technique. A clinical trial is being organized that should answer the questions of initial success, complication, and early patency. The long-term track record of these procedures will require several years to establish. Accordingly, the final analysis of the role of the TIPSS remains to be established.

Three reports totaling 11 patients have recorded the very early experience with the procedure.[159–161] Of these, three died in the early postshunt period, one from uncontrolled hemorrhage associated with a percutaneous embolization attempt. One shunt occluded at 3 months following creation, but was successfully reopened; another required redilatation. This initial experience served to establish the feasibility of the procedure, and has generated considerable enthusiasm.

The most recent report is from Ring and associates in San Francisco. They have described their initial experience with 25 patients who underwent the TIPSS procedure for active bleeding (12), recurrent bleeding (12), and ascites secondary to Budd-Chiari syndrome (1). They noted that they were able to place the shunts in all patients. Their 30-day mortality was 20 per cent. Eight of their patients eventually underwent liver transplantation. Of the 12 patients who were available for prolonged follow-up (average of 5.5 months), three suffered shunt occlusion. All three shunts were reopened. Notable complications included encephalopathy and the development of intima in the shunt. They concluded that the TIPSS procedures provide good reduction of portal hypertension and control of bleeding, but that their long-term efficacy is far from established.[162]

An informed survey of institutions where these procedures are being performed suggests that the exact indication for the TIPSS is not clear. They have been used in patients who are awaiting transplantation, in those who are very poor surgical candidates, and in Child's class A patients who did not want to undergo surgery. The TIPSS has been used in elective, urgent, and emergent circumstances. Early experience indicates that somewhere between 10 and 20 per cent of attempts to create these shunts may not succeed because of technical difficulties. The principal problem in these instances is the difficult anatomical relationship between the portal and hepatic veins. In centers with extensive experience, the number of technically impossible cases decreases toward zero. Another unexpected finding is a fairly significant incidence of encephalopathy following the TIPSS procedures.

The best current role of the TIPSS appears to be as an investigational procedure. While these shunts, on initial inspection, appear to be relatively safe and effective, early reported experience has revealed a considerable periprocedural morbidity and mortality. Most surgeons and radiologists who are involved with these procedures would agree that these shunts represent a significant advance in the care of portal hypertensive patients. The consensus appears to be forming that the number of these (TIPSS) shunts will increase, but that given the complexity of these patients and the difficulty of their care, the majority of them will probably be done at institutions with a specialized interest in hepatoportal procedures.

ORTHOTOPIC LIVER TRANSPLANTATION

With the advent of liver transplantation as an established modality for the care of patients with end-stage liver failure, the role of nontransplant procedures (shunt surgery in particular) has been the subject of considerable debate. Current best transplant survival rates are generally more favorable than most of the reported survival of Child's class C patients following the best care with combination of sclerotherapy and shunting. This issue has been the subject of two reports from Iwatsuki and colleagues at the University of Pittsburgh Liver Transplant Unit.[163,164] These reports have described the survival of 302 patients who presented with bleeding esophageal varices. According to the authors, these patients were all ranked as Child's class C with regard to their hepatic function. The survival of these patients is reported in a life-table format as 79 per cent at 1 year, 74 per cent at 2 years, and 71 per cent at 5 years. These authors then compared these results to shunt survival as reported in medical literature and concluded that in Child's class C patients who present with bleeding varices, liver transplantation should be considered as the treatment of choice—assuming that the patients are reasonable transplant candidates.

Our experience at UCLA has revealed that superior survival is afforded to Child's class C patients by transplantation (Table 40–4). In a series of 761 patients operated between January of 1986 and December of 1991, 77 underwent portosystemic shunting as their initial procedure, and 684 underwent hepatic transplantation. Of those transplanted, 86 per cent were Child's class C patients, whereas only 16 per cent of the shunt patients were Child's class C patients. Despite this, 15 per cent of shunt patients eventually required liver transplantation for progressive hepatic deterioration. Furthermore, the 5-year survival of the shunt group was 64 per cent, in contrast to a 73 per cent 5-year survival of the transplanted patients. These data support the impression that portosystemic shunting is an appropriate form of therapy for Child's class A and B patients, but that the Child's class C patients who are transplant candidates are best managed by liver transplantation.

Further complicating the issue is the effect of a prior shunt operation on a subsequent transplant operation. It has been reported that patients who must undergo a liver transplant following a prior portacaval shunt will have a considerably increased blood loss, longer operative procedure, increased morbidity, and a higher mortality.[165] The portacaval shunt is a particularly troublesome procedure to overcome, since the technical elements in performing a successful liver transplant in this situation require dissection through the scarred tissues about the portal structures, disconnection of the shunt, and reconstitution of the normal caval anatomy: only then may the liver transplant operation begin. This is in contrast to the peripheral shunt operations such as the mesocaval shunt or the DSRS. While these shunts will impact on the transplant procedure, they are not as difficult to manage as the central shunts. In the case of a mesocaval shunt, the shunt must be disconnected or occluded before the transplant operation is completed or the new liver may be deprived of portal nutrient blood flow. A similar problem may arise even with the DSRS, although by the nature of this shunt, the siphon effect (drainage of portal blood through peripancreatic collaterals into the shunt) is usually relatively minor and the shunt frequently does not require dismantling.

The essential feature of any consideration as to the role of shunting versus liver transplantation is the underlying cause of the hepatic disease, the current stage of hepatic dysfunction, and the expected progression (the natural and treated history) of the hepatic disease. Assuming that the patient is a reasonable transplantation candidate, and that the liver disease is approaching the end-stage (Child's class C), then transplantation should be strongly considered. If the patient requires an emergent procedure for control of bleeding before being able to be transplanted, then all efforts should be made to provide a peripheral shunt. The patient who is not a transplant candidate should then be treated with the best therapy available: sclerotherapy supported by either esophageal transection with devascularization or shunting.

TABLE 40–4. UCLA EXPERIENCE: RESULTS OF PORTOSYSTEMIC SHUNTING AND LIVER TRANSPLANTATION FROM JANUARY 1986 TO DECEMBER 1991[a]

	N	Child's Class C	5-Year Survival
Portosystemic shunt	77	16%	64
Liver transplant	684	87%	73
Total	761		

[a]50 per cent of shunt operations were DSRS; 15 per cent of shunt patients eventually underwent liver transplantation for deterioration of hepatic function.

VARICEAL SCLEROSIS

Esophageal variceal sclerosis was first introduced by Crafoord and Frenckner in 1939.[166] These authors demonstrated a single patient who underwent rigid endoscopic sclerotherapy to prevent further variceal bleeding. With the upsurge in the variety of surgical procedures for variceal hemorrhage in the 1940s, however, sclerotherapy was soon forgotten. Once it was recognized that therapeutic portacaval shunts were not the ultimate surgical procedure, with their inherent operative mortality and risk of encephalopathy, attention was redirected toward less invasive, more direct methods of treatment, and there was renewed interest in sclerotherapy, following the results of several controlled trials.

The first major review of sclerotherapy was by Johnston and Rodgers in 1973.[167] In certain patients, a shunt procedure is not possible. These include patients under 10 years of age with a thrombosed portal vein, acute variceal bleeders with poor liver function or advanced years, and postshunt recurrent bleeders. A rigid Negus esophagoscope was utilized to inject ethanolamine oleate into the varix. In 117 patients with 194 admissions for acute variceal hemorrhage, bleeding was initially controlled in 92 per cent and the hospital mortality per admission was 18 per cent. The average time to recurrence of variceal hemorrhage was 10 months. This group, however, made no attempt to perform sequential variceal sclerosis and recommended a shunt for long-term variceal control. Similar mortality and variceal hemorrhage control rates were reported by Terblanche from South Africa.[168-171]

Endoscopy is necessary to confirm the presence of varices and differentiate those who are actively bleeding from those who have ceased to bleed. The use of sclerotherapy to stop acute bleeding at the time of initial endoscopy has been recently advocated as the treatment of choice.[168,169] Urgent or emergent sclerotherapy is used in many institutions following stabilization with balloon tamponade or with failure of conservative supportive therapy and vasopressin. Several controlled trials have compared sclerotherapy to medical management with the Sengstaken-Blakemore tube in the acute setting.[172-175] Three studies demonstrated a significantly lower early rebleed rate,[172-174] and all the studies supported the use of sclerotherapy for acute bleeds. Only Paquet and Feussner demonstrated significantly improved overall survival with sclerotherapy.[172]

The ability of sclerotherapy to prevent recurrent variceal hemorrhage and improve long-term survival with extended treatment has been examined in numerous controlled trials[175-179] (Table 40–5). When sclerotherapy was performed to eradicate all varices and compared to conservative medical management, sclerotherapy patients had fewer recurrent bleeds[177,179] and improved long-term survival.[176] Terblanche et al. were able to demonstrate complete eradication of varices in 95 per cent of sclerotherapy patients; however,

they could not demonstrate a significant difference in survival, and varices recurred in greater than 60 per cent of the sclerosed patients.[177]

Only in the last 5 years has sclerotherapy been systematically compared to portosystemic shunts in the management of variceal hemorrhage. Cello et al. compared the portacaval shunt to sclerotherapy in Child's class C patients, showing greater rebleeding, increased rehospitalization, and higher blood transfusion requirements in the sclerotherapy group, with 40 per cent of the sclerotherapy patients ultimately requiring surgical therapy. However, they were unable to demonstrate any significant difference in survival (Table 40–6). It was concluded that in high-risk patients, sclerotherapy and portacaval shunting are equal in the acute setting, but one must consider shunt surgery if varices are not totally obliterated.[180,181]

With the resurgence of endoscopic sclerotherapy, the distal splenorenal shunt has recently been compared to this form of treatment for the long-term management of variceal bleeds in 3 controlled trials[172] (Table 40–7). The study by Warren and coworkers showed that although early mortality was the same, there was a higher rebleeding rate with sclerotherapy, and one third of the patients failed treatment and required surgery.[182] Treatment with sclerotherapy allowed significant improvement in liver function when successful, with less encephalopathy and improved survival when backed up by surgical therapy for patients with uncontrolled bleeding. Therefore, the improved survival in the sclerotherapy group actually represents a combination of sclerotherapy and surgical therapy. The study by Teres et al.[183] showed no difference in early and long-term mortality, as did the results of Rikkers et al.'s trial.[184] However, the rebleeding rate was greater in those patients who had sclerotherapy, and encephalopathy rates were higher in shunted patients in Teres et al.'s study.[183]

Burroughs et al. recently concluded a prospective randomized study comparing staple transection with sclerotherapy for emergency control of variceal bleeding. They found no difference in overall mortality and improved control of bleeding with esophageal transection when compared to a single injection, but a similar incidence of hemorrhage following three injection treatments.[185] Teres et al. randomized cirrhotic patients with uncontrolled bleeding to portacaval shunt or staple transection in low-risk patients and staple transection or sclerotherapy in high-risk patients.[186] Survival was similar in both comparisons. In the low-risk patients, portacaval shunt had a greater hemostatic effect but a greater incidence of encephalopathy. In high-risk patients, sclerotherapy and staple transection had similar rebleed rates and survival, but fewer complications were observed in the sclerotherapy group. The authors therefore recommended staple transection for low-risk patients and sclerotherapy for the initial management of high-risk patients. Although a consensus opinion on sclerotherapy has not yet been reached, sclerotherapy may well represent an appropriate alternative ablative pro-

TABLE 40–5. SCLEROTHERAPY VERSUS MEDICAL MANAGEMENT[a]

Study	Follow-up (Months)	Sclerotherapy			Control		
		N	Rebleed	Survival	N	Rebleed	Survival
Terblanche et al.[177]	60	37	43%	45% (5 yr)	38	73%	45% (5 yr)
Copenhagen project[175]	9–52	93	48%	36% (2 yr)	97	54%	25% (2 yr)
Westaby et al.[176]	3–60	56	55%	60% (4 yr)	60	80%	31% (4 yr)
Korula et al.[179]	3–35	63	[b]	60% (2 yr)	57	[b]	56% (2 yr)
Soderlund and Ihre[178]	12–48	57	[c]	49% (2 yr)	50	[c]	34% (2 yr)

[a]Controlled trials, long-term follow-up.
[b]There was a significant decrease in transfusion requirements in the sclerotherapy group as well as fewer rebleeding episodes per patient-month of follow-up.
[c]Overall recurrent hemorrhage was 3.6 times more frequent in the control group.

TABLE 40–6. SCLEROTHERAPY VERSUS PORTACAVAL SHUNT[a]

	Sclerotherapy	Portacaval Shunt	p
N	32	32	
Rebleed rate	50%	19%	<.009
Encephalopathy	13%	13%	NS
Not requiring surgery	7 (22%)		
Long-term cost	$23,000	$28,000	NS
18-month survival	28%	13%	NS

[a]Data from Cello et al.[181]; controlled trial, long-term follow-up.

TABLE 40–7. SCLEROTHERAPY VERSUS DISTAL SPLENORENAL SHUNT (DSRS)[a]

	Sclerotherapy	DSRS	p
Warren et al.[182]			
N	36	35	
Rebleed rate	53%	3%	<.05
Portal perfusion	95%	53%	<.05
No. requiring surgery	10 (28%)		
2-year survival	84%	59%	<.01
Rikkers et al.[184]			
N	30	27	
Rebleed rate	57%	19%	.003
Encephalopathy	7%	16%	
2-year survival	61%	65%	NS
Teres et al.[186]			
N	55	57	
Rebleed rate	37.5%	14.3%	<.02
Encephalopathy	8%	24%	<.05
2-year survival	68%	71%	NS

[a]Controlled trials.

cedure in selected patients with hepatic dysfunction.[157,172,186–193]

There are basically two methods of esophageal sclerotherapy, each advocated by different groups. Some prefer rigid Negus esophagoscope with injection of sodium morrhuate or ethanolamine oleate; others prefer a flexible endoscope. Each has its specific advantages.[167,190] A rigid scope requires general anesthesia with muscle relaxation and adequate neck extension. This, in a patient with varying degrees of liver failure, has obvious disadvantages. On the other hand, it allows direct tamponade of varices against its rigid structure to adequately stop bleeding. A flexible scope, on the other hand, permits performance

under topical anesthesia and intravenous sedation. It is simple and provides another distinct advantage in its ability to fully visualize the entire stomach and proximal duodenum at the same time in order to eliminate other sources of bleeding. Hence, it may be used as an adjunctive procedure rather than an additional procedure. Despite the ability to visualize gastric varices with the flexible scope, one is not capable of sclerosis.[189,194]

We prefer, for these reasons, to perform the technique using a flexible Olympus endoscope. A balloon inflated with 20 ml of air is impacted at the gastroesophageal junction in order to diminish blood flow and prevent rapid migration of the sclerosing solution. Once the site of bleeding has been visualized, 2 ml of sodium morrhuate is injected into the lumen of the varix approximately 1 to 2 cm distal to the bleeding point. The other visible varices are then injected in a similar manner. When hemorrhage has been arrested, the balloon is deflated and the endoscope removed.[191]

A number of complications of varying degrees of severity arise from esophageal variceal sclerosis. Frequently the patients complain of odynophagia lasting from hours to days. This may also be associated with retrosternal chest pain, lasting for several days. Not infrequently as a result of pyrogens within the sclerosing solution, a fever of greater than 101°F develops that abates within 2 to 3 days and is not associated with a leukocytosis. Bacteremias have been documented in as many as 50 per cent of procedures.[195] Pleural effusion sometimes occurs but does not necessarily indicate esophageal perforation.[196] Variceal ulceration of varying degrees, depending on the amount of sclerosant injected, is not uncommon and usually resolves spontaneously.[197] Rare serious complications, including esophageal perforation, spinal cord paralysis, and bradyarrhythmias, have also been described.[25,27,28,30,171,190,194]

Another technique of variceal sclerosis was developed by Lunderquist and Vang. This group developed a method consisting of percutaneous transhepatic portal venipuncture with manipulation of a catheter into the coronary vein and injection of a 50 per cent glucose and thrombin sclerosing solution (PTHCVO).[29,198] Widrich and associates utilized this technique in 38 patients with documented variceal bleeding. Eighty-seven per cent of the patients had successful coronary vein occlusion with cessation of bleeding. Approximately 19 per cent of patients undergoing PTHCVO suffered recurrent bleeding within 30 days, and 40 per cent of those not undergoing a shunt procedure subsequently developed hemorrhage. In the emergency group, 69 per cent of patients, all Child's class C, died within 30 days, six because of recurrent hemorrhage, and 17.6 per cent of elective PTHCVO patients died within 30 days. The most common minor complication of this procedure was a low-grade fever; however, portal vein thrombosis and intraperitoneal hemorrhage occurred in a significant number of patients.[199]

Mendez and Russell made the significant observation that in the presence of hepatofugal flow, embolization of varices is of no value because new collateral pathways develop from the splenic hilum almost immediately, preventing control of hemorrhage. Furthermore, they noted that in 6 of 10 patients coming to autopsy, Gelfoam particles were present in the lungs.[200]

Bengmark et al., in a follow-up of 43 patients, found that the overall rate of rebleeding was 55 per cent, and the incidence of portal vein thrombosis was 36 per cent in acutely bleeding patients.[198] The high incidence of portal vein thrombosis, 20 per cent, was also noted by Gembarowicz et al.,[201] eliminating subsequent portosystemic shunts.

At present, PTHCVO cannot be recommended as a definitive first-line procedure in the management of variceal hemorrhage. At best, catheterization of the coronary vein in an acutely bleeding patient is time consuming and demands significant technical skill. Furthermore, it is not usually possible to prevent recurrent variceal hemorrhage by repeated coronary vein occlusion because new collateral pathways may develop from the area of the splenic hilum, which is inaccessible by this method.[202,203] Additionally, the significant incidence of portal vein thrombosis dictates against this technique.

Endoscopic variceal sclerosis, however, has the distinct advantage of having no risk of portal vein thrombosis but good control of variceal hemorrhage and easy accessibility for recurrent sclerotherapy. There is no question that in patients presenting with an acute variceal bleed who have had a prior splenectomy or portosystemic shunt that has failed, variceal sclerosis is indicated. Because of the high mortality associated with emergency shunting procedures, variceal sclerosis in conjunction with vasopressin is probably indicated in the acute management of variceal hemorrhage, especially in Child's class C-minus patients. Sclerotherapy does not treat gastric varices, nor does it prevent the severe gastritis frequently associated with hemorrhage in these patients. Recurrent variceal hemorrhage is likely if follow-up routine sclerotherapy is not performed. Hence, sclerotherapy should be considered as an adjunctive therapeutic management tool for the acute control of variceal bleeding, rather than its definitive treatment.

TREATMENT PLAN FOR VARICEAL HEMORRHAGE

When a patient presents with an upper GI tract bleed, whose history and physical examination suggest esophageal varices in association with hepatic disease, a preset treatment plan should rapidly be followed. It is important to consider that in these patients time is of the essence, and that delays to consider, define, and formulate a new plan of action will frequently jeopardize the patient's life. The initial care of the bleeding portal hypertensive patient should be as routine as the initial care of a trauma patient. The A, B, and C steps should be routinely followed. Special variations are implemented because of the underlying hepatic disease and the associated risks that this presents.

Initial laboratory studies should include CBC; platelet count; electrolytes; blood type and cross-match; and determinants of liver function, including bilirubin, SGOT, LDH, SGPT, prothrombin time, partial thromboplastin time, albumin, total protein, and alkaline phosphatase. Nasogastric tubes must be placed in all of these patients; if blood is present in the stomach, then gastric lavage and emergency endoscopy are indicated. This will allow for the verification of the source of hemorrhage, and emergent sclerotherapy if required.

Initial fluid management is crucial. Treatment with fluids and blood products should be directed at maintaining adequate tissue perfusion. Resuscitation should include packed cells and fresh-frozen plasma as needed. Cryoprecipitates and calcium may be required in massive bleeds. It is generally preferable to resuscitate with a combination of crystalloid and blood components (albumin and PRBCs) rather than saline only. Thiamine should be administered to prevent Wernicke's encephalopathy. Propranolol or diazepam may be required for abatement of alcohol withdrawal.

If bleeding does not stop during the resuscitation and transfusion, vasopressin should be administered intravenously and repeated sclerotherapy performed. Balloon tamponade may be especially helpful at this juncture. If the patient fails to stop bleeding following injections and balloon tamponade, emergent intervention is indicated. Depending on the institutional resources, the patient should be considered for either a TIPSS, a portosystemic shunt, or an esophageal transection with devascularization. The choice of portosystemic shunt is largely dependent on the abilities of the surgeons involved. If the patient is a potential liver transplant candidate, then a peripheral shunt (DSRS or mesocaval) should be performed. The use of the TIPSS should probably be limited to investigation protocols in institutions with considerable expertise.

Once bleeding is controlled, patients with relatively good hepatic function (Child's class A or B) should undergo long-term sclerotherapy until varices are obliterated. If this is successful, then the patient should continue to be observed and no further interventions planned. If the patient has breakthrough bleeding from noncompliance, gastric varices, or hypertensive gastritis, and is an appropriate candidate for elective shunt, preoperative evaluation should be done (angiography, duplex scan) and a shunt performed.

Patients with poor hepatic function should be considered for transplant if they fulfill the appropriate criteria. While awaiting orthotopic liver transplant, a peripheral shunt may be necessary as a bridge to transplantation. Child's class C-minus patients with marked muscle wasting and obvious hyaline necrosis have a prohibitively high operative mortality rate and should undergo endoscopic sclerotherapy followed by transplant. If this technique is not available, esophageal transection with or without the EEA stapler and ligation of portoazygous collateral pathways is indicated, although the mortality can be expected to be greater than 60 per cent (Fig. 40–7).

MANAGEMENT OF ASCITES

Ascites predisposes these patients to potentially lethal complications, including renal failure, peritonitis, variceal hemorrhage, pleural effusions with respiratory insufficiency, abdominal wall hernias, anorexia, and generalized malaise. Most patients with ascites may be controlled with a restricted-salt diet and diuretic regimen. Only 5 per cent of ascitic patients can be considered to have truly intractable ascites, and it is these patients who may require surgical intervention.[204]

Patients who present with ascites related to liver disease should be admitted to the hospital for a complete evaluation and therapy. The admission workup should include a careful neurologic status examination as well as measurements of electrolytes and renal and liver function tests. These patients should be placed at strict bed rest, because this will increase the amount of diuresis. Encephalopathy should be monitored by checking for asterixis at least once or twice a day.

A fluid restriction of no more than 1 liter/day should be ordered in addition to a 20 mEq/day sodium diet. With this regimen, one would expect a diuresis of 500 ml to 1 liter/day.

If such a diuresis does not occur, then progressive diuretic therapy is indicated. This usually involves gradual increase in the dosages and varieties of diuretics. Frequently, the first diuretic used is spironolactone, a potassium-sparing diuretic. It should be started at a dosage of 100 mg/day and doubled at 2-day intervals until a maximum dosage is obtained. If further diuresis is required, the other agents such as metalazone, hydrochlorothiazide, and Lasix may be used.

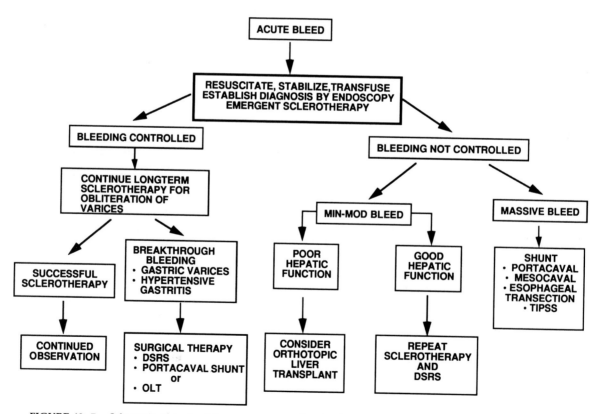

FIGURE 40–7. Schematic of protocol for management of variceal hemorrhage. *DSRS*, distal splenorenal shunt; *OLT*, orthotopic liver transplant; *TIPSS*, transjugular intrahepatic portosystemic shunt.

At the first sign of encephalopathy or elevation of blood urea nitrogen by 10 mg/dl or creatinine by 0.5 mg/dl, all diuretics must be discontinued to avoid development of the hepatorenal syndrome. If after such a trial of intensive nonsurgical therapy no significant response occurs, surgery is indicated.[205]

In 1974, LeVeen introduced the peritoneovenous shunt. This device consists of a Silastic tube that runs from the peritoneum to the superior vena cava. It is controlled by a one-way valve, so that a pressure gradient of 5 cm H_2O will suffice to transfer the ascitic fluid from the abdomen to the intravascular space.[206]

The Denver shunt is a variation on the LeVeen shunt that incorporates a pump in line with the shunt, and is implanted in the subcutaneous tissues on the chest wall. Its proposed benefit is its ability to clear the shunt of debris by using the pump mechanism.[127]

While a promising innovation, both of these shunts are dogged by complications. Early complications include congestive failure from the infusion of ascitic fluid, and disseminated intravascular coagulopathy (DIC). In 39 to 100 per cent of patients, changes consistent with DIC may be detected by laboratory studies. Clinically apparent DIC is much less common.[72,207] Coagulation parameters tend to improve after the first postoperative week, possibly related to diminished ascitic flow into the venous system.[208] If clinically apparent DIC develops, the only definitive treatment possible is shunt ligation.[207] Some authors have been concerned that the increased intravascular volume may result in increased variceal hemorrhage. Finally, a high perioperative mortality rate (20 per cent) has been reported from a number of institutions.[209]

Late complications include shunt infection, shunt occlusion, and death. Infection may occur in as many as 26 per cent of patients. Shunt occlusion is thought to result from the precipitation of the ascitic protein in the shunt tubing. Death related to inherent liver dysfunction is not uncommon.

Usually, the infusion of ascitic fluids will result in a brisk diuresis. The exact mechanism is not clear. Proposed mechanisms include the volume expansion, increased renin levels from the ascitic fluid, and the relief of intraabdominal pressure.[6] The hepatorenal syndrome is the name given to the concomitant loss of renal function in patients with hepatic failure and no intrinsic renal disease. While the cause is unknown, it may be related to a redistribution of blood within the cortex of the kidney. The mortality from untreated hepatorenal syndrome is usually 100 per cent.[210] The peritoneovenous shunt is considered a potential treatment of these cases. Successful resolution of the syndrome by placement of such a shunt has been reported.[210]

Contraindications to the placement of peritoneovenous shunts include the presence of infected ascitic fluid, recurrent sepsis, or encephalopathy. Another absolute contraindication includes a bilirubin greater than 6 or prolongation of prothrombin time more than 4 seconds. These have been shown to be associated with a prohibitively high incidence of postoperative coagulopathy, resulting in death. DIC resulting from an intravenous test infusion of ascitic fluid is another relative contraindication to peritoneovenous shunting. Finally, a large pleural effusion associated with an elevated intrathoracic pressure may preclude use of these shunts.[204]

In general, peritoneovenous shunting is an effective method to treat ascites. It should be kept in mind as an adjunct to the care of these patients, and may not be as simple in practice as it is in concept. It should not be expected to result in prolongation of survival or alteration of the natural course of their hepatic disease.

SUMMARY

The management of portal hypertension and its sequela of ascites, encephalopathy, and recurrent variceal hemorrhage continues to be a significant challenge to the clinician. Its etiology and pathogenesis have been well described. Alcoholic cirrhosis resulting in intrahepatic sinusoidal and postsinusoidal obstruction continues to be the most common cause.

Long-term survival depends on rapid control of hemorrhage and institution of the most appropriate care for the patient according to the nature and severity of their hepatic disease. A patient who presents with variceal hemorrhage should be quickly resuscitated, followed by endoscopy to establish the source of GI tract bleeding, and sclerotherapy. Initial management should include intravenous vasopressin followed by balloon tamponade. Angiography or duplex Doppler studies should be performed in patients to be considered for shunting. Emergent shunt surgery should be avoided if at all possible, because the mortality is excessive.

Selective shunt procedures (e.g., DSRS), while not extending the long-term survival, will produce less encephalopathy and stop bleeding. Patients should be considered for elective shunting if they cannot be controlled with sclerotherapy and have relatively good hepatic function (Child's class A or B). Child's class C patients and "unshuntable" patients are best initially treated with nonshunt procedures or transplantation. Esophageal variceal sclerosis provides effective control of acute variceal hemorrhage. If unsuccessful after several attempts, a portoazygous devascularization procedure should be attempted. Ultimately, the survival of these patients depends upon their degree of hepatic function. Patients with end-stage liver disease should be considered for liver transplantation.

Encephalopathy is a consequence of hepatic failure. If present it may be ameliorated by a medical regimen of neomycin, lactulose, and a low-protein diet. Ascites usually can be managed with salt restriction and diuretics. In patients with intractable ascites, a peritoneovenous shunt will provide effective control.

The best treatment for patients with portal hypertension relies on the recognition that the hepatic disease will dictate the progression of liver failure. Depending on the stage of hepatic dysfunction, different options are available for each patient. In deciding how best to manage these patients it is necessary to keep in mind that the goal is not merely survival; one must also consider quality of life.

REFERENCES

1. Malt R: Portasystemic venous shunts. N Engl J Med *295*:24–29, 1976.
2. Shaldon S, Sherlock S: Portal hypertension in the myeloproliferative syndrome and the reticuloses. Am J Surg *32*:758, 1962.
3. Shaldon S, Chiandussi L, Guevara L: The measurement of hepatic blood flow and intrahepatic shunted blood flow by colloid, heat denatured serum albumin labeled with I 131. J Clin Invest *40*:1038, 1969.
4. Gordon M, DelGuercio L: Late effects of portal systemic shunting procedures on cardiorespiratory dynamics in man. Ann Surg *176*:672–679, 1972.
5. Langer B, Stone R, Colapinto R: Clinical spectrum of the Budd-Chiari syndrome and its surgical management. Am J Surg *129*:137–145, 1975.
6. Ludwick J, Markel S, Child L: Chiari's disease. Arch Surg *91*:697–704, 1965.
7. Sherlock S: Classification and functional aspects of portal hypertension. Am J Surg *127*:121–128, 1974.
8. Ahn S, Yellin A, Sheng F, et al: Selective surgical therapy of the Budd-Chiari syndrome provides superior survival rates than conservative medical management. J Vasc Surg *5*:28–37, 1987.
9. Bosch J, Navasa M, Garcia-Pagan J, et al: Portal hypertension. Med Clin North Am *73*:931–953, 1989.
10. Bosch J, Mastai R, Kravetz D, et al: Hemodynamic evaluation of the patients with portal hypertension. Semin Liver Dis *6*:309–317, 1986.
11. Koslin D, Berland L: Duplex Doppler examination of the liver and portal system. Clin Ultrasound *15*:675–686, 1987.
12. Ohnishi K, Saito M, Koen H, et al: Pulsed Doppler flow as a criterion of portal venous velocity: Comparison with cineangiographic measurements. Radiology *154*:495–498, 1985.
13. Bolondi L, Gandolfi L, Arienti V, et al: Ultrasonography in the diagnosis of portal hypertension: Diminished response of portal vessels to respiration. Radiology *142*:167–172, 1982.
14. Cello J, Deveney K, Trunkey D: Factors influencing survival after therapeutic shunts. Am J Surg *141*:257–265, 1981.
15. Orloff M, Duguay L, Kosta L: Criteria for selection of patients for emergency portacaval shunt. Am J Surg *134*:146–152, 1977.
16. Schwartz S: Liver. *In* Schwartz S (ed): Principles of Surgery. New York, McGraw-Hill, 1984, pp 1257–1305.
17. Rueff B, Benhamou J: Management of gastrointestinal bleeding in cirrhotic patients. Clin Gastroenterol *4*(2):426–438, 1975.
18. Rikkers L: Operations for management of esophageal variceal hemorrhage. West J Med *136*:107–121, 1982.
19. Resnick R: Portal hypertension. Med Clin North Am *59*(4):945–953, 1975.
20. Phemister D, Humphreys E: Gastroesophageal resection and total gastrectomy in the treatment of bleeding varicose veins in Banti's syndrome. Ann Surg *125*:397, 1947.
21. Mikkelsen W: Therapeutic portacaval shunt. Arch Surg *108*:302–305, 1974.
22. Bell R, Miyai K, Orloff M: Outcome in cirrhotic patients with acute alcoholic hepatitis after emergency portacaval shunt for bleeding esophageal varices. Am J Surg *147*:78–84, 1984.
23. Eckhauser F, Appelman H, O'Leary T: Hepatic pathology as a determinant of prognosis after portal decompression. Am J Surg *139*:105–112, 1980.
24. Viamonte M, Warren W, Famon J: Angiographic investigations in portal hypertension. Surg Gynecol Obstet *130*:37–53, 1970.
25. Huizinga W, Keenan J, Marszaley A: Sclerotherapy for bleeding esophageal varices. A case report. S Afr Med J *65*:436–438, 1984.
26. Mikkelsen W, Turrill F, Kern W: Acute hyaline necrosis of the liver. A surgical trap. Am J Surg *116*:266–272, 1968.
27. Seidman E, Neber A, Morin C: Spinal cord paralysis following sclerotherapy for esophageal varices. Hepatology *4*:950–954, 1981.
28. Perakos P, Cirbus J, Camara D: Persistent bradyarrhythmia after sclerotherapy for esophageal varices. South Med J *77*:531–532, 1984.
29. Lunderquist A, Vang J: Transhepatic catheterization and obliteration of the coronary vein in patients with portal hypertension and esophageal varices. N Engl J Med *291*:646–649, 1974.
30. Abecossis M, Makowka L, Lanser B: Sclerotherapy for esophageal varices. Can J Surg *27*:561–566, 1984.
31. Reynolds T: The role of hemodynamic measurements in portasystemic shunt surgery. Arch Surg *108*:276–281, 1974.
32. Lebrec D, DeFleury P, Rueff B, et al: Portal hypertension, size of esophageal varices and risk of gastrointestinal bleeding in alcoholic cirrhosis. Gastroenterology *79*:1139–1144, 1980.
33. Paquet K: Prophylactic endoscopic sclerosing treatment of the esophageal wall varices. A prospective controlled randomized trial. Endoscopy *14*:4–5, 1982.
34. Witzel L, Wolbergs E, Merki H: Prophylactic endoscopic sclerotherapy of esophageal varices. A prospective controlled study. Lancet *1*:773–775, 1985.
35. The North Italian Endoscopic Club for the Study and Treatment of Esophageal Varices: Prediction of the first variceal hemorrhage in patients with cirrhosis of the liver and esophageal varices: A prospective multicenter trial. N Engl J Med *319*:983–989, 1988.
36. Dagradi A: The natural history of esophageal varices in patients with alcoholic cirrhosis. Am J Gastroenterol *57*:520–540, 1972.
37. Schenker S, Breen K, Hoyumpa A: Hepatic encephalopathy: Current status. Gastroenterology *66*:121–151, 1974.
38. Fischer J, James J, Jeppsson B: Hyperammonaemia, plasma amino acid imbalance and blood-brain amino acid transport. Lancet *2*:772–778, 1979.
39. Fischer J, Furovics J, Folcao H: L-Dopa in hepatic coma. Ann Surg *183*:386–391, 1976.
40. Waldram R, Davis M, Nunnerly H: Emergency endoscopy after gastrointestinal hemorrhage in 50 patients with portal hypertension. Br Med J *4*:94–96, 1974.
41. Maddrey W, Weber F: Chronic hepatic encephalopathy. Med Clin North Am *59*(4):937–944, 1975.
42. Elkington S: Lactulose. Gut *11*:1043–1048, 1970.
43. Bainbridge F, Trevan J: Some actions of adrenalin upon liver. J Physiol *51*:460–468, 1917.
44. Graszmann R, Kravetz D, Bosch J: Nitroglycerin improves the hemodynamic response to vasopressin in portal hypertension. Hepatology *2*:757–762, 1982.
45. Kehne J, Hughes F, Gompertz M: The use of surgical Pituitrin in the control of esophageal varix bleeding. Surgery *39*:917–925, 1956.

46. Conn H, Storer E: Intra-arterial vasopressin in the treatment of upper gastrointestinal hemorrhage: A prospective clinical trial. Gastroenterology *68*:211–221, 1975.

47. Nusbaum M, Younis M, Baum S: Control of portal hypertension. Arch Surg *108*:114–119, 1974.

48. Johnson W, Widrich W, Ansell J: Control of bleeding varices by vasopressin: A prospective randomized study. Ann Surg *186*:369, 1977.

49. Chandler J: Vasopressin and splanchnic shunting. Ann Surg *195*:543–553, 1982.

50. Sirinek K, Thomford N: Isoproterenol in offsetting adverse effect of vasopressin in cirrhotic patients. Am J Surg *129*:130–136, 1975.

51. Mols P, Hallemans R, Van Kuyk M: Hemodynamic effects of vasopressin alone and in combination with nitroprusside, in patients with liver cirrhosis and portal hypertension. Ann Surg *199*:176–181, 1984.

52. Gimson A, Westaby D, Hegarty J: A randomized trial of vasopressin and vasopressin plus nitroglycerin in the control of acute variceal hemorrhage. Hepatology *6*:410–413, 1986.

53. Kravetz D, Bosch J, Teres J, et al: A controlled comparison of continuous somatostatin and vasopressin infusions in the treatment of acute variceal hemorrhage. Hepatology *4*:442–446, 1984.

54. Bosch J, Kravetz D, Rodes J: Effects of somatostatin on hepatic and systemic hemodynamics in patients with cirrhosis of the liver. Comparison with vasopressin. Gastroenterology *80*:518–525, 1985.

55. Burroughs A, Jenkins W, Sherlock S: Controlled trial propranolol for the prevention of recurrent variceal hemorrhage in patients with cirrhosis. N Engl J Med *309*:1539–1542, 1983.

56. Fleig W, Stange E, Hunecke R, et al: Prevention of recurrent bleeding in cirrhotics with recent variceal hemorrhage: Prospective randomized comparison of propranolol and sclerotherapy. Hepatology *7*:355–361, 1987.

57. Lebrec D, Poynard T, Hillani P: Propranolol for prevention of recurrent gastrointestinal bleeding in patients with cirrhosis. N Engl J Med *805*:1371–1374, 1981.

58. Lebrec D, Bernjau J, Rueff B: Gastrointestinal bleeding after abrupt cessation of propranolol administration in cirrhosis. N Engl J Med *807*:560, 1982.

59. Maringhini A, Simonetti R, Marceno M: Propranolol for gastrointestinal bleeding in cirrhosis. N Engl J Med *307*:1710, 1982.

60. Poynard T, Lebrec D, Hillon P, et al: Propranolol for prevention of recurrent gastrointestinal bleeding in patients with cirrhosis: A prospective study of factors associated with rebleeding. Hepatology *7*:447–451, 1987.

61. Edlich R, Lande A, Goodale R: Prevention of aspiration pneumonia by continuous esophageal aspiration during esophagogastric tamponade and gastric cooling. Surgery *67*:405–408, 1968.

62. Burcharth F, Malmstrom J: Experience with the Linton-Nachlas and the Sengstaken-Blakemore tubes for bleeding esophageal varices. Surg Gynecol Obstet *142*:529–531, 1976.

63. Bauer J, Kreel I, Kark A: The use of the Sengstaken-Blakemore tube for the control of bleeding esophageal varices. Ann Surg *179*:273–277, 1974.

64. Hermann R, Traul D: Experience with the Sengstaken-Blakemore tube for bleeding esophageal varices. Surg Gynecol Obstet *130*:879–885, 1970.

65. Pitcher J: Safety and effectiveness of the modified Sengstaken-Blakemore tube: A prospective study. Gastroenterology *61*:291–298, 1971.

66. Johnson W, Nabseth D, Widrich W: Bleeding esophageal varices. Ann Surg *195*:893–400, 1982.

67. Conn H, Simpson J: Excessive mortality associated with balloon tamponade or bleeding varices. JAMA *202*:135, 1967.

68. Eck N: On the question of ligature of the portal vein. Voyenno Med *130*:1–2, 1877.

69. Warren W: Control of variceal bleeding. Reassessment of rationale. Am J Surg *145*:8–16, 1983.

70. Whipple A: The problem of portal hypertension in relation to the hepatosplenopathis. Ann Surg *122*:449–475, 1945.

71. Blakemore A, Lord JJ: The technique of using vitalium tubes in establishing portacaval shunts for portal hypertension. Ann Surg *122*:476–488, 1945.

72. Greig P, Langer B, Blendis L, et al: Complications of the peritoneovenous shunting for ascites. Am J Surg *139*:125–131, 1980.

73. Conn H, Lindemuth W: Prophylactic portacaval anastomosis in cirrhotic patients with esophageal varices: A progress report of a continuing study. N Engl J Med *272*:1255–1263, 1965.

74. Conn H, Lindemuth W, May L, et al: Prophylactic portacaval anastomosis: A tale of two studies. Medicine *51*:27–40, 1972.

75. Resnick R, Chalmers T, Ishihara A: The Boston Interhospital Liver Group: A controlled study of the prophylactic portacaval shunt. A final report. Ann Intern Med *70*:675–688, 1969.

76. Jackson F, Perrin E, Felix W, et al: A clinical investigation of the portacaval shunt. Ann Surg *174*:672–701, 1971.

77. Resnick R, Iber F, Ishihara A, et al: A controlled study of the therapeutic portacaval shunt. Gastroenterology *67*:843–857, 1974.

78. Reynolds T, Donovan A, Mikkelsen W, et al: Results of a 12-year randomized trial of portacaval shunt in patients with alcoholic liver disease and bleeding varices. Gastroenterology *80*:1005–1011, 1981.

79. Rueff B, Prandi D, Degos F, et al: A controlled study of portacaval shunt in alcoholic cirrhosis. Lancet *1*:655, 1976.

80. Conn H: Therapeutic portacaval anastomosis: To shunt or not to shunt. Gastroenterology *67*:1065–1071, 1974.

81. Zeppa R, Hensley G, Levi J: The comparative survivals of alcoholics versus nonalcoholics with the distal splenorenal shunts. Ann Surg *187*:510–514, 1978.

82. Sarfeh I, Carter J, Welch H: Analysis of operative mortality after portal decompressive procedures in cirrhotic patients. Am J Surg *140*:306–311, 1980.

83. Orloff M, Bell R, Hyde P, et al: Long-term results of emergency portacaval shunt for bleeding esophageal varices in unselected patients with alcoholic cirrhosis. Ann Surg *192*:325–340, 1980.

84. Villeneuve J, Pomier-Layrargues G, Duguay L, et al: Emergency portacaval shunt for variceal hemorrhage. A prospective study. Ann Surg *206*:48–52, 1987.

85. LeVeen H, Wapnick S, Grosberg S, et al: Further experience with peritoneovenous shunt for ascites. Ann Surg *184*:574–581, 1976.

86. Burchell A, Rousselot L, Panke W: A seven-year experience with side-to-side portacaval shunts for cirrhotic ascites. Ann Surg *168*:655–670, 1968.

87. Turcotte J, Wallin V, Child C: End-to-side versus side-to-side portacaval shunts in patients with hepatic cirrhosis. Am J Surg *117*:108–116, 1979.

88. Iwatsuki S, Mikkelsen W, Redeker A, et al: Clinical comparison of the end-to-side and side-to-side portacaval shunt. Ann Surg *178*:65–69, 1973.

89. Blakemore W: The technique of portal systemic shunt surgery. Surgery *57*:778–786, 1965.

90. Hermann R: Shunt operations for portal hypertension. Surg Clin North Am *55*:1073–1087, 1975.

91. Maillard J, Rueff B, Prandi D: Hepatic arterialization and portacaval shunt in hepatic cirrhosis. Arch Surg *108*:315–320, 1979.

92. Otte J, Reynaent M, Hemptinne B, et al: Arterialization of the portal vein in conjunction with a therapeutic portacaval shunt. Ann Surg *196*:656–663, 1982.

93. Sarfeh I, Rypins E, Mason G: A synthetic appraisal of portacaval H-graft diameters. Clinical and hemodynamic perspectives. Ann Surg *204*:356–363, 1986.

94. Clatworthy H, Wall T, Watman R: A new trial of portal-to-

systemic venous shunt for portal hypertension. Arch Surg 71:588, 1955.

95. Drapanas T, LoCicero J, Dowling J: Interposition mesocaval shunt for treatment of portal hypertension. Ann Surg 176:435, 1972.

96. Lord J, Rossi G, Daliana M, et al: Mesocaval shunt modified by the use of a Teflon prosthesis. Surg Gynecol Obstet 130:525–526, 1970.

97. Nay H, Fitzpatrick H: Mesocaval "H" graft using autogenous vein graft. Am Surg 183:114–119, 1976.

98. Read R, Thompson B, Wise W, et al: Mesocaval H venous homografts. Arch Surg 101:785, 1970.

99. Thompson B, Reed B, Casall R: Interposition grafting for portal hypertension. Am J Surg 130:733–739, 1975.

100. Drapanas T, LoCiciero J, Dowling J: Hemodynamics of the interposition mesocaval shunt. Ann Surg 181:523–532, 1975.

101. Smith R, Warren W, Salam A, et al: Dacron interposition shunts for portal hypertension. Ann Surg 92:9–17, 1980.

102. Fulenwider J, Nordlinger B, Millikan W: Portal pseudoperfusion: An angiographic illusion. Ann Surg 189:257, 1979.

103. Cargenas A, Busuttil R: A comparative analysis of the mesocaval H graft versus the distal splenorenal shunt. Curr Surg 39:151–157, 1982.

104. Malt R: Portasystemic venous shunts. N Engl J Med 295:80–86, 1976.

105. Cameron J, Zuidema G, Smith G, et al: Mesocaval shunts for the control of bleeding esophageal varices. Surgery 85:257–262, 1979.

106. Cameron J, Harrington D, Maddrey W: The mesocaval C shunt. Surg Gynecol Obstet 150:401, 1980.

107. Resnick R, Langer B, Taylor B, et al: Results and hemodynamic changes after interposition mesocaval shunt. Surgery 95:275–280, 1984.

108. Reichle F, Fahmy W, Golsorkhi M: Prospective comparative clinical trial with distal splenorenal and mesocaval shunts. Am J Surg 137:13–21, 1979.

109. Thompson B, Casall R, Reed R, et al: Results of interposition "H" grafts for portal hypertension. Ann Surg 187(5):515–522, 1978.

110. Mulcare R, Halleran D, Gardine R: Experience with 49 consecutive Dacron interposition mesocaval shunts. A unified approach to portasystemic decompression procedures. Am J Surg 147:393–399, 1984.

111. Linton R, Ellis D, Geary J: Critical comparative analysis of early and late results of splenorenal and direct portacaval shunts performed in 169 patients with portal cirrhosis. Ann Surg 154:446–449, 1961.

112. Pliam M, Adson M, Foulk W: Conventional splenorenal shunts. Arch Surg 110:588–599, 1975.

113. Bismuth H, Franco D, Hepp J: Portal-systemic shunt in hepatic cirrhosis: Does the type of shunt decisively influence the clinical result? Ann Surg 179:209–218, 1974.

114. Ottinger L: The Linton splenorenal shunt in the management of the bleeding complications of portal hypertension. Ann Surg 196:664–668, 1982.

115. Warren W, Zeppa R, Fomon J: Selective transsplenic decompression of gastroesophageal varices by distal splenorenal shunt. Ann Surg 166:431, 1967.

116. Langer B, Rotstein L, Stone R: A prospective randomized trial of the selective distal splenorenal shunt. Surg Gynecol Obstet 150:45–48, 1980.

117. Harley H, Morgan T, Redeker A, et al: Results of a randomized trial of end-to-side portacaval shunt and distal splenorenal shunt in alcoholic liver disease and variceal bleeding. Gastroenterology 91:802–809, 1986.

118. Resnick R, Atterbury L, Grace N, et al: Distal splenorenal shunt versus portal systemic shunt: Current status of a controlled trial. Gastroenterology 77:433, 1979.

119. Rikkers L, Rudman D, Galambos J: A randomized controlled trial of distal splenorenal shunts. Ann Surg 188:271–282, 1978.

120. Millikan W, Warren W, Henderson J, et al: The Emory prospective randomized trial: Selective versus nonselective

121. Busuttil R, Brin B, Tompkins R: Matched control study of distal splenorenal and portacaval shunts in the treatment of bleeding esophageal varices. Am J Surg 138:62–67, 1979.

122. Busuttil R: Selective and nonselective shunts for variceal bleeding. A prospective study of 103 patients. Am J Surg 148:27–35, 1984.

123. Hen R, Halbfass H, Rossle M, et al: Mesocaval and distal splenorenal shunts: Effect on hepatic function, hepatic hemodynamics, and portal systemic encephalopathy. Klin Wochenschr 63:409–413, 1985.

124. Adson M, Van Heerden J, Ilstrup D: The distal splenorenal shunt. Arch Surg 119:609–614, 1984.

125. Busuttil R, Maywood B, Tompkins R: The Warren shunt in treating bleeding esophageal varices. West J Med 130:304–308, 1979.

126. Fulenwider J, Smith R, Millikan W, et al: Variceal hemorrhage in the veteran population. To shunt or not to shunt? Am Surg 50:264–269, 1984.

127. Lund R, Newkirk J: Peritoneo-venous shunting system for surgical management of ascites. Contemp Surg 14:31–45, 1979.

128. Maksoud J, Mies S: Distal splenorenal shunt in children. Ann Surg 195:401–405, 1982.

129. Martin E, Molnar J, Cooperman M, et al: Observations of fifty distal splenorenal shunts. Surgery 84:379–383, 1978.

130. Mosimman R, Loup P: Efficacy and risks of the distal splenorenal shunt in the treatment of bleeding esophageal varices. Am J Surg 133:163–168, 1977.

131. Silver D, Puckett C, McNeer J: Evaluation of selective transsplenic decompression of gastroesophageal varices. Am J Surg 127:30–34, 1974.

132. Warren W, Millikan W, Henderson J: The years of portal hypertension surgery at Emory. Ann Surg 195:530–542, 1982.

133. Warren W, Henderson J, Millikan W, et al: Management of variceal bleeding in patients with noncirrhotic portal vein thrombosis. Ann Surg 207:623–634, 1988.

134. Warren W, Millikan W: Selective transsplenic decompression procedure: Changes in technique after 300 cases. Contemp Surg 18:11–29, 1981.

135. Henderson J, Millikan W, Chippani J: The incidence and natural history of thrombus in the portal vein following distal splenorenal shunts. Ann Surg 196:1–7, 1982.

136. Rousselot L: The role of congestion (portal hypertension) in so-called Banti's syndrome: A clinical and pathological study of thirty-one cases with late results following splenectomy. JAMA 107:1788–1793, 1936.

137. Thompson W: The pathogenesis of Banti's disease. Ann Intern Med 14:255–262, 1940.

138. Pemberton J, Kiernan P: Surgery of the spleen. Surg Clin North Am 25(4):880–890, 1945.

139. Suguira M, Futagawa S: A new technique for treating esophageal varices. J Thorac Cardiovasc Surg 66:677–685, 1973.

140. Strauch G: Supradiaphragmatic splenic transposition. Am J Surg 119:379–384, 1970.

141. McClelland R, Bashour F: Supradiaphragmatic transposition of the spleen in portal hypertension. Arch Surg 98:175–179, 1969.

142. Peters R, Womack N: Surgery of vascular distortions in cirrhosis of the liver. Ann Surg 154:432, 1961.

143. Keagy B, Schwartz J, Johnson G: Should ablative operations be used for bleeding esophageal varices? Ann Surg 203:463–469, 1986.

144. Boerema I: Surgical therapy of bleeding varices of esophagus during hepatic cirrhosis and Banti's disease. Ned Tijdschr Geneeskd 93:4174–4182, 1949.

145. Crile GJ: Transesophageal ligation of bleeding esophageal varices. Arch Surg 61:654–660, 1950.

146. Wirthlin L, Linton R, Ellis D: Transthoracoesophageal ligation of bleeding esophageal varices. Arch Surg 109:688–692, 1974.

147. Wexler M: Treatment of bleeding esophageal varices by

transabdominal esophageal transection with the EEA stapling instrument. Surgery *88*:406–416, 1980.

148. Cooperman M, Fabri P, Martin E, et al: EEA esophageal stapling for control of bleeding varices. Am J Surg *140*:821–824, 1980.

149. Delaney J: A method for esophagogastric devascularization. Surg Gynecol Obstet *150*:899–900, 1980.

150. Suguira M, Futagawa S: Further evaluation of the Suguira procedure in the treatment of esophageal varices. Arch Surg *112*:1317–1321, 1977.

151. Koyarna K, Takagi Y, Ouchi K, et al: Results of esophageal transection for esophageal varices. Am J Surg *139*:204–209, 1980.

152. Suguira M, Futagawa S: Results of six hundred thirty-six esophageal transections with paraesophagogastric devascularization in the treatment of esophageal varices. J Vasc Surg *1*:254–260, 1984.

153. Superina R, Weber J, Shandling B: A modified Suguira operation for bleeding varices in children. J Pediatr Surg *18*:794–799, 1983.

154. Weese J, Starling J, Yale C: Control of bleeding esophageal varices by transabdominal esophageal transection, gastric devascularization and splenectomy. Surg Gastroenterol *3*:31–36, 1984.

155. Wanamaker S, Cooperman M, Carey L: Use of the EEA stapling instrument for control of bleeding esophageal varices. Surgery *94*:620–626, 1983.

156. Wexler M: Esophageal procedures to control bleeding from varices. Surg Clin North Am *63*:905–914, 1983.

157. Spence R, Anderson J, Johnston G: Twenty-five years of injection sclerotherapy for bleeding varices. Br J Surg *72*:195–198, 1985.

158. Huizinga W, Angorn I, Baker L: Esophageal transection versus injection sclerotherapy in the management of bleeding esophageal varices in patients of high risk. Surg Gynecol Obstet *160*:539–546, 1985.

159. Colapinto R, Stronell R, Birch S, et al: Creation of an intrahepatic portosystemic shunt with a Gruntzig balloon catheter. Can Med Assoc J *126*:267–268, 1982.

160. Roberts J, Ring E, Lake JR, et al: Intrahepatic portacaval shunt for variceal hemorrhage prior to liver transplantation. Transplantation *52*:160–162, 1991.

161. Richter G, Noeledge G, Palmaz J, et al: The transjugular intrahepatic portosystemic stent-shunt (TIPSS): Results of a pilot study. Cardiovasc Int Radiol *13*:200–207, 1990.

162. LaBerge JM, Ring E, Lake J, et al: Transjugular intrahepatic portosystemic shunts: Preliminary results in 25 patients. J Vasc Surg *16*:258–267, 1992.

163. Iwatsuki S, Starzl T, Todo S, et al: Liver transplantation in the treatment of bleeding esophageal varices. Surgery *104*:697–705, 1988.

164. Reyes J, Iwatsuki S: Current management of portal hypertension with liver transplantation. Adv Surg *25*:189–208, 1992.

165. Brems J, Hiatt J, Klein A, et al: Effect of a prior portasystemic shunt on subsequent liver transplantation. Ann Surg *209*:51–56, 1989.

166. Crafoord C, Frencker P: New surgical treatment of varicose veins of the esophagus. Acta Otolaryngol *27*:422, 1939.

167. Johnston G, Rodgers H: A review of 15 years experience in the use of sclerotherapy in the control of acute hemorrhage for esophageal varices. Br J Surg *60*:797–799, 1973.

168. Paquet K, Kalk J, Koussouris P: Immediate endoscopic sclerosis of bleeding esophageal varices: A prospective evaluation over 5 years. Surg Endosc *2*:18–23, 1988.

169. Schubert T, Smith O, Kirkpatrick S, et al: Improved survival in variceal hemorrhage with emergent sclerotherapy. Am J Gastroenterol *82*:1134–1137, 1987.

170. Terblanche J, Northover J, Bornman P, et al: A prospective evaluation of injection sclerotherapy in the treatment of acute bleeding esophageal varices. Surgery *85*:239–245, 1979.

171. Terblanche J, Yakoob H, Bornman P, et al: Acute bleeding

172. Paquet K, Feussner H: Endoscopic sclerosis and esophageal balloon tamponade in acute hemorrhage from esophagogastric varices: A prospective controlled randomized trial. Hepatology *5*:580–583, 1985.

173. Larson A, Cohen H, Zweiban B, et al: Acute esophageal variceal sclerotherapy: Results of a prospective randomized controlled trial. JAMA *255*:497–500, 1986.

174. Barsoum M, Bolous F, El-Rooby A, et al: Tamponade and injection sclerotherapy in the management of bleeding oesophageal varices. Br J Surg *69*:76–78, 1982.

175. Project CEVS (Copenhagen Esophageal Varices Sclerotherapy Project): Sclerotherapy after first variceal hemorrhage in cirrhosis: A randomized multicenter trial. N Engl J Med *311*:1594–1600, 1984.

176. Westaby D, MacDougall B, Williams R: Improved survival following injection sclerotherapy for esophageal varices: Final analysis of a controlled trial. Hepatology *5*:827–830, 1985.

177. Terblanche J, Bornman P, Kahn D, et al: Failure of repeated injection sclerotherapy to improve long-term survival after esophageal variceal bleeding: A five year prospective controlled clinical trial. Lancet *2*(8363):1328–1332, 1983.

178. Soderlund C, Ihre T: Endoscopic sclerotherapy v. conservative management of bleeding oesophageal varices. Acta Chir Scand *151*:449–156, 1985.

179. Korula J, Balart L, Radvan G, et al: A prospective randomized controlled trial of chronic esophageal variceal sclerotherapy. Hepatology *5*:584–589, 1985.

180. Cello J, Grendell J, Crass R, et al: Endoscopic sclerotherapy versus portacaval shunt in patients with severe cirrhosis and variceal hemorrhage. N Engl J Med *311*:1589–1594, 1984.

181. Cello J, Grendell J, Crass R, et al: Endoscopic sclerotherapy versus portacaval shunt in patients with severe cirrhosis and acute variceal hemorrhage. Long-term follow-up. N Engl J Med *316*:11–15, 1987.

182. Warren W, Henderson J, Millikan W, et al: Distal splenorenal shunt versus endoscopic sclerotherapy for long-term management of variceal bleeding: Preliminary report of a prospective, randomized trial. Ann Surg *203*:454–462, 1986.

183. Teres J, Bordas J, Bravo D, et al: Sclerotherapy vs. distal splenorenal shunt in the elective treatment of variceal hemorrhage: A randomized controlled trial. Hepatology *7*:430–436, 1987.

184. Rikkers L, Burnett D, Volentine G, et al: Shunt surgery versus endoscopic sclerotherapy for long-term treatment of variceal bleeding: Early results of a randomized trial. Ann Surg *206*:261–271, 1987.

185. Burroughs A, Hamilton G, Phillips A, et al: A comparison of sclerotherapy with staple transection of the esophagus for the emergency control of bleeding from esophageal varices. N Engl J Med *321*:857–862, 1989.

186. Teres J, Baroni R, Bordas M, et al: Randomized trial of portacaval shunt, stapling transection and endoscopic sclerotherapy in uncontrolled variceal bleeding. J Hepatol *4*:159–167, 1987.

187. Terblanche J, Bornman P, Kirsch R: Sclerotherapy for bleeding esophageal varices. Annu Rev Med *35*:83–94, 1984.

188. Yassim Y, Sherif S: Randomized controlled trial of injection sclerotherapy for bleeding esophageal varices. Ann Br J Surg *70*:20–22, 1983.

189. Reilly J, Schade R, Roh M, et al: Esophageal variceal sclerosis. Surg Gynecol Obstet *155*:497–502, 1982.

190. Palani L, Abvabara S, Kraft A, et al: Endoscopic sclerotherapy in acute variceal hemorrhage. Am J Surg *141*:164–168, 1981.

191. Lewis J, Chung R, Allison J: Sclerotherapy of esophageal varices. Arch Surg *115*:476–480, 1980.

192. Johnston G: Bleeding esophageal varices: The management of shunt rejects. Ann R Coll Surg Engl *63*:3–8, 1981.

193. Goodale R, Silvis S, O'Leary J, et al: Early survival for bleed-

ing esophageal varices. Surg Gynecol Obstet *155*:523–528, 1982.

194. Lewis J, Chung R, Allison J: Injection sclerotherapy for control of acute variceal hemorrhage. Am J Surg *142*:592–595, 1981.

195. Cohen L, Rorsten M, Scherl E, et al: Bacteremia after endoscopic injection sclerosis. Gastrointest Endosc *29*:198–200, 1983.

196. Bacon A, Bauley-Newton R, Connors A: Pleural effusions after endoscopic variceal sclerotherapy. Gastroenterology *88*:1910–1914, 1985.

197. Tripodis S, Buenskin A, Wenser J: Gastric ulcers after endoscopic sclerosis of esophageal varices. J Clin Gastroenterol *7*:77–79, 1985.

198. Bengmark S, Borjesson B, Hoevels J, et al: Obliteration of esophageal varices by PTP. Ann Surg *190*:549, 1979.

199. Widrich W, Willard C, Robbins A, et al: Esophagogastric variceal hemorrhage: Its treatment by percutaneous transhepatic coronary vein occlusion. Arch Surg *113*:1331–1338, 1978.

200. Mendez G, Russell E: Gastrointestinal varices: Percutaneous transhepatic therapeutic embolization in 54 patients. AJR *135*:1045–1050, 1980.

201. Gembarowicz R, Kelly J, O'Donnell T, et al: Management

of variceal hemorrhage: Results of a standardized protocol using vasopressin and transhepatic embolization. Arch Surg *115*:1160–1164, 1980.

202. Yune H, O'Connor K, Klatte E, et al: Ethanol thrombotherapy of esophageal varices. AJR *144*:1049–1053, 1985.

203. Benner K, Keefe E, Keller E, et al: Clinical outcome after percutaneous transhepatic obliteration of esophageal varices. Gastroenterology *85*:146–153, 1983.

204. Stanley M: Treatment of intractable ascites in patients with alcoholic cirrhosis by peritoneovenous (LeVeen) shunting. Med Clin North Am *63*:523–536, 1979.

205. Frakes J: Physiologic considerations in the medical management of ascites. Arch Intern Med *140*:620–623, 1980.

206. LeVeen H, Christovadias G, Ip M, et al: Peritoneo-venous shunting for ascites. Ann Surg *180*:580, 1974.

207. Harman D, Demirjian Z, Ellman L, et al: Disseminated intravascular coagulation with the peritoneovenous shunt. Ann Intern Med *90*:774–776, 1979.

208. Reinhardt G, Stanley M: Peritoneovenous shunting for ascites. Surg Gynecol Obstet *145*:419–424, 1977.

209. Epstein M: Peritoneovenous shunt in the management of ascites and the hepatorenal syndrome. Gastroenterology *82*:790–799, 1982.

210. Fullen W: Hepatorenal syndrome: Reversal by peritoneovenous shunt. Surgery *83*:337–341, 1977.

REVIEW QUESTIONS

1. A 35-year-old female with a history of viral hepatitis and cirrhosis, status postcholecystectomy, presents with variceal hemorrhage unresponsive to medical therapy. Which surgical procedure is indicated if sclerotherapy fails?
   - (a) end-to-side portacaval shunt
   - (b) side-to-side portacaval shunt
   - (c) H mesocaval shunt
   - (d) EEA abdominal esophageal transection
   - (e) distal splenorenal shunt

2. A 10-year-old male with a history of omphalitis presents with his first episode of variceal hemorrhage. Which is the most appropriate therapy?
   - (a) distal splenorenal shunt
   - (b) medical regimen
   - (c) variceal sclerotherapy
   - (d) end-to-side portacaval shunt
   - (e) H mesocaval shunt

3. Specific contraindications to peritoneovenous shunts include all of the following except:
   - (a) hepatic necrosis
   - (b) bilirubin greater than 6
   - (c) hepatorenal syndrome
   - (d) infected ascitic fluid
   - (e) prothrombin time more than 4 seconds prolonged

4. Prophylactic portacaval shunts have been shown to:
   - (a) prolong longevity
   - (b) decrease encephalopathy
   - (c) have a greater than 50 per cent recurrent hemorrhage rate
   - (d) be associated with a prohibitively high operative mortality
   - (e) not be indicated

5. The Budd-Chiari syndrome may be treated by all of the following except:
   - (a) anticoagulants
   - (b) side-to-side portacaval shunt
   - (c) end-to-side portacaval shunt
   - (d) mesoatrial shunt
   - (e) mesocaval shunt

6. Technical considerations in favor of performing a distal splenorenal shunt include:
   - (a) cavernomatous transformation of the splenic vein
   - (b) acute hyaline necrosis
   - (c) splenic vein greater than 4 mm in diameter
   - (d) intractable ascites
   - (e) hepatopetal flow

7. False statements regarding sclerotherapy include:
   - (a) percutaneous transhepatic coronary vein occlusion is associated with a 20 per cent portal vein thrombosis rate
   - (b) sclerotherapy should not be used in the acute setting because of a higher mortality
   - (c) Sodium morrhuate and ethanolamine oleate are appropriate sclerosing agents
   - (d) repeated sclerotherapy is necessary for control of hemorrhage
   - (e) esophageal ulcerations usually resolve spontaneously without sequelae

8. Advantages of selective shunts are:
   - (a) continued portal perfusion
   - (b) gastric and esophageal varix decompression
   - (c) no greater incidence of shunt thrombosis than with portacaval shunts
   - (d) decreased incidence of encephalopathy
   - (e) all of the above

9. A 40-year-old male presents with hematemesis and

hypotension. Initial diagnostic measures to be performed after stabilization include:

(a) superior mesenteric arteriography
(b) splenoportography
(c) esophagogastroscopy
(d) celiac angiogram with venous phase
(e) upper gastrointestinal series

10. The most common site(s) of obstruction causing portal hypertension in the Western world is/are:

(a) portal vein thrombosis
(b) extrahepatic postsinusoidal
(c) intrahepatic presinusoidal
(d) intrahepatic sinusoidal and postsinusoidal
(e) extrahepatic presinusoidal

ANSWERS

1. c	2. b	3. c	4. e	5. c	6. e	7. b
8. e	9. c	10. d				

41
VENOUS THROMBOEMBOLIC DISEASE

LAZAR J. GREENFIELD

The critical connection between venous thrombosis and pulmonary thromboembolism was made by Virchow in 1856. He not only proved by experimental studies that venous thrombi would embolize to the lungs, but also defined the triad of mechanisms by which intravascular thrombosis could occur. This triad remains the basis of our understanding of the disorder and consists of stasis, vessel wall injury, and hypercoagulability of the blood. The importance of the disorder is reflected in the estimates of the development of deep venous thrombosis (DVT) in more than 500,000 hospital patients in the United States each year and a mortality rate of more than 50,000 deaths/year from pulmonary thromboembolism. Of the patients who survive their DVT, more than half will develop chronic venous insufficiency with its disabling edema and potential stasis ulcerations, representing a costly outcome in terms of lost productivity and demands on health care services. In the older patient with "idiopathic" DVT, there is increased likelihood that this presentation represents the first manifestation of a hidden malignancy as originally described by Trousseau.[1] Recently, it has been demonstrated in some tumors that this prothrombotic state is due to the elaboration of tissue factor, which may either activate procoagulant proteins or stimulate the release of a protease from circulating blood cells, thus activating the coagulation cascade.[2,3]

In postoperative and posttrauma patients, stasis is probably the most important and most treatable of the etiological factors. When venous contrast medium is injected into the feet of supine immobilized patients, it may remain in soleal vein valvular sinuses for as long as an hour. This is the favored location for the formation of a nidus of thrombus. The original thrombus may become attached to the opposite wall, causing interruption of flow, retrograde thrombosis, and signs of venous stasis in the extremity. Subsequent edema formation within the confines of the deep muscular fascia produces pain. However, the thrombus may propagate without interrupting flow and develop a long floating "tail" that is highly susceptible to breaking loose from its tenuous anchor

within the valvular sinus. It is this sequence of events that is the most dangerous aspect of the disorder, since major pulmonary embolism can occur without premonitory signs or symptoms at its point of origin.

The site of venous obstruction determines the level at which swelling is observed clinically. Swelling at the thigh level always implies obstruction at the level of the iliofemoral system, whereas swelling of the calf or foot suggests obstruction at the femoropopliteal level. Autopsies suggest that it is more common for thrombi to originate in the soleal veins, and then propagate proximally in 20 to 30 per cent of cases.[4,5] There is also evidence of primary thrombosis of femoral and iliac venous tributaries.

In addition to stasis, hypercoagulability must be considered as a causative factor. Earlier efforts to find differences in coagulation factors among patients with or without deep venous thrombosis were unrewarding, but there is a naturally occurring inhibitor of activated factor X called antithrombin III. Congenital deficiency in antithrombin III levels has been found to predispose patients to venous thrombosis and pulmonary embolism, and similar susceptibility occurs with deficiencies of protein C, protein S, or heparin cofactor II. Other unexplained hypercoagulable states seem to be associated with recent trauma, major surgical procedures, and sepsis. When stasis develops, the substances that promote platelet aggregation, including activated factor X, thrombin, fibrin, and catecholamines, remain at high concentration in a particular area. This leads to platelet aggregation, which initiates coagulation and thrombin generation with release of adenosine diphosphate (ADP), which further aggregates platelets as the fibrin complex propagates. Opposing this process is the fibrinolytic system of the blood and vein walls. The endothelium of the vein wall contains an activator that converts plasminogen to plasmin, which lyses fibrin. As might be expected, however, the fibrinolytic system is inhibited after surgery and trauma, and there is less activity in the veins of the lower extremity than in the upper extremity. Inadequate fibrinolytic activity has been associated both with adequate levels of nonfunctioning plasminogen and with low levels of adequately functioning plasminogen.[3] The third major causative factor of Virchow's triad is vessel wall damage, which usually is not demonstrable in areas of thrombosis. Obesity, aging, and malignancy also increase the risk of developing DVT by mechanisms that are not well understood.

DIAGNOSIS

Major venous thrombosis involving the deep venous system of the thigh and pelvis produces a characteristic but nonspecific clinical picture of pain, extensive pitting edema, and blanching that has been termed "phlegmasia alba dolens." Association with pregnancy may derive from hormonal effects on blood, relaxation of vessel walls, or mechanical compression of the left iliac vein at the pelvic brim, giving rise to the term "milk leg of pregnancy." It was originally believed that the blanching was due to spasm and compromise of arterial flow, but it is the subcutaneous edema that is responsible for the blanching. In addition to pregnancy, mechanical factors that can affect the left iliac vein include compression from the right iliac artery or an overdistended bladder and congenital webs within the vein. These factors are responsible for the observed 4:1 preponderance of left versus right iliac vein involvement.

With further progression of venous thrombosis to impede most of the venous return from the extremity, there is danger of limb loss from cessation of arterial flow. The clinical picture is characteristic, with sufficient congestion to produce phlegmasia cerulea dolens, or a painful blue leg. With the loss of sensory or motor function, venous gangrene is likely unless blood flow is restored. A variant of this disorder occurs peripherally in the leg and is associated with concurrent malignant disease and a high mortality rate.

As indicated earlier, these major complications represent less than 10 per cent of the patients with venous thrombosis. In fact, only 40 per cent of patients with venous thrombosis have any clinical signs of the disorder. In addition, false-positive clinical signs occur in up to 50 per cent of patients studied. Because of this there is a great deal of interest in the development of better diagnostic tests. Of course, contrast venography provides direct evidence of both occlusive and nonocclusive thrombi, but it is invasive and requires movement of the patient to a radiographic suite. In addition, there is interobserver disagreement regarding interpretation of the study in 10 per cent of cases, and in an additional 5 per cent, the study is not technically possible or the result is not diagnostic.[6]

Duplex Examination

The Doppler probe can be used at the bedside to detect major venous thrombi with a high degree of accuracy, but it is a subjective form of testing dependent on the examiner's experience. The principle is straightforward and is based on the impairment of an accelerated flow signal produced by intraluminal thrombi. The examination begins at the ankle with identification of the posterior tibial vein signal adjacent to the artery. The flow signal should be altered by distal and proximal compression producing, respectively, augmentation and interruption of flow. The same maneuvers are repeated over the superficial and deep femoral veins and can be done over the popliteal vein. Failure to augment flow on compression below or release of interruption of flow above the probe suggests venous thrombi. The sensitivity of the test exceeds 90 per cent, but the specificity is 5 to 10 per cent lower owing to the interference with venous flow by other mechanical problems (e.g., Baker's cyst, hematoma). A negative Doppler ultrasound examination is reassuring, but a positive or equivocal test should be confirmed by B-mode ultrasound imaging. A negative test is not reassuring when thromboembolism is suspected, because the thrombus may have been evacuated from the extremity. The test is also less sensitive to calf vein thrombi, but it can be used in patients who are wearing a plaster cast.

Real-time B-mode ultrasonography to visualize extremity veins has gained wide acceptance and offers a more direct technique to visualize intraluminal thrombus noninvasively.[7] The probe can visualize valvular movement and accelerated blood flow in the presence of a partially obstructing thrombus. When pressure is applied by the probe, normal vein walls are easily compressed, but resistance to compression is noted when thrombus is present, increasing with increased age of the thrombus. Chronic thrombi also show more bright echogenicity, heterogeneity, and an irregular surface. The addition of color to the duplex scan has increased the sensitivity and specificity of the study in symptomatic patients with proximal DVT to 96 and 100 per cent, respectively, with a negative predictive value of 98 per cent and accuracy of 99 per cent.[8] Acceptance of this technique has reduced the need for venography.

Plethysmography

Impedance plethysmography measures the volume response of the extremity to temporary occlusion of the venous system. The diagnosis of venous thrombosis depends on the changes in venous capacitance and rate of emptying after release of the occlusion. A proximal thigh cuff is inflated to 40 to 50 mm Hg pressure for 50 to 120 seconds or until maximum filling has occurred by plateau of the electrical signal. The inflation cuff is then rapidly deflated, allowing rapid outflow and reduction of volume in a normal limb. Prolongation of the outflow wave suggests major venous thrombosis with 95 per cent accuracy and is much more reliable than any voluntary technique of venous occlusion. The deficiency with this technique, as with all of the noninvasive methods, is in its detection of calf vein thrombosis or definition of new pathology in patients with old postthrombotic sequelae. The strain gauge plethysmograph can also be used to make therapeutic decisions in the absence of clinical conditions that can produce false-positive results, such as cardiac failure, constrictive pericarditis, hypotension, arterial insufficiency, or external compression of veins.

Air plethysmography is a noninvasive technique that measures absolute limb blood volume change. It provides quantification of venous reflux, muscle pump action, venous capacitance, and noninvasive ambulatory venous pressure, thus providing a useful index of the severity of venous disease. It is used primarily to quantitate chronic venous insufficiency.

Venography

The injection of contrast material for direct visualization of the venous system of the extremity is the most accurate method of confirming the diagnosis of venous thrombosis and the extent of the involvement. Injection is usually made into the foot while the superficial veins are occluded by a tourniquet. A supplementary injection into the femoral veins may be required to visualize the iliofemoral system. Both filling defects and nonvisualization can be found and provide an assessment of the threat of a thrombus, such as from one seen to be floating free and extending into the iliofemoral system. This finding has been associated with a greatly increased risk of thromboembolism despite anticoagulation.[9] Potential false-positive examinations may result from external compression of a vein or washout of the contrast material from collateral veins. This procedure can also be performed with isotope injection using a gamma scintillation counter to record flow of the isotope. Delayed imaging of persistent "hot spots" may also reflect isotope retention at the sites of thrombus formation. A perfusion lung scan can also be obtained for baseline comparison and to detect silent embolism. Recent experimental work with ^{99m}Tc-labeled Fab' fragments of antifibrin antibody in an animal model demonstrated visualization of fresh and aged thrombus. This technique employs antifibrin rather than antiplatelet monoclonal antibodies, which provides more direct targeting. The few clinical trials done to date are encouraging but not adequate.[10,11]

Assay of Fibrin/Fibrinogen Products

The degradation of intravascular fibrin can be detected by measuring the plasma products of the lysis of fibrin or fibrinogen. Both fibrinopeptide A and fibrin fragment E can be detected by radioimmunoassay, but these are not specific for acute venous thrombosis. A negative test result could conceivably

have some value in ruling out the diagnosis, but the tests are difficult and will require more investigation and simplification. D-Dimers or cross-linked degradation products serve as markers for the action of plasmin or fibrin. Thrombin–antithrombin III (TAT) complexes in plasma are correlated with activation of coagulation. These factors lack specificity as indicators of thromboembolic disease but, if sensitive enough, may be useful in ruling out DVT in certain subgroups.[12]

PROPHYLAXIS

In theory, the formation of venous thrombi should be prevented either by eliminating or reducing venous stasis or by altering blood coagulability. The belief that early ambulation prevents stasis and reduces the formation of thrombi has been controversial and is not supported by studies using tagged fibrinogen. One explanation of this is that early ambulation often consists of having the patient walk to a chair and sit, whereupon the legs are subjected to even more stasis.

There has been considerably more interest in the prophylactic use of anticoagulant drugs and drugs such as aspirin and dipyridamole that inhibit platelets, although most reports have shown no protection from the latter. However, there are strong data to support the use of preoperative oral anticoagulation therapy with coumarin derivatives in high-risk patients. Unfortunately, this increases the risk of hemorrhage, and with the added difficulties of laboratory control of prothrombin time, the approach has not been widely accepted. More recently the use of fixed "minidose" warfarin has been shown to be both safe and efficacious in various surgical and medical patients. This regimen offers protection against thromboembolism without the risks of hemorrhage or the cost of laboratory monitoring.[13-15] The administration of dextran 40, which produces a variety of effects on platelets and clotting factors, has been demonstrated to reduce the incidence of thrombi, but it too can produce hemorrhagic problems as well as allergic reactions and, in older patients, congestive failure.

In an effort to minimize the problems associated with anticoagulant prophylaxis, the current recommendation is to use heparin prior to and following surgery in low (minidose) doses that do not alter the laboratory clotting profile. Generally, a 5000-unit dose is given subcutaneously 2 hours preoperatively and then every 12 hours postoperatively for 5 days. This treatment has appeared to provide protection for most high-risk patients, with the exception of those undergoing orthopedic or urologic procedures. The beneficial effect may be due to the enhancement of heparin cofactor (antithrombin III) as a natural inhibitor of activated factor X. Kakkar and Lawrence showed protection against fatal pulmonary embolism in a randomized series of 4121 patients, as well as against DVT.[16]

For the general population of surgical patients under age 40 years, the risk of DVT is low, and prophylaxis can be limited to early ambulation with or without graduated compression stockings. For patients over age 40 undergoing major surgical procedures, the risk is moderate, and prophylaxis, such as intermittent pneumatic compression or low-dose heparin administered subcutaneously twice daily, should be considered. The patients at highest risk (age over 40 and obese, with malignant disease, history of DVT, or major trauma) need more protection, which might include low-dose heparin, sequential intermittent pneumatic compression, oral anticoagulants, or dextran. Low-dose heparin should not be used in neurosurgical patients, because of the consequences of any intracranial bleeding. For these patients, external pneumatic compression is the prophylaxis of choice.

As experience with use of the Greenfield vena caval filter has grown and percutaneous insertion has been facilitated by a no. 12-French carrier system, interest has increased in the prophylactic use of this device in high-risk patients who have additional risks from anticoagulants.[17-19] In many other countries the low molecular weight heparins (LMWHs) have been adopted as a primary method of prophylaxis in both general and orthopedic surgical patients.[20-22]

TREATMENT

Management of the patient with DVT must attempt to minimize the risk of pulmonary embolism, limit further thrombosis, and facilitate resolution of existing thrombi to avoid the postthrombotic syndrome. The patient is initially placed on bed rest, with the foot of the bed elevated 8 to 10 inches. Pain, swelling, and tenderness generally resolve over a 5- to 7-day period with anticoagulation, when ambulation with continued elastic stocking support can be permitted. Standing still and sitting should be prohibited in order to avoid increased venous pressure and stasis.

Anticoagulation

The foundation of therapy for DVT is adequate anticoagulation, initially with heparin and then with coumarin derivatives for prolonged protection against recurrent thrombosis. Unless there are specific contraindications, heparin should be administered in an initial dose of 100 to 150 units/kg intravenously. Heparin is an acid mucopolysaccharide that neutralizes thrombin, inhibits thromboplastin, and reduces the platelet release reaction. It may be administered by continuous or intermittent intravenous doses regulated by whole blood or activated partial thromboplastin clotting time. Bleeding complications can be minimized by doses of heparin that prolong the laboratory clotting determinations in the range of twice normal with no loss of effectiveness. Continuous intravenous

infusion regulated by an infusion pump seems to minimize the total dose required for control and is associated with a lower incidence of complications.

The LMWHs have also been used to treat thromboembolic disease. Early animal studies indicated that the LMWH fractions that are derived from standard heparin retained their ability to inhibit factor Xa while producing less bleeding. They also have a longer biologic half-life, making them an attractive alternative to unfractionated heparin. These LMWHs require additional testing as a therapeutic modality and are not available in the United States.[23-25]

The side effects associated with heparin treatment include bleeding, thrombocytopenia, hypersensitivity, arterial thromboembolism, and osteoporosis. Bleeding is more likely to occur in elderly females, in patients treated with aspirin, or in patients after recent surgery or trauma. It has been well demonstrated that bleeding can occur when the results of laboratory monitoring tests are within the therapeutic range, which may be due to the effect of heparin on platelets.

Arterial thromboembolism can complicate heparin administration by any route and is more common in the elderly. It tends to occur after 7 to 10 days of therapy and is associated with thrombocytopenia. This complication carries high morbidity and mortality rates and requires immediate cessation of heparin treatment. Thrombocytopenia is due to an immune reaction and is rapidly reversed when heparin is stopped, usually within 2 days. Hypersensitivity to heparin may take the form of a skin rash or, rarely, may produce anaphylaxis. Subcutaneous injections that show urticaria may become necrotic as an unusual form of sensitivity. Osteoporosis has been noted in patients on long-term heparin therapy in excess of 6 months. It is probably due to a direct effect on bone resorption and can be avoided by shorter periods of treatment and dosage less than 15,000 units/day.

Oral administration of anticoagulants is begun shortly after initiation of heparin therapy, since several days usually are required to bring the prothrombin time within the therapeutic range of 1.3 to 1.5 times the control value and to provide the optimal antithrombotic effect. It is also preferable to use a maintenance dose rather than a larger loading dose when initiating therapy, to avoid suppression of the natural anticoagulant, protein C. The coumarin derivatives block the synthesis of several clotting factors, and prolongation of the prothrombin time beyond the range suggested is associated with a high incidence of bleeding complications. Nonhemorrhagic side effects are uncommon but include skin necrosis, dermatitis, and a syndrome of painful erythema in areas of large amounts of subcutaneous fat. Most changes are reversible if the drug is stopped. Also, the administration of vitamin K or fresh-frozen plasma usually restores the prothrombin time. After an episode of acute DVT, anticoagulation should be maintained for a minimum of 3 months; some investigators favor 6 months for thrombi in the larger veins. Many drugs alter the pharmacodynamics of Coumadin by altering its metabolic clearance, rate of absorption, inhibition of vitamin K–dependent coagulation factor synthesis, or altering other hemostatic factors. Phenylbutazone, sulfinpyrazone, disulfiram, metronidazole, and trimethoprim sulfamethoxazole have all been shown to potentiate Coumadin's action.[26] Therefore a routine for regular monitoring of prothrombin time is essential after the patient leaves the hospital. In addition, levels of concurrent medications ought to be monitored, as Coumadin may compete for binding sites, thus altering plasma levels of these drugs. Oral anticoagulants are teratogenic and should not be used during established or planned pregnancy. In the pregnant patient, heparin is the drug of choice, and for long-term management subcutaneous self-administration should be taught. This regimen allows a normal delivery and can be continued postpartum.

Fibrinolysis

There has been great interest in the use of fibrinolytic agents to activate the intrinsic plasmin system. Tissue plasminogen activator, streptokinase, and urokinase have been used and found to be effective, although associated with a high incidence of hemorrhagic complications. Ten per cent of patients treated with streptokinase suffer allergic reactions, which vary from urticaria to anaphylaxis. In addition, streptokinase offers no advantage over heparin in the treatment of recurrent venous thrombosis or when thrombosis has existed for over 72 hours, and the lytic agents are contraindicated in the postoperative or posttraumatic patient. Rarely, the fibrinolytic agent has apparently lysed the attachment of the thrombus, allowing it to embolize. Even when thrombolysis is complete, preservation of valvular function does not occur.[27]

Regional intraarterial lysing of emboli has been demonstrated to be effective. Application of similar techniques to proximal deep venous thrombosis may offer the advantages of early thrombus resolution with long-term valve preservation, and a reduced incidence of the postthrombotic syndrome.[28–31] The use of new thrombolytic agents such as recombinant tissue-type plasminogen activator (rt-PA) and specialized catheters that allow localized administration of thrombolytics may provide improved therapy for deep vein thrombosis.

Surgical Approaches

Operative Thrombectomy

A direct surgical approach to remove thrombi from the deep veins of the leg by way of the common femoral vein has been employed and facilitated by the use of Fogarty venous balloon catheters and an elastic wrap for milking the extremity. Although the operative results are impressive, venograms obtained prior to discharge from the hospital show rethrombosis in most patients, and no reduction in the incidence of the postthrombotic syndrome. Consequently, the procedure is now usually reserved for limb salvage in the presence of phlegmasia cerulea dolens and impending venous gangrene.

Vena Cava Interruption

Adequate anticoagulation usually is effective in managing DVT, but if recurrent pulmonary embolism occurs during anticoagulant therapy or if there is a contraindication to anticoagulation, then a mechanical approach is necessary. Mechanical protection is also indicated as prophylaxis against recurrence of embolism for the patient who has required pulmonary embolectomy and for some high-risk patients who could not tolerate recurrence. There is current interest in extending prophylactic indications (Table 41–1).

Early surgical efforts to prevent recurrence of pulmonary embolism were directed toward bilateral ligation of the common femoral vein. The next approach was ligation of the inferior vena cava below the renal veins resulting in a sudden reduction in cardiac output. This effect, coupled with stasis sequelae and recurrent embolism through dilated collateral veins, led to efforts to compartmentalize the vena cava by means of sutures, staples, and external clips to provide filtration without occlusion.

The cone-shaped Greenfield filter was developed to prevent pulmonary embolism while maintaining caval patency, preventing lower extremity venous stasis and facilitating lysis of the embolus (Fig. 41–1). Prior to implementation of percutaneous placement techniques, the filter was commonly placed via the jugular vein; however, the femoral vein was used when the jugular vein was inadequate or there was an open neck wound. The recurrent embolism rate with this device has been 4 per cent, and its long-term patency rate exceeds 95 per cent.[32] The high caval patency rate makes it possible to position the

---

TABLE 41–1.   INDICATIONS FOR INSERTION OF A VENA CAVA FILTER

Recurrent thromboembolism in spite of adequate anticoagulation

Deep venous thrombosis or documented thromboembolism in a patient who has a contraindication to anticoagulation

Complication of anticoagulation forcing therapy to be discontinued

Chronic pulmonary embolism with associated pulmonary hypertension and cor pulmonale

Immediately following pulmonary embolectomy

Relative indications

    Patient who has more than 50 per cent of the pulmonary vascular bed occluded and who would not tolerate any additional embolism

    Patient with a propagating iliofemoral thrombus despite anticoagulation

    High-risk patient with a large free-floating iliofemoral thrombus on venogram

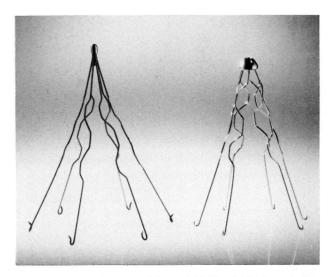

FIGURE 41–1.   The original Greenfield filter (*right*) is made from stainless steel and inserted via a no. 24-French carrier. The newer titanium model of the filter (*left*) is inserted via a no. 12-French carrier system.

filter above the renal vein when thrombus extends into the inferior vena cava or in young women of child-bearing potential. A long-term follow-up study of patients with suprarenal filters demonstrated the safety and efficacy of such placements.[32a]

The complications of filter insertion range in severity from minor wound hematoma due to early resumption of anticoagulation to potentially lethal migration of the device into the pulmonary artery, as documented with the Mobin-Uddin umbrella. The most common complication with the Greenfield filter has been misplacement, which has occurred in 7 per cent of cases. This rate fell to 4 per cent when the use of a guidewire became standard. When the filter is misplaced below the diaphragm, the patient has inadequate protection but the location (renal or iliac vein) poses no regional problem. A second filter can be placed in the appropriate location, or the misplaced filter can be retrieved using a modified guidewire,[33] which is always advocated if there has been misplacement into the right ventricle associated with a disturbance in cardiac rhythm or tricuspid insufficiency. Air embolism can occur during jugular insertion, but the risk is minimized by tilting the head down, or timing insertion with exhalation. In some patients, the veins may be too small or fragile to permit insertion of the carrier catheter, and rarely the patient may be too obese to permit fluoroscopy.

Recurrent embolism after filter placement has occurred in 2 to 4 per cent of cases and may be due to a source of thrombus outside of the filtered flow, such as the upper body veins or the right atrium. In one case, a tilted filter was found to have allowed proximal thrombus formation, but this responded to treatment with urokinase and oral anticoagulation.[32] Recurrent embolism is an indication for inferior venacavography to evaluate the filter for possible proximal thrombus. This is a rare finding and can be managed either by thrombolytic therapy if the amount of thrombus is small or by placement of a second filter in the suprarenal vena cava.

Secondary infection of captured thrombus within a Greenfield filter has been produced in the laboratory, but it was possible to sterilize the stainless steel filter and thrombus with a 2-week course of antibiotic therapy.[34] Sepsis is not a contraindication to filter insertion. The capture of a very large embolus within a filter may suddenly occlude the vena cava, with a precipitous fall in blood pressure. In a patient with known prior pulmonary embolism, this event can be mistaken for recurrent pulmonary embolism with disastrous results from vasopressor therapy. The basic distinction between functional hypovolemia of caval occlusion and right ventricular overload from recurrent pulmonary embolism can be made at the bedside by the measurement of central venous pressure and arterial oxygen tension. The response to volume resuscitation for the patient with sudden vena caval occlusion should be dramatic.

There is one circumstance in which migration of a Greenfield filter is possible after discharge; that is, when heparinized saline is not flushed through the cylindrical carrier and a thrombus forms within it during the period of positioning under fluoroscopy. The thrombus can then tether the limbs of the filter, preventing their expansion and fixation to the wall of the vena cava. Only one such episode has been reported to the author, and it remains a complication that can be completely avoided. For optimal protection, a continuous drip of heparinized saline can be attached by intravenous tubing directly to the insertion catheter. The improved technique of insertion over a guidewire should minimize this complication.[35]

PERCUTANEOUS FILTER INSERTION

Favorable experience with the Seldinger technique for percutaneous introduction of catheters and devices has led to considerable enthusiasm on the part of radiologists for utilizing this approach to insert a variety of innovative vena caval filter devices (Fig. 41–2). As early as 1977, a device was described made from Nitinol, which is a nickel/titanium alloy that exists as a pliable wire when cool, but rapidly transforms into a previously imprinted rigid shape when warmed.[36] The Nitinol filter has a cone shape with an overlying dome. Clinical experience with follow-up in 102 of 224 patients demonstrated a 4 per cent incidence of recurrent pulmonary embolism. There was a caval occlusion rate of 19 per cent. Insertion site thrombosis was observed in 11 per cent (Table 41–2). In a review of 20 patients there was a 25 per cent incidence of penetration, a 20 per cent incidence of occlusion, and a 10 per cent incidence of filter leg fracture.[37]

Another device, the Bird's Nest filter,[38] has also become popular because of its ease of insertion and consists of four stainless steel wires, each of which

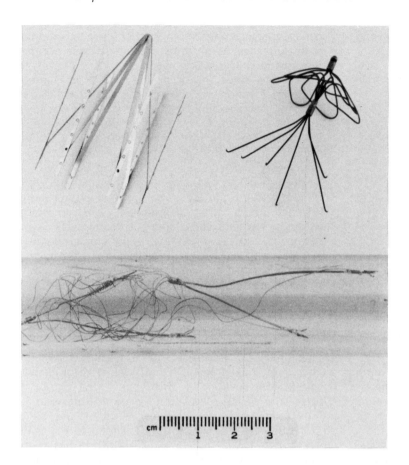

FIGURE 41–2. Alternative vena caval filters that have been developed for percutaneous introduction: Venatech filter (*top left*), Simon Nitinol filter (*top right*), and Bird's Nest filter (*bottom*).

is 25 cm long and 0.18 mm in diameter. The wires are intended to be packed into a 7-cm length of the vena cava to trap thromboemboli. In the largest series of patients, only 37 of the 481 patients in whom the filter had been in place for 6 months or more had objective evaluation at follow-up by means of cavography or ultrasound. Seven of them (19 per cent) had caval occlusion. A more significant problem with this device has been migration proximally after what appeared to be secure placement. This has been seen both experimentally and clinically, with published reports in five patients, including one death. Subsequent to this there had been a change in hook design in an effort to provide better fixation. Despite its small introducer system, the deployment of the device is more operator dependent than other vena caval filters. In addition, it requires 6 to 7 cm for adequate deployment, which is not always possible when the infrarenal caval segment is short, thus requiring placement extension into the iliac veins.[39]

Another recently introduced cone-shaped device known as the Venatech filter has added hooked stabilizers with sharp ends intended to center and fix the device. The initial experience was from France and consisted of 100 attempted insertions resulting in 98 filters discharged, 82 of which were positioned correctly.[40] Eight filters had a 15-degree tilt or more, five opened incompletely, and an additional three were both incompletely opened and tilted. Nine of

the filters migrated distally and four in a cephalad direction for a 13 per cent migration rate. At follow-up at 1 year there were seven occlusions (8 per cent), and recurrent pulmonary embolism occurred in two patients with incompletely opened filters. At later follow-up, 13 filters were observed to have migrated, nine to the iliac vein and four to the renal veins. More recent studies indicate a 2 per cent rate of recurrent pulmonary embolism, an 8 per cent caval occlusion rate, insertion site thrombosis in 23 per cent, migration greater than 10 mm in 14 per cent of those studied, and a 6 per cent incidence of incomplete opening (Table 41–2).

Although it is technically possible to insert the standard stainless steel Greenfield filter (SGF) percutaneously using a no. 28-French sheath, there is a higher incidence of insertion site venous thrombosis, in the range of 30 to 40 per cent.[41] However, the advantages of the percutaneous technique have prompted the development of a titanium Greenfield filter (TGF) that can be inserted through a no. 14-French sheath or operatively (Fig. 41–3). Clinical experience in 52 patients resulted in 51 placements (98 per cent), with the majority below the renal veins (90 per cent).[42] There was a 4 per cent recurrent embolism rate. At follow-up of 30 patients, averaging 5.2 months, all filters were patent and there were no proximal migrations. However, there was distal migration of 9 to 64 mm in nine patients (30 per cent)

TABLE 41–2.   COMPARISON OF INFERIOR VENA CAVAL FILTERS[a]

Characteristic	Greenfield Stainless Steel	Greenfield Titanium	Venatech	Bird's Nest	Simon Nitinol
Evaluation	Registry (1988)	Clinical trial (1991)	Clinical trial (1990)	Clinical trial (1988)	Clinical trial (1990)
Duration	12 years	30 days	1 year	6 months	6 months
Number	469	186 (123 at FU)	97 (77 at FU)	568 (440 at 6 months)	224 (102 at FU)
Recurrent PE	4%	3%	2%	2.7% (33–67% in subset with objective FU)	4% based upon those who had FU
Caval patency	98%	100%	92%	97%	81%
Filter patency	98%	Not reported	63% without thrombus	81%	Not reported
Insertion site DVT	41% (Percutaneous)	8.7%	23%	"Few" none objective	11%
Migration	35% > 3 mm	11% > 9 mm	14% > 10 mm	9% with original model	1.2% of those with FU
Penetration	Not reported	1%	Not reported	Not reported	0.6% of those with FU
Misplacement	4%	0.5%	Not reported	Not reported	Not reported
Incomplete opening	Not seen	2%	6%	Not reported	Not reported
Means of follow-up	PE, IVC scan, x-ray, noninvasive vascular exam	PE, x-ray, CT, (noninvasive vascular exam 2 sites)	Objective data are variable by site (cavagram, duplex, CT, x-ray)	Phone interview, objective data random & available for 40/440	Clinical, x-ray, lab

[a]FU, follow-up; PE, pulmonary embolism; DVT, deep venous thrombosis; IVC, inferior vena cava; CT, computed tomography.

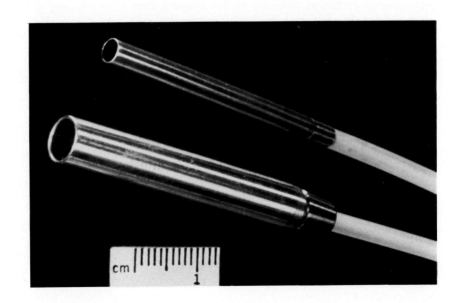

FIGURE 41–3. Comparison of the carrier systems used for the titanium Greenfield filter (*top*) and the standard stainless steel filter (*bottom*).

and tilting that increased from eight patients at insertion to 12 at follow-up. Insertion site venous thrombosis occurred in two patients (7 per cent) who were asymptomatic. Limb penetration of the vena cava was suspected in nine patients (30 per cent), but there were no clinical sequelae from this or the distal migrations. Although the clinical results of the TGF are comparable to the SGF, modifications of hook design were required to correct the tendency for wall penetration and distal migration. The filter was subsequently modified by adding an 80-degree angle to the hook, which provided greater stability in the vena cava. A multicenter study was completed in 186 patients, with a 3 per cent rate of recurrent pulmonary embolism. Initial incomplete opening was noted in 2 per cent of the cases and asymmetry of the legs in 5 per cent. Apparent movement of the filter greater than 9 mm occurred in 11 per cent of the patients and increased filter base diameter occurred in 14 per cent. Insertion site thrombosis was noted by duplex scanning in 9 per cent. The use of a sheath during insertion reduced the incidence of premature discharge, and the modification of the hook reduced migration and penetration noted with the initial titanium design.[43]

PULMONARY THROMBOEMBOLISM

The most serious complication of DVT is pulmonary thromboembolism, which is estimated to cause more than 50,000 deaths per year in the United States. It is difficult to know the exact incidence of the disorder, since the clinical diagnosis is inherently inaccurate and often confused with myocardial infarction, pneumothorax, sepsis, or pneumonia. Management of acute, massive pulmonary thromboembolism depends on an accurate diagnosis that documents the presence and location of intravascular thrombus. This usually requires angiography, which has the added advantage of allowing pressure measurement in the pulmonary circulation. Because of the inherent nonspecificity of the perfusion lung scan, scans are most useful as a screening test to exclude the diagnosis in patients with minor degrees of embolism. In suspected massive embolism, the patient should receive heparin sodium (150 to 200 units/kg) and be taken directly to the angiographic suite for selective pulmonary angiography. In addition to insertion of the angiographic catheter, usually through the femoral vein, a radial artery cannula is inserted for monitoring arterial blood gases, and anesthesia standby is requested should the patient require intubation and ventilatory control. If the patient's condition is too unstable for angiography and there are other objective signs of venous thrombosis or embolism, such as a prior scan showing large or multiple defects, it is reasonable to proceed to the operating room where the diagnosis can be confirmed under fluoroscopy by injection of contrast material through an embolectomy catheter.

Pulmonary Embolectomy

For those patients who sustain massive embolism producing systemic hypotension, management must be a coordinated and rapidly responsive effort, since survival may be only a matter of minutes. The initial approach to thromboembolism in patients who have either transient collapse or persistent systemic hypotension should include full heparinization and administration of inotropic drugs if necessary to support the circulation while the diagnosis is confirmed angiographically. For the patient with thromboembolism who responds to heparin sodium and does not require vasopressors to maintain systemic blood pressure or urine output, careful monitoring is essential to determine whether anticoagulation alone will control the disorder. Often the additional protection of a vena caval filter is indicated in the high-risk patient who would not tolerate another embolic event.

The high mortality associated with the Trendelenburg procedure of thoracotomy for pulmonary embolectomy prompted the use of extracorporeal circulation to bypass the impacted pulmonary circulation. Further experience showed that partial bypass support under local anesthesia using the femoral artery and vein could provide initial support to allow general anesthesia. Once the sternotomy was accomplished, the partial bypass could be converted to total bypass by insertion of a superior vena caval catheter. Then the pulmonary emboli could be removed through a pulmonary arteriotomy.

Although it is effective, open pulmonary embolectomy still has high mortality, and the most serious complication is uncontrollable pulmonary parenchymal hemorrhage, which may follow restoration of pulmonary perfusion. Consequently, open pulmonary embolectomy is most appropriate for patients who require closed cardiac massage to maintain blood pressure or for patients in whom the catheter embolectomy procedure fails to remove thrombi.

Transvenous Catheter Embolectomy

Access for insertion of the catheter is obtained by isolation of either the jugular or the common femoral vein (Fig. 41–4). It is technically easier and quicker to use the jugular vein, although in some patients the straighter route from the femoral vein and the opportunity to perform local thrombectomy may be advantageous. The absence of projecting thrombi in the pelvis above the level of insertion is confirmed by injection of contrast medium prior to advancement of the catheter. If thrombi are encountered, they can be extracted readily with a Fogarty catheter. The embolectomy catheter is filled with heparinized saline through an intravenous extension tube attached to the handle, and a guidewire may be used during introduction to facilitate positioning in the pulmonary artery, although it is rarely necessary. The cup-

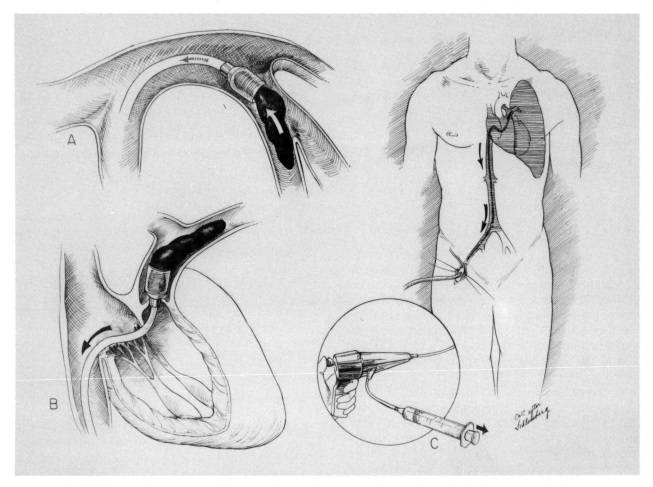

FIGURE 41–4. Technique of catheter embolectomy based on positioning the steerable cup catheter (*A*) adjacent to the embolus and using syringe suction to aspirate a portion of the embolus into the cup. The catheter is then withdrawn (*B*), maintaining syringe vacuum (*C*) as the embolus is removed. Repeated insertions are usually necessary to clear the pulmonary circuit and improve cardiac output.

catheter is inserted through a transverse venotomy, and the radiopaque cup is readily visualized under fluoroscopy as it is guided in the vena cava with the left hand while the right hand holds the control unit to provide tip deflection. Passage into the right ventricle is aided by medial angulation and anterior deflection, which then allow the cup to enter the pulmonary artery. Electrocardiographic monitoring should be maintained to detect premature ventricular contractions and other rhythm disturbances. The arrhythmias that occur during passage almost always respond to withdrawal or change in position of the catheter. The left main pulmonary artery is entered most easily, and the cup may then be positioned according to the angiographic location of the major embolus on that side (usually the left lower lobe). Entry into the right main pulmonary artery requires deflection of the cup in that direction as it reaches the superior edge of the heart shadow. Rotation of the tip also aids in advancement of the catheter. Juxtaposition of the cup and the embolus is confirmed by injection of 5 to 10 ml of contrast medium through the catheter.

A large syringe is attached to the control handle via the intravenous extension tubing, and the barrel is pulled back sharply by the assistant. A sustained jet of blood in the syringe can result if the cup is not in apposition to the thrombus, and a vacuum is produced if the embolus is suctioned into the cup. Sustained vacuum is used to hold the embolus in the cup as the entire catheter and attached embolus are withdrawn through the right ventricle, down the inferior vena cava or up the superior vena cava and out of the venotomy (Fig. 41–4). Multiple retrievals are usually necessary to remove additional emboli or fragments if the embolus cannot be withdrawn intact (Fig. 41–5). Any blood that is aspirated in the syringe can be returned to the patient. The cup should be cleansed for free passage of fluid and effective suctioning prior to each attempted retrieval. Although access and extraction from the jugular vein are easier technically in most patients, severe dyspnea in some patients may preclude this approach.

Emboli that are refractory to extraction are usually found in patients with a history of embolism of more than 72 hours and consequent fixation of the embolus

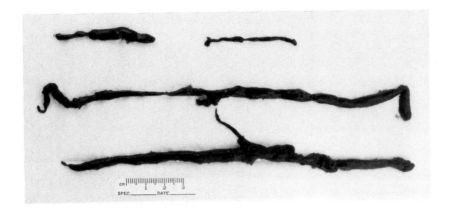

FIGURE 41–5. Specimens obtained during suction pulmonary embolectomy.

to the pulmonary arterial wall. In these patients, however, subsequent embolism usually is responsible for acute decompensation, and the unfixed emboli can often be retrieved to allow hemodynamic stabilization. If the patient remains in shock and no emboli have been extracted after 30 to 40 minutes, an inferior vena cava filter should be inserted and the patient taken to the operating room for open embolectomy on cardiopulmonary bypass.

Our recent clinical experience with the technique in 35 patients showed that emboli could be extracted in 32 (91 per cent), with overall survival of 77 per cent, which is similar to our earlier report.[44] In this series, open embolectomy during bypass also was performed for acute thromboembolism in nine patients, five of whom survived (55 per cent). The most common complication after catheter embolectomy is wound hematoma, due usually to resumption of heparin sodium administration within 12 hours of operation. Pulmonary infarctions occurred in two patients but not in areas where perfusion had been restored. Preventable deaths occurred in three patients, one from Swan-Ganz balloon rupture of the pulmonary artery and two from large-bolus contrast medium injection in the main pulmonary artery at the time of angiography. No myocardial damage has been seen with the steerable catheter. The procedure is always completed by insertion of a Greenfield filter to prevent recurrent embolism.

OTHER TYPES OF VENOUS THROMBOSIS

The term "thrombophlebitis" is usually applied to the disorder of the superficial veins characterized by a local inflammatory process that is usually aseptic. The cause in the upper limb is usually acidic fluid infusion or prolonged cannulation. In the lower extremities, it is usually associated with varicose veins and may coexist with DVT. The association with the injection of contrast material can be minimized by washout of the contrast material with heparinized saline.

Thrombophlebitis Migrans

Thrombophlebitis migrans, a condition of recurrent episodes of superficial thrombophlebitis, has been associated with visceral malignancy, systemic collagen vascular disease, and blood dyscrasias. Involvement of the deep veins and the visceral veins has also been described.

Subclavian Vein Thrombosis

Subclavian vein thrombosis is most likely to be secondary to an indwelling catheter and can occur in children. It may also occur as a primary event in a young, athletic person ("effort thrombosis"), presumably as a result of chronic compressive injury at the thoracic outlet. If the patient is seen late, there is usually a satisfactory response to elevation and anticoagulation, although some venous insufficiency and discomfort with exercise may persist. Pulmonary thromboembolism can occur from these thrombi, with an incidence of 12 per cent reported in two series. Although rarely necessary, we have inserted a Greenfield filter in the superior vena cava in an inverted position in two patients.

Increased use of the axillary and subclavian veins for diagnostic and therapeutic procedures has resulted in a higher incidence of traumatic and foreign body thrombosis. Often these thrombi are asymptomatic because of gradual onset, short segment involvement, or only partial occlusion. Thrombolytic therapy may be of value and should be considered with any acute subclavian vein thrombosis occurring within 3 to 4 days of onset.[45] If the thrombus lyses, a contrast venogram should be obtained to outline any anatomic site of compression that could be treated surgically. Direct venolysis with first rib or medial clavicular excision can be employed and should be considered for younger patients and manual laborers. Thrombectomy should always be performed in conjunction with creation of an ipsilateral arteriovenous fistula for angioaccess if there is proximal venous thrombosis. If the fistula is made without recognizing the proximal occlusion, the extremity may be endangered by massive edema. Operative correction is still possible without loss of the fistula, however, even if a jugular venous bypass is necessary, because the fistula will assist in maintaining patency of the repair or bypass.

Abdominal Vein Thrombosis

Thrombosis of the inferior vena cava can result from tumor invasion or propagating thrombus from the iliac veins. Most often, however, it results from ligation, plication, or insertion of occluding caval devices. Thrombosis of the renal vein is most likely to be associated with the nephrotic syndrome. It can be a source of thromboembolism and has been treated successfully by suprarenal placement of the Greenfield filter.[46]

Portal vein thrombosis may occur in the neonate, usually secondary to propagating septic thrombophlebitis of the umbilical vein. Collateral development leads to the occurrence of esophageal varices. Thrombosis of the portal, hepatic, splenic, or superior mesenteric vein in an adult can occur sponta-

neously, but usually it is associated with hepatic cirrhosis. Thrombosis of mesenteric or omental veins can simulate an acute abdomen but usually results in prolonged ileus rather than intestinal infarction.

Hepatic vein thrombosis (Budd-Chiari syndrome) usually produces massive hepatomegaly, ascites, and liver failure. It can be associated with a congenital web, endophlebitis, or polycythemia vera. Although some success has been reported using a direct approach to the congenital webs, the usual treatment is a side-to-side portacaval shunt to allow decompression of the liver or liver transplantation. The development of pelvic sepsis after abortion, tubal infection, or puerperal sepsis can lead to septic thrombophlebitis of the pelvic veins and septic thromboembolism. Ovarian vein and caval ligation has been the traditional treatment, but the emphasis should be on drainage or excision of the abscesses and appropriate antibiotic therapy. We have also used the Greenfield filter for septic thrombosis because the filter is inert stainless steel and does not lead to the development of an intraluminal abscess, which could occur after the traditional approach of ligation of the vena cava.[47] Long-term follow-up of patients with suprarenal filters has shown no obstruction and consequently no interference with renal function.

REFERENCES

1. Trousseau A: Phlegmasia Alba Dolens. Clinique Medicale de l'Hotel-Dieu de Paris, vol 3. Paris, JB Balliere et Fils, 1865, pp 654–712.
2. Maruyama M, Yagawa K, Kinjo M, et al: Presence of thrombosis inducing activity in plasma from patients with lung cancer. Am Rev Resp Dis *140*:778–781, 1989.
3. Perler B: Review of hypercoagulability syndromes: What the interventionalist needs to know. JVIR *2*:183–193, 1991.
4. Lohr JM, Kerr TM, Lutter KS, Cranley RD, Spirtoff K, Cranley JJ: Lower extremity calf thrombosis—to treat or not to treat. J Vasc Surg *14*:618–623, 1991.
5. White R, McGahan J, Daschbach M, Hartling R: Diagnosis of deep-vein thrombosis using duplex ultrasound. Ann Intern Med *111*:297–304, 1989.
6. Naidich J, Feinberg A, Karp-Harman H, Karmel M, Tyma C, Steink H: Contrast venography: Reassessment of its role. Radiology *168*:97–100, 1988.
7. Flanagan LD, Sullivan ED, Cranley JJ: Venous imaging of the extremities using real-time B-mode ultrasound. *In* Bergan JJ, Yao JST (eds): Surgery of the Veins. Orlando, FL, Grune & Stratton, 1985, p 89.
8. Rose S, Zwiebel W, Nelson B, et al: Symptomatic lower extremity deep venous thrombosis: Accuracy, limitations, and role of color duplex flow imaging in diagnosis. Radiology *175*:639–644, 1990.
9. Norris CS, Greenfield LJ, Barnes RW: Free-floating iliofemoral thrombosis: A risk of pulmonary embolism. Arch Surg *120*:806–808, 1985.
10. Walker KZ, Boniface GR, Phippard AF, Harewood W, Bautovich G, Bundesen P: Preclinical evaluation of 99m technetium-labeled DD-3B6/22 FAB for thrombus detection. Thromb Res *64*(6):691–701, 1991.
11. Pinson A, Becker D, Philbrick J, Pareckh J: Technetium-99m-RBC venography in the diagnosis of deep venous thrombosis of the lower extremity: A systemic review of the literature. J Nucl Med *32*(12):2324–2328, 1991.
12. Paiement GD, Desautels C: Deep vein thrombosis: Prophy-

laxis, diagnosis, and treatment-lessons from orthopedic studies. Clin Cardiol *13*:19–22, 1991.
13. Poller L, McKernan A, Thomson J, Elstein M, Hirsch P, Jones J: Fixed minidose warfarin: A new approach to prophylaxis against venous thrombosis after major surgery. Br Med J *295*:1309–1312, 1987.
14. Bern M, Lokich J, Wallach S, et al: Very low doses of warfarin can prevent thrombosis in central venous catheters. Ann Intern Med *112*:423–428, 1990.
15. MacCallum P, Thomson J, Poller L: Effects of fixed minidose warfarin on coagulation and fibrinolysis following major gynaecological surgery. Thromb Haemost *64*(4):511–515, 1990.
16. Kakkar VV, Carrigan TP, Spindler JR, et al: Efficacy of low doses of heparin in prevention of deep vein thrombosis after major surgery. A double-blind, randomized trial. Lancet *2*:101, 1972.
17. Walker H, Pennington D: Inferior vena caval filters in heart transplant recipients with perioperative deep vein thrombosis. J Heart Transplant *9*(5):579–580, 1990.
18. Fink J, Jones B: The Greenfield filter as the primary means of therapy in venous thromboembolic disease. Surg Gynecol Obstet *172*(4):253–256, 1991.
19. Brenner D, Brenner C, Scott J, Wehbert K, Granger J, Schellhammer P: Suprarenal Greenfield filter placement to prevent pulmonary embolus in patients with vena caval tumor thrombi. J Urol *147*:19–23, 1992.
20. Hirsh J: Rationale for development of low-molecular-weight heparins and their clinical potential in the prevention of postoperative venous thrombosis. Am J Surg *161*(4):512–518, 1991.
21. Haas S, Blumel G: An objective evaluation of the clinical potential of low molecular weight heparin in the prevention of thromboembolism. Semin Thromb Hemost *15*(4):424–434, 1989.
22. Hass S, Blumel G: Prophylaxis of thromboembolism with various low-molecular-weight heparins. Haemostasis *18*:82–87, 1988.

23. Kakkar V, Adams P: Preventive and therapeutic approach to venous thromboembolic disease and pulmonary embolism—can death from pulmonary embolism be prevented? J Am Coll Cardiol 8:146–158, 1986.

24. Nieuwenhuis H, Albada J, Banga JD, Sixma J: Identification of risk factors for bleeding during treatment of acute venous thromboembolism with heparin or low molecular weight heparin. Blood 78:2337–2343, 1991.

25. Albada J, Nieuwenhuis H, Sixma J: Treatment of acute venous thromboembolism with low molecular weight heparin (Fragmin). Circulation 80(4):935–940, 1989.

26. Hirsh J: Oral anticoagulant drugs. N Engl J Med 324(26):1865–1875, 1991.

27. Kakkar VV, Lawrence D: Hemodynamic and clinical assessment after therapy for acute deep vein thrombosis: A prospective study. Am J Surg 150:54, 1985.

28. Levine M, Weitz J, Turpie A, Andrew M, Cruickshank M, Hirsh J: Recombinant tissue plasminogen activator in patients with venous thromboembolic disease. Chest 97(4):168–171, 1990.

29. Valji K, Roberts A, Davis G, Bookstein J: Pulsed-spray thrombolysis of arterial and bypass graft occlusions. AJR 156:617–621, 1991.

30. Bookstein J, Fellmeth B, Roberts A, Valji K, Davis G, Machado T: Pulsed-spray pharmacomechanical thrombolysis: Preliminary clinical results. AJR 152:1097–1100, 1989.

31. Valji K, Bookstein J: Fibrinolysis with intrathrombic injection of urokinase and tissue-type plasminogen activator. Results in a new model of subacute venous thrombosis. Invest Radiol 22:23–27, 1987.

32. Greenfield LJ, Peyton R, Crute S, et al: Greenfield vena caval filter experience: Late results in 156 patients. Arch Surg 116:1451, 1981.

32a. Greenfield LJ, Cho KJ, Proctor MC, Sobel M, Shah S, Wingo J: Late results of suprarenal Greenfield filter placement. Arch Surg 127:969–973, 1992.

33. Greenfield LJ, Crute SL: Retrieval of Kimray-Greefield vena caval filter. Surgery 88:719, 1980.

34. Peyton JWR, Hylemon MB, Greenfield LJ, Crute SL, Sugarman JH, Qureshi GD: Comparison of Greenfield filter and vena caval ligation for experimental septic thromboembolism. Surgery 93:533–537, 1983.

35. Greenfield LJ, Stewart JR, Crute SL: Improved technique for Greenfield vena caval filter insertion. Surg Gynecol Obstet 156:217, 1983.

36. Simm M, Athanasoulis CA, Kim D, Steinberg FL, Porter DH, Byse BH, Kleshinski S, Geller S, Orran DE, Waltman AC: Simon Nitinol inferior vena cava filter: Initial clinical experience. Radiology 172:99–103, 1989.

37. McCowan T, Ferris E, Carver D, Molphus M: Complications of the Nitinol vena caval filter. JVIR 3:401–408, 1992.

38. Roehm JOF Jr, Johnsrude IS, Barth MH, Gianturco C: The bird's nest inferior vena cava filter progress report. Radiology 168:745–749, 1988.

39. Vesely T, Darcy M, Picus D, Hicks M: Technical problems associated with placement of the Bird's Nest inferior vena cava filter. Am J Roentgenol 158:875–880, 1992.

40. Ricco JB, Crochet D, Sebilotte P, Serradimigni A, Lefebvre JM, Barisson E, Geslin P, Virot P, Vaislic C, Gallet M, Biron Y, Lefant D, Dosmarq JM, DeLaFaye D: Percutaneous transvenous caval interruption with the "LGM" filter: Early results of a multicenter trial. Ann Vasc Surg 3:142–147, 1988.

41. Kantor A, Glanz S, Gordon DH, Sclafani SJA: Percutaneous insertion of the Kimray-Greenfield filter: Incidence of femoral vein thrombosis. Am J Roentgenol 149:1065–1066, 1987.

42. Greenfield LJ, Cho KJ, Tauscher JR: Limitations of percutaneous insertion of Greenfield filters. J Cardiovasc Surg 31:344–350, 1990.

43. Greenfield L, Cho KJ, Proctor M, et al: Results of a multicenter study of the modified hook titanium Greenfield filter. J Vasc Surg 14:253–257, 1991.

44. Greenfield LJ: Complications of venous thrombosis and pulmonary embolism. In Greenfield LJ (ed): Complications in Surgery and Trauma, 2nd ed. Philadelphia, JB Lippincott Company, 1989, pp 430–438.

45. Mealy K, Shanik DG: Axillary vein thrombosis—local treatment with streptokinase. Ir Med J 78:289, 1985.

46. Greenfield LJ, Peyton R, Crute SL: Hemodynamics and renal function following experimental suprarenal vena caval occlusion. Surg Gynecol Obstet 155:37, 1982.

47. Greenfield LJ, Michna BA: Twelve-year experience with the Greenfield vena caval filter. Surgery 104:706–712, 1988.

42

VARICOSE VEINS: Chronic Venous Insufficiency

JOHN J. BERGAN

In organizing knowledge of vascular surgery, it is important to categorize problems as they appear in a given patient. For example, arterial disease must be separated from venous problems. Venous problems divide themselves into acute thromboembolic events as opposed to chronic venostasis. This chapter treats the latter subject. Chronic venostasis disease is best divided into primary varicose veins, superficial venous incompetence, and deep venous incompetence, because primary varicose veins can be treated for cure, whereas chronic venous insufficiency due to deep vein pathophysiology is treatable but not curable.

VARICOSE VEINS

Varicose veins are a disease of western civilization in which more than half of adult men and two thirds of adult women have physically identifiable varicosities. More severe chronic venous insufficiency is found in nearly 20 per cent of working men and women. Varicose veins themselves range in severity from the undesirable appearance of venectasia or telangiectasia to protuberant, tortuous varicosities with or without associated dermatitis, cutaneous ulcerations, and severe pigmentation. Chronic venous insufficiency produces findings identical to primary venostasis.

The cause of varicose veins is linked to genetics and exacerbated by hormonal influence. Strangely, the appearance of varicose veins in childhood is rare, although examination in adolescents with a strong family history of varicosities reveals that some have venous valves that are incompetent. Primary varicose veins in the young adult are common. As with many common conditions, the precise etiology is difficult to define and must be multifactorial. The present state of knowledge of varicosities does not allow selection of treatment on the basis of etiology. Therefore, identification of precise cause is less important than careful planning and selection of treatment for an individual. It is sufficient to know that genetics is important in genesis of varicosities and that female hormones in general, and progesterone in particular, affect varicosities profoundly. For example, progesterone, the hormone of the second phase of a menstrual cycle and the principal hormone of pregnancy, causes passive dilation of varicosities under the influence of venous hypertension.

This fact is of importance in explaining clinical symptomatology. Observant women will know that their leg aching, heaviness, and tiredness caused by venous insufficiency is worse in the second 14 days of a menstrual cycle, and peaks just before a menstrual period or during the first 2 days of such period. Furthermore, the multiparous woman who is a good observer will note the appearance or exacerbation of symptoms of varicosities when she becomes pregnant, sometimes even before the first menstrual period is missed.

Cutaneous venectasias develop under the same influences and may become symptomatic similarly. It is important to know this because textbooks of venous disease in the past and recent present have referred to venectasias as cosmetic and not symptomatic. Ample documentation exists that this is not true. Effective treatment of venectasias can relieve symptoms of venostasis.

Primary varicosities consist of elongated, tortuous, superficial veins that are protuberant and contain incompetent valves. These produce the symptoms of mild swelling, heaviness, and easy fatigability. In this situation, the skin and subcutaneous tissue is normal and edema, when present, is mild.

Primary varicose veins merge imperceptibly into more severe, chronic venous insufficiency when swelling is moderate to severe, and there is an increased sensation of heaviness with larger varicosities, and early skin changes of mild pigmentation and subcutaneous induration appear. The induration is termed "liposclerosis" by the English. Here, edema is regularly present.

When chronic venous insufficiency becomes severe, there is marked swelling and calf pain following standing, sitting, or ambulation. Multiple, dilated veins are seen associated with varicose clusters and heavy, medial and lateral, supramalleolar skin pigmentation. Marked liposclerosis and scars from previously healed ulcerations or current ulceration are also noted.

The description above lends itself to anatomic classification in which grade 0 is asymptomatic, grade I is mild symptoms and findings, grade II is moderate symptoms and findings, and grade III is severe symptoms and findings.[2]

PATHOGENESIS

Fundamental defects in the strength and characteristics of the venous wall enter into the pathogenesis of varicose veins. These may be generalized or localized and consist of deficiencies in elastin and collagen. Furthermore, anatomic differences in the location of the superficial veins of the lower extremities also contribute to pathogenesis. For example, the main saphenous trunk is not always involved in varicose disease. This is because it contains a well-developed, medial fibromuscular layer and also is supported by fibrous connective tissue that binds it to the deep fascia. In contrast, tributaries to the long saphenous vein are less well supported in the subcutaneous fat superficial to the membranous layer of superficial fascia. These tributaries also contain less muscle mass in their walls. Thus these, and not the main trunk, become varicose regularly.[3]

When those fundamental anatomic peculiarities are recognized, then the intrinsic competence or incompetence of the valve system becomes important. For example, failure of a valve protecting a tributary vein from the pressures of the long saphenous vein will allow a cluster of varicosities to develop. This is the common history found in pregnant women who describe a sudden development of a cluster of varicosities of unknown cause. Failure of the protective valve is the mechanism for such development.

Furthermore, communicating veins connecting the deep with the superficial compartment may exhibit valve failure. If a perforating vein valve fails, high pressure developed within the muscular compartments during exercise, ranging from 150 to 200 mm Hg, are transmitted directly to the superficial venous system. Here the sudden pressure transmitted causes dilatation and lengthening of the superficial veins. Progressive distal valvular incompetence may occur. If proximal valves such as the saphenofemoral valve become incompetent, systolic muscular contraction pressure is supplemented by the weight of the static column of blood from the heart. Furthermore, this static column becomes a barrier. Blood flowing proximally through the femoral vein spills into the saphenous and flows distally. As it refluxes distally through progressively incompetent valves, it is returned through perforating veins to the deep veins.

Here, it is conveyed once again to the femoral veins, only to be recycled distally.

Changes occur at the cellular level as well. In the distal liposclerotic area, capillary proliferation is seen and extensive capillary permeability occurs as a result of widening of interendothelial cell pores. Transcapillary leakage of osmotically active particles is noted. The principal one is fibrinogen. In chronic venous insufficiency, venous fibrinolytic capacity is diminished and the extravascular fibrin remains to prevent the normal exchange of oxygen and nutrients in the surrounding cells.[4,5] However, there is little proof that there is an actual abnormality in the delivery of oxygen to the tissues.[6] Instead, recent research suggests that many pathological processes are involved and at present there is difficulty in identifying which are active and which are bystanders. Fundamental investigations into this problem in the future should improve the care of patients with severe venous stasis disease.[7]

PRECISE SYMPTOMATOLOGY

There are many causes of leg pain, most of which coexist. Therefore, it is necessary to define the precise symptoms of venostasis. These symptoms may be of gradual onset or initiated by a lancinating pain followed by appearance of varicosities. The initial symptomatology may vary from a pulsating pressure or burning to a feeling of heaviness. The pain is characteristically dull, does not occur during recumbency or early in the morning, and is exacerbated in the afternoon, especially after long standing. It is of importance to recognize that the discomforts of aching, heaviness, fatigue, or burning pain are relieved by recumbency, leg elevation, or elastic support.

A further level of increased symptomatology includes nocturnal cramps.

Cutaneous itching is also a sign of venostasis and is often the hallmark of inadequate external support. It is a manifestation of local congestion and may precede the onset of dermatitis. This and nearly all the symptoms of stasis disease can be explained by irritation of superficial nerve fibers by local pressure or accumulation of metabolic end products with a consequent pH shift. Finally, external hemorrhage may occur as superficial veins press on overlying skin within this protective envelope. These are the facts that aid in differential diagnoses.

NONINVASIVE ASSESSMENT

The most important, and perhaps least expensive, of noninvasive tests available to study the venous system are the physical examination and a careful history that elucidates the symptoms indicated earlier. Clinical examination of the patient in a good light provides nearly all the information necessary. It determines the nature of the venostasis disease and ascertains the presence of intercutaneous venous blemishes and subcutaneous protuberant varicosities, the location of principal points of control or perforating veins that feed clusters of varicosities, the presence and location of ankle pigmentation and its extent, and the presence and severity of subcutaneous induration (liposclerosis). After facts described previously are noted, the physician may turn to noninvasive techniques to supplement his knowledge and corroborate his preliminary diagnosis.

Instruments to be used in assessment of the venous system can be divided into those that assess physiologic function and those that image the pathologic anatomy. Physiologic assessment can be performed with the Doppler ultrasonic blood flow detector, the photoplethysmograph, light reflection rheograph, or mercury strain gauge plethysmograph. It is a common misconception to believe that the Doppler instrument is used to locate perforating veins. Instead, it is used in specific locations to detect incompetent valves (e.g., the hand-held, continuous-wave, 8-MHz flow detector placed over the greater and lesser saphenous veins near their terminations). With distal augmentation of flow and release, with normal deep breathing, and with performance of a Valsalva maneuver, accurate identification of valve reflux is ascertained.[8] An example of the usefulness of this technique is finding greater saphenous valvular competence above midthigh varicosities or anteromedial calf varicosities. Such a finding has immediate therapeutic implications.

The photoplethysmograph, light reflection rheograph, and mercury strain gauge plethysmograph have similar objectives: they attempt to quantitate the venous pool.[8–11] Quantitating the venous pool implies that manipulation of the pool will give quantitative information. For example, exercise-induced emptying and passive refilling will give a pool recovery time. This correlates well with recovery time obtained on dynamic venous pressure determinations. Both of the light techniques transmit light through the epidermal barrier to be reflected off the subcutaneous pool of blood vessels.[12] This is largely venous, and the amount of light reflected from the red blood cell content of the pool determines the reading of the instrument. In practice, muscular exercise empties the venous pool, and during relaxation the venous pool is refilled slowly through the arterial side of the circulation. If refill is rapid, reflux is assumed. Repetition of the test with placement of superficial tourniquets at the ankle, below-knee, or above-knee position allows differentiation of reflux from superficial or deep sources. Tourniquet techniques are subject to error because of differences in pressure exerted by the tourniquet and inadequate knowledge about completeness of obstruction of superficial flow.

Strain gauge plethysmography acts similarly. The sensor quantitates the leg volume that it encircles. This volume is decreased by exercise and then allowed to refill. Refill volume and time become end points of measurements.

Another instrument reintroduced to assess physiologic function of the muscle pump and the venous valves is the air displacement plethysmograph.[13,14] Originally, this instrument was discarded after its use in the 1960s because of its cumbersome nature. Computer technology has allowed its reintroduction as championed by Nicolaides and his coworkers.[15] It consists of an air chamber that surrounds the leg from knee to ankle. During calibration, leg veins are emptied by leg elevation and then the patient is asked to stand so that leg venous volume can be quantitated and the time for filling recorded. The filling rate is then expressed in milliliters per second, thus giving readings similar to those obtained with the mercury strain gauge technique.

Imaging of the venous system by noninvasive techniques is achieved by B-mode ultrasound scanning. This can be black and white, with or without frequency spectral analysis, or color (duplex or triplex scans). Noninvasive imaging is reliable in finding occluded venous segments, which are usually highly echoic and without blood flow. In addition, careful examination of valve function will reveal valve competency and incompetency.[8] The hemodynamic function of the valves is assessed by calf muscle augmentation and Valsalva maneuvers.

Imaging is obtained with a 10- or 7.5-MHz probe and the pulsed Doppler consists of a 3.0-MHz probe. The patient is examined in the standing position with the probe placed longitudinally on the groin. After imaging, sample volumes can be obtained from the femoral and/or saphenous vein. This flow can be observed during quiet respiration or by distal augmentation. Sudden release of augmentation allows assessment of valvular competence. The short saphenous vein and popliteal veins are similarly examined. Imaging improves accuracy of the Doppler examination. For example, short saphenous venous incompetence can be differentiated from gastrocnemius venous valvular incompetence by the imaging and flow detection of the duplex or triplex scans.

Quantitation of reflex can be obtained by application of standard compression, sudden release, Doppler spectrum recordings, and vein diameter measurement. Flow at peak reflex is obtained by multiplying cross-sectional area by mean velocity at peak reflux.[16]

PHLEBOGRAPHY

In general, phlebography is unnecessary in treatment of primary venostasis disease and varicose veins.[17] In the complex problems of severe chronic venous insufficiency, phlebography has specific utility.[18,19] Ascending phlebography defines obstruction. Descending phlebography identifies specific valvular incompetence suspected on B-mode scanning and clinical examination.

SURGICAL TREATMENT

Indications for treatment are pain, easy fatigability, heaviness, recurrent superficial thrombophlebitis, external bleeding, and appearance.[20] Treatment of venous insufficiency is similar to surgical treatment elsewhere; that is, it may be ablative or restorative. Since restorative venous surgery is so new, most of its methods remain somewhat experimental and only a few can be considered to be standard therapy. On the other hand, ablative treatment has been utilized for such a long time that the operations have undergone marked improvement and modernization in recent time.[21-25]

Venous Ablation

Cutaneous venectasias with vessels smaller than 1 mm in diameter do not lend themselves to surgical treatment. If their cause is saphenous or tributary venous incompetence, these conditions can be treated surgically. The venectasias themselves can be ablated successfully using modern sclerotherapy technique. Dilute solutions of sclerosant (e.g., 0.2 per cent sodium tetradecyl) can be injected directly into the vessels of the blemish.[26] Care should be taken to ensure that no single injection dose exceeds 0.1 ml but that multiple injections completely fill all vessels contributing to the blemish. When all of the ramifications of the blemish have been filled with sclerosant, and before the subsequent inflammatory reaction has progressed, a pressure dressing can be applied to keep vessels free of return blood for 24 to 72 hours. At 14 to 21 days postinjection, incision and drainage of entrapped blood are performed and a second pressure dressing applied for 12 to 18 hours. This liberation of entrapped blood is as important to success as the primary injection. Such therapy is remarkably successful in achieving an excellent cosmetic result and in relief of stasis symptomatology.

In hyperallergic patients, a solution of hypertonic saline can be used for sclerotherapy.[27] On the other hand, the use of new technology such as the laser in treatment of telangiectasias has proven to be disappointing.[28]

Venules larger than 1 mm and less than 3 mm in size can also be injected with sclerosant of slightly greater concentration (e.g., 0.5 per cent sodium tetradecyl) but limiting the amount injected to less than 0.5 ml. Pressure dressings for these venules must be in place for 72 hours or more. Evacuation of entrapped blood is of paramount importance to prevent recanalization of these vessels after treatment.

Surgical treatment may be used to remove clusters with varicosities greater than 4 mm in diameter. This is performed using stab avulsion technique with preservation of the greater and lesser saphenous veins if they are unaffected by valvular incompetence.[29,30] When greater or lesser saphenous incompetence is present, the removal of clusters of varicosities is preceded by limited removal of the saphenous vein(s) (stripping). Stripping techniques are best done from above downward to avoid lymphatic and cutaneous nerve damage. The stripper head should be retrieved proximally to avoid creation of a large, anticosmetic, distal incision (Fig. 42–1). Further details on performance of stripping operation for saphenous insufficiency have been described elsewhere.[31]

Surgery of Severe Venous Insufficiency

The mainstay of therapy for chronic, severe venous insufficiency is the elastic stocking.[32] At this point in our knowledge of the condition we cannot say that perforator interruption techniques are obsolete, but we can say with some definiteness that they are disappointing.[33,34] The traditional Linton medial long calf incision down to and through deep fascia with reflection of the fascia to identify perforating veins has been virtually abandoned (Fig. 42–2). In its place the posterior stocking seam incision has achieved the same purpose.[35] However, a disappointingly small number of perforating veins have been encountered using those techniques, and very few are done today.

In the most severe chronic venous insufficiency problems, a wide excision of skin, liposclerotic subcutaneous tissue, and fascia has been performed. Forty-eight hours later, sheet skin grafting or mesh grafting is done to achieve coverage.[36] Recurrent ulcerations are found with this technique, but such ulcers are smaller and are limited to the graft–normal skin borders, where they can be controlled by conservative techniques.

At this time, surgical treatment for venous ulceration is reserved for those ulcers that are resistant to outpatient techniques. When a decision is made that outpatient techniques are failing, the patient is admitted to the hospital, the legs are placed on a foam rubber block to elevate them 10 to 20 inches above heart level, and Betadine wet-to-dry dressings are applied to the leg ulcerations and overwrapped with tight, elastic bandages and changed every 8 hours (Fig. 42–3). Mechanical débridement is carried out daily during dressing changes when slough and necrotic debris is removed. If the granulation tissue begins to look healthy, direct skin grafting can be done. However, in many resistant ulcerations, excision of the ulcer, its bed, and surrounding liposclerotic and pigmented tissue is done. Mesh grafting, postage-stamp grafting, and pinch grafting have been done to cover such wound excisions. However, sheet grafting with multiple perforations conveys the best cosmetic result.

Venous ulcer healing is inseparable from attempts to correct the abnormal pathophysiology that underlies the ulcer[6,7] (Fig. 42–4). This is achieved by obliteration of perforating veins by sclerotherapy and surgical ligation of the superficial and lower leg communicating veins, usually combined with the wearing of tight, elastic compression stockings.

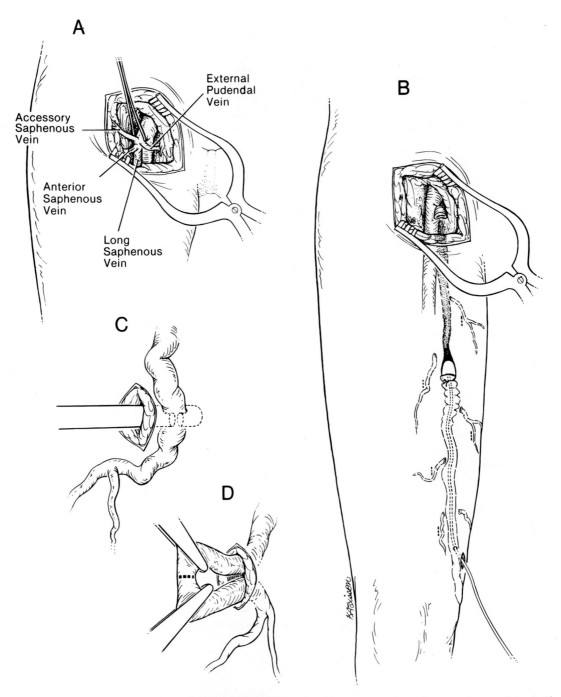

FIGURE 42–1. These diagrams illustrate the essentials of modern surgery for primary varicose veins. *A,* If preoperative gross saphenofemoral valvular incompetence is present on Doppler examination, a proximal ligation or limited saphenous stripping is indicated. A 2-cm groin crease incision will prove sufficient to identify, ligate, and divide the greater saphenous vein and each of its tributaries. *B,* Depending upon the location of the thigh or calf perforating vein that is to be interrupted, the distal incision can be placed appropriately. It can be limited in length to 4 to 5 mm. The stripper is pulled downward, the saphenous vein ligated over the stripper distally, divided, and removed from below upward as illustrated. An umbilical tape tied to the stripper head allows retrieval of the device and the vein. *C,* Individual varices are exposed through 2- to 3-mm stab incisions, grasped with hemostats or hooks, and delivered externally. *D,* Each varix is divided and carefully avulsed proximally and distally without ligation. An inverted, dermal stitch of absorbable suture material then effects wound closure.

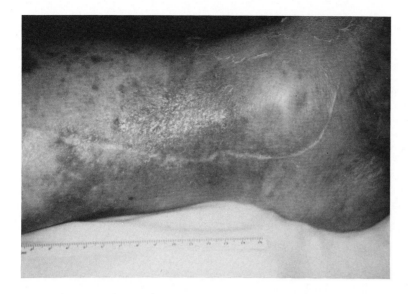

FIGURE 42–2. Correct placement of the incision to perform subfascial perforator interruption according to the modified Linton technique. Note the retromalleolar, medial, posterior tibial extension and the evidence of primary healing achieved by a plaster, posterior-mold immobilization of the ankle.

Reports from centers employing sclerotherapy plus compression and those reporting surgical interruption of perforating veins and superficial veins plus compression are uncontrolled.[23] Although these reports imply that the method being described is better than any other, it is impossible to render an objective view because of the lack of controls in the various studies. At this time, it is best to consider such reports as being anecdotal. Until conclusive proof is established, a policy of outpatient healing of ulcerations or inpatient skin grafting prior to performance of operations to correct abnormal calf pump mechanisms seems to be a good one. This allows operation on incompetent veins in a sterile field.

Because ablative techniques have been disappointing, with an ulcer recurrence rate ranging from 20 to 100 per cent, direct venous reconstructive procedures have been advocated.

Direct Venous Reconstruction

Historically, the first successful procedures done to reconstruct major veins were the femorofemoral crossover graft of Eduardo Palma, and the saphenopopliteal bypass described by him and employed also by Richard Warren of Boston.[38-40] These operations were elegant in their simplicity, use of autogenous tissue, and reconstruction by a single venovenous anastomosis.[41,42]

With regard to femorofemoral crossover grafts, the only group to provide long-term physiologic study of a large number of patients is Halliday, Harris, and May from Sydney.[43] Although phlebography was used in selecting patients for surgery, no other details of preoperative indications are given. They were able to document that 34 of 50 grafts remained patent in

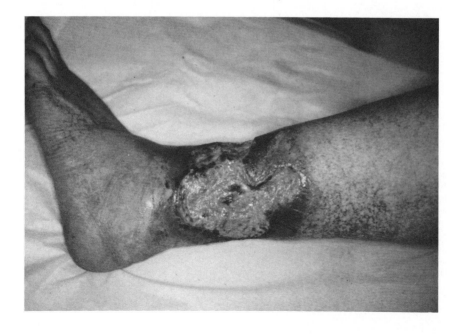

FIGURE 42–3. Grossly infected, circumferential venous ulcers as shown here may require inpatient therapy as described in the text. Outpatient care demands more of the patient than he can deliver.

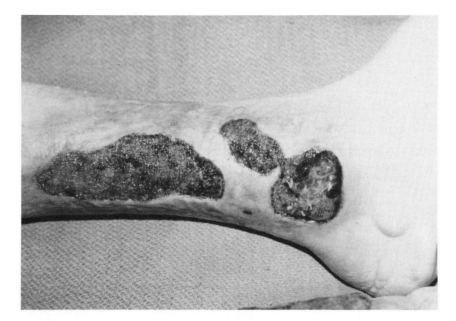

FIGURE 42–4. Attempts to correct venous pathophysiology must not ignore correct diagnosis. Note that atypical location (over pressure points), absence of cutaneous pigmentation, and presence of exuberant granulation tissue in these ulcers caused by rheumatoid arteritis.

the long term as assessed by postoperative phlebography. They believed the best clinical results were achieved in relief of postexercise calf pain, but had the impression that a patent graft also slowed the progression of distal liposclerosis and controlled recurrent ulceration. No proof of this was given in their report.

The other operation invented by Eduardo Palma was the saphenopopliteal bypass.[39,42] In a large series of patients, Gruss noted the results of this procedure were much less favorable than those of the cross-femoral bypass. Furthermore, there was seldom either a morphologic or functional indication for this operation.[44]

Kistner and Taheri have described venous valve surgery and venous valve transplantation.[45–48] Kistner summarized his view of valve surgery by saying, "The ultimate place of proximal venous valve surgery will be determined in the light of future experience."[45] He further stated that "Surgery on the incompetent deep veins deserves a place in the management of chronic venous insufficiency states as an adjunctive measure to be used in highly selected cases." It should be remembered that valvuloplasty techniques are for primary valvular incompetence and not for correction of the postthrombotic destroyed valves. Objectivity is necessary in evaluating these techniques.[49–51]

Taheri et al. have reported on 67 limbs operated upon by valvuloplasty, first with transplantation to the femoral vein and later to the popliteal vein.[48] Follow-up by questionnaire, office visits, and telephone inquiry was obtained in 70 per cent of patients, with 17 of 18 leg ulcers healed and 75 per cent of the other patients receiving a satisfactory result. This procedure must be considered investigational at this time until other surgical teams duplicate Taheri's results.

CONCLUSION

Sclerotherapy and surgical treatments of primary venous insufficiency manifested by venectasias and varicose veins have proven satisfactory. Treatment of severe chronic venous insufficiency is less so. However, long-term palliation can be achieved by outpatient treatment combined with carefully selected operations to improve pathologic venous physiology.

REFERENCES

1. Struckmann JR, Meiland H, Bagi P, Juul-Jorgensen B: Venous muscle pump function during pregnancy. Acta Obstet Gynecol Scand *69*:209–215, 1990.
2. Porter JM, Rutherford RB, Clagett GP, et al: Reporting standards in venous disease. J Vasc Surg *8*:172–181, 1988.
3. Mashiah A, Rose SS, Hod I: The scanning electron microscope in the pathology of varicose veins. Isr J Med Sci *27*:202–206, 1991.
4. Burnand KG, O'Donnell TF, Thomas ML, et al: The relative importance of incompetent communicating veins in the production of varicose veins and venous ulcers. Surgery *82*:9–14, 1977.
5. Burnand KG, Whimster IW, Clemenson G, et al: The relationship between the number of capillaries in the skin of the venous ulcer-bearing area of the lower leg and the fall in foot vein pressure during exercise. Br J Surg *68*:297–300, 1981.
6. Scurr JH, Coleridge Smith PD: Pathogenesis of venous ulceration. Phlebologie (suppl) *1*:13–16, 1992.

7. Scott HJ, McMullin GW, Coleridge Smith PD, Scurr JH: Histological study of white blood cells and their association with lipodermatosclerosis and venous ulceration. Br J Surg 78:210–211, 1991.
8. Nicolaides A, Christopoulos DG, Vasdekis S: Progress in investigation of chronic venous insufficiency. Ann Vasc Surg 3:278–292, 1989.
9. Nicolaides A, Christopoulos DG: Diagnosis and quantitation of venous reflux. Angiologie 13:391–393, 1988.
10. O'Donnell TF, Shepard AD, et al: Chronic venous insufficiency. *In* Jarett F, Hirsch J (eds): Vascular Surgery of the Lower Extremity. St. Louis, CV Mosby Company, 1985.
11. Schanzer H, Peirce EC: A rational approach to surgery of the chronic venous stasis syndrome. Ann Surg 195:25–29, 1982.
12. O'Donnell TF, Mackey WC, Shepard AD, et al: Clinical, hemodynamic, and anatomic followup of direct venous reconstruction. Arch Surg 122:474–482, 1987.
13. Christopoulos DG, Nicolaides AN: Noninvasive diagnosis and quantitation of popliteal reflux in the swollen and ulcerated leg. J Cardiovasc Surg 29:535–539, 1988.
14. Christopoulos DG, Nicolaides AN, Szendro G, Irvine AT, Bull M-L, Eastcott HHG: Air plethysmography and the effect of elastic compression on the venous hemodynamics of the leg. J Vasc Surg 5:148–157, 1987.
15. Christopoulos DG, Nicolaides AN, Szendro G: Venous reflux: Quantification and correlation with the clinical severity of chronic venous disease. Br J Surg 75:352–356, 1988.
16. Moulton S, Bergan J, Beeman S, Poppiti R: Quantification of gravitational venous reflux in lower extremity venous stasis. Phlebologie (in press), 1992.
17. Wesolowski SA, Greenfield H, Sawyer PN, et al: Diagnostic value of phlebography in venous disorders of the lower extremity. J Cardiovasc Surg 8(suppl):133–135, 1965.
18. Darke SG, Andress MR: The value of venography in the management of chronic venous disorders of the lower limb. *In* Greenhalgh RM (ed): Diagnostic Techniques and Assessment Procedures in Vascular Surgery. London, Grune & Stratton, 1985.
19. Lea Thomas M, McDonald LM: Complications of phlebography of the leg. Br Med J 2:307–315, 1978.
20. Bergan JJ: Surgical treatment of the veins. *In* Nora PJ (ed): Operative Surgery. Philadelphia, Lea & Febiger, 1991.
21. Doran FSA, White M: A clinical trial designed to discover if the primary treatment of varicose veins should be Fegan's method or by an operation. Br J Surg 62:72–76, 1975.
22. Editorial: The treatment of varicose veins. Lancet 1:311–312, 1975.
23. Fegan WG: Continuous compression technique of injecting varicose veins. Lancet 1:109–112, 1963.
24. Hobbs JT: Surgery and sclerotherapy in the treatment of varicose veins. Arch Surg 109:793–796, 1974.
25. Marston A: Treatment of varicose veins. Lancet 1:453, 1975.
26. Goldman MP: A comparison of sclerosing agents. Clinical and histologic effects of intravascular sodium morrhuate, ethanolamine oleate, hypertonic saline (11.7%), and Sclerodex in the dorsal rabbit ear vein. J Dermatol Surg Oncol 17:354–362, 1991.
27. Sadick NS: Sclerotherapy of varicose and telangiectatic leg veins. Minimal sclerosant concentration of hypertonic saline and its relationship to vessel diameter. J Dermatol Surg Oncol 65:65–70, 1991.
28. Goldman MP, Martin DE, Fitzpatrick DE, Ruiz-Esparza J: Pulsed dye laser treatment of telangiectasias with and without subtherapeutic sclerotherapy. J Am Acad Dermatol 23:23–30, 1991.
29. Bishop CCR, Jarrett PEM: Outpatient varicose veins surgery under local anesthesia. Br J Surg 73:821–822, 1986.
30. Large J: Surgical treatment of saphenous varices with preservation of the main great saphenous trunk. J Vasc Surg 2:886–891, 1985.
31. Bergan JJ, Kistner RL: Surgical procedures for varicose veins: Axial stripping and stab avulsion. *In* Atlas of Venous Surgery. Philadelphia, WB Saunders Company, 1992, pp 61–77.
32. Ruckley CV: Treatment of venous ulceration—compression therapy. Phlebologie (suppl) 1:22–26, 1992.
33. O'Donnell TF: Popliteal vein valve transplantation. *In* Bergan JJ, Yao JST (eds): Venous Disorders. Philadelphia, WB Saunders Company, 1990.
34. O'Donnell TF, Burnand KG, Browse NL: Is interruption of incompetent perforating veins really important to the management of chronic venous insufficiency? Surgery 82:9–14, 1977.
35. Johnson WC, O'Hara ET, Corey C, Widrich WC, Nabseth DC: Venous stasis ulceration—effectiveness of subfascial ligation. Arch Surg 120:797–800, 1985.
36. Scurr JH: Wide excision and skin grafting: *In* Bergan JJ, Kistner RL (eds): Atlas of Venous Surgery. Philadelphia, WB Saunders Company, 1992, pp 165–173.
37. Moore DJ, Himmel PD, Sumner DS: Distribution of venous valvular incompetence in patients with postphlebitis syndrome. J Vasc Surg 3:49–57, 1986.
38. Palma EC, Riss F, Del Campo F, Tobler H: Tratamiento de los trastornos postflebiticos mediante anastomosis venosa safenofemoral controlateral. Bull Soc Surg Uruguay 29:135–145, 1958.
39. Palma EC, Esperon R: Vein transplants and grafts in the surgical treatment of the postphlebitic syndrome. J Cardiovasc Surg 1:94–107, 1960.
40. Warren R, Thayer TR: Transplantation of the saphenous vein for postphlebitic stasis. Surgery 35:867–976, 1964.
41. Dale WA: Crossover vein grafts for iliac and femoral venous occlusion. Resident Staff Phys June:58–64, 1983.
42. Danza R, Navarro T, Baldizan J, Olivera D: Injerto venovenoso libre. Indicaciones, tecnica y resultados (11 anos de experiencia). Cir del Uruguay 50:485–494, 1980.
43. Halliday P, Harris J, May J: Femorofemoral crossover grafts (Palma operation): A long-term followup study. *In* Bergan JJ, Yao JST (eds): Surgery of the Veins. Orlando, FL, Grune & Stratton, 1985, pp 241–245.
44. Gruss JD: The saphenopopliteal bypass for chronic venous insufficiency (May-Husni operation). *In* Bergan JJ, Yao JST (eds): Surgery of the Veins. Orlando, FL, Grune & Stratton, 1985, pp 255–265.
45. Kistner R: Surgical repair of the incompetent femoral vein valve. Arch Surg 110:1336–1343, 1975.
46. Kistner RL: Surgical repair of a venous valve. Straub Clin Proc 34:41–43, 1968.
47. Kistner RL: Surgical repair of the incompetent femoral valve. Arch Surg 110:1336–1342, 1975.
48. Taheri SA, Pendergast DR, Lazar E: Vein valve transplantation. Am J Surg 150:201–202, 1985.
49. Husni EA: Reconstruction of veins: The need for objectivity. J Cardiovasc Surg 24:525–528, 1983.
50. Johnson HD, Queral LA, Flinn WR, et al: Late objective assessment of venous valve surgery. Arch Surg 116:1461–1466, 1981.
51. Raju S: Venous insufficiency of the lower limb and stasis ulceration: Changing concepts and management. Ann Surg 197:688–697, 1983.

REVIEW QUESTIONS

True or False:

1. Varicose veins are distinctly separable from the postthrombotic syndrome.

2. Varicose veins are distinctly hereditary.

3. Cutaneous venous blemishes may be symptomatic.

4. Surgical removal of spider veins is justified by their symptomatology.

5. Clinically, chronic venous insufficiency and varicose veins are easily separable.

6. Aching, fatigue, night cramps, and distal swelling may be associated with venectasias.

7. Night cramps are indicative of arterial insufficiency in association with varicose veins.

8. Venography performed preoperatively aids in planning varicose vein surgery.

9. The hand-held, continuous-wave Doppler defines communicating vein locations reliably and determines surgical therapy.

10. Sclerotherapy is unwarranted except for cosmetic indications.

ANSWERS

1. false   2. false   3. true   4. false   5. false   6. true   7. false
8. false   9. false   10. false

43

LYMPHEDEMA AND TUMORS OF THE LYMPHATICS

ERIC R. ASHBY, SAMY ABDOU, and TIMOTHY A. MILLER

In this day of rapidly advancing medical knowledge, our understanding of the lymphatic system lags far behind. Medical and surgical therapy of lymphatic diseases is still delivered on an empiric basis. The numerous different approaches to the treatment of lymphedema and lymphangiomas document our frustration in finding an effective way to deal with these problems.

Lymphangiomas, cystic hygromas, and a significant portion of lymphedema are probably due to embryologic aberrations in the lymphatic system. Surgical trauma to the lymphatic system likewise can produce lymphedematous problems for the surgeon.

ANATOMY

Although lymphatic vessels were first observed over 2200 years ago, recognition of the lymphatics as a discrete system did not occur until the 17th century. It is now generally agreed that lymphatics and lymph nodes arise from endothelial sprouting of the primordial venous system.[1,2] This development begins in four areas: the paired jugular and iliac systems, the cisterna chyli, and the retroperitoneal system. Between the third and eighth weeks of gestation, these sprouting endothelial sacs develop peripherally and invade almost all tissues of the body with the exception of the epidermis, central nervous system, bone marrow, muscle, cartilage, tendon, coats of the eye, internal ear, and intralobar portions of the liver. The thoracic duct arises from fusion of the cisterna chyli and left jugular buds. The lymphatic channels and regional nodes of each extremity are eventually formed by this peripheral growth and drain into either the cisterna chyli (lower extremities) or directly into the thoracic duct (upper extremities), thereby returning lymph to the venous system. Variations in the communications between the major lymphatic trunks and the subclavian veins are relatively common.[3]

The lymphatic system is composed of three major components: initial lymphatics (also referred to as terminal lymphatics), collecting ducts, and lymph nodes. The initial lymphatic vessels are similar to capillaries, except their basement membrane is absent or poorly defined, facilitating the absorption of lymph fluid from the interstitial space. The lymphatic capillaries progress in size, becoming collecting lymphatics. A valved system of collecting lymphatics normally ascends alongside the primary blood vessels of an extremity and transports lymph to regional lymph nodes. Collecting lymphatics have intimal, medial, and adventitial layers. The elastic fibers and smooth muscle in the media vary in direct proportion to lymphatic size.

Lower Extremity Lymphatics

The lower extremity lymphatics consist of separate *superficial* and *deep* systems. In the *superficial lymphatic system*, medial and lateral pathways of lymphatic vessels exist that closely correspond to the venous drainage of the leg. The *medial superficial pathway* contains five or more vessels that follow the course of the greater saphenous vein and subsequently drain into the superficial inguinal lymph nodes. The *lateral superficial pathway* consists of three or four vessels that follow the course of the lesser saphenous vein and then drain into the popliteal lymph nodes or join the medial pathway in the thigh. The superficial lymphatics normally drain the subcutaneous compartment, the site of fluid accumulation in lymphedema.

The *deep lymphatic system* of the lower extremities consists of several vessels that run parallel to the anterior and posterior tibial veins and the peroneal vein. Normally, the four vessels drain into the popliteal lymph nodes, while four to six vessels ascend the thigh medially, following the course of the superficial femoral vein and subsequently draining into the inguinal nodes.

The inguinal nodes are divided into a superficial group (around the fossa ovalis) and a deep group (within the fatty tissues of the femoral sheath). These

792

nodes (approximately 15) drain into the iliac lymph nodes. Although virtually all lymph flow from the lower extremities passes through the inguinal nodes, studies have shown that lymph drainage can bypass these nodes and drain directly into the iliac area.[4] Lymph from these nodes is subsequently returned to the venous circulation via the cisterna chyli.

Upper Extremity Lymphatics

The anatomy of the upper extremity lymphatics is similar to that of the lower extremities. The *superficial lymphatic system* consists of medial and lateral groups of vessels. The medial group of lymphatics parallels the basilic vein and then drains into the axillary lymph nodes. The lateral group of vessels follows the course of the cephalic and median veins and drains primarily into the supraclavicular lymph nodes. (This lateral group of lymphatics may serve as a collateral path of lymph drainage in patients who have undergone axillary lymph node dissection.) The *deep lymphatic system* of the arms parallels the brachial vessels and also drains into axillary lymph nodes.

Regional Lymphatic Drainage

Lymphatic drainage of the extremities is generally a regional process. Normally, the superficial and deep lymphatic systems do not communicate until the vessels drain into common lymph nodes. Only under abnormal conditions, such as with proximal obstruction, do the two systems communicate.[5,6] There are no significant direct lymphovenous communications in the extremities.[7] There is also little communication between the medial and lateral superficial pathways distal to the knee.[8] Some evidence exists that lymphatic channels draining the lower leg do not receive tributaries from the thigh. Lymphangiographic studies have shown that the thigh drains into the superior inguinal lymph nodes, whereas the lower leg drains into the more inferior inguinal nodes.[9] Because of this, in some patients with acquired lymphedema, the swelling may be limited to the lower leg.

PHYSIOLOGY

The normal lymphatic system clears the interstitial space of macromolecular protein and accompanying fluid lost from the capillary circulation, infectious agents and other foreign material, and substances absorbed by the gastrointestinal tract. When the formation of protein-rich interstitial fluid exceeds the lymphatic transport capacity (the maximum lymph flow per unit time), edema results. Several factors influence the rate of lymph formation and the lymphatic transport capacity.

Formation of Interstitial Fluid and Lymph

Interstitial fluid is essentially an ultrafiltrate of plasma, formed by capillary filtration. According to Starling's law, the rate of capillary filtration is determined by the difference in hydrostatic and colloid osmotic pressures between the intravascular/capillary space and the interstitial space. Under normal physiologic conditions, the larger hydrostatic pressure in the capillaries is opposed by a comparably large capillary osmotic pressure. This allows relatively small net amounts of fluid and protein to enter the interstitial space. An abnormally elevated venous pressure can increase capillary hydrostatic pressure and subsequently increase fluid shift into the interstitial space.[10] However, the lymphatic system compensates by increasing lymph flow to return this interstitial fluid to the systemic circulation.[8,11,12]

Lymph is formed primarily by absorption of interstitial fluid by the initial lymphatic vessels. The basement membrane of these vessels is absent or poorly organized, which may allow interstitial fluid and macromolecules to pass through open junctions between endothelial cells.[13] Pinocytosis and phagocytosis do not contribute substantially to the formation of lymph.[14-16] After passing through the initial lymphatics, lymph is not appreciably altered or concentrated, as all other lymphatic vessels are relatively impermeable.[17-19] The concentration of protein within the interstitial fluid depends on the permeability of capillaries and the ability of the lymphatics to clear excessive interstitial protein. Over a 24-hour period, the capillaries normally allow 40 to 80 per cent of intravascular protein to enter the interstitial space, where it is then transported via the lymphatics back to the circulation.[20]

Lymphatic Function/Transport Capacity

The propulsion of lymph proximally results from a combination of several factors. Muscular contractions adjacent to lymphatic vessels increase the surrounding interstitial tissue pressure, which propels lymph proximally. Lymphatic valves prevent the regress of lymph upon subsequent muscle relaxation and in general encourage the unidirectional flow of lymph by lowering lymphatic pressure relative to interstitial pressure. Proximal lymph flow has also been shown to be promoted by adjacent arterial pulsations.[21] Additionally, the alternating negative then positive intrathoracic and intraabdominal pressures associated with respiration and Valsalva maneuvers act to pump lymph through the thoracic and abdominal cavities.[20]

In addition to the extrinsic factors promoting lymph flow, considerable evidence supports an intrinsic contractile mechanism that promotes the flow of lymph. All lymphatics, except for terminal lymphatics, have smooth muscle fibers and nerve endings in their walls and have been shown to contract spontaneously and rhythmically.[22,23]

Lymph flow can be impeded by abnormalities in lymphatic anatomy that increase resistance (which will be discussed later), by gravity, and by an elevated central venous pressure, which impedes the return of lymph to the left innominate vein by increasing the thoracic duct pressure.[24]

Pathophysiology of Lymphedema

Lymphedema, a contraction of the term lymphostatic edema, results from an impaired capacity of the lymphatics to transport interstitial fluid back to the circulation. This lymphatic insufficiency results in a low-lymph-flow state and in the accumulation of protein-rich edema fluid. A normal, healthy lymphatic system is able to compensate for an increase in the rate of lymph formation by increasing the rate of lymph flow up to 10 times the resting flow rate.[25] However, a substantial increase in interstitial flow fluid formation may overwhelm normal lymphatic compensation and lead to the accumulation of interstitial fluid. Because this accumulated fluid has a *low protein concentration*, this type of edema is not considered lymphedema. Thus, an increase in the rate of interstitial fluid formation by itself does *not* produce lymphedema.[26] Lymphatic dysfunction is a prerequisite for lymphedema formation. Irrespective of an increase in the rate of interstitial fluid formation, lymphatic dysfunction can lead to the interstitial accumulation of *protein-rich* edema fluid. This type of edema constitutes lymphedema.[27]

In the lymphedematous extremity there is a 20 to 30 per cent increase in venous flow, presumably as a compensatory mechanism.[8] In lymphedema, a new balance of pressure is established at a higher level. The increase in interstitial pressure in surrounding tissue tends to increase lymph flow.

Early in the course of lymphedema, the accumulation of protein-rich interstitial fluid results only in a soft, pitting edema. As the disease progresses, the protein concentration within the interstitium gradually increases and accelerates the rate of subcutaneous inflammation and fibrosis. Subcutaneous fibrosis invariably involves the remaining functional lymphatics and leads to valvular incompetence as well as a decrease in vessel wall permeability and intrinsic contractility. Moreover, this protein-rich fluid combined with lymphatic stasis provides an ideal environment for bacterial proliferation. Recurrent episodes of lymphangitis are a common complication, involving approximately 25 per cent of lymphedema patients.[28] Lymphangitis and cellulitis further accelerate the rate of subcutaneous fibrosis and subsequent lymphatic obstruction.

In summary, lymphatic obstruction leads to the accumulation and concentration of protein-rich interstitial fluid, which accelerates the rate of subcu-

taneous fibrosis, and produces further lymphatic obstruction, thus establishing a vicious cycle.

PRIMARY LYMPHEDEMA

All forms of primary lymphedema result from some congenital abnormality in the anatomy and/or function of the lymphatic system. Primary lymphedema has generally been classified on the basis of the age of onset, but can also be classified by lymphangiographic findings.

Classification by Age of Onset

Primary lymphedema is classically subdivided into three groups on the basis of the age of disease onset.[29,30]

Congenital lymphedema presents at birth and accounts for approximately 10 to 15 per cent of patients with primary lymphedema. Milroy's disease is a specific congenital form of lymphedema characterized by aplasia of the lymphatic trunks and a familial, sexlinked incidence. A family history is present in less than 5 per cent of patients with congenital lymphedema.[31,32] This congenital form can be associated with other diseases of the lymphatic system, such as cystic hygroma and lymphangiectasia.

Lymphedema praecox presents during adolescence and accounts for approximately 80 per cent of patients with primary lymphedema. This represents another form of congenital lymphatic system disease but with a later onset of symptoms.

Lymphedema tarda generally presents after age 35 and constitutes approximately 10 to 15 per cent of patients. It is unclear why normal middle-aged adults would suddenly develop lymphedema without any known precipitating event. Nor can we adequately explain (1) why women are afflicted at least three times more frequently than men, (2) why the left leg is affected significantly more often than the right, or (3) why the upper extremities are seldom involved. The general category designated as "primary lymphedema" encompasses several conditions with varying and incompletely understood etiologies.

Classification by Lymphangiographic Findings

The development of lymphography advanced a clinically more descriptive classification. Based on lymphangiographic findings, primary lymphedema can be divided into two major categories: hypoplastic and hyperplastic.

Hypoplastic Lymphedema

Ninety-two per cent of all cases of primary lymphedema show a hypoplastic pattern on lymphangiogram.[33] The hypoplasia can be further classified as distal, proximal, or both distal and proximal. In distal hypoplasia, usually less than five vessels are visualized at the thigh. If any lymphatics are seen, they are narrow and few. A *distal hypoplastic pattern* is most often seen in female adolescents with lymphedema praecox, which may be related to puberty or pregnancy. The associated lymphedema is mild and nonprogressive and generally affects both lower legs. *Aplasia* is an extreme form of distal hypoplastic lymphedema that is usually seen in congenital lymphedema and accounts for 15 per cent of all cases of primary lymphedema. In these patients, lymphangiography reveals no lymphatic trunks.

A *proximal hypoplastic pattern* is seen in patients with pelvic obstruction. This is a less common but more severe form of primary hypoplastic lymphedema. Its incidence is equal in males and females, and it constitutes 17 to 34 per cent of patients with primary lymphedema.[34–36] In these patients, lymphangiography reveals only a few small lymph nodes and vessels in the groin and pelvis, with numerous distended lymphatics distal to the site of hypoplasia. The edema is generally unilateral but most often affects the entire lower extremity.[37]

In *combined proximal and distal hypoplasia* the lymphangiographic findings and clinical characteristics are a combination of those of the two categories previously described.

Hyperplastic Lymphedema

Lymphangiography reveals a hyperplastic pattern in approximately 8 per cent of primary lymphedema patients.[33] Hyperplastic lymphedema can be further categorized as *bilateral hyperplasia* or *megalymphatics*.[38] Bilateral hyperplasia is presumed to be secondary to obstruction caused by an abnormal thoracic duct or cisterna chyli. Lymphangiogram demonstrates numerous, slightly dilated lymphatics distal to the obstruction. Large edematous pelvic lymph nodes are seen bilaterally. Mediastinal and intercostal lymph nodes may also be visualized, but the thoracic duct is seldom seen.

In patients with a megalymphatic pattern, lymphangiogram demonstrates large tortuous, varicose-like lymphatics. Edema of the extremity is often mild or absent. More importantly, the incompetent lymphatic valves allow the reflux of chyle into the pelvis. This pattern may be associated with angioma of the lower extremity or trunk or bowel lymphangiectasia.

SECONDARY (ACQUIRED) LYMPHEDEMA

In secondary lymphedema, damage to previously normal lymph nodes and/or vessels results in lymphatic dysfunction. This damage can be caused by surgery, trauma, irradiation, infection (filariasis, tuberculosis, lymphogranuloma, actinomycosis, cat scratch fever–*Afipia felis* infection), inflammation (chronic lymphangitis, snake bite, or insect bite) or tumor invasion. On a worldwide basis, secondary lymphedema is significantly more common than primary lymphedema and is most frequently caused by lymphatic infection by the parasite *Wuchereria bancrofti* (filariasis).[39,40] In the civilized world, secondary lymphedema is usually related to regional lymph node dissection in the treatment of malignant disease, especially when combined with radiation therapy.

Approximately 10 to 15 per cent of patients undergoing radical mastectomy will develop significant postoperative arm swelling.[41,42] A study of 200 operable breast cancer patients found that radiation to the axilla after radical node dissection significantly increased the risk of postmastectomy lymphedema in the ipsilateral extremity.[43] In addition to patients undergoing radiation therapy, obese patients and patients with postmastectomy wound healing problems exhibit a higher incidence of lymphedema. In these patients the swelling may not become clinically evident for as long as 1 year. This delay is a result of ongoing soft tissue fibrosis, which compresses the remaining lymphatics and possibly acts as a barrier to the regeneration of new lymphatic vessels. Factors that increase the formation of fibrous tissue, such as irradiation and infection, increase the chances that lymphedema will develop.

Lymphedema due to malignant disease occurs late in the disease process after there is extensive spread of tumor.

Lymphedema may also develop following lower extremity arterial reconstruction and appears to be more frequent after using an autologous vein graft.[44] During dissection of arterial segments or during harvest of the greater saphenous vein, lymphatic vessels may be damaged. To reduce lymphatic injury some surgeons have proposed careful dissection with the aid of a diffusible dye to directly visualize the lymphatics.[45] In patients with secondary lymphedema, lymphangiography reveals a varicose-type pattern with dilation of the distal lymphatics and obstruction at the operative site.

DIAGNOSIS

Patient Presentation and History

In the vast majority of patients the diagnosis of lymphedema can and should be made by the history and physical examination alone. The gradual ascent of a soft pitting edema beginning at the ankle and proceeding proximally over a period of several months, unassociated with other symptoms, is characteristic. An increase in limb diameter produces an even greater increase in limb weight, causing lymphedema patients to often complain of fatigue in the involved extremity. As the subcutaneous fibrosis progresses, the limb becomes indurated and develops a nonpitting, spongy edema. Eventually, the skin becomes thick and hyperkeratotic.

The patient with lymphedema may present at any age. Patients with primary lymphedema classically present at birth, puberty, or middle age. In women the onset of lymphedema is often at menarche or pregnancy. Patients with secondary lymphedema present sometime after the inciting event, such as surgery, irradiation, infection, trauma, or tumor growth. The time interval between the occurrence of the inciting event and the onset of disease is variable and may range from weeks to years.

Laboratory Studies

Initial laboratory studies should include a differential white blood cell count to detect the eosinophilia often seen with filariasis and a peripheral blood smear to search for *Wuchereria bancrofti* microfilaria. Serum albumin, total protein, electrolytes, renal function tests, liver function tests, and urinalysis should be obtained to rule out other causes of limb edema.

Lymphangiography and Lymphoscintigraphy

Lymphedema can usually be diagnosed on the basis of history and physical examination alone. Laboratory tests can help exclude other causes of extremity edema. If the diagnosis is still in doubt, then lymphoscintigraphy is indicated. Lymphangiography should be avoided, as it can lead to further lymphatic damage.

Lymphangiography is an anatomical study that provides some function information. In contrast, lymphoscintigraphy is a functional study that can provide some anatomical information. In the lower extremities, lymphangiography is performed by injecting a blue dye into the first intradigital web space bilaterally. The web spaces are massaged and the extremity moved to promote dye dispersion. Dye uptake and proximal movement through the subcutaneous lymphatics can be easily visualized through intact skin of the normal extremity. In the lymphedematous extremity, dye diffusion may be limited to the dermal lymphatic plexus and gives the foot a diffuse bluish tinge ("dermal backflow"). If any subcutaneous lymphatic channels are identified by dye uptake, they are canalized directly and a radiopaque dye is injected. Dye progression is followed radiographically. While informative, lymphangiography may damage remaining lymphatics and exacerbate existing lymphedema. Other potential complications include wound infection, skin staining, allergic reaction, and pulmonary or cerebral embolization. Because lymphangiography seldom influences the medical or surgical management of the lymphedematous patient, it should not be routinely performed.

Lymphoscintigraphy assesses lymphatic function by quantitating the rate of lymphatic isotope clearance. This study has emerged as the diagnostic study of choice for lymphedema and has been used by some to select patients for microsurgical lymphatic reconstruction.[46] Several radioisotopes (such as radioiodinated (^{131}I) human serum albumin (RIHSA), gold (^{198}Au) colloid, and ^{99}Tc-labeled colloid) have been used to study lymphatic function. RIHSA is now rarely used, since approximately 10 per cent of the isotope will enter the vascular system after subdermal injection. This reduces the study's ability to differentiate between lymphatic and other causes of edema. Lymphoscintigraphy with radiolabeled colloidal suspensions can more accurately quantitate lymphatic function. The beta emitter colloidal gold (^{198}Au) was used initially but then abandoned in favor of ^{99}Tc-labeled sulphide colloid. Lymphoscintigraphy is performed by measuring the amount of radioactivity at the inguinal nodes at 30 minutes and 1 hour after bipedal isotope injection. The normal range of inguinal node uptake is 0.6 to 1.6 per cent. Uptake values below 0.3 per cent are considered abnormal and most patients with distal hypoplasia lymphedema exhibit uptake values less than 0.1 per cent.[47,48] Parameters such as time of first isotope appearance, lymph speed, change in the rate and isotope uptake before and after exercise, and condensed image and factorial analysis techniques have been developed to derive even more information from lymphoscintigraphy. Variables such as the actual tissue depth of radioisotope injection, the volume injected, the patient's activity during the test, and the position of the extremity must be controlled. Fortunately, variation in the interstitial fluid content (degree of swelling) does not significantly change the rate of isotope clearance.

Differential Diagnosis

Lymphedema can usually be differentiated from other causes of limb edema on a clinical basis (see Table 43–1). The most common causes of bilateral edema are systemic (e.g., cardiac, renal, or hepatic insufficiency). These are easily differentiated from lymphedema by history and physical findings or occasionally with the aid of laboratory tests. Venous disease is the most common cause of unilateral limb edema. The characteristic atrophic skin and brawny pigmentation make long-standing venous stasis easy to differentiate from lymphedema. Additionally, edema secondary to venous disease demonstrates decreased capillary perfusion, characteristic dark brawny edema, and ulceration of the skin secondary to impaired perfusion and tissue anoxia. In lymphedema, capillary perfusion is unimpaired, ulceration is extremely rare, and the deep brown discoloration of venous diseases is unusual. While limb elevation rapidly improves venous edema, usually within hours, lymphedema resolves more slowly, often requiring days of limb elevation.

Left leg swelling (which is seen in 60 per cent of lymphedema patients) has also been attributed to obstruction of the left iliac vein produced by crossing the right iliac artery. This has been termed the "iliac

TABLE 43–1.   DIFFERENTIAL DIAGNOSIS OF CHRONIC LEG EDEMA

	Lymphatic Insufficiency	Venostasis	Cardiac, Renal, or Hepatic Insufficiency	Lipedema (Not True Edema)
Consistency of edema	Initially soft & pitting Eventually spongy & firm	Brauny & pitting	Pitting	Nonpitting
Distribution of edema	Diffuse, greatest distally Usually unilateral	Greatest at ankles & legs, feet spared Usually unilateral	Diffuse, greatest distally Always bilateral	Greatest at ankles & legs, feet spared Always bilateral
Resolution with elevation	Mild, over several days	Complete, within hours	Complete, within hours	Minimal
Skin changes	Initially none Eventually hypertrophic, hyperkeratotic & thick Ulceration is rare	Atrophic with brawny pigmentation Possible ulceration	Shiny, no trophic changes	None

compression syndrome" and is proposed as an explanation of the lymphedema.[49] However, few of these patients demonstrate any classical evidence of peripheral venous disease, and it is difficult to see how venous hypertension can be reflected as lymphedema without a high incidence of chronic skin changes and ulceration. Venography in such cases is useful but not always easily interpreted.[50] Doppler findings are valuable in differentiating *acute venous thrombosis* from lymphedema.[39]

Two additional uncommon conditions are *lipedema* and the *yellow nail syndrome* (YNS). Lipedema is a relatively rare condition generally affecting women. This lipodystrophy is characterized by diffuse, symmetric, nonpitting enlargement of the subcutaneous tissue of the extremity. A weight-reduction regimen often has limited effectiveness, and surgery can be helpful in selected cases. Yellow nail syndrome was first described in patients with lymphedema and yellow nails.[51] The triad of yellow dystrophic nails, primary lymphedema, and bilateral effusions is also associated with an increased incidence of maxillary sinusitis. One report of YNS included a refractory pericardial effusion.[52] The etiology of YNS remains obscure.[53,54]

TREATMENT

Lymphatic insufficiency leads to the interstitial accumulation of protein-rich fluid, with subsequent stagnation, inflammation, and eventual fibrosis of the subcutaneous tissue. Elevation, compression, and other means that remove the interstitial fluid without removing a significant fraction of the accumulated interstitial proteins will only provide transient relief and must be maintained indefinitely. To effect a cure, lymphatic drainage must be restored in order to effectively remove the protein-rich fluid prior to the onset of significant subcutaneous fibrosis. Unfortunately, this objective is largely unattainable. The patient must understand that lymphedema is a chronic condition and that none of the available medical or surgical treatment options will completely restore the affected limb.

Medical Management

Medical therapy is the initial form of treatment for all lymphedema patients. Many patients can be adequately managed without subsequent surgical intervention. The medical management of the lymphedematous limb is accomplished through (1) the prevention of skin infection and the prompt treatment of all cutaneous complications, (2) the mechanical reduction of the interstitial fluid content, and (3) the pharmacologic reduction of interstitial proteins. Of course, identifiable conditions such as filariasis or tuberculosis, which can damage the remaining lymphatics, must be appropriately treated.

Cutaneous infection leads to increased fibrosis and must be avoided. All patients must be taught meticulous hygiene and skin care. Fungal infection of the web space can precipitate skin breakdown and must be avoided. Careful drying of the toes and web space after washing and use of an antifungal powder are important preventative measures. Some physicians advocate the use of a low-pH, lanolin-based skin lotion to prevent skin cracking and subsequent infection.[55] However, lotions with additives should be avoided, since they can sensitize the skin and trigger an inflammatory reaction.[38]

When infections occur, they must be treated immediately and aggressively. The patient should receive a systemic antistaphylococcal and antistreptococcal agent and be restricted to bed rest with the extremity elevated until the infection subsides. Urgent care is necessary because the infection can be fulminant, and each inflammatory episode leads to more subcutaneous fibrosis. In patients with recurrent infectious episodes of unknown origin, a prophylactic penicillin is the drug of choice; *Streptococcus* is the most common etiologic agent.

Reduction of interstitial fluid is the mainstay of medical therapy. Several treatment modalities are available to mechanically reduce the accumulation of interstitial fluid in the lymphedematous limb. In the United States, compression garments and pneumatic compression pumps are the most common treatments. In Europe, a special massage technique called manual lymph drainage (MLD) and compressive bandaging therapy (CBT) are popular.

Pneumatic compression pump therapy has proven to be an effective method of reducing the volume of interstitial fluid in the lymphedematous limb. An inflatable sleeve or stocking is placed over the edematous limb and intermittently inflated, thus forcing edema fluid proximally. These pneumatic devices vary from the single-chamber, single-pressure type to the segmental, sequential, adjustable pressure gradient pump (Lympha Press, Biocompression Pump).[56] These more sophisticated pumps use multiple chambers to sequentially compress the extremity. The pump pressure decreases as the "wave" advances proximally, thus "milking" the edema fluid out of the limb. Studies have shown that pump compression therapy is effective in reducing limb volume by 30 to 47 per cent.[57-59] Compression pump therapy must be continued or else the limb edema rapidly reaccumulates. In order to maintain the newly reduced limb volume, elastic support garments should be worn continuously between treatment sessions. Ideally, the garments should be custom fitted with a 30 to 60 mm Hg gradient pressure at the ankle.[38,60]

Compressive garments (support stockings, sleeves, gloves, pantyhose, etc.) should not be prescribed as the sole treatment for nonpitting lymphedema. In the nondecompressed lymphedematous limb, the constant compression delivered by these garments may collapse and occlude the few existing lymphatic vessels and restrict lymphatic return. Support garments are best used to maintain a normal or near-normal limb volume.[38,55,61] Pump therapy and compression garments are most effective in the early stages of lymphedema before the onset of significant subcutaneous fibrosis.

Manual lymph drainage and CBT have been popular treatment modalities in Europe for several years.[61] They have been introduced in the United States and are gaining in popularity. Manual lymph drainage is a superficial massage technique of lymphatic vessels developed in 1936 by Vodder to promote lymph drainage.[62,63] Generally, normal functioning lymphatic vessels immediately adjacent to the lymphedematous limb are first massaged to promote lymph flow. Then the edematous limb is massaged repeatedly in a distal to proximal direction beginning with the proximal part of the limb and finishing with the distal end. This reportedly increases the function of existing lymphatics and directs lymph past the diseased or obstructed lymphatic vessels to the functional vessels that were previously "cleared" by massage. Subsequent European studies have reported that MLD increases lymph flow in collecting channels, increases local blood flow, increases the rate of

contraction of lymphatic vessels, and promotes protein reabsorption.[64-66]

Compressive bandaging therapy was first described by Winiwater in 1892 for the treatment of elephantiasis.[67] It entails wrapping the lymphedematous limb with several layers of a minimal-stretch (nonelastic) bandage, such that distal pressure is greater than proximal pressure. This reportedly reestablishes the tissue pressure and subcutaneous mechanical support, which is compromised as a result of the destruction of subcutaneous elastic fibers. Moreover, this bandaging reportedly prevents the reaccumulation of lymph fluid and increases lymph flow. During normal activities or while performing prescribed exercises, the patient contracts the muscles of the bandaged limb within an almost nonyielding space. This reportedly increases tissue pressure and also promotes lymph flow. Most practitioners who use CBT apply the bandages after MLD. In one study, MLD combined with CBT over a 3-week period resulted in a 20 per cent reduction of arm volume in postmastectomy lymphedema patients.[68] In 1989 Földi described his experience treating 399 patients with benign, postmastectomy lymphedema. Ninety-five per cent of his patients had a significant reduction in limb volume, and 56 per cent of his patients had a greater than 50 per cent reduction. At 3-year follow-up, 54 per cent had fully maintained their therapeutic results.[27]

Although diuretics have been used widely in the past, they are of little value in the treatment of lymphedema. In fact, some physicians believe they may be harmful. By decreasing limb water content, diuretics may increase the interstitial protein concentration, accelerating the rate of subcutaneous fibrosis.[27,38,55]

Reduction of interstitial protein can be accomplished pharmacologically. The benzopyrones are a family of diverse compounds that increase the number of macrophages in the interstitium of lymphedematous tissue as well as the rate of protein breakdown by macrophages.[69,70] In clinical trials, benzopyrones given orally for 6 months produced a 15 to 20 per cent decrease in excess limb volume, a decrease in perceived limb heaviness and discomfort, and an increase in skin softness.[71] Multiple clinical trials in both Europe and Australia have documented moderate improvement in lymphedema patients.[71-75]

Benzopyrones are inexpensive oral agents with little demonstrable toxicity. They do not offer rapid relief but can slowly improve clinical high-protein lymphedema.[71,72] Although they are not currently available in the United States, they have been used as adjuvant therapy in other affluent countries.[76] They may be most useful, however, in impoverished nations where filariasis is widespread and where patient access to more effective treatment modalities is limited.

Limb hyperthermia has been reported as a treatment for lymphedema.[77] An electric oven is used to heat the leg to approximately 40°C (1 hr/day for 20 days). Following treatment, the leg is tightly wrapped in elastic bandage. In a series of 1000 patients, good results have been reported, with the improvement attributed to lymphatic regeneration.[78]

Surgical Management

Surgical intervention should be considered only after medical management has been maximized. The aim of surgical therapy is to drain or excise the lymphedematous skin and subcutaneous tissue and thereby improve function and appearance as well as decrease the frequency of recurrent infection. All patients must understand that surgery is palliative and that a cosmetically perfect result is unattainable. Functional impairment caused by the inability to control the size of the extremity is the best indication for surgery. The patient with restricted movement secondary to gross extremity enlargement is most likely to benefit from surgical intervention. Those with primary hypoplastic lymphedema of moderate severity who seek surgical correction for cosmetic reasons are less likely to be satisfied.

The frustration encountered in the surgical management of lymphedema is reflected in the numerous procedures described over the past 80 years. In general, these operations can be divided into physiologic procedures and excisional procedures (see Table 43–2). The physiologic operations attempt to reconstruct lymphatic drainage either by (1) establishing communication between a lymphatic-rich flap and the edematous limb or (2) bypassing a segmental lymphatic obstruction by introducing a lympholymphatic or lymphovenous shunt. The excisional operations remove varying amounts of subcutaneous tissue and skin. Most pedicle flap procedures also include a significant amount of excision. Thompson's buried dermis flap is intended to be both an excisional and a physiologic operation.

Physiologic Operations

Lymphangioplasty was first proposed by Handley in 1908. He implanted silk threads in the subcutaneous tissues in lymphedematous limbs (lymphangio-plasty).[79] He argued that fibrous channels would form around the foreign body and transport lymph by capillary action. While some patients who underwent lymphangioplasty had early postoperative improvement, no patient demonstrated long-term benefit.[80] Clearly, any channel that forms around an alloplastic implant will fibrose with time.

As new and less immunogenic implant materials become available, interest in this operation is periodically renewed.[81-83] In the most recent report, 16 patients underwent multifilament Teflon-wick lymphangioplasty and were followed for 10 years.[81] In this report, several patients experienced an initial reduction in limb circumference lasting as long as 13 months, and all patients had returned to their baseline or a worse state by the fifth postoperative year.

Lymphangioplasty is a very simple but ineffective operation. This procedure should play no role in the long-term management of either primary or secondary lymphedema.

Microsurgical Lymphatic Reconstruction

Microsurgical procedures designed to reestablish lymphatic drainage to an affected extremity can be divided into two operative categories: (1) lymphonodal-venous shunts or lymphovenous shunts and (2) lympholymphatic shunts. The aim of each procedure is to reroute lymphatic flow around the diseased lymphatic vessels or nodes. As with arterial reconstruction, a limited segmental obstruction with good distal vessel function provides the optimal setting in which to perform a bypass procedure.

Lymphonodal-venous and lymphovenous shunts were first reported in the early 1960s.[89,90] In the lower extremity, a lymphonodal-venous shunt is created by identification and transection of a lymph node (usually femoral), removal of the lymphoid pulp, and anastomosis of the transected node onto the anterior surface of a neighboring vein (usually femoral or saphenous). Care is taken to avoid injuring the afferent lymphatic vessels entering the node. Alternatively, a lymphovenous shunt is established by identification of patent functional lymphatic vessels in the proximal medial thigh and creation of an end-to-end anastomosis with a branch of the saphenous vein immediately distal to the saphenofemoral junction (a complete description of these operations is provided by Olszewski[91] and Gloviczki[46]).

By the late 1960s, Nielubowicz and Olszewski had performed these operations in patients with lymphedema.[92] Their operative results were described as "fair" to "very good," in 74 per cent of patients with secondary lymphedema and in 55 per cent of patients with primary hyperplastic lymphedema. However, the reduction in limb circumference was modest. Furthermore, in patients with primary hypoplastic lymphedema, these procedures were ineffective. Only 24 per cent of these patients who underwent surgery improved, whereas 28 per cent improved with conservative therapy alone. More recent studies have reported even better results.[93-95]

TABLE 43–2. OPERATIONS FOR LYMPHEDEMA

Physiologic operations
  Alloplastic implants (lymphangioplasty)
  Pedicle flap operations
    Skin pedicle flap
    Omental pedicle flap
    Enteromesenteric pedicle flap (small bowel flap)
  Microsurgical reconstruction
    Lymphonodal-venous or lymphovenous anastomoses
    Lympholymphatic anatomoses

Excisional operations
  Total subcutaneous excision (Charles procedure)
  Buried dermis flap (Thompson procedure)[a]
  Subcutaneous excision underneath flaps (modified Homans procedure)

---
[a]This operation is intended to be both "excisional" and "physiologic."

After more than 25 years of clinical experience, the question of long-term anastomotic patency remains unsettled. Sequential limb volume determination continues to be one of the predominant methods of perioperative patient assessment, and it only provides indirect evidence of anastomotic function. While lymphangiography is capable of visualizing the anastomosis directly, this method has been shown to damage residual lymphatics and should not be used in postoperative patient evaluation. Lymphoscintigraphy can estimate the rate of lymphatic flow and document perioperative changes in the flow rate. It cannot directly demonstrate flow across a lymphonodal-venous or lymphovenous shunt, since any radiolabeled colloid that enters the vein is rapidly diluted. Lymphoscintigraphy, however, can demonstrate flow across a lympholymphatic anastomosis, since rapid colloid washout does not occur.

Lympholymphatic shunts are promising procedures that were developed in the late 1970s. These procedures use functional, autologous lymphatic vessels harvested from a nondiseased extremity to bypass a segmental lymphatic obstruction.[84–87] Baumeister and associates have the most experience with this operation and have recently published their experience with 55 patients.[88] A segmental lymphatic obstruction is the principal indication for surgery; patients with primary hypoplastic lymphedema are not operative candidates. Of the 55 patients studied, only 4 had primary lymphedema (unilateral pelvic lymphatic atresia with functional distal lymphatics). Eighty per cent of study patients had achieved significant postoperative volume reduction of the affected extremity when followed for more than 3 years. Anastomotic patency was demonstrated in several patients using lymphoscintigraphy, although the patency rate was not cited. Overall, the lymphatic transport index was improved by 30 per cent in the recipient limb, while none of the donor extremities developed lymphedema.

In summary, shunt procedures in general are most likely to benefit patients with a limited segmental lymphatic obstruction and good distal lymphatic vessel function. Secondary lymphedema of short duration (less than 5 years) provides the best indication for microsurgical reconstruction. Clearly, however, it is the functional state of the distal lymphatic vessels and not the duration of disease that best predicts the probability of shunt success. Primary lymphedema patients with distal hypoplasia (most common form) are unlikely to significantly benefit from microsurgical reconstruction.[96]

Pedicle flap operations juxtapose lymphatic-rich pedicle flaps and lymphedematous tissue in hopes of inducing lymphatic communication and providing drainage for the lymphedematous tissue. To date, skin, omentum, and small bowel have been used as pedicle flaps.

Gilles was first to use the skin pedicle flap to drain lymphedematous tissue.[97] Significant volume reduction was achieved in a patient with secondary lymph-edema where a tubed skin flap presumably functioned as a lymphatic bridge across a segmental obstruction. However, subsequent attempts to drain the affected limbs of patients with primary lymphedema met with predictable failure. Other surgeons have tried to provide drainage by rotating an inguinal skin flap from an uninvolved extremity to the contralateral lymphedematous limb.[98] This approach is usually not effective and may threaten the lymphatic function of the uninvolved limb. Other skin flap procedures have been devised, but they are usually unsuccessful.

Use of the omental pedicle flap was popularized by Goldsmith in the 1960s.[77,99] Although initial reports were encouraging, the omental pedicle flap provides little long-term benefit.[100] The omentum is rich in lymphatics, but the vessels are small and the lymphatic flow rate is low. Experimental studies have failed to demonstrate any postoperative lymphatic connections between the omental flap and the lymphedematous tissue.[101,102] In addition, at reoperation a bursa-like sac is often found to have formed around the flap that may act as a physical barrier against lymphatic anastomoses. Because this operation is largely ineffective and may result in serious complications (abdominal wall hernia, intestinal obstruction, or gangrene), it has been abandoned.

A small bowl pedicle flap has been developed and successfully used in the laboratory.[103] The operation is performed by raising an ileal flap on its mesenteric pedicle and stripping the mucosa to expose the submucosal lymphatics. The iliac or inguinal lymph nodes are transected (depending on the obstruction site) and sutured onto the denuded submucosa.[104] Early clinical results have been encouraging.[105] However, the mesenteric pedicle is of limited length and the operation must be limited to patients with a very proximal segmental obstruction.

Excisional Operations

Total subcutaneous excision was originally described by Charles in 1912 and is the most extensive of the excisional procedures.[106] In the lower extremity, all of the skin and subcutaneous tissues are excised from the tibial tuberosity to the malleoli (except for tissue overlying the tendo calcaneus). While some surgeons remove the deep fascia in its entirety, others resect only heavily fibrosed segments. Tapering of tissue at the proximal and distal margins is performed in order to prevent a step deformity. The defect is closed using a split-thickness or a full-thickness skin graft from the resected specimen or a split-thickness skin graft from an uninvolved donor site (the operative procedure is described in detail by Hoopes[107]). Coverage with a split-thickness skin graft is technically easier and gives a satisfactory initial appearance. However, these grafts are easily injured, ulcerate frequently, scar extensively, become hyperpigmented, and may develop a severe hyperkeratotic, weeping chronic dermatitis. The end result is almost always far worse than the original problem. We strongly oppose the use of split thickness graft resurfacing after subcutaneous excision.[108] Coverage with a full-thickness skin graft is technically more demanding but produces a more durable graft site. Nevertheless, regions of graft breakdown and substantial scar formation can also occur with full-thickness grafts.

The long-term efficacy of the Charles procedure has been evaluated in very few studies. Preliminary results of patients who had undergone the operation at the Johns Hopkins Hospital were reported in 1959,[109] with a long-term follow-up study of the same patients in 1977.[110] Some degree of hyperpigmentation and hyperkeratosis of the grafted skin was reported in all 10 patients in the follow-up study. However, both conditions were more frequently observed in areas covered with split-thickness skin grafts than with full-thickness grafts. Two of the 10 patients had recurrent cellulitis that required hospitalization. Two had notable swelling of the extremity distal to the graft and two required a subsequent procedure to revise scars or release contractures, but none of the patients required a second operation for recurrent lymphedema. All patients had mild to moderate swelling after prolonged standing that was well controlled by compression stockings. Overall, all patients were "pleased" with the improved appearance and function.

In 1965, Taylor reported a series of 34 patients who had undergone total subcutaneous excision followed by a split-thickness skin graft.[111] Thirty-six per cent of patients had a "good" result, 36 per cent had a "satisfactory" result, and 28 per cent had an "unsatisfactory" result. Despite its obvious limitations, this procedure is sometimes the only surgical option for patients with very extensive swelling and extreme skin changes.

Suction curettage has been reported as a useful adjunct to the surgical management of primary and secondary lymphedema.[112,113] This method is useful for debulking lymphedematous limbs but cannot be used to treat extremity lymphedema of any significant magnitude without a concomitant resection of the expanded skin envelope. Excisional procedures continue to be the mainstay of surgical treatment for chronic, whole-limb edema with poor distal lymphatic function.

Thompson's buried dermis flap is an operation in which a portion of the lymphedematous subcutaneous tissue is resected beneath flaps, a flap edge is deepithelized, and the resulting dermis flap is buried into the underlying muscle compartment. Thompson's operation has three theoretical advantages: (1) The buried dermis permits the formation of lymphatic connections between the subdermal lymphatic plexus of the flap and the deep lymphatics of the muscle compartment, (2) muscle contraction will increase the lymphatic flow rate through the subdermal plexus, and (3) the buried flap provides a physical barrier against deep fascia regeneration.[114] The operation is intended to be both excisional and physiologic in approach.

In the thigh, a medial incision is made approximately 3 cm posterior to the course of the femoral vessels and carried distally about 1 cm behind the posterior border of the tibia. The posterior flap is elevated and a 4- to 5-cm-wide split-thickness skin graft is harvested from the flap edge. The subcutaneous tissue and the underlying fascia are excised, and the shaved flap edge is buried beneath the anterior flap. The buried segment lies next to the femoral vessels in the thigh and next to the tibial vessels in the leg. If required, a lateral operation is performed at a later date. (The operation is presented in more detail by Thompson.[114])

In 1980, Thompson published his long-term results using this procedure.[115] One hundred fifty-one operations were performed on 140 patients (11 were bilateral). Of these, 88 operations were performed for primary lymphedema of the leg, 14 for secondary lymphedema of the leg, and 49 for secondary lymphedema of the arm. One third of patients were followed for 5 years, one third for 5 to 10 years, and the remainder for 10 to 20 years. Operative results were reported as "good," "satisfactory," or "unimproved." A good result indicated reduction of excess swelling by more than 75 per cent, a return to normal activity, and relief from the main complaints. A satisfactory outcome indicated a significant but less than 70 per cent reduction of swelling, a return to moderate activity, and alleviation of most complaints.

In patients with primary lymphedema, 51 per cent of the limbs had a good surgical result and another 32 per cent had a satisfactory outcome. Comparable results were reported for patients with secondary lymphedema of the lower extremity. In the upper extremity, 61 per cent had a good result and 14 per cent were satisfactory. Flap necrosis was the most common complication and occurred in 47 per cent of all operative patients. While most areas of tissue loss were small, 12 per cent of patients had significant tissue necrosis (exceeding 10 sq cm) and required excision and skin grafting under anesthesia. An additional 14 per cent of patients developed a draining sinus at the surgical incision. Two patients had inadvertent nerve injury during dissection.

Although operative success is attributed to the formation of lymphatic connections between the flap and the muscle compartment, postoperative lymphangiography has failed to demonstrate any lymphatic anastomosis. RIHSA clearance studies have demonstrated postoperative improvement in the rate of lymphatic isotope clearance. However, comparable improvement in RIHSA clearance was noted after skin and subcutaneous excision alone, suggesting that the tissue excision may account for postoperative improvement.[116]

Staged subcutaneous excision underneath flaps was first described by Sistrunk in 1918[117] and later popularized by Homans.[118] In our opinion, this approach provides the most reasonable surgical compromise of the excisional procedures. It offers reliable improvement and a minimum of unfavorable postoperative complications. It produces results comparable to those of Thompson's operation but has a lower complication rate. (The third excisional operation, the Charles procedure, should be reserved for patients with severe skin changes.)

Improvement is directly related to the amount of skin and subcutaneous tissue removed and the postoperative care. The surgical procedure is offered to patients as a means of managing their lymphedema and not as a cure.[119] During the operation, as much subcutaneous tissue and skin as possible are removed while attempting to maintain a viable skin flap and achieve primary skin closure.[119–121] An experience with 652 cases over 40 years demonstrated the safety and efficacy of this approach.[122] The following section describes our preferred surgical approach.

PREOPERATIVE CARE.

All patients are placed at bed rest, and the extremity is elevated. Although this step can be started at home, the patient is usually admitted to the hospital 1 to 3 days preoperatively, and the lower extremity is elevated using a modified Thomas orthopedic splint suspended from an overhead frame. The rate of edema resolution depends on the chronicity of the condition and the amount of subcutaneous fibrosis. While in the hospital, the extremity is washed daily. Other than a single preoperative dose, antibiotics are not routinely used.

OPERATIVE TECHNIQUE.

The procedure is done in two stages. The medial side is usually done first and involves the largest amount of tissue resection. A pneumatic tourniquet is placed as proximally as possible.

Lower Extremity.   A medial incision is made in the leg approximately 1 cm posterior to the tibial border and extended proximally into the thigh. Flaps about 1.5 cm thick are elevated anteriorly and posteriorly to the midsagittal plane of the calf (Fig. 43–1). The dissection is less extensive in the thigh and ankle. All subcutaneous tissue underneath the flap is removed. After excising the subcutaneous fat from the periosteum of the tibia, the deep fascia is incised, permitting an easy plane of dissection to develop. The sural nerve is identified and preserved. All of the attached subcutaneous fat and deep fascia along the medial aspect of the calf are removed (Fig. 43–2). The dissection is kept superficial to the deep fascia at the knee and ankle. Flaps in the ankle are rarely longer than 6 cm. The redundant skin is excised after removal of the subcutaneous fat (Fig. 43–3). A suction catheter is placed in the dependent portion of the posterior flap and is left in place for 5 days. Interrupted and continuous 4-0 nylon is employed for skin closure. No subcutaneous or dermal sutures are placed. The extremity is immobilized with a posterior splint and gauze dressing and kept elevated. Sutures are usually removed on the eighth day. The patient is measured for an elastic stocking and dependency of the leg is begun on the ninth day. Am-

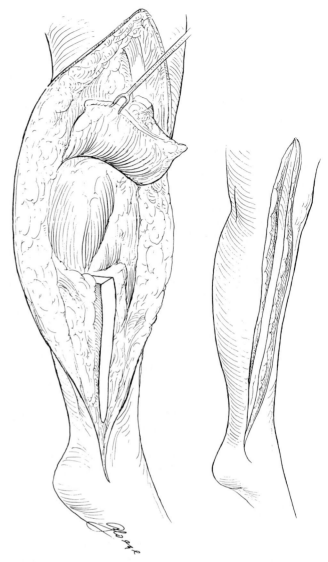

FIGURE 43–1.   The incision is made along the midmedial aspect of the leg extending from the midthigh to the area posterior to the medial malleolus. Flaps are elevated anteriorly and posteriorly. All of the underlying fatty tissue beneath the flaps, including the deep muscle fascia investing the gastrocnemius and soleus muscles, is removed.

bulation is started on the 11th postoperative day, but only with the leg tightly wrapped.

The second stage is performed on the lateral aspect of the limb 3 months later. The operation is essentially identical, except that the deep fascia is not removed. Great care is taken to avoid damaging the peroneal nerve.

Upper Extremity.   A medial incision is made from the distal ulna across the medial epicondyle of the humerus to the posterior, medial upper arm. Flaps approximately 1 cm thick are elevated to the midsagittal aspect of the forearm and the dissection is tapered distally and proximally. The edematous subcutaneous tissue is removed, but the deep fascia is not spared. The ulnar nerve is identified in the region of the medial epicondyle and preserved. The redun-

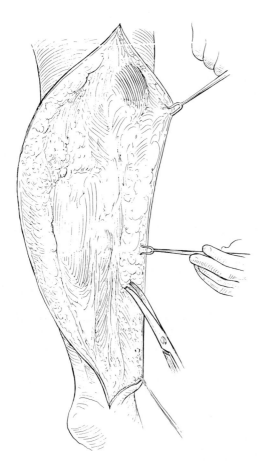

FIGURE 43-2. Additional amounts of subcutaneous tissue are removed from the skin flaps with scissors, thinning them to approximately 1.75 cm in thickness. The flaps are thinner around the ankle but are undermined only 4 to 8 cm. Hemostasis is accomplished after release of the pneumatic tourniquet.

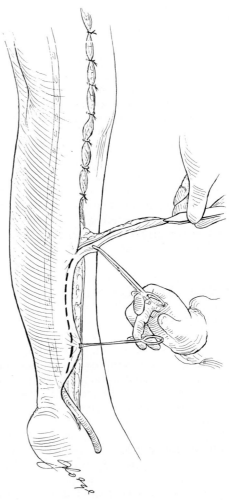

FIGURE 43-3. Upon closure, additional amounts of skin can be removed. As shown in Figure 43-1, some of the skin can be excised at the time of initial incision. The closure should leave no redundant skin. Large drains, placed in the most dependent position, are left in place to drain blood and lymph for at least a 5-day period. During this time the leg is immobilized in a posterior, well-padded plaster splint and elevated. The patient walks on the ninth postoperative day, at which time the leg is wrapped securely with elastic bandage.

dant skin is excised. If necessary, the tourniquet can be removed, the area prepped, and the operation continued into the axilla. A suction catheter is placed, and the skin is closed with 4-0 nylon suture. No subcutaneous or dermal sutures are used. The arm is immobilized and elevated for 5 days. The suction catheter can often be removed after the third day. Otherwise, the postoperative management is similar to that described for the leg.

Operative results. Eighty-two lower extremity operations were performed on 49 patients. Sixty-five per cent of patients had a significant reduction in extremity size. Of the remaining patients, 10 per cent have had some improvement that has lasted through 2 years of follow-up. The remainder have returned to postoperative levels of swelling or continued to progress. Men have a worse prognosis than women, although the explanation for this is unclear. Only three postoperative complications related to ischemic necrosis of the flap have occurred. All have healed by secondary intention, and none have required further surgery. Although many patients experience decreased sensation at the incision site, this has not been a source of complaint. None of these patients had inadvertent nerve injury, nor has any alteration

in hand or foot sensation been observed. All patients have some recurrence of swelling and must continue to wear support stockings.

The operative results for postmastectomy lymphedema have been more varied. In patients with massive swelling, the postoperative improvement is usually significant, and function can often be restored. In 10 patients, the postoperative arm volume was reduced by 250 to 1200 ml; the reduced volume was maintained through 6 years of follow-up. In the remaining four patients, arm swelling continued to progress despite the initial surgical reduction. Three of these patients had a progressive increase in hand edema following surgery. Whether this was the result of surgery or merely a continued progression of the underlying disease is unclear. The mechanism of improvement with staged subcutaneous excision underneath flaps is unclear. Extensive surgical dissection may establish lymphatic venous anastomoses during the process of healing, and the procedure may favorably alter the balance of lymph flow by reducing the amount of lymph-forming tissue. The excision of substantial tissue and skin may result in external compression effecting an increase in interstitial pressure much like an elastic stocking, thus improving lymph flow.

The discouraging fact remains that no procedure cures lymphedema. A degree of edema inevitably follows any operative procedure. In our opinion, compared to all available methods of surgical management, skin and subcutaneous excision is the most reliable, consistently beneficial, and uncomplicated means of surgically managing the symptoms of lymphedema.

TUMORS OF LYMPHATICS

Lymphangioma

Lymphangiomas are generally divided into three types: lymphangioma simplex, composed of small capillary–sized lymphatic channels; cavernous lymphangioma, composed of dilated lymphatic channels, often with fibrous adventitial covering; and cystic lymphangioma or cystic hygroma. All three are thought to have their origin in the embryologic development of the lymphatic system. Sabin[123] and, later, Goetsch[124] postulated that during the development of the lymphatic system, cell buds of lymphatic primordium occasionally fail to establish communication with veins, resulting in isolated lymphatic spaces. Portions of the lymphatic system can become sequestered and retain the ability to produce lymph and form endothelial cysts. These lymphatic cysts slowly enlarge and infiltrate the surrounding tissues by pushing other structures aside.

These tumors are all benign. The majority are present at birth, and 90 per cent can be identified by the end of the first year of life.[98,125] They tend to grow in proportion to the growth of the child and can greatly enlarge at times of infection.

The most common of the three types of lymphangioma is the cystic hygroma. The hygromas appear as soft, cystic, discrete, nontender masses that transilluminate. They vary in size from a few millimeters to several centimeters. They can be located on any portion of the body; however, the majority are found in the head and neck region. Hygromas of the neck, tongue, and intraoral regions can present significant respiratory problems in the newborn and on occasion require emergent excision. These lesions must be distinguished from hemangiomata, branchial cleft cysts, lipomas, and occasionally, neoplasms such as rhabdomyosarcoma.[126]

Treatment

Spontaneous remission of cystic hygromas is extremely rare. Percutaneous aspiration of hygromas is usually followed by prompt recurrence and, occasionally, hemorrhage or development of infection. Introduction of sclerosing agents has been proposed, but the multiloculated nature of most hygromas makes this therapy unfeasible. Excision subsequent to sclerosis is technically difficult.[126] Radiation therapy has no place in the treatment of cystic hygroma.

Treatment of cystic hygromas should be surgical excision, taking care to preserve all normal structures in the area. At times a staged excision is appropriate. These lesions are nonmalignant and care should be taken to preserve all normal anatomy. Excision is usually deferred until the age of 6 months if there is no compression of the trachea or respiratory difficulty.[125,127]

Lymphangioma simplex is similar in behavior to the cystic hygroma; however, it appears in a more even distribution throughout the body, occurring more frequently in the extremities and trunk. Treatment is the same as for the cystic hygroma. Cavernous lymphangiomas likewise are amenable to surgical resection, usually when the child is a few years old. Lymphangiomas have also been reported in the small bowel, lungs, and solid viscera of the abdomen. Resection is necessary only if the lesions produce symptoms.

Lymphangiosarcoma

Stewart and Treves described the association between postmastectomy lymphedema and lymphangiosarcoma in 1948.[128] This malignant lesion of the lymphatics is nearly always associated with lymphedema, most commonly with postmastectomy lymphedema, but also with filariasis.[39,129–131] The lesion generally appears 10 years after the onset of lymphedema and pursues an aggressive malignant course. Average survival is 19 months following initiation of treatment. The lesion is described as a reddish purple discoloration or nodule, and has been confused with Kaposi's sarcoma. Satellite lesions are occasionally found, but the tumor spreads primarily by a hematogenous route.

Treatment

The mainstay of therapy has traditionally been early radical amputation.[131–133] Because of the very small number of these tumors, it has been impossible to study the effects of various forms of therapy in a randomized fashion.

Successful treatment of other soft-tissue sarcomas with preoperative radiation therapy and chemotherapy, surgical excision, and postoperative adjunct chemotherapy makes a similar approach in lymphangiosarcoma justified.[134] However, insufficient evidence exists to strongly recommend any one form of therapy for this highly malignant tumor, and the prognosis remains poor.

REFERENCES

1. Crockett DJ: Lymphatic anatomy and lymphoedema. Br J Plast Surg 18:12, 1965.
2. Sabin FR: The development of the lymphatic system. In Keibel F, Mall FP (eds): Manual of Human Embryology, vol 2. Philadelphia, JB Lippincott, 1992.
3. Anson BJ: Atlas of Human Anatomy. Philadelphia, WB Saunders Company, 1950.
4. Selkurt E (ed): Physiology. Boston, Little, Brown & Co, 1966.
5. Melak P, Belan A, Kocandrle VL: The superficial and deep lymphatic system of the lower extremities and their mutual relationship under physiological and pathological conditions. J Cardiovasc Surg 5:686, 1964.
6. Thompson N: The surgical treatment of chronic lymphoedema of the extremities. Surg Clin North Am 47:445, 1967.
7. Futrell JW, Pories W: Physiologic and immunologic considerations of the lymphatic system in tumours and transplants. Surg Gynaecol Obstet 140:273, 1975.
8. Pflug JJ, Calnan JS: The normal anatomy of the lymphatic system in the human leg. Br J Surg 58:925–930, 1971.
9. Rodbard S, Feldman P: Functional anatomy of the lymphatic fluids and pathways. Lymphology 8:49, 1975.
10. Baylis W, Starling EH: Observations on venous pressure and their relationship to capillary pressures. J Physiol 16:159, 1894.
11. Field M, Drinker C: The rapidity of interchanges between the blood and the lymph in the dog. Am J Physiol 98:378, 1931.
12. Jacobson S: Studies of the blood circulation in lymphedematous limbs. Scand J Plast Reconstr Surg 3(suppl), 1967.
13. Smith JB, McIntosh G, Morris B: The migration of cells through chronically inflamed tissues. J Pathol 100:21, 1970.
14. Casley-Smith J: The lymphatic system in inflammation. In Zweitach BB (ed): The Inflammatory Process. New York, Academic Press, 1973.
15. Casley-Smith J, Florey H: The structure of normal small lymphatics. J Exp Physiol 46:101, 1961.
16. Leak L, Burke J: Fine structure of the lymphatic capillary and adjoining connective tissue area. Am J Anat 118:785, 1966.
17. Nicoll P: Permeability of lymphatic vessels in the bat wing. In Conference on Microcirculation. Aurlborg, Denmark, European Society for Microcirculation, 1970.
18. Olszewski W: Pathophysiology and clinical observations of obstructive lymphedema of the limbs. In Clodius L (ed): Lymphoedema. Stuttgart, Georg Thieme, 1977.
19. Taylor A, Gibson H: Concentrating ability of lymphatic vessels. Lymphology 8:43, 1975.
20. Yoffey JM, Courtice FC: Lymphatics, Lymph and the Lymphomyeloid Complex. London, Academic Press, 1970.
21. Parsons R, McMaster P: The effect of pulse upon the formation and flow of lymph. J Exp Med 68:353, 1938.
22. Kinmonth JB, Taylor GW: Spontaneous rhythmic contractility in human lymphatics. J Physiol (Lond) 133:3, 1956.
23. Olszewski WL, Engaset A: Intrinsic contractility of prenodal lymphatic vessels and lymph flow in human leg. Am J Physiol 239:H775, 1980.
24. Wegria R, Zekert H, Walter K, et al: Effect of systemic venous pressure on drainage of lymph from the thoracic duct. Am J Physiol 204:284, 1963.
25. Olszewski W: Peripheral Lymph: Formation and Immune Function. Boca Raton, FL, CRC Press, 1985.
26. Kirk RM: Capillary filtration rates in normal and lymphedematous legs. Clin Sci 27:363, 1964.
27. Földi E, Földi M, Clodius L: The lymphedema chaos: A lancet. Ann Plast Surg 22(6):505, 1989.
28. Schirger A, Harrison E, Janes J: Idiopathic lymphedema: Review of 131 cases. JAMA 182:14, 1962.
29. Allen E: Lymphedema of the extremities. Classification, etiology, and differential diagnosis: Study of 300 cases. Arch Intern Med 54:606, 1934.
30. Kinmonth JB, Taylor GW, Tracey GD, et al: Primary lymph-edema: Clinical and lymphangiographic studies of a series of 107 patients in which the lower limbs were affected. Br J Surg 45:1, 1957.
31. Milroy WF: An undescribed variety of hereditary oedema. NY Med J 56:505, 1892.
32. Ersek RA, Danese CA, Howard J: Hereditary congenital lymphedema (Milroy's disease). Surgery 50:1098, 1966.
33. Kinmonth JB: Primary lymphedema: Classification and other studies based on oleolymphography and clinical features. J Cardiovasc Surg (Torino) (special ed. for 27th Congress of European Society of Cardiovascular Surgery), p 65, 1969.
34. Olszewski W, Mackowshki J, Sawicki Z, Nielubowicz J: Clinical studies in primary lymphedema. Pol Med J 11:1560, 1972.
35. Thompson N: Buried dermal flap operation for chronic lymphedema of the extremities. Ten year survey of results in 79 cases. Plast Reconstr Surg 45:541, 1970.
36. Wolfe JHN, Kinmonth JB: The outcome of primary lymphedema of the leg. Arch Surg 116:1157, 1981.
37. Kinmonth JB, Wolfe JHN: Fibrosis in the lymph nodes in primary lymphedema. Ann R Coll Surg Engl 62:344, 1980.
38. Wolfe JHN: The management of lymphedema. In Rutherford RB (ed): Vascular Surgery, 3rd edition. Philadelphia, WB Saunders Company, 1989.
39. Dale A: The swollen leg. Curr Probl Surg 140:1, 1973.
40. Stone E, Hugo N: Lymphedema. Surg Gynecol Obstet 135:635, 1972.
41. Fitts WT, Keuhnelian JG, Ravdin IS, Schor S: Swelling of the arm after radical mastectomy. Surgery 35:460, 1954.
42. Treves N: An evaluation of the etiological factors of lymphedema following radical mastectomy. Cancer 10:444, 1957.
43. Kissin MW, della Rovere GQ, Easton D, et al: Risk of lymphoedema following the treatment of breast cancer. Br J Surg 73:580, 1986.
44. Person NH, Takolander R, Bergovist D: Edema after lower limb arterial reconstruction: Influence of background factors, surgical technique and potentially prophylactic methods. Vasa 20(1):57–62, 1991.
45. Leaper D, Evans M, Pollock A: Colour lymphography in clinical surgery. Br J Surg 66:51, 1979.
46. Gloviczki P: Microsurgical treatment for chronic lymphedema: An unfilled promise? In Bergan JJ, Yao JST (eds): Venous Diseases. Philadelphia, WB Saunders Company, 1991.
47. Beaulieu F, Vaillant L, Bealieu JL, et al: The current role of lymphoscintigraphy in the study of lymphedema of the limbs. J Mal Vasc 15:152, 1990.
48. Browse NL: The diagnosis and management of primary lymphedema. J Vasc Surg 3:181, 1986.
49. Crockett F: The iliac compression syndrome. Br J Surg 52:391, 1967.
50. Yoffey JM, Courtice FC: Lymphatics, Lymph and Lymphoid Tissue. Cambridge, Harvard University Press, 1956.
51. Samman PD, White WF: The "yellow nail" syndrome. Br J Dermatol 76:153, 1964.
52. Wakasa M, Imaizumi T, Suymama A, Takeshita A, Nakamura M: Yellow nail syndrome associated with chronic pericardial effusion. Chest 92:366, 1987.
53. David I, Crawford FA Jr, Hendrix GH, et al: Thoracic surgical implications of the yellow nail syndrome. Thorac Cardiovasc Surg 91:788, 1986.
54. Gupta AK, Davies GM, Haberman HF: Yellow nail syndrome. Cutis 37:371, 1986.
55. Lerner R: Complete decongestive physiotherapy (CDP): The ideal treatment for lymphedema. Massage Ther J Winter: 37, 1992.
56. Zelikovski A, Manoach M, Giler S, Urca I: Lympha-Press, a new pneumatic device for the treatment of lymphedema of the limbs. Lymphology 13:68, 1980.
57. Baulieu F, Baulieu JL, Vaillant L, Secchi V, Barso HJ: Factorial analysis in radionuclide lymphography: Assessment

of the effects of sequential pneumatic compression. Lymphology 22(4):178, 1989.

58. Raines JK, O'Donell TR, Kalisher L, et al: Selection of patients with lymphedema for compression therapy. Am J Surg 133:430–437, 1977.

59. Richman DM, O'Donnell TF, Zelikovski A: Sequential pneumatic compression for lymphedema. Arch Surg 120:1116, 1985.

60. Van der Molen HR: Compression in lymphedema. Plebologie 41(2):391–396, 1988.

61. Földi M: Lymphedema. In Foldi M, Casley-Smith JR (eds): Lymphangiology. Stuttgart-New York, Schattaner, 1983, pp 667–668.

62. Vodder E: Le drainage lymphatique, une rouvelle methode therapeutique. Soute' pour tons, 1936.

63. Vodder E: Foreword. In Wittlinger H, Wittlinger G (eds): Textbook of Dr. Vodder's Manual Lymph Drainage, Vol 1: Basic Course, 3rd revised edition (translated by RH Harris).

64. Hutzschenreuter P, Bruemmer H, Epperfeld K: Experimentelle und Klinische Untersuchungen Zur Wirkungsweise der manuellen Lymphdrainage-Therapie. Lymphol 13(1):62–64, 1989.

65. Hutzschenreuter P, Bruemmer H: Influence of complex physical decongesting therapy on positive interstitial pressure and on lymphangiomotor activity. In Progress in Lymphology. Amsterdam-New York-Oxford, Excerpta Medica 11:557–560, 1988.

66. Leduc O, Bourgeois P, Leduc A: Manual lymphatic drainage: Scintigraphic demonstration of its efficacy on colloidal protein reabsorption. In Partsch H (ed): Progress in Lymphology. Amsterdam-New York-Oxford, Excerpta Medica 11:551, 1988.

67. Winiwater A: Die Elephantiasis. In Deutsche Chirugie. Stuttgart, Enke, 1892.

68. Hutzschenreuter P, Wittlinger H, Wittlinger G, Kurz I: Postmastectomy arm lymphedema: Treated by manual lymph drainage and compression bandage therapy. Eur J Phys Med Rehabil 1(16):161–170, 1991.

69. Piller NB, Morgan G, Casley-Smith JR: A double-blind trial of 5,6 benzo-[alpha]-pyrone in human lymphoedema. In Casley-Smith JR, Piller NB (eds): Progress in Lymphology X. University of Adelaide Press, 1985.

70. Piller NB: Macrophage and tissue changes in the developmental phases of secondary lymphoedema and during conservative therapy with benzopyrone. Arch Histol Cytol 53(suppl):209, 1990.

71. Piller NB, Morgan RG, Casley-Smith JR: A double-blind, cross-over trial of O-(β-hydroxyethyl)-rutosides (benzopyrones) in the treatment of lymphoedema of the arms and legs. Br J Plast Surg 41:20, 1988.

72. Casley-Smith JR, Casley-Smith JR: The pathophysiology of lymphedema and the action of benzopyrones in reducing it. Lymphology 21(3):190, 1988.

73. Jamal S, Casley-Smith JR, Casley-Smith JR: The effects of 5,6 benzo-[a]-pyrone (coumarin) and DEC on filaritic lymphoedema and elephantiasis in India. Preliminary results. Trop Med Parasitol 83:287, 1989.

74. Clodius L, Piller NB: The conservative treatment of postmastectomy lymphoedema in patients with coumarin results in a marked continuous reduction in swelling. In Bartos V, Davidson JW (eds): Advances in Lymphology. Prague, Avicenum, 1982.

75. Knight KR, Khazanchi RK, Pederson WC, McCann JJ, Coe SA, O'Brien BM: Coumarin and 7-hydroxycoumarin treatment of canine obstructive lymphoedema. Clin Sci 77:69, 1989.

76. Pecking A: Medical treatment of lymphedema with benzopyrones. Experimental basis and application. J Mal Vasc 15:157, 1990.

77. Goldsmith HS, de los Santos R: Omental transposition in primary lymphedema. Surg Gynecol Obstet 125:607, 1967.

78. Lin WY: Heating and bandage treatment for treating chronic lymphedema of the extremity. Unpublished report from the department of plastic and reconstructive surgery. The Ninth People's Hospital, Shanghai's Second Medical College, 1982.

79. Handley WS: Lymphangioplasty: A new method for the relief of the brawny edema of breast cancer and for similar conditions of lymphatic oedema: Preliminary note. Lancet 1:783, 1908.

80. Handley WS: Hunterian lectures on the surgery of the lymphatic system. Br Med J 1:853, 1910.

81. Silver D, Puckett CL: Lymphangioplasty: A ten year evaluation. Surgery 80:748, 1976.

82. O'Reilly K: Treatment by nylon setons of lymphoedema of the arm following radical mastectomy. Med J Aust 59:1269, 1972.

83. Degni M: New technique of drainage of the subcutaneous tissue of the limbs with nylon net for the treatment of lymphedema. Vasa 3:329, 1974.

84. Acland RD, Smith P: Experimental lymphatico-lymphatic anastomoses. In Abstract Book of the VIIth International Congress of Lymphology, Florence, 1979.

85. Baumeister RG, Seifert J, Wiebecke B: Homologous and autologous experimental lymph vessel transplantation: Initial experience. Int J Microsurg 3:19, 1981.

86. Baumeister RG, Seifert J, Wiebecke B: Experimental basis and first application of clinical lymph vessel transplantation of secondary lymphedema. World J Surg 5:401, 1981.

87. Baumeister RG, Seifert J, Wiebecke B: Transplantation of lymph vessels on rats as well as a first therapeutic application on the experimental lymphedema of the dog. Eur Surg Res 12(suppl 2):7, 1980.

88. Baumeister RG, Siuda S: Treatment of lymphedemas by microsurgical lymphatic grafting: What is proved? Plast Reconstr Surg 85:64, 1990.

89. Laine JB, Howard JM: Surg Forum 14:111, 1963.

90. Nielubowicz J, Olszewski W: Experimental lymphovenous anastomosis. Br J Surg 55:440, 1968.

91. Olszewski WL: The treatment of lymphedema of the extremities with microsurgical lymphovenous anastomosis. Int Angiol 7:312, 1988.

92. Nielubowicz J, Olszewski WL, et al: Late results of lymphovenous anastomosis. J Cardiovasc Surg (Torino) 14 (special issue):113, 1973.

93. Nieuborg L: The role of lymphatico-venous anastomoses in the treatment of postmastectomy oedema. Alblasserdam, Holland, Offsetdrukkerij Kanters BV, 1982.

94. O'Brien BMcC, Mellow CG, Khazanchi RK, et al: Long-term results after microlymphaticovenous anastomoses for the treatment of obstructive lymphedema. Plast Reconstr Surg 85:562, 1990.

95. Gong-Kang H, Ru-Qi H, Zong-Zhao L, et al: Microlymphatico-venous anastomosis in the treatment of lower limb obstructive lymphedema: Analysis of 91 cases. Plast Reconstr Surg 76:671, 1985.

96. Gloviczki P, Fisher J, Hollier LH, Pairolero PC, et al: Microsurgical lymphovenous anastomosis for treatment of lymphedema: A critical review. J Vasc Surg 7:647, 1988.

97. Gillies H, Fraser FR: The treatment of lymphoedema by plastic operation: A preliminary report. Br Med J 1:96, 1935.

98. Clodius L, Piller NB: Conservative therapy for postmastectomy lymphedema. Chir Plast 4:193, 1978.

99. Goldsmith HS, de los Santos R, Beattie EJ: Relief of chronic lymphedema by omental transposition. Ann Surg 166:572, 1967.

100. Goldsmith HS: Long term evaluation of omental transposition for chronic lymphedema. Ann Surg 180:847, 1974.

101. Kinmonth JB: The Lymphatics: Diseases, Lymphograph and Surgery. Baltimore, Williams & Wilkins Company, 1972.

102. Danese CA, Papioannou AN, Morales LE, et al: Surgical approaches to lymphatic blocks. Surgery 56:821, 1968.

103. Hurst PA, Kinmonth JB, Rutt DL: A gut and mesentery pedicle for bridging lymphatic obstruction. J Cardiovasc Surg 19:589, 1978.

104. Kinmonth JB, Hurst PAE, Edwards JM, Rutt DL: Relief of lymph obstruction by use of a bridge of mesentery and ileum. Br J Surg 65:829, 1979.
105. Hurst P, Stewart G, Kinmonth J, et al: Long term results of the entero-mesenteric bridge operation in treatment of primary lymphoedema. Br J Surg 72:272, 1985.
106. Charles RH: Elephantiasis scroti. *In* Latham A (ed): A System of Treatment, vol 3. London, Churchill, 1912.
107. Hoopes JE: Lymphedema of the extremity. *In* Cameron JL (ed): Current Surgical Therapy, 3rd edition. Philadelphia, BC Decker, 1989.
108. Miller TA: Charles procedure for lymphedema: A warning. Am J Surg 139:290, 1980.
109. McKee DM, Edgerton MT: The surgical treatment of lymphedema of the lower extremities. Plast Reconstr Surg 23:480, 1959.
110. Dellon AL, Hoopes JE: The Charles procedure for primary lymphedema. Plast Reconstr Surg 60:589, 1977.
111. Taylor GW: Surgical management of primary lymphedema. Proc R Soc Med 58:1024, 1965.
112. Louton RB, Terranova WA: The use of suction curettage as adjunct to the management of lymphedema. Ann Plast Surg 22:354, 1989.
113. Nava VM, Lawrence WT: Liposuction on a lymphedematous arm. Ann Plast Surg 21:366, 1988.
114. Thompson N: Surgical treatment of chronic lymphedema of the lower limb. With preliminary report of new operation. Br Med J II:1566, 1962.
115. Thompson N, Wee JTK: Twenty years' experience of the buried dermis flap operation in the treatment of chronic lymphedema of the extremities. Chir Plast 5:147, 1980.
116. Kondoleon E: Die operative behandlung der elephantiastichen Oedeme. Zentralbl Chir 39:1022, 1912.
117. Sistrunk WE: Further experiences with the Kondoleon operation for elephantiasis. JAMA 71:800, 1918.
118. Homans J: The treatment of elephantiasis of the legs: A preliminary report. N Engl J Med 215:1099, 1936.
119. Miller TA: Surgical management of lymphedema of the extremity. Plast Reconstr Surg 56:633, 1975.
120. Fonkalsrud EW, Coulson WF: Management of congenital lymphedema in infants and children. Ann Surg 177:280, 1973.
121. Miller TA: Surgical approach to lymphedema of the arm after mastectomy. Am J Surg 148:152, 1984.
122. Servelle M: Surgical treatment of lymphedema: A report on 652 cases. Surgery 101:484, 1987.
123. Sabin FR: Direct growth of veins by sprouting. *In* Contributions to Embryology. Washington, DC, Carnegie Institution of Washington 14:1, 1933.
124. Goetsch E: Hygroma colli cysticum and hygroma axillere: Pathologic and clinical study and report of twelve cases. Arch Surg 36:394, 1938.
125. Fonkalsrud EW: Surgical management of congenital malformations of the lymphatic system. Am J Surg 128:152, 1974.
126. Fonkalsrud EW: Malformation of the lymphatic system and hemangiomas. *In* Holder TH, Ashcraft KW (eds): Pediatric Surgery. Philadelphia, WB Saunders Company, 1980.
127. Bill AH Jr, Summer DS: A united concept of lymphangioma and cystic hygroma. Surg Gynecol Obstet 120:79, 1965.
128. Steward FW, Treves N: Lymphangiosarcoma in postmastectomy lymphedema: A report of six cases in elephantiasis chirurgica. Cancer 1:64, 1948.
129. Unruh H, Robertson DI, Karasewich E: Postmastectomy lymphangiosarcoma. Can J Surg 22:586, 1979.
130. Shafiroff BB, Nightingale G, Baxter JJ, O'Brien B: Lymphatico lymphatic anastomosis. Ann Plast Surg 3:199, 1979.
131. Woodward AH, Ivins JC, Soule EH: Lymph angiosarcoma arising in chronic lymphedematous extremities. Cancer 30:562, 1972.
132. Sordillo PP, Chapman R, Haidu SI, et al: Lymphangiosarcoma. Cancer 48:1674, 1981.
133. Tomita K, Yokogawa A, Oda Y, et al: Lymphangiosarcoma in postmastectomy lymphedema (Stewart-Treves syndrome): Ultrastructural and immunohistologic characteristics. J Surg Oncol 38:275, 1988.
134. Rosenberg SA, Suit HD, Baker LH, Rosen E: Sarcomas of the soft tissues and bone. *In* Devita VT Jr, Hellman S, Rosenberg SA (eds): Cancer: Principles and Practice of Oncology. Philadelphia, JB Lippincott, 1982.

REVIEW QUESTIONS

1. All of the following lymphatic structures have valves except:
   (a) interdermal lymphatics
   (b) dermal level lymphatics
   (c) collecting channels
   (d) main lymphatic trunks

2. Lower leg lymphatics drain principally into:
   (a) superior inguinal nodes
   (b) iliac nodes
   (c) inferior inguinal nodes
   (d) periaortic nodes

3. There is communication between superficial and deep vein lymphatics in:
   (a) normal extremities
   (b) 50 per cent of normal extremities
   (c) only under abnormal conditions
   (d) only after trauma

4. Complications of lymphangiography include all except:
   (a) lymphangitis
   (b) pulmonary embolus
   (c) fever
   (d) pancytopenia

5. Normal lymph contains what concentration of protein?
   (a) 0.01 to 0.05 gm/dl
   (b) 0.1 to 0.5 gm/dl
   (c) 1.0 to 5.0 gm/dl
   (d) 5.0 to 10.0 gm/dl

6. Lymphedema is characterized by all of the following except:
   (a) nonpitting edema
   (b) reduction of edema with elevation over days
   (c) skin ulceration
   (d) normal skin color

7. What percentage of patients with primary lymphedema present during adolescence (lymphedema praecox)?
   (a) 10 per cent
   (b) 40 per cent
   (c) 60 per cent
   (d) 80 per cent

8. "Staged subcutaneous excision" of lymphedematous tissue:
   (a) decreases postoperative lymphangitis and cellulitis
   (b) doesn't change RIHSA clearance
   (c) involves extensive skin grafting
   (d) cures lymphedema in the affected extremity

9. Therapy for congenital cystic hygroma causing respiratory obstruction in the neonatal period is:
   (a) sclerosis of the hygroma
   (b) radiation therapy
   (c) simple surgical excision
   (d) radical surgical excision

10. Lymphangiosarcoma:
    (a) arises only after radical mastectomy
    (b) occurs within 2 to 3 years of onset of lymphedema
    (c) has 80 per cent 5-year survival
    (d) responds poorly to currently available therapy

ANSWERS _____

1. a	2. c	3. c	4. d	5. b	6. c	7. d
8. a	9. c	10. d				

44

LOWER EXTREMITY AMPUTATION

JAMES M. MALONE

OVERVIEW AND HISTORICAL PERSPECTIVE

Amputation surgery is thought to be one of the oldest surgical procedures.[1] The earliest artificial limb dates from the Samnite wars of 300 B.C. Until the time of Ambroise Paré (1510–1590), the techniques for amputation surgery and amputation level selection were extremely crude. Paré not only improved the surgical technique of amputation through the use of vascular ligatures, but he also developed many guidelines for the selection of appropriate levels of amputation. Since many of his original drawings and descriptions are not greatly different than our surgical and prosthetic practices of today, he is considered to be the originator of the modern principles of amputation surgery. Paré's work was expanded by Dominique Jean Larrey (1776–1842) during the Napoleonic wars. Larrey advocated early amputation for traumatic limb injuries and was instrumental in the acceptance of both complete stump débridement and modern surgical techniques, whereby bone was buried deep in the amputation stump, rather than the previous method of suturing skin tightly over the bone. Larrey was also involved in developing methods of early mobilization of war amputees.[2]

The idea of immediate or rapid fitting of an artificial leg after lower extremity amputation is relatively recent. Credit for the concept of rapid fit is generally given to Berlemont (France, 1958) based on his work with patients with delayed healing after lower extremity amputation,[3] while the concept of immediate postsurgical prosthetic fitting was developed by Weiss (Poland, 1963).[4] In 1965, Burgess et al. noted accelerated rehabilitation, increased acceptance of a prosthesis, and less psychological trauma associated with loss of a limb when a prosthesis was applied immediately after lower extremity amputation.[5] In the last decade, advances in lower extremity amputation have included the development of new techniques for amputation level selection, the extension of the frontiers for limb salvage, and the fabrication of prosthetic limbs that have incorporated new designs and materials as well as energy storage.

Despite the long and colorful history attached to amputation surgery, amputation has been considered by most surgeons as a surgical defeat and an uninteresting and unrewarding surgical procedure. In many surgical institutions, amputation surgery has traditionally been passed down to the youngest and most inexperienced member of the surgical team, who often operated without senior supervision. A recent report from the European surgical literature suggests that amputation failure is statistically linked to the amputation experience of the surgeon.[6]

Recently, there has been a resurgence of interest in amputation surgery and rehabilitation. It is the view of the author that amputation surgery is not a failure; it is clearly a reconstructive surgical technique. In addition, the surgeon who performs the amputation *owes the patient the debt of rehabilitation* following surgery.

Historically, amputations were performed by orthopedic rather than general surgeons. However, since two thirds of all lower extremity amputations are now performed as a result of complications of peripheral vascular disease and/or diabetes mellitus, it is not surprising that the majority of lower extremity amputations are now performed by general and vascular surgeons. Unfortunately, most general surgical training programs fail to provide education in prosthetics, prosthetic design, biomechanics, and rehabilitation. The qualifications of the surgeon performing the amputation are not nearly as important as the interest of the surgeon in providing postoperative rehabilitation for the newly amputated patient.

This chapter will review important features of lower extremity amputation surgery and amputation rehabilitation that include detailed subsections on patient evaluation and preparation for amputation; techniques of amputation level selection; the indications, surgical techniques, and prosthetic requirements for each level of amputation; a review of surgical morbidity and mortality; an overview of common principles of lower extremity prosthetics; a discussion on techniques of postsurgical rehabilitation; and finally, some thoughts on future trends.

PATIENT EVALUATION AND PREPARATION FOR AMPUTATION

A review of the literature suggests that the mortality rates for below-knee and above-knee amputation are 4 to 16 per cent and 12 to 40 per cent, respectively.[7-12] It has been estimated that two thirds of patients undergoing lower extremity amputation have diabetes mellitus and that one half to two thirds have symptoms of cardiorespiratory diseases.[7,9,13] A review of the causes of late mortality following successful amputation surgery discloses that two thirds of the patients die from cardiovascular diseases, approximately one half of whom die from myocardial infarction.[7,14]

There are between 30,000 and 50,000 new lower extremity amputations performed in the United States each year.[7,9] At the present time, the data are unclear with respect to the question of whether the increase in distal revascularization has decreased the number of amputations. The indications for lower extremity amputation are listed in Table 44-1. For those patients with diabetes mellitus, it has been estimated that the risk of losing their second leg in the ensuing 5 years after amputation of the first leg ranges from 15 to 33 per cent (3 to 7 per cent/yr)[16-18]; however, one third to one half of amputees with diabetes mellitus die of complications of diabetes or cardiorespiratory diseases prior to undergoing an amputation of their second extremity.[16,18,19]

In view of the mean age of patients undergoing lower extremity amputation (62 years),[7,8,13-15] the incidence of associated diseases, and the morbid and nonmorbid complications associated with surgery, the importance of a careful preoperative physical examination cannot be overly stressed. The physical examination should include a search for physical signs and/or symptoms suggestive of cardiorespiratory diseases. Documentation of all pulses, as well as careful assessment of the presence or absence of physical findings suggestive of extremity ischemia (pain, paresthesias, elevation pallor, rubor, alteration of sensory or motor function) should be clearly documented. The extent and depth of infection and/or gangrene should be noted. The presence of malnutrition or systemic diseases such as diabetes mellitus, collagen vascular diseases, and immunodeficiency

syndromes or the systemic administration of antiinflammatory drugs, such as steroids, should be noted, since their presence may have a major influence on the preoperative preparation and timing of lower extremity amputation, as well as postsurgical recovery. A recent paper by Pinzur et al. reinforces the concept that multidisciplinary presurgical evaluation helps correct amputation level selection, correct prosthetic limb fitting, and improves patient rehabilitation.[20]

The presence of lower extremity infection in a diabetic patient requires special mention. Historically, most studies have suggested that the primary organisms were *Staphylococcus aureus* and/or enteric gramnegative bacilli. More recent information, however, suggests that 60 per cent of lower extremity infections in patients with diabetes mellitus involve both obligate and facultative anaerobic organisms.[21] Fierer et al. also pointed out that patients with mixed infections required more operations than those with simple staphylococcal infections and that their surgical wounds tended to heal more slowly.[21] We therefore recommend that appropriate antibiotic coverage for diabetics with lower extremity infections should include drugs that provide broad-spectrum bactericidal aerobic and anaerobic coverage.

In the absence of acute arterial embolization, diabetes mellitus, immunodeficiency syndromes, collagen vascular diseases, or drugs that inhibit the immune system, it is unusual to see tissue loss with or without infection in patients without multilevel vascular occlusive disease. Chronic single-level arterial obstruction is not usually associated with limb loss. As a general guideline, chronic occlusion of the superficial femoral artery will not cause limb loss without outflow (tibial trifurcation) or inflow (iliofemoral or profunda) occlusive disease.

The aims of the surgeon when recommending amputation are the following: to remove gangrenous tissues, to relieve pain, to obtain primary healing of the most distal amputation possible, and to obtain maximum rehabilitation after amputation. For purposes of further discussion, indications and management of patients undergoing amputation are divided into three general categories: (1) acute ischemia; (2) progressive chronic ischemia; and (3) ischemia complicated by infection.

Acute Ischemia

The choice of amputation for the management of acute ischemia in a patient whose arterial tree is considered unreconstructable or in a patient who presents late in the course of acute ischemia, such that arterial reconstruction may be contraindicated, is a decision that will tax the judgment of even the most experienced surgeon. In addition, urgent or emergent amputation following acute arterial occlusion is generally associated with the greatest risk of morbidity and mortality for the entire field of amputation surgery. The degree of urgency for amputation in the

TABLE 44-1.   INDICATIONS FOR LOWER EXTREMITY AMPUTATION[a]

	Percentage (Range)
Complications of diabetes mellitus	60–80
Nondiabetic infection with ischemia	15–25
Ischemia without infection	5–10
Chronic osteomyelitis	3–5
Trauma	2–5
Miscellaneous (neuroma, frostbite, tumor, pain, nonhealing)	5–10

[a]Data from Huston et al.,[7] Malone et al.,[9,15] Otteman and Stahlgren,[13] and Roon et al.[14]

face of acute arterial ischemia is governed by multiple factors that include, but are not limited to, the following: the extent of extremity ischemia, especially the muscle mass; the pain the patient is experiencing from the ischemic tissues; and the presence of signs of systemic toxicity resulting from products of necrotic muscle or bacteria reaching the general circulatory system. If the affected ischemic area is small, such as toes or forefoot, the pain is relatively moderate, and there are no signs of supervening infection or systemic toxicity, then amputation can and should be postponed as long as possible to allow maximum development of collateral circulation. Delay of amputation in such a case will improve the likelihood that a more distal limited amputation will heal. Mild to moderate pain can be controlled with narcotics. Adjunctive therapy, including systemic heparin, low-molecular-weight dextran, or the use of fibrinolytic agents, may be valuable in preventing progression of thrombus within capillary beds during the period of reduced blood flow, thus maintaining viability of marginally ischemic tissues during the time the collateral channels are beginning to enlarge. The presence of severe pain, extensive muscle necrosis, or systemic toxicity may require more emergent amputation with less patient preparation preoperatively. If muscle necrosis is extensive, the need for urgent or emergent amputation is critical because of the risk of renal damage that may occur secondary to circulating myoglobin. In addition to renal dysfunction, necrotic muscle tissue may cause cardiovascular or respiratory compromise and further push the need for emergent amputation. The presence of systemic toxicity, especially a necrotizing infection, often necessitates emergent amputation. For those patients with significant medical comorbidities and/or systemic toxicity, cryologic or physiologic amputation allows extended time for patient preparation for surgery and decreases mortality.[22]

Several features of patient evaluation and clinical progression are helpful in this decision-making process. The first consideration is the extent of nonviable skin. While discoloration or gangrene is readily apparent, hyposensitive areas due to severe skin ischemia will not allow adequate healing and may not be so easily identified. Excluding patients with diabetic neuropathy, sensation to pinprick and light touch is a useful discriminant. If there is diminished sensation below the knee, for example, the chances of being able to perform a successful below-knee amputation are small and morbidity may be avoided by proceeding expeditiously to an above-knee amputation. The presence of significant calf muscle swelling or muscle rigidity is an ominous sign suggestive of myonecrosis. Careful monitoring of calf circumference, skin sensation, urine color and output, and signs of systemic toxicity such as lethargy, confusion, or hallucinations must be employed on an hourly basis. The presence of systemic toxicity or significant changes in physical examination represent indications for proceeding with immediate amputation or

physiologic amputation.[22] Similarly, the presence of myoglobinuria or cardiovascular instability represents an indication for immediate amputation. It is generally impossible to obtain rapid myoglobin determinations in serum or urine, but the presence of urinary heme (blood)-positive dipstick in the absence of red cells under microscopic examination or pink serum (hemoglobin) is consistent with a diagnosis of myoglobinuria. In addition, the presence of markedly elevated creatine phosphokinase and lactate dehydrogenase isoenzymes in the serum is suggestive of myonecrosis in the absence of trauma, myocardial infarction, or recent surgery. If continued observation is elected, prophylaxis against renal damage from myoglobin pigment is recommended and includes maintenance of a diuresis in the range of 75 to 100 ml/hr by the administration of osmotic diuretics such as mannitol and fluids. In addition, the urine should be maintained at an alkaline pH, since myoglobin precipitates in the renal tubules at a pH less than 7. Usually a mixture of mannitol and sodium bicarbonate in a balanced salt solution can be used to titrate urine output and pH. Finally, the presence of infection in the ischemic extremity is an ominous complication requiring very careful consideration. The presence of such an infection in a diabetic is even more ominous because of the sometimes rapid progression of seemingly innocuous infections. Any evidence of systemic toxicity or progressive infection is an indication for immediate surgical débridement, which may be in the form of a débriding amputation or a physiologic amputation followed later by a formal surgical amputation.

As long as there is continued improvement in collateral blood supply to an acutely ischemic extremity, and there is absence of signs of systemic or renal toxicity, observation may be continued. As soon as circulatory improvement ceases or signs of toxicity develop, amputation should be performed promptly. An alternative to amputation in an unstable or high-risk patient is physiologic amputation as previously discussed.

Evaluation for potential vascular reconstruction in a patient with clear-cut demarcation of a nonviable area of a lower extremity after a period of observation for acute ischemia is not likely to be beneficial; however, if there is a question of marginal viability of tissue above an area that is believed to be nonviable, and the questionably viable tissue might permit a lower amputation level, then evaluation for vascular reconstruction may be beneficial.[23] For example, the presence of a nonviable forefoot and a marginal lower extremity between the knee and ankle may be an indication for evaluation for vascular reconstruction in an attempt to salvage a below-knee rather than an above-knee amputation.

Progressive Chronic Ischemia

The patient with progressive chronic ischemia who ultimately presents for amputation has experienced one or more of the following problems: rest pain, nonhealing skin lesion or ulceration, gangrene, or gangrene with superimposed infection. Gangrene complicated by infection is a special problem and will be discussed in a separate section.

From the patient's point of view, ischemic rest pain is one of the most compelling indications for amputation. Characteristically, the patient will seek relief by sitting up and allowing his/her leg(s) to hang over the side of the bed or by ambulation. The dependent position provides relief of ischemic rest pain because gravity favors improved collateral blood flow, which augments arterial perfusion pressure. In its more severe forms, ischemic rest pain forms part of a vicious cycle. As the patient more frequently uses dependency to achieve pain relief, the extremity becomes edematous and lymphatic return decreases, which eventually results in more ischemia. The end result of this vicious cycle is a massively swollen, very painful ischemic extremity. Mild to moderate rest pain may often be successfully managed with narcotics. There have been reports that early mild rest pain may be relieved by sympathectomy. As long as there are no signs of systemic toxicity or supervening infection and if mild ischemic rest pain can be controlled with medication, then a patient can be followed and amputation postponed.

Another manifestation of chronic ischemia is the presence of ischemic skin ulceration or nonhealing skin lesions on the lower extremity. Unfortunately, many of these skin ulcers occur in hospitalized patients as a result of abrasion of the foot or pressure necrosis (due to poor foot protection in the hospital bed). In the diabetic patient, ulceration usually occurs at pressure points and the patient will often be unaware of the problem because of diabetic neuropathy. Patients without peripheral neuropathy will be very much aware of these ischemic ulcers because they are typically extremely painful. Besides obvious areas of pressure necrosis such as the heel and the lateral and medial malleoli, other common points of ulceration include the bony prominences over the metatarsal heads and midphalangeal joints or between the toes.

Fortunately, most patients with chronic progressive ischemia come to medical attention before the presence of frank tissue loss. Even patients with tissue loss usually present early with involvement of one or more toes, or under more severe circumstances, the entire forefoot. Under these circumstances, there is usually ample opportunity to fully prepare and evaluate the patient for lower extremity amputation or arterial reconstruction if possible. Preoperative evaluation and management should include proper medical attention to all associated diseases and a careful evaluation for potential critical organ dysfunction, especially the heart, lungs, and kidneys.

All patients with chronic ischemia should undergo consideration for vascular reconstruction for limb salvage. Angiographic evaluation from the infrarenal abdominal aorta down to and including the pedal arches is mandatory. In general, the surgeon should ensure good inflow to the level of the profunda femoris artery. Reconstruction distal to the level of the profunda femoris artery should be done only if chances for success are reasonably high and if a successful procedure would obviate the need for a major amputation. There is continuing controversy on the effect of prior revascularization on amputation level.[24–32] In the author's opinion revascularization should always be attempted unless contraindicated by the patient's medical condition. If vascular reconstruction is brought below the knee, the incision required for approaching the distal popliteal artery and tibial trifurcation vessels should be planned along the lines of the posterior skin flap that might be required for a subsequent below-knee amputation. Techniques for evaluating amputation level selection will be discussed in a subsequent section. However, one of the interesting spin-offs from studies of amputation level selection is the identification of patients who are not able to heal a low-level amputation and in whom the chance for rehabilitation at a high level of amputation is unlikely. When such objective information is available, attempts at proximal and/or extended distal extremity bypass, to salvage a knee joint, for example, may be indicated in order to keep a patient ambulatory.[23,25,26]

Gangrene Complicated by Infection

The presence of dry gangrene is not an emergent surgical problem, nor necessarily the hallmark of an ominous clinical situation. Dry gangrene, limited to the toes, for example, may be treated conservatively and require little, if any, surgical or ancillary medical support; however, infection complicating dry gangrene (i.e., wet gangrene), especially in a diabetic patient, is a limb- and life-threatening emergency. Control of sepsis may sometimes be achieved with antibiotic therapy plus limited débridement and drainage, or it may require radical excision and débridement; however, antibiotic therapy alone is seldom adequate treatment for gangrene complicated by infection. Failure to institute prompt therapy, especially in diabetic patients, will result in rapid ascension of the infectious process, the loss of potentially salvageable tissue, and a large increase in patient mortality. As noted earlier, in patients with systemic toxicity, cryoamputation prior to definitive surgical amputation will help decrease mortality.

The first step in the management of infected or wet gangrene is identification of the infecting organisms. Usually the urgency of the clinical situation does not allow the time required for identification of specific organisms by culture, although culture should be obtained and submitted for both anaerobic and aerobic organisms. It has been our practice to assume that gangrene complicated by infection of necessity includes a mixture of aerobic and anaerobic organisms and, therefore, broad-spectrum bactericidal antibiotic coverage is used.[21]

Once antibiotic therapy has been started, the patient must be very carefully monitored. The indicators usually followed include pulse rate, white blood cell count, blood pressure, temperature, extent of infection, severity of pain, and diffuse signs of systemic toxicity such as lethargy, hallucinations, and general mental status. In a diabetic patient, serum glucose and insulin requirements are additional useful monitoring parameters. If a prompt response to antibiotic therapy is noted, therapy should be continued for maximum effect and a definitive amputation then performed. If the patient does not respond promptly to antibiotic management or if undrained purulent material was initially evident, débridement of gangrenous tissue and establishment of drainage should be employed as an early adjunct to antibiotic therapy.

If the gangrenous infection extensively involves the foot and contaminates tendon and tissue spaces, especially in a diabetic patient, then radical débridement should be performed. One of the better methods to obtain radical débridement and establish open drainage is a guillotine amputation of the foot carried out at the level of the malleoli (Fig. 44–1). Guillotine amputation will eliminate the septic focus, and allow drainage of contaminated lymphatics and tissue spaces in the lower leg. The presence of cellulitis and lymphangitis at the level of ankle guillotine is not a contraindication for this type of débridement technique.

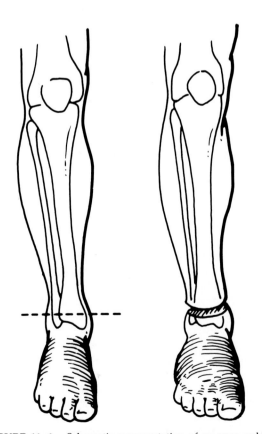

FIGURE 44–1. Schematic representation of an open ankle guillotine or preparatory amputation in a patient with a septic foot.

After performance of a guillotine-type amputation for débridement, systemic antibiotics are continued until the definitive amputation is performed. Definitive amputation is performed after ascertaining that, in fact, the infection has been controlled and the patient's preoperative status has been optimized.

The incidence of stump infection in patients who present with a septic foot is decreased if a preparatory ankle guillotine amputation is performed prior to definitive amputation. In our experience such a two-stage surgical approach decreased the stump infection rate from 22 per cent to 3 per cent ($p \leq .01$).[33] This approach was reaffirmed in a prospective randomized study by Fischer et al.,[34] in which the incidence of stump infection was decreased from 21 per cent (one stage) to 0 per cent (two stage) ($p \leq .05$).

Amputation for Trauma

In general, patients undergoing traumatic lower extremity amputation tend to be young and in good medical health, so patient evaluation and preparation for amputation is easier than that described for the geriatric patient with peripheral vascular disease and diabetes. As a general principle, formal traumatic amputation is performed to achieve healing at the lowest amputation level possible and amputation level selection is usually predetermined by the injury. Adequate débridement of dead tissue is mandatory. The presence of a large amount of marginally viable tissue or potentially infected tissue may be indications for débridement and open amputation followed at a later date by formal amputation with skin closure. A special effort should be made to rule out proximal bony or ligamentous injuries. Careful attention must be paid to looking for other potentially life- or limb-threatening injuries, and management of such injuries must be handled in a sequence that is appropriate for the best overall salvage of the patient. The use of a proximal extremity tourniquet for control of bleeding is optional but to be discouraged in a dysvascular patient. The use of drains after traumatic amputation is controversial, although there is some evidence to suggest that drainage after traumatic amputation results in a more rapid resolution of post-amputation stump edema. If drains are used they should be of the closed-system type (and not open Penrose drains).

AMPUTATION LEVEL DETERMINATION

The objective of preoperative amputation level selection is to determine the most distal amputation site that will heal. The general requirements are as follows: (1) the amputation must remove all necrotic, painful, or infected tissue; (2) the amputation stump must be able to be fitted with a functional and easily applied prosthesis; and (3) the blood supply at the level of proposed amputation must be sufficient to allow primary skin healing. Appropriate amputation level selection is of critical importance. If the surgeon elects too proximal an amputation, such as a mid-thigh amputation, the patient may be deprived of the opportunity for subsequent ambulation and rehabilitation although the amputation might heal without difficulty. If a distal amputation site is selected and the blood supply is inadequate for amputation healing, further surgery will be required in order to achieve healing of an amputation at a higher level. This latter approach may result in increased morbidity and mortality and, in addition, may ultimately result in rehabilitation failure.

The inherent advantages of a below-knee amputation as opposed to an above-knee amputation should be obvious. It is easier to ambulate on a below-knee prosthesis, a fact that is extremely important, especially in geriatric patients. In general, a unilateral below-knee amputee requires a 10 to 40 per cent increase in energy expenditure for ambulation compared to the energy required for walking with an intact extremity. In contrast, a unilateral above-knee amputee (using a prosthesis with a locked or unlocked knee) requires approximately a 50 to 70 per cent increase in energy expenditure. Crutch walking without a lower extremity prosthesis utilizes approximately a 60 per cent increase in energy expenditure, whereas wheelchair use necessitates only a small increase in energy expenditure (9 per cent). Patients with severe coronary artery disease and/or severe chronic obstructive pulmonary disease may be physically unable to provide the additional energy expenditure required for ambulation on an above-knee compared to below-knee prosthesis.

It is usually possible for the surgeon to decide on an amputation level that will remove necrotic, painful, or infected tissue as well as to plan an amputation stump that can be fit with a prosthesis. However, the decision regarding the adequacy of blood supply at the proposed amputation level has been one of the most difficult problems facing the amputation surgeon.

The earliest attempts at amputation level selection utilized presence of pulses in the affected extremity, skin temperature, correlation of arteriographic findings, and "clinical judgment." It has been well documented that none of these selection techniques has a consistent enough correlation with amputation healing to provide a sound basis for clinical decision making. In a study by Robbs and Ray,[35] the morbidity, mortality, and rates of healing of lower limb amputations in 214 patients, wherein the amputation level was determined by nonobjective criteria, were retrospectively analyzed. Six of 67 (8.9 per cent) primary above-knee amputations and 37 of 147 (25 per cent) primary below-knee amputations had to be revised to a higher level. The authors concluded "that flap viability could not be predicted by the extent of ischemic lesion in relation to the ankle joint, the popliteal pulse status or lower limb angiography."[35] In

a recent study comparing clinical parameters and skin perfusion pressure for amputation level selection, Dwars et al. noted that the presence of palpable pulses immediately above the selected level correlated well with primary healing. However, the absence of palpable pulses and angiographic patency scores were of no clinical value in amputation level selection.[36] However, Golbranson et al. have recently presented promising data on improved methods of skin temperature measurement that had a high degree of accuracy (90 per cent) for selecting below- versus above-knee amputation levels.[37] In addition, Spence and Walker[38] have recently demonstrated a clear correlation between three different temperature isotherms (1.8°C separation) and isotopically derived skin blood flow ($p < .001$). Stoner et al. recently reported that when the ratio of temperatures at the posterior and anterior incision sites (Burgess posterior flap below-knee amputation) was greater than 0.98, healing was improved.[39] In a study comparing several modalities for amputation level selection, Wagner et al. noted (for above- and below-knee amputations) that the average skin temperature at the amputation site was higher (34.3°C) in the group that healed primarily compared to those that required operative stump revision (33.3°C) ($p \leq .001$).[40] One physical finding that has some value in differentiating proposed amputation levels is the presence of dependent rubor. Skin that develops dependent rubor is clearly ischemic and hence skin with dependent rubor, like gangrenous tissue, is an absolute contraindication to amputation at that level; however, the absence of dependent rubor does not necessarily ensure healing ability. Early workers in the field of amputation surgery solved the problem of level selection by performing above-knee amputations on almost all patients. In the 1960s, Lim and coworkers demonstrated that 83 per cent of all patients requiring a lower extremity amputation would heal a below-knee amputation.[41] However, using empiric below-knee amputation selection potentially deprives some patients who might have healed a more distal amputation, such as transmetatarsal or Syme's. In addition, identifying the 20 to 30 per cent of patients in whom a below-knee amputation is doomed to failure would be advantageous so that either a knee disarticulation or above-knee amputation could be performed primarily, saving the patient additional surgical procedures.

The need for more sensitive and objective methods for preoperative amputation level selection has led to the development of numerous noninvasive techniques including Doppler ankle and calf systolic blood pressures, with or without pulse volume recordings,[42-49] xenon-133 skin blood flow studies,[50-56] digital or transmetatarsal photoplethysmographic pressures,[47] transcutaneous oxygen determination,[56-64] skin fluorescence after intravenous fluorescein dye,[65-68] laser Doppler skin blood flow[52,69] (F. A. Matsen, personal communication), pertechnetate skin blood pressure studies,[70,71] and photoelectrically measured skin color changes.[72]

An overview of the various selection criteria for prediction of healing of digit and forefoot amputations is shown in Table 44–2. Totals from Table 44–2 suggest that preoperative amputation level selection techniques correctly predicted primary healing in 174 out of 180 toe and forefoot amputations (97 per cent). Similar data for preoperative below-knee amputation level selection are summarized in Table 44–3. Excluding empiric below-knee selection, the tests shown in Table 44–3 were able to correctly predict primary healing of below-knee amputations in 522 out of 554 elective amputations (94 per cent). Clearly, objective amputation level selection is able not only to predict potential healing of a more distal level of amputation (Table 44–2), but also to accurately assess the likelihood of healing of a below-knee compared to an above-knee amputation (Table 44–3). It is my opinion that elective lower extremity amputation should not be performed without some type of preoperative testing in order to ensure primary healing of the most distal amputation possible.

The techniques for the use of ankle, calf, and popliteal Doppler systolic blood pressure determinations have been well described[42–46,48,49] and will not be covered in the text of this chapter. Similarly, use of the photoplethysmograph for determination of digit and transmetatarsal blood pressures has been well described by Schwartz et al.[47] and will not be presented in this chapter. The potential advantages of both the Doppler and the photoplethysmograph are that they are relatively simple, inexpensive, and totally noninvasive. The problem with the use of these instruments is that the presence of a blood pressure less than a predetermined level does not necessarily guarantee failure of amputation healing at that level (negative predictive value). This problem was nicely summarized by Verta et al., who noted that "for forefoot amputation a high Doppler ankle pressure did not guarantee successful healing and a low ankle pressure did not contraindicate primary healing."[48] In an effort to increase the accuracy of Doppler ankle pressures, both Gibbons et al. and Raines et al. have suggested the ancillary use of pulse volume recordings.[45,46] Although Raines et al. quoted 100 per cent successful healing in 27 below-knee amputations where Doppler systolic ankle pressure was greater than 30 mm Hg, calf pressure was greater than 65 mm Hg, and there was a pulsatile pulse volume recording in the foot,[46] Gibbons et al. were unable to duplicate those results, and concluded that "we find no consistent criteria which are more accurate and reliable than clinical judgment and no ankle pressure above which primary healing was guaranteed."[45] Gibbons et al. also noted decreased accuracy in amputation level prediction using pulse volume recording and Doppler ankle systolic pressures in patients with diabetes mellitus. Most probably, the problem with diabetic patients (falsely high systolic pressure measurements) is due to medical calcinosis of their vessels. More recently, Wagner et al. reported that Doppler pressures at the thigh, popliteal, midcalf, or ankle levels were unreliable in predicting healing of a below-knee amputation.[40]

Theoretically, the measurement of skin fluorescence with a Wood's ultraviolet lamp after intravenous injection of fluorescein dye (Funduscen) should form the basis for a reliable test for amputation level selection. Although this technique is somewhat more invasive than Doppler ankle systolic pressure measurements or pulse volume recordings, it is less complicated and noninvasive than xenon-133 skin blood flow or pertechnetate skin perfusion measurements. The commercial availability of two new types of fluorometers (Fiberoptic Perfusion Fluorometer, Diversatronics, Broomall, PA; and Fluoroscan, V. Elings, Ph.D, University of California, Santa Barbara), which are able to provide objective numerical readings quickly and in the absence of a Wood's lamp, may further enhance the use of this technique.[65,67,68] More recent development of a computerized video camera system to analyze skin perfusion after the oral ingestion of fluorescein obviates the risk of intravenous injection and allows easy data manipulation for limb mapping. Such a system is now under study at Maricopa Medical Center in Phoenix. McFarland and Lawrence[66] reported an accuracy rate of 80 per cent for skin fluorescence compared to 47 per cent for Doppler popliteal systolic blood pressure (50 mm Hg) for prediction of healing of below-knee amputation (Table 44–3). In addition, when skin fluorescence and Doppler pressure did not agree on the level of amputation, fluorescein always predicted a more distal level.[66]

TABLE 44–2.   TOE AND FOREFOOT AMPUTATION SELECTION CRITERIA

Selection Criteria[a]	Reference	Amputation Level	Healing Patients	
Doppler ankle systolic pressure				
70 mm Hg	42	Forefoot	38/44	(86%)
	47	Digit/forefoot	25/27	(93%)
35 mm Hg	48	Digit	44/46	(96%)
Fiberoptic fluorometry DFI >44	68	Foot forefoot	18/20	(90%)
Photoplethysmographic digit or TMA pressure				
20 mm Hg	47	Digit	20/20	(100%)
Xenon skin clearance >2.6 ml/100 gm tissue/min	54	Digit/forefoot	25/28	(89%)
TcpO$_2$ >20 mm Hg	62	Forefoot	4/4	(100%)
		TOTAL	174/180	(97%)

[a]*DFI*, dye fluorescence index; *TMA*, transmetatarsal-ankle; *TcpO$_2$*, transcutaneous partial pressure of oxygen.

TABLE 44–3.   BELOW-KNEE AMPUTATION SELECTION CRITERIA

Selection Criteria[a]	Reference	Healing Patients	
Doppler systolic ankle pressure 30 mm Hg + calf pressure 65 mm Hg + pulsatile PVR	46	27/27	(100%)
Doppler systolic calf pressure 70 mm Hg	43	32/32	(100%)
Doppler systolic thigh pressure 80 mm Hg or calf pressure 50 mm Hg	49	36/36	(100%)
Empiric below knee	41	38/46	(83%)[b]
Fiberoptic fluorometry DFI >44	68	12/12	(100%)
Fluorescein dye	66	24/30	(80%)
99mTc-pertechnetate skin blood pressure	82	24/26	92%
Laser Doppler velocimetry > 20 mV	74	25/26	96%
Photoelectric skin pressure 20–100 mm Hg	72, 83	60/71	85%
TcpO2 >10 mm Hg or >10 mm Hg increase on 100% oxygen	59, 76	76/80	95%
>35 mm Hg	57, 61, 64	51/51	100%
>20 mm Hg	62	16/16	(100%)
>0<40 mm Hg	57	17/19	89%
0 mm Hg	57	0/3	0%[b]
index >0.59	61	17/17	100%
index >0.20	73	33/34	97%
Xenon skin clearance =3.1 ml blood flow/100 gm tissue/min	51	23/26	88%
>2.6 ml blood flow/100 gm tissue/min	54	35/36	97%
Epicutaneous >0.9 ml/100 gm tissue/min	50, 53	14/15	93%
	TOTAL	522/554	94%

[a]*PVR*, pulse volume recording; *DFI*, dye fluorescence index; *TcpO2*, transcutaneous partial pressure of oxygen.
[b]Excluded from total.

Silverman et al.[68] recently reported their data on fiberoptic fluorometry for amputation level selection at the below-knee, below-ankle, and above-knee levels in dysvascular limbs. The overall success rate was 92 per cent (36 of 39), and individual levels were 18 of 20 below-ankle (90 per cent); 12 of 12 below-knee (100 per cent); and 6 of 7 above-knee (86 per cent). Discriminate analysis demonstrated an optimum reference point between healing and nonhealing amputations, and a dye fluorescence index (DFI) of greater than 44 had 93 per cent accuracy. Two more recent studies, however, did not demonstrate such promising results.[73,74] In a blinded prospective review of 56 patients undergoing below-knee amputation, objective measurement of fluorescein perfusion did not correlate with amputation healing.[75] In a study comparing multiple methods of amputation level selection, Wagner et al.[40] found that qualitative skin fluorescence was not as successful as cutaneous oxygen measurement.

Promising work with a modified Clark-type oxygen electrode (with a heating element and thermostat for temperature control) (Transoxode, Hellige-Orager, FRG; U.S. manufacturer, Litton Industries) for amputation level selection has been reported by several groups.[57,59,61,62,64,76] Franzeck et al. reported that the mean transcutaneous pO2 values of patients who primarily healed a lower extremity amputation compared to those that failed to heal were 36.5 ± 17.5 and less than 0.3 mm Hg, respectively.[59] However, in those patients with a transcutaneous pO2 less than 10 mm Hg, 6 of 9 failed to heal while 3 of 9 healed primarily. In a study on below-knee amputations, Burgess et al. found that 15 of 15 amputations healed primarily if the transcutaneous pO2 was greater than 40 mm Hg, 17 of 19 healed if the transcutaneous pO2 was greater than 0 mm Hg but less than 40 mm Hg, and none of the three amputations with a pO_2 of 0 mm Hg healed.[57] Katsamouris et al.[61] reported that 17 of 17 lower extremity amputations healed if the pO_2 was greater than 38 mm Hg or if the pO_2 index (chest wall control site) was greater than 0.59. Ratliff et al.[64] noted that 18 below-knee amputations healed if the pO_2 was greater than 35 mm Hg, while 10 of 15 failed if the pO_2 was less than 35 mm Hg. Kram et al.[73] noted success in 33 of 34 (97 per cent) below-knee amputations with multisensor transcutaneous oxygen mapping when the critical pO_2 index was greater than 0.20. In addition, none of the six patients healed with an index of less than 0.20. All investigators have reported that some patients heal an amputation with low pO_2 values. A partial explanation of this observation might be the nonlinear relationship between pO_2 and cutaneous blood flow. In a very careful study, Matsen et al.[63] reported that pO_2 measurements are most dependent on arterial-venous gradients and cutaneous vascular resistance. Techniques to improve the accuracy of transcutaneous pO_2 probes include local heating (44°C) (minimizes local vascular resistance and makes pO_2 more linear with respect to cutaneous blood flow), measurements before and after oxygen administration, oxygen isobar extremity mapping, and transcutaneous oxygen recovery half-time (TORT).[77] Oishi et al.[78] noted—in a study comparing skin temperature, Doppler pressure, and transcutaneous oxygen—that after the inhalation of oxygen, if the pO_2 increased 10 mm Hg or more, the pO_2 predicted amputation healing with a sensitivity of 98 per cent. In a recent study, the author and his associates prospectively compared the following tests for their accuracy in amputation level selection: transcutaneous oxygen, transcutaneous carbon dioxide, transcutaneous oxygen–to–transcutaneous carbon dioxide, foot–to–chest transcutaneous oxygen, intradermal xenon-133, ankle-brachial index, and absolute popliteal artery pressure.[62] All metabolic parameters had a high degree of statistical accuracy in predicting amputation healing, whereas none of the other tests had statistical reliability. All amputations, transmetatarsal, below-knee, and above-knee, healed primarily if the transcutaneous pO_2 level was greater than 20 mm Hg and there was a 0 per cent incidence of false-positive and false-negative studies. Also of importance was the observation that amputation site healing was not affected by the presence of diabetes mellitus, nor were the test results for any of the metabolic parameters. Similar data have recently been reported by Bacharach et al.,[79] where 51 of 52 limbs healed (primary and delayed) (98 per cent) with a pO_2 greater than or equal to 40 mm Hg and a pO_2 of less than 20 mm Hg was associated with universal failure. In that study, pO_2 measurements during limb elevation improved predictability of outcome for patients with supine

pO_2 values greater than 20 mm Hg but less than 40 mm Hg.

Theoretically, laser Doppler velocimetry should be an ideal tool for skin blood flow determination, since it is noninvasive and "measures" capillary blood flow (good correlation between laser Doppler blood flow measurements using microspheres and electromagnetic flow probes and xenon-133 clearance[80]); however, data by Holloway et al.[51,52,80] and Matsen (personal communication) suggest that although there is a linear relationship among techniques, there is a fair amount of variance. These groups, however, have noted that the use of local skin heating may enhance the accuracy of the laser Doppler and make it a more valuable adjunct for amputation level selection.[80] Holloway and Burgess[69] reported their experience with laser Doppler velocimetry in 20 lower extremity amputations at the foot, forefoot, below- and above-knee levels, and the accuracy rates were as follows: foot/forefoot 2 of 6 (33 per cent); below-knee 8 of 8 (100 per cent); and above-knee 6 of 6 (100 per cent).

The author's greatest postsurgical experience was with the use of xenon-133 skin clearance for amputation level selection.[54,55] The techniques for utilization of xenon-133 skin blood flow have been well described by Moore,[51] Daly and Henry,[81] and subsequently Malone et al. One of the major difficulties with the application of xenon skin clearance for amputation level selection is its reproducibility by other investigators. In an earlier publication, Holloway and Burgess were not able to document a clear-cut end point above which all amputations healed.[51] On the other hand, Silberstein et al.[56] reported that 38 of 39 patients (11 above-knee and 18 below-knee/transmetatarsal amputations, and 9 no amputation) healed when xenon-133 skin blood flow was greater than 2.4 ml/100 gm tissue/min and that when flow was less than 2.4 ml/100 gm tissue/min only 4 of 7 patients healed. One significant advantage of xenon-133 clearance techniques that may offset both of these problems, if its ultimate reliability is demonstrated in other centers, is its potential ability to successfully predict healing at all levels of lower extremity amputation.[54] A final problem with the intradermal use of xenon-133 for skin blood flow measurements is that the manufacturer no longer supplies xenon-133. The product must be made by nuclear medicine departments. This limitation may further preclude widespread use of the intradermal xenon-133 technique. Finally, in spite of past publications[54,55,81] and previously published excellent results, the author no longer uses xenon-133 skin clearance for amputation level selection. In part this change was made because of the enumerated difficulties; however, for the most part this change was made as a result of a recently published study[62] wherein xenon-133 was not found to be statistically reliable as a selection method for amputation level determination (as noted previously, transcutaneous oxygen was very reliable).

Using the disappearance of intradermal ^{99m}Tc-pertechnetate, Na [^{131}I], ^{131}I-antipyrine, or xenon-133 in the presence of external pressure, Holstein[70] and Holstein and Lassen[82] have reported amputation level selection data comparable to that reported by Moore, Daly, Henry, Malone, et al. Because xenon-133 is trapped in subcutaneous fat, there are solid theoretical issues that support the use of an isotope other than xenon-133. In a recent publication, Holstein et al.[71] found no significant difference among Na[^{131}I], ^{131}I-antipyrine, and ^{99m}Tc-pertechnetate for the measurement of skin perfusion pressure.

Stockel et al.[72] and Oveson and Stockel[83] have reported preliminary data that correlate well with the xenon-133 skin perfusion pressure techniques of Holstein and Holstein et al.[70,71] on the use of a photodetector and plethysmography (Medimatic, Denmark) for amputation level selection. This technique uses a blood pressure cuff placed over a photoelectric detector, which is connected to a plethysmograph, to measure the minimal external pressure required to prevent skin reddening after blanching. To date, 66 of 71 (85 per cent) below-knee amputations healed with skin pressures between 20 and 100 mm Hg. Most recently, Dwars et al.[36] reported that skin perfusion pressure measurements were of excellent predictive value for the healing of lower extremity amputations (positive predictive value 89 per cent, negative predictive value 99 per cent).

In summary, it is the opinion of the author that elective lower extremity amputation should not be performed in the absence of objective testing in order to perform the most distal amputation that will primarily heal, yet allow removal of infected, painful, or ischemic tissue. A variety of techniques are available and which of the various techniques are chosen depends upon available equipment, amputation level under consideration, and the current accuracy rates for the reported techniques.

LOWER EXTREMITY AMPUTATION LEVELS: INDICATIONS, CONTRAINDICATIONS, TECHNIQUE, ADVANTAGES, DISADVANTAGES, PROSTHETIC REQUIREMENTS, AND REHABILITATION POTENTIAL

This section will discuss only those amputation levels that are relevant for patients with peripheral vascular disease and/or diabetes mellitus. Amputation levels that are less desirable from the standpoint of healing or rehabilitation, or those that present specific prosthetic fitting problems, will be omitted. In the experience of the author and others, Chopart, Lisfrank, and Boyd forefoot amputations have been fraught with controversy because of healing problems, prosthetic fitting problems, and equinus deformities.[84] Since these amputation levels are seldom

used by vascular surgeons they will not be reviewed in the text.

Toe Amputation

Toe amputation is the most frequently performed peripheral amputation. It is especially common in patients with diabetes mellitus, since these patients are prone to lesions that necessitate amputation (ulceration, osteomyelitis, and gangrene).

Patients who present with dry gangrene allow the surgeon a choice between direct surgical intervention and autoamputation. In the absence of supervening infection or pain, expectant management permits epithelialization to take place under the dry gangrenous eschar. As soon as epithelialization is complete, the toe will drop off, leaving a cleanly healed stump. Autoamputation is preferable to direct surgical intervention because it removes the necessity for healing after amputation and probably results in a more distal site of healing than would be achieved after surgical intervention. However, this process often requires months before it is complete.

Indications

The gangrene, infection, neuropathic ulceration, or osteomyelitis should be confined to the mid- or distal phalanx. There must be no dependent rubor and venous filling time should be less than 20 to 25 seconds. Sizer and Wheelock have demonstrated that the presence of pedal pulses, even in patients with diabetes, is associated with a very high rate of healing after toe amputation (98 per cent).[85]

Contraindications

Cellulitis proximal to the area of proposed toe excision, the presence of dependent rubor, forefoot infection, and involvement of the metatarsophalangeal joint or (distal) metatarsal head all represent specific contraindications for toe amputation.

Surgical Technique

A single toe should never be amputated by disarticulation, but should be transected through the proximal phalanx, leaving a small button of bone to protect the metatarsal head. Skin flaps can be of any design, so long as they obey basic surgical principles and have adequate base for length of flap. The flaps can be fish mouth, plantar base, dorsal base, side to side, or any variation or combination: however, they must be long enough to close without tension. The most commonly used incision is circular (Fig. 44–2). Amputation through the metatarsophalangeal joint or an interphalangeal joint should be avoided because of the avascular nature of cartilage and the likelihood of supervening infection or failure to heal.

Careful atraumatic edge-to-edge skin closure without the use of forceps will maximize the chances of primary healing. Suture material that produces minimal reaction when left in place for long periods of

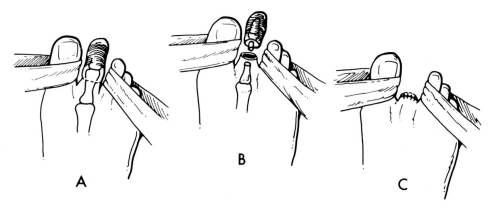

FIGURE 44–2. Artist's conception of a single-toe amputation using a circular incision and transverse wound closure.

time should be employed, such as monofilament wire or plastic. A soft postoperative dressing, which provides gentle wound compression, should be applied.

Chronic osteomyelitis of the great toe without gangrene in a diabetic patient presents a difficult surgical problem. Since complete healing is not common and since total resection of the great toe will result in some imbalance in walking (which can be accommodated with proper shoe orthotics), débridement and resection of the infected phalanges through a medial or lateral incision, leaving a soft tissue toe remnant in place, is probably the best surgical procedure from a functional standpoint.

Advantages and Disadvantages

The primary advantage of toe amputation is the lack of requirement for prosthetic rehabilitation and the fact that minimal tissue is excised.

Except for the risk of nonhealing of secondary infection and stump breakdown, requiring a higher level of amputation, there are no disadvantages to this level of amputation.

Rehabilitation Potential

Rehabilitation potential is 100 per cent. However, the performance of a toe amputation in a patient with peripheral vascular disease, especially with concomitant diabetes, is an ominous sign with respect to long-term prognosis. Little et al. found that by 3.5 years after toe amputation, almost three quarters of their patients required a more proximal major amputation.[86]

Ray Amputation

Indications

If the gangrenous skin or infectious process approaches the phalangeal-metatarsal crease or includes the (distal) metatarsal head, this precludes a toe amputation. A conservative partial distal forefoot amputation can still be performed by extending the toe amputation to include the distal metatarsal shaft and head.

Contraindications

Gangrene, infection, cellulitis, and dependent rubor involving skin proximal to the metatarsal-phalangeal crease are contraindications to the ray amputation. In addition, involvement of multiple toes is a relative contraindication, since a transmetatarsal amputation would be a more suitable surgical procedure. Ray amputation for gangrene or infection of the great toe also is a relative contraindication, since removal of the first metatarsal head leads to unstable weight bearing and difficulties with ambulation; however, with proper shoe orthotics, ray amputation of the first or great toe results in an excellent foot salvage and provides patients with a stable gait pattern.

Surgical Technique

The incision begins vertically on the dorsum of the foot, bifurcates laterally and medially to encircle the toe, meets on the plantar aspect of the foot, and extends for a variable distance on the plantar aspect of the foot. The plantar incision is extended proximally as needed to allow removal of the toe and distal metatarsal head. Care should be taken not to injure the digital arteries or nerves adjacent to the metatarsal bone and not to enter into the deep tension or joint spaces of the medial and lateral toes. The distal metatarsal shaft is divided at its neck and soft tissues are removed by sharp dissection. The surgical specimen consists of the toe, metatarsophalangeal joint, and distal portion of the metatarsal shaft and head. If possible, the surgical specimen should be removed in continuity. The metatarsal shaft must be transected in an area of normal bone. "Soft bone" suggests osteomyelitis, especially in diabetic patients, and mandates higher (i.e., more proximal) bone division.

We recommend that the surgical wound be generously irrigated with an antibiotic solution (the content of which is based upon preoperative cultures, if available). Once again, attention is paid to meticulous hemostasis and an atraumatic deep tissue and skin closure. Interrupted monofilament sutures that achieve edge-to-edge skin coaptation (without the use of forceps) should be placed (Fig. 44–3). The postoperative dressing can either be a soft dressing with an outer elastic wrap (which will allow compression of the forefoot and remove tension from the suture line) or a combination of a soft dressing with foot and lower leg plaster cast that will provide maximum skin and wound protection. In the event that adequate hemostasis cannot be obtained, the use of a drain is suggested. In the presence of infection in either the phalangeal-metatarsal joint or skin flaps, consideration should be given to leaving the wound open and doing a delayed primary closure or allowing secondary healing.

Advantages and Disadvantages

This relatively conservative amputation results in minimal cosmetic deformity and maximum (100 per cent) rehabilitation potential. There are no prosthetics required; however, ray resection of the first metatarsal head will cause some walking imbalance and the foot/patient should be fit with a specially constructed shoe to minimize foot trauma and improve ambulatory balance.

There are no disadvantages except for the risk of hematoma formation, nonhealing, secondary infection, or chronic osteomyelitis of the remaining metatarsal shaft.

Transmetatarsal Amputation

Indications

The indication for transmetatarsal amputation is gangrene or infection involving several toes and/or the great toe (on the same foot). This amputation may also be used if the gangrenous or infectious process extends a small distance on the dorsal skin past the metatarsal-phalangeal crease (but not up to the distal third/midthird junction of the forefoot), provided that the plantar skin is uncompromised.

Contraindications

Deep forefoot infection, cellulitis, lymphangitis, or dependent rubor involving the dorsal forefoot proximal to the metatarsal-phalangeal crease all represent contraindications to amputation at this level. In addition, gangrenous changes on the plantar skin of the foot, even those extending only a small distance past the metatarsal-phalangeal crease, is a specific contraindication to amputation at this level. Foot pulses are not necessary for healing and venous refill should probably be less than 25 seconds.

Surgical Technique

An excellent description of the technique for transmetatarsal amputation was presented by McKittrick et al. in 1949.[87] A skin incision is designed that uses a total plantar flap. A slightly curved dorsal incision is carried from side to side of the foot at the level of the midmetatarsal shafts. The incision extends to the base of the toes medially and laterally in the midplane axis of the foot and then across the plantar surface at the metatarsal-phalangeal crease. It is important to place the dorsal skin incision slightly distal to the anticipated line of bone division. The dorsal skin incision is carried down to the metatarsal bones and each metatarsal shaft is transected with an air-driven oscillating saw approximately 4 mm to 1 cm proximal to the skin incision (Fig. 44–4).

The plantar tissues in the distal forefoot are separated from the metatarsal shafts with a scalpel. The tissues of the plantar flap are thinned sharply, excising exposed tendons and leaving the underlying musculature attached to the skin flap. The plantar flap is then rotated dorsally for closure. Further tailoring or thinning of the plantar flap may be necessary to achieve good skin coaptation.

Attention to absolute hemostasis cannot be overemphasized. A simple closure with a deep layer of absorbable interrupted sutures and a skin closure

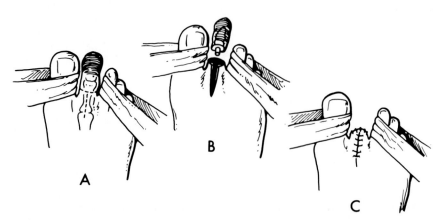

FIGURE 44–3. Artist's conception of a single-digit ray amputation of the foot. The dorsal and plantar incisions are closed in their original direction; the toe incision can be closed either vertically or transversely.

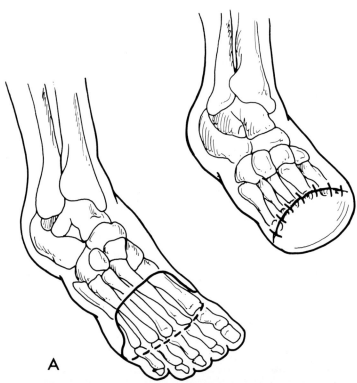

FIGURE 44–4. *A,* Illustration of the planned transmetatarsal plantar-based skin flap and appearance of the completed closure. *B,* A healed right transmetatarsal amputation treated with immediate postsurgical prosthetic fitting, 1 month after amputation.

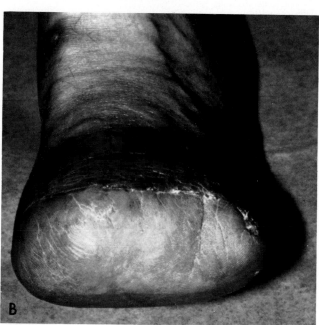

with a monofilament suture utilizing a vertical mattress technique is used. Once again, careful approximation of skin edges is important, and the author recommends that forceps not be used on the skin.

If adequate hemostasis cannot be readily achieved, use of a closed drainage system is suggested. Bone wax should not be used to control bleeding from the metatarsal shafts; however, the use of electrocautery to achieve hemostasis is preferable.

A well-padded short leg plaster cast is the best postoperative dressing, since it will control edema and prevent stump trauma. I do not prefer early ambulation after transmetatarsal amputation because of problems with flap necrosis and stump healing. If wound healing is satisfactory at the first cast change (7 to 10 days after surgery) and if the surgeon chooses, then a rubber heel may be incorporated into the second cast for ambulation. Subsequent casts are changed when they become loose, generally once every 7 to 14 days, and a rigid dressing is used until the transmetatarsal flap is well healed, usually 3 to 4 weeks after surgery.

Advantages and Disadvantages

Transmetatarsal amputation provides an excellent result compared to more proximal foot or lower extremity amputations. Disability is minimal and there are relatively simple prosthetic requirements.

The primary disadvantages of a transmetatarsal amputation are the risks of nonhealing, infection, hematoma formation, and the resultant necessity for a secondary higher level amputation.

Prosthetic Requirements and Rehabilitation Potential

In order to achieve maximum ambulation potential there are minor prosthetic requirements that should be considered. Shoe modification that incorporates a steel shank in the sole of the shoe will allow normal toe-off during ambulation. The spring steel shank reproduces the action of the longitudinal arch of the foot during ambulation. A custom-molded foam pad or lamb's wool can be used to fill the toe portion of the shoe. An alternative approach is a custom-molded shoe that utilizes a roller-shaped sole to provide toe-off motion during walking.

There are relatively few, if any, limitations in rehabilitation for a transmetatarsal amputation. With proper shoe modification, there should be no discernible physical disability for a transmetatarsal amputee during ambulation. It is important, however, that a shoe or other prosthetic device be properly constructed in order to avoid stump ulceration and breakdown. There are increased numbers of anecdotal reports combining guillotine forefoot amputation with secondary distal split-thickness skin graft(s) in order to achieve successful healing at this amputation level. While this latter technique will allow salvage of more proximal transmetatarsal amputations, it is not a technique that the author favors, because of frequent problems with distal stump (skin graft) breakdown in active patients.

Syme's Amputation

James Syme first described this amputation in 1843.[88] Then, as now, there have been arguments as to its merit. Harris (Toronto) has championed Syme's amputation and has written several excellent articles concerning its development and the surgical technique necessary for successful results.[89,90] We believe the Syme's amputation level to be the most technically demanding lower extremity amputation and that attention to surgical detail is crucial for its success.

Indications

If the gangrenous or infectious process precludes transmetatarsal amputation, then the next level to be considered is an ankle disarticulation or Syme's amputation.

Contraindications

If the gangrenous or infectious process involves the heel, if there are open lesions on the heel or about the ankle, if there is cellulitis or lymphangitis ascending up the distal leg, or if dependent rubor is present at the heel, then Syme's amputation is contraindicated. The presence of a neuropathic foot in a diabetic patient, where there is absence of heel sensation, is also a relative contraindication to a Syme's amputation. A high rate of primary healing for a Syme's amputation demands the use of preoperative objective noninvasive amputation level selection techniques and preservation of the posterior tibial artery (if patent).

Surgical Technique

The skin incision is placed to construct a posterior flap using the heel pad. The dorsal incision extends across the ankle from the tip of the medial malleolus to the tip of the lateral malleolus. The plantar incision begins at a 90-degree angle from the dorsal incision and progresses around the plantar aspect of the foot distal to the heel pad (Fig. 44–5). The dorsal incision is deepened through subcutaneous tissues and carried down to bone without dissection in the tissue planes. The anterior tendons (tibialis anterior, extensor hallucis longus, and extensor digitorum longus) are pulled down into the wound, transected, and allowed to retract. The anterior tibial artery is identified, clamped, divided, and suture ligated. The incision is then deepened and the capsule of the tibial-talar joint is opened. The posterior tibialis tendon is divided and the foot is forced into plantar flexion to provide increased visualization of the tibial-talar joint. Great care should be taken during medial dissection to preserve the posterior tibial artery. The joint is further dislocated by incising the posterior capsule. The peroneus brevis and tertius tendons are transected. The plantar aspect of the incision is deepened through all layers of the sole of the foot down to the neck of the calcaneus. The calcaneus is then carefully and sharply dissected from the heel pad. Dissection of the calcaneus is the most difficult part of the operation and great care is taken to maintain the dissection on the bony surface of the calcaneus in order to avoid damaging the soft tissues of the heel, prevent injury to the posterior tibial artery, and prevent button-holing of the posterior skin as the Achilles tendon is transected. Performance of the Syme's amputation by the one-stage and two-stage techniques is identical to this point.

If the surgeon chooses the one-stage technique, then the lateral and medial malleoli are transected flush with the articular surface of the tibial-talar joint with an air-driven reciprocating saw. Once again, the importance of hemostasis cannot be overemphasized. If adequate hemostasis cannot be achieved, then a closed drainage system should be incorporated. Even in dry surgical wounds the use of a drain is advocated by some authors.[84,89,90] I prefer to irrigate the surgical

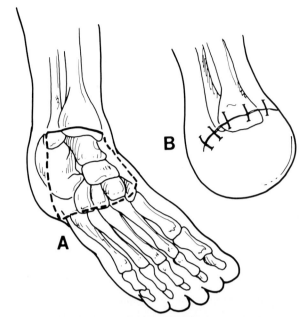

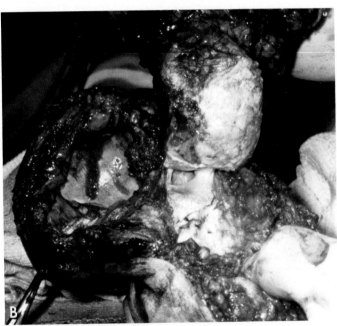

FIGURE 44–5. *A,* Artist's conception of the Syme's level amputation with the posterior heel-based skin flap performed with the one-stage surgical technique. *B,* Intraoperative photograph of a Syme's amputation showing the Achilles attachment of the calcaneus (midsuperior portion of picture), the tibial plateau, and the heel flap (lower left corner).

wound with copious amounts of antibiotic solution prior to closure. The heel pad is rotated anteriorly and sutured to the proximal dorsal skin edge with a single layer of interrupted vertical mattress sutures. Once again, atraumatic placement of skin sutures is mandatory and forceps should not be used on the skin edges.

If the two-stage technique is selected,[84] the lateral and medial malleoli are not transected. A drain is placed and the wound is closed as previously described. Approximately 6 weeks after performance of the first stage, the patient is returned to surgery for the second stage (which can be done under local anesthesia). Medial and lateral incisions are made

over the dog ears on the amputation stump and the incisions carried down to bone with sharp dissection. The malleoli are removed flush with the ankle joint. The tibial articular cartilage is not disturbed. The distal tibia and fibula are exposed subperiosteally approximately 6 cm above the ankle joint and the tibial and fibular flares are removed with an osteotome and a smooth rongeur. This latter procedure produces a relatively square stump that simplifies postoperative prosthetic fitting and improves cosmesis. If the heel pad is loose after removal of the malleoli, it can be secured to the tibia and fibula through drill holes in the bones.

The postoperative dressing for a Syme's amputation stump for both the one- and two-stage surgical procedures is extremely important because it is critical to maintain correct alignment of the heel pad over the end of the tibia/fibula during healing. Either a soft compression dressing or a rigid plaster cast can be used as a postoperative dressing; however, most authors prefer the application of a short-leg plaster cast. If a cast is used, great care must be taken to avoid injury to the medial and lateral skin flaps (dog-ears). Weight bearing should not occur during the early phases of healing of a Syme's amputation because of the risks of nonhealing and flap necrosis. When the first cast is removed, usually 7 to 10 days after surgery, a second cast that incorporates a walking heel can be applied if healing is satisfactory. I prefer to keep Syme's amputee patients nonambulatory for 3 weeks after amputation in order to allow good heel pad fixation/healing. After ambulation begins, the patients are kept in a short-leg walking cast for an additional 3 to 4 weeks prior to construction of a temporary removable prosthesis.

Advantages and Disadvantages

The Syme's amputation stump is extremely durable, because it is end–weight bearing. It provides minimal disability from the standpoint of walking. Performance of a one-stage Syme's amputation procedure results in a somewhat bulbous distal stump compared to a two-stage Syme's amputation. For cosmetic reasons, a two-stage procedure is probably preferable in female patients, although I, generally, will not perform a Syme's amputation in young female patients because of concerns about cosmesis. Clinical evaluation by patients, prosthetists, and surgeons have consistently shown Syme's amputation to be superior to levels above the ankle. Oxygen uptake, gait velocity, cadence, and stride length are significantly better in patients with Syme's amputation compared to patients with higher level amputations.[91]

Delayed healing or healing complications due to hematoma formation or infection are not uncommon. Careful preoperative amputation level selection will help ensure primary healing of the Syme's amputation. Failure to heal a Syme's amputation almost always results in performance of a more proximal amputation. Long-term follow-up of our diabetic patients, in whom a Syme's level was chosen with normal or "almost normal" sensation, has demonstrated a high incidence of revision to the below-knee level because of problems resulting from a progressive insensate Syme's stump (i.e., progressive neuropathy). Other authors have not reported similar problems.

Prosthetic Requirements and Rehabilitation Potential

Ambulation in the home can be achieved without the application of a prosthetic appliance; however, ambulation outside the home requires some type of prosthetic device. The usual cosmetic prosthesis consists of a foot and a plastic shell that incorporates

the lower leg. A typical prosthesis for a patient with a one-stage Syme's amputation is shown in Figure 44–6. Ambulation in the home or for limited distances can be achieved with the application of a simple strap on a cup slipper with a built-up heel.

A patient with a successful Syme's amputation and an appropriately fitted prosthesis can expect a minimal degree of disability. Energy consumption compared to a nonamputee is, at most, 10 per cent above normal. Many patients with Syme's amputations continue to be employed, including some who perform heavy manual labor activities. The salvage of a Syme's amputation, especially in those patients who are likely to become bilateral amputees, may be the ultimate difference for continued ambulation and nonambulation.

Below-Knee Amputation

Indications

Below-knee amputation is the most common amputation level selected for management of lower extremity gangrene, infection, or ischemia with nonhealing lesions that preclude more distal amputations. When the blood supply is inadequate to heal at more

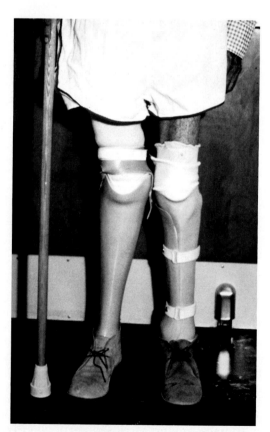

FIGURE 44–6.   A bilateral lower extremity amputee with a right below-knee and left Syme's amputation. The Syme's prosthesis is a standard medial window design for a one-stage Syme's amputation. Notice the bulbous distal ankle on the Syme's (L) compared to the cosmetic ankle on the below-knee (R).

distal levels, amputation at the below-knee level can be expected to have adequate blood supply for healing in the majority of cases. In fact, as previously noted, 83 per cent of all patients undergoing lower extremity amputation can be expected to heal a below-knee amputation (Table 44–3).[41] Through the use of objective amputation level selection, primary healing of below-knee amputation in excess of 94 per cent can be expected.

Contraindications

A below-knee amputation is contraindicated if the gangrenous or infectious process extends to involve skin on the anterior portion of the lower extremity within 4 to 5 cm of the tibial tuberosity or to involve the skin that would be used to construct the posterior flap. A flexion contracture of the knee greater than 20 degrees also represents a contraindication to below-knee amputation. Great caution should be used in attempting below-knee amputation in patients with an occluded profunda femoris artery (the superficial femoral is almost always occluded) in the absence of objective amputation level selection data that suggest that the amputation will heal. Finally, a patient with stroke or neurologic dysfunction on the side of proposed amputation, in whom muscle spasticity or rigidity is marked, should not have a below-knee amputation, because following amputation, spastic muscles will force the knee into flexion and result in ultimate amputation failure.

Surgical Technique

There have been two significant advances in amputation technique that have contributed to better results after below-knee amputation: use of a long posterior flap and the application of a rigid dressing in the immediate postoperative period. There is considerable clinical and theoretical information available to support the use of a long posterior flap. The gastrocnemius and soleus muscles and the overlying posterior calf skin derive their major blood supply through the sural arteries, which originate proximal to the knee joint. Blood flow is maintained to this area in many patients, particularly diabetic patients, in whom flow through the popliteal artery and its major branches is restricted. Blood supply via the anterior tibial artery and geniculate collaterals to the skin and soft tissues of the anterior lower leg is so poor that even if equal anterior and posterior below-knee skin flaps are utilized, there is a high incidence of rehabilitation failure due to wound necrosis of the anterior skin flap.

The operation can be performed under general or spinal anesthesia, with the patient in the supine position on the operating table. If there are open infected lesions on the foot, a plastic bag or plastic adherent drape can be placed over the open infected portion of the extremity to isolate it. As mentioned previously, in patients with a septic foot, a preparatory ankle guillotine amputation followed by a delayed primary below-knee amputation will result in

a higher rate of healing and less stump infections than the performance of a one-stage primary below-knee amputation.[33,34] An alternative to the two-stage approach (one-stage technique with delayed primary closure) that works well for all diabetic patients except those with Wagner grade 5 foot infection was reported by Kerner and Rozzi.[92]

We prefer to use a long posterior flap and no anterior flap for reasons previously stated; however, there is at least one prospective randomized study comparing sagittal technique and long posterior musculocutaneous flaps that shows no significant difference with respect to healing, limb fitting, ambulation, and ultimate rehabilitation.[93] Another report of sagittal incisions for below-knee amputation by Persson points out the utility of this type of incision in patients in whom a long posterior flap may be contraindicated because of infection or skin necrosis.[94] A more recent report by Rockley et al. notes that, for below-knee amputations in patients with end-stage peripheral vascular disease, the skew flap is an excellent option to the long posterior flap.[95] The techniques for construction of a long posterior flap in below-knee amputation have been well documented in many previous publications[10,96–98]; however, the salient features of the amputation are outlined below.

For a standard below-knee amputation, I select a point of bone division approximately a hand's breadth, including the thumb, below the tibial tuberosity. In those patients in whom there is concern that the posterior flap may impinge upon distal infection or ischemia, a palm's breadth (minus the thumb) can be used for a point of division below the tibial tuberosity. The absolute minimum length for a below-knee amputation is three fingers' breadth (7 to 8 cm) below the tibial tuberosity. The skin incision should be approximately 1 cm distal to the intended point of bone division. The transverse diameter of the midshaft calf at the level of the anterior incision, plus 1 inch, represents the approximate length of the posterior skin flap. It is usually my preference to outline the flap with a marking pencil prior to making a skin incision. The anterior skin incision represents the anterior half of the circumference of the extremity. The skin incision then abruptly turns distally with gentle curves and proceeds down the medial and lateral aspects of the extremity, in the midplane axis of the leg, to the point of distal extent of the posterior skin flap. The two lateral incisions are then connected posteriorly. My preference is to then incise the flap through skin and fascia in all areas prior to muscle transection. Use of a proximal tourniquet for hemostatic control is optional in patients undergoing traumatic below-knee amputation, but is relatively contraindicated in patients undergoing elective below-knee amputation for ischemia. Use of electrocautery is preferred for division of all muscles. The anterior tibial muscle is divided at the level of bone division and the anterior tibial neurovascular bundle is identified, clamped, divided, and suture ligated. Electrocautery is used to incise the tibial periosteum circumferentially and a periosteal elevator is used to mobilize the periosteum of the tibia proximal to the point of proposed bone division. The tibia is then divided with an air-driven reciprocating saw. Using electrocautery, the fibula is isolated at the level of the transected tibia and divided approximately one quarter of an inch proximal to the tibia using the saw. Following division of fibula and tibia, proximal traction is placed on the transected tibia (use of a bonehook is easiest) and the lower extremity is bent at 90 degrees and retracted distally. The posterior tibial artery and vein and the common peroneal artery and vein are identified, clamped, transected, and individually suture ligated. The posterior tibial nerve is identified, pulled into the wound, ligated, transected, and allowed to retract out of the area of surgical incision. The posterior calf musculature is transected, leaving the gastrocnemius muscle as part of the posterior skin flap. The surgical specimen is then divided at the same point as the posterior flap skin incision, which permits removal of the surgical specimen. Care should be taken not to thin the posterior flap so much as to provide inadequate coverage for the tibia when the flap is closed. The saw is used to bevel the tibia at a 45- to 60-degree angle and bony edges are filed smooth. Care is also taken to make sure that the distal ends of the fibula are smooth (Fig. 44–7).

The wound is copiously irrigated with an antibiotic solution. Once again, the importance of meticulous hemostasis cannot be stressed enough. Generally, drains are not necessary on below-knee amputations for peripheral vascular disease; however, drains are frequently used in below-knee amputations performed for trauma or reasons other than peripheral vascular insufficiency. If a drain is required, I prefer a closed suction drain, which is brought through a separate stab wound in the lateral aspect of the lower leg. The sural nerve (posterior flap) is identified, pulled down, ligated, transected, and allowed to retract back from the edge of the flap. The flap is rotated anteriorly and the muscle fascia of the posterior flap is approximated to anterior fascia with interrupted absorbable sutures. The skin is carefully approximated with interrupted vertical mattress sutures using a monofilament plastic or metal suture. I avoid the use of tissue forceps and believe that the closure of the below-knee stump, especially in patients with peripheral vascular disease, should be performed with the care of a plastic surgical procedure. Tailoring the corner of the skin flap may be required in order to prevent excessive dog-ears.

The use of a rigid plaster of Paris dressing incorporating the knee is ideal, regardless of whether or not an immediate postoperative prosthesis is to be used. A rigid dressing will control edema, promote healing, and protect the stump during the postoperative period. In addition, a rigid dressing will prevent a flexion contracture. Application of an immediate postoperative prosthesis as part of the rigid dressing will be described in detail in a subsequent section of this chapter.

Advantages and Disadvantages

The below-knee amputation has been shown to be an extremely durable amputation. The likelihood of primary healing is very good and the ability to rehabilitate a patient on a below-knee prosthesis is excellent. In a report by Kim et al. in 1976, 90 per cent of their patients with unilateral below-knee amputations were able to ambulate.[99] Roon et al. achieved a 100 per cent ambulation rate with unilateral below-knee amputation and a 93 per cent ambulation rate in patients with bilateral below-knee amputations.[14] In addition, 91 per cent of the patients reported by Roon et al. were still ambulatory an average of 44 months following amputation.[14]

In the absence of the ability to perform a more distal amputation, there are no specific disadvantages for a below-knee amputation.

Prosthetic Requirements and Rehabilitation Potential

A below-knee prosthesis is required for ambulation at this level of amputation. A variety of prostheses are available, but in general involve total stump contact (with or without a prosthesis liner) with weight bearing on the patellar tendon and tibial-fibular condyles. Newer types of below-knee prostheses incorporate total contact/total weight bearing designs. The prosthesis can be suspended with a variety of techniques, including thigh lacer with external joints, Silastic sleeve suspension, standard PTB (patella tendon-bearing) strap, supracondylar medial clip, suction, and self-suspension secondary to muscle control. These prostheses can incorporate a variety of feet, some of which have flexion/extension motion or "ankle rotation" (with weight loading) or energy storage (Seattle Foot; Flex-Foot). The energy requirement for a unilateral below-knee amputee is increased approximately 40 to 60 per cent compared to normal (energy consumption with an energy-storing leg has not yet been reported).

It has been our experience, as well as that of others, that any patient, irrespective of age, who was ambulatory prior to below-knee amputation and who undergoes amputation within 30 days of hospital entrance can ambulate successfully on a below-knee prosthesis. In fact, most patients who require bilateral below-knee amputations can ambulate successfully, as shown by Roon et al.[14] The importance of aggressive rehabilitation after unilateral below-knee amputation in patients who are high risk for bilateral lower extremity amputation was stressed in a recent report by Inderbitzi et al.[100] Delay in rehabilitation resulted in a high rate of nonambulatory patients after their second amputation. The time required for gait training for a unilateral below-knee amputee approximates 2 to 3 weeks and the gait pattern most patients develop is very good. There are some physical limitations for a geriatric below-knee amputee;

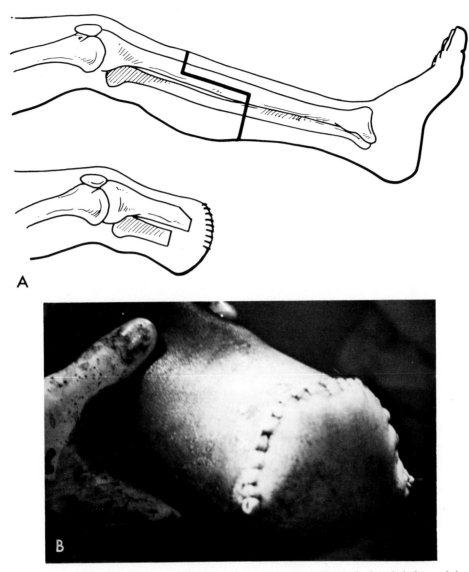

FIGURE 44–7. *A*, The standard posterior flap below-knee amputation. Notice the beveled tibia and the proximal shortening of the fibula compared to the tibia. *B*, An intraoperative photograph showing a below-knee amputation. Notice the skin coaptation with interrupted sutures and the minimal dog-ears.

however, young below-knee amputees are able to negotiate ladders, stairs, and other obstacles with minimal difficulty.

Knee Disarticulation

Indications

The indications for knee disarticulation amputation are limited and it is primarily performed on young active males for whom the advantages of strength and serviceability outweigh prosthetic cosmesis. Disarticulation amputation of the knee is the second most technically difficult lower extremity amputation procedure following the Syme's amputation. Successful performance of a knee disarticulation amputation with a high degree of primary healing usually requires some type of preoperative objective amputation level selection technique. The primary indication for knee disarticulation is when the gangrenous process, infection, trauma, tumor, or orthopedic disability encroaches too close to the anterior and posterior (or sagittal) limits of a below-knee amputation flap or has resulted in a nonsalvageable knee joint. Another potential indication for knee disarticulation is a patient who has had either acute or chronic failure of a below-knee amputation in whom skin flaps at the knee are viable enough to consider knee disarticulation. In general, British surgeons have been more enamored with knee disarticulation than their American colleagues. Recent interest in this level of amputation has arisen as a result of advances in cosmetic prosthetic components and prosthetic fitting techniques. Moreover, in a study of 169 unilateral lower extremity amputees, Houghton et al. found that rehabilitation results were better for thru-knee amputation (62 per cent) than for above-knee (33 per cent) ($p < .02$) or for Gritti-Stokes amputations (44 per cent).[101]

Contraindications

Contraindications to knee disarticulation are primarily inadequate blood flow of the skin in the region and/or ulceration, gangrene, or infection involving tissues about the knee joint or the joint space.

Surgical Technique

There are two excellent reviews that describe the advantages and disadvantages and surgical techniques of disarticulation of the knee and, therefore, the techniques will be only briefly described in the following paragraphs.[102,103] We prefer the knee disarticulation technique described by Burgess,[102] having reached this conclusion after failures with other types of knee disarticulation amputation and success using the modified Burgess technique.

Anesthetic management for knee disarticulation is best handled with either spinal or general anesthesia with the patient in the prone position. The operation can be performed, but is more difficult, with the patient in the supine position. At the discretion of the surgeon, a gown or pack can be placed beneath the thigh to hyperextend the hip joint and provide an easier working surface on the anterior portion of the knee and lower leg. The leg is held in a flexed position. Depending upon the availability of suitable skin, either a classic long anterior, equal flap, or sagittal flap–type incision can be used (Fig. 44–8). A marking pencil should be used to outline the skin flaps prior to making the skin incision. Construction of the knee disarticulation skin flaps is crucial in order to avoid tension on the skin suture line when the amputation stump is closed. Dissection is first carried anteriorly down to the insertion of the patellar tendon on the tibia. The tendon is severed at its insertion and sharply dissected proximally. Deep dissection on the medial side of the knee results in exposure of the hamstring muscles. The tendons are sectioned and allowed to retract. The deep fascia is reflected with the overlying tendon/skin flap. On the lateral side of the knee, the tendon of the biceps femoris muscle and iliotibial band are sectioned low. The knee joint is entered anteriorly, the knee is flexed, and the cruciate ligaments are transected at their tibial insertion. The posterior knee capsule structures are divided and the individual members of the popliteal vascular sheath are clamped, transected, and suture ligated. The tibial and peroneal nerves are identified, retracted under moderate tension, ligated, sectioned with a sharp knife, and allowed to retract into the proximal amputation stump. The patella is removed subperiosteally and the fascial defect in the patellar tendon is closed with interrupted sutures.

The femoral condyles are now transected transversely, approximately 1.5 cm above the level of the knee joint (Fig. 44–9A). Sharp distal femoral margins are carefully contoured. The patellar tendon is pulled down into the intracondylar notch under moderate tension and sewn to the stump of the crus ligaments. The semitendinosus and biceps tendons are likewise pulled into the notch, tailored, and sewn to the stump of the patellar tendon and cruciate ligaments. This approximation of the tendons and ligaments allows muscle stability. The superficial skin fascia is approximated with interrupted absorbable sutures and, once again, the skin is meticulously closed using a vertical mattress technique with monofilament metal or plastic sutures, but without use of forceps. Alternatively, skin staples may be used. The use of a through-and-through or a suction drain is optional and left to the discretion of the surgeon. A rigid dressing, with or without the incorporation of an immediate postoperative prosthesis, should be applied.

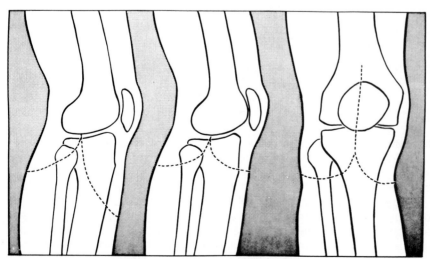

Classical long anterior   Equal flaps   Sagittal flaps

FIGURE 44–8. The three types of skin incision commonly used for knee disarticulation amputation. (From Burgess EM: Disarticulation of the knee. A modified technique. Arch Surg *117*:1251, 1977.)

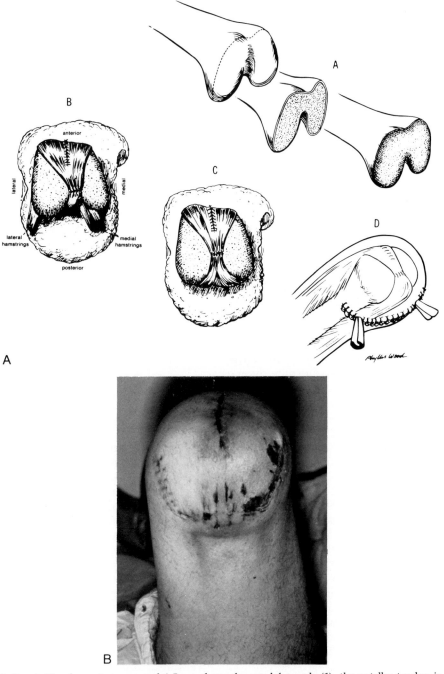

FIGURE 44–9. *A*, The femur is transected 1.5 cm above the condylar ends (*1*), the patellar tendon is sewn to the cruciate ligaments (*2*), hamstring tendons are sutured to the cruciate/patellar ligaments (*3*), and the wound is closed over a drain (*4*). (From Burgess EM: Disarticulation of the knee. A modified technique. Arch Surg *117*:1253, 1977.) *B*, An anterior flap knee disarticulation amputation at the first immediate postoperative cast change (7 to 10 days) with the patient in the supine position (in this case, the patella was removed transcutaneously).

Advantages and Disadvantages

The advantages of a knee disarticulation amputation include excellent durability and end–weight bearing capacity; retention of a long and powerful, muscle-stabilized femoral lever arm; improved proprioception; and a limb-socket interface with improved prosthetic suspension and rotational control (compared to an above-knee amputation). This amputation level is almost as good as a below-knee amputation, and therefore is a tremendous benefit to the patient in comparison to the next higher level, the above-knee amputation.

The absence of a knee joint and increased energy expenditure make this amputation level less advantageous than a below-knee amputation.

Prosthetic Requirements and Rehabilitation Potential

Historically, knee disarticulation amputations were not well liked in the prosthetic community because of cosmetic and knee/thigh length problems resulting from existing prosthetic components (nonequal knee centers); however, the availability of lightweight polycentric hydraulic knee joints and endoskeletal systems has helped to solve these problems. The usual knee disarticulation socket incorporates some type of medial window to allow the bulbous stump to pass through the smaller lower thigh portion of the socket.

Knee disarticulation level amputation probably has its greatest usefulness in a young, active, nonperipheral vascular amputee. However, this amputation is also an excellent choice for a geriatric patient. Patient performance is better than that of a mid to high above-knee amputation, although not nearly as good as a standard below-knee amputation. There are some limitations of physical activities resulting from the absence of a knee joint, and they specifically involve those tasks such as stair climbing, ladder climbing, or physical abilities that require rotational or flexion/extension knee motions.

Above-Knee Amputation

Indications

The indications for an amputation at the above-knee level are inadequate blood flow to heal at a more distal level, a disabled patient who is not expected to walk again, profound life-threatening infection with questionable viability of the lower extremity, and/or extensive infection or gangrene that would preclude a knee disarticulation or below-knee level amputation. Historically, above-knee amputation has been the operation of choice for many surgeons because greater than 90 per cent primary healing can be anticipated regardless of the vascular status of the patient.

Contraindications

Extension of the infectious or gangrenous process to the level of proposed above-knee amputation is the most common contraindication. Severe necrotizing lower extremity infection is a relative contraindication unless a high above-knee amputation is performed.

Surgical Technique

There are three basic levels for above-knee amputation (Fig. 44–10). In general, the longer the above-knee amputation stump the more likely the patient is to ambulate, so the stump should be as long as possible. If an amputation is being performed to con-

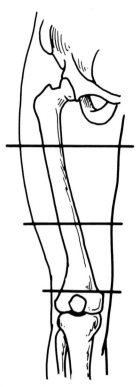

FIGURE 44–10. Artist's schematic conception of the three common levels of above-knee amputation.

trol sepsis or toxicity, a midthigh or high-thigh amputation will provide better assurance of healing and control of systemic toxicity, although the chances of rehabilitation are lessened.

Either a circular or a sagittal-type incision can be used. I prefer the use of a circular (or fish mouth) incision appropriate for the level of anticipated bone division. A circumferential line of incision is drawn with a marking pen 2 to 3 cm below the level of proposed bone transection. The incision is then carried down through skin and fascia. The skin and fascia are retracted superiorly to allow more proximal muscle division. I prefer the use of electrocautery for muscle division. The femoral artery and vein are identified, clamped, divided, and suture ligated in the subsartorial canal. All the muscles of the anterior, medial, and lateral thigh are transected. The muscle mass is then retracted proximally, the proposed line of bone transection is exposed, and the periosteum is cut using electrocautery. An air-driven reciprocating saw is then used to transect the femur. The posterior muscles are transected using electrocautery. The sciatic nerve is identified, pulled down into the wound, ligated, transected, and allowed to retract into the proximal amputation stump. The rough edges of the femur are filed smooth. Again, the amputation stump should be irrigated with an antibiotic solution, especially if the amputation is being performed for infection. The soft tissues and skin are drawn distally to ensure adequacy of soft tissue coverage for the femur. If soft tissue coverage is adequate, the wound is closed in two layers. The fascia is closed with an interrupted absorbable suture and the skin is closed with interrupted vertical mattress sutures of monofilament plastic or metal. Again, good skin coaptation is important and the use of forceps on the skin is to be avoided. If the soft tissue coverage for the bone is inadequate, then the femur is shortened as required, so as to allow adequate soft tissue coverage without tension on the skin suture line (Fig. 44–11).

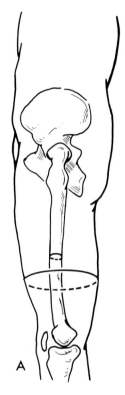

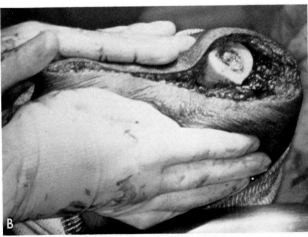

FIGURE 44–11. *A,* The standard circular incision technique for above-knee amputation. Sagittal flaps can be used if appropriate. The key to closure is adequate femur shortening to avoid later bone protrusion through the distal end of the stump. *B,* This intraoperative photograph of an above-knee amputation stump demonstrates why skin/soft tissue length for bone coverage should be checked prior to closure. Proximal femur shortening was required to decrease wound tension.

If the amputation is being performed for infection, especially a necrotizing infection, then the wound should be left open. If a fish mouth incision is used then the apex of the "angle of the mouth" approximates the point of bony division. Closure, although spatially different, encompasses the careful atraumatic technique described above.

A rigid dressing can be applied, and is advantageous for control of stump edema, but it is much more cumbersome and less valuable than a rigid dressing used at lower amputation levels. I prefer to use a soft dressing suspended with a silesian type of elastic bandage or a modified waist suspension belt.[104] After the wound has healed satisfactorily (1 to 2 weeks after surgery), a temporary removable prosthesis can be provided if appropriate.

Advantages and Disadvantages

The primary advantage of an above-knee amputation is the very high likelihood of primary healing. Prosthetic rehabilitation is very difficult at this level of amputation. Whereas 80 to 90 per cent of all patients with unilateral or bilateral below-knee amputations can be expected to ambulate, only 40 to 50 per cent of unilateral above-knee amputees can be expected to ambulate. It has been the author's experience that less than 10 per cent of bilateral lower extremity amputees, where one side is an above-knee amputation, will successfully ambulate.

Prosthetic Requirements and Rehabilitation Potential

A variety of prostheses are available for the above-knee amputee. Newer prosthetic devices incorporate contoured axially aligned sockets, ultralightweight materials, endoskeletal design, hydraulic-assisted knee joints, the use of ankle rotators and/or motion feet, and energy storage. There is a direct correlation between successful ambulation at this level of amputation and the weight of the prosthesis because of the energy expenditure required for walking. Compared to normal, the energy expenditure of an above-knee amputee is increased 80 to 120 per cent.

As noted, the rehabilitation potential for a unilateral above-knee amputee is only fair and averages 10 to 50 per cent.

Hip Disarticulation Amputation

In general, hip disarticulation amputation is not an amputation that the usual general or vascular surgeon will perform, since almost all patients will heal a high above-knee amputation.

Indications

The indications for hip disarticulation are inadequate blood flow (usually in patients with occlusion of both the profunda femoris and superficial femoral arteries) to heal a more distal amputation, a life-threatening infection or extensive gangrene that precludes amputation at a lower level, trauma, tumor, and failed hip reconstruction.[105] Wound complications occur frequently and their incidence is increased for urgent/emergent operations and prior above-knee amputations.[106] In addition, both limb ischemia and infection increase the mortality rate.

Contraindications

In our experience, infection that precludes hip disarticulation amputation is almost a uniformly fatal event. There are no contraindications to this level of amputation, except infection and gangrene (or tumor) that extends above the level of the proposed amputation.

Surgical Technique

Since this procedure is performed only occasionally by the general and vascular surgeon and since there are excellent articles published describing this operation, the surgical technique for performance of this level of amputation will not be presented in the present chapter.[105–109] Based on a limited experience, I favor a posterior flap technique (Fig. 44–12A).

Advantages and Disadvantages

In the absence of healing at an above-knee level, there is a higher likelihood of primary healing.

Prosthetic rehabilitation at this level of lower extremity amputation is uncommon (less than 10 per cent) even with unilateral amputation in geriatric patients.

Prosthetic Requirements

Various types of prostheses have been described and created for the hip disarticulation amputation. Most of them entail a pelvic bucket (Canadian-type) prosthesis (Fig. 44–12B). Most prostheses are endoskeletal in construction (in order to save weight) and very few involve the use of sophisticated knee joints, ankle joints, or motion feet. A full discussion of prosthetic requirements for this level of amputation is beyond the scope of most general and vascular surgeons and the interested reader is referred to appropriate references.[105–108] Compared to normal, the energy expenditure of a hip disarticulation amputee is increased 1.5 to 2.5 times.

COMPLICATIONS OF LOWER EXTREMITY AMPUTATION

Historically, postoperative morbidity and mortality following major lower extremity amputation were unacceptably common and the incidence of fatal com-

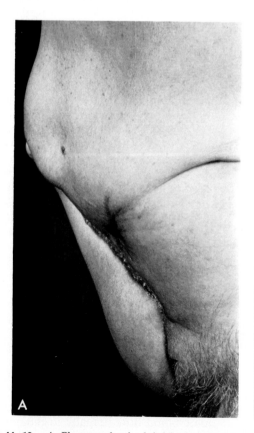 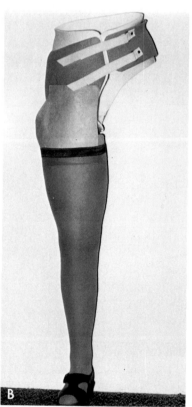

FIGURE 44–12.   *A,* Photograph of a left hip disarticulation stump 6 months after amputation. The operation was performed with a posterior/gluteal flap technique. *B,* An ultralightweight (4.5 pounds) left hip disarticulation prosthesis based on an Aqualite plastic endoskeletal system with cosmetic cover and Scotchcast Canadian-type socket (bucket).

plications was high enough that there was considerable debate as to the optimum preoperative, operative, and postoperative management. In general, however, the morbidity and mortality following a major lower extremity amputation have decreased with time.[110–112]

The major postoperative complications following lower extremity amputation with ranges of frequency of occurrence are listed in Table 44–4. Each of these complications will be addressed separately in the following paragraphs.

Early Postoperative Complications

Pain

The literature suggests that the incidence of disabling stump pain and phantom limb pain following major lower extremity amputation ranges from 5 to 30 per cent.[113–118] In a retrospective random survey of 5000 Veterans Administration (VA) amputees, Sherman et al. noted that 85 per cent of the amputees responding to their survey noted significant phantom limb pain.[119,120] Their explanation for the high incidence of pain problems was, in part, based on the fact that most reports, especially those citing pain treatment modalities, do not have adequate post-treatment follow-up. In addition, Sherman et al. suggested that most amputees quickly learn that physicians are not interested in pain problems and, therefore, fail to give accurate responses when questioned, often in order to protect their credibility and relationship with their physicians (thereby guaranteeing long-term care).[119,120] Of more concern was the fact that statistical analysis of 42 of the most common treatment modalities for phantom limb pain, including drug therapy, local injections, and surgery, failed to show that any treatment gave satisfactory results.[119,120] At most, 8.4 per cent of survey respondents could be said to have been helped to any real extent. In my experience, based upon an amputation program that uses immediate postsurgical prosthetic fitting and aggressive postamputation rehabilitation, the incidence of disabling pain problems following major lower extremity amputations is less than 5 per cent. I have no objective explanation for the difference between reports in the surgical literature and our personal experience, but I believe that the rap-

idity and success of rehabilitation, as well as postoperative rigid dressings, with or without a pylon, have a positive impact in decreasing postamputation pain problems.

Death

The incidence of death following major lower extremity amputation ranges from 0 to 35 per cent.[7,9,15,17,110,111,121,122] Although the postoperative death rate has decreased each decade since the 1950s, an overall death rate of 6 to 10 per cent is still the average for centers treating large numbers of amputees.[9,14,15] As might be expected, the postoperative death rate for above-knee amputation (20 to 40 per cent) exceeds that for below-knee amputation (3 to 10 per cent).[9,14,15,91,110,111,122] Two thirds of all postoperative deaths are due to cardiovascular complications, including myocardial infarction, stroke, congestive heart failure, and visceral ischemia, with approximately one third to one half of these deaths due to myocardial infarction alone. Death following lower extremity amputation is related to patient age. In my experience and that of others the mortality increases for patients over the age of 75.

Nonhealing

Nonhealing of an amputation stump represents a major complication, since it almost always results in an amputation at a higher level. Nonhealing represents failure due either to inadequate blood supply at the level selected for amputation, to rough or traumatic intraoperative handling of marginally vascularized tissue, or to a stump hematoma with or without secondary infection. The incidence of nonhealing after major lower extremity amputation ranges from 3 to 28 per cent.[9,14,15,110,111,121] In other words, the primary healing rate after major lower extremity amputation ranges from 63 to 97 per cent. Since, in previous sections, we have shown that the literature suggests an overall healing rate of 97 per cent for digit and forefoot amputations (Table 44–2) and 94 per cent for below-knee amputations (Table 44–3) when objective amputation level selection techniques were used, it can be anticipated that the failure of an amputation stump to heal is probably directly related to the methods used for amputation level selection. In a modern amputation program using objective preoperative amputation level selection

TABLE 44–4. POSTOPERATIVE COMPLICATIONS

	Incidence	References
Stump pain/phantom pain	5–80%	9, 14, 15, 113–120
Death	0–35%	7, 9, 15, 91, 110, 111, 121, 122
Pulmonary complications	8%	14
Stump infection	12–28%	111, 122
Nonhealing stump	3–28%	9, 14, 15, 110, 111, 121
Pulmonary embolus	4–38%	7, 14
Deep venous thrombosis	1–3%	9, 14, 15
Flexion contracture	1–3%	9, 14, 15, 54
Renal insufficiency	1–3%	9, 14, 15

techniques, the rate of nonhealing should not be greater than 4 to 8 per cent. In my last 134 consecutive lower extremity amputations there has been one failure (0.8 per cent) due to nonhealing from ischemia.

The literature is somewhat controversial on healing differences between patients with and without diabetes mellitus. However, it has been my experience, as well as that of others, that there is no significant difference in the healing rates of major lower extremity amputation between the diabetic and nondiabetic patient.[9,15,51,54,57,62,72,125] The rate of infectious stump complications might be slightly higher in diabetics; however, this has not been my experience.

In a review of 59 consecutive lower extremity amputations in diabetics, Bailey et al. noted that the preoperative hemoglobin level was statistically significantly lower in patients whose amputations healed primarily.[126] Eighteen amputations done in patients with a preoperative hemoglobin less than 12 gm healed primarily, whereas all 30 amputations in patients with a hemoglobin level greater than 13 gm failed to heal.

It seems reasonable to consider isovolemic hemodilution in patients with marginally viable skin or borderline values by amputation level selection techniques. In a study on skin flap survival, Gatti and colleagues suggested that isovolemic hemodilution might be a valuable technique for the salvage of marginally ischemic tissues.[127]

Stump Infection

The incidence of infection in an amputation stump following major lower extremity amputation ranges from 12 to 28 per cent.[9,15,18,54,111] As might be expected, the incidence of postoperative stump infection is directly related to the reason for performing the amputation. The incidence of this complication can be reduced by appropriate management of preexisting infections, including the use of perioperative antibiotic therapy, as well as wide débridement and/or drainage of infection prior to definitive amputation. Recent reviews by McIntyre et al. and Fischer et al. noted a statistically significant decrease in the rate of stump infection in patients undergoing definitive below-knee amputation for a septic foot in whom prior ankle guillotine amputation was performed to control infection.[33,34] The incidence of below-knee stump infection in patients managed with a one-stage surgical procedure was 22 and 21 per cent, respectively, while the incidence in those patients who had undergone preparatory guillotine ankle amputation was 3 and 0 per cent, respectively ($p < .05$).[33,34] My most recent incidence of stump infection is 3 per cent (4 of 134) and most of these infections represent aggressive closure of contaminated wounds or amputations in limbs with distal ipsilateral septic foci.

I do not recommend the use of prophylactic systemic antibiotics in the absence of established infection. It has been my practice to treat patients with preoperative infections with broad-spectrum antibiotics that provide bactericidal aerobic and anaerobic coverage. The necessity for aerobic and anaerobic coverage is especially important in diabetic patients, in whom the incidence of mixed facultative and obligative anaerobic infections may be as high as 60 per cent.[21]

Once an infection is established in an amputation stump, the wound must be opened widely to provide adequate drainage. In general, this means that amputation will have to be revised to a higher level, so that, for example, a stump infection in a below-knee amputation usually results in an above-knee amputation. The importance of this complication is emphasized by the fact that for a geriatric patient, conversion from a below-knee to an above-knee amputation is often the difference between successful ambulation and nonwalking.

Stump hematoma after lower extremity amputation is a catastrophic complication, especially when the amputation has been performed for distal extremity infection. Although the correlation between stump hematoma and stump infection is not 1 : 1, it is high enough to make the avoidance of a postamputation stump hematoma highly desirable. The importance of meticulous hemostasis after amputation cannot be emphasized enough. If an amputation is not dry, then the wound should be closed with drains (closed drainage system, not Penrose drains), although several studies have suggested that the use of drains increases the risk of infection.[128]

Pulmonary Embolism and Deep Venous Thrombosis

The incidence of pulmonary embolism and deep venous thrombosis following major lower extremity amputation is 1 to 3 per cent[7,14] and 4 to 38 per cent,[9,14] respectively. The postoperative lower extremity amputee is at high risk for venous thromboembolic complications. Usually, these patients have had a prolonged period of hospitalization and bed rest prior to amputation. In addition, many have undergone attempts at prior vascular surgical reconstruction that may cause injury to the deep veins in the leg and prolong preamputation immobilization. The amputation itself involves division of veins, which may result in stagnation and thrombosis in these vein segments postoperatively. When an active rehabilitation program is not begun on the first day after surgery, an additional period of inactivity or immobilization may follow the amputation and further predispose the patient to venous thromboembolic complications. The morbidity and mortality from venous thromboembolic complications may be significant and, in addition, impairment of blood oxygenation may further compromise the healing of ischemic tissues.

For those patients undergoing elective major lower extremity amputation in whom major risk factors for venous thromboembolic complications exist, appropriate prophylaxis for pulmonary embolism should be instituted. Since there is a slight increase in stump hematoma formation, the use of a closed suction drainage system in those patients is advisable. Probably the most important factor in preventing thromboembolic complications is not to allow patients undergoing major lower extremity amputation to become bedridden either preoperatively or postoperatively. The patient being prepared for lower extremity amputation should be undergoing preoperative physical therapy for range of motion and strengthening of the contralateral leg and upper extremities. The postoperative amputee, even if an immediate postoperative prosthesis is not used, should be going to physical therapy for similar body conditioning. Attention should be paid to the nonamputated extremity, and the use of thromboembolic elastic stockings is recommended during the perioperative period. A final factor that must be considered is state of hydration in the amputee patient, both preoperatively and postoperatively. This is especially true in those patients who have undergone prior attempts at vascular reconstruction or angiography.

Pulmonary Complications

The incidence of pulmonary complications, including pneumonia, atelectasis, and sepsis, has been estimated to approximate 8 per cent in patients undergoing a major lower extremity amputation.[14] These complications will be significantly higher in patients undergoing above-knee amputation, as noted by Huston et al.,[7] in whom the incidence of pneumonia and sepsis ranged from 8 to 60 per cent. The same conditions of bed rest, inactivity, dehabilitation, and dehydration that predispose to thromboembolic complications also predispose a patient to atelectasis and pneumonia. Next to myocardial infarction, pulmonary complications are probably the biggest problem with geriatric patients undergoing lower extremity amputation. Attention to good pulmonary toilet, increased muscular activity, and active exercise (physical therapy) are all valuable adjuncts in the preoperative and perioperative care.

Flexion Contractures

Flexion contractures of the knee or hip joint can occur quite rapidly following major lower extremity amputation, especially in geriatric patients. In my experience, the incidence of such postoperative flexion contracture has been 1 to 3 per cent.[9,14,15,54]

Irreversible flexion contracture will prohibit successful fitting of a prosthesis and subsequently successful patient ambulation. Such a problem may also necessitate amputation at a higher level. The use of a rigid postoperative dressing, with or without an immediate postoperative pylon, will help decrease the incidence of this complication. In those patients not being treated with immediate postoperative prosthesis, physical therapy directed toward range of motion and muscle strengthening should be instituted preoperatively if possible, and as rapidly as possible after amputation.

Renal Insufficiency

Renal insufficiency represents a low-frequency complication following major lower extremity am-

putation, with an incidence of 1 to 3 per cent.[9,54] This complication is, for the most part, avoidable if proper attention is paid to adequate preoperative and postoperative hydration. In addition, in patients requiring prolonged antibiotic therapy for perioperative infections, attention must be paid to antibiotic dosage in order to avoid renal insufficiency as a complication of antibiotic therapy.

Long-Term Complications

Stump Revision

There is little information available in the literature regarding the frequency of stump revision in those patients who have been successfully discharged from the hospital following lower extremity amputation. A previous report by Malone et al., in which there was a 97 per cent rate of primary healing after lower extremity amputation, noted that 88 per cent of their lower extremity amputees were followed without stump revision for up to 18 months after surgery.[15] The incidence of prosthesis use in those patients was 100 per cent. Similar information was reported by Roon et al., who noted that 91 per cent of their patients were ambulatory on their prostheses 44 months following amputation.[14] I believe that the frequency of stump revision is probably related to methods of amputation level selection, the quality of prosthesis fit, and careful postoperative follow-up. My current incidence of late stump revision is 2.3 per cent (10 of 450).

Death

Approximately one third of all lower extremity amputees will die within 5 years of their amputation, and two-thirds of these deaths will be due to cardiovascular causes.[111] Roon et al. reported a 45 per cent overall 5-year survival following lower extremity amputation, compared to an expected 85 per cent 5-year survival for the age-adjusted normal population.[14] More striking, however, was Roon et al.'s analysis of the projected 5-year survival following lower extremity amputation for diabetic and nondiabetic amputees. They reported a 5-year survival for nondiabetics of 75 per cent and only a 39 per cent 5-year survival for patients with diabetes mellitus (Fig. 44–13).[14] Analysis of the cause of death for patients in the series reported by Roon et al. disclosed that 35 per cent were due to myocardial infarction and two thirds were due to cardiovascular causes.

Contralateral Limb Loss

It can be estimated that the rate of contralateral limb loss ranges from 15 to 33 per cent in 5 years following major lower extremity amputation.[16–18] In all probability, however, the diabetic amputee is likely to die prior to contralateral limb loss.[14,111] Because of the risk of contralateral limb loss, significant care and attention should be paid to examination of the contralateral limb as well as education of the patient in

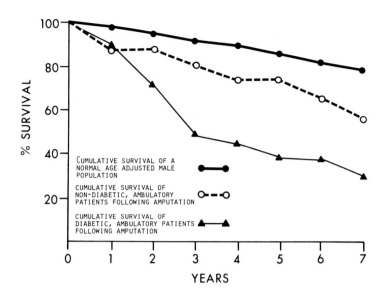

FIGURE 44–13. Life-table representation of survival after lower extremity amputation for both diabetic and nondiabetic amputees compared to the age-adjusted normal population. (From Roon AJ, Moore WS, Goldstone J: Below knee amputation: A modern approach. Am J Surg *134*:153–158, 1977.)

prophylactic skin and foot care. Patient instructions for the care of diabetic feet that are used at the Tucson VA Medical Center and Maricopa Medical Center (Phoenix) are shown in Figure 44–14.

Data from a randomized prospective educational study at the Tucson VA in diabetics who present with foot ulcers, infection, prior amputation, or high-risk lesions suggest that an audiovisual education program decreased the incidence of subsequent amputation significantly (at 1 year).[16] That prospective randomized study evaluated the influence of a simple education program on the incidence of lower extremity amputation in diabetic patients. Two hundred three patients were randomized into two groups: education and no education. There were no significant differences in medical management or clinical risk factors between the two groups. There was no significant difference in the incidence of infection; however, the rate of ulceration and amputation was three times higher in the no-education subgroup (26 of 177 versus 8 of 177 ulceration, $p \leq .005$; 21 of 177 versus 7 of 177 amputation, $p \leq .025$). That study demonstrated that a simple education program significantly reduced the incidence of ulcer or foot and limb amputation in diabetic patients.[16] Other studies have documented the importance of diabetes education, protective footwear, and preventative footcare.[129,130]

PROSTHETIC CONSIDERATIONS FOLLOWING MAJOR LOWER EXTREMITY AMPUTATION

In general, as the level of amputation moves proximally up the lower extremity and the age of the patient increases, the success rates for rehabilitation decline and the length of time required to achieve ambulation increases.[17,131–137] Prior to discussions on prosthetic considerations after major lower extremity

amputation, a review of some of the problems with rehabilitation of geriatric amputees is worthwhile.

Rehabilitation of Elderly Amputees

In the mid to late 1960s, the literature was replete with reports on problems with rehabilitation of geriatric amputees. Many of these reports have been forgotten; however, the information they presented is still valid. Among the most important surveys of that period was that of Mazet et al. involving a 10-year follow-up of 1770 geriatric patients from the Veterans and county hospitals in Los Angeles.[17] Among the findings from that study was the fact that 60 per cent of patients who were given limbs discarded them within 6 months. Thirteen years later, Jamieson and Hill reported, in their review of amputation for peripheral vascular disease, that over half the patients fitted with an artificial leg never used it effectively.[138] In addition, they reported that if the rehabilitation process was not started for 2 or more months after amputation, the likelihood of ultimate ambulation was very poor. In a more recent review on the delays in rehabilitation following lower extremity amputation, Kerstein et al. noted that it required an average of 27 weeks (189 days) to achieve maximum benefits of rehabilitation and it was approximately 6 months before the successfully rehabilitated amputee was returned to society.[139] In an earlier article analyzing the influence of age on rehabilitation, Kerstein et al. found that many patients over age 65 required a year to achieve maximum benefit from the rehabilitation process.[133] Malone et al. analyzed contemporary series on below-knee amputation in patients treated with conventional rehabilitation techniques and found that the average rate of rehabilitation was 64 per cent and the average time from operation to rehabilitation (ambulation) was 133 days[9] (Table 44–5). In a more recent review, Malone

---

Patient Instructions for Care of the Diabetic Foot

1. Inspect your feet daily for blisters, cuts, scratches, and areas of possible infection. Do not miss looking between your toes. A mirror can help you see the bottom of your feet or between the toes. If it is not possible for you to inspect your feet yourself, seek the help of a family member or friend.

2. Wash your feet and toes daily, and dry very carefully, especially between the toes. It is also important to dry carefully after showering or swimming.

3. Avoid extreme temperatures for your feet. Test bath water with your hand to ensure that it is not too hot, and be extremely careful of hot pavement or concrete during the summer.

4. If your feet feel cold at night, wear socks. Do not apply hot water bottles or heating pads.

5. Do not use chemical agents to remove corns or calluses.

6. Inspect your shoes daily for foreign objects, nail points, torn linings, or other problems that might damage your feet.

7. Wear properly fitting stockings, and try to avoid stockings with seams and stockings that are mended. It is important to change stockings daily.

8. All shoes should be comfortable and loose fitting at the time of purchase. Do not depend on shoes to stretch or break in. Try to avoid shoes that are pointed or apply pressure on the toes.

9. Do not wear shoes without stockings.

10. Do not wear sandals with thongs between the toes. Never walk barefoot, especially on hot surfaces. Be extremely careful of walking barefoot at home owing to danger from pins, tacks, or other items dropped on the floor.

11. Toenails should be cut straight across, and if there is a question, please consult your physician or podiatrist.

12. Do not cut corns or calluses yourself; seek counseling from your physician or podiatrist. See your physician or podiatrist regularly, and be sure that your feet are examined on each visit.

13. If your vision is impaired or you have other difficulties with examining your feet, have a family member or friend inspect your feet, trim nails, and otherwise ensure adequate foot care.

14. Be sure to tell your podiatrist or physician that you are diabetic.

15. Do not smoke.

16. Remember that even minor infections can cause significant problems in diabetics, and a physician or podiatrist should be consulted when infection occurs.

FIGURE 44–14. Patient instruction sheet for care of the diabetic foot.

et al. noted that the rehabilitation times for patients treated with conventional techniques versus accelerated rehabilitation techniques (including amputation level selection and immediate postoperative prosthesis) were 128 and 31 days, respectively[15] (Table 44–6). The same review pointed out that the success rate for ambulation after amputation with conventional rehabilitation techniques was 70 per cent, whereas it was 100 per cent for amputees treated with accelerated rehabilitation techniques.[15] In addition, it has been my experience with geriatric amputees that if a patient is nonambulatory for either a month before amputation or a month after amputation (rehabilitation is delayed), the likelihood for rehabilitation is significantly less than if the patient is maintained in an ambulatory status in the perioperative period.

Part of the problem with rehabilitation of geriatric amputees is their decreased cardiorespiratory reserve and the increased energy expenditures required after lower extremity amputation, especially at more proximal amputation levels. These problems are complicated by the fact that individual surgeons probably see too few amputees to treat them with maximum efficiency and the few patients they see create a large burden on beds, resources, and physician time.

TABLE 44–5. OVERVIEW OF POSTSURGICAL AND REHABILITATION OUTCOME FOR SEVERAL SERIES[a]

Authors	Number of Amputations	Primary Healing (%)	Eventual Healing (%)	Mortality Rate (%)	Rehab With Prosthesis (%)	Average Time Operation to Rehabilitation (Days)
Warren & Kihn	121	48.8	66.9	4.1	69.4	180–270
Chilvers et al.	53	50.0	67.9	7.5	60.4	—
Robinson	47	77.0	—	17.0	83.0	—
Bradham & Smoak	84	85.7	88.0	—	—[c]	—
Block & Whitehouse	43	88.0	95.0	0.0[b]	53.5	120–180
Cranley et al.	101	76.0	86.0	7.0	73.3	—
Lim et al.	55	53.0	83.0	16.0	51.0	70
Ecker & Jacobs	69	77.0	85.0	8.7	52.2	201
Wray et al.	174	92.0	—	3.5	70.0	49–77
Nagrendran et al.	174	80.5	91.4	—	—	—
Berardi & Keonin	44	—	61.4	4.5	29.5	111
Averaged totals	965	74.9	82.0	6.7	63.8	133

[a]Series reporting their results with conventional techniques of rehabilitation after below-knee amputation. Notice that the overall rehabilitation rate was 64 per cent and the average time to achieve ambulation was 133 days. (From Malone JM, Moore WS, Goldstone J, Malone SJ: Therapeutic and economic impact of a modern amputation program. Ann Surg *189*:801, 1979.)
[b]Two patients died before discharge, and were not included as postoperative deaths.
[c]Authors commented that very few patients attained ambulation; however, no numbers were given.

TABLE 44–6. COMPARISON OF REHABILITATION TIME WITH CONVENTIONAL AND ACCELERATED TECHNIQUES[a]

Level of Amputation	Group 1, Days Range	Group 1, Days Mean	Group 2, Days Range	Group 2, Days Mean	*p* Value
Transmetatarsal	20–60	47.0	10–24	18.4	NS
Syme's	—	—	15–17	23.0	—
Below-knee	60–330	132.0	18–140	32.5	.0001
Knee disarticulation	—	—	15–140	60.7	—
Above-knee	360	—	27–30	28.5	NS
Hip disarticulation	—	—	35	—	—
Overall	20–360	128.4	10–140	30.8	.0001

[a]Rehabilitation time following lower extremity amputation for patients treated with conventional surgical and prosthetic techniques (Group 1: 128 days) and accelerated techniques incorporating immediate postoperative prostheses (Group 2: 31 days) (*p* < .001). (From Malone SM, Moore WS, Leal JM, Childers SJ: Rehabilitation for lower extremity amputation. Arch Surg *116*:97, 1981.)

In a review on the energy cost of walking for amputees, Waters et al. found that in both unilateral traumatic and vascular amputees, performance was directly related to the level of amputation.[136] Walking velocity, cadence, and stride length were all decreased in amputation patients compared to control groups. In a detailed analysis of velocity of ambulation, rate of oxygen uptake, respiratory quotient, and heart rate, these authors concluded that amputees adjust their gait velocity to keep their rate of energy expenditure within normal limits.[136] The approximate energy expenditures (compared to control) after lower extremity amputation are shown in Table 44–7.[136,140–142] Notice that the energy expenditures for both unilateral and bilateral below-knee amputees are less than those of unilateral above-knee amputees. This clearly demonstrates the importance of the knee joint in terms of energy used for ambulation. The additional effort for walking with an above-knee prosthesis is accomplished by the use of small muscles, which are poorly designed for locomotion.[142]

Decreased physical strength due to increasing age, decreased cardiorespiratory reserve due to the rav-

ages of cardiovascular and/or pulmonary disease, and increased energy expenditures for ambulation after lower extremity amputation can all be seen to have an additive effect that complicates the rehabilitation of geriatric amputees. It is in this setting that the salvage of the most distal amputation that will heal may establish the difference between ambulation and independence and nonambulation and dependence

TABLE 44–7. ENERGY EXPENDITURE (COMPARED TO CONTROLS) AFTER LOWER EXTREMITY AMPUTATION[a]

	% Increase in Energy Expenditure
Unilateral below-knee	9–25
Bilateral below-knee	41
Unilateral above-knee	25–100
Bilateral above-knee	280

[a]As measured by oxygen utilization per minute (Gonzalez et al.,[140] Kavanagh and Shephard,[142] and Waters et al.[136]) or indirect calorimetry (Huang et al.[141]). Measured at comfortable walking speeds that averaged 22 per cent of normal.

for the elderly amputee. These factors also explain the higher likelihood of ambulation for a young high-level amputee as contrasted to an elderly high-level or bilateral amputee. In their evaluation of 113 amputations in 103 patients, most of whom underwent amputation for peripheral vascular disease and/or diabetes (mean age of 61 years), Roon et al. found the following rates of success for rehabilitation for below-knee, above-knee, and combination bilateral amputations: 100 per cent for unilateral below-knee amputation; 93 per cent for bilateral below-knee amputations; 17 per cent for a combination of above-knee and below-knee amputations; and no success for patients with bilateral above-knee amputations.[14]

Postoperative Prosthetic Techniques

After major lower extremity amputation, the surgeon has three choices for prosthetic management: soft dressings or conventional technique; constant environmental treatment (CET) (which at this point is probably only of historical interest); and rigid dressings with or without a postoperative prosthesis. In addition, the surgeon may choose delayed (conventional), rapid, or immediate postoperative rehabilitation.

Conventional Stump Wrap (Soft Dressing)

The historical standard, and a technique that is still used in many institutions, is the application of a soft postoperative dressing. Cotton gauze or fluffs are used to pad the amputation stump and the stump is wrapped with elastic bandages (Fig. 44–15). The advantage of this technique is that it does not require a prosthetist to be present in the operating room or at the time of dressing changes. The disadvantages are that it does not readily control stump edema, the

dressings are difficult to maintain in place (especially for high-level amputees), there is minimal stump protection from postoperative trauma, the dressing will not prevent knee flexion contracture, and ambulation may be delayed as a result of the prolonged time period required for stump maturity (6 months).

Except for the above-knee and hip disarticulation amputation levels, where it is technically difficult to maintain a rigid dressing in good stump contact, we do not believe that there are valid reasons to continue the use of this postoperative dressing technique.

CET Unit

Developed and used almost exclusively in Great Britain, the CET unit consists of a control console containing a multistage centrifugal air compressor. The air passes through pressure control valves, a pressure cycle timing device, a bacteriologic filter, and a thermostatically controlled heating element that controls heat and relative humidity. The dressing on the patient consists of a transparent flexible polyvinyl bag. The bag is not in direct contact with the residual limb except on the resting surface. A pleated airseal is incorporated into the proximal end of the bag in order to maintain a pressure seal. A sterile CET bag is placed over the amputation stump in the operating room. The amputation stump is in essence "enclosed" in a sterile environment with cyclical pressure (which controls stump edema) and airflow set to desired temperature and humidity (Fig. 44–16).

The CET unit was designed for use in a setting in which a prosthetist was not immediately available to the surgeon or one in which the surgeon wishes to be able to control stump edema and yet have easy ability to examine the surgical wound. The system incorporates a long flexible hose so that the patient can undergo rehabilitation training at the bedside. The use for the CET unit is relatively limited and it

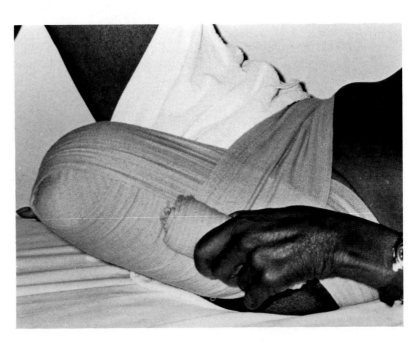

FIGURE 44–15. The standard conventional soft dressing and stump wrap being applied by a patient on his right above-knee amputation.

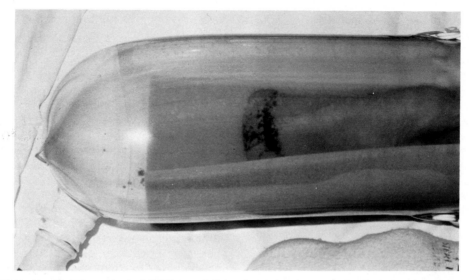

FIGURE 44–16. The clear polyvinyl CET bag, which has been placed over a left below-knee amputation. Notice the air supply hose at the distal end of the bag.

is probably best used on those patients in whom there is some risk of stump infection and the ability to have continuous observation of the wound without dressing changes is desirable. Because of its limited application, high cost, and poor patient acceptance due to noise, the CET unit, although successful, has seen limited use in the United States.[143]

Rapid and Immediate Postoperative Prostheses

The application of an immediate postoperative prosthesis has received considerable attention, support, credit, and discredit in the past 15 years. Proponents of the technique have waxed eloquently on the benefit to the patient, while opponents of the technique have cautioned about the potential complications to the amputation stump from the casting technique.

Berlemont is generally credited with the early work that led to establishment of the technique based upon his application of temporary prostheses to patients with delayed (secondary) amputation stump healing.[3] Professor Marion Weiss from Poland is credited with adapting this technique for stumps undergoing primary healing (i.e., immediate postoperative prosthesis). The latter technique proved highly successful and Weiss reported his initial results at the 6th International Prosthetic Course in Copenhagen in July of 1963. This early presentation and a subsequent publication in 1966[4] came to the attention of surgeons worldwide. The Prosthetic and Sensory Aids Service of the VA was especially interested in the application of this technique for the management of veteran amputees and was instrumental in bringing this procedure to the American surgical theatre. Working with the VA, Dr. Ernest Burgess, an orthopedic surgeon in Seattle, Washington, refined and developed the application of the immediate postoperative

prosthetic technique for the American surgical field.[5,125,144–146] Burgess and his team performed most of the early work in the United States on the use of immediate postoperative prosthetic techniques and he was instrumental in training other investigators in its use. In the late 1960s and early 1970s there were multiple reports extolling the virtues and possible pitfalls of the immediate postoperative prosthetic (IPOP) technique (also called IPPF, immediate postoperative prosthetic fitting).

Initially, there was general agreement that the immediate postoperative prosthetic technique was ideally suited for the nondiabetic, nondysvascular amputee. Subsequent reports in the literature, however, have shown that if properly used the technique works perhaps ideally in the geriatric dysvascular amputee because of its ability to shorten hospitalization time and increase rates of rehabilitation.[9,14,15]

In general, proponents of the technique note that its benefits include an increased rate of healing, decreased hospital time, decreased rehabilitation time, decreased psychological trauma to the patient, control of stump edema, protection from trauma to the stump in the early postoperative period, and perhaps an increased rate of rehabilitation.[9,14,15,84,147–150] The paper most commonly quoted against the use of immediate postoperative prosthesis is that by Cohen et al.[151] Using conventional surgical/prosthetic techniques, Cohen and colleagues were able to achieve 97 per cent amputation stump healing, whereas only two of nine amputation stumps treated with immediate postoperative prostheses healed. They noted no rehabilitation advantage to the immediate postoperative prosthetic technique and recommended caution in the application of this technique. The experience reported by Cohen and coworkers is not matched by other similar reports in the literature. There are reports that notice no change in the rate of wound healing,[147] but in general most papers find no deleterious effect to the stump from the use of a rigid postoperative dressing (with or without a prosthesis), decreased hospitalization time, and decreased rehabilitative time.[9,14,15,147,149,150] Importantly, Cohen and colleagues suggested that their problems with the immediate postoperative prosthetic technique might be in the plaster technique itself or in the application of the technique. A review of their paper shows that four patients sustained what are described as second-degree blisters, which almost certainly indicate problems with plaster fabrication and application rather than problems with the immediate postoperative technique itself. In my own experience with 600 consecutive major lower extremity amputations during the past 12 years, there has been only one stump problem related to the use of an immediate postoperative prosthesis and that problem was directly caused by improper application of an immediate postoperative cast.

An overview of data on use of the immediate postoperative prosthesis technique reported from the San Francisco VA Hospital, the Tucson VA Hospital, and Maricopa Medical Center by Roon and Malone and associates are summarized in Table 44–8.[9,14,15] A more recent paper by Folsom et al.[152] documents the overall rate of rehabilitation at 80 per cent and the interval from amputation to ambulation at 15.2 days and 9.3 days for below-knee and above-knee amputees, respectively. Information not tabulated in Table 44–8 suggests that the ambulatory status of the patient prior to surgery was one of the most important predeterminants of postoperative ambulation. Essentially, 100 per cent of patients undergoing unilateral major lower extremity amputation who ambulated prior to surgery were successfully rehabilitated after amputation, whereas less than 15 per cent of the patients who were nonambulatory prior to amputation surgery were successfully rehabilitated.[9,14,15]

The advantages of immediate or early postoperative prostheses can be divided into two categories: those derived from the rigid dressing and those derived from early weight bearing and ambulation. The advantages of the rigid dressing include edema control, stump immobilization, perhaps improved healing, prevention of joint flexion contracture, and protection to the amputation stump from external trauma. There may not be a difference between soft and rigid

TABLE 44–8. OVERVIEW: SAN FRANCISCO & TUCSON, VA MARICOPA MEDICAL CENTER IMMEDIATE PROSTHESIS DATA[a]

Stump healing	138/153	(90%)
Rehabilitation time	15–32 days	
Rate of rehabilitation	155/175	(88%)
Unilateral BK below-knee	128/129	(99%)
Bilateral BK below-knee	17/19	(89%)
Bilateral (above/below-knee or above/above-knee	6/23	(26%)
Unilateral above-knee	4/4	(100%)

[a]Data from Roon et al.,[14] Malone et al.,[9,15] and Malone unpublished.

dressings with respect to the time required to reach eventual stump maturity (6 months), although postoperative stump edema resolves much more quickly with a rigid dressing. The advantages of immediate or early ambulation include decreased hospital time, shortened time from surgery to ambulation, increased rates of rehabilitation compared to patients managed in a more conventional manner, a reduction in morbid and nonmorbid complications of amputation, and an improvement in the psychological outlook of the patient after amputation.[9,14,15,114]

In summary, then, there is general agreement upon both the benefits and pitfalls of the immediate postoperative prosthetic technique. We agree with Friedmann's conclusions: "immediate postoperative prosthetic fitting should be confined to large centers with medical and prosthetic facilities available on short notice." In other circumstances, he believed that the use of conventional amputation rehabilitation was indicated, but specified that conventional amputation management should include modern postoperative techniques, specifically including the early use of temporary prostheses for evaluation and training.[76] The best solution to the problem of choosing a postoperative prosthetic technique would be the routine use of a rigid dressing and the application or use of a temporary prosthesis when the surgeon thinks that adequate wound healing has occurred (usually 1 to 2 weeks after amputation), thereby avoiding some of the potential hazards of immediate ambulation.[153–155]

Another variant of a postoperative rigid dressing that allows early postsurgical ambulation is the air splint.[132,156] This device may be a practical alternative for a surgeon who wants to achieve early postoperative amputation, but does not have access to a prosthetist skilled in the application of immediate postoperative prostheses or temporary removable prostheses.

Techniques of Immediate Postoperative Prosthetic Application

Immediate postoperative prosthetic use has been described for all levels of major lower extremity amputation from the transmetatarsal through the high above-knee; however, it is best suited to below-knee amputation. Specific technical details regarding application of immediate postoperative prostheses have been well described and will therefore be only briefly outlined in the present chapter.[98]

Transmetatarsal and Syme's Amputation

A rigid cast with felt padding for bony prominence relief is used as the first dressing for these distal levels of lower extremity amputation; however, ambulation is not allowed until adequate primary healing has been obtained (3 weeks). Early ambulation for the transmetatarsal and Syme's amputation patients results in a higher incidence of wound complications. It is extremely important for the Syme's amputation that the posterior heel flap be held in good approximation and alignment by the cast, and that great care be taken to pad the distal stump and dog-ears as well as the bony prominences. If a two-stage surgical approach for Syme's amputation is used,[84] it is probably best to avoid weight bearing until completion of the second stage of the surgical procedure (6 to 8 weeks). Both transmetatarsal and Syme's amputees will ultimately ambulate well and a short delay in the ambulation process has essentially no impact on their overall rehabilitation. Avoidance of stump trauma to ensure primary wound healing during the early postoperative period is of paramount importance, and rehabilitation efforts can be confined to range of motion and strengthening of the opposite leg and upper extremities during the early postoperative period.

Below-Knee Amputation Level

Following completion of the amputation, a thin sheet of fine mesh material (Owen's silk) is moistened in antibiotic solution or saline and applied over the suture line with care taken to avoid wrinkling (Fig. 44–17). Next, lamb's wool or polyurethane foam is placed over the end of the stump to provide stump compression and padding (Fig. 44–18). A Spandex stump sock is then carefully rolled over the stump with care taken to avoid displacement of the distal stump padding (Fig. 44–19). Relief pads made from nonporous foam are fashioned and glued to the stump sock with Dow-Corning medical adhesive. These pads can be obtained precut or can be hand fashioned in the operating room. They are placed so as to pad the bony prominences, specifically including the fibular head, the tibial condyles, and the patella. Care is taken to leave a relief area between the medial and lateral tibial pads (Fig. 44–20). Next, elastic plaster is used to form the inner layer of the immediate postoperative prosthesis. It is important that an assistant maintain traction on the stump sock during plaster application. Care is taken to maintain compression from posterior to anterior (direction of the posterior skin flap) and to grade compression from the distal end of the stump to the more proximal thigh (Fig. 44–21). The suspension assembly of the immediate postoperative pylon is then contoured to the inner cast after the cast has dried (Fig. 44–22). The pylon can then be attached and static alignment achieved before incorporating the suspension assembly into the cast. The pylon is removed and the suspension assembly is secured to the inner cast using fiberglass casting tape. The use of lightweight casting tape decreases the weight of the immediate postoperative prosthesis and significantly increases its durability.[154] A completed immediate postoperative prosthesis, waist suspension belt, pylon, and foot are shown in Figure 44–23. If a drain is employed, the drain should be brought out proximally (and laterally) through a separate hole made in the cast during the fabrication process. The drain should not be secured to the skin so that it can be pulled out through the cast when appropriate.

Most surgical pain is gone within 36 to 48 hours after surgery. Significant pain more than 48 hours after surgery is an indication that the cast is too tight or that there is a wound complication, and the cast should be removed, the wound inspected, and the cast reapplied if appropriate. Almost all patients comment that their postoperative stump pain diminishes if the heel of the prosthesis is weight loaded (when they are in the supine position) and this test can be used as a further check for stump swelling/prosthesis fit. One of the most important principles in the post-

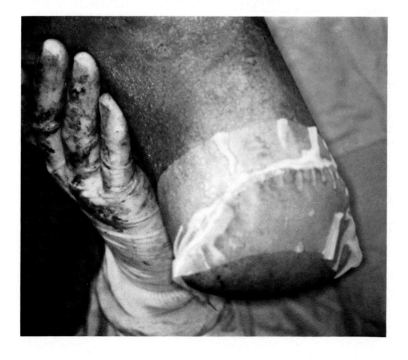

FIGURE 44–17. A single sheet of moistened Owen's silk is placed over the suture line on the below-knee amputation stump. Care is taken to avoid wrinkling of the silk material.

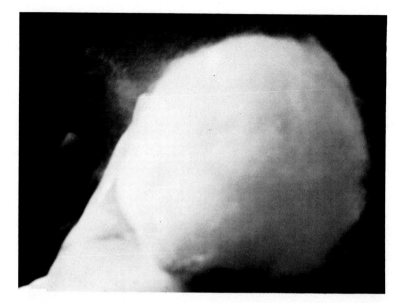

FIGURE 44–18. Lamb's wool, Dacron waste, or prefabricated polyurethane foam can be placed over Owen's silk to provide distal stump padding. Care is taken to place padding material both above and below skin dog-ears, if they exist.

operative management of these patients is that if there is any question about prosthesis fit or healing of the surgical wound, the prosthesis should be removed, the wound inspected by the surgeon and the prosthetist, and the cast reapplied at the discretion of the surgeon.

On the first postoperative morning, the patient is helped into a standing position at the bedside and he/she is instructed in techniques of touchdown weight bearing. At this time, the prosthetist will complete

his initial static alignment. On the second postoperative morning, the patient will go to the physical therapy department, where he/she is taught touchdown weight bearing using the bathroom scale technique (Fig. 44–24). An alternative to the scale technique is the load cell, which is a pressure-sensing

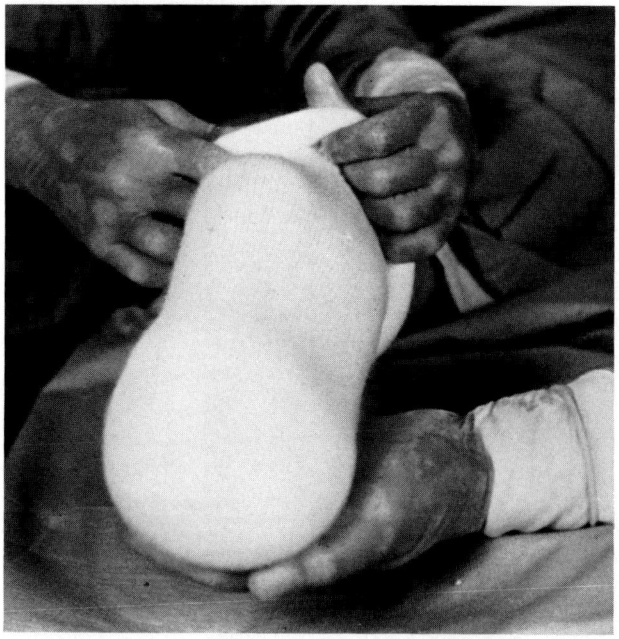

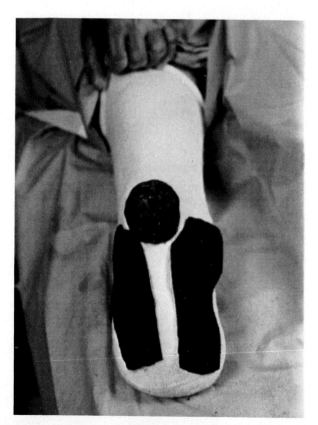

FIGURE 44–19. A Spandex stump sock is carefully pulled over the distal end of the below-knee stump and rolled proximally up the leg. Care is taken to not displace distal end stump padding during application of the sock. Until the postoperative cast is dry, it is necessary for an assistant to maintain traction on the stump sock.

FIGURE 44–20. Felt relief pads are measured, trimmed, and glued to the Spandex stump sock over the bony prominences of the knee and lower leg. Care is taken to leave a relief area between the medial and lateral tibial pads.

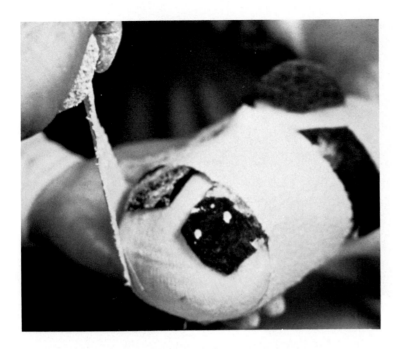

FIGURE 44–21. The inner layer of the postoperative rigid cast is made using elastic plaster. Elastic plaster provides good control of stump compression. Compression should be from posterior to anterior, in the direction of the posterior flap, and distal to proximal so that the compression decreases as the cast moves higher on the upper leg.

device built into the prosthetic pylon.[157] During the first 7 to 10 days after surgery, the patient will ambulate in parallel bars with a maximum of 10 to 15 pounds touchdown weight bearing (10 per cent of body weight). After application of the second postoperative prothesis, the patient will increase his/her weight bearing to approximately 50 per cent of total body weight. At the end of 14 to 21 days, upon removal of the second postoperative prosthesis, a decision is made to place the patient either in a third postoperative prosthesis (if there is a question of wound healing) or in a removable temporary prosthesis (if the wound appears to be healing satisfactorily).[154,155] At this time the patient begins full weight bearing. By approximately 30 to 35 days after amputation surgery, most patients have achieved either independent ambulation or ambulation with some type of ancillary walking aid (cane, walker). If a patient lives close to the hospital and is able to come to daily physical therapy training as an outpatient, he/she may be discharged from the hospital shortly after receiving his/her second postoperative pros-

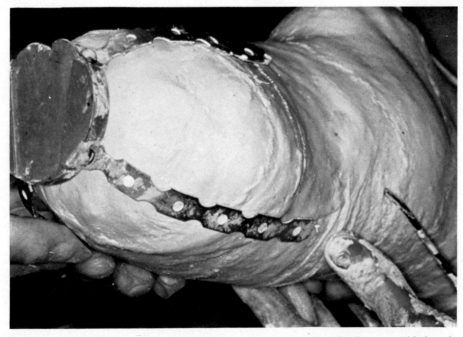

FIGURE 44–22. The metal arms of the immediate postoperative prosthetic bucket are molded to the contours of the inner plaster shell after the cast has dried.

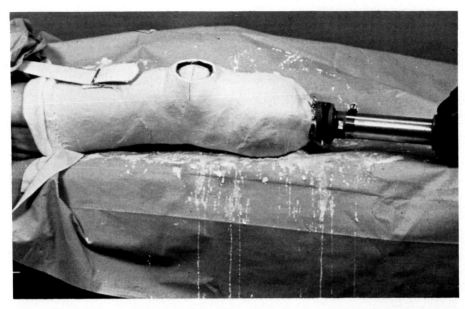

FIGURE 44–23. Intraoperative photograph of a completed immediate postoperative below-knee prosthesis with pylon, foot, and waist suspension belt. Note that a relief window has been placed over the area of the patella.

thesis (5 to 10 days); however, if the patient lives a great distance from the hospital, then discharge is usually delayed until surgeon, prosthetist, and therapist are happy with the rehabilitation process (4 to 5 weeks). This approach may, however, have to be modified under the economic restraints that surround current medical care. Reasonable alternatives include transfer to a rehabilitation unit/service or early discharge with outpatient care. In either case, careful follow-up by the surgeon, prosthetist, and therapist is mandatory, especially in patients undergoing early ambulation/rehabilitation.

It can be anticipated that between discharge from the hospital and construction of the first permanent

prosthesis (average 6 months after amputation), approximately three to six changes in the socket on the temporary prosthesis will be required as a result of progressive stump shrinking. A typical lightweight removable temporary below-knee prosthesis is shown in Figure 44–25. The same pylon and foot can be used throughout all intermediate (temporary) cast changes, so that the only new prosthetic requirement is the prosthetic socket and realignment of the prosthesis. Prosthetic fit is maintained with stump socks and the primary indication for change of the temporary prosthesis is when the patient has reached a total of 15-ply stockings in order to maintain a good prosthetic fit. Obviously, great care is taken to ed-

FIGURE 44–24. In order to control the amount of postoperative weight bearing by the patient, a bathroom scale is used to teach them distribution of body weight. During the first week after surgery, weight bearing is limited to 10 to 15 pounds. After the second cast change, weight bearing is limited to 50 per cent of total body weight.

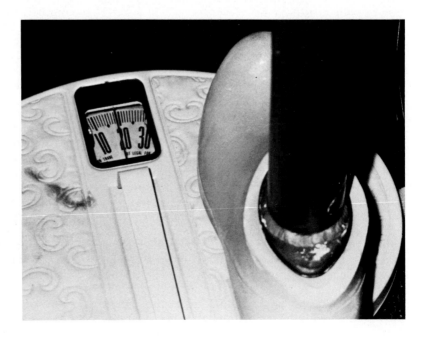

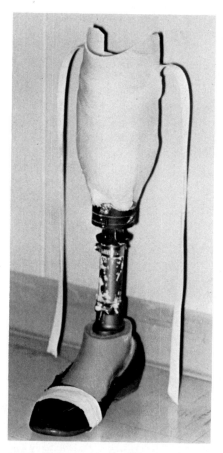

FIGURE 44–25. Standard removable lightweight below-knee temporary/intermediate prosthesis. This prosthesis is prescribed after removal of the last immediate postoperative prosthesis. The particular prosthesis in the photograph is constructed with 3M Scotchcast. Fabrication with Scotchcast allows construction of a lightweight, cool, yet durable prosthesis.

ucate the patient about the use of the prothesis and stump care in order to avoid any stump problems due to poor prosthetic fit.

Knee Disarticulation Amputation

The techniques for the application of an immediate postoperative prosthesis for the knee disarticulation amputation are essentially the same as those for the below-knee amputation. Because of the bulbous distal end of the knee disarticulation stump, the immediate postoperative prosthesis for this amputation level is self-suspending. Great care should be taken during cast fabrication to carefully contour the femoral flares and to bring the proximal end of the cast to at least the upper third of the thigh to minimize distal end–weight bearing. Our preference is to incorporate a polypropylene quadralateral above-knee brim into the knee disarticulation cast so as to provide ischial weight bearing. The stump should be well padded, since there is more stump weight bearing with this level of amputation than with a below-knee amputation. At the choice of the surgeon and prosthetist, polycentric hydraulic knee units can be incorporated with the initial immediate postoperative

prosthesis or be incorporated anytime during postoperative follow-up. The times for cast change, rehabilitation techniques, and use of a temporary prosthesis are approximately the same as those for a below-knee amputation.

Above-Knee Amputation

Immediate postoperative prosthetic techniques for above-knee amputation require more prosthetic attention to detail in order to maintain adequate suspension and socket fit. Although techniques using a modified silesian suspension (contralateral hip sling) or waist suspension belt are described and are simple to use,[104] we believe that the difficulties encountered when using immediate postoperative prostheses at the above-knee level are not offset by significant improvements in the overall rehabilitation process so as to make the effort worthwhile. Our use of immediate postoperative prostheses at this amputation level is reserved for young amputees. For the dysvascular amputee, a temporary above-knee prosthesis is prescribed when primary wound healing has been achieved (2 to 3 weeks). During the postoperative period, the above-knee amputee goes to rehab daily in order to achieve upper extremity strengthening, balance, and to practice ambulation with parallel bars or other walking aids. Once a temporary prosthesis has been constructed, the times for prosthesis modification and rehabilitation techniques are similar to those for below-knee or knee disarticulation amputation postsurgical management.

Overview of Prostheses and Prosthetic Techniques

There is not one type of standard prosthetic prescription for any level of lower extremity amputation, and knowledge of available components is crucial in developing the proper prescription for each amputee based upon his or her activities and lifestyle. A more complete discussion of prosthetic components is beyond the scope of this chapter; however, the interested surgeon is referred to the local prosthetist or prosthetic facility with whom he/she should be working.

Immediate postoperative prosthetic techniques will not work in all clinical settings. The success of the technique is based upon the experience and dedication of the team and there is no question that if the immediate postoperative prosthesis is improperly applied, significant damage to the amputation stump can and will occur. In the absence of the availability of an experienced prosthetist and therapist to help the surgeon, we suggest that a rigid postoperative dressing be applied and, when primary stump healing has occurred, an appropriate temporary prosthesis can be prescribed and the rehabilitation process can be initiated. A week or two delay in the rehabilitation process is meaningless in the overall context of amputee rehabilitation; however, it has been the author's experience that if the rehabilitation process is delayed for a month or more, the ultimate success of rehabilitation, especially for high-level amputations in geriatric patients, is severely compromised. It is therefore logical and reasonable to provide a temporary prosthesis sometime between wound healing (7 to 10 days after surgery) and 1 month after surgery. Using this "between" type of approach (i.e., a rigid dressing with early prosthetic application), maximum rehabilitation results can be achieved even in the absence of a formalized rehabilitation team.

Prosthetic Components

For the occasional amputation surgeon, the number and types of prostheses and prosthetic components for lower extremity amputees can be bewildering and probably of little interest. Therefore, a general overview of prosthetic components and specific combinations of components for certain levels of lower extremity amputation may be of value.

Transmetatarsal Amputation

In general, there is minimal, if any, prosthetic requirement for a transmetatarsal amputation. A steel shank placed in the sole of the shoe will allow near-normal toe-off and the void spot in the shoe can be filled with cotton, lamb's wool, or a soft foam material. The other available option is construction of a specially designed shoe molded to the patient's foot where toe-off is built into the shoe during construction.

Syme's Amputation

Depending upon whether the Syme's amputation has been performed with a one- or two-stage surgical procedure, the cosmetic quality of the prosthesis will be different (two-stage is more cosmetic). In general, this is an end–weight bearing stump and a prosthetic foot is attached to the leg shaft portion of the prosthesis. Because of the bulbous nature of the stump, a medial window has to be cut into the prosthesis to allow the stump to pass through the narrow midportion of the prosthesis. These prostheses are usually built with a nonmotion SACH (solid ankle–cushion heel) foot. The presence of a particularly bulbous distal end will preclude a very cosmetic prosthesis and, particularly in young women, this type of amputation may be contraindicated for cosmetic reasons alone.

Below-Knee Amputation

In general, the below-knee prosthesis consists of a prosthetic socket that is attached to a pylon/ankle block (endoskeletal system) and a foot. The prosthetic shell can be composed of plastic laminate, wood, or some of the newer lightweight-rolled fiberglass materials such as 3M Scotchcast. The socket may use no liner (skin-socket interface) or may use a liner composed of lightweight plastic such as pelite, silicone gel bonded between two sheets of soft leather, or stump socks. The prosthesis can be suspended in

a variety of manners, the most common of which include a standard patella tendon-bearing (PTB) strap, a supracondylar clip, Silastic sleeve suspension, suction, or a thigh lacer with external hinges (Fig. 44–26). Self-suspending prosthesis or physiologic suspension (prosthesis is held in place by changes in muscle shape/contour with contraction) may be used in young active amputees. In a young, highly active amputee, an ankle rotating unit may be placed between the prosthesis and the foot. The feet currently in use include the SACH foot, which is a nonmotion foot, the stationary attachment flexible endoskeletal (SAFE) foot, or the Griesinger 5-Way foot. Both of the latter two feet incorporate flexion, extension, and internal/external rotation when the foot is stressed under weight. The drawback to either of those motion feet is increased weight and perhaps decreased life expectancy compared to the SACH foot. The most popular motion foot, the Seattle foot, overcomes the drawbacks of the previously mentioned motion feet, and has a cosmetic design that incorporates toes. A hydraulic ankle unit has recently been developed, but the unit is quite heavy and there are still problems with oil leakage. New energy-storing feet (energy is

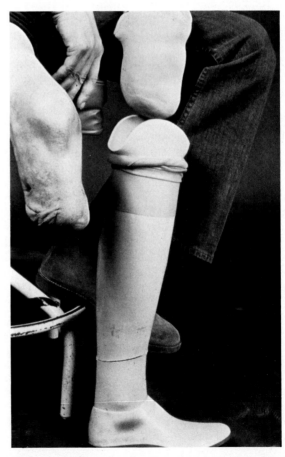

FIGURE 44–26. The below-knee prosthesis shown in this photograph is an ultralightweight patellar tendon weight-bearing–type prosthesis using a Silastic sleeve for suspension, a Silastic gel insert, and a SAFE motion–type foot. This is an ideal prosthetic prescription for a young active amputee.

"stored" by deformation of carbon-plastic composites and "released" on toe-off), such as the Seattle-Boeing-Burgess Foot and the Flex-Foot, offer significant improvements in gait and activity levels (such as running), especially for the young active amputee. The combination of a motion foot and a lightweight prosthesis provides a very high degree of function for an active amputee.

Knee Disarticulation

Historically, knee disarticulation amputations were a prosthetic nightmare because the knee centers (thigh/knee length) could not be matched; however, the availability of polycentric knee joints has allowed construction of a cosmetic knee disarticulation prosthesis. In general, this prosthesis is similar to the Syme's type prosthesis in that the distal bony end of the stump is passed through the proximal portion of the prosthesis via a window cut in the medial portion of the prosthesis. The prosthetic shell can again be constructed of plastic or wood. In general, the prosthetic shell extends from the end of the stump up to the ischium in order to provide both distal end and ischial weight bearing. Most knee disarticulation prostheses incorporate some type of hydraulic knee unit for both cosmetic and functional reasons. The lower part of the leg can be constructed of either solid wood, plastic laminate, or a metal or plastic endoskeletal system for connection to the ankle block and foot. Again, ankle rotators and energy-storing motion or nonmotion feet can be used at the discretion of the prosthetist and surgeon.

Above-Knee Amputation

The above-knee prosthesis can be constructed of plastic or wood. Suspension techniques include an external hip joint with belt, shoulder suspension, or suction socket suspension. The prosthesis is not an end–weight bearing prosthesis and all the weight is borne by the proximal socket quadralateral brim design (the soft tissues of the thigh and ischium). Newer prosthetic designs for above-knee sockets include the CAT-CAM design (which holds the stump laterally and medially providing rigid support for the femur, in contrast to the quad socket, which holds the stump anteriorly and posteriorly with poor femur support) and a variety of new flexible socket and strut designs (outer rigid strut attached to the knee joint with an inner soft flexible inner socket). These new designs significantly enhance function for above-knee amputees. A hydraulic, passive, or manual lock knee joint can be incorporated as required by the needs of each individual patient. The lower part of the prosthesis is constructed as outlined in the section for knee disarticulation prostheses.

Hip Disarticulation Prostheses

In general, the hip disarticulation prostheses are built along the lines of the Canadian system, which incorporates a pelvic bucket, an endoskeletal upper and lower leg, simple spring-assisted hip and knee joints, and a nonmotion foot.

AMPUTATION REHABILITATION TEAM

It is exceedingly difficult to achieve consistently reliable rehabilitation results in the absence of a formal centralized, dedicated rehabilitation team that includes active participation by a prosthetist and members of the physical medicine and therapy department. Just as some surgical procedures are confined to regional centers because of cost and necessity of skilled manpower, it is our feeling that under the best of circumstances, amputation rehabilitation should be a centralized resource in a community or among communities in order to achieve the best results. Our concept of the structure of the amputation rehabilitation team is shown in Figure 44–27. Notice that the center of the rehabilitation team is the patient and that other members of the team interface with the patient through or with an amputation coordinator. This coordinator could be a physical therapist, occupational therapist, nurse, or lay person. In the opinion of the author, this person is the key in maintaining coordination and especially long-term follow-up among members of the team. It has been our experience that one break in this rehabilitation circle results in at least a 50 per cent failure in amputee rehabilitation. This fact (i.e., a break in the rehabilitation circle) may explain why the average rate of rehabilitation after lower extremity amputation is 60 per cent or less.

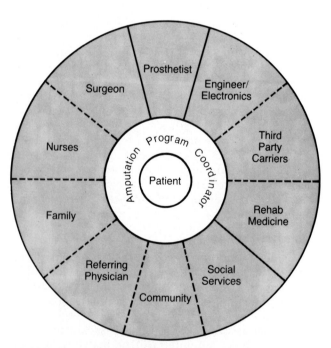

FIGURE 44–27. The rehabilitation team or circle of resources required for successful amputation rehabilitation. Notice the patient is at the center and the surgeon is only one of many coequal team members.

There are five primary areas of concern in successful amputee rehabilitation: (1) coordination of care, (2) education of patient and family, (3) directed access to community resources, (4) discharge planning, and (5) centralized follow-up. In essence, the coordination of health care and mobilization of resources is under the direct control of the physician; however, in actual fact, once surgery is completed this task is best organized by the amputation program coordinator. Discharge planning for the patient should start, if possible, prior to amputation. Education of the patient and family and evaluation of financial and social resources available to the patient should also begin prior to amputation or as soon as possible after amputation. Centralized follow-up probably is only important if the team is interested in evaluating specific treatment techniques or prosthetic components. However, long-term follow-up is mandatory if reliable information on rehabilitation and postoperative complications is to be obtained.

The role of the physician is that of a team director and a provider of health care. The enthusiasm and interest of the physician will be reflected by all other members of the health care team. In the absence of an interested physician, it can be expected that many rehabilitation failures will be common.

It is my personal feeling that the prosthetist should be seen as coequal to the physician in the amputation rehabilitation process. From a practical standpoint, most patients identify with their prosthetist, not their physician (in the absence of medical problems) once the acute phase of rehabilitation is completed.

The therapist is in the unique position of being able to make or break all of the efforts of the surgeon and prosthetist. Only if the rehabilitation process runs smoothly and if attention is paid to small details during the rehabilitation process will the patient successfully regain ambulation. The greatest surgery in the world or the best limb in the world can meet defeat at the hands of an unskilled therapist. The therapist is the third coequal in the rehabilitation team with the physician and prosthetist.

Finally, the patient is the most important member of the rehabilitation team. The team can provide the patient with the tools and techniques for rehabilitation, but it cannot provide the patient with motivation. It is of the utmost importance that the patient be taught to take primary control of the rehabilitation process. Included in this learning process are care of the amputation stump, care of the nonamputated contralateral leg, and care of the prosthesis. Failure of the patient to take an active role in the rehabilitation process will necessarily doom it to ultimate failure.[158]

One of the areas in which we as physicians and rehabilitation team members fail our patients is in the area of posthospital discharge follow-up and home care. There is an excellent review article on this topic that appeared in the February 1979 issue of the *ONA Journal*. All interested rehabilitation physicians and team members are advised to review this information and pass it on to their patients.[112]

WHAT'S NEW IN AMPUTATION SURGERY

Instrumentation

As noted in earlier sections, many new instruments are currently undergoing evaluation for amputation level selection. In addition to amputation level selection, many of these instruments are now being evaluated for their discriminate role in arterial insufficiency. Once again, early information is available, but the definitive place for these instruments is undecided. Perhaps more promising than any of the specific instruments for amputation level selection will be the availability of computer software/microprocessors to integrate results from several different types of noninvasive amputation level selection techniques, resulting, in essence, in the era of the "limb viability lab." It can be anticipated that multiinstrument testing will have greater accuracy than single instrument evaluation. In addition, many of these instruments will find use in the evaluation of limb ischemia, especially in the perioperative period.

Prosthetics

Three current areas of prosthetic development that are showing promising results are: the emergence of

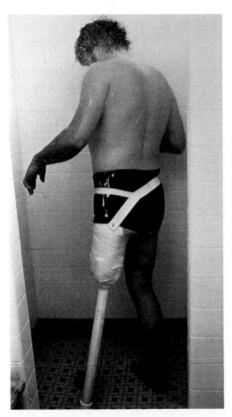

FIGURE 44–28. Patients with lower extremity amputations usually sit on a stool when taking a shower. The left above-knee amputee shown here is wearing an Aqualite above-knee shower prosthesis (US Manufacturing Co, Pasadena, CA).

ultralightweight/throwaway or temporary/intermediate prostheses (Fig. 44–28); the design and development of energy-absorbing/energy-returning prosthetic components (designed to return energy on toe-off), as exemplified by the Burgess-Seattle-Boeing foot and the Flex-Foot; and new fabrication techniques such as flexible sockets (ISNY socket), flexible suction sockets (OCERPSS and ICEPOSS sockets), and non-quadralateral or medial-lateral contoured above-knee sockets (CAT-CAM). The use of new plastics, fiberglass casting tapes, and carbon fiber polymers is allowing the construction of ultralightweight, yet rugged, durable prostheses. These prostheses have obvious value for the geriatric amputee in terms of energy-saving characteristics, especially for the high-level amputee, but they also have value for the young active amputee for sports or water-related activities. Lightweight prostheses constructed with these new materials are often easier to fabricate than standard plastic laminate prostheses. Artificial limbs con-

structed with fiberglass casting tapes, such as 3M Scotchcast, allow a decrease in skin temperature at the socket-skin interface because of the porous nature of the casting material. Preliminary work by our group demonstrated a 5° to 7°C drop in skin temperature with 3M Scotchcast PTB below-knee prostheses, compared to standard plastic laminant PTB below-knee prostheses. The importance of decreased skin temperature is unknown with respect to stump durability, but there is no question these prostheses result in improved patient comfort in hot, humid climates.

Increasing numbers of studies are now being done with young active amputees to improve their performance abilities in activities such as running, jumping, and other sports functions.[159] Projects such as this point not only toward directions for improvements in existing prosthetic devices, but also toward directions for future research efforts and perhaps improving the efficiency with which amputees conduct their physical activities.

REFERENCES

1. Wangensteen OH, Wangensteen SD: The Rise of Surgery from Empiric Craft to Scientific Discipline. Minneapolis, University of Minnesota Press, 1978, p 18.
2. Boedner CW: Baron Dominique Jean Larrey, Napoleon's surgeon. ACS Bull, 18–21, July, 1982.
3. Berlemont M: Notre experience de l'appareillage precoce des amputes des membres inferieurs aux establissements helioMarins de Berk. Ann Med Phys Med 5(4), 1961.
4. Weiss M: The prosthesis on the operating table from a neurophysical point of view. Report of a workshop panel on lower extremity prosthetic fitting. Committee on Prosthetics Research Development, presented to the National Academy of Sciences, Feb, 1966.
5. Burgess EM, Tramb JE, Wilson AB Jr: Immediate Postsurgical Prosthetics in the Management of Lower Extremity Amputees. TR 10-5, Washington, DC, Veterans Administration, 1967.
6. Falstie-Jensen N, Christensen KB: A model for prediction of failure in amputation of the lower limb. Dan Med Bull 37:283–286, 1990.
7. Huston CC, Bivins BA, Ernst CB, Griffen WO Jr: Morbid implications of above-knee amputations. Report of a series and review of the literature. Arch Surg 115:165–167, 1980.
8. Kerstein MD, Zimmer H, Dugdale FE, Lerner E: Associated diagnoses complicating rehabilitation after major lower extremity amputation. Angiology 25:536–547, 1974.
9. Malone JM, Moore WS, Goldstone J, Malone SJ: Therapeutic and economic impact of a modern amputation program. Ann Surg 189:798–802, 1979.
10. Moore WS, Hall AD, Lim RC: Below the knee amputation for ischemic gangrene. Comparative results of conventional operation and immediate postoperative fitting technic. Am J Surg 124:127–134, 1972.
11. Porter JM, Baur GM, Taylor LM Jr: Lower-extremity amputation for ischemia. Arch Surg 116:89–92, 1981.
12. Towne JB, Condon RE: Lower extremity amputation for ischemic disease. Adv Surg 13:199–227, 1979.
13. Otteman MG, Stahlgren LH: Evaluation of factors which influence mortality and morbidity following major lower extremity amputation for arteriosclerosis. Surg Gynecol Obstet 120:1217–1220, 1965.
14. Roon AJ, Moore WS, Goldstone J: Below-knee amputation: A modern approach. Am J Surg 134:153–158, 1977.
15. Malone JM, Moore WS, Leal JM, Childers SJ: Rehabilitation

for lower extremity amputation. Arch Surg 116:93–98, 1981.
16. Malone JM, Synder M, Anderson GG, Bernhard VM, Holloway GA, Bunt TJ: Prevention of amputation by diabetic education. Am J Surg 158:520–524, 1989.
17. Mazet R Jr, Schiller FJ, Dunn OJ, Alonzo NJ: The influence of prosthesis wearing on the health of the geriatric patient. Project 431. Dept HEW, Office of Voc Rehab., Washington, DC, Office of Vocational Rehabilitation, Department of Health, Education and Welfare (unpublished), March 1963.
18. Whitehouse FW, Jurgensen C, Block MA: The later life of the diabetic amputee. Another look at fate of the second leg. Diabetes 17:520–521, 1968.
19. Malone JM, Moore WS, Goldstone J: Life expectancy following aortofemoral arterial grafting. Surgery 81:551–555, 1977.
20. Pinzur MS, Littooy F, Daniels J, Arney C, Reddy NK, Graham G, Osterman H: Multidisciplinary preoperative assessment and late function in dysvascular amputees. Clin Orthop 281:239–243, 1992.
21. Fierer J, Daniel D, Davis C: The fetid foot: Lower-extremity infections in patients with diabetes mellitus. Rev Infect Dis 1:210–217, 1979.
22. Brinker MR, Timberlake GA, Goff JM, Rice JC, Kerstein MD: Below knee physiologic cryoanesthesia in the critically ill patient. J Vasc Surg 7:433–438, 1988.
23. Johansen K, Burgess EM, Zorn R, et al: Improvement of amputation level by lower extremity revascularization. Surg Gynecol Obstet 153:707–709, 1981.
24. Kazmers M, Satiani B, Evans WE: Amputation level following unsuccessful distal limb salvage operations. Surgery 87:683–687, 1980.
25. Samson RH, Gupta SK, Scher LA, Veith FJ: Treatment of limb threatening ischemia despite a palpable popliteal pulse. J Surg Res 32:535–539, 1982.
26. Samson RH, Gupta SK, Scher LA, Veith FJ: Level of amputation after failed limb salvage procedures. Surg Gynecol Obstet 154:56–58, 1982.
27. Stoney RJ: Ultimate salvage for the patient with limb threatening ischemia: Realistic goals and surgical considerations. *In* Bergan JJ, Yao JST (eds): Gangrene and Severe Ischemia of the Lower Extremities. New York, Grune & Stratton, 1978, pp 383–392.
28. Stirneman P, Walpoth B, Wiursten VH, Graber P, Parli R,

Althaus V: Influence of failed arterial reconstruction on the outcome of major limb amputation. Surgery 111:363–368, 1992.

29. Tsang GM, Crowson MC, Hickey NC, Simms MH: Failed femorocrural reconstruction does not prejudice amputation level. Br J Surg 78:1479–1481, 1991.

30. Evans WE, Hayes JP, Vermilion BD: Effect of a failed distal reconstruction on the level of amputation. Am J Surg 160:217–220, 1990.

31. Epstein SB, Worth MH Jr, e Ferzli G: Level of amputation following failed vascular reconstruction for lower limb ischemia. Curr Surg 46:185–192, 1989.

32. Bloom RJ, Stevick CA: Amputation level and distal salvage of the limb. Surg Gynecol Obstet 166:1–5, 1988.

33. McIntyre KE Jr, Bailey SA, Malone JM, Goldstone J: The nonsalvageable infected lower extremity: A new look at guillotine amputation. Am J Surg 117:58–64, 1985.

34. Fischer DF, Clagett GP, Fry RE, Humble TH, Fry WJ: One-stage versus two-stage amputation for wet gangrene of the lower extremity: A randomized study. J Vasc Surg 8:428–433, 1988.

35. Robbs JV, Ray R: Clinical predictors of below knee stump healing following amputation for ischemia. S Afr J Surg 20:305–310, 1982.

36. Dwars BJ, Van Den Broek TA, Ravwerda JA, Bakker FC: Criteria for reliable selection of the lowest level of amputation in peripheral vascular disease. J Vasc Surg 15:536–542, 1992.

37. Golbranson FL, Yu EC, Gelberman RH: The use of skin temperature determinations in lower extremity amputation level selection. Foot Ankle 3:170–172, 1982.

38. Spence VA, Walker WF: The relationship between temperature isotherms and skin blood flow in the ischemic limb. J Surg Res 36:278–281, 1984.

39. Stoner HB, Taylor L, Marcuson RW: The value of skin temperature measurements in forecasting the healing of below-knee amputation for end stage ischemia of the leg in peripheral vascular disease. Eur J Vasc Surg 3:355–361, 1989.

40. Wagner WH, Keagy BA, Kotb MN, Burnham JJ, Johnson G Jr: Noninvasive determination of healing of major lower extremity amputation: The continued role of clinical judgment. J Vasc Surg 8:703–710, 1988.

41. Lim RC Sr, Blaisdell FW, Hall AD, et al: Below knee amputation for ischemic gangrene. Surg Gynecol Obstet 125:493–501, 1967.

42. Baker WH, Barnes RW: Minor forefoot amputation in patients with low ankle pressure. Am J Surg 133:331–332, 1977.

43. Barnes RW, Shanik GO, Slaymaker EE: An index of healing in below-knee amputation: Leg blood pressure by Doppler ultrasound. Surgery 79:13–20, 1976.

44. Bernstein EF: The noninvasive vascular diagnostic laboratory. In Najarian JS, Oelaney JP (eds): Vascular Surgery. Miami, Symposia Specialists Stratton Intercontinental Medical Book Corp, 1978, pp 33–46.

45. Gibbons GW, Wheelock FC Jr, Siembieda C, et al: Noninvasive prediction of amputation level in diabetic patients. Arch Surg 114:1253–1257, 1979.

46. Raines JK, Darling RC, Buth J, et al: Vascular laboratory criteria for the management of peripheral vascular disease of the lower extremities. Surgery 79:21–29, 1976.

47. Schwartz JA, Schuler JJ, O'Connor RJA, Flanigan DP: Predictive value of distal perfusion pressure in the healing of amputation of the digits and the forefoot. Surg Gynecol Obstet 154:865–869, 1982.

48. Verta MJ, Gross WS, Van Bellan B, et al: Forefoot perfusion pressure and minor amputation surgery. Surgery 80:729–734, 1976.

49. Yao JST, Bergan JJ: Application of ultrasound to arterial and venous diagnosis. Surg Clin North Am 54:23–38, 1974.

50. Cheng EY: Lower extremity amputation level: Selection using noninvasive hemodynamic methods of evaluation. Arch Phys Med Rehabil 63:475–479, 1982.

51. Holloway GA Jr, Burgess EM: Cutaneous blood flow and its relation to healing of below knee amputation. Surg Gynecol Obstet 146:750–756, 1978.

52. Holloway GA Jr, Watkins BW: Laser Doppler measurement of cutaneous blood flow. J Invest Dermatol 69:300–309, 1977.

53. Kostuik JP, Wood D, Hornby R, et al: Measurement of skin blood flow in peripheral vascular disease by the epicutaneous application of xenon-133. J Bone Joint Surg 58:833–837, 1964.

54. Malone JM, Leal JM, Moore WS, et al: The "gold standard" for amputation level selection: Xenon-133 clearance. J Surg Res 30:449–455, 1981.

55. Moore WS: Determination of amputation level. Measurement of skin blood flow with xenon-133. Arch Surg 107:798–802, 1973.

56. Silberstein EB, Thomas S, Cline J, et al: Predictive value of intracutaneous xenon clearance for healing of amputation and cutaneous ulcer sites. Radiology 147:227–229, 1983.

57. Burgess EM, Matsen FA, Wyss CR, Simmons CW: Segmental transcutaneous measurements of P0$_2$ in patients requiring below the knee amputation for peripheral vascular insufficiency. J Bone Joint Surg [Am] 64:378–382, 1982.

58. Clyne CAC, Ryan J, Webster JHH, Chant AOB: Oxygen tension on the skin of ischemic legs. Am J Surg 143:315–318, 1982.

59. Franzeck UK, Talke P, Berstein EF, et al: Transcutaneous P0$_2$ measurement in health on peripheral arterial occlusive disease. Surgery 91:156–163, 1982.

60. Harward TRS, Volny J, Golbranson F, et al: Oxygen-inhalation induced transcutaneous P0$_2$ changes as a predictor of amputation level. J Vasc Surg 2:220–227, 1985.

61. Katsamouris A, Brewster DC, Megerman J, et al: Transcutaneous oxygen tension in selection of amputation level. Am J Surg 147:510–516, 1984.

62. Malone JM, Anderson GG, Halka SC, Hagaman RM, Henry R, McIntyre KE, Bernhard VM: Prospective comparison of noninvasive techniques for amputation level selection. Am J Surg 154:179–184, 1987.

63. Matsen FA, Wyss CR, Robertson CL, et al: The relationship of transcutaneous P0$_2$ and laser Doppler measurements in a human model of local arterial insufficiency. Surg Gynecol Obstet 159:418–422, 1984.

64. Ratliff DA, Clune CAC, Chant ADB, Webster JHH: Prediction of amputation healing: The role of transcutaneous P0$_2$ assessment. Br J Surg 71:219–222, 1984.

65. Graham BH, Walton RL, Elings VB, Lewis F: Surface quantification of injected fluorescein as a predictor of flap viability. Plast Reconstr Surg 71:826–833, 1983.

66. McFarland DC, Lawrence PF: Skin fluorescence. A method to predict amputation site healing. J Surg Res 32:410–415, 1982.

67. Silverman DG, Hurford WE, Cooper HS, et al: quantification of fluorescein distribution to strangulated reticulum. J Surg Res 34:179–186, 1983.

68. Silverman DG, Rubin JM, Reilly CA, et al: Fluorometric prediction of successful amputation levels in the ischemic limb. J Rehab Res Dev 22:29–34, 1985.

69. Holloway GA Jr, Burgess EM: Preliminary experiences with laser Doppler velocimetry for the determination of amputation levels. Prosthet Orthot Int 7:63–66, 1983.

70. Holstein P: Level selection in leg amputation for arterial occlusive disease: A comparison of clinical evaluation and skin perfusion pressure. Acta Orthop Scand 53:821–831, 1982.

71. Holstein P, Trap-Jensen J, Bagger H, Larsen B: Skin perfusion pressure measured by isotope wash out in legs with arterial occlusive disease. Clin Physiol 3:313–324, 1983.

72. Stockel M, Ovesen J, Brochner-Morstensen J, Emneus H: Standardized photoelectric technique as routine method for selection of amputation level. Acta Orthop Scand 53:875–878, 1982.

73. Kram HB, Appel PL, Shoemaker WC: Multisensor trans-

cutaneous oximetric mapping to predict below-knee amputation wound healing: Use of critical pO_2. J Vasc Surg 9:796–800, 1989.

74. Kram HB, Appel PL, Shoemaker WC: Prediction of below-knee amputation wound healing using noninvasive laser Doppler velocimetry. Am J Surg 158:29–31, 1989.

75. Burnham ST, Wagner WH, Keagy BH, Johnson G Jr: Objective measurement of limb perfusion by dermal fluorometry. A criterion for healing of below knee amputation. Arch Surg 125:104–106, 1990.

76. Friedmann LW: The prosthesis—immediate or delayed fitting? Angiology 23:513–524, 1972.

77. Durham JR, Anderson GG, Malone JM: Methods of preoperative selection of amputation level. *In* Flanigan P (ed): Modern Methods of Perioperative Assessment in Peripheral Vascular Surgery. New York, Marcel Dekker, 1986.

78. Oishi CS, Fronek A, Golbranson FL: The role of noninvasive vascular studies in determining levels of amputation. J Bone Joint Surg [Am] 70:1520–1530, 1988.

79. Bacharach JM, Rooke TW, Osmundson PJ, Gloviczki P: Predictive value of transcutaneous oxygen pressure and amputation success by use of supine and elevation measurement. J Vasc Surg 15:558–563, 1992.

80. Holloway GA Jr: Cutaneous blood flow responses to infection trauma measured by laser Doppler velocimetry. J Invest Dermatol 74:1–4, 1980.

81. Daly MJ, Henry RE: Quantitative measurement of skin perfusion with xenon-133. J Nucl Med 21:156–160, 1980.

82. Holstein P, Lassen NA: Assessment of safe level of amputation by measurement of skin blood pressure. *In* Rutherford R, et al (eds): Vascular Surgery. Philadelphia, WB Saunders Company, 1977, pp 105–111.

83. Ovesen J, Stockel M: Measurement of skin perfusion pressure by photoelectric technique: Aid to amputation level selection in arteriosclerotic disease. Prosthet Orthot Int 8:39–41, 1984.

84. Wagner FW Jr: Amputation of the foot and ankle. Current Status. Clin Orthop Rel Res 122:62–69, 1977.

85. Sizer JS, Wheelock FC: Digital amputations in diabetic patients. Surgery 72:980–989, 1972.

86. Little JM, Stephen MS, Zylstra PL: Amputation of the toes for vascular disease: Fate of the affected leg. Lancet 2:1318–1319, 1976.

87. McKittrick LS, McKittrick MB, Risby TS: Transmetatarsal amputation for infection of gangrene in patients with diabetes mellitus. Ann Surg 130:825–842, 1949.

88. Syme J: On amputation at the ankle joint. London and Edinburgh Monthly J Med Sci 3(26):93, 1843.

89. Harris RI: Syme's amputation, the technical details essential for success. J Bone Joint Surg [Br] 38:614–632, 1956.

90. Harris RI: The history and development of Syme's amputations. Artif Limbs 6:4–43, 1961.

91. Warren R, Kihn RB: A survey of lower extremity amputations for ischemia. Surgery 63:107–120, 1968.

92. Kernek CB, Rozzi WB: Simplified two stage below-knee amputation for unsalvageable diabetic foot infections. Clin Orthop 261:251–256, 1990.

93. Termansen NB: Below-knee amputation for ischaemic gangrene. Prospective, randomized comparison of a transverse and a sagittal operative technique. Acta Orthop Scand 48:311–316, 1977.

94. Persson BM: Sagittal incision for below-knee amputation in ischaemic gangrene. J Bone Joint Surg [Br] 56:110–114, 1974.

95. Ruckley CV, Stonebridge PA, Prescott RJ: Skewflap versus long posterior flap in below-knee amputations: Multicenter trial. J Vasc Surg 13:423–427, 1991.

96. Block MA, Whitehouse FW: Below-knee amputation in patients with diabetes mellitus. Arch Surg 87:682–689, 1963.

97. Dellon AL, Morgan RF: Myodermal flap closure of below the knee amputation. Surg Gynecol Obstet 153:383–386, 1981.

98. Moore WS: Immediate postoperative prothesis. *In* Ruther-

ford R, Bernhard V, et al (eds): Vascular Surgery. Philadelphia, WB Saunders Company, 1977, pp 1333–1343.

99. Kim GE, Imparato AM, Chu DS, Davis SW: Lower limb amputation for occlusive vascular disease. Am Surg 42:589–601, 1976.

100. Inderbitzi R, Biuttiker M, Pfluger D, Nachbur B: The fate of bilateral lower limb amputees in end stage disease. Eur J Vasc Surg 6:321–326, 1992.

101. Houghton A, Allen A, Luff R, McColl I: Rehabilitation after lower extremity amputation: A comparative study of above-knee, through knee and Gritti-Stokes amputations. Br J Surg 76:622–624, 1989.

102. Burgess EM: Disarticulation of the knee. A modified technique. Arch Surg 112:1250–1255, 1977.

103. Doran J, Hopkinson BR, Making GS: The Gritti-Stokes amputation in ischaemia: A review of 134 cases. Br J Surg 65:135–137, 1978.

104. Puddifoot PC, Weaver PC, Marshall SA: A method of supportive bandaging for amputation stumps. Br J Surg 60:729–731, 1973.

105. Ford LT, Holder BR: Disarticulation for failed surgical procedures about the hip. South Med J 70:1293–1296, 1977.

106. Endean ED, Schwarz TH, Barker DE, Munfakh NA, Wilson-Neely R, Hyde GL: Hip disarticulation: Factors affecting outcome. J Vasc Surg 14:398–404, 1991.

107. Boyd HB: Anatomic disarticulation of the hip. Surg Gynecol Obstet 84:346–349, 1947.

108. Hogshead HP: Experience with hip disarticulation and hemipelvectomy procedure. J Bone Joint Surg [Am] 53:1031, 1971.

109. Wu KK, Guise ER, Frost HM, Mitchell CL: The surgical technique for hindquarter amputation. Report of 19 cases. Acta Orthop Scand 48:479–486, 1977.

110. Baur GM, Porter JM, Axthelm S, et al: Lower extremity amputation for ischemia. Am Surg 44:472–477, 1978.

111. Berardi RS, Keonin Y: Amputations in peripheral vascular occlusive disease. Am J Surg 135:231–234, 1978.

112. Home instructions: Amputee with prosthesis. Orthop Nurses Assoc J 6:73–77, 1979.

113. Abramson AS, Feibel A: The phantom phenomenon: Its use and disuse. Bull NY Acad Med 57:99–112, 1981.

114. Bradway JR, Racy J, Malone JM: Psychological adaptation to amputation. Orthot Prosthet 38:46–50, 1984.

115. Parkes CM: Factors determining persistence of phantom pain in the amputee. J Psychosom Res 17:97–108, 1973.

116. Sherman RA: Published treatment of phantom pain. Am J Phys Med 59:232–244, 1980.

117. Sherman RA, Tippens JK: Suggested guidelines for treatment of phantom limb pain. Orthopedics 5:1595–1600, 1982.

118. Solomon GF, Schmidt KM: A burning issue. Phantom limb pain and psychological preparation of the patient for amputation. Arch Surg 113:185–186, 1978.

119. Sherman RA, Sherman CJ, Gall NG: A survey of current phantom limb pain treatment in the United States. Pain 8:85–99, 1980.

120. Sherman RA, Sherman CJ, Parker L: Chronic phantom and stump pain among American veterans: Results of a survey. Pain 18:83–95, 1984.

121. Nagendran T, Johnson G Jr, McDaniel WJ, et al: Amputation of the leg: An improved outlook. Ann Surg 175:994–999, 1972.

122. Wray CH, Still JM Jr, Moretz WH: Present management of amputations for peripheral vascular disease. Am Surg 38:87–92, 1972.

123. Bertin VJ, Plechia FR, et al: The early results of vascular surgery in patients 75 years of age or older: An analysis of 3,259 cases. J Vasc Surg 2:769–774, 1985.

124. Gregg RO: Bypass or amputation? Concomitant review of bypass arterial grafting and major amputation. Am J Surg 149:397–401, 1985.

125. Burgess EM, Romano RL, Aettl JH, Schrock Jr: Amputation

of the leg for peripheral vascular ischemia. J Bone Joint Surg [Am] 53:874–890, 1971.

126. Bailey MJ, Johnston CLW, Yates CJP, et al: Preoperative haemoglobin as predictor of outcome of diabetic amputations. Lancet 2:168–170, 1979.

127. Gatti JE, LaRossa D, Neff SR, Silverman DG: Altered skin flap survival and fluorescein kinetics with hemodilution. Surgery 92:200–205, 1982.

128. Malone JM: Complications of lower extremity amputation. *In* Bernhard VM, Towne J (eds): Complications in Vascular Surgery. Orlando, FL, Grune & Stratton, 1985, pp 445–470.

129. Reiber GE, Pecoraro RE, Koepsell TD: Risk factors for amputation in patients with diabetes mellitus. A case control study. Ann Intern Med 117:97–105, 1992.

130. Ebskou LB: Epidemiology of lower limb amputations in Denmark. (1980 to 1989). Int Orthop 15:285–288, 1991.

131. Harris PL, Read F, Eardley A, et al: The fate of elderly amputees. Br J Surg 61:665–668, 1974.

132. Kerstein MD: Utilization of an air splint after below knee amputation. Am J Phys Med 53:119–126, 1974.

133. Kerstein MD, Zimmer H, Dugdale FE, Lerner E: The delays in the rehabilitation in lower extremity amputees. Conn Med 41:549–551, 1977.

134. Kihn RB, Warren R, Beebe GW: The "geriatric" amputee. Ann Surg 176:305–314, 1972.

135. Reyes RL, Leahey EB, Leahey EB Jr: Elderly patients with lower extremity amputations: Three year study in a rehabilitation setting. Arch Phys Med Rehabil 58:116–123, 1977.

136. Waters RL, Perry J, Antonelli D, Hislop H: Energy cost of walking of amputees: The influence of level of amputation. J Bone Joint Surg [Am] 58:42–46, 1976.

137. Weaver PC, Marshall SA: A functional and social review of lower-limb amputees. Br J Surg 60:732–737, 1973.

138. Jamieson CW, Hill D: Amputation for vascular disease. Br J Surg 63:693–690, 1976.

139. Kerstein MD, Zimmer H, Dugdale FE, Lerner E: What influence does age have on rehabilitation of amputees? Geriatrics 30:67–71, 1975.

140. Gonzalez EG, Corcoran PH, Reyes RL: Energy expenditure in below-knee amputees: Correlation with stump length. Arch Phys Med Rehabil 55:111–119, 1974.

141. Huang CT, Jackson JR, Moore NB, et al: Amputation: Energy cost of ambulation. Arch Phys Med Rehabil 60:18–24, 1979.

142. Kavanagh T, Shephard RJ: The application of exercise testing to the elderly amputee. J Can Med Assoc 108:314–317, 1973.

143. Kegel B: Controlled environment treatment (CET) for patients with below-knee amputations. Phys Ther 56:1366–1371, 1976.

144. Burgess EM, Romano RL: The management of lower extremity amputees using immediate postsurgical prosthesis. Clin Orthop 57:137–146, 1968.

145. Burgess EM, Romano RL, Zettl JH: The Management of Lower Extremity Amputation Surgery. Immediate Postsurgical Prosthetic Fitting. Patient Care, Washington, DC, US Government Printing Office, 1969.

146. Burgess EM, Zettl JH: Amputations below the knee. Artif Limbs 13:1–12, 1969.

147. Baker WH, Barnes RW, Shurr OG: The healing of below-knee amputations. A comparison of soft and plaster dressings. Am J Surg 133:716–718, 1977.

148. Kraeger RR: Amputation with immediate fitting prostheses. Am J Surg 120:634–636, 1970.

149. Ruoff AC, Smith AG, Thoroughman JC, et al: The immediate postoperative prosthesis in lower extremity amputations. Arch Surg 101:40–44, 1970.

150. Thorpe W, Gerber LH, Lampert M, et al: A prospective study of the rehabilitation of the above-knee amputee with rigid dressings. Comparison of immediate and delayed ambulation and the role of physical therapists and prosthetists. Clin Orthop Rel Res 143:133–137, 1979.

151. Cohen SI, Goldman LO, Salzman EW, Glotzer OJ: The deleterious effect of immediate postoperative prosthesis in below-knee amputation for ischemic disease. Surgery 761:992–1001, 1974.

152. Folsum D, King T, Rubin J: Lower extremity amputation with immediate postoperative prosthetic placement. Am J Surg 164:370–322, 1992.

153. Leal JM, Malone JM, Moore WS, Malone SJ: For accelerated postamputation rehabilitation: Zoroc intermediate protheses. Orthot Prosthet 34:3–12, 1980.

154. Seery J, Leal JM, Malone JM: Impact of new casting tapes on prosthetic fabrication. Paper presented to the International Society for Prosthetics and Orthotics 4th World Congress, London, England, September, 1983.

155. Wu Y, Brncick MD, Krick HJ, et al: Scotchcast® P.V.C. interim prosthesis for below-knee amputees. Bull Prosthet Res Fall:40–45, 1981.

156. Sher MH: The air splint. An alternative to the immediate postoperative prosthesis. Arch Surg 108:746–747, 1974.

157. Kegel B, Moore AJ: Load cell. A device to monitor weight bearing for lower extremity amputees. Phys Ther 57:652–654, 1977.

158. Lipp MR, Malone SJ: Group rehabilitation of vascular surgery patients. Arch Phys Med Rehabil 57:180–183, 1976.

159. Enoka RM, Miller DI, Burgess EM: Below-knee amputee running gait. Am J Phys Med 61:66–84, 1982.

REVIEW QUESTIONS

1. The best overall approach to postamputation prosthetic care and rehabilitation is:

   (a) conventional soft dressings
   (b) rigid dressings
   (c) immediate postoperative prosthetics
   (d) rigid dressings with early ambulation
   (e) soft dressings with early ambulation

2. The advantages of a rigid dressing (without an attached prosthesis) after major lower extremity amputation include all of the following except:

   (a) control of stump edema
   (b) protection of the wound from trauma
   (c) stump immobilization
   (d) prevention of joint flexion contracture
   (e) accelerated stump maturity

3. Which of the following statements about amputees or amputation rehabilitation is false?

   (a) the risk of contralateral limb loss in the 5 years following major lower extremity amputation is greater than 25 per cent
   (b) the 5-year life expectancy for patients with diabetes after major lower extremity amputation is less than 50 per cent
   (c) above-knee amputations should be performed in all geriatric patients because of their poor prognosis for successful rehabilitation

(d) using noninvasive amputation level selection techniques, primary healing can be expected in greater than 90 per cent of all below-knee amputations

(e) none of the above

4. Which of the following statements about amputation surgery or amputees is true?
   (a) clinical judgment is the best technique for amputation level selection
   (b) there is no benefit to the patient in performing a knee disarticulation amputation
   (c) amputees decrease their walking speed to control energy expenditure
   (d) the successful rehabilitation of bilateral above-knee amputees is common
   (e) none of the above

5. The following therapeutic maneuvers are often successful for the treatment of phantom pain:
   (a) surgical stump revision
   (b) psychotherapy
   (c) narcotics
   (d) physical therapy
   (e) none of the above

6. Amputation level selection techniques such as transcutaneous oxygen measurement can also be used:
   (a) intraoperatively
   (b) postoperatively
   (c) to evaluate or quantitate the degree of ischemia
   (e) all of the above

7. Which statement about major lower extremity amputation is false?
   (a) eighty per cent of all patients will heal a below-knee amputation
   (b) two thirds of patients undergoing amputation surgery have other cardiovascular diseases
   (c) the best amputation level selection technique is a combination of clinical judgment and preoperative arteriography

(d) it takes at least twice as much energy for an above-knee amputee to walk as a below-knee amputee

(e) any patient ambulating prior to amputation can ambulate after amputation, irrespective of age

8. The most common cause of major lower extremity amputation is:
   (a) a failed vascular reconstruction
   (b) trauma
   (c) ischemia
   (d) tumor
   (e) complications of diabetes mellitus

9. Which of the following statements about major lower extremity amputation is false?
   (a) most amputations are caused by complications of peripheral vascular disease and/or diabetes mellitus
   (b) the average rate of ambulation after major lower extremity amputation is 60 per cent
   (c) occlusion of the superficial femoral artery is the most common arterial lesion that leads to below-knee amputation
   (d) patients, especially those with diabetes mellitus, who have undergone successful amputation have a decreased life expectancy
   (e) there is no difference in healing between patients with diabetes mellitus and those without diabetes

10. Which of the following statements are true?
    (a) amputation surgery is reconstructive surgery
    (b) amputation surgery may be the preferred procedure compared to extended distal bypass or multiple revisions of below-knee distal bypass if good amputee rehabilitation treatment is available
    (c) patient education and foot care of the contralateral nonamputated extremity is important
    (d) optimum results after lower extremity amputation require amputation level selection techniques and early or rapid postamputation rehabilitation
    (e) all of the above

ANSWERS

1. d	2. e	3. c	4. c	5. e	6. d	7. c
8. e	9. c	10. e				

INDEX

Note: Page numbers in *italics* refer to illustrations; page numbers followed by t refer to tables.

Myocardial ischemia, pathophysiology of, 648

Myointimacyte, 372

Myointimal hyperplasia, 673. See also *Intimal hyperplasia.*

Myonephropathic metabolic syndrome, 650–651, 667–668, 668t

Nafcillin, prophylactic, 380

Naftidrofuryl (Praxilene), for chronic lower extremity ischemia, 230–231, 231t

Neck, traumatic vascular injury to, 638, *639*

Necrotizing arteritis, 109, 112

Neonate. See also *Child.*
    portal vein thrombosis in, 781

Nephrectomy, in renovascular hypertension, 515

Nephropathy, ischemic, renal revascularization and, 516–517, *517*, 517t

Nerve(s). See also specific nerve.
    peripheral, ischemia in, 648–649

Neurofibromatosis, *138*, 138

Neuropathy, diabetic, 493, 497
    ischemic optic, 547

Nicotinic acid, for hyperlipidemia, 94

Nifedipine, for lower extremity ischemia, 231t
    for upper extremity ischemia, 596

Nimodipine, to suppress intimal hyperplasia formation, 682t

Nitroglycerin, for chronic lower extremity ischemia, 231t

Nitroprusside, for chronic lower extremity ischemia, 231t

Nonsteroidal antiinflammatory drugs, 84

No-reflow phenomenon, 649–650

Norepinephrine, as relaxing agent, 39

North American symptomatic carotid endarterectomy trial, 564

Nuclear imaging, to diagnose arterial infection, 153

Nutrition, total parenteral
    for chylous ascites, 722–723
    vascular access for, 622–625, *623, 625*

Nylidrin, for chronic lower extremity ischemia, 231t

Occlusive arterial disease. See also specific artery.
    history of, 6–9

Oculopneumoplethysmography, *594*, 594

Omega-3 polyunsaturates, to suppress intimal hyperplasia formation, 682t, 683

Omega-6 polyunsaturates, atherosclerosis and, 91, 94

Omphalitis, portal vein thrombosis from, 736

Ophthalmic artery pressure, measurement of, 208, *594*, 594

Optical thermal laser, 284–285

Ornithine decarboxylase inhibitors, 682t, 687

Oscillation, of blood flow, plaque formation and, 99–101, *100*

Osteogenesis imperfecta, 75t

Osteomyelitis, arterial infection from, 149

Oudot, Jacques, 5, 7

Oxacillin, prophylactic, 362t

Oxygen radical injury, in ischemia, 649

Pachon, V., 12–13

Paget-Schroetter syndrome, *595*, 600, *601*

Palm, arteriovenous malformation of, *164–165*

Palmaz stent, 267–268, 295

Palpation, in upper extremity examination, 593

Pancreatic arterial aneursym, 442–443

Pancreaticoduodenal arterial aneursym, 442–443

Pancreatitis, hyperlipidemia and, 92–93
    splenic aneurysm formation and, 435–436, *439*

Papaverine, for chronic lower extremity ischemia, 231t
    for vasculogenic impotence, 177t

Paraplegia
    after abdominal aortic aneurysm repair, 415
    after thoracoabdominal aortic aneurysm repair, 396t, 398, *399*

Parkes-Weber syndrome, 161, 163

Patch angioplasty, 664

Patent ductus arteriosus, division of, history of, 4

Pedicle flap operations, for lymphedema, 800

Pefloxacin, prophylactic, 363

Penetrating injury, 630, 630t
    ischemia after, 652
    to abdominal aorta, 638–640

Penicillin, prophylactic, 362t, 363

Penile brachial index, 172–173

Penile erection. See also *Impotence.*
    aortofemoral reconstruction interference with, 455
    physiology of, 171

Pentoxifylline, for chronic lower extremity ischemia, 229–230, 230t
    for vasculogenic impotence, 177t
    hemodyamics of, 195

Peptide growth factors, in intimal hyperplasia, 678–679

Percutaneous transluminal angioplasty. See *Transluminal angioplasty, percutaneous.*

Peroneal artery, exposure of, 67

Peyronie's disease, 172t, 173

Phantom limb pain, 833, 833t

Phenoxybenzamine, for chronic lower extremity ischemia, 231t

Phentolamine, for lower extremity ischemia, 231t
    for vasculogenic impotence, 177t

Phlebography, 215–216, *216*, 218–219, 785

Phleborheography, 13

Phlegmasia alba dolens, 771

Phlegmasia cerulea, thrombolytic therapy for, 324

Photodynamic therapy, for intimal hyperplasia, 687–688

Photoplethysmography
    in determining lower extremity amputation level, 815
    of varicose veins, 785
    venous reflux, 217–218, *218*

Pituitrin. See *Vasopressin.*

Plantar arteries, exposure of, *67–68*, 67, 69

Plaque. See also *Atherosclerosis.*
    duplex scan of, 209–210
    embolization from, to lower extremity, 652, *653*
    localization of, artery wall susceptibility to, 101–103, 102t
        hemodynamic factors in, 96–101, *97–100*
        in abdominal aorta, 105
        in carotid bifurcation, 103–104, *104*
        in coronary arteries, 104–105

Plasma, fresh-frozen, 80

Plasmin, functions of, 314–316
    in intimal hyperplasia, 679–680

Plasmin b-chain streptokinase complex, 319

Plasminogen, 74, 313, *314*. See also *Fibrinolytic agents.*

Plasminogen activator. See also *Tissue plasminogen activator.*
    deficiency of, 80

Plasminogen activator inhibitors, 74, 315

Plasminogen streptokinase activator complex, anisoylated, 319

Plastic prosthesis, 8

Platelet activation, in hemostasis, 72–73
    intimal hyperplasia and, 676–677

Platelet derived growth factor, in intimal hyperplasia, 676–678
    in vascular wall thickening, 40, 42, *43*, 90

Platelet disorders, 76–77

Platelet function-inhibiting drugs. See *Antiplatelet agents.*

Plethysmography, impedance, 13, 771–772
    of varicose veins, 785
    segmental, 212–213, *213*

Pneumatic compression, to prevent venous thromboembolism, 81

Pneumonia, after lower extremity amputation, 835

Poiseuille's law, 180–181, *181*, 183, 185
    in arterial stenosis, 187–188
    rheologic agents and, 195

Polyarteritis nodosa, 109–115, *111*, *113–114*

Polycythemia vera, hyperviscosity in, 138t
    vascular occlusion in, 239
    venous thrombosis and, 81

Polyethylene terephthate graft. See *Dacron graft.*

Polygenic hyperlipidemia, 92

Polymyalgia rheumatica, 117

Polytetrafluoroethylene graft. See also *Graft* entries.
    bacterial resistance of, 357, 360, 363
    bonding antibiotic to, 364, 704
    compliance mismatch with, 675
    cross-section of, *43*
    dilatation of, 729
    failure of, 656–657
    for bypass from ascending aorta, 584–585
    for infected artery, 156
    for infrapopliteal bypass, 471–472
    for vascular trauma surgery, 635
    infected, removal of, 699
    occlusion of, lytic therapy for, 330–331
    patency of, *611*
    portacaval, 750

ISBN 0-7216-4841-X

9 780721 648415

90038